Lawrence S. Chin, M.D.
Assistant Professor, Department of Surgery, Division of
Neurosurgery, University of Maryland School of Medicine,
Baltimore, Maryland
Principles of Stereotactic Neurosurgery

Cindy Christian, M.D.
Assistant Professor of Pediatrics, University of Pennsylvania
School of Medicine; Medical Director, Child Abuse
Program, Children's Hospital of Philadelphia, Philadelphia,
Pennsylvania
Child Abuse

Charles S. Cobbs, M.D.
Resident, Department of Neurological Surgery, University
of California, San Francisco, San Francisco, California
Ependymomas

Robert J. Coffey, M.D.
Associate Professor, and Consultant of Neurological
Surgery, Mayo Medical Center, Rochester, Minnesota
Neurosurgical Management of Intractable Pain

Edward S. Connolly, M.D.
Professor of Neurosurgery, Louisiana State University
School of Medicine; Clinical Professor of Neurosurgery,
Tulane University School of Medicine; Chief, Neurosurgery,
Alton Ochsner Medical Foundation, New Orleans,
Louisiana
Metabolic and Other Nondegenerative Causes of Low Back Pain

Shlomo Constantini, M.D.
Lecturer, Department of Neurosurgery, Hebrew
University–Hadassah Medical School, Jerusalem, Israel
Intraspinal Tumors in Infants and Children

Charles F. Contant, Jr., Ph.D.
Assistant Professor, Department of Neurosurgery, Baylor
College of Medicine, Houston, Texas
Prognosis After Head Injury

Paul R. Cooper, M.D.
Professor of Neurosurgery, Department of Neurosurgery,
New York University Medical Center, New York, New York
*Treatment of Disc and Ligamentous Diseases of the Cervical
Spine by the Anterior Approach*

James J. Corbett, M.D.
Professor of Neurology, and Professor of Ophthalmology,
University of Mississippi School of Medicine; Chairman of
Neurology, University of Mississippi Medical Center,
Jackson, Mississippi
Neuro-Ophthalmology; Pseudotumor Cerebri

Daniel M. Corcos, M.D., Ph.D.
Associate Professor, School of Kinesiology, University of
Illinois at Chicago, and Department of Neurological
Sciences, Ruth Medical College of Rush University, Chicago,
Illinois
*Management of Spasticity by Central Nervous System Infusion
Techniques*

Kerry R. Crone, M.D.
Associate Professor of Neurosurgery and Pediatrics,
University of Cincinnati College of Medicine, Children's

Hospital Medical Center, and the Mayfield Neurological
Institute, Cincinnati, Ohio
Neuroendoscopy

Carlos David, M.D.
Chief Resident, Department of Neurological Surgery,
Jackson Memorial Hospital, Miami, Florida
Spinal Cord Injuries in Adults

Arthur L. Day, M.D.
Professor, Department of Neurological Surgery, Shands
Teaching Hospital, University of Florida College of
Medicine, Gainesville, Florida
Management of Aneurysms of the Anterior Circulation

J. Diaz Day, M.D.
Clinical Instructor, Department of Neurological Surgery,
University of Southern California School of Medicine, Los
Angeles, California
Posterior Circulation Aneurysms; Cavernous Sinus Neoplasms

Johnny B. Delashaw, Jr., M.D.
Associate Professor, Division of Neurosurgery, Oregon
Health Sciences University, Portland, Oregon
Repair of Cranial Defects

Ramon del Busto, M.D.
Assistant Professor of Medicine, Case Western Reserve
University, Cleveland, Ohio; Senior Staff Physician, Division
of Infectious Diseases, Henry Ford Hospital, Detroit,
Michigan
Cranial and Intracranial Bacterial Infections

Robert J. Dempsey, M.D.
Professor of Neurosurgery, and Director of the Stroke
Program of the Sanders-Brown Center on Aging, University
of Kentucky School of Medicine, Lexington, Kentucky
Neurosonology

Fernando G. Diaz, M.D., Ph.D.
Professor and Chairman, Department of Neurosurgery,
Wayne State University School of Medicine, Detroit,
Michigan
Extracranial Occlusive Disease of the Vertebral Artery

Curtis A. Dickman, M.D.
Associate Chief, Spine Section, and Director, Spinal
Research, Barrow Neurological Institute, Phoenix, Arizona
Posterior Instrumentation of the Cervical Spine

Peter B. Dirks, M.D.
Resident, Division of Neurosurgery, University of Toronto
Faculty of Medicine, Toronto, Ontario, Canada
*The Genetic Basis of Neurosurgical Disorders; Intracranial Germ
Cell Tumors: Classification, Diagnosis, and Management*

Concezio Di Rocco, M.D.
Associate Professor of Pediatric Neurosurgery, Catholic
University Medical School; Consultant, "Bambino Gesù"
Pediatric Hospital, Rome, Italy
Arachnoid Cysts

Nikolas H. Blevins, M.D.
Assistant Professor of Otolaryngology, Tufts University
School of Medicine–New England Medical Center Hospitals,
Boston, Massachusetts
*Facial, Auditory, and Vestibular Nerve Injuries Associated with
Basilar Skull Fractures*

Jeffrey P. Blount, M.D.
Resident in Neurological Surgery, University of Minnesota,
Minneapolis, Minnesota
Infections of Cerebrospinal Shunts

James E. Boggan, M.D.
Professor and Acting Chairman, Department of
Neurological Surgery, University of California, Davis,
School of Medicine, Sacramento, California
Use of Lasers in Neurological Surgery

Guy Bouvier, M.D.
Professor of Neurosurgery, Université de Montréal; Chief,
Division of Neurosurgery, Hôpital Notre-Dame, Montréal,
Québec, Canada
Surgical Treatment of Spasmodic Torticollis

Frank J. Bova, Ph.D.
Professor, Department of Radiation Oncology, University of
Florida College of Medicine, Gainesville, Florida
Radiosurgery for Arteriovenous Malformations

John Brick, M.D.
Associate Dean of Hospital Affairs and Professor,
Department of Neurology, West Virginia University School
of Medicine; Vice President, Medical Affairs, Hospital
Administration, Ruby Memorial Hospital, Morgantown,
West Virginia
Brain Death

Jason A. Brodkey, M.D.
Resident, Department of Neurosurgery, University of
Tennessee College of Medicine, Memphis, Tennessee
Glomus Jugulare Tumors

Dennis E. Bullard, M.D.
Assistant Clinical Professor of Neurosurgery, University of
North Carolina at Chapel Hill School of Medicine, Chapel
Hill; Chief of Surgery, Rex Hospital, Raleigh, North
Carolina
Mesencephalotomy and Other Brain Stem Procedures for Pain

Kim J. Burchiel, M.D.
John Raaf Professor and Head, Division of Neurosurgery,
Oregon Health Sciences University; Head, Neurosurgery
Service, Oregon Health Sciences University Hospitals,
Portland, Oregon
*Physiological Anatomy of Pain; Alternative Treatments for
Trigeminal Neuralgia and Other Cranial Neuralgias*

Peter C. Burger, M.D.
Professor of Pathology, Department of Pathology, The Johns
Hopkins Medical Institutions, Baltimore, Maryland
Classification and Biology of Brain Tumors

Charles V. Burton, M.D.
Medical Director, The Institute for Low Back Care,
Minneapolis, Minnesota
Lumbosacral Arachnoiditis

Paul J. Camarata, M.D.
Assistant Professor, Department of Neurosurgery,
University of Minnesota Medical School, Minneapolis,
Minnesota
Arteriovenous Malformations of the Brain

Martin B. Camins, M.D.
Associate Clinical Professor of Neurosurgery, Mount Sinai
School of Medicine of the City University of New York,
New York, New York
*Tumors of the Vertebral Axis: Benign, Primary Malignant, and
Metastatic Tumors*

Michael E. Carey, M.D.
Professor of Neurosurgery, Louisiana State University
Medical Center, New Orleans, Louisiana
Infections of the Spine and Spinal Cord

Peter W. Carmel, M.D., D.Med.Sc.
Professor of Neurological Surgery, and Chief, Division of
Neurosurgery, University of Medicine and Dentistry of
New Jersey, New Jersey Medical School; Director of
Neurosurgical Service, UMDNJ–University Hospital,
Newark, New Jersey
Brain Tumors of Disordered Embryogenesis

Don E. Carpenter, M.D.
Clinical Assistant Professor, Department of Neurology,
University of Mississippi Medical Center, Jackson,
Mississippi
Electromyography

Parakrama Chandrasoma, M.D.
Professor Associate of Pathology, University of Southern
California School of Medicine; Chief of Anatomic Pathology,
Los Angeles County–University of Southern California
Medical Center, Los Angeles, California
Neoplasms of the Pineal and Third Ventricular Region

Susan Chang, M.D.
Assistant Professor, Department of Neurological Surgery,
University of California, San Francisco, School of Medicine;
Neuro-Oncology Service, Brain Tumor Research Center of
the Department of Neurological Surgery, University of
California, San Francisco, School of Medicine, San
Francisco, California
Chemotherapy of Brain Tumors

Thomas C. Chen, M.D.
Clinical Instructor, Department of Neurological Surgery,
University of Southern California School of Medicine, Los
Angeles, California
Diagnostic Biopsy for Neurological Disease

Lawrence Cher, M.B.B.S.
Neuro-Oncology Fellow, Massachusetts General Hospital,
Boston, Massachusetts
Primary Central Nervous System Lymphoma

FOURTH EDITION

Neurological Surgery

A Comprehensive Reference Guide to the Diagnosis and Management of Neurosurgical Problems

Editor-in-Chief
JULIAN R. YOUMANS, M.D., Ph.D.
Professor Emeritus, Department of Neurological Surgery
School of Medicine, University of California
Davis, California

VOLUME

2

W.B. SAUNDERS COMPANY
A Division of Harcourt Brace & Company
Philadelphia   London   Toronto   Montreal   Sydney   Tokyo

W.B. SAUNDERS COMPANY
A Division of Harcourt Brace & Company

The Curtis Center
Independence Square West
Philadelphia, Pennsylvania 19106

Library of Congress Cataloging-in-Publication Data

Neurological surgery: a comprehensive reference guide to the
diagnosis and management of neurosurgical problems/
editor-in-chief, Julian R. Youmans.—4th ed.

p. cm.

Includes bibliographical references and index.

ISBN 0–7216–5141–0 (set)

1. Nervous system—Surgery.   I. Youmans, Julian R.   [DNLM:
   1. Neurosurgery.   WL 368 N4945 1996]

RD593.N4153 1996   617.4'8–dc20

DNLM/DLC   94–33455

Neurological Surgery: A Comprehensive Reference Guide
to the Diagnosis and Management of Neurosurgical
Problems, fourth edition

Volume 1	ISBN	0–7216–5142–9
Volume 2	ISBN	0–7216–5143–7
Volume 3	ISBN	0–7216–5144–5
Volume 4	ISBN	0–7216–5145–3
Volume 5	ISBN	0–7216–6421–0
Five-Volume Set	ISBN	0–7216–5141–0

Printed in the United States of America.

Last digit is the print number: 9   8   7   6   5   4   3   2

Neurological
Surgery

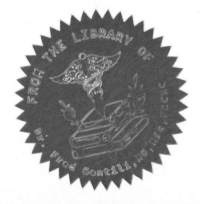

The Editor dedicates these volumes to his children,
Reed Nesbit, Susan Hare, John Edward,
Julian Milton, and Lawson Nesbit,

and to

All contributors to this Edition and the previous ones.

Contributors

A. A. Abla, M.D.
Assistant Professor of Neurosurgery, The Medical College of Pennsylvania, Philadelphia; Neurosurgeon, Department of Neurosurgery, Allegheny General Hospital, Pittsburgh, Pennsylvania
Tumors of the Orbit

P. David Adelson, M.D.
Assistant Professor of Pediatric Neurosurgery, University of Pittsburgh School of Medicine; Attending Pediatric Neurosurgeon Children's Hospital of Pittsburgh; Presbyterian University Hospital, Pittsburgh, Pennsylvania
Diseases of the Intervertebral Disc in Children

Arvind Ahuja, M.D.
Clinical Instructor of Neurosurgery, School of Medicine and Biomedical Sciences, State University of New York at Buffalo, Buffalo, New York
Endovascular Techniques to Treat Brain Tumors

Timothy E. Albertson, M.D., Ph.D.
Professor of Medicine and Pharmacology, University of California, Davis, School of Medicine, Davis; Chief, Division of Pulmonary and Critical Care Medicine, University of California, Davis, Medical Center, Sacramento, California
Pulmonary Considerations and Complications in the Neurosurgical Patient

A. Leland Albright, M.D.
Professor of Neurosurgery, University of Pittsburgh School of Medicine; Chief of Pediatric Neurosurgery, Children's Hospital of Pittsburgh, Pittsburgh, Pennsylvania
Brain Stem Gliomas

E. Francois Aldrich, M.D.
Associate Professor, Department of Surgery, Division of Surgery, University of Maryland School of Medicine, Baltimore, Maryland
Mild Head Injury in Children; Sequelae of Traumatic Brain Injury and Their Management

Lon F. Alexander, M.D.
Staff Neurosurgeon, Methodist Medical Center, Jackson, Mississippi
Endovascular Management of Intracranial Aneurysms; Post-Traumatic Syndrome

Ossama Al-Mefty, M.D.
Professor and Chairman, Department of Neurosurgery, University of Arkansas for Medical Sciences, Little Rock, Arkansas
Aneurysms of the Cavernous Sinus: Treatment Options and Considerations

Wayne M. Alves, Ph.D.
Associate Professor of Research in Neurosurgery, University of Virginia School of Medicine; Executive Director, Neuroclinical Trials Center, The Virginia Neurological Institute, Charlottesville, Virginia
Mild Head Injury in Adults

Michael L. J. Apuzzo, M.D.
Edwin M. Todd/Trent H. Wells, Jr. Professor, Department of Neurological Surgery and Radiation Oncology, Biology, and Physics, University of Southern California School of Medicine; Director of Neurosurgery, Kenneth R. Norris, Jr. Cancer Hospital and Research Institute, Los Angeles, California
Diagnostic Biopsy for Neurological Disease; Principles of Stereotactic Neurosurgery; Neoplasms of the Pineal and Third Ventricular Region

E. Joy Arpin-Sypert, M.D.
Chief, Neurosurgery, Cape Coral Hospital, Cape Coral, Florida
Evaluation and Management of the Failed Back Syndrome

John L. D. Atkinson, M.D.
Assistant Professor, Department of Neurosurgery, Mayo Medical School, Mayo Clinic, Rochester, Minnesota
Operative Management of Intracranial Arterial Occlusive Disease

Roy A. E. Bakay, M.D.
Professor of Neurological Surgery, Emory University School of Medicine; Attending Physician, Emory University Hospital, Crawford Long Hospital, and Egleston Children's Hospital, Atlanta, Georgia
Central Nervous System Transplantation

Stanley L. Barnwell, M.D., Ph.D.
Associate Professor of Neurosurgery, Radiology, and The Dotter Interventional Institute, Oregon Health Sciences University School of Medicine, Portland, Oregon
Lesions of Cerebral Veins and Dural Sinuses

Daniel L. Barrow, M.D.
Vice Chairman, Department of Neurosurgery, Emory University School of Medicine; Associate Chief of Neurosurgery, Emory University Hospital, Atlanta, Georgia
Tumors of the Sellar and Parasellar Area in Adults

H. Hunt Batjer, M.D.
Professor, Department of Neurological Surgery, University of Texas Southwestern Medical Center, Dallas, Texas
Spontaneous Intracerebral and Intracerebellar Hemorrhage

Ulrich Batzdorf, M.D.
Professor of Neurosurgery, University of California, Los Angeles, School of Medicine; Attending Neurosurgeon, University of California, Los Angeles, Medical Center, Los Angeles, California
Syringomyelia, Chiari Malformation, and Hydromyelia

Thomas K. Baumann, Ph.D.
Assistant Professor, Division of Neurosurgery and Department of Pharmacology, Oregon Health Sciences Center, Portland, Oregon
Physiological Anatomy of Pain

Donald P. Becker, M.D.
Professor and Chief, Division of Neurosurgery, University of California, Los Angeles, School of Medicine, Los Angeles, California
Pathology and Pathophysiology of Head Injury; Diagnosis and Treatment of Moderate and Severe Head Injuries in Adults

Lawrence E. Becker, M.D.
Professor of Pathology, Division of Neuropathology, University of Toronto; Chief of Pathology, Hospital for Sick Children, Toronto, Ontario, Canada
Intracranial Germ Cell Tumors: Classification, Diagnosis, and Management

Martin Bednar, M.D., Ph.D.
Assistant Professor, Neurosurgery, and Director of Surgical Research, University of Vermont College of Medicine, Burlington, Vermont
Medical Management of Acute Cerebral Ischemia

Reina Benabou, M.D.
Assistant Neurologist, Division of Functional Neurosurgery, University of São Paulo Medical School, São Paulo, Brazil; Research Fellow, Division of Neurosurgery, Hôpital Notre-Dame, Montreal, Québec, Canada
Surgical Treatment of Spasmodic Torticollis

Gregory J. Bennett, M.D.
Assistant Professor of Neurosurgery, State University of New York at Buffalo; Director of Spine Research, Millard Fillmore Hospital, Buffalo, New York
Spondylolysis and Spondylolisthesis

John R. Bentson, M.D.
Associate Professor of Radiology, University of California, Los Angeles, School of Medicine; Chief of Section of Neuroradiology, University of California, Los Angeles, Medical Center, Los Angeles, California
Magnetic Resonance Imaging

Mitchel S. Berger, M.D.
Associate Professor, Department of Neurological Surgery, University of Washington School of Medicine; Chief, Neurosurgical Oncology, University of Washington and Children's Hospital Medical Center, Seattle, Washington
Lipomyelomeningocele and Myelocystocele; Cerebellar Astrocytomas; Sarcomas and Neoplasms of Blood Vessels

Thomas A. Bergman, M.D.
Assistant Professor, Department of Neurosurgery, University of Minnesota Medical School; Assistant Chief, Division of Neurosurgery; Hennepin County Medical Center, Minneapolis, Minnesota
Cerebrospinal Fluid Fistulae

Marvin Bergsneider, M.D.
Assistant Professor, Division of Neurosurgery, University of California, Los Angeles, School of Medicine; Harbor–University of California, Los Angeles, Medical Center, Los Angeles, California
Pathology and Pathophysiology of Head Injury

Claude M. Bertrand, M.D.
Emeritus Professor of Surgery, Université de Montréal; Emeritus Chief of Neurosurgery, Hôpital Notre-Dame, Montréal, Québec, Canada
Surgical Treatment of Spasmodic Torticollis

Siegfried Bien, M.D.
Professor and Head, Department of Neuroradiology, University of Marburg, Marburg, Germany
Arteriovenous Malformations of the Spinal Cord

Juan Bilbao, M.D.
Associate Professor of Neuropathology, University of Toronto; Associate Pathologist, St. Michael's Hospital, Toronto, Ontario, Canada
Tumors of the Peripheral Nervous System

Keith Black, B.S., M.D.
Professor of Neurosurgery, University of California, Los Angeles, School of Medicine; Head, Neurosurgical Oncology, University of California, Los Angeles, Medical Center, Los Angeles, California
Blood-Brain Barrier

Peter McL. Black, M.D., Ph.D.
Franc D. Ingraham Professor of Neurosurgery, Harvard Medical School, Neurosurgeon-in-Chief, Children's Hospital, Brigham and Women's Hospital, Boston, Massachusetts
Hydrocephalus in Adults

Susan Blaser, M.D.
Assistant Professor, Department of Radiology, University of Toronto; Staff Neuroradiologist, Hospital for Sick Children, Toronto, Ontario, Canada
Choroid Plexus Papillomas and Carcinomas

Cheryl L. Dixon, M.D.
Anesthesiologist, Anesthesia Consultants, PA, Memorial Medical Center at Jacksonville, Jacksonville, Florida
Management of Pain by Anesthetic Techniques

Curt Doberstein, M.D.
Assistant Professor, Department of Clinical Neurosciences, Brown University School of Medicine; Head, Section of Cerebrovascular Surgery, Department of Neurosurgery, Rhode Island Hospital, Providence, Rhode Island
Cerebral Blood Flow in Clinical Neurosurgery

Stephen E. Doran, M.D.
Instructor, Section of Neurosurgery, University of Michigan Medical Center, Ann Arbor, Michigan
Tumors of the Skull

Nicholas W. C. Dorsch, M.D.
Clinical Associate Professor, University of Sydney Medical School, Sydney; Staff Neurosurgeon, Westmead Hospital, Westmead, New South Wales, Australia
Special Problems Associated With Subarachnoid Hemorrhage

James M. Drake, M.D.
Associate Professor, University of Toronto Faculty of Medicine; Staff Neurosurgeon, Hospital for Sick Children, Toronto, Ontario, Canada
Birth Trauma

Ann-Christine Duhaime, M.D.
Assistant Professor of Neurosurgery, University of Pennsylvania School of Medicine; Associate Neurosurgeon, and Associate Director of Trauma, Children's Hospital of Philadelphia, Philadelphia, Pennsylvania
Child Abuse

Stewart B. Dunsker, M.D.
Professor and Director of Spinal Neurosurgery, University of Cincinnati College of Medicine, Cincinnati, Ohio

Michael S. B. Edwards, M.D.
Professor and Vice Chairman, Department of Neurological Surgery, University of California, San Francisco, School of Medicine, San Francisco, California
Ependymomas

Marc E. Eichler, M.D.
Assistant Professor, Department of Neurosurgery, Washington University School of Medicine; Attending Physician, Barnes Hospital, The Jewish Hospital of St. Louis, and Christian Hospital, St. Louis, Missouri
Cervical Spine Trauma

Howard M. Eisenberg, M.D.
Professor, Department of Surgery, Division of Neurosurgery, University of Maryland School of Medicine; Chief, Division of Neurosurgery; Chief, Division of Neurotrauma, MIEMSS; Director of Medical Services, Shock Trauma Center; University of Maryland Medical System, Baltimore, Maryland
Mild Head Injury in Children; Sequelae of Traumatic Brain Injury and Their Management

Frank J. Eismont, M.D.
Professor and Vice Chairman, Department of Orthopaedics and Rehabilitation, University of Miami; Co-Director, Acute Spinal Cord Injury Unit, Jackson Memorial Hospital, Miami, Florida
Diagnosis and Management of Thoracic Spine Fractures

Amr O. El-Naggar, M.D.
Neurosurgeon, Lake Cumberland Regional Hospital, Somerset, Kentucky
Dorsal Root Entry Zone Lesions for Pain

Dominique Engel, M.D.
Instructor, Northwestern University School of Medicine; Chief Resident, Department of Surgery, Neurosurgery, Northwestern Memorial Hospital, Chicago, Illinois
Viral Infections of the Central Nervous System: Neurosurgical Considerations

Fred J. Epstein, M.D.
Professor and Director, Pediatric Neurosurgery, New York University School of Medicine; Professor and Director, Pediatric Neurosurgery, Tisch Hospital, New York, New York
Intraspinal Tumors in Infants and Children

Joseph E. Epstein, M.D.
Clinical Professor of Neurological Surgery, Albert Einstein College of Medicine, Bronx; Honorary Attending Physician, Divisions of Neurosurgery, Long Island Jewish Medical Center, New Hyde Park, and North Shore University Hospital, Manhassett, New York
Lumbar Spinal Stenosis

Nancy E. Epstein, M.D.
Clinical Associate Professor in Surgery–Neurosurgery, Cornell University Medical College, New York; Chief, Division of Neurosurgery, North Shore University Hospital, Manhasset, New York
Lumbar Spinal Stenosis

Steven F. Falcone, M.D.
Assistant Professor, Clinical Radiology and Neurological Surgery, University of Miami School of Medicine; Director of Magnetic Resonance Center, Department of Radiology, Jackson Memorial Hospital, Miami, Florida
Spinal Cord Injuries in Adults

Richard G. Fessler, M.D., Ph.D.
Dunspaugh-Dalton Chair in Brain and Spinal Surgery, University of Florida Medical School, University of Florida, Gainesville, Florida
Benign Extradural Lesions of the Dorsal Spine

Paul C. Francel, M.D., Ph.D.
Resident, Department of Neurosurgery, University of Virginia School of Medicine, Charlottesville, Virginia
Mild Head Injury in Adults; Diagnosis and Treatment of Moderate and Severe Head Injuries in Infants and Children

Lars Friberg, M.D.
Professor, Department of Neurosurgery, University of Texas Southwestern Medical Center, Dallas, Texas
Spontaneous Intracerebral and Intracerebellar Hemorrhage

Matthew Frick, M.D.
Professor and Chairman, Department of Radiology, West
Virginia University School of Medicine, Morgantown, West
Virginia
Brain Death

Alan H. Friedman, M.D.
Professor of Surgery, Department of Surgery, Division of
Neurosurgery, Duke University, Durham, North Carolina
Dorsal Root Entry Zone Lesions for Pain

William A. Friedman, M.D.
Edward Shedd Wells Professor of Stereotactic and
Functional Neurosurgery; Residency Program Coordinator;
and Associate Chairman, Department of Neurological
Surgery and Neuroscience, University of Florida College of
Medicine, Gainesville, Florida
*Monitoring the Nervous System; Radiosurgery for Arteriovenous
Malformations*

Takanori Fukushima, M.D., D.M.Sc.
Professor of Neurosurgery, Medical College of
Pennsylvania, and Hahnemann University School of
Medicine, Philadelphia; Director, Allegheny Neuroscience
Institute Center for Skull Base Surgery, Allegheny General
Hospital, Pittsburgh, Pennsylvania
Cavernous Sinus Neoplasms

Gregory N. Fuller, M.D., Ph.D.
Assistant Professor of Pathology, Department of Pathology,
The University of Texas M. D. Anderson Cancer Center,
Houston, Texas
Classification and Biology of Brain Tumors

Michael Gallagher, M.D.
Instructor, Spine Fellow, Department of Neurosurgery, The
Medical College of Wisconsin, Milwaukee, Wisconsin
Spondyloarthropathies, Including Ankylosing Spondylitis

Stephen S. Gebarski, M.D.
Associate Professor, Division of Neuroradiology and
Magnetic Resonance Imaging, University of Michigan
Medical Center, Ann Arbor, Michigan
Tumors of the Skull

William O. Geisler M.D.
Professor Emeritus of Medicine, University of Toronto
Faculty of Medicine; Senior Physician, Lyndhurst Spinal
Injury Hospital, Toronto, Ontario, Canada
Rehabilitation After Central Nervous System Lesions

Steven L. Giannotta, M.D.
Professor of Neurosurgery, University of Southern
California School of Medicine; Chief of Neurosurgery, USC
University Hospital, Los Angeles, California
Posterior Circulation Aneurysms

Kevin J. Gibbons, M.D.
Assistant Professor of Neurosurgery, State University of
New York at Buffalo; Attending Neurosurgeon, Millard
Fillmore Hospital, Buffalo General Hospital, Erie County
Medical Center, and Children's Hospital of Buffalo, Buffalo,
New York
Endovascular Techniques to Treat Brain Tumors

Philip L. Gildenberg, M.D., Ph.D.
Clinical Professor of Neurosurgery and Radiation Oncology,
Baylor College of Medicine; Clinical Professor of
Neurosurgery and Psychiatry, University of Texas Medical
School; Director, Houston Stereotactic Center, Houston,
Texas
Medical Management of Chronic Pain

Ryan S. Glasser, M.D.
Resident, Department of Neurosurgery, University of
Florida College of Medicine, Gainesville, Florida
Cerebrovascular Diseases in Children

Ziya L. Gokaslan, M.D.
Assistant Professor, Department of Neurosurgery,
University of Texas M. D. Anderson Cancer Center; Clinical
Assistant Professor, Department of Neurosurgery, Baylor
College of Medicine, Houston, Texas
*Treatment of Disc and Ligamentous Diseases of the Cervical
Spine by the Anterior Approach*

William B. Gormley, M.D.
Chief Resident, Department of Neurosurgery, Henry Ford
Hospital, Detroit, Michigan
Cranial and Intracranial Bacterial Infections

Liliana C. Goumnerova, M.D.
Assistant Professor of Surgery, Harvard Medical School;
Associate in Neurosurgery, Children's Hospital, Boston,
Massachusetts
Diseases of the Intervertebral Disc in Children

Barth A. Green, M.D.
Professor and Chairman, Department of Neurological
Surgery, University of Miami School of Medicine; Chief of
Neurosurgery Service, Jackson Memorial Hospital, Miami,
Florida
*Spinal Cord Injuries in Adults; Diagnosis and Management of
Thoracic Spine Fractures*

Cordell E. Gross, M.D.
Chairman and Professor, Neurological Surgery, University
of Vermont College of Medicine, Burlington, Vermont
Medical Management of Acute Cerebral Ischemia

Ernst H. Grote, M.D.
Professor and Head, Department of Neurosurgery,
University of Tübingen; Neurosurgeon, University Hospital,
Tübingen, Germany
Arteriovenous Malformations of the Spinal Cord

Abhijit Guha, M.D.
Assistant Professor of Neurosurgery and Surgical Oncology,
University of Toronto Faculty of Medicine; Attending
Neurosurgeon, Toronto Hospital, Toronto, Ontario, Canada
Tumors of the Peripheral Nervous System

Nalin Gupta, M.D.
Research Fellow, Brain Tumor Research Center, Department
of Neurological Surgery, University of California, San
Francisco, School of Medicine, San Francisco, California
Choroid Plexus Papillomas and Carcinomas

Lee R. Guterman, Ph.D., M.D.
Clinical Instructor of Neurosurgery, School of Medicine and Biomedical Sciences, State University of New York at Buffalo, Buffalo, New York
Endovascular Treatment of Arteriovenous Malformations

Philip H. Gutin, M.D.
Professor and Chairman, Department of Neurological Surgery, University of California, San Francisco, School of Medicine, San Francisco, California
Interstitial and Intracavitary Irradiation of Brain Tumors

Michael Haglund, M.D., Ph.D.
Acting Instructor, Senior Epilepsy Fellow, Department of Neurological Surgery, University of Washington School of Medicine, Seattle, Washington; Assistant Professor, Departments of Neurosurgery (Surgery) and Neurobiology, Duke University Medical Center, Durham, North Carolina
Post-Traumatic Seizures

Joseph F. Hahn, M.D.
Chairman, Division of Surgery, Chairman, Department of Neurosurgery, Cleveland Clinic Foundation, Cleveland, Ohio
General Methods of Clinical Examination

Regis W. Haid, M.D.
Associate Professor, Department of Neurosurgery, and Director, Center for Neurosurgical Spinal Research, Emory Clinic, Emory University School of Medicine, Atlanta, Georgia
Spondyloarthropathies, Including Ankylosing Spondylitis

Stephen J. Haines, M.D.
Professor of Neurosurgery, Otolaryngology, and Pediatrics, University of Minnesota Medical School, Minneapolis, Minnesota
Infections of Cerebrospinal Shunts

H. Bruce Hamilton, M.D.
Neurosurgery Resident, Louisiana State University Medical Center, New Orleans, Louisiana
Metabolic and Other Nondegenerative Causes of Low Back Pain

Mark G. Hamilton, M.D.C.M.
Assistant Professor, Division of Neurosurgery, Department of Clinical Neurosciences, University of Calgary Faculty of Medicine; Neurosurgeon, Alberta Children's Hospital, Foothills Hospital, Tom Baker Cancer Center, Calgary, Alberta, Canada
Aneurysms of the Vein of Galen

Russell W. Hardy, M.D.
Professor of Neurosurgery, Case Western Reserve University School of Medicine, and University Hospitals of Cleveland, Cleveland, Ohio
Extradural Cauda Equina and Nerve Root Compression from Benign Lesions of the Lumbar Spine

Marwan I. Hariz, M.D., Ph.D.
Associate Professor of Neurosurgery, University of Umeå; Consultant Neurosurgery, Department of Neurosurgery, University Hospital, Umeå, Sweden
Movement Disorders

Griffith R. Harsh, IV, M.D.
Associate Professor, Department of Surgery, Harvard Medical School; Director, Neurosurgical Oncology, Massachusetts General Hospital, Boston, Massachusetts
Neuroepithelial Tumors of the Adult Brain

Samuel J. Hassenbusch, M.D., Ph.D.
Associate Surgeon, and Director, Section of Neurosurgical Pain Management, University of Texas M. D. Anderson Cancer Center, Houston, Texas
Intracranial Ablative Procedures for Pain; Intracranial Procedures for Affective Disorders

M. Peter Heilbrun, M.D.
Joseph J. Yager Professor and Chair, Department of Neurosurgery, University of Utah School of Medicine, Salt Lake City, Utah
Frameless Stereotactic Localization and Guidance

Martin M. Henegar, M.D.
Department of Neurosurgery, Washington University School of Medicine; Resident in Neurosurgery, Washington University Medical Center, St. Louis Children's Hospital, St. Louis, Missouri
Occult Spinal Dysraphism

James M. Herman, M.D.
Community Memorial Hospital of San Buenaventura, Ventura County Medical Center, St. John's Regional Medical Center, Ventura; Pleasant Valley Hospital, Camarillo, California
Aneurysms of the Vein of Galen

Roberto C. Heros, M.D.
Professor and Co-Chairman, Department of Neurosurgery, University of Miami School of Medicine; Director, University of Miami International Neurosurgical Institute, Miami, Florida
Arteriovenous Malformations of the Brain

David R. Hinton, M.D.
Associate Professor, Pathology and Neurosurgery, University of Southern California School of Medicine, Los Angeles, California
Diagnostic Biopsy for Neurological Disease

Fred H. Hochberg, M.D.
Associate Professor of Neurology, Harvard Medical School; Neurologist, Massachusetts General Hospital, Boston, Massachusetts
Primary Central Nervous System Lymphoma

Julian T. Hoff, M.D.
Richard C. Schneider Professor of Neurosurgery, Professor of Surgery, and Section Head, Neurosurgery, University of Michigan Medical School, Ann Arbor, Michigan
Intracranial Pressure; Tumors of the Skull; Treatment of Intractable Vertigo

Harold J. Hoffman, M.D.
Professor of Surgery, Division of Neurosurgery, University of Toronto Faculty of Medicine; Chief of Neurosurgery, The Hospital for Sick Children, Toronto, Ontario, Canada
Optic Pathway and Hypothalamic Gliomas in Children; Intracranial Germ Cell Tumors: Classification, Diagnosis, and Management

William Y. Hoffman, M.D.
Associate Professor of Clinical Surgery (Plastic and Reconstructive Surgery), University of California, San Francisco, School of Medicine, San Francisco, California
Scalp Injuries and Their Management; Tumors of the Scalp

James Hollowell, M.D.
Assistant Professor of Neurosurgery, Department of Neurosurgery, Medical College of Wisconsin; Staff Neurosurgeon, Department of Veterans Affairs Medical Center, and Froedtert Memorial Lutheran Hospital, Milwaukee, Wisconsin
Biomechanics of the Spine

Leo N. Hopkins, M.D.
Professor and Chairman of Neurosurgery, and Professor of Radiology, School of Medicine and Biomedical Sciences, State University of New York at Buffalo; Head, Department of Neurosurgery, Buffalo General Hospital; Chairman, Department of Neurosurgery, Millard Fillmore Hospitals; and Department Head, Children's Hospital of Buffalo and Erie County Medical Center, Buffalo, New York
Endovascular Treatment of Arteriovenous Malformations; Endovascular Techniques to Treat Brain Tumors

Alan R. Hudson, M.B., Ch.B.
Professor of Neurosurgery, University of Toronto Faculty of Medicine; President and Chief Executive Officer, The Toronto Hospital, Toronto, Ontario, Canada
Acute Injuries of Peripheral Nerves; Tumors of the Peripheral Nervous System

R. P. Humphreys, M.D.
Professor, Division of Neurosurgery, University of Toronto Faculty of Medicine; Staff Neurosurgeon, Hospital for Sick Children, Toronto, Ontario, Canada
Choroid Plexus Papillomas and Carcinomas

Michael Hutchinson, D.Phil., M.D.
Assistant Professor, Departments of Neurology and Radiology, New York University School of Medicine; Assistant Attending in Neurology, New York University Hospital, Bellevue Hospital, New York, New York
Neurosurgical Applications of Positron Emission Tomography

Robert K. Jackler, M.D.
Professor of Otolaryngology, and Professor of Neurosurgery, University of California, San Francisco, School of Medicine, San Francisco, California
Facial, Auditory, and Vestibular Nerve Injuries Associated with Basilar Skull Fractures

R. Patrick Jacob, M.D.
Assistant Professor, Department of Neurological Surgery, University of Florida College of Medicine; Chief, Neurosurgery Service, Veterans Affairs Medical Center, Gainesville, Florida
Diagnosis and Nonoperative Management of Trigeminal Neuralgia

John A. Jane, M.D., Ph.D.
David D. Weaver Professor and Chairman, Department of Neurosurgery, University of Virginia School of Medicine, Charlottesville, Virginia
Craniosynostosis; Mild Head Injury in Adults; Diagnosis and Treatment of Moderate and Severe Head Injuries in Infants and Children

Peter J. Jannetta, M.D.
Walter E. Dandy Professor and Chairman, Department of Neurological Surgery, University of Pittsburgh School of Medicine; Attending Neurosurgeon, Presbyterian University Hospital, University of Pittsburgh Medical Center, Pittsburgh, Pennsylvania
Microvascular Decompression of the Trigeminal Nerve for Tic Douloureux; Cranial Rhizopathies

V. Jay, M.D.
Assistant Professor, Department of Pathology, University of Toronto Faculty of Medicine; Staff Neuropathologist, Hospital for Sick Children, Toronto, Ontario, Canada
Choroid Plexus Papillomas and Carcinomas

Robert R. Johnson, II, M.D.
Assistant Professor and Vice-Chief, Department of Neurological Surgery, Wayne State University School of Medicine, Detroit, Michigan
Extracranial Occlusive Disease of the Vertebral Artery

A. T. Jousse, M.D.
Professor Emeritus of Rehabilitation Medicine, University of Toronto Faculty of Medicine, Toronto, Ontario, Canada
Rehabilitation After Central Nervous System Lesions

Paul M. Kanev, M.D.
Director of Pediatric Neurosurgery, Department of Surgery, Henry Ford Hospital, Detroit, Michigan
Lipomyelomeningocele and Myelocystocele; Occult Spinal Dysraphism

Neal F. Kassell, M.D.
Distinguished Professor and Vice Chairman, Neurosurgery, University of Virginia School of Medicine; President, Virginia Neurological Institute, Charlottesville, Virginia
Nonoperative Treatment of Aneurysmal Subarachnoid Hemorrhage

Bruce A. Kaufman, M.D.
Professor of Neurological Surgery, Washington University School of Medicine; Attending Neurosurgeon, St. Louis Children's Hospital, St. Louis, Missouri
Occult Spinal Dysraphism

Howard H. Kaufman, M.D.
Professor and Chairman, Department of Neurosurgery, Residency Program, West Virginia University School of Medicine, Morgantown, West Virginia
Brain Death; Trauma to the Carotid Artery and Other Cervical Vessels

Daniel F. Kelly, M.D.
Assistant Professor of Neurosurgery, University of California, Los Angeles, School of Medicine, Los Angeles; Assistant Professor of Neurosurgery, Harbor–University of

California, Los Angeles, Medical Center, Torrance,
California
Diagnosis and Treatment of Moderate and Severe Head Injuries in Adults

Mazen H. Khayata, M.D.
Division of Neurological Surgery, Barrows Neurological
Institute, St. Joseph's Hospital and Medical Center, Phoenix,
Arizona
Aneurysms of the Vein of Galen

Steven P. Kiefer, M.D.
Senior Resident in Neurosurgery, University Hospitals of
Cleveland, Cleveland, Ohio
*Pathophysiology and Clinical Evaluation of Ischemic
Cerebrovascular Disease*

Glen W. Kindt, M.D.
Professor, Neurosurgery, University of Colorado School of
Medicine, Denver, Colorado
Medical Management of Acute Cerebral Ischemia

Wesley A. King, M.D.
Associate Professor of Clinical Neurosurgery, University of
Medicine and Dentistry of New Jersey, Newark, New Jersey
Neuro-Otology

David G. Kline, M.D.
Professor and Chairman, Department of Neurosurgery,
Louisiana State University School of Medicine in New
Orleans; Attending Neurosurgeon, University Hospital,
Ochsner Foundation Hospital, and Charity Hospital at New
Orleans, New Orleans, Louisiana
*Acute Injuries of Peripheral Nerves; Tumors of the Peripheral
Nervous System*

K. John Klose, Ph.D.
Research Associate Professor, Department of Neurological
Surgery, University of Miami School of Medicine;
Neurosurgeon, Jackson Memorial Hospital, Miami, Florida
Spinal Cord Injuries in Adults

Thomas A. Kopitnik, Jr., M.D.
Assistant Professor, Department of Neurological Surgery,
University of Texas Southwestern Medical Center at Dallas,
Dallas, Texas
Spontaneous Intracerebral and Intracerebellar Hemorrhage

Johan M. Kros, M.D., Ph.D.
Department of Pathology/Neuropathology, University
Hospital Rotterdam–Dijkzigt, Rotterdam, The Netherlands
Sarcomas and Neoplasms of Blood Vessels

Lauri V. Laitinen, M.D., Ph.D.
Associate Professor of Neurosurgery, Umeå University,
Consultant Neurosurgeon, Sophiahemmet Hospital,
Stockholm, Sweden
Movement Disorders

Giuseppe Lanzino, M.D.
Resident, Department of Neurosurgery, University of
Virginia School of Medicine, Charlottesville, Virginia
*Nonoperative Treatment of Aneurysmal Subarachnoid
Hemorrhage*

David A. Larson, Ph.D., M.D.
Associate Professor and Vice Chairman, Department of
Radiation Oncology, University of California, San Francisco,
School of Medicine, San Francisco, California
*Radiation Therapy and Radiosurgery for Brain Tumors; Radiation
Therapy of Pituitary Tumors; Radiation Therapy of Tumors of the
Spine*

Sanford J. Larson, M.D., Ph.D.
Professor and Chairman, Department of Neurosurgery,
Medical College of Wisconsin, Milwaukee, Wisconsin
Concepts and Biomechanics of Instrumentation of the Spine

Kevin R. Lee, M.D.
Department of Surgery, University of Michigan Medical
School, Ann Arbor, Michigan
Intracranial Pressure

Thomas T. Lee, M.D.
Resident Surgeon, University of Miami/Jackson Memorial
Hospital, Miami, Florida
Diagnosis and Management of Thoracic Spine Fractures

Harvey S. Levin, Ph.D.
Professor, Division of Neurological Surgery, University of
Maryland School of Medicine; Professor, Shock Trauma
Center, Baltimore, Maryland
*Mild Head Injury in Children; Sequelae of Traumatic Brain
Injury and Their Management*

Michael L. Levy, M.D., Ph.D.
Assistant Professor, Department of Neurological Surgery,
University of Southern California School of Medicine,
Children's Hospital, Los Angeles, California
Principles of Stereotactic Neurosurgery

Robert M. Levy, M.D., Ph.D.
Associate Professor, Departments of Surgery
(Neurosurgery) and Physiology, Northwestern University
Medical School; Acting Chief, Division of Neurological
Surgery, Northwestern University Medical School and
Northwestern Memorial Hospital, Chicago, Illinois
*Viral Infections of the Central Nervous System: Neurosurgical
Considerations*

Adam I. Lewis, M.D.
Chief Resident in Neurosurgery, University of Cincinnati
College of Medicine, Cincinnati, Ohio
Neuroendoscopy

Linda M. Liau, M.D.
Resident, University of California, Los Angeles, School of
Medicine, Los Angeles, California
Pathology and Pathophysiology of Head Injury

William J. Logan, M.D.
Professor of Paediatrics and Medicine, University of
Toronto Faculty of Medicine; Chief of Neurology, Hospital
for Sick Children, Toronto, Ontario, Canada
Neurological Examination in Infancy and Childhood

Stephen P. Lownie, M.D.
Assistant Professor, Department of Clinical Neurological Sciences (Neurosurgery) and Department of Radiology (Neuroradiology), University of Western Ontario Faculty of Medicine; Attending Neurosurgeon, University and Victoria Hospitals, London, Ontario, Canada
Cerebral Angiography

R. Loch Macdonald, M.D., Ph.D.
Assistant Professor, Section of Neurosurgery, Pritzker School of Medicine, University of Chicago Medical Center, University of Chicago Hospitals, Chicago, Illinois
Pathophysiology and Clinical Evaluation of Subarachnoid Hemorrhage

Chriss A. Mack, M.D.
Neurosurgeon, Neurological Associates, Missoula, Montana
Benign Extradural Lesions of the Dorsal Spine

Ellen E. Mack, M.D.
Assistant Clinical Professor, Department of Neurological Surgery, School of Medicine, University of California, San Francisco, San Francisco, California
Chemotherapy of Brain Tumors

Parley W. Madsen, III, M.D., Ph.D.
Assistant Professor, Department of Neurological Surgery, and Staff Scientist, The Miami Project to Cure Paralysis, University of Miami School of Medicine; Associate Director, Acute Spinal Cord Injury Unit, Jackson Memorial Hospital; Consulting Neurosurgeon, Surgery Service, Veterans Administration Medical Center, Miami, Florida
Diagnosis and Management of Thoracic Spine Fractures

Michael E. Mahla, M.D.
Associate Professor, Departments of Anesthesiology and Neurosurgical Surgery and Neuroscience; Assistant Chairman for Education, Department of Anesthesiology, University of Florida College of Medicine, Member, Brain Institute, University of Florida; Director, Intraoperative Neurologic Monitoring Laboratory, Shands Hospital at the University of Florida, Gainesville, Florida
Monitoring the Nervous System

Dennis Jay Maiman, M.D., Ph.D.
Professor of Neurosurgery, Medical College of Wisconsin; Medical Director, Spinal Cord Injury Center, Froedtert Memorial Hospital; Chief, Spinal Cord Injury Center, Department of Veterans Affairs Medical Center; Medical Director, Medical College of Wisconsin Spine Care, Milwaukee, Wisconsin
Biomechanics of the Spine

Daniel Marchac, M.D.
Professor, Collège de Médecine des Hôpitaux de Paris; Plastic Surgeon, Center for Craniofacial Anomalies, Department of Pediatric Neurosurgery, Hôpital Necker Enfants Malades, Paris, France
Congenital Craniofacial Malformations

Joseph C. Maroon, M.D.
Professor of Surgery (Neurosurgery), Medical College of Pennsylvania, Philadelphia; Chairman, Department of

Neurosurgery, Allegheny General Hospital, Pittsburgh, Pennsylvania
Intradiscal Treatment of Lumbar Disc Disease; Tumors of the Orbit

Lawrence F. Marshall, M.D.
Professor and Chief, Division of Neurosurgical Services, University of California, San Diego, School of Medicine, San Diego, California
Differential Diagnosis of Altered States of Consciousness

Sharon Bowers Marshall, B.S.N.
Assistant Clinical Professor, Neurosurgery, University of California, San Diego, School of Medicine, San Diego, California
Differential Diagnosis of Altered States of Consciousness

Neil A. Martin, M.D.
Professor, Division of Neurosurgery; Head, Vascular Neurosurgery Section, University of California, Los Angeles, School of Medicine; Director, Cerebral Blood Flow Laboratory; Medical Director, Neurosurgery Intensive Care Unit, UCLA Medical Center, Los Angeles, California
Cerebral Blood Flow in Clinical Neurosurgery

Timothy J. Martin, M.D.
Assistant Professor of Surgical Sciences, Ophthalmology, and Neuro-Ophthalmology, Department of Ophthalmology, Bowman Gray School of Medicine (Wake Forest University Eye Center), Winston-Salem, North Carolina
Neuro-Ophthalmology; Pseudotumor Cerebri

P. Mathew, B.M.B.S.
Honorary Clinical Lecturer, Senior Registrar in Neurosurgery, Institute of Neurological Sciences, Southern General Hospital, Glasgow, Scotland, United Kingdom
Mechanisms of Cerebral Concussion, Contusion, and Other Effects of Head Injury

Yoshiharu Matsushima, M.D., D.M.Sc.
Associate Professor, Department of Neurosurgery, Faculty of Medicine, Tokyo Medical and Dental University, and University Hospital, Tokyo, Japan
Moyamoya Disease

Marc R. Mayberg, M.D.
Professor, Department of Neurological Surgery, University of Washington School of Medicine; Chief, Neurosurgery Clinical Services, University of Washington Medical Center, Seattle, Washington
Extracranial Occlusive Disease of the Carotid Artery

John C. Mazziotta, M.D., Ph.D.
Professor of Neurology, Radiological Sciences, and Pharmacology, University of California, Los Angeles, School of Medicine; Director, Division of Brain Mapping, Neuropsychiatric Institute and Hospital, Los Angeles, California
Neurosurgical Applications of Positron Emission Tomography

J. Gordon McComb, M.D.
Professor of Neurological Surgery, University of Southern California School of Medicine; Head, Division of

Neurosurgery, Children's Hospital of Los Angeles, Los Angeles, California
Encephaloceles

Bruce McCormack, M.D.
Assistant Professor of Neurosurgery, University of California, San Francisco, School of Medicine, San Francisco, California
Diagnosis and Management of Thoracolumbar and Lumbar Spine Injuries

Paul C. McCormick, M.D.
Associate Professor of Clinical Neurosurgery, Columbia University College of Physicians and Surgeons; Associate Attending Physician, Columbia Presbyterian Medical Center, New York, New York
Indications and Techniques of Lumbar Spine Fusion; Spinal Cord Tumors in Adults

Michael W. McDermott, M.D.
Assistant Clinical Professor, Department of Neurological Surgery, University of California, San Francisco, School of Medicine; Attending Neurosurgeon, University of California, Moffitt Hospital, San Francisco, California
Meningiomas; Interstitial and Intracavitary Irradiation of Brain Tumors

Jeffrey D. McDonald, M.D., Ph.D.
Assistant Professor, Department of Neurological Surgery, University of Utah School of Medicine, Salt Lake City, Utah
Ependymomas

David G. McLone, M.D., Ph.D.
Professor, Department of Surgery, Division of Neurosurgery, Northwestern University Medical School; Division Head, Pediatric Neurosurgery, Children's Memorial Hospital, Chicago, Illinois
Myelomeningocele

Arnold H. Menezes, M.D.
Professor and Vice Chairman, Division of Neurosurgery, University of Iowa College of Medicine, University of Iowa Hospitals and Clinics, Iowa City, Iowa
Congenital and Acquired Abnormalities of the Craniovertebral Junction; Tumors of the Craniovertebral Junction

J. Parker Mickle, M.D.
Professor of Neurosurgery, University of Florida College of Medicine, Gainesville, Florida
Cerebrovascular Diseases in Children

David W. Miller, M.D.
Chief Resident, Cleveland Clinic Foundation, Cleveland, Ohio
General Methods of Clinical Examination

Jimmy D. Miller, M.D.
Clinical Associate Professor, Department of Neurosurgery, University of Mississippi School of Medicine, Jackson; Staff Neurosurgeon, Department of Neurosurgery, North Mississippi Medical Center, Tupelo, Mississippi
Post-Traumatic Syndrome

Pedro Molina-Negro, M.D.
Professor of Neurosurgery, Université de Montréal; Director, Laboratory of Neurophysiology, Hôpital Notre-Dame, Montréal, Québec, Canada
Surgical Treatment of Spasmodic Torticollis

Jacques J. Morcos, M.D.
Cerebrovascular and Skull Base Fellow, Barrow Neurological Institute, Phoenix, Arizona
Management of Aneurysms of the Anterior Circulation

Donald E. Morgan, Ph.D.
Professor of Otolaryngology, Department of Otorhinolaryngology: Head and Neck Surgery, University of Pennsylvania Medical School; Director, Division of Audiology and Speech-Language Pathology, University of Pennsylvania Medical Center, Philadelphia, Pennsylvania
Neuro-Otology

John S. Myseros, M.D.
Resident in Neurosurgery, Virginia Commonwealth University, Medical College of Virginia, Richmond, Virginia
Problems Associated with Multiple Trauma

Raj K. Narayan, M.D.
Professor and Chairman, Department of Neurosurgery, Temple University School of Medicine, Philadelphia, Pennsylvania
Prognosis After Head Injury

Blaine S. Nashold, Jr., M.Sc., M.D.
Emeritus Professor of Neurosurgery, Duke University Medical Center, Durham, North Carolina
Dorsal Root Entry Zone Lesions for Pain; Mesencephalotomy and Other Brain Stem Procedures for Pain

James R. B. Nashold, M.D., M.Phil.
Chief Resident, Department of Surgery, Division of Neurosurgery, Duke University School of Medicine, Durham, North Carolina
Dorsal Root Entry Zone Lesions for Pain

Lucien Nedzi, M.D.
Assistant Professor, Department of Radiation Therapy, University of Southern California School of Medicine, Los Angeles, California
Neoplasms of the Pineal and Third Ventricular Region

Valeriy Nenov, M.D., Ph.D.
Assistant Professor-in-Residence, Division of Neurosurgery, University of California, Los Angeles, School of Medicine, Los Angeles, California
Neurosurgical Applications of Positron Emission Tomography

Diana L. Nikas, R.N., M.N.
Assistant Clinical Professor, University of California, Los Angeles, School of Nursing, Los Angeles; Neurosurgical Clinical Nurse Specialist, Harbor-UCLA Medical Center, Torrance, California
Diagnosis and Treatment of Moderate and Severe Head Injuries in Adults

Russ P. Nockels, M.D.
Director of Spine and Trauma, Department of Neurosurgery, Henry Ford Hospital, Detroit, Michigan
Diagnosis and Management of Thoracolumbar and Lumbar Spine Injuries

Richard B. North, M.D.
Associate Professor of Neurosurgery, Johns Hopkins
University School of Medicine, Baltimore, Maryland
*Spinal Cord and Peripheral Nerve Stimulation for Chronic,
Intractable Pain*

James W. Ogilvie, M.D.
Vice Chairman, Department of Orthopaedic Surgery,
University of Minnesota Medical School—Minneapolis; Staff
Surgeon, Twin Cities Scoliosis–Spine Center, Minneapolis,
Minnesota
Scoliosis, Kyphosis, and Lordosis

George A. Ojemann M.D.
Professor, Department of Neurological Surgery, University
of Washington School of Medicine; Attending Physician,
Department of Neurosurgery, University of Washington
Medical Center, and Department of Neurosurgery,
Harborview Medical Center, Seattle, Washington
Surgical Treatment of Epilepsy in Adults

Robert G. Ojemann, M.D.
Professor of Surgery, Harvard Medical School; Visiting
Neurosurgeon, Massachusetts General Hospital, Boston,
Massachusetts
Acoustic Neuroma (Vestibular Schwannoma)

Oisin R. O'Neill, M.D.
Clinical Instructor of Neurosurgery, Oregon Health Sciences
University School of Medicine, Portland, Oregon
Lesions of Cerebral Veins and Dural Sinuses

Jeffrey S. Oppenheim, M.D.
Instructor in Clinical Neurosurgery, Columbia University
College of Physicians and Surgeons, Columbia Presbyterian
Medical Center; Attending Physician, Nyack Hospital,
Nyack, New York, and Good Samaritan Hospital, Suffern,
New York
*Tumors of the Vertebral Axis: Benign, Primary Malignant, and
Metastatic Tumors*

Thomas C. Origitano, M.D., Ph.D.
Assistant Professor of Neurological Surgery and Physiology,
Loyola University Medical Center, Maywood, Illinois
*Aneurysms of the Cavernous Sinus: Treatment Options and
Considerations*

Linda Ott, M.S.
Consultant, University of Kentucky Chandler Medical
Center, Division of Neurosurgery, Lexington, Kentucky
Nutrition and Parenteral Therapy

Dachling Pang, M.D.
Professor, Neurological Surgery, University of California,
Davis, School of Medicine, Davis; Chief, Division of
Pediatric Neurosurgery, University of California, Davis,
Medical Center, Sacramento, California
Pediatric Spinal Cord and Vertebral Column Injuries

Tae S. Park, M.D.
Professor of Neurosurgery and Pediatrics, Washington
University School of Medicine; Neurosurgeon-in-Chief, St.
Louis Children's Hospital, St. Louis, Missouri
*Occult Spinal Dysraphism; Diagnosis and Treatment of Moderate
and Severe Head Injuries in Infants and Children*

Alberto Pasqualin, M.D.
Assistant Professor of Neurosurgery, Verona School of
Medicine; Vice-Chief, Second Division of Neurosurgery,
Verona City Hospital, Verona, Italy
Cerebral Metabolism

Roy A. Patchell, M.D.
Associate Professor of Surgery (Neurosurgery) and
Neurology, University of Kentucky; Chief of Neuro-
Oncology, University of Kentucky Chandler Medical Center,
Lexington, Kentucky
Brain Metastases

Warwick J. Peacock, M.B., Ch.B.
Professor of Surgery (Neurosurgery), and Chief of Pediatric
Neurosurgery, University of California, Los Angeles, School
of Medicine, Los Angeles, California
*Neurosurgical Aspects of Epilepsy in Children; Management of
Spasticity by Ablative Techniques*

Richard D. Penn, M.D.
Professor, Department of Neurosurgery, Rush Medical
College; Associate Attending Physician, Department of
Neurosurgery, Rush-Presbyterian-St. Luke's Medical Center,
Chicago, Illinois
*Intrathecal Drug Infusion for Pain; Management of Spasticity by
Central Nervous System Infusion Techniques*

Noel I. Perin, M.D.
Assistant Professor and Director, Division of Spinal
Surgery, Department of Neurosurgery, Mount Sinai
Medical Center, New York, New York
Sacral Fractures

Richard G. Perrin, M.D.
Associate Professor, Department of Surgery, Division of
Neurosurgery, University of Toronto Faculty of Medicine;
Head, Division of Neurosurgery, Wellesley Hospital,
Toronto, Ontario, Canada
*Tumors of the Vertebral Axis: Benign, Primary Malignant, and
Metastatic Tumors*

John A. Persing, M.D.
Professor of Plastic Surgery and Neurosurgery, Yale
University School of Medicine; Chief of Plastic Surgery,
Yale-New Haven Hospital, New Haven, Connecticut
Craniosynostosis; Repair of Cranial Defects

Keith R. Peters, M.D.
Assistant Professor, Departments of Radiology and
Neurological Surgery, University of Florida College of
Medicine; Director, Interventional Neuroradiology, Shands
Hospital, Gainesville, Florida
Computed Tomography

David G. Piepgras, M.D.
Professor and Chairman, Department of Neurosurgery,
Mayo Medical School, Mayo Clinic, Rochester, Minnesota
Operative Management of Intracranial Arterial Occlusive Disease

Frank Pintar, Ph.D.
Associate Professor, Medical College of Wisconsin;
Biomedical Engineer, Clement J. Zablocki Veterans Affairs
Medical Center, Milwaukee, Wisconsin
Biomechanics of the Spine

Stephen K. Powers, M.D.
Professor and Chief, Division of Neurological Surgery,
Hershey Medical Center, Hershey, Pennsylvania
Use of Lasers in Neurological Surgery

Michael D. Prados, M.D.
Associate Clinical Professor, Department of Neurological
Surgery, and Head, Neuro-Oncology Service, Brain Tumor
Research Center of the Department of Neurological Surgery,
University of California, San Francisco, School of Medicine,
San Francisco, California
Chemotherapy of Brain Tumors

Donald J. Prolo, M.D.
Clinical Associate Professor of Neurosurgery, Stanford
University School of Medicine, Stanford; Attending
Neurosurgeon, Good Samaritan Hospital, San Jose,
California
Morphology and Metabolism of Fusion of the Lumbar Spine

Matthew R. Quigley, M.D.
Assistant Professor, Medical College of Pennsylvania,
Philadelphia, Pennsylvania; Assistant Professor, Department
of Surgery (Neurosurgery), West Virginia University School
of Medicine, Morgantown, West Virginia; Staff
Neurosurgeon, Allegheny General Hospital, Pittsburgh,
Pennsylvania
Intradiscal Treatment of Lumbar Disc Disease

Ronald Q. Quisling, M.D.
Professor of Radiology, University of Florida College of
Medicine; Chief of Neuroradiology, Shands Hospital,
Gainesville, Florida
Computed Tomography

Frank A. Raila, M.D.
Associate Professor, Department of Radiology, University of
Mississippi School of Medicine, Jackson, Mississippi
Radiology of the Skull

Robert A. Ratcheson, M.D.
The Harvey Huntington Brown, Jr., Professor and
Chairman, Department of Neurological Surgery, Case
Western Reserve University School of Medicine; Director,
Department of Neurological Surgery, University Hospitals
of Cleveland, Cleveland, Ohio
*Pathophysiology and Clinical Evaluation of Ischemic
Cerebrovascular Disease*

Shlomo Raz, M.D.
Professor of Surgery and Urology, University of California,
Los Angeles, Center for Health Sciences, Los Angeles,
California
*Urological Problems Associated with Central Nervous System
Disease*

Nizam Razack, M.D.
Resident, Department of Neurological Surgery, Jackson
Memorial Hospital, Miami, Florida
Spinal Cord Injuries in Adults

Dominique Renier, M.D.
Pediatric Neurosurgeon, Center for Craniofacial Anomalies,
Department of Pediatric Neurosurgery, Hôpital Necker
Enfants Malades, Paris, France
Congenital Craniofacial Malformations

Daniel Resnick, M.D.
Resident in Neurological Surgery, Department of
Neurological Surgery, University of Pittsburgh School of
Medicine, Pittsburgh, Pennsylvania
Cranial Rhizopathies

Francisco Revilla, M.D.
Professor and Neurosurgeon, The American British
Cowdray Hospital; Specialty Hospital, National Medical
Center, IMSS, Mexico City, Mexico
Management of Aneurysms of the Anterior Circulation

Albert L. Rhoton, Jr., M.D.
R. D. Keene Family Professor of Neurological Surgery,
University of Florida College of Medicine; R. D. Keene
Family Professor and Chairman, Department of
Neurological Surgery, Shands Hospital at the University of
Florida, Gainesville, Florida
*General and Micro-operative Techniques; Diagnosis and
Nonoperative Management of Trigeminal Neuralgia*

Jon H. Robertson, M.D.
Associate Professor, Department of Neurosurgery,
University of Tennessee, Memphis, College of Medicine,
and The Health Science Center, Memphis, Tennesssee
Glomus Jugulare Tumors

Jack P. Rock, M.D.
Senior Staff, Department of Neurosurgery, Henry Ford
Hospital, Detroit, Michigan
Primary Central Nervous System Lymphoma

Gaylan L. Rockswold, M.D., Ph.D.
Professor, Department of Neurosurgery, University of
Minnesota Medical School—Minneapolis; Chief, Division of
Neurosurgery, Hennepin County Medical Center,
Minneapolis, Minnesota
Cerebrospinal Fluid Fistulae

Juan F. Ronderos, M.D.
Spine Fellow, Division of Neurological Surgery, Barrow
Neurological Institute, and St. Joseph's Hospital and
Medical Center, Phoenix, Arizona
Posterior Instrumentation of the Cervical Spine

Mark L. Rosenblum, M.D.
Professor of Neurosurgery, Case Western Reserve
University School of Medicine, Cleveland, Ohio; Chairman,
Department of Neurosurgery, and Director, Henry Ford
Midwest Neuro-Oncology Center, Henry Ford Hospital,
Detroit, Michigan
*Primary Central Nervous System Lymphoma; Cranial and
Intracranial Bacterial Infections*

Michael J. Rosner, M.D.
Professor of Neurological Surgery and of Anesthesiology,
School of Medicine, University of Alabama at Birmingham;
Attending Physician, University of Alabama Hospital,

Children's Hospital of Alabama, Veterans Affairs Medical Center; Medical Director, Neurosciences Intensive Care Unit, University of Alabama Hospital, Birmingham, Alabama
Preoperative Evaluation: Complications, Their Prevention and Treatment

James T. Rutka, M.D., Ph.D., F.R.C.S.(C.)
Assistant Professor, Division of Neurosurgery, University of Toronto Faculty of Medicine; Staff Neurosurgeon, Hospital for Sick Children, Toronto, Ontario, Canada
The Genetic Basis of Neurosurgical Disorders; Intracranial Germ Cell Tumors: Classification, Diagnosis, and Management; Choroid Plexus Papillomas and Carcinomas

Kamran Sahrakar, M.D.
Senior Resident, University of California, Davis, School of Medicine; Resident Physician, University of California, Davis, Medical Center, Sacramento, California
Pediatric Spinal Cord and Vertebral Column Injuries

Christian Sainte-Rose, M.D.
Professor, Paris V University; Neurosurgeon, Hôpital Necker des Enfants Malades, Paris, France
Hydrocephalus in Childhood

Madjid Samii, M.D.
Professor, Hannover Medical School; Chairman and Chief, Neurosurgery Department, Nordstadt Hospital, Hannover, Germany
Neurosurgical Aspects of Tumors of the Base of the Skull

John H. Sampson, M.D.
Senior Resident in Neurosurgery, Department of Surgery, Division of Neurosurgery, Duke University Medical Center, Durham, North Carolina
Dorsal Root Entry Zone Lesions for Pain

Louis D. Saravolatz, M.D.
Professor of Medicine, Case Western Reserve University–Henry Ford Health Sciences Center; Division Head, Infectious Diseases, Henry Ford Hospital, Detroit, Michigan
Cranial and Intracranial Bacterial Infections

John H. Schneider, Jr., M.D.
Attending Neurosurgeon, Department of Neurosurgery, Wilford Hall Medical Center, Lackland Air Force Base, San Antonio, Texas
Neoplasms of the Pineal and Third Ventricular Region

Richard C. Schultz, M.D.
Clinical Professor of Surgery, Division of Plastic and Reconstructive Surgery, University of Illinois College of Medicine, Chicago; Attending Surgeon, Lutheran General Hospital, Park Ridge, Northwest Community Hospital, Arlington Heights, and Holy Family Hospital, Des Plaines, Illinois
Maxillofacial Injuries

Warren R. Selman, M.D.
Associate Professor of Neurological Surgery, Case Western Reserve University School of Medicine; Vice Chairman,

Department of Neurological Surgery, University Hospitals of Cleveland, Cleveland, Ohio
Pathophysiology and Clinical Evaluation of Ischemic Cerebrovascular Disease

Christopher I. Shaffrey, M.D.
Fellow, Department of Neurosurgery, University of Virginia School of Medicine, Charlottesville, Virginia
Nonoperative Treatment of Aneurysmal Subarachnoid Hemorrhage

Mark E. Shaffrey, M.D.
Assistant Professor, Department of Neurosurgery, University of Virginia School of Medicine, Charlottesville, Virginia
Nonoperative Treatment of Aneurysmal Subarachnoid Hemorrhage; Diagnosis and Treatment of Moderate and Severe Head Injuries in Infants and Children

Masato Shibuya, M.D.
Associate Professor, Department of Neurosurgery, Nagoya University School of Medicine, Nagoya, Japan
Intracranial Giant Aneurysms

Shah N. Siddiqi, M.B., B.Chir.
Neurosurgery Resident, Division of Neurosurgery, University of Toronto, Faculty of Medicine; Hospital for Sick Children, Toronto, Ontario, Canada
Birth Trauma

Robert R. Smith, M.D.
Professor Emeritus, University of Mississippi School of Medicine; Director of Neurosciences, Methodist Medical Center, Jackson, Mississippi
Endovascular Management of Intracranial Aneurysms

Penny K. Sneed, M.D.
Assistant Professor, Department of Neurological Surgery, University of California, San Francisco, School of Medicine, San Francisco, California
Interstitial and Intracavitary Irradiation of Brain Tumors

Volker K. H. Sonntag, M.D.
Professor of Surgery (Neurosurgery), University of Arizona College of Medicine, Tucson; Vice Chairman, Division of Neurological Surgery, Barrow Neurological Institute, Phoenix, Arizona
Posterior Instrumentation of the Cervical Spine

Robert F. Spetzler, M.D.
Professor, Section of Neurosurgery; University of Arizona School of Medicine; Director and J. N. Harber Chairman of Neurological Surgery, Barrow Neurological Institute, Phoenix, Arizona
Aneurysms of the Vein of Galen

Scott C. Standard, M.D.
Clinical Instructor, Department of Neurosurgery, Vanderbilt University School of Medicine, Nashville, Tennessee
Endovascular Treatment of Arteriovenous Malformations

Michael I. Stanley, M.D.
Attending Neurosurgeon, Neurosurgical Practice Associates, Crozer-Chester Medical Center, Upland, Pennsylvania
Sacral Fractures

Loretta A. Staudt, M.S., P.T.
Clinical Research Physical Therapist, Division of Neurosurgery, University of California, Los Angeles, Los Angeles, California
Management of Spasticity by Ablative Techniques

Stephen N. Steen, Sc.D., M.D.
Professor of Anesthesiology, University of Southern California School of Medicine; Director of Research/Anesthesiology, Los Angeles County–University of Southern California Medical Center, Los Angeles, California
Neuroanesthesia

Bennett M. Stein, M.D.
Byron Stookey Professor and Chairman, Department of Neurological Surgery, Columbia University College of Physicians and Surgeons; Director of Service, Neurological Surgery, Presbyterian Hospital in The City of New York, New York, New York
Spinal Cord Tumors in Adults

S. H. Subramony, M.D.
Professor and Vice Chairman, Department of Neurology, University of Mississippi Medical Center; Attending Neurologist, University Hospital, Jackson, Mississippi
Electromyography

Kenichiro Sugita, M.D.
Professor, Department of Neurosurgery, Nagoya University School of Medicine, Nagoya, Japan
Intracranial Giant Aneurysms

Peter P. Sun, M.D.
Resident, Department of Neurosurgery, Yale University School of Medicine, New Haven, Connecticut
Pediatric Spinal Cord and Vertebral Column Injuries

Leslie N. Sutton, M.D.
Professor, Department of Neurosurgery, University of Pennsylvania School of Medicine; Associate Neurosurgeon, Division of Neurosurgery, Children's Hospital of Philadelphia, Philadelphia, Pennsylvania
Child Abuse

George W. Sypert, M.D.
Chairman, Neurological Institute, and Chief, Neurological Surgery, Southwest Florida Regional Medical Center, Fort Myers, Florida
Evaluation and Management of the Failed Back Syndrome

Jamal M. Taha, M.D.
Chief Resident, Department of Neurosurgery, University of Cincinnati College of Medicine, Cincinnati, Ohio
Treatment of Trigeminal Neuralgia, and Other Facial Neuralgias by Percutaneous Techniques

Edward C. Tarlov, M.D.
Physician, Department of Neurosurgery, Lahey Hitchcock Clinic, Burlington, Massachusetts
Extradural Spinal Cord and Nerve Root Compressions from Benign Lesions of the Cervical Area and Their Management by the Posterior Approach

Ronald R. Tasker, M.D.
Professor, Division of Neurosurgery, Department of Surgery, University of Toronto Faculty of Medicine; Neurosurgeon, Division of Neurosurgery, The Toronto Hospital, Western Division, Toronto, Ontario, Canada
Cordotomy for Pain; Deep Brain Stimulation for the Control of Intractable Pain

Marcos Tatagiba, M.D.
Associate, Neurosurgery Department, Nordstadt Hospital, Hannover, Germany
Neurosurgical Aspects of Tumors of the Base of the Skull

Stephen B. Tatter, M.D., Ph.D.
Clinical Fellow in Surgery, Harvard Medical School; Resident in Neurosurgery, Massachusetts General Hospital, Boston, Massachusetts
Neuroepithelial Tumors of the Adult Brain

Graham Teasdale, M.B.B.S.
Professor of Neurosurgery, University of Glasgow; Consultant Neurosurgeon, Institute of Neurological Sciences, Southern General Hospital, Glasgow, Scotland, United Kingdom
Mechanisms of Cerebral Concussion, Contusion, and Other Effects of Head Injury

Steven A. Telian, M.D.
Associate Professor, Department of Otolaryngology–Head and Neck Surgery, University of Michigan Medical School, Ann Arbor, Michigan
Treatment of Intractable Vertigo

Nancy R. Temkin, Ph.D.
Associate Professor, Departments of Neurological Surgery and Biostatistics, University of Washington School of Medicine, Seattle, Washington
Post-Traumatic Seizures

John M. Tew, Jr., M.D.
Frank H. Mayfield Professor and Chairman, Department of Neurosurgery, University of Cincinnati College of Medicine; Chief of Neurosurgery, Children's Hospital Medical Center, University of Cincinnati Hospital, and Department of Veterans Affairs Medical Center; Attending Physician, Christ Hospital, and Good Samaritan Hospital, Cincinnati, Ohio
Treatment of Trigeminal Neuralgia and Other Facial Neuralgias by Percutaneous Techniques

George T. Tindall, M.D.
Chairman, Department of Neurosurgery, Emory University School of Medicine; Chief, Neurosurgery, Emory University Hospital, Atlanta, Georgia
Tumors of the Sellar and Parasellar Area in Adults

Suzie C. Tindall, M.D.
Professor of Neurological Surgery, Emory University School of Medicine, Atlanta, Georgia
Chronic Injuries of Peripheral Nerves by Entrapment

Samuel Tobias, M.D.
Resident, Department of Neurosurgery, National Institute of Neurology and Neurosurgery "Manuel Velasco-Suarez," Mexico City, Mexico
Granulomatous Diseases of the Central Nervous System

Tadanori Tomita, M.D.
Associate Professor of Surgery, Northwestern University
Medical School; Attending Pediatric Neurosurgeon, and
Director of Brain Tumor Center, Children's Memorial
Hospital, Chicago, Illinois
Medulloblastomas

Bruce Tranmer, M.D.
Associate Professor, University of Calgary Faculty of
Medicine; Foothills Hospital, Calgary, Alberta, Canada
Medical Management of Acute Cerebral Ischemia

Russell L. Travis, M.D.
Neurosurgeon, Neurosurgical Associates, Lexington,
Kentucky
Hypertension and Hyperflexion Injuries of the Cervical Spine

Vincent C. Traynelis, M.D.
Associate Professor of Surgery, Division of Neurosurgery,
University of Iowa College of Medicine, and Division of
Neurosurgery, University of Iowa Hospital and Clinics,
Iowa City, Iowa
Tumors of the Craniovertebral Junction

Brent E. Van Hoozen, M.D.
Assistant Clinical Professor, Division of Pulmonary and
Critical Care Medicine, University of California, Davis,
School of Medicine, Davis, California
*Pulmonary Considerations and Complications in the
Neurosurgical Patient*

Chi M. Van Hoozen, M.D.
Postdoctoral Fellow, University of California, Davis, School
of Medicine, Division of Pulmonary and Critical Care
Medicine, Davis, California
*Pulmonary Considerations and Complications in the
Neurosurgical Patient*

Javier Verdura, M.D.
Clinical Visiting Professor of Neurosurgery, Department of
Neurosurgery, University of Virginia School of Medicine,
Charlottesville, Virginia; Attending Neurosurgeon,
American British Cowdray Hospital, Mexico City, Mexico
*Parasitic Diseases of the Central Nervous System; Granulomatous
Diseases of the Central Nervous System*

Osvaldo Vilela Filho, M.D.
Attending Neurosurgeon, Division of Neurosurgery,
Hospital das Clínicas, and Researcher, Department of
Physiology and Pharmacology, Universidade Federal de
Goiás; Head, Department of Neurosurgery and Neurology,
and Director, Center of Pain, Movement Disorders, and
Epilepsy Surgery, Instituto Ortopédico de Goiânia, Goiânia,
Goiás, Brazil
Deep Brain Stimulation for the Control of Intractable Pain

Dennis G. Vollmer, M.D.
Assistant Professor of Neurological Surgery, Washington
University School of Medicine; Attending Physician, Barnes
Hospital, The Jewish Hospital of St. Louis, and St. Louis
Children's Hospital, St. Louis, Missouri
Cervical Spine Trauma

Phillip A. Wackym, M.D.
Professor, Department of Otolaryngology, Mount Sinai
School of Medicine of the City University of New York,
New York, New York
Neuro-Otology

Gregory R. Wahle, M.D.
Assistant Professor of Urology, Indiana University Medical
Center, Indianapolis, Indiana
*Urological Problems Associated with Central Nervous System
Disease*

Ajay K. Wakhloo, M.D., Ph.D.
Research Assistant Professor of Neurosurgery, School of
Medicine and Biomedical Sciences, State University of New
York at Buffalo, Buffalo, New York
Endovascular Treatment of Arteriovenous Malformations

B. A. Ward, M.D.
Chief Resident, Department of Neurosurgery, University of
Mississippi School of Medicine, Jackson, Mississippi
Post-Traumatic Syndrome

Karen Weingarten, M.D.
Associate Professor of Clinical Radiology, Cornell
University Medical College; Attending Radiologist, Division
of Neuroradiology, The New York Hospital-Cornell Medical
Center, New York, New York
Neuroradiology of the Spine

Philip R. Weinstein, M.D.
Professor of Neurological Surgery, Department of
Neurological Surgery, University of California, San
Francisco, School of Medicine, San Francisco, California
*Ossification of the Posterior Longitudinal Ligament and Other
Enthesopathies*

Bryce Weir, M.D.
Maurice Goldblatt Professor, Surgery and Neurology,
Pritzker School of Medicine, University of Chicago; Chief,
Section of Neurosurgery, University of Chicago Medical
Center, Chicago, Illinois
*Pathophysiology and Clinical Evaluation of Subarachnoid
Hemorrhage*

Harold A. Wilkinson, M.D., Ph.D.
Professor of Neurosurgery, and Professor of Anatomy and
Cell Biology, University of Massachusetts Medical School;
Professor, Chairman, and Program Director, University of
Massachusetts Medical Center, Worcester, Massachusetts
Sympathectomy for Pain

Charles B. Wilson, M.D.
Professor of Neurosurgery, Department of Neurological
Surgery, University of California, San Francisco, School of
Medicine, San Francisco, California
Neuroepithelial Tumors of the Adult Brain; Meningiomas

H. Richard Winn, M.D.
Professor and Chairman, Department of Neurological
Surgery, University of Washington School of Medicine,
Seattle, Washington
Post-Traumatic Seizures

Narayan Yoganandan, Ph.D.
Professor, Department of Neurosurgery, Medical College of Wisconsin, and Professor, Marquette University, Milwaukee, Wisconsin
Biomechanics of the Spine

Julian R. Youmans, M.D., Ph.D.
Professor Emeritus, Department of Neurological Surgery, University of California, Davis, School of Medicine, Davis, California

Byron Young, M.D.
Professor of Neurosurgery, University of Kentucky College of Medicine; Johnston-Wright Chair of Surgery, Chief of Neurosurgery, University of Kentucky Chandler Medical Center, Lexington, Kentucky
Nutrition and Parenteral Therapy; Brain Metastases

George Pei Herng Young, M.D.
Assistant Professor of Surgery, Department of Urology, Cornell University Medical College; Assistant Attending Surgeon (Urology), Director of Female Urology, Neurourology, Urodynamics, and Reconstructive Urology Unit, The New York Hospital, New York, New York
Urological Problems Associated with Central Nervous System Disease

Harold F. Young, M.D.
Professor and Chairman, Department of Neurosurgery, Virginia Commonwealth University, Medical College of Virginia, Richmond, Virginia
Problems Associated with Multiple Trauma

Ronald F. Young, M.D.
Clinical Professor of Neurosurgery, University of California, Irvine, School of Medicine, Orange; Medical Director, Northwest Neurosciences Institute, and Northwest Hospital Gamma Knife Center, Seattle, Washington
Dorsal Rhizotomy and Dorsal Root Ganglionectomy; Periacqueductal and Periventricular Stimulation for Pain

Vladimir Zelman, M.D., Ph.D.
Professor of Anesthesiology, Neurological Surgery, and Neurology, University of Southern California School of Medicine; Interim Chairman, Department of Anesthesiology, Director of Neuroanesthesia, Los Angeles County–USC Medical Center, Los Angeles, California
Neuroanesthesia

Robert D. Zimmerman, M.D.
Professor of Radiology, Cornell University Medical College; Director of Neuroradiology and of Radiology Residency Training, The New York Hospital, New York, New York
Neuroradiology of the Spine

Yuri N. Zubkov, M.D., D.M.Sc.
Professor, A. L. Polenov Neurosurgical Research Institute, St. Petersburg, Russia
Endovascular Management of Intracranial Aneurysms

Preface to the Fourth Edition

The preface to the first edition appearing on the following pages outlines the goals of and hopes for *Neurological Surgery*. The succeeding three editions have reflected the changing practice and scope of our specialty. Chapters were deleted as techniques became obsolete, new chapters were added as new areas of knowledge emerged, and all chapters have been altered appropriately for the discipline covered. A perusal of the table of contents reveals more than a dozen new chapter titles in this Edition.

An important change in the fourth edition is the addition of Associate Editors, whose expertise in their areas of interest has contributed immeasurably toward the assembly of a prime, worldwide faculty of authors. The Editor would like to express his appreciation to Drs. Donald P. Becker, Stewart B. Dunsker, William A. Friedman, Harold J. Hoffman, Robert R. Smith, and Charles B. Wilson for their contributions to this Edition.

A major production such as a multivolume reference text requires the efforts of a dedicated team. The Editor wishes to express his appreciation to the many at the W. B. Saunders Company who produced these volumes. In particular, he would like to thank Richard Zorab, Senior Medical Editor; Sandra Valkhoff, Developmental Editor; Linda R. Garber, Senior Production Manager; Gina Scala, Copy Editing Supervisor; Frank Messina, Senior Copy Editor; and Karen O'Keefe, Designer. Also, he owes special thanks and appreciation to Bobbi Catton of Davis, California, who worked cheerfully, tirelessly, and effectively despite the many demands of contributors, the publisher, and the Editor.

A comprehensive reference text is never complete. Each edition grows from prior ones, and all contributors to each edition aid in its evolution. The Editor wishes to thank all contributors to this Edition and the previous ones.

JULIAN R. YOUMANS

Preface to the First Edition

Like other medical sciences, neurological surgery has undergone rapid changes in recent years. New techniques and entire areas of new knowledge have been developed. The knowledge that a competent neurosurgeon must master has increased vastly. As a result, no individual or small group can be expert in all areas. The only means of making a book authoritative in every area, and especially in the paraneurosurgical areas in which a neurosurgeon must be knowledgeable, is to use multiple authors from all over the world. The concept of *Neurological Surgery* came with the recognition of this problem and the need for a comprehensive reference volume that would include the more usual areas of concern to a neurosurgeon and also the allied areas in which he must be informed if he is going to give his patients the best care that is possible.

Neurological Surgery is intended for use by the surgeon in practice, the trainee who is beginning to assume responsibility for patient care, and the allied specialist who works with neurosurgical patients. Emphasis is placed on fundamental knowledge concerning etiology, pathogenesis, diagnosis, treatment, and prognosis for each disease entity of concern to the neurosurgeon. Essentials of operative technique are discussed and special techniques are evaluated and put into perspective with the more usual ones. Where appropriate, special sections or chapters are devoted to the basic aspects of neurobiology.

In addition to attempting to fill the need for a comprehensive reference source, *Neurological Surgery* has been set up so as to recognize ongoing problems and divergent views within our specialty. Wherever there are major differences in the points of view concerning methods of diagnosis or treatment, each viewpoint is presented by a recognized proponent. This approach avoids the inevitable dilution that occurs when a conflicting view is evaluated and summarized by an individual, regardless of his fairness and integrity, who does not believe in the merits of the opposing view. A perusal of the chapter titles will show numerous examples of this approach.

Many chapters are included that usually have not been present in previous texts of neurological surgery. Examples are chapters that discuss the psychological evaluation of the neurosurgical patient, neuro-otology, mechanisms of coma, hyperextension-flexion injuries of the neck, the post-traumatic syndrome, cerebral blood flow in clinical problems, the biology of brain tumors, affective disorders, the physiological and the psychiatric aspects of pain, and the principles of stereotaxic surgery. Special emphasis is given to preoperative evaluation and prevention and treatment of complications.

Like the shakedown cruise of a ship, the first edition of a text such as *Neurological Surgery* will have omissions and errors that will be revealed as the book is put to the scrutiny of those interested in our queen specialty. Mr. John Dusseau and his staff at the W. B. Saunders Company have been dedicated to producing a publication of quality, and I wish to give my wholehearted expression of appreciation to them. In particular, Mr. Raymond Kersey has given care and attention to reproducing the illustrations with accuracy and clarity, and

Miss Ruth Barker has worked with enthusiasm and dedication throughout the years from inception to the publication. To her, I owe especial thanks for her patient help in the editing and indexing and otherwise shepherding of this book to publication.

A book such as *Neurological Surgery* can be produced only with capable secretarial help. Miss Georgene Pucci has been invaluable to me in handling the thousands of pages of manuscripts, galley proofs, page proofs, and correspondence. Only with assistance of the type given by Miss Barker in Philadelphia and Miss Pucci in Davis could *Neurological Surgery* have become a reality. Finally, I would like to thank the contributors to *Neurological Surgery* for their cooperation and help in achieving for our joint effort the degree of success that it may enjoy.

JULIAN R. YOUMANS

Contents

VOLUME I

VOLUME II

VOLUME III

PART IX

Benign Spine Lesions 2219

VOLUME IV

VOLUME V

Color Plates

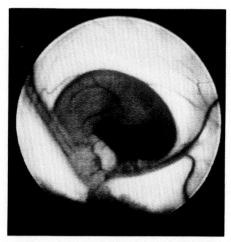

Figure 36–18

Endoscopic view of the right foramen of Monro in a 10-year-old female with hydrocephalus due to a pineal tumor.

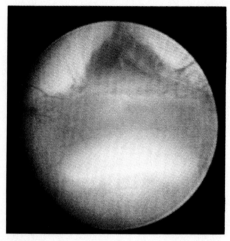

Figure 36–19

Landmarks on the floor of the third ventricle can be more or less obvious, depending on the degree of attenuation. Visualization and "palpation" of the posterior clinoid recesses is the safest way of avoiding arterial injury.

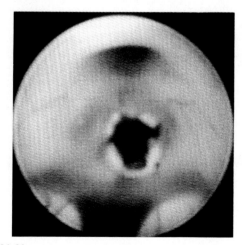

Figure 36–20

The risk of secondary obliteration of the hole in the floor of the third ventricle is almost nil because of the amplitude of the pulsatile flow at this level.

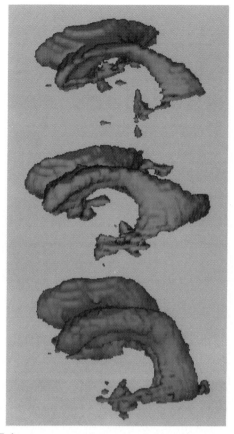

Figure 37–4

Three-dimensional reconstruction of the ventricular system in a normal patient *(top)*, a patient with Alzheimer's disease *(middle)*, and a patient with idiopathic normal-pressure hydrocephalus *(bottom)*. (Courtesy of Ron Kikinis, John Martin, and Mitsunori Matsumae, Surgical Planning Laboratory, Brigham and Women's Hospital, Boston.)

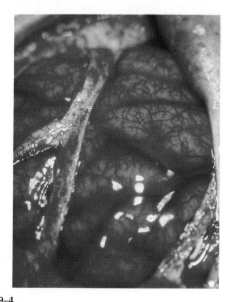

Figure 49–4

Marked leptomeningeal anastomosis of the surface of the brain observed in a moyamoya patient. This picture was taken during encephalomyosynangiosis. (From Matsushima, Y., and Inaba, Y.: The specificity of the collaterals to the brain through the study and surgical treatment of moyamoya disease. Stroke, *17*:117–122, 1986. Reproduced by permission. Copyright 1986 American Heart Association.)

PLATE IV

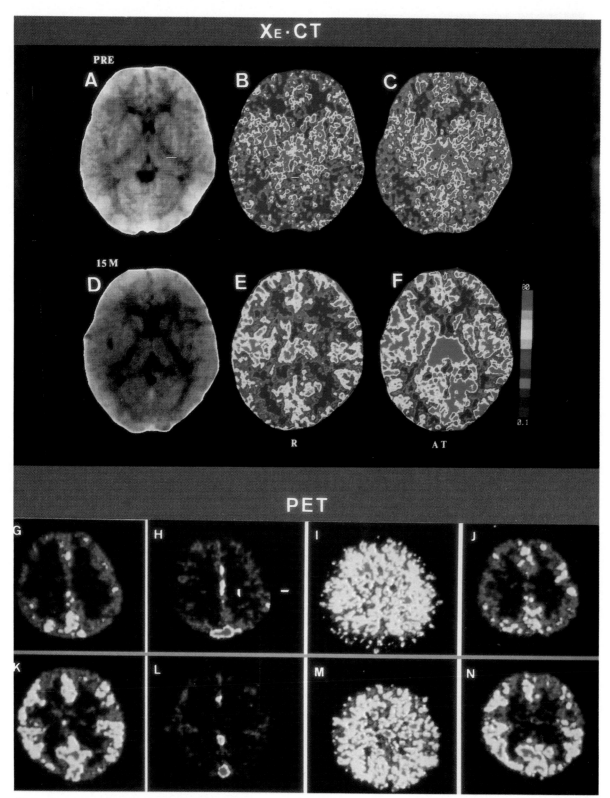

Figure 49–8

Preoperative and 15 months postoperative xenon-enhanced computed tomography and positron emission tomography of a 16-year-old girl with symptomatic onset of type II disease at 11 years of age. Xenon-enhanced cerebral blood flow studies: before *(A through C)* and 15 months after encephaloduroarteriosynangiosis *(D through F). A and D.* Plain scans. *B and E.* Xenon-enhanced scans at rest. *C and F.* Xenon-enhanced scans with acetazolamide challenge test. PET studies: before *(G through J)* and 15 months after encephaloduroarteriosynangiosis *(K through N). G and K.* Cerebral blood flow studies. *H and L.* Cerebral blood volume studies. *I and M.* Oxygen extraction factor. *J and N.* Cerebral metabolic rate for oxygen (CMRO$_2$).

PLATE V

B

C

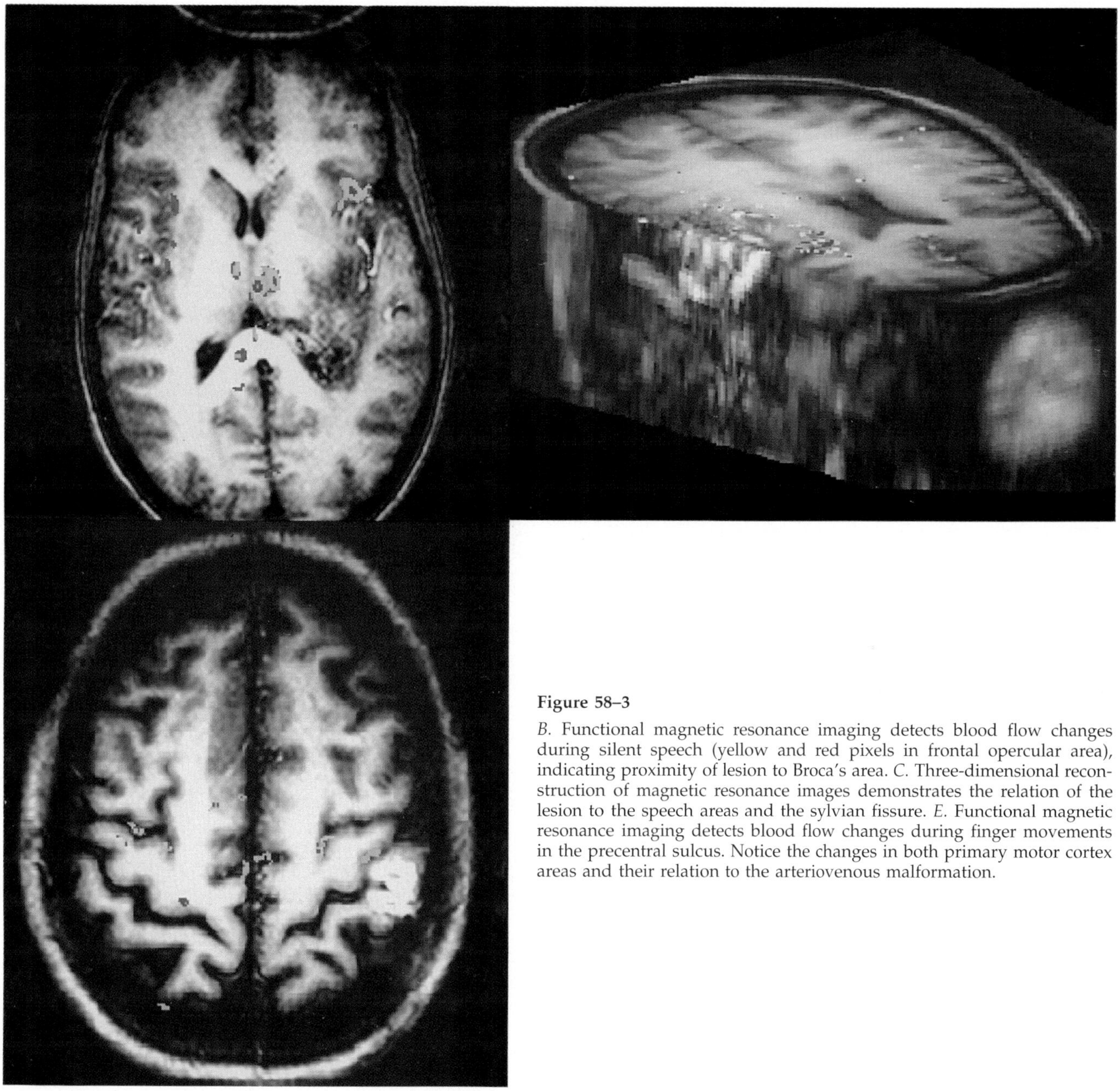

E

Figure 58–3

B. Functional magnetic resonance imaging detects blood flow changes during silent speech (yellow and red pixels in frontal opercular area), indicating proximity of lesion to Broca's area. *C.* Three-dimensional reconstruction of magnetic resonance images demonstrates the relation of the lesion to the speech areas and the sylvian fissure. *E.* Functional magnetic resonance imaging detects blood flow changes during finger movements in the precentral sulcus. Notice the changes in both primary motor cortex areas and their relation to the arteriovenous malformation.

PLATE VI

PART VI

Developmental and Acquired Anomalies

The Genetic Basis of Neurosurgical Disorders

The human genome project is rapidly approaching completion. Soon the entire human genome will be mapped. Approximately 738 human diseases have been ascribed to specific chromosomal loci.[78] In the past 5 years, the identification of the genes responsible for neurofibromatosis types 1 and 2 and the von Hippel–Lindau syndrome have opened new vistas in understanding of the fundamental molecular changes that occur in these disorders. As a result, a working knowledge of the principles of genetics has become essential for the neurosurgeon who wishes to understand the pathogenesis of the many disorders affecting the central and peripheral nervous systems.

Although the identification of a specific genetic locus or gene sequence is an important initial step in the characterization of the molecular pathogenesis of a disease, the transcription of genetic information to messenger RNA and the coordinated translation of messenger RNA to protein are equally important events that control vital cell functions. After the completion of the human genome project, a greater understanding of a disease phenotype is likely to follow only from careful and in-depth analyses of aberrant protein structure and function.

The pathogenesis of some inherited diseases, such as tuberous sclerosis, is extremely complex. Numerous chromosomal loci have been linked to this disorder. Only now is it being appreciated how apparently different chromosomal aberrations lead to phenotypically similar diseases. In many other disorders, such as neural tube defects and intracranial saccular aneurysms, genetic changes alone seem to play a less prominent role. An understanding of how hereditary susceptibility to an environmental factor leads to disease may open the way to a better understanding of the pathogenesis of these conditions.

Disorders inherited in a mendelian fashion have been catalogued by McKusick.[74] His text serves as an excellent reference for several thousands of genetically linked disorders and describes in detail the principles of mendelian inheritance. Much of our knowledge of genetics has come from the study of families with recognizable patterns of inheritance.

Many genes have been identified through linkage studies of these families. A linkage study assesses the inheritance of two genetic loci in a pedigree. Two loci are said to be linked if they segregate together more often than by chance alone, and linkage occurs if the two loci are close together on the same chromosome. Linkage studies have been based on restriction fragment length polymorphisms (RFLPs). A restriction enzyme is an enzyme that cleaves internal phosphodiester bonds of double-stranded DNA at a specific sequence (Table 31–1). Because DNA sequences vary slightly among individuals, different numbers of recognition sites for restriction enzymes may be found in different persons. This variability in restriction enzyme cleavage sites produces different patterns of DNA fragmentation after the DNA is segregated by gel electrophoresis and thus reveals the presence of restriction fragment length polymorphisms. Restriction fragment length polymorphisms are stably inherited variations in chromosome structure that can be investigated by restriction digestion and Southern blot analysis of the DNA of normal cells. Molecular geneticists have developed a bank of probes that frequently reveal restriction fragment length polymorphisms, and these probes have been mapped to specific chromosomes in the human genome.

Genetically inherited diseases may be studied by restriction fragment length polymorphism analysis. If a specific disease is associated with a known DNA marker sequence, then a restriction fragment length polymorphism for the marker may be inherited with the disease, suggesting that the gene of interest is located nearby. Further studies can then be performed to more precisely identify the site of the disease gene.

P. B. Dirks • J. T. Rutka

Table 31–1
RESTRICTION ENDONUCLEASES

A restriction endonuclease is an enzyme that recognizes specific double-stranded DNA sequences and cleaves DNA in a precise and reproducible fashion. Usually, the double-stranded DNA molecule is cleaved in a staggered fashion, creating single-stranded DNA overhangs (sticky ends). These sticky ends may associate by complementary base pairing. Restriction endonucleases have allowed the controlled manipulation of DNA that is essential to most techniques in molecular biology, including gene cloning. Restriction enzymes are found in bacteria, where they act as a protective mechanism against viral infection. This table lists several common enzymes, the bacterium from which they were isolated, their specific sequence recognition sites, and the sticky ends created after cleavage.

Organism	Enzyme	Cleavage Sequence	Ends After Cleavage
Escherichia coli	EcoRI	5′...G|AATTC...3′ 3′...CTTAA|G...5′	G + AATTC CTTAA G
Haemophilus influenzae	Hind III	5′...A|AGCTT...3′ 3′...TTCGA|A...5′	A + AGCTT TTCGA C
Bacillus amyloliquefaciens	BamHI	5′...G|GATCC...3′ 3′...CCTAG|G...5′	G + GATCC CCTAG G

Identifying the locus of the disease gene is an essential first step in knowing the DNA sequence of the gene. One problem with this type of analysis is that it requires the study of large families and the assessment of many different markers. One purpose of the human genome project is to determine markers for every region of each human chromosome.

A concept called loss of heterozygosity has also been important for determining potential genetic loci for disease processes. Often, normal individuals are heterozygous for a specific chromosome marker by restriction fragment length polymorphism analysis, because a different restriction enzyme site is inherited from each parent. If a parent has a mutation in a gene on one chromosome that results in a loss of a restriction enzyme site, loss of heterozygosity of the normal restriction fragment length polymorphism is said to occur. Several tumor suppressor genes have been discovered as a consequence of detection of loss of heterozygosity.

Physical assessment of chromosomes by analysis of Giemsa-stained metaphase chromosomal preparations has also been important in identifying possible loci of genetically inherited diseases. The identification of chromosome breaks that lead to translocations has been an important initial step in the cloning of a disease gene. However, the limit of resolution with this technique is 1 megabase of deletion, insertion, or translocation.[33] More recently, fluorescence in situ hybridization has allowed mapping of a specific fluorescent-tagged, cloned complementary DNA fragment to a specific chromosome. Fluorescence in situ hybridization is capable of detecting aneuploidy, microdeletions or duplications, and complex rearrangements.[33] An example of fluorescence in situ hybridization is shown in Figure 31–1.

The development of the polymerase chain reaction, which allows enzymatic amplification of DNA, has led to many new methods of detection of structural alterations of DNA, down to a single base alteration. Although a discussion of polymerase chain reaction methods is beyond the scope of this chapter, determin-ing the sequence of DNA using polymerase chain reaction–based techniques is a fundamentally important step in the final characterization of the gene of interest. A study of the factors controlling gene transcription and protein formation must follow to fully understand the impact of a disease gene on phenotype.

Developmental Disorders

NEURAL TUBE DEFECTS

Neural tube defects are a group of common congenital malformations that includes craniorachischisis totalis, anencephaly, myelomeningocele, and encephalocele. These malformations are believed to be caused by failure of the neural tube to close. The anterior and posterior neuropores are the last regions of the neural tube to close and, for poorly understood reasons, are the most vulnerable to malformation, resulting in anencephaly and myelomeningocele. Encephalocele probably represents a defect that occurs after the completion of neurulation.[13] Despite the prevalence of these malformations, their causes are still poorly understood. An understanding of the origins of these disorders is made difficult because many reports in the literature refer to this potentially heterogeneous group of disorders collectively as neural tube defects without further definition. The fact that myelomeningocele can have varied pathology also complicates the issue.[13] Neural tube defects may represent a diverse group of malformations with many different causes, linked only by a common clinical appearance.[13]

A multitude of environmental and genetic factors have been implicated in the pathogenesis of neural tube defects. Genetic susceptibility to environmental agents has also been suggested.[13] An astounding number of environmental factors, including geography, season of conception, maternal age (both older and younger), socioeconomic class, zinc deficiency, folic acid deficiency, maternal diabetes, elevated maternal

Figure 31–1

The figure shows a fluoresence in situ hybridization image of an interphase nucleus and chromosomal spread from a tumor cell line established from a childhood neuroblastoma outside the central nervous system. The *MYCN* proto-oncogene has been used as a molecular probe to determine whether it has been amplified in this tumor. Amplification of *MYCN* correlates with poor prognosis in neuroblastoma. The bright spots (*arrows*) identify the location of the amplified *MYCN* gene in these two nuclear preparations (amplified *MYCN* is identified as a homogeneously staining region on chromosome 7). There is an increased amount of bright signal, suggesting that the *MYCN* gene is amplified. Southern analysis of tumor DNA confirms that *MYCN* is amplified 70-fold in this tumor. This method may be a rapid means of screening for genetic alterations in cancer. (Courtesy of Jeremy Squire, Ph. D., Department of Pathology, Hospital for Sick Children, Toronto.)

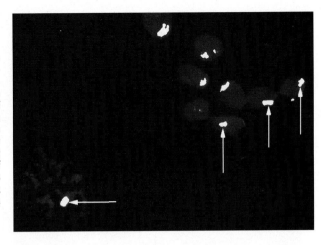

temperature during the first month of gestation, alcohol abuse during the first month of pregnancy, and maternal use of valproic acid, have been associated with neural tube defects.[13, 20, 60] Encephaloceles do not exhibit ethnic, geographical, or gender variation, as other neural tube defects do.[86]

Genetic factors alone are probably only rarely the cause of neural tube defects. Concordance between monozygotic twins is low.[86] More likely, genetic predisposition to an environmental factor is responsible. If genetic factors alone are involved, they are probably polygenic.[13, 60] An increased prevalence in certain ethnic groups, a slight female preponderance, and an increased incidence in offspring of consanguineous marriages are traits of neural tube defects that have suggested a genetic basis. Female predominance is more pronounced in anencephaly.[13, 60] Females are also more commonly afflicted with neural tube defects above the thoracolumbar junction. Mariman and Hamel have reported that affected females with neural tube defects often inherit the trait from their mothers, implying a possible anomalous X-inactivation mechanism.[67] Studies of families with neural tube defects have shown an increased risk in sibs and offspring of affected individuals (1 to 2 per cent and 3 per cent, respectively).[13] That the genetic mechanisms underlying neural tube defects are complex is well illustrated by a myriad of reports that describe autosomal dominant, autosomal recessive, and X-linked recessive patterns of inheritance in some families.[5, 27, 48, 131, 132] These families are very rare, and within each family, phenotypic expression of the neural tube defect may be highly variable. Chromosomal abnormalities, such as trisomy 13, 18, and 21, have also been associated with neural tube defects.[13, 105]

In animals, neural tube defects have occurred with various mutations.[20, 125] Mutations in 13 genetic loci and three chromosomal aberrations have been identified in rodents with neural tube defects.[20] The mouse sploch (Sp) mutation that causes neural tube defects maps to a region that is homologous to the human gene for Waardenburg's syndrome type 1 on the long arm of chromosome 2. One report has described a family with two members affected with both Waardenburg's syndrome and myelomeningocele.[15]

HYDROCEPHALUS

Hydrocephalus is commonly a congenital disorder that can occur as an isolated finding or as part of a complex congenital malformation syndrome. Congenital or primary hydrocephalus, with an incidence of 1 in 1,000 births, is usually a sporadic condition, but families with X-linked and autosomal recessive patterns of inheritance have been reported.[77] The X-linked form is more common and is estimated to occur in 1 in 30,000 male births.[36] This condition accounts for an estimated 25 per cent of male hydrocephalus not associated with myelomeningocele.[11] The clinical features of this disorder are hydrocephalus, mental retardation, adducted thumbs, and spastic paraplegia. Hydrocephalus is usually caused by aqueductal stenosis, and other cerebral anomalies have been described, including agenesis of the corpus callosum and defects of the septum pellucidum.[49] Clinical features can be extremely heterogeneous within and between families.[36, 49] Genetic linkage studies have assigned the locus for X-linked hydrocephalus to the chromosomal band Xq28.[49, 137] A gene (*L1CAM*) for a neural cell adhesion molecule, L1, has also been localized to the same site.[108] This molecule is a cell surface glycoprotein that may play a role in neuronal cell migration, neurite outgrowth, and development of the neuromuscular junction.[108] Abnormal L1 messenger RNA has been found in three members of a family with X-linked hydrocephalus.[108] The *L1CAM* gene has been confirmed as the responsible gene through the finding of different aberrantly spliced messenger RNA molecules in other families.[134] Hydrocephalus that follows an autosomal recessive pattern has been described much less frequently.[17, 36] Computed tomography and magnetic resonance imaging of a child with autosomal recessive hydrocephalus are depicted in Figure 31–2.

DANDY-WALKER SYNDROME

The cause of Dandy-Walker syndrome is unknown. Despite the common association of other congenital anomalies with this syndrome (including other central nervous system, cardiac, gastrointestinal, urogenital,

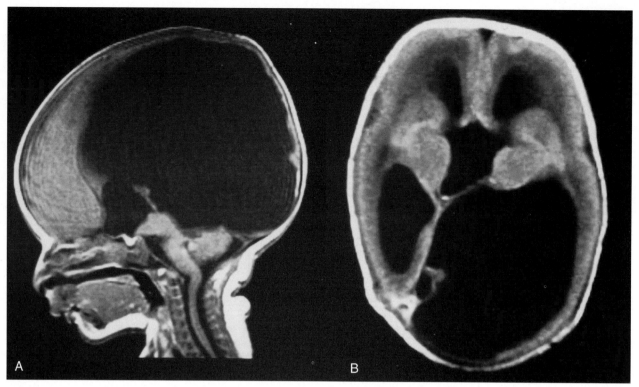

Figure 31–2

A sagittal magnetic resonance image (*A*) and an axial computed tomogram (*B*) of a child with Walker-Warburg syndrome and hydrocephalus are shown. Walker-Warburg syndrome is a neurodevelopmental condition characterized by severe cerebral dysgenesis and hydrocephalus. Even after cerebrospinal fluid diversionary procedures, the mortality rate from neurological decline is exceptionally high. Family studies have shown that Walker-Warburg syndrome is inherited on an autosomal recessive basis.

facial, and skeletal anomalies), this condition has been only occasionally described in families, most often as part of a syndrome inherited in an autosomal recessive manner.[12, 99, 103] This syndrome may also occur in the context of chromosomal aberrations.[85] Other associated nervous system abnormalities may include agenesis of the corpus callosum, aqueductal stenosis, cerebral heterotopias, holoprosencephaly, neural tube defects, and rachischisis. Before 1984, with 300 reported cases of Dandy-Walker syndrome in the literature, only 16 had been described in families, suggesting that a genetic predisposition to this syndrome probably is uncommon.[41] The syndrome probably represents a nonspecific central nervous system malformation, which may occur alone or with other malformations and which may occur in single gene disorders, in chromosomal aberrations, or as a consequence of an environmental insult.[85]

CRANIOSYNOSTOSIS

The craniosynostoses comprise a heterogeneous group of disorders of multifactorial origin. The incidence of craniosynostosis has been estimated to be 1 in 2,500 live births.[43] Primary, or simple, craniosynostosis is familiar to most neurosurgeons; the term refers to single- or multiple-suture synostosis in children who are otherwise neurologically normal. Synostosis that occurs as part of a syndrome of complex

congenital malformations is frequently called complex, or syndromic, craniosynostosis.[18, 21] The term "secondary craniosynostosis" refers to craniosynostosis caused by teratogens, metabolic disorders, and hematological disorders. Secondary craniosynostosis can also occur as the consequence of lack of growth at the suture lines because of microcephaly, encephalocele, or shunted hydrocephalus.[18, 21]

Genetic causes of primary craniosynostosis include mendelian (monogenic) disorders and chromosomal aberrations. Mendelian disorders may cause simple or complex craniosynostosis, but craniosynostosis associated with chromosomal aberrations is usually part of a syndrome.[19] Most cases of simple craniosynostosis, however, are sporadic. It has been estimated that approximately 8 per cent of coronal synostosis cases and 2 per cent of sagittal synostosis cases (the most common type of primary synostosis) are familial.[42, 43] Affected families may have members with involvement of different sutures, and, in the case of familial coronal synostosis, family members may have unilateral or bilateral involvement.[42] Dominant inheritance is more common than recessive inheritance. Approximately 27 different chromosomal aberrations have been reported for craniosynostosis, and more continue to be described each year.[19]

Scaphocephaly

Premature fusion of the sagittal suture is the most common form of primary craniosynostosis, accounting for approximately 45 to 50 per cent of cases.[21, 121] From 73 to 80 per cent of scaphocephaly patients are males.[21] Familial cases are unusual (2 per cent) so the risk of recurrence is thought to be extremely low.

Plagiocephaly

Frontal plagiocephaly, caused by unilateral coronal suture synostosis, is the second most common type of craniosynostosis (20 to 25 per cent of cases).[21] This type of synostosis is more commonly associated with a clinical syndrome than is scaphocephaly, but the majority of cases remain sporadic. If it is inherited in families, other family members tend to have bilateral coronal synostosis, suggesting that the two conditions may have a similar genotype.[21, 42] A family with monozygotic twins with mirror-image unilateral coronal synostosis is depicted in Figure 31–3.

Occipital plagiocephaly, or unilateral lambdoid synostosis (1.3 per cent of all synostoses), has been described as an isolated abnormality in two members of the same family.[21] A review of 74 patients with this condition revealed two patients with first-degree relatives with sagittal synostosis.[84] Males are affected twice as often as females.[84] Occipital plagiocephaly may be seen as a part of a complex craniofacial syndrome.

Trigonocephaly

Isolated metopic suture synostosis (5 per cent of craniosynostoses) has rarely been described in families.[21] It may be associated with Christian syndrome II, an X-linked, semidominant syndrome consisting of hypertelorism, clinodactyly, vertebral anomalies, and imperforate anus. Metopic synostosis is one of many different suture synostoses seen in Carpenter's syndrome.[21]

Turricephaly

This type of craniosynostosis is characterized by a tall, broad head, and as an isolated entity it represents 5 to 10 per cent of primary craniosynostoses.[121] Typically, the coronal sutures are involved bilaterally, along with the sphenofrontal sutures. Familial forms have been described, with a possible autosomal dominant pattern.[21] More commonly, this type of synostosis is the type found in the autosomal dominant Apert's syndrome (100 per cent of cases) and in Crouzon's syndrome (50 to 60 per cent of cases).[121]

Oxycephaly

Simultaneous fusion of multiple sutures may produce a conical-shaped head and is seen in 5 to 10 per cent of primary craniosynostoses.[121] This condition is heterogeneous in origin and may be seen in Crouzon's syndrome.[21]

Crouzon's Syndrome

Crouzon's syndrome is the most common craniofacial syndrome. It is characterized by calvarial deformity, facial deformity, and exophthalmos. The calvarial deformities always involve more than one suture and consist of oxycephaly, turricephaly, and dolichocephaly. In 5 per cent of cases, the calvaria is normal.[21] Cloverleaf skull deformity may also occur. The skull base is implicated, and sphenofrontal synostosis is a factor involved in producing exophthalmos. Maxillary hypoplasia, the characteristic facial deformity, is a more important cause of exophthalmos. Hydrocephalus is more common in Crouzon's syndrome than in simple craniosynostoses.[31]

This condition is inherited in an autosomal dominant fashion, but there is an equal incidence of sporadic cases, which probably represent new mutations. Pene-

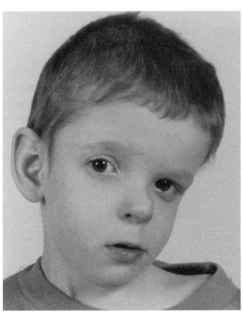
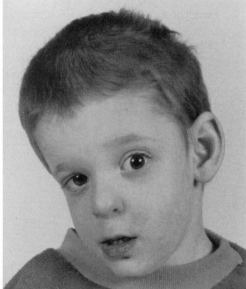

Figure 31–3

Monozygotic twins 3 years of age show untreated mirror-image unilateral coronal synostoses. Although the vast majority of unilateral coronal synostoses are thought to be sporadic in origin, the presence of identical cranial vault deformities in these twins suggests a possible genetic basis of inheritance.

trance is high, although severity is variable.[21] Within the same family, members tend to have similar facial deformities but variable calvarial deformities.[21] This phenotypic heterogeneity makes genetic counseling difficult.

Apert's Syndrome

Apert's syndrome, the second most common craniofacial syndrome, is characterized by turricephaly, mental retardation, maxillary hypoplasia, orbital hypertelorism, syndactyly, and vertebral and skeletal abnormalities. Usually, cases are sporadic, but the syndrome may be inherited in an autosomal dominant fashion.

Other Acrocephalosyndactyly Syndromes

Three of the less common craniofacial disorders that may be encountered by the neurosurgeon are Carpenter's syndrome, Saethre-Chotzen syndrome, and Pfeiffer's syndrome. All types may occur sporadically, but mendelian inheritance may also occur in a recessive fashion for Carpenter's syndrome and in a dominant fashion for the other two. In Carpenter's syndrome, the calvarial deformity is variable and is less striking than the facial and digital anomalies. Mental retardation, cardiac anomalies, and hypogonadism are also common. Saethre-Chotzen syndrome is a relatively benign condition. The features of this condition include brachycephaly or plagiocephaly, facial asymmetry with hypertelorism and orbital dystopia, low frontal hairline, ptosis, and mild maxillary hypoplasia. Syndactyly is usually mild, and mental retardation is much less common. Pfeiffer's syndrome is characterized by turricephaly, hypertelorism, slanted palpebral fissures, and broad thumbs and toes; mentation is usually normal.[21]

Vascular Disorders

Most of the vascular disorders with which neurosurgeons are familiar are thought to be acquired. However, genetic factors may play a role in certain vascular disorders, such as intracranial aneurysms and cavernous malformations. Cerebral arteriovenous malformation is a congenital disorder but is not believed to be genetically inherited. Cerebral arteriovenous malformations occasionally occur in the context of Rendu-Osler-Weber syndrome, a genetic disorder with predominantly systemic consequences.

CEREBRAL ANEURYSMS

Observations from cases of subarachnoid hemorrhage that have occurred in families and in association with heritable diseases have led to speculation that intracranial saccular aneurysms may form as the consequence of a genetic defect in the arterial wall of a basal intracranial vessel. However, this theory of aneurysmal formation has been strongly disputed.[123] Others vehemently support the notion that intracranial aneurysms are degenerative lesions that arise as a consequence of hemodynamic stress.[123] Certainly, the occurrence of cerebral aneurysms has been well documented in families in the literature, but a familial association does not necessarily imply a congenital cause or inherited condition.[94, 107, 136] However, findings from reported cases among families suggest that a certain subpopulation of patients may have an inherited predisposition to cerebral aneurysm formation. In addition, Weir has speculated that the incidence of familial aneurysms may be under-reported because most patients with ruptured intracranial aneurysms present in extremis in a state not conducive to detailed family history-taking.[136]

Familial aneurysms are estimated to represent 2 to 10 per cent of all cases of cerebral aneurysms.[94, 107, 128, 136] The highest incidence has been reported in a population from eastern Finland.[107] In most of these cases, a single sib is the other affected family member, and it is difficult to be certain whether this incidence exceeds occurrence by chance alone. In families with more than two affected members, the suggestion of a possible genetic basis is more convincing. In these families, an autosomal dominant pattern of inheritance has usually been suspected.[39, 119] In other large families, the mode of inheritance has been indeterminate.[35]

Familial cases of aneurysms seem to have some unique clinical features compared with sporadic cases. Familial aneurysms rupture at a younger age (42 years versus mid-50s) and are less often seen in the anterior communicating complex than are sporadic aneurysms.[35, 61] Some authors have found that patients with multiple aneurysms frequently have a family history of aneurysms, and others have suggested that these patients have aneurysms that may rupture at a smaller size.[35, 94] Aneurysms tend to occur more often in the same site or a mirror site, and in reports of identical twins with aneurysms, all aneurysms occur at the same sites or at mirror sites.[35] In addition, sibling pairs are more likely to have aneurysms rupture in the same decade, and twins to have rupture within 2 to 5 years of each other.[35] The existence of a collagen type III deficiency in patients with familial aneurysm is controversial.

In a very small percentage of cases, cerebral aneurysms are associated with a known hereditary condition. Cerebral aneurysms have been described with Marfan's syndrome, Ehlers-Danlos syndrome, pseudoxanthoma elasticum, polycystic kidney disease, tuberous sclerosis, hereditary hemorrhagic telangiectasia, Anderson-Fabry disease, and neurofibromatosis.[136] Steubens has argued that the coexistence of congenital anomalies and cerebral aneurysms is statistically insignificant.[123] Steubens found a higher incidence of cerebral aneurysms in polycystic kidney disease (and also in aortic coarctation), and severe secondary hypertension was thought to have been responsible.[123] Cerebral aneurysms that affect children also appear to be a distinct clinical entity, with male predominance, posterior circulation involvement, and a high frequency of giant aneurysms.[80, 124] However, as with other subpopulations of patients with aneurysms, the cause in these patients remains uncertain.

CAVERNOUS MALFORMATIONS

With the improvement in neuroimaging techniques, a familial association of patients with cavernous malformations has been recognized with increased frequency. The inheritance pattern is autosomal dominant, lesions are often multiple, and an increased frequency of occurrence among Latino families has been noted.[23, 40, 71, 102, 111] Most patients are asymptomatic.[102] An understanding of the natural history of this condition awaits further study. A pedigree of a family with familial cavernous malformations is shown in Figure 31–4.

Phakomatoses

NEUROFIBROMATOSIS

Neurofibromatosis, one of the most common autosomal dominant inherited disorders, is characterized by a predisposition to tumors of the nervous system. Two clinically and genetically distinct forms of neurofibromatosis have been recognized, neurofibromatosis type 1 (von Recklinghausen's neurofibromatosis) and neurofibromatosis type 2 (bilateral acoustic neurofibromatosis). The genes for both disorders have been identified, and it appears that they act as tumor suppressor genes. The gene for neurofibromatosis type 1 resides on chromosome 17, and the gene for neurofibromatosis type 2 is located on chromosome 22; their protein products have been characterized and named neurofibromin and merlin (schwannomin), respec-

tively. These discoveries have opened up an exciting era in the study of cancer genetics. It remains to be discovered how perturbations of these genes lead to the characteristic cancers seen in these conditions. A comparison of the two types of neurofibromatosis is presented in Table 31–2.

Neurofibromatosis Type 1

Neurofibromatosis type 1 has an incidence of 1 in 4,000 individuals. Although the gene is transmissible in an autosomal dominant fashion, a very high rate of spontaneous mutation exists. The new mutation rate for the neurofibromatosis type 1 gene has been estimated at 1×10^{-4}, which is one of the highest rates for any human disorder.[44] Approximately 50 per cent of individuals with neurofibromatosis type 1 do not have a family history of the disorder, and the disease is thought to arise sporadically. Neurofibromatosis type 1 is also characterized by 100 per cent penetrance; all patients with the genetic defect have at least some of the clinical manifestations of the disorder. However, the expressivity of the neurofibromatosis type 1 defect is extremely variable, and the severity of the disease in individuals even within the same family is unpredictable.

Clinical Manifestations

The clinical manifestations of neurofibromatosis type 1 are characterized primarily, but not exclusively, by abnormalities in tissues derived from the neural crest. Because of the variable expressivity of the disorder, a clinical diagnosis can be difficult. Diagnostic criteria have been firmly established[89] (Table 31–3). Skin lesions are the most common manifestations, consisting of multiple café au lait spots, cutaneous neurofibromas,

FAMILY C

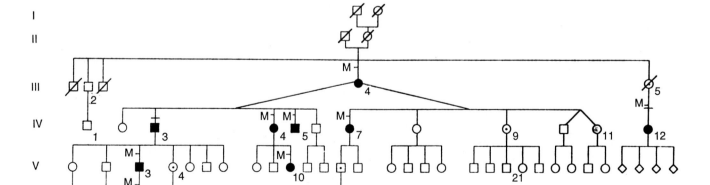

Figure 31–4

The pedigree of a Mexican American family with cavernous malformations is shown. Solid black symbols represent affected individuals confirmed by magnetic resonance imaging or by pathology. Multiple generations are involved, and males and females are affected equally. (From Rigamonti, D., Hadley, M. N., Drayer, B. P., et al.: Cerebral cavernous angiomas: Incidence and family occurrence. N. Engl. J. Med., *319*:343–347, 1988. Reprinted by permission. Copyright 1988 Massachusetts Medical Society.)

Table 31–2

COMPARISON OF NEUROFIBROMATOSIS TYPE 1 AND NEUROFIBROMATOSIS TYPE 2

Characteristic	Neurofibromatosis Type 1	Neurofibromatosis Type 2
Incidence	1 in 4000	1 in 40,000
Inheritance	Autosomal dominant	Autosomal dominant
Chromosome locus	17q11.2	22q12
Complementary DNA	13 kilobases	1.8 kilobases
Protein	Neurofibromin	Merlin or schwannomin
Protein function	GAP-like function downregulates proto-oncogene *RASA*	Links cell membrane proteins to cytoskeleton
Mutation rate	1 in 10,000	Uncertain
Penetrance	100%	95% for VS
Expressivity	Variable	Not variable for VS
Clinical onset	First decade	Second to third decade
Intellectual deficit	>25%	None
Café au lait macules	99% by adulthood	Not uncommon
Cutaneous neurofibromas	Frequent	Few
Lisch nodules	100% in patients older than 20 years of age	None
Posterior lens opacities	None	>85%
Skeletal abnormalities	Not uncommon	Rare
Nervous system tumors		
Vestibular schwannoma	Occasionally	95%
Optic nerve glioma	15%	Very rare
Cerebral gliomas	Common	Occasionally
Meningioma	Few	>50%, 30% multiple
Spinal neurofibroma	Common	Absent
Spinal schwannoma	Absent	Common
Plexiform neurofibroma	Common	Uncommon
Other tumors	Not rare	Rare

GAP, guanosine triphosphatase–activating protein; VS, vestibular schwannoma.

and intertriginous freckling. Café au lait spots are found in 99 per cent of patients and are usually present at birth, but they may take months to years to appear.[101] Café au lait spots vary from 2 to 15 mm in size and may be found anywhere on the skin, but they are rarely present on the face.[101] Café au lait spots may occur in unaffected individuals, but more than three café au lait macules should arouse suspicion for neurofibromatosis type 1.[63] Prepubertal patients with five or more café au lait spots greater than 5 mm in diameter, and postpubertal patients with six macules larger than 15 mm, fulfill the criteria for the diagnosis of neurofibromatosis type 1. Other types of macular lesions may be seen in patients with neurofibromatosis type 1, including hyperpigmentation of skin overlying a plexiform neurofibroma, axillary freckling, and small areas (1 to 2 mm) of hyperpigmentation in the groin, in the inframammary region, and in the skin folds associated with obesity.

Cutaneous and subcutaneous neurofibromas, which arise from distal cutaneous nerve endings, are other hallmarks of neurofibromatosis type 1. These lesions vary in number from a few to thousands and in size from a few millimeters to a few centimeters. They may occur anywhere on the body, but there is a predilection for the breast areolar region in women and for the thoracoabdominal region in all patients.[63, 101] Lesions tend to enlarge with age and may also increase in number at puberty and during pregnancy, at which time they may also become pruritic. Cutaneous neurofibromas rarely undergo malignant transformation. Plexiform neurofibromas usually develop on the larger peripheral nerves, particularly the cervical, brachial, and lumbosacral plexuses, as well as the sympathetic chain.[10] These lesions are of particular concern because they have a 5 to 10 per cent incidence of malignant transformation; this possibility should be suspected in any patient with neurofibromatosis type 1 in whom rapid growth of a subcutaneous lesion is found.

Lisch nodules are an extremely important manifestation of neurofibromatosis type 1. These lesions are mel-

Table 31–3

DIAGNOSTIC CRITERIA FOR NEUROFIBROMATOSIS TYPE 1 AND NEUROFIBROMATOSIS TYPE 2

Neurofibromatosis Type 1

A diagnosis is established if any two of the following features exist:
1. Six café au lait macules more than 5 mm in greatest diameter if prepubertal, or more than 15 mm if postpubertal
2. Two or more neurofibromas of any type, or one plexiform neurofibroma
3. Axillary or inguinal freckling
4. A distinctive osseous lesion, such as sphenoid dysplasia, congenital bowing, or thinning of long bone cortex, with or without pseudarthrosis
5. Bilateral optic nerve gliomas
6. Two or more iris Lisch nodules
7. A first-degree relative with neurofibromatosis type 1, diagnosed by the above criteria

Neurofibromatosis Type 2

1. Bilateral vestibular schwannomas demonstrated by computed tomography or magnetic resonance imaging

OR

2. A first-degree relative with bilateral vestibular schwannomas *and* either a unilateral vestibular schwannoma *or* any two of the following: neurofibroma, meningioma, glioma, schwannoma, posterior lens opacity

anocytic hamartomas that appear as well-circumscribed, domelike elevations on the surface of the iris.[62] They may be clear, yellow, or brown. In patients older than 20 years of age with neurofibromatosis type 1, Lisch nodules are present in 100 per cent of cases.[62] There has been only one case report of a patient with neurofibromatosis type 2 who had a Lisch nodule[14]; therefore, Lisch nodules are considered to be a very sensitive clinical marker for neurofibromatosis type 1.

Central nervous system tumors are also prevalent in neurofibromatosis type 1. Optic gliomas are the most common brain tumor in these patients, with an incidence of approximately 15 per cent. These tumors usually involve the anterior visual system and frequently are bilateral. It is controversial whether they have a natural history different from that of the optic gliomas that occur in patients without neurofibromatosis.[22] Other brain tumors, such as low-grade gliomas of the hypothalamus, cerebellum, brain stem, and spinal cord, as well as ependymomas, meningiomas, and primitive neuroectodermal tumors, have been reported with increased frequency in patients with neurofibromatosis type 1 compared with the general population.[129] Although rare, unilateral vestibular schwannomas can also occur in neurofibromatosis type 1.[101] Since the advent of magnetic resonance imaging, a common finding in many of these patients is "bright" lesions on T2-weighted images in the basal ganglia and brain stem, possibly representing hamartomas.[100, 118]

Patients with neurofibromatosis type 1 are also susceptible to developing tumors outside the nervous system. Pheochromocytomas, Wilms' tumor, rhabdomyosarcoma, and leukemia all have been implicated.[8, 101] Neurofibromas may also arise within solid viscera of the abdominal cavity.[101]

Finally, sphenoidal bone dyplasia, pseudoarthrosis of the tibia or radius, scoliosis, short stature, learning disabilities, seizures, and macrocephaly are other possible clinical features of neurofibromatosis type 1. Some reports have also suggested that patients with this disorder may have underlying vascular anomalies.[101, 115] Stroke may be caused by fusiform aneurysmal dilatation of the intracranial carotid or basilar arteries, which can lead to thrombosis, luminal obliteration, and the development of extracranial-intracranial anasomotic channels (moyamoya disease). Rarely, neurofibromas have been found to arise in the cerebral arterial tree, causing cerebral ischemia.[101] A higher incidence of moyamoya phenomenon has also been observed in patients with neurofibromatosis type 1 who received radiation therapy for optic pathway gliomas.[55]

Molecular Genetics

The gene for neurofibromatosis type 1 (NF1) has been cloned, and the locus resides on the long arm of chromosome 17. NF1 functions as a tumor suppressor gene, and in the most typical mode of transmission, affected patients inherit a mutated form of the gene from an affected parent. However, a mutation of one of the neurofibromatosis type 1 alleles may also be the consequence of a new paternal mutation within a spermatogonial stem cell or a mature sperm.[47] Irrespective of the mode of inheritance, a second somatic mutation within the remaining normal NF1 locus in neural crest tissues is postulated to be the mechanism by which tumors occur in the neurofibromatosis patient, because absence of normal NF1 expression leads to the loss of growth suppression and to uncontrolled proliferation. Many different types of mutations have been observed in neurofibromatosis type 1, from large megabase deletions of the whole NF1 locus to smaller kilobase deletions, translocations, and nucleotide substitutions.[34] Large deletions are typically found in patients with classic neurofibromatosis type 1. Cognitive and intellectual impairment, which is frequently seen in these patients, may ultimately map to as yet unidentified gene sequences adjacent to the NF1 locus.[34] However, it has been very difficult to correlate the heterogeneity of gene mutations in patients with this disorder with the variability in phenotypic manifestations seen in families.[34]

The neurofibromatosis 1 gene product, neurofibromin, is ubiquitously expressed, with predominance in brain, kidney, spleen, white blood cells, and neural crest–derived tissues.[34] Neurofibromin is localized to the cell cytoplasm and is intimately associated with cytoskeletal elements. It is believed that neurofibromin may act as a tumor suppressor because its complementary DNA sequence shares sequence homology with a gene encoding for a guanosine triphosphatase–activating protein (often abbreviated as GAP), which causes inactivation of the RASA oncoprotein (formerly p21-ras). The RASA oncoprotein is believed to play an important role in growth factor–mediated cellular proliferation and has been implicated as a mechanism for tumorigenesis in some human malignancies. Thus, a major function of neurofibromin may be to downregulate RASA expression and keep cell proliferation in check. Basu and colleagues showed that neurofibrosarcomas from patients with neurofibromatosis type 1 express wild-type RASA proteins in a constitutively activated state in cells that do not express neurofibromin.[6] It has been suggested that the interaction of neurofibromin with key cytoskeletal proteins plays an important role in limiting cellular proliferation.[34]

Further evidence that supports the notion that the NF1 gene functions as a tumor suppressor gene includes experiments demonstrating its homozygous deletion in malignant melanoma cell lines and in a neurofibrosarcoma from a patient with neurofibromatosis type 1.[4, 59] Alterations in this gene's locus have also been identified in other cancers.[116] However, not all tumors from patients with neurofibromatosis type 1 exhibit mutations in both copies of the gene. In some patients with neurofibromatosis type 1 malignancies, a mutation in the P53 gene has been found, which emphasizes the fact that multiple mechanisms of tumorigenesis may be operational.[79]

Preclinical genetic diagnosis remains based on linkage analysis because of the absence of consistent recognizable mutational patterns in the NF1 gene and the frequency of spontaneous mutations. The large size of the gene makes the search for causative mutations difficult. Prenatal diagnosis is possible with chorionic villus sampling.

Neurofibromatosis Type 2

Clinical Manifestations

Neurofibromatosis type 2 is much less common than neurofibromatosis type 1 with an incidence of approximately 1 in 40,000 births. Compared with neurofibromatosis type 1, neurofibromatosis type 2 is less heterogeneous clinically and is characterized by the presence of bilateral vestibular schwannomas. The diagnostic criteria are given in Table 31–3. The occurrence of vestibular schwannomas in affected families is 95 per cent.[69] Neurofibromatosis type 2 is clearly distinct from unilateral sporadic vestibular schwannomas, which are not inherited and tend to occur in older individuals. In neurofibromatosis type 2, patients typically become symptomatic from their vestibular schwannomas in the second or third decade and present with hearing loss.[69]

Tumors of the nervous system other than bilateral vestibular schwannomas are common in patients with neurofibromatosis type 2. Schwann cell tumors are the most common, but meningiomas and gliomas may also develop. The schwannomas involve other cranial and spinal nerves, and meningiomas may be cranial or spinal, with a tendency toward multiplicity of lesions and en plaque formation.[129] Meningiomas of the cranium or spine may occur in as many as one half of patients with neurofibromatosis type 2.[26] Most ependymomas and astrocytomas in these patients are intraspinal, but astrocytomas may also involve the brain stem or cerebellum. Optic nerve gliomas are not seen in patients with this disorder.

Café au lait spots, cutaneous neurofibromas, and intertriginous freckling are much less common in neurofibromatosis type 2 than in neurofibromatosis type 1, but they may be found through careful clinical examination.[69] The most common type of cutaneous lesion consists of a well-circumscribed, slightly raised, roughened, pigmented area of skin often associated with excess hair.[70] Cutaneous tumors are more likely to be schwannomas than neurofibromas.[26] Posterior capsular lens opacities are a characteristic finding in neurofibromatosis type 2. They occur in 85 per cent of patients and frequently have bilateral involvement.[50] These opacities can occur at a young age and may be the initial presentation in a patient with this disease. Progressive visual loss may occur, warranting surgical removal of the affected lens. A gene for a lens protein localizes to the same region on chromosome 22 on which the NF2 gene resides.[50] Skeletal anomalies are rare in neurofibromatosis type 2, and, in contrast to neurofibromatosis type 1, clinical features appear to be confined to the nervous system.[26]

The diagnosis of neurofibromatosis type 2 is difficult in the absence of bilateral vestibular schwannomas. A diagnosis should be suspected in any first-degree relative of an affected patient, any patient younger than 30 years old with a unilateral vestibular schwannoma, any child with a meningioma or a schwannoma, and any patient with multiple neurogenic tumors.[129] A detailed screening proposal has been outlined by Evans and associates.[26]

Molecular Genetics

The gene for neurofibromatosis type 2 (NF2) has been identified on chromosome 22. The gene product, named merlin (or schwannomin), has been localized to the cell membrane. Merlin belongs to a family of proteins that act as membrane organizers, linking integral membrane proteins with cytoskeletal elements.[109, 133] It is possible that merlin contributes to the maintenance of cell shape, participates in cell adhesion to the extracellular matrix, and is involved in intercellular communication. Mutations have been identified in the NF2 region in the germ line of patients with this disorder.[109] In addition, somatic mutations have been identified in schwannomas and meningiomas in neurofibromatosis type 2 patients with an identified germ line mutation, supporting the hypothesis that the NF2 gene has tumor suppressor function.[109] Inactivation of this gene may be a common occurrence in sporadic meningiomas and has also been identified in other tumor types.[7, 112]

Presymptomatic diagnosis became feasible after development of genetic linkage analysis, and, because of the identification of the gene for neurofibromatosis type 2, specific DNA diagnosis may be forthcoming.[88]

VON HIPPEL–LINDAU DISEASE

Von Hippel–Lindau disease is an autosomal dominant inherited disorder characterized by a hereditary predisposition to benign and malignant tumors in multiple organ systems. The gene for this disease (VHL) has been mapped to the short arm of chromosome 3 and appears to act as a tumor suppressor gene. Like neurofibromatosis, von Hippel–Lindau disease is characterized by variable expressivity and a high degree of penetrance. Younger patients may be asymptomatic, but penetrance is believed to be 100 per cent by 65 years of age. The mean age at diagnosis is 26.3 years. The incidence is estimated at 1 in 36,000 live births. The spontaneous mutation rate is estimated at 4.4×10^{-6}, much lower than that in neurofibromatosis type 1.[64]

Clinical Manifestations

The principal features of von Hippel–Lindau disease are retinal angiomas, hemangioblastomas of the central nervous system, renal cysts and renal cell carcinoma, pancreatic cysts, pheochromocytoma, and epididymal cystadenoma. There is a tendency toward familial clustering of features of this disease, suggesting that different mutations within the VHL locus may be responsible for different phenotypes.[30, 93] Patients with pheochromocytomas from families with von Hippel–Lindau disease frequently develop retinal angiomas but rarely develop central nervous system hemangioblastomas.[30, 92] Renal lesions and hemangioblastomas commonly occur together in kindred from von Hippel–Lindau families.[93]

Central nervous system hemangioblastomas are the most common lesions seen in von Hippel–Lindau disease.[57, 91] These lesions are most commonly found in the cerebellum, followed closely by the spinal cord (usually intramedullary) and, less commonly, the medulla and cerebrum. Approximately 25 per cent of all central nervous system hemangioblastomas occur in association with von Hippel–Lindau disease.[92] With the disease, hemangioblastomas occur at a younger age (29 versus 47 years) and are more often multiple than with sporadic tumors.[92] The peculiar association of cystic cerebellar hemangioblastomas (as well as renal cell carcinoma) and polycythemia has long been recognized, the latter being caused by the release of an erythropoietin-like substance by the tumor cells.[57] Approximately one quarter to one half of all central nervous system hemangioblastomas arise in the spine. These lesions are most commonly found in the thoracic and cervical regions and are prone to bleeding, resulting in subarachnoid hemorrhage. Syringomyelia, causing dissociated sensory symptoms, frequently accompanies intramedullary spinal hemangioblastomas. In general, hemangioblastomas are benign tumors, and patients can be cured with total excision. Historically, cerebellar hemangioblastomas were considered treacherous lesions because of their extreme vascularity, and they were associated with a high perioperative mortality rate. However, since the advent of microneurosurgical technique, hemangioblastomas can be safely removed with minimal morbidity.

The manifestations of von Hippel–Lindau disease outside the central nervous system are protean. Retinal angiomas are seen in 60 per cent of patients with the disease.[57] These lesions appear as a red spot on funduscopy with an associated dilated, tortuous artery and vein. In half of affected patients, both eyes are involved, and half develop unilateral or bilateral blindness secondary to glaucoma or retinal detachment. Renal cell carcinoma affects 25 per cent of von Hippel–Lindau patients and may be becoming the leading cause of death among them.[57] Renal cysts and pancreatic cysts are frequently asymptomatic, but renal cysts may become malignant. Pancreatic adenocarcinomas and islet cell tumors have been rarely reported. Pheochromocytoma is seen in approximately 20 per cent of patients. Epididymal cystadenomas are found in 17 per cent of male patients with this disease, and they are frequently bilateral.

Molecular Genetics

Linkage analysis of affected families established that the gene for von Hippel–Lindau disease is located on chromosome 3p. Clues that this chromosome was the correct site came from studies that demonstrated alterations in chromosome 3p in renal cell carcinoma and pheochromocytoma in patients with the disease.[56, 117] Linkage analysis remains the method for diagnosis of apparently unaffected family members.

TUBEROUS SCLEROSIS

Tuberous sclerosis is a disease with variable features that affect multiple organ systems. Hamartomas are the characteristic pathological lesion. The estimated incidence of the disease is 1 in 27,000 overall, with an incidence in children of 1 in 12,000.[76] Because of the highly variable clinical features, the actual incidence of the disease may be as high as 1 in 5,800.[98] Familial cases are inherited in an autosomal dominant fashion, but most cases probably arise sporadically. Expressivity is extremely variable even within families. As a result, diagnosis of affected members of the family of a patient with tuberous sclerosis is difficult. The clinical features of tuberous sclerosis may be so mild that the diagnosis may not be made until the patient is of middle age. Affected family members may completely lack the characteristic external stigmata of tuberous sclerosis.[96] This extreme variability has also made the understanding of its molecular pathogenesis elusive. Linkage analysis of families has led to the identification of genetic loci on chromosomes 9 and 16, but other chromosomal sites have been implicated in different families, including chromosomes 11 and 14.[51, 52, 95, 113] A 1993 collaborative study identified a gene at the chromosome 16 locus called *TSC2* (the candidate gene on chromosome 9 is referred to as *TSC1*) that contains deletions in patients with tuberous sclerosis. This finding is an important advance that represents the beginning of an understanding of the molecular pathogenesis of this disorder.[90]

Clinical Manifestations

The traditional clinical triad of adenoma sebaceum, seizures, and mental retardation has been refined with appreciation of the complexity of the disorder. Diagnostic criteria have been established by the National Tuberous Sclerosis Association (Table 31–4).[104] No single clinical feature is always present, although some are highly specific, such as multiple facial angiofibromas (previously referred to as adenoma sebaceum).[104] Mental retardation and seizures are extremely common in this disease, but because of their lack of specificity they are not included as diagnostic criteria. Many of the clinical features, such as facial angiofibromas, ungual fibromas, and subependymal nodules, are not apparent until adulthood.

The clinical manifestations of tuberous sclerosis involve skin, nervous system, eyes, heart, kidneys, and bone. Depigmented nevi or white patches characteristically of "ash-leaf" shape are the earliest sign of the disease, but these may require use of an ultraviolet lamp in a dark room for visualization.[97] Angiofibromas are found on the cheeks, nasal folds, and chin but spare the upper lip. Fibromas are also seen in the periungual and subungual regions. A shagreen patch is a leathery, discolored patch found on the trunk or the lumbar region. A fibrous plaque on the forehead may also be an early sign.[97] Fibromas may also occur on the gums, and the teeth may be pitted.

Seizures are the most common presenting feature

Table 31–4

DIAGNOSTIC CRITERIA FOR TUBEROUS SCLEROSIS COMPLEX

Definite tuberous sclerosis: Either one primary feature, two secondary features, or one secondary plus two tertiary features.
Probable tuberous sclerosis: Either one secondary plus one tertiary, or three tertiary features.
Suspect tuberous sclerosis: Either one secondary or two tertiary features.

Primary Features
    Facial angiofibromas
    Multiple ungual fibromas
    Cortical tuber, subependymal nodule, or giant cell astrocytoma (pathology confirmed)
    Multiple retinal astrocytomas

Secondary Features
    Affected first-degree relative
    Cardiac rhabdomyoma
    Cerebral tubers or subependymal nodules (radiologically confirmed)
    Shagreen patch
    Forehead plaque
    Pulmonary lymphangiomyomatosis (pathology confirmed)
    Renal angiomyolipoma
    Renal cyst (pathology confirmed)

Tertiary Features
    Hypomelanotic macules
    Confetti skin lesions
    Enamel pits
    Hamartomatous renal polyps (pathology confirmed)
    Bone cysts
    Pulmonary lymphangiomyomatosis by radiography
    Cerebral white matter migration tracts or heterotopias
    Gingival fibromas
    Other hamartomas
    Infantile spasms

Modified from Roach, E. S., Smith, M., Huttenlocher, P., et al.: Report of the Diagnostic Criteria Committee of the National Tuberous Sclerosis Association. J. Child Neurol., 7:221, 1992.

of tuberous sclerosis, and infantile spasms are both common in and fairly specific for tuberous sclerosis.[104] Approximately 20 per cent of patients with infantile spasms have tuberous sclerosis.[97] Myoclonic seizures are also commonly found. Cognitive delay is seen in about 60 per cent of patients with this disorder.[87] Children often appear to be neurologically normal during infancy, but with time they fall behind in achieving the developmental milestones and develop mental retardation and seizures.[68] The classic brain lesion in tuberous sclerosis consists of focal areas of gliosis with giant neurons and astrocytes. Known as "tubers," these lesions occur on the cortex and subependymal regions of the lateral ventricles, where they have been referred to as "candle drippings." Frequently, these lesions are calcified and are easily seen on computed tomography. Subependymal giant cell astrocytomas are thought to arise from these hamartomas, and they can reach considerable size and may cause obstructive hydrocephalus because of their proximity to the foramen of Monro.[110] The histological appearance of subependymal giant cell astrocytomas is characterized by large cells containing an abundance of eosinophilic cytoplasm on a coarse fibrillary background.[9] It is not clear whether the cell of origin in this tumor is a neoplastic astrocyte. The giant cells are variably positive for glial fibrillary acidic protein and neurofilaments, suggesting the presence of astrocytic and neuronal elements in the lesion and supporting their hamartomatous nature.[9] On occasion, malignant astrocytomas may occur in patients with tuberous sclerosis, possibly representing malignant degeneration of a subependymal giant cell astrocytoma.

Visceral abnormalities are also most frequently hamartomatous in nature. Renal cysts and angiomyolipomas of the kidney may occur. Multiple renal angiomyolipomas are considered diagnostic.[97] Cardiac rhabdomyomas also occur, along with pulmonary hamartomas. Retinal lesions may resemble those of the subependymal giant cell astrocytomas seen in the brain.

Molecular Genetics

Linkage analysis first localized tuberous sclerosis to the ABO blood group at chromosome 9q34.[28] Several years later, linkage to chromosome 11q was identified, but this latter finding has not been confirmed. Other possible sites have not been confirmed, and many families remain unlinked.[51] Linkage to chromosome 16p13, in the region of the gene for autosomal dominant polycystic kidney disease type 1 (*PKD1*), has been reported.[51] Polycystic kidneys are common in patients with tuberous sclerosis, and any patient with polycystic kidneys should be investigated for the diagnosis of tuberous sclerosis.[51] The gene at 16p13 has been cloned, and the protein product has been named tuberin.[90] This protein has sequence homology to guanosine triphosphatase–activating proteins, which are important components of intracellular signal transduction pathways (RASA and NF1 gene products are also involved in these pathways, as has been discussed). A variety of deletions in this gene have been identified in unrelated tuberous sclerosis patients, and it is possible that this gene product may also have tumor suppressor function.[90] Loss of heterozygosity for DNA markers at chromosome 16p13 in hamartomas from tuberous sclerosis patients supports its putative tumor suppressor function.[32] Our understanding of the molecular biology of this condition is in the very early stages, and much further study is necessary.

Neurocutaneous Angiomatoses

ATAXIA TELANGIECTASIA

Ataxia telangiectasia is an autosomal recessive disorder characterized by cerebellar ataxia, oculocutaneous telangiectases, immune deficiency, extreme sensitivity to ionizing radiation, and a high incidence of cancer. The incidence of ataxia telangiectasia is estimated at 1 in 20,000 to 100,000 births, but the prevalence of heterozygous carriers in the United States white population has been estimated at 0.68 to 7.7 per cent.[29, 127]

Cerebellar ataxia, the most common presenting

symptom, is noticed within the first 2 years of life.[29] Ataxia is predominantly truncal at younger ages and becomes more appendicular at later ages. Dysarthria, muscle hypotonia, and slow initiation of movement also occur. Choreoathetosis and dystonia occur in older patients. The ataxia is progressive, and the child is usually confined to a wheelchair by 10 years of age. Abnormalities of voluntary conjugate gaze and peripheral neuropathy (in older patients) are other common neurological features of the disease. Mental retardation may occur, but most patients have normal or above average intelligence quotient scores.[29]

Telangiectases do not appear until the child is 3 to 5 years of age, but they then progressively involve the conjunctivae, face, arms, legs, and hard and soft palate. These abnormal capillary vessels rarely hemorrhage. Telangiectases are not common in visceral organs or the brain.[29] Other cutaneous lesions, resembling those found in the elderly, also occur. Senile keratosis and basal cell carcinomas of the face may occur in patients in their twenties.[29]

Patients with ataxia telangiectasia are immune deficient and highly susceptible to infections. Pneumonia is a common cause of death. Diminished immunoglobulin levels, decreased response to skin testing, and lymphopenia occur.[29] The thymus is commonly absent. Endocrine changes are also common, including gonadal hypoplasia or dysplasia, diminished secondary sexual characteristics, and short stature. Glucose intolerance affects more than half of patients.[73]

Neoplasms are the second most common cause of death in patients with ataxia telangiectasia.[29] More than one third of ataxia telangiectasia patients develop malignancy. Patients are susceptible to leukemia, lymphoma, gastrointestinal epithelial neoplasms, breast carcinoma, medulloblastomas, and astrocytomas. The incidence of cancer is also increased in heterozygous carriers of ataxia telangiectasia, particularly for breast carcinoma in women (relative risk 6.8).[127] This increased risk may be related to exposure to low levels of ionizing radiation.[126] Treatment of cancers in patients with ataxia telangiectasia must be performed with great care because of inherited radiation susceptibility.

Cells from patients with ataxia telangiectasia exhibit sensitivity to a number of factors, including ionizing radiation and multiple chemotherapeutic agents.[73] Ionizing radiation damages DNA by creating single- and double-strand breaks, cross-links, and modification of bases.[73] The extreme sensitivity to radiation in ataxia telangiectasia is believed to result from an inability of ataxia telangiectasia cells to cease their replication after radiation exposure, because the cells retain the ability to repair strand breaks.[73] A delay in cell cycle progression after DNA damage is a normal mechanism for preventing replication of a damaged DNA template (arrest in the first gap phase, G_1, of the cell cycle) and for preventing passage of damaged chromosomes on to daughter cells (arrest in the second gap phase, G_2, of the cell cycle).[53] Presumably, the delays allow time for DNA repair. In addition, ataxia telangiectasia cells have been shown to lack the radiation-induced increase in P53 protein levels seen in normal cells.[53] It appears that P53, a transcription factor that activates genes involved in slowing cell proliferation, plays an important role in G_1 arrest after irradiation. Possibly, the normal ataxia telangiectasia gene product is responsible for activating the P53 product.[53]

Chromosomal abnormalities are frequent in ataxia telangiectasia. An increase in random chromosomal breaks and rearrangements and an increase in balanced translocations have been observed in lymphocytes and fibroblasts of patients with this condition.[29] Elevated rates of mitotic recombination between homologous chromosomes have also been observed and may contribute to tumorigenesis in ataxia telangiectasia patients.[81]

RENDU-OSLER-WEBER DISEASE

This generalized vascular disorder, also called hereditary hemorrhagic telangiectasia, is an autosomal dominant disorder characterized by telangiectasia of the skin, mucous membranes, and viscera. The incidence is estimated at 1 to 2 in 100,000, with 97 per cent penetrance by 40 years of age.[75] A imperfection in the vessel wall causing mechanical fragility is believed to be the underlying defect. These lesions may be small, 1 mm in size; they first appear in childhood and increase in number with age. Bleeding episodes are the principal presenting features, including epistaxis, hemoptysis, hematuria, and melena. Patients may present with chronic iron deficiency anemia.

In the central nervous system, telangiectases and arteriovenous malformations have been reported in the brain and spinal cord and may cause clinical bleeding. Multiple cerebral arteriovenous malformations in a patient should lead to consideration of a diagnosis of hereditary hemorrhagic telangiectasia.[3] Pulmonary arteriovenous fistulae are common and render the patient susceptible to brain abscess.[1, 106] A clinical diagnosis is based on the presence of at least two of the following characteristics: telangiectasia (most commonly on the face and lips), recurrent epistaxis, and a family history of the disorder.[106] There is a very wide spectrum of clinical severity. Neurological symptoms do not occur exclusively as the result of anatomical lesions in the central nervous system. A wide variety of symptoms may occur as the result of systemic vascular shunts, including cerebral ischemia from polycythemia or paradoxical emboli, both caused by pulmonary arteriovenous fistulae.[106]

The molecular pathogenesis of this disorder is not well understood, but linkage analysis has now mapped the gene to 9q33–q34.[72, 120] A candidate gene for this disorder is the type V collagen gene, found at the 9q33–q34 locus. Collagen type V is an important component of the blood vessel extracellular matrix.

STURGE-WEBER SYNDROME

Clinically, Sturge-Weber syndrome is characterized by the presence of a unilateral port-wine nevus in the

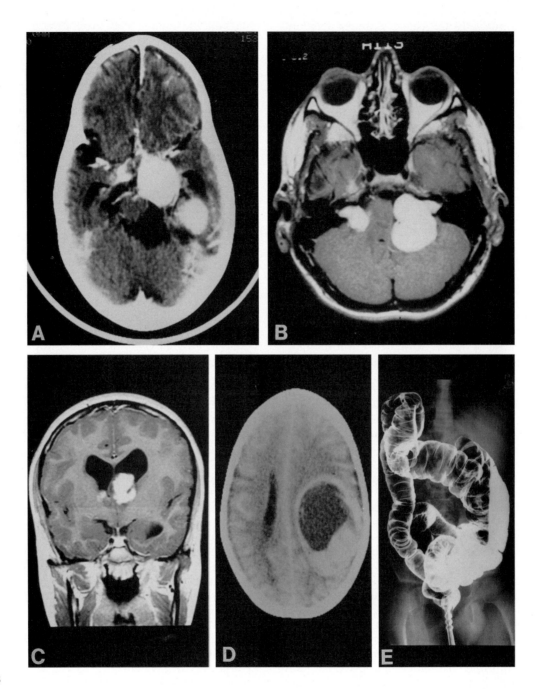

Figure 31–5

Studies of neurogenetically linked syndromes with tumor formation in the central nervous system are shown. *A.* Contrast-enhanced computed tomography demonstrates an optic pathway glioma in a young male with neurofibromatosis type 1 who presented with visual failure and macrocephaly. A large mass lesion is seen arising from the left optic tract and is compressing the brain stem and extending posteriorly along the optic radiation. The large lesion was excised surgically, and in follow-up at 2 years, there was no new growth in tumor. *B.* Gadolinium-enhanced axial magnetic resonance image demonstrates bilateral vestibular schwannomas in a 14-year-old male with neurofibromatosis type 2 who presented with left-sided hearing loss. Treatment was directed toward excising the larger symptomatic left vestibular schwannoma. *C.* Gadolinium-enhanced coronal magnetic resonance image demonstrates a large left enhancing lateral ventricular tumor taking origin from the region of the caudate nucleus in a 14-year-old female with tuberous sclerosis who presented with headaches and papilledema. The tumor is obstructing the interventricular foramen or Monro, and the third ventricle is small. A subependymal giant cell astrocytoma was completely excised via a transcallosal approach through the left lateral ventricle. The child was well 2 years after surgery and did not require a ventriculoperitoneal shunt. *D and E.* Patient with Turcot's syndrome. At 5 years of age, he developed seizures and a right hemiparesis. Contrast-enhanced computed tomography showed a large left cystic parietal brain tumor (*D*), and the tumor was radically excised via a left parietal craniotomy. The patient received postoperative radiation therapy and has remained disease-free for 7 years. At 11 years of age, rectal bleeding led to investigation with double-contrast barium enema. A large polyp was identified and was completely excised (*E*). The patient has remained free from gastrointestinal symptoms. (From Laws, E. L., and Kaye, A., eds.: The Encyclopedia of Human Brain Tumours. Edinburgh, Churchill Livingstone, 1994, p. 24. Reprinted by permission.)

ophthalmic division of the trigeminal nerve, along with seizures, contralateral hemisensory and motor deficit, and cortical tramline calcification on computed tomography. The nevus is present at birth, and involvement of the upper eyelid is a strong clue to cerebral involvement.[2] Abnormal meningeal vessels overlie atrophic, calcified, dysfunctional cerebral cortex, and these vessels do not have a tendency to bleed. Most cases are sporadic, and chromosomes are normal. A similar disorder, Klippel-Trenaunay-Weber syndrome, is characterized by a hemangioma of the spinal cord with corresponding unilateral dermatomal skin hemangioma; this syndrome is believed to be of sporadic origin.

Genetic Aspects of Brain Tumors

Most brain tumors occur sporadically, and those in families are usually associated with another disease or syndrome.[16] A number of neurogenetically linked central nervous system tumors are depicted in Figure 31–5. Numerous case reports in the literature describe apparently isolated brain tumors, particularly gliomas, in families. In a report of 178 consecutive, newly diagnosed patients with gliomas, without evidence of neurofibromatosis or other predisposing condition, 6.7 per cent had a pathologically verified history of glioma.[45] In addition to the genetic disorders mentioned in this chapter, brain tumors appear to have a particularly high incidence in Turcot's syndrome, in which there is an association with clonic polyposis, and in Li-Fraumeni syndrome, in which a germ line mutation in the P53 suppressor gene predisposes individuals to multiple types of cancer.

TURCOT'S SYNDROME

Turcot's syndrome is a rare inherited disorder in which multiple colonic polyps are associated with malignant astrocytomas and medulloblastomas. Because of its rarity, there has been controversy as to whether this condition is merely a phenotypic variant of familial adenomatous polyposis, an autosomal dominant condition. The gene for familial adenomatous polyposis has been cloned, and it resides on chromosome 5. Some authors believe that the high association of brain tumors, different numbers of colonic polyps, and autosomal recessive inheritance in Turcot's syndrome distinguish it from familial adenomatous polyposis.[46] A report of a patient with a colonic polyp and a frontal lobe astrocytoma, in a family with several members affected with colon carcinoma or polyps, did not suggest linkage with markers for familial adenomatous polyposis.[130] The molecular pathogenesis of Turcot's syndrome remains to be discovered.

LI-FRAUMENI SYNDROME

Mutations in the P53 suppressor gene are seen in approximately half of all types of cancer arising from a variety of tissues.[38] The discovery that patients with Li-Fraumeni syndrome have a germ line mutation in the P53 tumor suppressor gene has been very important for the understanding of the role of tumor suppressor genes in oncogenesis. Patients with this syndrome are susceptible to a variety of tumors at a young age, including breast carcinoma, soft tissue sarcomas, brain tumors, osteosarcoma, leukemia, and adrenocortical carcinoma.[66] Multiple primary tumors are common. Patients with a P53 germ line mutation have a 50 per cent chance of developing a malignancy by 30 years of age, and 90 per cent by 65 years of age.[66] Treatment of the primary tumor with radiation therapy or chemotherapy may increase the risk of a second neoplasm.[65] In addition, P53 mutations have been identified in 6.8 per cent of children who had second malignant neoplasm but were not considered to have the Li-Fraumeni syndrome.[65]

The P53 gene is believed to encode for a protein that is involved in control of cellular proliferation through regulation of gene transcription. It has also been implicated in DNA repair and synthesis, cell differentiation, and programmed cell death.[38] Normal P53 probably helps control the "inherent mutability" of the human genome.[38] Binding of the P53 protein to specific DNA sequences has been demonstrated.[54] This binding leads to regulation of gene expression adjacent to the binding site, and these genes probably control cell growth.[54] Binding of the P53 protein to DNA can cause induction or repression of gene transcription, depending on the sequence of the binding site.[38] Mutations in P53 may occur in four characteristic "hotspots" that affect binding to DNA and interfere with adjacent gene expression.[24] Other mutations alter the conformation of the P53 protein molecule and susequently interfere with wild-type P53 protein function.[82] This effect has been described as the dominant negative effect of mutated P53. Mutations that cause P53 conformational changes have been shown to cause neoplastic transformation of cells. Other mechanisms that alter the P53 gene's control of cell growth have also been postulated, including degradation of the P53 protein by viral oncoproteins, and interference by overexpression of cellular genes (MDM2).[83, 114] The role that normal P53 may play in growth control in situations of stress has already been discussed (see the section on ataxia telangiectasia), and patients with Li-Fraumeni syndrome have neoplasms related to previous ionizing radiation.[122] The identification of genes regulated by the wild-type P53 protein and better understanding of the P53 gene structure should clarify its role in growth control.[135] For example, a possible mechanism of P53 suppression of cell growth has been proposed: in conditions of stress, P53 expression is increased, and P53, in turn, stimulates the expression of a 21-kilodalton protein. This protein binds to the cell cycle regulatory proteins cyclins and cyclin-dependent kinases and thereby inhibits progression through the cell cycle.[25, 37, 138]

REFERENCES

1. Adams, H. P., Subbiah, B., and Bosch, E. P.: Neurologic aspects of hereditary hemorrhagic telangiectasia: Report of two cases. Arch. Neurol., 34:101, 1977.

2. Adams, R. D., and Victor, M.: Principles of Neurology. New York, McGraw-Hill, 1989, p. 988.

3. Aesch, B., Lioret, E., de Toffol, B., et al.: Multiple cerebral angiomas and Rendu-Osler-Weber disease: Case report. Neurosurgery, 29:599, 1991.

4. Anderson, L. B., Fountain, J. W., Gutmann, D. H., et al.: Mutations in the neurofibromatosis 1 gene in sporadic malignant melanoma cell lines. Nat. Genet., 3:118, 1993.

5. Baraitser, M., and Burn, J.: Neural tube defects as an X-linked condition. Am. J. Med. Genet., 17:383, 1984.

6. Basu, T. N., Gutmann, D. H., and Fletcher, J. A.: Aberrant regulation of ras proteins in malignant tumour cells from type 1 neurofibromatosis. Nature, 356:713, 1992.

7. Bianchi, A. B., Hara, T., Ramesh, V., et al.: Mutations in transcript isoforms of the neurofibromatosis II gene in multiple human tumor types. Nat. Genet., 6:185, 1994.

8. Blatt, J., Jaffe, R., Deutch, M., et al.: Neurofibromatosis and childhood tumors. Cancer, 57:1225, 1986.

9. Burger, P. C., Scheithauer, B. W., and Vogel, F. S.: Surgical Pathology of the Nervous System and Its Coverings. New York, Churchill Livingstone, 1991, pp. 248–251.

10. Burger, P. C., Scheithauer, B. W., and Vogel, F. S.: Surgical Pathology of the Nervous System and Its Coverings. New York, Churchill Livingstone, 1991, pp. 682–694.

11. Burton, B. K.: Recurrence risk for congenital hydrocephalus. Clin. Genet., 16:47, 1979.

12. Buttiens, M., Fryns, J. P., and van den Berghe, H.: An apparently new autosomal recessive syndrome with facial dysmorphism, macrocephaly, myopia and Dandy-Walker malformation. Clin. Genet., 36:451, 1989.

13. Campbell, L. R., Dayton, D. H., and Sohal, G. S.: Neural tube defects: A review of human and animal studies on the etiology of neural tube defects. Teratology, 34:171, 1986.

14. Charles, S. J., Moore, A. T., Yates, J. R., et al.: Lisch nodules in neurofibromatosis type 2. Arch. Ophthalmol., 107:1571, 1989.

15. Chatkupt, S., Chatkupt, S., and Johnson, W. G.: Waardenburg syndrome and myelomeningocele in a family. J. Med. Genet., 30:83, 1993.

16. Chemke, J., Katznelson, D., and Zucker, G.: Familial glioblastoma without neurofibromatosis. Am. J. Med. Genet., 21:731, 1985.

17. Chow, C. W., McKelvie, P. A., Anderson, R. M., et al.: Autosomal recessive hydrocephalus with third ventricle obstruction. Am. J. Med. Genet., 35:310, 1990.

18. Cohen, M. M.: Craniosynostosis: Diagnosis, Evaluation, and Management. New York, Raven Press, 1986, pp. 59–79.

19. Cohen, M. M.: Etiopathogenesis of craniosynostosis. Neurosurg. Clin. North Am., 2:507, 1991.

20. Copp, A. J., Brook, F. A., Estibeiro, P., et al.: The embryonic development of mammalian neural tube defects. Prog. Neurobiol., 35:363, 1990.

21. David, D. J., Poswillo, D., and Simpson, D.: The Craniosynostoses: Causes, Natural History, and Management. Berlin, Springer-Verlag, 1982.

22. Dirks, P. B., Jay, V., Becker, L. E., et al.: Development of anaplastic change in low-grade astrocytomas of childhood. Neurosurgery, 34:68, 1994.

23. Dobyns, W. B., Michels, V. V., Groover, R. V., et al.: Familial cavernous malformations of the central nervous system and retina. Ann. Neurol., 21:578, 1987.

24. El-Deiry, W. S., Kern, S. E., Pietenpol, J. A., et al.: Definition of a consensus binding site for p53. Nat. Genet., 1:45, 1992.

25. El-Deiry, W. S., Tokino, T., Velculescu, V. E., et al.: WAF 1, a potential mediator of p53 tumor suppression. Cell, 75:817, 1993.

26. Evans, D. G., Huson, S. M., Donnai, D., et al.: A genetic study of type 2 neurofibromatosis in the United Kingdom: II. Guidelines for genetic counselling. J. Med. Genet., 29:847, 1992.

27. Fineman, R. M., Jorde, L. B., and Martin, R. A., et al.: Spinal dysraphism as an autosomal dominant defect in four families. Am. J. Med. Genet., 12:457, 1982.

28. Fryer, A. E., Connor, A. E., Povey, S., et al.: Evidence that the gene for tuberous sclerosis is on chromosome 9. Lancet, 1:659, 1987.

29. Gatti, R. A., Boder, E., Vinters, H. V., et al.: Ataxia telangiectasia: An interdisciplinary approach to pathogenesis. Medicine (Baltimore), 70:99, 1991.

30. Glenn, G. M., Daniel, L. N., Choyke, P., et al.: Von Hippel-Lindau (VHL) disease: Distinct phenotypes suggest more than one mutant allele at the VHL locus. Hum. Genet., 87:207, 1991.

31. Golabi, M., Edwards, M. S., and Ousterhout, D. K.: Craniosynostosis and hydrocephalus. J. Neurosurg., 21:63, 1987.

32. Green, A. J., Smith, M., and Yates, J. R.: Loss of heterozygosity on chromosome 16p13 in hamartomas in tuberous sclerosis. Nat. Genet., 6:193, 1994.

33. Grompe, M.: The rapid detection of unknown mutations in nucleic acids. Nat. Genet., 5:111, 1993.

34. Guttman, D. H., and Collins, F. S.: Recent progress toward understanding the molecular biology of von Recklinghausen neurofibromatosis. Ann. Neurol., 31:555, 1992.

35. Halal, F., Mohr, G., Toussi, T., et al.: Intracranial aneurysms: A report of a large pedigree. Am. J. Med. Genet., 15:89, 1983.

36. Halliday, J., Chow, C. W., Wallace, D., et al.: X-linked hydrocephalus: A survey of a 20-year period in Victoria, Australia. J. Med. Genet., 23:23, 1986.

37. Harper, J. W., Adami, G. R., Wei, N., et al.: The p21 Cdk-interacting protein cip1 is a potent inhibitor of G_1 cyclin–dependent kinases. Cell, 75:805, 1993.

38. Harris, C. C., and Hollstein, M.: Clinical implications of the p53 tumor suppressor gene. N. Engl. J. Med., 229:1318, 1993.

39. Hashimoto, I: Familial intracranial aneurysms and cerebrovascular anomalies. J. Neurosurg., 46:419, 1977.

40. Hayman, L. A., Evans, R. A., Ferrell, R. E., et al.: Familial cavernous angiomas: Natural history and genetic study over a 5-year period. Am. J. Med. Genet., 11:147, 1982.

41. Hirsch, J. F., Pierre-Kahn, A., Renier, D., et al.: The Dandy-Walker malformation: A review of 40 cases. J. Neurosurg., 61:515, 1984.

42. Hunter, A. G., and Rudd, N. L.: Coronal synostosis: Its familial characteristics and associated clinical findings in 109 patients lacking bilateral polysyndactyly or syndactyly. Tetralogy, 15:301, 1977.

43. Hunter, A. G., and Rudd, N. L.: Craniosynostosis: Sagittal synostosis: Its genetics and associated clinical findings in 214 patients who lacked involvement of the coronal sutures. Tetralogy, 14:185, 1977.

44. Huson, S. M., Compston, D. A., Clark, P., et al.: A genetic study of von Recklinghausen neurofibromatosis in south east Wales: I. Prevalence, fitness, mutation rate, and effect of paternal transmission on severity. J. Med. Genet., 26:704, 1989.

45. Ikzler, Y., van Meyel, D. J., Ramsay, D. A., et al.: Gliomas in families. Can. J. Neurol. Sci., 19:492, 1992.

46. Itoh, H., Ohsato, K., Iida, M., et al.: Turcot's syndrome and its mode of inheritance. Gut, 20:414, 1979.

47. Jadayel, D., Fain, P., Upadhyaya, M., et al.: Paternal origin of new mutations in von Recklinghausen neurofibromatosis. Nature, 343:559, 1990.

48. Jensson, O., Arnason, A., Gunnarsdottir, H., et al.: A family showing apparent X-linked inheritance of both anencaphaly and spina bifida. J. Med. Genet., 25:227, 1988.

49. Jouet, M., Feldman, E., Yates, J., et al.: Refining the genetic location of the gene for X-linked hydrocephalus within Xq28. J. Med. Genet., 30:214, 1993.

50. Kaiser-Kupfer, M. I.: Ophthalmic manifestations. In Mulvihill, J. J., moderator. Neurofibromatosis 1 (Recklinghausen disease) and neurofibromatosis 2 (bilateral acoustic neurofibromatosis): An update. Ann. Intern. Med., 113:39, 1990.

51. Kandt, R. S., Haines, J. L., Smith, M., et al.: Linkage of an important gene locus for tuberous sclerosis to a chromosome 16 marker for polycystic kidney disease. Nat. Genet., 2:37, 1992.

52. Kandt, R. S., Pericak-Vance, M. A., Hung, W. Y., et al.: Linkage analysis in tuberous sclerosis: Chromosome 9?, 11?, or maybe 14! Ann. N. Y. Acad. Sci., 615:284, 1991.

53. Kastan, M. B., Zhan, Q., El-Deiry, W. S., et al.: A mammalian cell cycle checkpoint pathway utilizing p53 and GADD45 is defective in ataxia telangiectasia. Cell, 71:587, 1992.

54. Kern, S. E., Pietenpol, J. A., Thiagalingam, S., et al.: Oncogenic forms of p53 inhibit p53-regulated gene expression. Science, 256:827, 1992.

55. Kestle, J. R., Hoffman, H. J., and Mock, A. R.: Moyamoya phenomenon after radiation for optic glioma. J. Neurosurg., 79:32, 1993.

56. Kiechle-Schwarz, M., Neumann, H. P., Decker, H. J., et al.: Cytogenetic studies on three pheochromocytomas derived from patients with von Hippel–Lindau syndrome. Hum. Genet., 82:127, 1989.

57. Lamiell, J. M., Salazar, F. G., and Hsia, E.: Von Hippel–Lindau disease affecting 43 members of a single kindred. Medicine (Baltimore), 68:1, 1989.

58. Latif, F., Tory, K., Gnarra, J., et al.: Identification of the von Hippel–Lindau disease tumor suppressor gene. Science, 260:1317, 1993.

59. Leigus, E., Marchuk, D. A., Collins, F. S., et al.: Somatic deletion of the neurofibromatosis type 1 gene in a neurofibrosarcoma supports the tumour suppressor gene hypothesis. Nat. Genet., 3:122, 1993.

60. Lemaire, R. J.: Neural tube defects. J.A.M.A., 259:558, 1988.

61. Lozano, A. M., and Leblanc, R.: Familial intracranial aneurysms. J. Neurosurg., 66:522, 1987.

62. Lubs, M. L., Bauer, M. A., Formas, M. E., et al.: Lisch nodules in neurofibromatosis 1. N. Engl. J. Med., 324:1256, 1991.

63. Mackool, B. T., and Fitzpatrick, T. B.: Diagnosis of neurofibromatosis by cutaneous examination. Semin. Neurol., 12:358, 1992.

64. Maher, E. R., Iselius, Yates, J. R., et al.: Von Hippel–Lindau disease: A genetic study. J. Med. Genet., 28:443, 1991.

65. Malkin, D., Jolly, K. W., Barbier, N., et al.: Germline mutations of the p53 tumor suppressor gene in children and young adults with second malignant neoplasms. N. Engl. J. Med., 326:1309, 1992.

66. Malkin, D., Li, F. P., Strong, L. C., et al.: Germ line p53 mutations in a familial syndrome of breast cancer, sarcomas, and other neoplasms. Science, 250:1233, 1990.

67. Mariman, E. C., and Hamel, B. C.: Sex ratios of affected and transmitting members of multiple case families with neural tube defects. J. Med. Genet., 29:695, 1992.

68. Martuza, R. L.: Neurofibromatosis and other phakomatoses. In Rengachary S. S., and Wilkins R. H., eds.: Neurosurgery. New York, McGraw-Hill, 1985, pp. 511–521.

69. Martuza, R. L., and Eldridge, R: Neurofibromatosis 2. N. Engl. J. Med., 318:684, 1988.

70. Martuza, R. L., and Ojemann, R. G.: Bilateral acoustic neuromas: Clinical aspects, pathogenesis, and treatment. Neurosurgery, 10:1, 1982.

71. Mason, I., Aase, J. M., Orrison, W. W., et al.: Familial cavernous angiomas of the brain in an Hispanic family. Neurology, 38:324, 1988.

72. McDonald, M. T., Papenberg, K. A., Ghosh, S., et al.: A disease locus for hereditary hemorrhagic telangiectasia maps to chromosome 9q33–34. Nat. Genet., 6:197, 1994.

73. McKinnon, P. J.: Ataxia telangiectasia: An inherited disorder of ionizing-radiation sensitivity in man. Hum. Genet., 75:197, 1987.

74. McKusick, V. A.: Mendelian Inheritance in Man. 10th ed. Baltimore, The Johns Hopkins University Press, 1992.

75. McKusick, V. A.: Mendelian Inheritance in Man. 10th ed. Baltimore, The Johns Hopkins University Press, 1992, pp. 1064–1066.

76. McKusick, V. A.: Mendelian Inheritance in Man. 10th ed. Baltimore, The Johns Hopkins University Press, 1992, p. 1117.

77. McKusick, V. A.: Mendelian Inheritance in Man. 10th ed. Baltimore, The Johns Hopkins University Press, 1992, p. 1449.

78. McKusick, V. A., and Amberger, J. S.: The morbid anatomy of the human genome: Chromosomal locations of mutations causing disease. J. Med. Genet., 30:1, 1993.

79. Menon, A. G., Anderson, K. M., Riccardi, V. M., et al.: Chromosome 17p deletions and p53 gene mutations associated with the formation of malignant neurofibrosarcomas in von Recklinghausen neurofibromatosis. Proc. Natl. Acad. Sci. U. S. A., 87:5435, 1990.

80. Meyer, F. B., Sundt, T. M., Fode, N. C., et al.: Cerebral aneurysms in childhood and adolescence. J. Neurosurg., 70:420, 1989.

81. Meyn, M. S.: High spontaneous intrachromosomal recombination rates in ataxia telangiectasia. Science, 260:1327, 1993.

82. Milner, J., and Medcalf, E. A.: Cotranslation of activated mutant p53 with wild type drives the wild-type p53 protein into the mutant confirmation. Cell, 65:765, 1991.

83. Momand, J., Zambetti, G. P., Olson, D. C., et al.: The mdm-2 oncogene product forms a complex with the p53 protein and inhibits p53-mediated transactivation. Cell, 69:1237, 1992.

84. Muakkassa, K. F., Hoffman, H. J., Hinton, D. R., et al.: Lambdoid synostosis: Part 2. Review of cases managed at the Hospital for Sick Children, 1972–1982. J. Neurosurg., 61:340, 1984.

85. Murray, J. C., Johnson, J. A., and Bird, T. D.: Dandy-Walker malformation: Etiologic heterogeneity and empiric recurrence risks. Clin. Genet., 28:272, 1985.

86. Myrianthopolous, N. C., and Melnick, M.: Studies in neural tube defects: I. Epidemiologic and etiologic aspects. Am. J. Med. Genet., 26:783, 1987.

87. Nagib, M. G., Haines, S. J., Erickson, D. L., et al.: Tuberous sclerosis: A review for the neurosurgeon. Neurosurgery, 14:93, 1984.

88. Narod, S. A., Parry, D. M., and Parboosingh J.: Neurofibromatosis 2 appears to be a genetically homogeneous disease. Am. J. Med. Genet., 51:486, 1992.

89. National Institutes of Health Consensus Development Conference: Neurofibromatosis. Conference statement. Arch. Neurol., 45:575, 1988.

90. Nellist, M., Janssen, B, Brook-Carter, P. T., et al.: Identification and characterization of the tuberous sclerosis gene on chromosome 16. Cell, 75:1305, 1993.

91. Neumann, H. P., Eggert, H. R., and Scheremet, R.: Central nervous system lesions in von Hippel–Lindau syndrome. J. Neurol. Neurosurg. Psychiatry, 55:898, 1992.

92. Neumann, H. P., Eggert, H. R., Weigel, K., et al.: Hemangioblastomas of the central nervous system: A 10-year study with special reference to von Hippel–Landau syndrome. J. Neurosurg., 70:24, 1989.

93. Neumann, H. P., and Wiestler, O. D.: Clustering of features for von Hippel–Lindau syndrome: Evidence for a complex genetic locus. Lancet, 337:1052, 1991.

94. Norrgaard, O., Angquist, K. A., Fodstad, H., et al.: Intracranial aneurysms and heredity. Neurosurgery, 20:236, 1987.

95. Northrup, H.: Tuberous sclerosis complex: Genetic aspects. J. Dermatol., 19:914, 1992.

96. Northrup, H., Wheless, J. W., Bertin, T. K., et al.: Variability of expression in tuberous sclerosis. J. Med. Genet., 30:41, 1993.

97. Osborne, J. P.: Diagnosis of tuberous sclerosis. Arch. Dis. Child., 63:1423, 1988.

98. Osborne, J. P., Fryer, A., and Webb, D.: Epidemiology of tuberous sclerosis. Ann. N. Y. Acad. Sci., 615:125, 1991.

99. Pierquin, G., Deroover, J., Levi, S., et al.: Dandy-Walker malformation with post-axial polydactyly: A new syndrome? Am. J. Med. Genet., 33:483, 1989.

100. Raffel, C., McComb, J. G., Bodner, S., et al.: Benign brain stem lesions in pediatric patients with neurofibromatosis: Case reports. Neurosurgery, 25:959, 1989.

101. Riccardi, V. M.: Von Recklinghausen neurofibromatosis. N. Engl. J. Med., 305:1617, 1981.

102. Rigamonti, D., Hadley, M. N., Drayer, B. P., et al.: Cerebral cavernous angiomas: Incidence and familial occurrence. N. Engl. J. Med., 319:343, 1988.

103. Ritscher, D., Schinzel, A., Boltshauser, E., et al.: Dandy-Walker (like) malformation, atrioventricular septal defect and a similar pattern of minor anomalies in two sisters: A new syndrome. Am. J. Med. Genet., 26:481, 1987.

104. Roach, E. S., Smith, M., Huttenlocher, P., et al.: Report of the Diagnostic Criteria: Committee of the National Tuberous Sclerosis Association. J. Child Neurol., 7:221, 1992.

105. Rodriguez, J. I., Garcia, M., Morales, C., et al.: Trisomy 13 and neural tube defects. Am. J. Med. Genet., 36:513, 1990.

106. Roman, G., Fisher, M., Perl, D. P., et al.: Neurological manifestations of hereditary hemorrhagic telangiectasia (Rendu-Osler-Weber disease): Case report and review of the literature. Ann. Neurol., 4:130, 1978.

107. Ronkainen, A., Hernesniemi, J., and Ryynanen, M.: Familial subarachnoid hemorrhage in east Finland, 1977–1990. Neurosurgery, 33:787, 1993.

108. Rosenthal, A., Jouet, M., and Kenwrick, S.: Aberrant splicing of neural cell adhesion molecule L1 mRNA in X-linked hydrocephalus. Nat. Genet., 2:107, 1992.

109. Rouleau, G. A., Merel, P., Lutchman, M., et al.: Alteration in a new gene encoding a putative membrane-organizing protein causes neurofibromatosis type 2. Nature, 363:515, 1993.

110. Russell, D. S., and Rubenstein, L. J.: Pathology of Tumors of the

Nervous System. 5th ed. Baltimore, Williams & Wilkins, 1989, pp. 766–769.

111. Rutka, J. T., Brandt-Zawadski, M., Wilson, C. B., et al.: Familial cavernous malformations: Diagnostic potential of magnetic resonance imaging. Surg. Neurol., *29*:467, 1988.

112. Ruttedge, M. H., Sarrazin, J., Rangaratnam, S., et al.: Evidence for complete inactivation of the *NF2* gene in the majority of sporadic meningiomas. Nat. Genet., *6*:180, 1994.

113. Sampson, J. R., Janssen, L. A., Sandkuijil, et al.: Linkage analysis of three putative tuberous sclerosis–determining loci on chromosomes 9q, 11q, and 12q. J. Med. Genet., *29*:861, 1992.

114. Scheffner M., Werness, B. A., Huibregtse, J. M., et al.: The E6 oncoprotein encoded by human papillomavirus types 16 and 18 promotes the degradation of p53. Cell, *63*:1129, 1990.

115. Schievink, W. I., and Piepgras, D. G.: Cervical vertebral artery aneurysms and arteriovenous malformations in neurofibromatosis type 1: Case reports. Neurosurgery, *29*:760, 1991.

116. Seizinger, B. R.: NF-1: A prevalent cause of tumorigenesis in human cancers. Nat. Genet., *3*:9, 1993.

117. Seizinger, B. R., Rouleau, G. A., Ozelius, L. J., et al.: Von Hippel–Lindau disease maps to region of chromosome 3 associated with renal cell carcinoma. Nature, *332*:268, 1988.

118. Sherman, J. L.: Imaging. *In* Mulvihill, JJ, moderator. Neurofibromatosis 1 (Recklinghausen disease) and neurofibromatosis 2 (bilateral acoustic neurofibromatosis): An update. Ann. Intern. Med., *113*:39, 1990.

119. Shinton, R., Palsingh, and Williams, B.: Cerebral haemorrhage and berry aneurysm: Evidence from a family for a pattern of autosomal dominant inheritance. J. Neurol. Neurosurg. Psychiatry, *54*:838, 1991.

120. Shovlin, C. L., Hughes, J. M., Tuddenham, E. G., et al.: A gene for hereditary hemorrhagic telangiectasia maps to chromosome 9q3. Nat. Genet., *6*:205, 1994.

121. Simpson, D. A., and David, D. J.: Craniosynostosis. *In* Hoffman, HJ, and Epstein, F., eds.: Disorders of the Developing Nervous System: Diagnosis and Treatment. Boston, Blackwell Scientific Publications, 1986, pp. 323–346.

122. Srivastava, S., Zou, Z., Pirollo, K., et al.: Germ-line transmission of a mutated *p53* gene in a cancer-prone family with Li-Fraumeni syndrome. Nature, *348*:747, 1990.

123. Steubens, W. E.: Etiology of intracranial aneurysms. J. Neurosurg., *70*:823, 1989.

124. Storrs, B. B., Humphreys, R. P., Hendrick, E. B., et al.: Intracranial aneurysms in the pediatric age group. Child's Brain, *9*:358, 1982.

125. Sulik, K. K., and Sadler, T. W.: Postulated mechanisms underlying the development of neural tube defects: Insights from in vitro and in vivo studies. Ann. N. Y. Acad. Sci., *678*:8, 1993.

126. Swift, M., Morrell, D., Massey, R. B., et al.: Incidence of cancer in 161 families affected by ataxia telangiectasia. N. Engl. J. Med., *325*:1831, 1991.

127. Swift, M., Reitnauer, P. J., Morrell, D., et al.: Breast and other cancers in families with ataxia telangiectasia. N. Engl. J. Med., *316*:1289, 1987.

128. Ter Berg, H. M., Diederik, D. W., Limburg, M., et al.: Familial intracranial aneurysms: A review. Stroke, *32*:1024, 1992.

129. Thapar, K., Fukuyama, K., and Rutka, J. T.: Neurogenetics and the molecular biology of human brain tumors. *In* Laws, E. L., and Kaye, A., eds.: Encyclopedia of Human Brain Tumours. Edinburgh, Churchill Livingstone, 1994.

130. Tops, C. M., Vasen, H. F., van Berge Henegouwen, G., et al.: Genetic evidence that Turcot syndrome is not allelic to familial adenomatous polyposis. Am. J. Med. Genet., *43*:888, 1992.

131. Toriello, H. V.: Report of a third kindred with X-linked anencephaly/spina bifida. Am. J. Med. Genet., *19*:411, 1984.

132. Toriello, H. V., Warren, S. T., and Lindstrom, J. A.: Possible X-linked anencephaly and spinal bifida: Report of a kindred. Am. J. Med. Genet., *6*:119, 1980.

133. Trofatter, J. A., MacCollin, M. M., Rutter, J. L., et al.: A novel moesin-, ezrin-, radixin-like gene is a candidate for the neurofibromatosis 2 tumor suppressor. Cell, *72*:791, 1993.

134. Van Camp, G., Vits, L., Coucke, P., et al.: A duplication in the L1CAM gene associated with X-linked hydrocephalus. Nat. Genet., *4*:421, 1993.

135. Vogelstein, B., and Kinzler, K. W.: p53 function and dysfunction. Cell, *70*:523, 1992.

136. Weir, B.: Aneurysms Affecting the Nervous System. Baltimore, Williams & Wilkins, 1987, pp. 54–74.

137. Willems, P. J., Vits, L., Raeymaekers, P., et al.: Further localization of X-linked hydrocephalus in the chromosomal region Xq28. Am. J. Med. Genet., *51*:307, 1992.

138. Xiong, Y., Hannon, G. J., Hui, H., et al.: p21 is a universal inhibitor of cyclin kinases. Nature, *366*:701, 1993.

Encephaloceles

An encephalocele is a cystic congenital malformation in which central nervous system structures, in communication with cerebrospinal fluid pathways, herniate through a defect in the cranium. If the cranial herniation contains only cerebrospinal fluid and meninges, it is by definition a craniomeningocele or, more commonly, a meningocele. If the cystic lesion also contains neural tissue, it is called a meningoencephalocele. Additional subclassifications of meningoencephaloceles have been made (e.g., hydromeningoencephalocele, encephalocystocele), but they have little clinical relevance. They are not considered further here, because the most important distinction is whether or not neural tissue is present within the lesion and, if so, how much. Encephalocele and cephalocele are the terms most frequently used to include all of these lesions because, before recent developments in imaging techniques, it was not possible to distinguish among them preoperatively. Other midline lesions of the skull that are not cystic include rudimentary encephaloceles, congenital defects of the scalp or skull, and congenital dermal sinuses. Terms that can be used to include all of the above are cranial dysraphism or cranium bifidum.

CLASSIFICATION OF ENCEPHALOCELES

Encephaloceles are classified as to structure and location (Table 32–1). With posteriorly located encephaloceles, their size, whether there is neural tissue, and how much neural tissue is contained within the lesion have overwhelming bearing on outcome (Fig. 32–1). Anterior lesions are quite distinct from those located on the posterior portion of the calvaria. The neurological outcome with most anterior lesions is normal and hydrocephalus is unusual, but the associated craniofacial disruption can vary from minimal to massive. Anterior encephaloceles can be classified into three categories:

frontal, sincipital (those located about the midface), and basal (those located at the base of the skull). Almost all of these lesions contain neural tissue and thus are meningoencephaloceles. Later in this chapter, attention is given to those lesions of the calvaria that are other forms of dysraphism or that simulate encephaloceles (see section on other dysraphic lesions involving the cranium).

EMBRYOLOGY

A dysraphic lesion is one that relates to the midline closure of the neural tube, which is complete in the human embryo by the 25th day of intrauterine development. Contrary to what is often thought to be the case, encephaloceles probably occur at some time after neural tube closure. Like open neural tube defects that are spinal in location, the vast majority of encephaloceles contain neural tissue. As several authors have pointed out, these cystic lesions very often contain cerebral cortex or cerebellum, both of which form after neural tube closure.[17, 20, 23] By a mechanism not well understood, central nervous system herniation occurs at the site of local mesenchymal disruption 8 to 12 weeks into gestation. Those lesions without a cystic component, such as congenital absence of the scalp or skull, could occur at an even later date. Some evidence also suggests that encephaloceles in the midface and cranial base regions result from a different mechanism than that which leads to posterior encephaloceles. Congenital dermal sinuses, most frequently associated with one or more dermoid cysts, represent a failure of neuroectoderm to completely separate from cutaneous ectoderm; only a minute disruption of the mesoderm occurs, as evidenced by the minimal disturbance of the surrounding skin and cranium. It has also been pointed out that all congenital dermal sinuses of the calvaria occur in either the nasal or subtorcular region and none

J. G. McComb

Table 32–1
CLASSIFICATION OF ENCEPHALOCELES

By Structure
Meningocele
Meningoencephalocele

By Location
Posterior
  Supratorcular
  Infratorcular
Anterior
  Frontal
  Sincipital
    Nasofrontal
    Nasoethmoidal
    Naso-orbital
  Basal
    Transethmoidal
    Transsphenoidal

cross the area occupied by the superior sagittal sinus.[8] Although the reason for this is unknown, it certainly relates to embryological development.

INCIDENCE

Encephaloceles are between one fifth and one tenth as common as myelomeningoceles, and they occur in roughly 1 of every 5,000 to 10,000 live births.[25, 28, 46, 47] In the Western hemisphere, more than three quarters are posterior in location, but in southern Asia, the majority of lesions are located anteriorly.[44, 45] The proportion of posterior encephaloceles in some parts of northern Asia, such as Japan, appears to be similar to

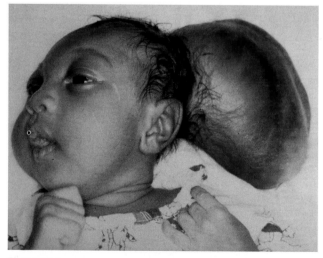

Figure 32–1
This neonate was microcephalic and had a large supratorcular encephalocele filled with dysplastic brain. Although the skin was malformed, it was fully epithelialized, and cerebrospinal fluid did not leak from the lesion. Maternal serum and amniotic alpha-fetoprotein levels would have been normal if tested. The patient developed progressive hydrocephalus after resection and required the insertion of a ventriculoperitoneal shunt. This infant's neurological development was severely delayed.

that in the Western hemisphere.[11] The reason for the geographical differences is unknown.

The gender ratio of anterior lesions is roughly equal, whereas a female predominance is present with posterior lesions.[28, 41] Most cases of encephalocele are sporadic, with only a few patients having a positive family history for neural tube defects involving either the cranium or the spine. This may be similar to the situation with open neural tube defects involving the spine, and, if so, the likelihood of a woman bearing a second child with an encephalocele would be roughly 20 times that of the general population. The role of other factors, such as nutrition, folic acid, and increased body temperature of the mother, are not known because the rarity of this lesion makes it difficult to obtain the appropriate epidemiological information.[32, 35, 37]

DIAGNOSTIC EVALUATION

With the exception of the rare occult basal lesion, the cystic form of this congenital defect is obvious and the neonate is referred for neurosurgical evaluation soon after birth. Physical examination alone in many cases yields a good approximation as to the treatment needed and the eventual outcome. The diagnostic study of choice for both posterior and anterior lesions is magnetic resonance imaging, supplemented by magnetic resonance angiography if the vascularity and its relation to the lesion need to be better defined.[5] With sincipital and basal encephaloceles, computed tomography studies, sometimes including three-dimensional reconstruction, may be of aid in determining the need for, and planning the extent of, craniofacial reconstruction.[43] Plain radiographs are of limited value and are rarely obtained. After repair of a posterior encephalocele, cranial ultrasound is an effective way of following the size of the ventricles for development of progressive hydrocephalus, which requires the placement of a shunt for diversion of cerebrospinal fluid.

IN UTERO EVALUATION

With the use of fetal ultrasound and maternal blood sampling for alpha-fetoprotein as a part of routine prenatal screening, a progressively higher proportion of encephaloceles is being diagnosed in utero.[7, 15, 34, 46] A large posterior encephalocele is easily seen on ultrasound, which could also determine the presence or absence of solid tissue within the sac. If the lesion is fully epithelialized, even though the skin is dysplastic, the alpha-fetoprotein levels for both maternal serum and amniotic fluid are normal (see Fig. 32–1); it is necessary for the lesion to be leaking tissue fluid and cerebrospinal fluid to produce an abnormal alpha-fetoprotein level (Fig. 32–2).

Depending on the size, a frontal lesion may or may not be visible on fetal ultrasound. Because these lesions are fully epithelialized, the alpha-fetoprotein determinations are normal. Hydrocephalus on prenatal ultrasound is not an expected finding even with large poste-

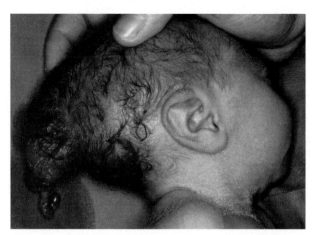

Figure 32–2

This newborn, like the neonate in Figure 32–1, had a large supratorcular encephalocele filled with dysplastic brain. This lesion was not fully epithelialized, with visible dysplastic brain, and was leaking cerebrospinal fluid. The maternal serum and amniotic fluid alphafetoprotein levels would have been elevated if tested. This patient's lesion was repaired, and progressive hydrocephalus ensued, requiring the insertion of a shunt as expected. This patient's development was also markedly impaired.

rior lesions. In fact, hydrocephalus is rarely present at birth and usually does not develop until after repair of a larger posterior lesion. The only confusion with an encephalocele on ultrasound could be with a tumor involving the skull, scalp, or high cervical region.[34] These lesions are even more rare than encephaloceles and, if fully epithelialized, they have normal alphafetoprotein levels.

Posterior encephaloceles are occasionally seen with other neural tube defects, Dandy-Walker malformation, or Meckel's syndrome (which involves polycystic kidneys, polydactyly, microgenitalism in males, and other defects).[2, 10] Those encephaloceles located anteriorly are often accompanied by varying degrees of midline facial deformity. The increased resolution of fetal ultrasound has improved prenatal assessment of these central nervous system malformations and could play a role in deciding whether or not to terminate the pregnancy.[7]

GENERAL CONSIDERATIONS

The temperature in the operating room should be raised to 80° F or higher to provide a warm environment for the neonate, who is placed on a heating pad and kept warm during induction by overhead warming lights or radiant warming elements. Ideally, the patient's temperature should be kept in the range of 36 to 37° C. Shortly after the infant's arrival in the operating room, either a rectal or an esophageal temperature probe is placed, and the patient's temperature is carefully monitored throughout the operative procedure. After the appropriate intravenous lines and monitoring devices have been placed on the extremities, the limbs are wrapped with either cotton or a plastic material to conserve body heat. The addition of a humidifier to the anesthesia circuit also helps keep the

patient's temperature in the normal range. A hypothermic infant tolerates general anesthesia poorly.

In addition to blood pressure, pulse, and electrocardiography monitoring, pulse oximetry has become standard. Changes in oxygen saturation may be the first sign of a life-threatening problem. Even if the patient is placed in the prone or lateral decubitus position, some anesthesiologists prefer to attach a Doppler ultrasound unit on the chest and to monitor end-expiratory carbon dioxide levels to detect the presence of air in the circulatory system during procedures that involve the dural sinuses. The author has never encountered such a complication but has no objection to the use of these monitoring techniques.

In addition to allowing the neonate to become hypothermic, the other most common intraoperative problem is an inadequate estimation of blood loss that leads to hypotension. Because the tolerances are small, fluid balance and blood loss must be monitored closely in these infants. Careful attention must be given to hemostasis and, in some cases, blood replacement may be avoided. Because much of the blood that is lost can accumulate in the surgical drapes and may not be readily apparent to the anesthesiologist, the surgeon should carefully estimate the blood loss and frequently notify the anesthesiologist so that blood replacement, if indicated, can proceed at the same rate. This reduces the risk of unexpected hypotensive episodes during the procedure.

Posterior encephaloceles require the patient to be placed in either a prone or lateral decubitus position, with the prone position being used most often. The neonate is situated face down with the neck flexed on a horseshoe support that has been padded to protect against pressure injury to the face. After the infant has been taped securely to the operating room table, the head of the table is elevated to approximately 15 to 30 degrees to reduce venous bleeding but not so high as to increase the risk of venous air emboli.

For large posterior lesions that are leaking cerebrospinal fluid and for lesions requiring craniofacial reconstruction, broad-spectrum perioperative antibiotics are usually given, but for small, fully epithelialized lesions this is probably not necessary.

Posterior Encephaloceles

The neurological prognosis with a posteriorly located encephalocele is predetermined by the size of the encephalocele, the amount of neural tissue in the sac, and the degree of microcephaly.[19, 25, 26, 30] Ventricular dilatation is usually not significant before repair, but if progressive hydrocephalus develops postoperatively, it is a reflection of a more severe malformation and its presence correlates with a poorer prognosis. The dysplastic tissue removed during repair has no bearing on subsequent neurological function. In addition to the general risks of operative intervention such as side effects of anesthesia, hemorrhage, and infection, the specific risks of repairing an encephalocele relate to the

contents of the sac and their relation to vital neural and vascular structures, which is best evaluated with magnetic resonance or computed tomography imaging.

Not all children with encephalocele should undergo repair. Neonates with meningocele should, because the outcome is usually favorable. In those infants with a meningoencephalocele, the severity of additional anomalies must be considered as well as the size of the lesions, amount of neural tissue within the sac, and degree of microcephaly.[4, 11, 42] If the amount of dysplastic brain within the sac exceeds that within the cranium, the likelihood of the infant's realizing any meaningful neurological development is nil, and the option of not closing the lesion can be considered (Fig. 32–3). Fortunately, this rarely arises, but if it does, extensive discussions with the family and medical personnel connected with the infant's care are necessary before deciding to withhold therapy, especially because the course on some occasions may be protracted. The decision not to treat can be made only if everyone involved is in agreement. If there are any significant differences of opinion, the best course is to repair the encephalocele. The goals of the operation are to remove the sac, to preserve functional neural tissue, and to obtain closure with nondysplastic skin.

Posterior meningoencephaloceles can be divided into supratorcular and subtorcular types.[5] Lesions that are located above the torcular most often contain dysplastic neural tissue, the resection of which does not influence neurological outcome (Fig. 32–4). Rarely, the cerebral tissue appears normal, in which case every effort should be made to preserve it intact. This may require removal of the surrounding bone so as to expand the cranial vault to accommodate the volume of the neural tissue. Lesions below the torcular pose problems similar to those found above, with the additional possibility of inclusion of brain stem and cerebellum in the encephalocele (Fig. 32–5).[18] Imaging studies should give good guidance as to the anticipated anatomy so that

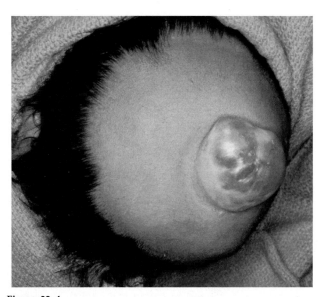

Figure 32–4

Only a small amount of dysplastic neural tissue was present in this meningoencephalocele. The overlying skin was fully epithelialized, although malformed, and without leakage of cerebrospinal fluid. The patient's development was almost normal, and cerebrospinal fluid diversion was not required.

there will be few, if any, surprises at the time of resection. Damage to the brain stem rarely results in intraoperative death. A more likely complication is inability to extubate the child postoperatively. If the neonate remains respirator-dependent for several weeks postoperatively, the likelihood that the infant will be able to breathe unassisted subsequently is quite remote.

A horizontal incision is usually preferred, but in low-lying lesions in which the bony defects include the foramen magnum or cervical vertebrae, a vertical incision is often more suitable. The extent of scalp resection should be marked at the beginning of the procedure so that the skin left for closure is neither too abundant nor too scant. Additional skin can always be removed,

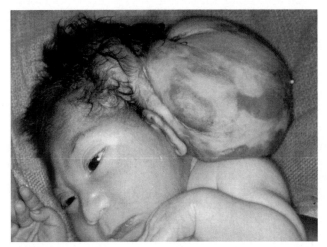

Figure 32–3

This newborn's malformation was much more extensive than those shown in Figures 32–1 and 32–2. With agreement from the family and medical staff, the lesion was not repaired, and the patient subsequently died.

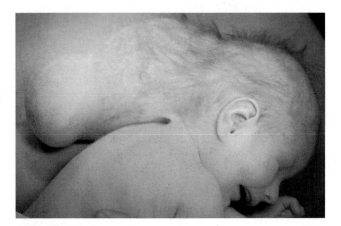

Figure 32–5

This infratorcular lesion at the cranial-cervical junction contained the cerebellum and brain stem, which were carefully protected at the time of repair. Postoperative cerebrospinal fluid diversion was required. The neurological outcome of this infant was very poor.

but this adds to operating time and increases blood loss. The skin is circumferentially incised about the base of the encephalocele, and blunt dissection from the underlying dura mater to the cranial defect is undertaken. The sac is then opened and drained of cerebrospinal fluid, and the contents are inspected. If neural tissue is present and dysplastic, it is resected flush with the bony opening. Redundant dura mater is excised, and that remaining is approximated. The dura mater and skin should be closed without tension; this is easily accomplished in most of these cystic lesions. Too much tension at the site of closure can lead to its breakdown, leakage of cerebrospinal fluid, and infection; redundant tissue produces dead space and a protuberance filled with cerebrospinal fluid. The dura mater is closed with a running absorbable suture, and the subcutaneous and subcuticular layers are closed with similar running or interrupted sutures. The skin edges are further approximated with Steri-Strips. Wound closure in such a fashion diminishes the possibility of a cerebrospinal fluid leak.

The primary intraoperative complications are bleeding and resection of functional neurological tissue, particularly portions of the brain stem. Large lesions can be associated with a significant arterial supply and venous drainage. The vessels therefore must be identified and coagulated before being divided, and the sagittal, transverse, and occipital sinuses as well as the torcular must be located before dural resection. If bleeding occurs from the major venous sinuses, the main consideration is to apply pressure to control bleeding before an attempt is made to close the rent by suture. Care should be taken when suturing a dural laceration not to occlude the sinus and thus produce a venous outflow obstruction. Air embolism, a potential problem when major venous sinuses are opened, can be minimized by elevating the head to only 15 to 30 degrees above the horizontal. Excision of functional brain tissue is avoided by carefully identifying neural structures during the repair and by assessment of its location preoperatively with imaging studies.

Craniomeningoceles are much less common than meningoencephaloceles but are usually easy to repair and have a more favorable prognosis. Craniomeningoceles tend to be smaller than those containing neural tissue, and they are less likely to be associated with hydrocephalus. The technique for repair of a craniomeningocele is the same as for a meningoencephalocele except that there is no neural tissue in the sac and often the bony defect tends to be smaller.

Although the incidence of hydrocephalus is much greater with meningoencephaloceles than with meningoceles, the treatment of hydrocephalus in either case is the same. Seizures may occur and are probably related to the degree of dysgenesis of the central nervous system as a whole than to the repair of the encephalocele.

In the immediate postoperative period, additional complications are hydrocephalus and infection. If cerebrospinal fluid absorption is impaired, fluid frequently accumulates at the site of repair and could compromise its closure. This can temporarily be controlled with intermittent aspiration. Sometimes, however, fluid build-up does not occur and progressive hydrocephalus is detected by an abnormal increase in head circumference, full fontanelle, and increased ventricular size on follow-up cranial ultrasound imaging. The treatment for progressive hydrocephalus is the placement of a ventriculoperitoneal shunt.

The best way to minimize the complications of shunting is not to insert the shunt until its necessity has been established. No harm ensues to the brain by waiting to confirm that hydrocephalus is progressive before the shunt is placed. If fluid accumulation develops under the scalp at the site of repair, it can be aspirated as a temporizing measure before the insertion of a ventriculoperitoneal shunt. If an infection of the cerebrospinal fluid pathways occurs, it is necessary to place the neonate on external ventricular drainage to control the hydrocephalus, allow the wound to heal, and clear the infection before placement of the cerebrospinal fluid diverting shunt.

The bony defects associated with posterior encephaloceles are often not large and tend to be low in the occipital region (i.e., similar to the defect created by a posterior fossa craniectomy). Because the lack of bone at this location is not of functional or cosmetic significance, nothing need be done. Regardless of the lesion site in a neonate, if the repair is made with normal dura mater there is often enough new bone formation to significantly reduce or even close the area of missing bone. A large bony defect at the vertex, with little chance for new bone formation, can be closed with bone harvested from an adjacent region of the skull; normal dura mater at the harvest site regenerates new bone. Bone defects can also be filled with flexible tantalum mesh whose edges are tucked beneath the bony margins of the defect to lock it into place and eliminate the possibility of erosion through the skin. The added risk of infection with the use of tantalum mesh alone is minimal. The resulting fibrosis about the mesh provides for a solid cranioplasty.

Anterior Encephaloceles

Anterior encephaloceles are quite distinct from lesions that are posterior in location. The neurological outcome in most instances is normal, any facial defect is usually covered with fully epithelialized, nondysplastic skin, and hydrocephalus is unusual. However, the associated craniofacial disruption can vary from minimal to massive.[21] Almost all of these encephaloceles, whether frontal, sincipital, or basal, contain neural tissue and thus are meningoencephaloceles.

FRONTAL ENCEPHALOCELES

Encephaloceles in a frontal location frequently consist of lipomatous and connective tissue as well as malformed neural elements, and they often involve the corpus callosum.[50] These lesions seem to be somewhat

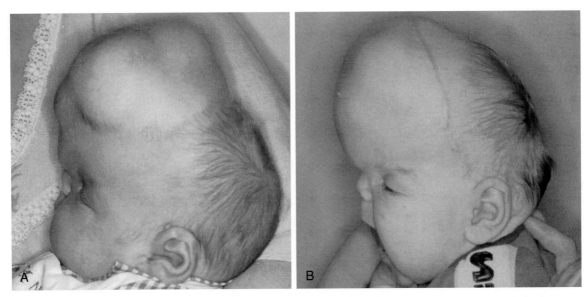

Figure 32–6

A. A massive lipomatous malformation of both frontal lobes to, and including, the corpus callosum was present in this infant. The lesion was fully epithelialized, and the skin was not significantly dysplastic. *B.* Only a limited amount of lipomatous tissue could be resected because it blended into the frontal lobes. Because of the extensive dysgenesis of both the hemispheres, the patient's neurological function was severely delayed and was accompanied by seizures. Because the patient's function was so poor, additional craniofacial reconstruction was not undertaken. This patient is now a teenager, lives in an extended-care facility, and is markedly retarded.

analogous to lipomatous malformations involving the spinal cord. Indications for repair of frontal encephaloceles are usually cosmetic, no attempt being made to remove the intracranial portion of the lipoma; the lipoma enlarges only in proportion to the growth of the patient, and therefore a true neoplasm is not a consideration. With the rare huge lipomatous malformation, the brain can be severely malformed, resulting in marked mental retardation, seizures, and even hydrocephalus (Fig. 32–6).

The imaging findings are quite typical. The rim of lipomatous mass may show calcification, a feature not found in lipomatous malformations involving the spine. The anterior cerebral arteries may be dilated and their lumina distorted within the lipomatous mass in an odd fusiform aneurysmal fashion.[50]

Smaller lesions in this location are easily repaired (Fig. 32–7); the superior sagittal sinus, which can bifurcate to lie on the lateral margin of the lesion, must be identified early in the procedure. The size and location of the lesion determine the nature of the incision used for repair. Every attempt is made to provide for an optimal cosmetic result. Encephaloceles that are massive cause significant deformity, and a combined cra-

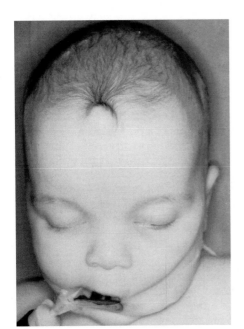

Figure 32–7

This infant had a small bony defect, through which herniated a mass containing malformed neural tissue, lipoma, and connective tissue. The encephalocele was continuous with a lipomatous mass that extended between the frontal lobes to the corpus callosum, as with the patient in Figure 32–6, but on a much reduced scale. Only the portion of the mass external to the calvaria was removed. This patient's neurological development has been completely normal.

niofacial approach is needed. With huge lesions, the lipomatous tissue blends imperceptibly with the parenchyma of the frontal lobes, and aggressive resection would add to the neurological deficit. An attempt to normalize the infant's appearance is certainly warranted, but numerous operative procedures may not be indicated if the patient is severely retarded.

SINCIPITAL ENCEPHALOCELES

Sincipital encephaloceles exit the cranium at the fronto-midfacial junction and can be classified as nasofrontal (Fig. 32–8), nasoethmoidal, or naso-orbital (Fig. 32–9), depending on the exact site of exit.[45] Because the prognosis and operative approach are similar for all three forms of sincipital encephalocele, the subclassifications, although relevant from an anatomical standpoint, have only minor clinical significance. Three-dimensional computed tomography reconstruction, although elegant, usually adds little to preoperative assessment except in the most complex lesions.[33]

In addition to the psychosocial implications, sincipital encephaloceles should be repaired, all else being equal, within the first few weeks of life to prevent progression of the bony deformities that occurs with growth and to enhance the development of binocular vision.[13, 44] Most infants with these lesions have displacement of the medial-orbital walls rather than true hypertelorism (Fig. 32–10). Correction should be undertaken by a craniofacial team at the time of the encephalocele repair.[6, 12, 38] Early repair can obviate the need for a second operative procedure to correct what would have been a more extensive facial deformity had the encephalocele not been removed.[36] Infants with midline facial deformities should routinely have imaging studies to determine the presence or absence of intracranial abnormalities (Fig. 32–11).

Intracranial repair with craniofacial reconstruction is preferred in most, if not all, sincipital encephaloceles.

The infant is placed in the supine position with the neck in a neutral position. A midcalvarial incision, beginning and ending near the junction of the ear with the temporal region, is used. Good access to the cranial base can be obtained while minimizing the cosmetic impact of the incision. Burr holes are placed in the temporal regions bilaterally, and the dura mater is separated from the overlying frontal bones at the open anterior fontanelle. The frontal bones are removed together, just above the floor of the anterior fossa. Frontal sinuses are nonexistent in infants. In some cases, a completely extradural approach is sufficient, and in others an intradural and extradural approach is indicated. If intradural visualization is needed, the dura mater is opened on either side of the superior sagittal sinus, which is ligated and divided. This allows good access to the floor of the anterior fossa. The dura mater on the floor of the anterior fossa is carefully conserved for use in closure of the defect. No attempt is made to save the brain within the encephalocele, because this tissue is dysplastic and nonfunctional. If possible, the olfactory tracts are left undisturbed.

If the calvarial defect is small, no bony repair is required. If the bony defect is large, bone can be removed from an area behind the hairline and secured at its new location. Placement of oxidized cellulose on one or both sides of the dural repair helps decrease the possibility of a cerebrospinal fluid leak. Because most of these patients do not develop hydrocephalus, cerebrospinal fluid leakage is not common, and, if present, it usually ceases spontaneously. A persistent leakage of cerebrospinal fluid could result in meningitis and further increase resistance to its drainage.

BASAL ENCEPHALOCELES

Basal encephaloceles differ from sincipital encephaloceles in that the bony defect is more posteriorly located on the cranial base. These lesions are usually

Figure 32–8

A. This infant had a nasofrontal encephalocele excised and a concomitant craniofacial reconstruction completed at the same operative procedure. *B.* The patient is older than 1 year of age in this postoperative photograph. The patient did not develop hydrocephalus, and the neurological development has been normal. (Courtesy of Gerald Sloan, M.D., Los Angeles, California.)

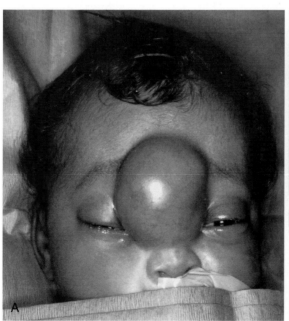
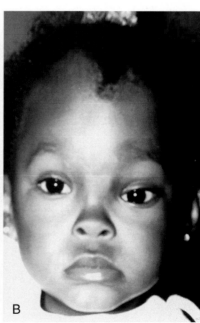

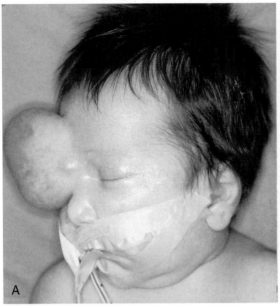

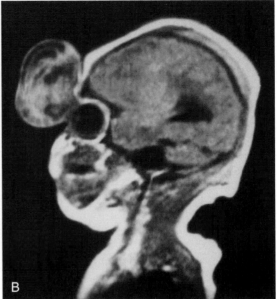

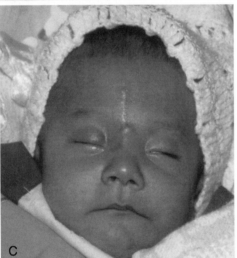

Figure 32–9

A. This infant had a naso-orbital encephalocele that was large enough to have impaired the development of vision if it was not corrected early. *B.* Magnetic resonance study shows the encephalocele exiting through the right orbit. *C.* Following intracranial excision of the encephalocele, facial repair was accomplished. Because the bony defect was small, it was not necessary to restructure any of the facial bones. The intraorbital distance is normal and the nasal bridge is forming appropriately in this photograph taken 1 month after operation. (Courtesy of Gerald Sloan, M.D., Los Angeles, California.)

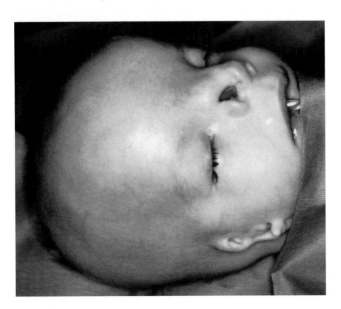

Figure 32–10

This patient had a wide nasal bridge, a defect of the nares, and a rudimentary right ear associated with a nasoethmoidal encephalocele. Intracranial repair was accomplished, followed by craniofacial reconstruction. The patient's development has been normal.

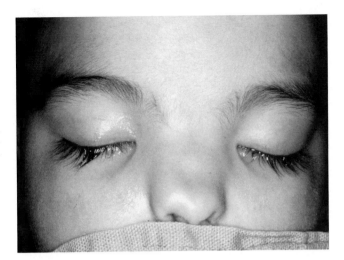

Figure 32–11

Although this patient has a wide nasal bridge and nasal deformity, an encephalocele was not present. Imaging studies are needed to determine the presence or absence of intracranial abnormalities in patients with midline facial abnormalities as part of the diagnostic evaluation.

classified as transethmoidal (Fig. 32–12), transsphenoidal, or a combination of both, according to the bony defect.[48] These more posteriorly located lesions, especially those involving the sphenoid, are more likely to contain structures such as the hypothalamus, pituitary gland and stalk, optic nerves, optic chiasm, and anterior cerebral arteries within the herniation. Associated malformations of the face include hypertelorism, cleft lip, cleft palate, cleft nose, optic nerve abnormality, absent optic chiasm, and micro-ophthalamus. In infants, the presence of a basal encephalocele may be heralded by nasal obstruction. As the mass presents in the nose, it may be mistaken for a nasal polyp, the biopsy of which can lead to cerebrospinal fluid rhinorrhea.[3, 14, 27, 40] The differentiation between a polyp and encephalocele is that an encephalocele pulsates, presents medially from the nasal septum, and widens the nasal bridge, while a polyp does not pulsate, is located laterally, emanates from the turbinates, and does not widen the nasion.[9] The only lesion in this region that could be mistaken for an encephalocele is a teratoma. Diagnostic imaging studies, including either magnetic resonance or computed tomography studies,

are needed for accurate definition of the lesion and are indicated to rule out the presence of an encephalocele with many midline craniofacial abnormalities.

The operative approach to a basal encephalocele is similar to that for the sincipital type; however, with basal encephaloceles, the contents of the herniation may need to be preserved if it contains vital structures. The dura mater of the sac can be densely adherent to the underlying mucosa, which is often entered during the course of the dissection and repair.[31] Because the herniation is more posteriorly located, more brain retraction is needed to expose the area of involvement, making it important to provide for brain protection and shrinkage by appropriate measures. Often, a craniofacial approach is not needed for these lesions because the degree of bony involvement is small. In the presence of a large cleft palate, an extracranial transpalatal repair can be considered whereby the herniation is reduced and bone is placed into the defect to keep the herniation permanently reduced.[24]

The complications associated with repair at this site are similar to those mentioned for the sincipital lesions, although injudicious brain retraction because of the

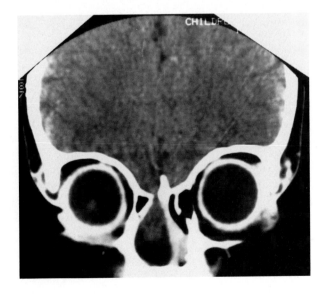

Figure 32–12

Computed tomography scan of a patient with a transethmoidal encephalocele shows a small defect in the floor of the cranial base. The patient presented with a partial nasal obstruction. The correct diagnosis was made, and the defect was repaired without incident.

more posterior location of the lesion can lead to cerebral swelling. Additional problems to consider include hypothalamic dysfunction, which would be most readily manifested as diabetes insipidus in the immediate postoperative period. The neurological prognosis for these infants can be quite good. The very rare anterobasotemporal encephalocele may be associated with seizures, which can be cured by resection of the encephalocele.[22]

Other Dysraphic Lesions Involving the Cranium

Rudimentary encephaloceles are midline lesions that are usually found at the vertex and are associated with various skin changes, which can include cutis aplasia, abnormal hair and hair pattern, telangiectasia, excessive fibrous tissue, and dysplastic glial elements.[1, 16, 39, 49] Because these lesions are usually flaccid and have no observable pulsations, they can be considered as a category separate from the encephaloceles described in the previous sections. Although these rudimentary encephaloceles can be associated with other intracranial abnormalities, most affected infants are neurologically normal, and hydrocephalus is very unusual. Although some lesions have no intracranial connection, most do have a stalk that enters through a small bony defect to connect with the cerebrospinal fluid pathways and thus are true encephaloceles (Fig. 32–13). With those lesions that do connect intracranially, computed tomography or magnetic resonance imaging frequently shows an underlying tract of cerebrospinal fluid density, which is related to the falx cerebri and may even extend into the region of the quadrigeminal cisterns. These tracts frequently have close proximation to, and may even bisect, the superior sagittal sinus. Any attempt to remove the intracranial portion of such a lesion could

lead to opening of the superior sagittal sinus with resultant hemorrhage; however, in reality there is no reason to trace these lesions intracranially, and one can therefore avoid this complication. The dysplastic skin is removed for cosmesis as well as to eliminate the local irritation and pain that can accompany these defects (Fig. 32–14). Satisfactory closure can be accomplished with elliptical removal of the lesion and undermining of the skin. Because these lesions are usually small in diameter, a tension-free closure can usually be accomplished.

Congenital defects of the scalp and cranium can vary from minimal to life-threatening and can be associated with additional congenital abnormalities. Small defects of the scalp may occur in the parietal or occipital region; most are in the midline and can easily be closed during the neonatal period. If not surgically closed, they epithelialize, leaving a scarred region without hair. Larger scalp defects associated with the absence of underlying bone can also occur and are usually in the same region. The scalp defect can be satisfactorily closed if it is small, but rotational flaps are needed for larger defects. Another possibility is to let the region epithelialize completely and then use tissue expanders to develop adequate full-thickness skin for better closure at a later date. The bony defect remains and, if small, is of no consequence. If large, it can be corrected by placement of tantalum mesh under the bone edges.

A more significant lesion, which can be life-threatening, is one in which the dura mater, bone, and scalp are missing so that the leptomeninges, superior sagittal sinus, and brain are exposed (Fig. 32–15). The area must be kept moist, because desiccation results in injury to the underlying brain or rents in the superior sagittal sinus, which can lead to exsanguination. The exposed brain is also vulnerable to direct trauma and to infection. The best method of providing coverage is with full-thickness skin. The use of split-thickness skin

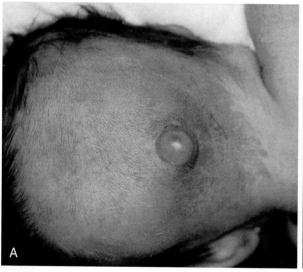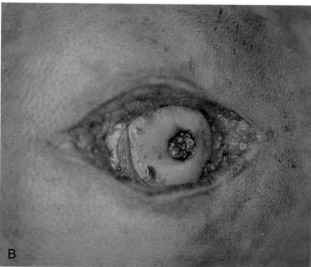

Figure 32–13

A. This patient has a rudimentary encephalocele near the torcular. The overlying skin is dysplastic, and the lesion contains malformed glial elements, skin, and connective tissue. This patient was neurologically normal and without hydrocephalus. *B.* Although the lesion was not pulsatile, there was a small stalk that extended through a small opening in the bone to connect with the subarachnoid space.

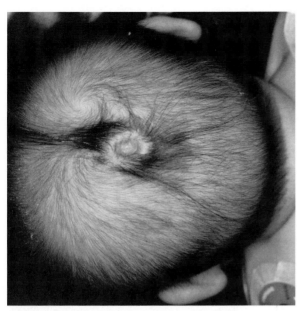

Figure 32–14

This rudimentary encephalocele was associated with cutis aplasia and abnormality of the adjacent hair and hair pattern. This lesion also connected to the intracranial space through a small bony defect. This patient was neurologically normal and without hydrocephalus. The lesion was excised to eliminate local irritation and discomfort as well as for cosmesis.

grafts or simply allowing the area to epithelialize would make it virtually impossible to perform a cranioplasty at a later date.

Other lesions that can be confused with encephaloceles are dermal inclusion cysts, hemangiomas, and lipomas of the scalp. With these lesions, there is no dysplasia of the overlying skin, as almost always oc-

curs with encephaloceles. Dermoid cysts can occur anywhere, but those that can be confused with encephaloceles are usually in the region of the anterior fontanelle (Fig. 32–16) or vertex (Fig. 32–17). These dermoids are extradural with no intracranial connection or bony defect, and if they are cystic, the fluid within is the result of the degeneration of the keratin debris and is not cerebrospinal fluid. Capillary hemangiomas (Fig. 32–18) and lipomas can occur at any place about the calvaria but are more frequently located off the midline; once again, they have no dysplasia of the overlying skin.

The remaining dysraphic lesion of the calvaria to be considered in this section is a congenital dermal sinus that is very often associated with a dermal inclusion cyst. This lesion is most likely to be found in the occipital location (Fig. 32–19), with the remainder presenting in the midline nasal region (Fig. 32–20). No congenital dermal sinus has been reported to be present in an area beneath which resides the superior sagittal sinus. Although some congenital dermal sinuses are inconspicuous, a definite tract is present and may contain hair or keratin debris. Local inflammation is sometimes present. The degree of dysplasia in the surrounding skin is minimal, with only telangiectasia being a common accompaniment. A congenital dermal sinus, if in an occipital location, is directed inferiorly and if intracranial, crosses below the level of the tentorium. The congenital dermal sinus tract is usually associated with a dermoid cyst, which may lie extradurally or, if it is intradural, may be located within the cerebel-

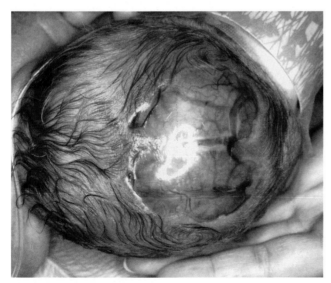

Figure 32–15

This newborn infant had a congenital absence of a large area of the scalp, bone, and dura mater so that the underlying brain and superior sagittal sinus are exposed. In addition, the infant had a myelomeningocele and a hypoplastic left heart. The patient died of the congenital heart anomaly within the first few days of life.

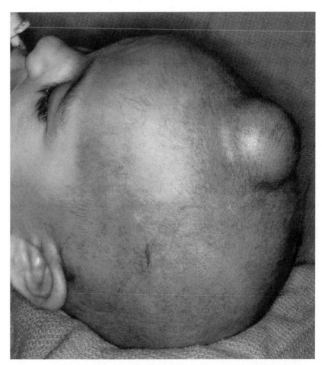

Figure 32–16

This patient had a large dermoid inclusion cyst in the region of the anterior fontanelle. The overlying scalp was not dysplastic and was without any additional cutaneous markers for a midline fusion defect. Although this lesion was not significantly pulsatile, transmission from an underlying open fontanelle could make it appear so. The underlying bone and dura mater were intact.

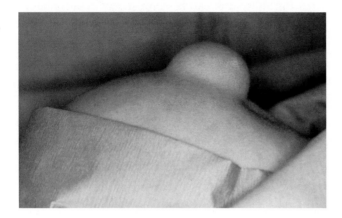

Figure 32–17

This patient has a dermal inclusion cyst at the vertex that is slowly enlarging. The skin over the lesion is not at all dysplastic and is nonpulsatile. The bone under the lesion is intact. The lesion is cystic because it contains fluid from the breakdown of the keratin debris.

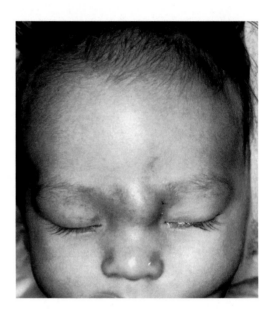

Figure 32–18

This patient had a capillary hemangioma of the nasal bridge. The overlying skin was not dysplastic, and the nasal bridge was not widened. Imaging studies found no bony defect and no intracranial abnormality. (With permission from Raffel, C., and McComb, J. G.: Encephalocele. *In* Apuzzo, M. L. J., ed.: Brain Surgery: Complication Avoidance and Management. New York, Churchill-Livingstone, 1993, pp. 1433–1447.)

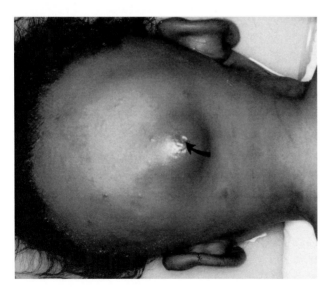

Figure 32–19

A midline occipital mass is present and consists of a congenital dermal sinus associated with an infected dermoid. The arrow points to the cutaneous opening of the sinus. Imaging studies showed the presence of a hole in the underlying bone and an intracranially located dermoid. (With permission from Raffel, C., and McComb, J. G.: Encephalocele. *In* Apuzzo, M. L. J., ed.: Brain Surgery: Complication Avoidance and Management. New York, Churchill-Livingstone, 1993, pp. 1433–1447.)

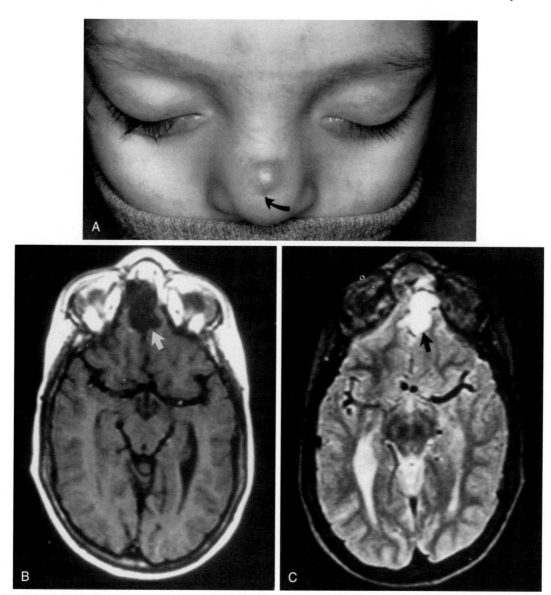

Figure 32–20

A. This infant has an infected congenital dermal sinus associated with a localized abscess. The sinus extends through a small defect at the foramen cecum. A dermoid or a localized abscess can enlarge the soft tissues over the nasal bridge and appear to be a more substantial midline defect that could be mistaken for an encephalocele. The differentiating features are the opening of the sinus tract on the nose *(arrow)* and the findings on imaging studies. *B.* T1-weighted magnetic resonance image shows an intracranial dermoid from the nasal congenital dermal sinus that extends through the formen cecum with an attenuation that is low but greater than that of cerebrospinal fluid *(arrow)*. *C.* T2-weighted image shows an intracranial dermoid from the nasal congenital dermal sinus that extends through the foramen cecum with high attenuation *(arrow)*.

lum, fourth ventricle, or cisterna magna.[29] Those sinuses that are in the nasal region can enter the cranium through a defect in the crista galli by means of a patent foramen cecum. Magnetic resonance and computed tomography studies can determine the intracranial extent of these dysraphic conditions.

REFERENCES

1. Bale, P. M., Hughes, L., and DeSilva, M.: Sequestrated meningoceles of scalp: Extracranial meningeal heterotopia. Hum. Pathol., 21:1156–1163, 1990.
2. Bindal, A. K., Storrs, B. B., and McLone, D. G.: Occipital meningoceles in patients with the Dandy-Walker syndrome. Neurosurgery, 28:844–847, 1991.
3. Blumenfeld, R., and Skolnik, E. M.: Intranasal encephaloceles. Acta Otolaryngol. (Stockh.), 82:527–531, 1965.
4. Brown, M. S., and Sheridan-Pereira, M.: Outlook for the child with a cephalocele. Pediatrics, 90:914–919, 1992.
5. Chapman, P. H., Swearingen, B., and Caviness, V. S.: Subtorcular occipital encephaloceles: Anatomic considerations relevant to operative management. J. Neurosurg., 71:375–381, 1989.
6. Charoonsmith, T., and Suwanwela, C.: Fronto-ethmoidal encephalomeningocele with special reference to plastic reconstruction. Clin. Plast. Surg., 1:27–47, 1974.
7. Chatterjee, M. S., Bondoc, B., and Adhate, A.: Prenatal diagnosis of occipital encephalocele. Am. J. Obstet. Gynecol., 153:646–647, 1985.
8. Cheek, W. R., and Laurent, J. P.: Dermal sinus tracts. Concepts Ped. Neurosurg., 6:63–75, 1985.

9. Choudhury, A. R., and Taylor, J. C.: Primary intranasal encephalocele: Report of 4 cases. J. Neurosurg., *57*:552–555, 1982.

10. Cohen, M. M., Jr., and Lemire, R. J.: Syndromes with cephaloceles. Teratology, *25*:161–172, 1982.

11. Date, I., Yagyu, Y., Asari, S., et al.: Long-term outcome in surgically treated encephalocele. Surg. Neurol., *40*:125–130, 1993.

12. David, D. J., Sheffield, L., Simpson, D., et al.: Fronto-ethmoidal meningoencephaloceles: Morphology and treatment. Br. J. Plast. Surg., *37*:271–284, 1984.

13. Dhawan, I. K., and Tandon, P. N.: Excision, repair and corrective surgery for fronto-ethmoidal meningocele. Childs Brain, *9*:126–136, 1982.

14. Dodge, H. W., Jr., Love, J. G., and Kerndhan, J. W.: Intranasal encephalomeningoceles associated with cranium bifidum. Arch. Surg., *79*:75–84, 1959.

15. Donnenfeld, A. E., Hughes, H., and Weiner, S.: Prenatal diagnosis and perinatal management of frontoethmoidal meningoencephalocele. Am. J. Perinatol., *5*:51–53, 1988.

16. Drapkin, A. J.: Rudimentary cephalocele or neural crest remnant? Neurosurgery, *26*:667–674, 1990.

17. Emery, J. L., and Kalhan, S. C.: The pathology of exencephalus. Dev. Med. Child. Neurol. Suppl., *22*:51–64, 1970.

18. Fenstermaker, R. A., Roessmann, V., and Rekate, H. L.: Fourth ventriculoceles with extracranial extension. J. Neurosurg., *61*:348–350, 1984.

19. Guthkelch, A. N.: Occipital cranium bifidum. Arch. Dis. Child., *45*:104–109, 1970.

20. Hendrick, E. B.: Encephaloceles. *In* Wilkins, R. H., and Rengachary, S. S., eds.: Neurosurgery. New York, McGraw-Hill, 1985, pp. 2087–2091.

21. Hockley, A. D., Goldin, J. H., and Wake, M. J. C.: Management of anterior encephalocele. Childs Nerv. Syst., *6*:444–446, 1990.

22. Leblanc, R., Tampieri, D., Robitaille, Y., et al.: Developmental anterobasal temporal encephalocele and temporal lobe epilepsy. J. Neurosurg., *74*:933–939, 1991.

23. Lemire, R. J., Loesser, J. D., Leech, R. W., et al.: Normal and Abnormal Development of the Human Nervous System. Hagerstown, MD, Harper & Row, 1975.

24. Lewin, M. L.: Sphenoethmoidal cephalocele with cleft palate: Transpalatial versus transcranial repair. Report of 2 cases. J. Neurosurg., *58*:924–931, 1983.

25. Lorber, J.: The prognosis of occipital encephalocele. Dev. Med. Child. Neurol. Suppl., *13*:75–86, 1967.

26. Lorber, J., and Schofield, J. K.: The prognosis of occipital encephalocele. Kinder Chirurgie, *28*:347–351, 1979.

27. Luyendijk, W.: Intranasal encephaloceles: A survey of 8 neurosurgically treated cases. Psychiatr. Neurol. Neurochir., *72*:77–87, 1969.

28. Mealey, J., Jr., Dzenitis, A. J., and Hockey, A. A.: The prognosis of encephalocele. J. Neurosurg., *32*:209–218, 1970.

29. McComb, J. G.: Congenital dermal sinus and dermoid/epidermoid tumors. *In* Cohen, A., ed.: Surgery of the Fourth Ventricle. Cambridge, Blackwell Scientific (in press).

30. McLaurin, R. L.: Encephalocele and related anomalies. *In* Hoffman, H. J., and Epstein, F., eds.: Disorders of the Developing Nervous System: Diagnosis and Treatment. Boston, Blackwell Scientific. 1986, pp. 153–174.

31. Modesti, L. M., Glasauer, F. E., and Terplan, K. L.: Sphenoethmoidal encephalocele: A case report and review of the literature. Childs Brain, *3*:140–153, 1977.

32. MRC Vitamin Study Research Group: Prevention of neural tube defects: Results of the medical research council vitamin study. Lancet, *338*:131–137, 1991.

33. Naidich, T. P., McLone, D. G., Bauer, B. S., et al.: Midline craniofacial dysraphism. Concepts Ped. Neurosurg., *4*:186–207, 1983.

34. Pilu, G., Rizzo, N., Orsini, L. F., et al.: Antenatal recognition of cerebral anomalies. Ultrasound Med. Biol., *12*:319–326, 1986.

35. Rapport, R. L., II, Dunn, R. C., Jr., and Alhady, F.: Anterior encephalocele. J. Neurosurg., *54*:213–219, 1981.

36. Rhaman, N.-V.: Nasal encephalocele. Treatment by transcranial operation. J. Neurol. Sci., *42*:73–85, 1979.

37. Sandford, M. K., Kissling, G. E., and Joubert, P. E.: Neural tube defect etiology: New evidence concerning maternal hyperthermia, health and diet. Dev. Med. Child. Neurol., *34*:661–675, 1992.

38. Sargent, L. A., Seyfer, A. E., and Gunby, E. N.: Nasal encephaloceles: Definitive one-stage reconstruction. J. Neurosurg., *68*:571–575, 1988.

39. Schlitt, M., Williams, J. P., Bastian, F. O., et al.: The small midline occipital encephalomeningocele: Definition of a syndrome. Neurosurgery, 24: 613–616, 1989.

40. Schmidt, P. H., and Luyendijk, W.: Intranasal meningoencephalocele. Arch. Otolaryngol., *99*:402–405, 1974.

41. Sever, L. E.: An epidemiologic study of neural tube defects in Los Angeles County: II. Etiologic factors in an area with low prevalence at birth. Teratology, *25*:323–334, 1982.

42. Shokunbi, T., Adeloye, A., and Olumide, A.: Occipital encephaloceles in 57 Nigerian children: A retrospective analysis. Childs Nerv. Syst., *6*:99–102, 1990.

43. Simpson, D. A., David, D. J., and White, J.: Cephaloceles: Treatment, outcome, and antenatal diagnosis. Neurosurgery, *15*:14–21, 1984.

44. Suwanwela, C., and Hongsaprabhas, C.: Frontoethmoidal encephalocele. J. Neurosurg., *25*:172–182, 1966.

45. Suwanwela, C., and Suwanwela, N.: A morphological classification of sincipital encephaloceles. J. Neurosurg., *36*:201–211, 1972.

46. Winsor, E. J. T., and St. John Brown, B.: Prevalence and prenatal diagnosis of neural tube defects in Nova Scotia in 1980–84. Can. Med. Assoc. J., *135*:1269–1273, 1986.

47. Wiswell, T. E., Tuttle, D. J., Northam, R. S., et al.: Major congenital neurologic malformations. Am. J. Dis. Child, *144*:61–67, 1990.

48. Yokota, A., Matsukado, Y., Funa, I., et al.: Anterior basal encephalocele of the neonatal and infantile period. Neurosurgery, *19*:468–477, 1986.

49. Yokuta, A., Kajiwara, H., Kohchi, M., et al.: Parietal cephalocele: Clinical importance of its atretic form and associated malformations. J. Neurosurg., *69*:545–551, 1988.

50. Zee, C. S., McComb, J. G., Segall, H. D., et al.: Lipomas of the corpus callosum associated with frontal dysraphism. J. Comput. Assist. Tomogr., *5*:201–205, 1981.

Myelomeningocele

More children are crippled by myelomeningocele than by polio, muscular dystrophy, or traumatic paraplegia. As a consequence, many physicians must confront this disease and help determine the proper management of the affected child and family. Until recently, there has been little solid information about the long-term prognosis for children with myelomeningocele. The medical, social, and ethical issues provoked heated debate. Within the last couple of decades, significant new data have emerged to provide the physician with a scientific basis for guiding patient management.[33, 34, 36, 40] There is now a consensus that children with myelomeningocele should be treated aggressively and that such treatment benefits most, but not all, affected children. It seems clear that no criteria can predict successfully the children for whom there will be a favorable long-term result.[2, 30, 31, 36] So-called "selection criteria" are simply invalid.[25]

It seems equally clear that the physician must avoid making a decision about treating the child based solely on a personal bias about what constitutes an acceptable quality of life. The author's experience with more than 1,000 families indicates that the family's view often differs from the physician's. The physician must review current knowledge regarding the outcome and late complications of myelomeningocele and must make this information available to the family to assist the parents in deciding these issues for their child.[30, 34]

Historical Perspective

The medical and social problems facing the patient with myelomeningocele are not new. Hippocrates and the Arabic physicians knew this lesion. Aristotle "resolved" the social problem by recommending infanticide. Tulpius, De Ruysch, and Morgagni first noted the relationship of paralysis of the legs to the sac and advised against ligation.[9, 42, 65] Trowbridge, 150 years later, continued to recommend ligation, although all his patients died with fever.[64] Morton treated the back with an iodine sclerosing solution that was later found to be more hazardous than doing nothing or performing minimal surgical repair.[43]

From the early 1900's onward, steady progress was made toward closure of the back without infection. Individual patients began to survive. Laurence reviewed the effect of closing the myelomeningocele by deflating the sac with a wide-bore needle and then laying on a skin graft.[24] He detailed the natural history of spina bifida cystica and documented the poor outcome in children not treated for hydrocephalus.

Hippocrates and Galen described children with large heads, but Vesalius was the first to note the large accumulation of water within the ventricular system of the brain.[68] In the early 1900's, Dandy and Blackfan produced hydrocephalus in a dog by plugging the aqueduct.[8] Later, Dandy demonstrated that the choroid plexus produced cerebrospinal fluid and performed choroid plesectomies to treat hydrocephalus.[7] In 1952, Holter, and also Nulsen and Spitz, initiated modern management of hydrocephalus by developing one-way shunt valves for the controlled drainage of cerebrospinal fluid.[41, 50]

Normal Development of the Mammalian Spinal Cord

Understanding congenital lesions is best achieved with a knowledge of normal embryology and fetal development. This knowledge of the developmental sequence is necessary for interpreting the relationships of mature structures. Likewise, an understanding of the structure of a congenital lesion affords insight into the time and the stage of development at which the

D. G. McLone

sequence was altered. The relationship of primitive cell layers limits the form that the embryopathy can take.

By day 17, ectodermal cells have migrated into the primitive pit and have advanced cephalically, in the midline, to create a column of cells that is situated between the ectoderm and the entoderm. This column of cells, called the notochordal process, extends from Hensen's node caudally to the prochordal plate cephalically. The primitive pit then deepens and invaginates into the previously solid notochordal process, lengthening it into a hollow notochordal canal, which quickly fuses with the entoderm. At the points of fusion, breakdown of cells opens the notochordal canal to the yolk sac. As a result, there is a transient communication from the amnion through the notochordal canal to the yolk sac. This is the neurenteric canal of Kovalevsky. Soon thereafter, the notochordal canal undergoes complex changes that close the communication with the yolk sac, re-establish complete layers of entoderm and ectoderm, and re-form a solid core of tissue designated the true notochord. The entoderm ultimately forms gut. The notochord induces formation of the neural plate and guides formation of the vertebral bodies. The ectoderm forms spinal cord and skin.

The greatest portion of the spinal cord, essentially all of the functional spinal cord, forms by an orderly sequence of steps designated neurulation. This mechanism establishes the brain, the cervical and thoracic segments of the spinal cord, and the upper portion of the lumbar enlargement. The smaller, distal portion of the spinal cord forms by a process that is much less well organized, a sequence of agglomeration of cells, vacuolation, and involution that is designated canalization and retrogressive differentiation, a cumbersome term. A better term is *secondary neurulation*. This process establishes the distal conus medullaris and the filum terminale.

Initially, the immature spinal cord extends to the distal end of the tail fold of the embryo. In a full-term infant, the tip of the spinal cord typically lies at the L2–L3 interspace (98 per cent) or overlies the L3 vertebra (1.2 per cent of cases).[3] By 3 months postpartum, the tip of the conus medullaris is almost at the adult level of the L1–L2 interspace. This apparent ascent of the cord results from disproportionately greater growth of the vertebral column.

Formation of the vertebrae proceeds along with formation of the neural elements. By day 17, mesodermal cells at the cephalic end of the embryo form a thick mass of paraxial mesoderm situated lateral to the notochord and ventrolateral to the neural plate. This paraxial mesoderm forms bilaterally symmetrical longitudinal columns of solid mesoderm. By day 20, these columns begin to segment into paired blocks called somites. Somites first form in the future occipital region. They continue to take shape as the embryo lengthens until, ultimately, 42 to 44 pairs are formed: 4 occipital, 8 cervical, 12 thoracic, 5 lumbar, 5 sacral, and 8 to 10 coccygeal. Later, the first occipital and the last five to seven coccygeal pairs disappear.

The ventromedial portion of each somite differentiates into a sclerotome that ultimately forms the carti-

lage, bone, and ligament of the vertebral column. During the fourth week of development, the notochord separates from the ectoderm and the entoderm. Cells from the sclerotomes then migrate medially, surround the notochord, and form a dense longitudinal column of mesenchyme about the notochord. After the neural tube closes and separates from the superficial ectoderm, cells from the sclerotomes also migrate dorsal to the neural tube, between future cord and future skin, to establish the precursors of the neural arches of the vertebrae. Migration of sclerotomic cells ventrolaterally forms the costal processes and ribs. These elements then undergo a complex resegmentation, chondrification, and ossification, creating the spinal column. These diverse processes are addressed in greater detail in the following sections.

NEURULATION

By the end of the third week, the notochord induces formation of a slipper-shaped plate of ectodermal cells in the midline, just cephalic to Hensen's node. This neural plate is directly contiguous laterally with the superficial ectoderm from which it differentiated (Fig. 33–1). During the next days, the lateral portions of the neural plate elevate to form the neural folds, while the midline portion remains depressed as the ventral neural groove. Progressive elevation and rolling over causes the left and the right neural folds to approximate each other and fuse together in the midline. This process forms a neural tube (future spinal cord) with a central channel (future central canal of the spinal cord) (Fig. 33–2). The folds first meet and fuse in the future

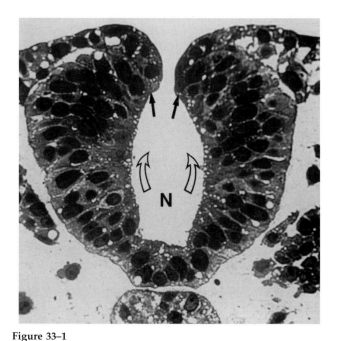

Figure 33–1

A light micrograph of a neurulating embryo is shown. The superficial ectoderm (*solid arrows*) is attached to the neuroectoderm; N is the neurocele of the future neural tube; the open arrows point to the apposing neural folds.

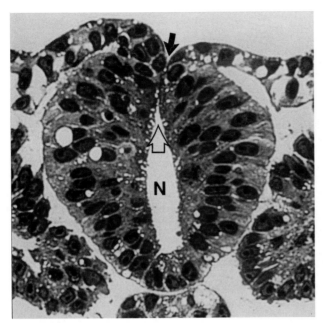

Figure 33–2

A light micrograph of a neurulating embryo is shown. The superficial ectoderm *(solid arrow)* is dorsal to the apposing neural folds *(open arrow)* of the neural tube (N).

cervical region. Thereafter, the process proceeds both cranially and caudally as a wave so that the level of fusion corresponds to the level of the most recently formed somite. At approximately 23 days and 25 days of gestation, respectively, the cephalic and caudal ends of the neural tube close at the anterior and posterior neuropores.

Immediately after fusion of the neural folds into the neural tube, the two portions of superficial ectoderm fuse together in the midline, dorsal to the neural tube, to establish the integrity of the superficial ectoderm (future skin). Only then does the superficial ectoderm of each side separate from the neural ectoderm in a process designated dysfunction (Fig. 33–3). As mesenchyme migrates dorsally between the neural tube and the skin, the entire cord becomes buried beneath a thick layer that ultimately forms the meninges, neural arches, and paraspinal muscles.

SECONDARY NEURULATION

After primary neurulation is complete, on approximately day 25, the distal spinal cord has yet to be formed. The caudal end of the neural tube and the caudal end of the notochord remnants of Hensen's node blend into a large aggregate of undifferentiated cells (the caudal cell mass) that extends into the tail fold, adjacent to the distal end of the developing hindgut and the mesonephros. This juxtaposition of developing genitourinary, notochordal, and neural structures within the tail fold appears to account for the common concurrence of distal vertebral, neural, anorectal, renal, and genital anomalies.

Within the caudal cell mass, small vacuoles form,

coalesce, and eventually connect with the central canal of the spinal cord above, thus "canalizing" the caudal cell mass. Because vacuoles form at many sites and link up variably, accessory central canals are commonly observed in the distal cords of embryos (35 per cent) and, occasionally, in otherwise normal adults.

As the vacuoles form, groups of cells orient themselves around the vacuoles and begin to differentiate into glial cells. By this method, the distal spinal cord and the canal of the cord elongate far into the tail fold. The most cephalic portion of this distal spinal cord forms the tip of the conus medullaris. The major portion of the distal spinal cord involutes to form the filum terminale. A portion of the lumen persists into adulthood as the terminal ventricle that lies within the distal-most conus or the proximal filum terminale.

The process of involution of the distal spinal cord has in the past been designated retrogressive differentiation. It begins even before canalization is complete. The embryonic tail disappears first. The lumen distal to future C2 becomes progressively narrower than the lumen above. The cells surrounding the narrowing distal lumen differentiate less completely than do those above and then involute further, to leave only the pial-ependymal strand, designated filum terminale. A small portion of the distal-most involuting spinal cord frequently remains within the connective tissue dorsal to the last two vertebrae for long periods, as the coccygeal medullary vestige.

After the distal spinal cord involutes, or rather, fails to differentiate into spinal cord, the newly formed conus medullaris lies opposite C2 or C3. Thereafter, the spinal cord does not shorten further, but it elongates with growth. The vertebral column also elongates

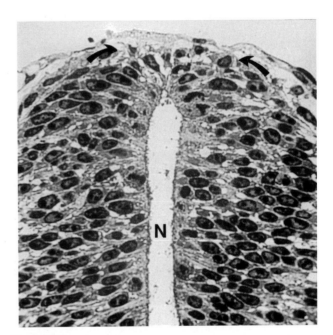

Figure 33–3

The figure shows a light micrograph of a closed neural tube (N) with the superficial ectoderm separated from the neural ectoderm. Mesenchyme *(curved arrows)* streams in to form the dorsal vertebral elements and paraspinous muscles.

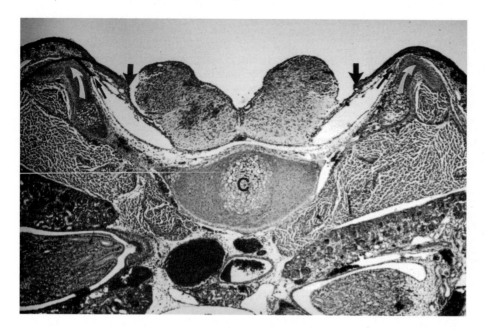

Figure 33–4

A photomicrograph of a transverse section of a dysraphic mouse embryo shows neural tissue open to the amniotic cavity. Notice that the skin edges *(large arrows)* stop before reaching the neural tissue. The dura mater joins the skin lateral to the open edges *(thin arrows)*. Curved arrows indicate everted lamina; C is the developing centrum of the vertebral body.

with growth—faster than the spinal cord. All further "ascent" of the spinal cord results from disproportionate longitudinal growth of the vertebrae: the bones grow away from the spinal cord.[3]

At this point, it is sufficient to understand that the caudal spinal column also forms by a less well organized process than that responsible for the more cephalic portions of the spine above. The caudal cell mass formed by notochord, mesoderm, and neural tissue simply segments into somites to form the sacral, coccygeal, and tail vertebrae. Secondary neurulation then leads to reduction of most of these segments, with loss of the tail.

Embryopathy

MYELOMENINGOCELE

A myelomeningocele (myelocele) is a form of spina bifida in which a focal segment of spinal cord appears as a flat plate of neural tissue that is exposed to view in the midline of the back. Such an anatomical derangement could result from either a primary failure of neurulation or a secondary disruption and splitting of a normally formed spinal cord.[37]

If the neural folds fail to roll up and fuse into a tube, they persist instead as a flat plate of neural tissue (Fig. 33–4). Because the tube does not close, the superficial ectoderm does not separate from the neural ectoderm and remains in a lateral position. Therefore, the skin that develops from the ectoderm is also lateral in position, leaving a midline defect. Mesenchyme cannot migrate between the neural tube and the superficial ectoderm, so it remains in an abnormal lateral position. Therefore, the bony, cartilaginous, muscular, and ligamentous elements that develop from the mesenchyme also remain in abnormal lateral positions. They are

deficient in the midline. Because the laminae and muscles develop in an abnormal lateral position, they appear bifid and everted. The unfused neural plate is exposed to view in the midline of the back, at the site of midline deficiency of skin, bone, cartilage, muscle, and ligament. This state is designated myelomeningocele. Myelomeningocele is the most common form of spinal dysraphism.

In myelomeningocele, the exposed surface of the neural plate appears as a raw, reddish, vascular, oval plate in the midline of the back (Fig. 33–5). The raw surface represents the interior of what should have been the closed spinal cord. A midline groove runs down the center of this plate. This groove is the residuum of the ventral neural groove and is directly continuous with the central canal of the normally formed cord above (and sometimes below) the plate.

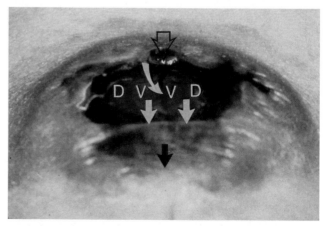

Figure 33–5

A lumbar myelomeningocele of a newborn infant is shown. The open arrow indicates the opening into the central canal of the closed portion of the spinal cord. *Curved arrow,* ventral sulcus; V, ventral (motor), and D, dorsal (sensory) plates of the open neural tube. Solid straight arrows show the partial epithelial covering of the neural tissue.

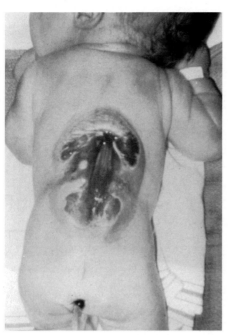

Figure 33–6

A photograph of an infant with a large thoracolumbar myelomeningocele is shown. Notice the midline ventral sulcus. The anatomical relationships are preserved in all these lesions.

The neural plate floats on closed subarachnoid space lined with arachnoid. The size of this membranous ring varies. If the subarachnoid space is small, the membranous ring is narrow, and the neural plate lies flush with the back (Fig. 33–6). If the subarachnoid space is very large, the membranous ring is wide, and the neural plate is elevated far above the skin surface (Fig. 33–7). In myelomeningocele, the neural plate and the membranous ring are surrounded by normal skin. With time, the membranous ring and the neural plate may become partially epithelialized by cells that grow medially from the skin margins to cover the midline defect.

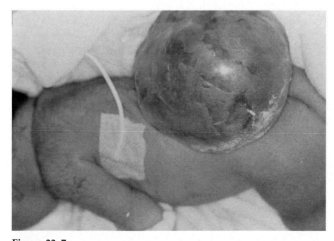

Figure 33–7

In this infant, an extremely large meningocele elevates the open neural tissue, but the relation of the neural tissue to the meningocele is the same.

Deep to the surface, the ventral face of the neural plate represents the neural tissue that should have formed the entire outer circumference of the spinal cord. The two ventral nerve roots arise from the ventral surface, just to each side of the midline sulcus. The left and right dorsal roots also arise from the dorsal root ganglion and enter the ventral surface of the neural plate, lateral to the corresponding ventral roots. These roots traverse the subarachnoid space and exit through the neural foramina, in the usual fashion.

The pia-arachnoid membrane continues medially over the ventral surface of the neural plate and around the entire subarachnoid space as one continuous sheet. This membrane is given the name pia mater where it is contiguous with neural tissue and the name arachnoid mater where it is separate from the neural tissue (Fig. 33–8). The dura mater lies peripheral to the arachnoid and becomes lost in the margins of the skin defect dorsally. Because the neural plate and meninges are anchored to the skin surface, the spinal cord is tethered and is relatively immobile.

PATHOGENESIS

The exact abnormality of embryogenesis that creates myelomeningocele is unknown. Two basic theories of its pathogenesis have been proposed: (1) the neural tube fails to close properly, and (2) the once-closed neural tube ruptures open.[13, 69] Experimental data suggest that both mechanisms may lead to myelomeningocele.[37, 38]

The best data strongly suggest that myelomeningocele represents a disturbance in the closure of the neural placode at or before the time the embryo reaches 3 to 5 mm (crown-rump length), leaving the neural tissue in its embryonal, plaquelike state (Fig. 33–9). The author's experiments with neurulating mouse embryos explanted into in vitro culture indicate that addition of

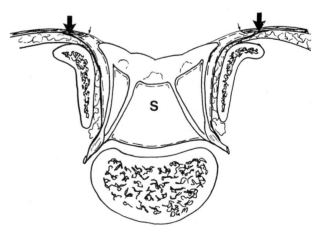

Figure 33–8

A drawing shows the constant relationship between tissues in a myelomeningocele. S is the subarachnoid space that determines the size of the meningocele. The dotted line indicates the pia-arachnoid lining of this space. The large arrows indicate where the dura mater joins the skin, and the small arrows indicate the junction of the skin with the epithelial layer that surrounds the neural tissue.

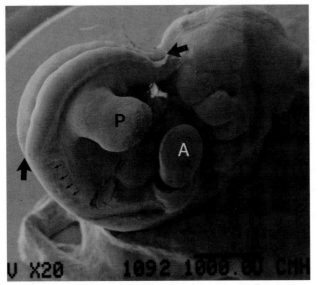

Figure 33–9

A scanning electron micrograph of an 11-day-old mouse embryo with an extensive neural tube defect *(large arrows)*. Small arrows indicate somites adjacent to the closed neural tube. A, anterior limb; P, posterior limb.

toxins such as tunicamycin interferes with the normal formation of glycosaminoglycans and prevents the neural tube from closing. This creates spina bifida.[37] Hydrocephalus and the Chiari II deformity at the cervicomedullary junction do not develop in the embryonic period but appear later, during fetal life.[51]

Also in the author's laboratory, addition of vitamin A to the same in vitro culture of a mouse embryo had no apparent effect on the developing embryo. However, injection of vitamin A into the pregnant mouse before or during the period of neurulation caused neural tube defects in some embryos and a remarkable increase in the volume of the neural tube in other embryos. In these latter embryos, the central canal appeared grossly distended. Light microscopy of the sectioned embryos documented marked distention of the neural tube. The neuroepithelia showed evidence of toxicity, with multiple intracellular inclusions.

In this experimental arrangement, the two portions of the neural tube that appeared to be the most thinned were the ventral and the dorsal sulci. In some embryos, the ventral sulcus of the neural tubes gaped. Because the ventral neural tube is normally never open, vitamin A–induced distention of the central canal must have caused the spinal cord to rupture.[37] The results of the vitamin A study support the postulate advocated by Padget and by Gardner and provide the first experimental evidence that the neural tube did, in fact, close and then reopen secondarily because of distention and rupture.[13, 52]

Other theories of the origin of myelomeningocele probably reflect secondary phenomena.[11, 13]

The studies of Osaka and colleagues of the incidence and distribution of myeloschisis in 92 human embryos and 4 human fetuses document that, in utero, diffuse myeloschisis is common (13 per cent), cervical myeloschisis is frequent (29 per cent), and holoprosencephaly is commonly associated with myeloschisis (20 per cent).[51] Embryos with diffuse myeloschisis, focal cervical myeloschisis, and concomitant holoprosencephaly are likely to be extruded by spontaneous abortion. Thus, the increased frequency of lumbosacral myelomeningocele in newborns does not indicate a greater occurrence of myelomeningocele in the lumbosacral area. Rather, it reflects the milder nature of lumbosacral myelomeningoceles, which permits fetuses affected with this relatively infrequent form to live to full term.

Closure of Myelomeningocele

PREPARATION OF THE NEONATE FOR SURGERY

Although it is important for the parents of an affected neonate to have some time to grapple with the many new issues facing them, it is equally important to proceed with definitive treatment in a timely fashion. The idea that, by significantly delaying closure of the myelomeningocele, the parents may be instructed about the nuances of this birth defect so that they can better make an informed consent is preposterous.[32] Unless the child is critically ill, repair of the myelomeningocele should proceed immediately. Significant delays increase both morbidity and mortality.

Optimally, the child is operated on soon after birth, preferably on the first postnatal day. Prenatal diagnosis now makes this increasingly more possible. However, operation may safely be deferred for up to 72 hours without an increase in complications. This delay is particularly important for the unstable or critically ill infant. Such infants can usually be stabilized within 72 hours. A search for coexistent anomalies of other organ systems should be undertaken during this time. Unrepairable cardiac defects or severe anomalies or absence of other vital organs may portend a poor outcome. Renal anomalies are common but are not usually life-threatening. Although the child may not produce significant amounts of urine during the first 24 hours, the presence of urine in the bladder implies the presence of functioning kidneys. An ultrasound study can delineate most major renal anomalies. Syndromes related to chromosomal anomalies may not be obvious on initial inspection but should be sought.

Although most coexisting anomalies are not immediately life-threatening and may be dealt with without much difficulty, a few children with myelomeningocele have fatal associated malformations and cannot be saved. Intervention to prolong the lives of these infants in the setting of a dismal outlook makes little sense; they should be kept comfortable and their families should be supported.

The preparation of the neonate with a myelomeningocele for surgery is usually not difficult. Most have a high hematocrit and an adequate intravascular volume; fluid resuscitation is therefore usually unnecessary. Common perioperative complications include hypothermia and hypoglycemia, both of which are easily prevented through the judicious use of heating lamps and the monitoring of serum glucose.

The placode may become desiccated with prolonged exposure to the air and should therefore be protected. Covering the placode with sterile saline-soaked gauze is preferable; the dressing may be covered with plastic wrap to avoid rapid evaporation of the saline. Betadine is toxic to tissues and results in inhibition and delay of wound healing; it should not be used directly on the malformation. The use of perioperative antibiotics is left to the discretion of the surgeon.

PRESERVATION OF NEUROLOGICAL FUNCTION

Preservation of Neural Tissue. It has clearly been shown that the exposed neural tissue of myelomeningoceles is functional. Movement of muscles subserved by spinal cord segments involved in the placode and the presence of somatosensory potentials conducted through the placode both point to the functional nature of this tissue.[28] Even if the initial examination fails to demonstrate movement of muscles innervated by the placode, the placode should still be considered functional, because more than one third of children with these deformities subsequently gain motor functions not previously detected.[29] Therefore, all neural tissue must be preserved.

Preservation of Vascular Supply. Preservation of the vascular supply to the placode is essential if this tissue is to survive. Unlike that to the normal spinal cord, the blood supply to the placode does not enter exclusively through the vertebral foramina along the nerve roots. Many large vessels pass directly through the laterally reflected dura mater to supply the myelomeningocele. Those that supply the junction between the neurulated spinal cord and the placode seem to be at greatest risk. Rarely is it possible to preserve all of these vessels, but they can sometimes be sacrificed if necessary without apparent injury to the placode. Nonetheless, great care must be exercised to preserve these vessels while mobilizing the dura for closure.

Inclusion Dermoid. Great care should be exercised

in separating the edge of the placode from the contiguous cutaneous epithelium; magnification is often very helpful. Retained fragments, possibly even a single cell, could, if imbricated within the closure, produce an inclusion dermoid. Not only do inclusion dermoids produce tumors, but associated desquamative debris may also stimulate an intense arachnoiditis. Tethered cord release in the face of the scar produced by this inflammatory process can be difficult.

MISSED ABNORMALITIES

Diastematomyelia. Both the cranial and caudal ends of the closure site should be closely inspected before closure of the placode to identify associated tethering, bony spurs, or fibrous bands (Fig. 33–10). Cranially, removal of an additional lamina may be necessary to adequately visualize the adjacent spinal cord. Hemimyelomeningoceles may also be readily visualized by examining the adjacent spinal cord. The presence of an asymmetrical neurological deficit preoperatively should alert the surgeon to the presence of a hemimyelomeningocele or an associated split-cord malformation.

Thickened Filum Terminale. Caudal to the placode, a thickened filum terminale may often be found; this should be sectioned if it is present. Spinal cord tethering may occur as often from a missed thickened filum as from adhesions directly related to the placode repair.

OPERATIVE CONSIDERATIONS

Retethering. After the neural tissue has been freed, every attempt should be made to prevent later retethering of the placode. Although pia-to-pia closure of the placode into a tubular structure may not always prevent retethering, it may reduce the incidence of this complication (Fig. 33–11).[28] More importantly, it makes later untethering considerably easier to perform because the reapproximated neural tube is usually adherent only along the dorsal closure line. In contrast, unclosed neural tissue is often densely adherent along the entire exposed ependymal area of the placode; the

Figure 33–10

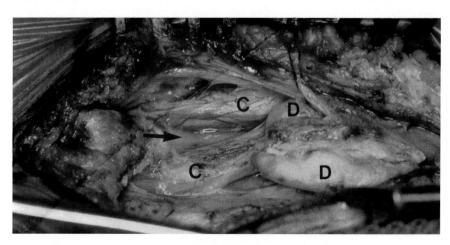

A child with a myelomeningocele was reoperated on for a diastematomyelia and bony spur *(arrow)* splitting the cord into two hemicords (C). Notice the inclusion dermoids (D).

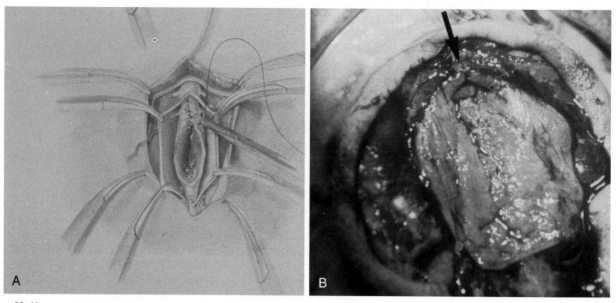

Figure 33–11

A. A drawing shows the dissected dura mater, the transected thickened filum, and the suturing of neural placode into a tube. *B.* An operative photograph shows the initial placement of sutures *(arrow)* for the repair of a myelomeningocele.

laterally displaced dorsal roots are usually caught in the scar, and it requires tedious dissection to free them. Unfortunately, even after reapproximation of the neural placode, the dura may occasionally be inadvertently sutured to the underlying neural tissue; great care should be taken to avoid this preventable complication.

Neural Compression During Closure. Dural closure is an important part of the myelomeningocele repair. Most pediatric neurosurgeons advocate a watertight dural closure. However, a more important consideration is creating enough space to house the neural placode. It makes no sense to preserve the placode through careful dissection and then strangulate it with a tight, constricting dural closure. To avoid neural compression, a dural patch graft may be used. Although the number of repairs that leak cerebrospinal fluid postoperatively may be increased by this type of closure, the ultimate functional outcome is better.

Wound Closure. Wound closure is fairly straightforward, although several controversies exist. Mobilization of the paraspinal muscles and overlying fascia to cover the closure is desirable but not always possible. Moreover, the frequency of complications is the same whether or not this layer is included in the closure.[58]

The method of skin closure is also a matter of debate. Although some authors have advocated complex plastic surgical closures, this is rarely necessary.[59] A linear, midsagittal closure is most satisfactory and provides easy access to the placode should later untethering or spinal stabilization procedures become necessary. In contrast, cutting across complex wound closures carries the potential risk of devascularizing segments of skin. In the author's experience, cutting across such incisions has occasionally been necessary at reoperation, but fortunately, in none of these cases has a portion of the closure been lost.

A significant kyphosis may preclude a simple wound closure. In addition, almost all kyphotic deformities are progressive and are associated with a sequential loss of neural function below the level of the kyphosis by 3 or 4 years of age. If significant kyphosis is present at birth, a kyphectomy may be performed at the time of closure (Fig. 33–12).

Hydrocephalus. The timing of shunt placement is a matter of some debate. Because about 10 per cent of children with myelomeningocele do not need a shunt, delaying a shunt procedure until well after the initial closure is reasonable if the ventricles are only slightly dilated. However, in the presence of obvious hydrocephalus at birth, it makes little sense to subject the infant to a second anesthetization. Placement of the shunt at the time of initial closure is safe and reduces the risks of fluid leakage and wound breakdown postoperatively.

Outcome

SURVIVAL

Between 1947 and 1956, 89 per cent of English children born with a myelomeningocele died before the age of 6 months.[24] In 1964, Laurence reviewed the outcome of 407 children cared for at a large children's hospital just before effective shunting devices became available.[24] In this group, the myelomeningocele was repaired in only 160 of the 407 children (39 per cent). Seventy-three per cent of the children had clinical evidence of hydrocephalus. Intracranial infection was the most common cause of death. In Laurence's study, a newborn infant with myelomeningocele had a 29 per cent chance of living to 12 years of age. Infants who survived 4 months had a 51 per cent chance of living

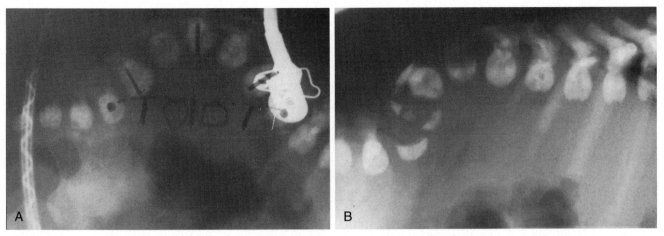

Figure 33–12

A. A lateral radiograph of the lower spine of a child with a large kyphosis is shown. The marked vertebral bodies are to be subperiosteally resected. *B.* After resection, the vertebrae are pushed ventrally and held with a dorsally placed suture.

that long. Those who survived to the age of 1 year had a 77 per cent chance of surviving to 12 years of age. The mortality rate began to level off at about 48 months. Similar leveling of the mortality rate has also been observed in more recent studies of children treated aggressively.[36] It may be a natural part of the disease course.

During the period from the middle of the 1950's to 1985, effective methods were developed for treating hydrocephalus. In 1971, Lorber reported the use of selection criteria to assign children with myelomeningocele to two groups: one with poor prognosis and the other with good prognosis.[25] Long-term follow-up of Lorber's selected series indicates that the overall mortality rate of the two groups approached 70 per cent, mostly because of the selection process itself.[26] The mortality rate in the group with a bad prognosis was almost 100 per cent. The mortality rate in the group with a good prognosis, selected to have the best chance of surviving, was 14 per cent.

In contrast, the author and his co-workers began in the 1980's treating all patients with myelomeningocele, without applying any selection criteria.[36] The overall mortality rate for the initial group of 100 unselected patients followed for 8 to 12 years after closure of the back was 15 per cent. Mortalities continued to occur through adolescence, and by 13 to 17 years after closure, the mortality rate had increased to 19 per cent. An unrecognized shunt malfunction was the most common cause of late mortality.[34] Two of the children (2 per cent) did not survive to leave the hospital, despite initial closure of the back and shunting procedures. A total of 10 per cent died by the end of the third year, and a total of 14 per cent died by the end of 5 years. The most common cause of death in these young children was hindbrain dysfunction, with stridor, apneic spells, and reflux aspiration. Eleven (11 per cent) of the deaths in the first group of 100 patients were from hindbrain dysfunction. Death was caused by central nervous system infection in 1 per cent.

In evaluating the selection process, one must weigh the differences in mortality rates (68 per cent versus 19 per cent) and in the number of children who survived with and without certain problems. Only 29 of 100 children in a selected series reported by Lorber and Salfield, versus 61 children in the author's nonselected series, survived with an intelligence quotient higher than 80.[26, 36] Moreover, 20 children survived with an IQ lower than 80 in the nonselected series, versus only 2 in the selected series. A similar situation results when one looks at ambulation.[26, 36]

The mortality rate in unselected patients with myelomeningocele is not statistically different from the survival rate in Lorber's best selected cases. For this reason, most major centers now treat almost all newborn children with myelomeningocele. Only the small number of children who are already agonal at birth (approximately 1 to 2 per cent) are cared for without surgery. This number will probably decrease with time as obstetrical ultrasound and fetal surgery improve.

HINDBRAIN DYSFUNCTION

Almost all children with myelomeningocele have occasional problems from hindbrain dysfunction. Thirty-two per cent of the first 100 patients in the author's series had serious sequelae of such dysfunction.[29, 36] Eleven per cent died of hindbrain dysfunction, which was the major cause of all deaths in this series.

In the first group of 100 patients, 13 patients suffered severe problems (apnea, cyanosis, gastric reflux with aspiration) during the neonatal period and required repeated hospitalizations and surgical procedures to manage the sequelae. One of these 13 children was born with vocal cord paralysis; the other 12 developed problems in the neonatal period. Four of the 13 underwent posterior cervical decompression to treat progressive respiratory pauses and apnea.[4] Two of the four died, one still requires a tracheostomy, and one has recovered. Of the 13 patients, 11 (85 per cent) have died.

Of the 32 children with significant hindbrain dysfunction, 4 were treated surgically.[29, 36] Two of the four died—a 50 per cent operative mortality rate. Of the remaining 28 patients, 9 died—a 32 per cent nonoperative mortality. Of the 19 survivors, one required a tracheostomy, and 18 have recovered. In this group of 32 children with serious hindbrain dysfunction, managed as described, the overall mortality rate was 34 per cent (11 of 32 patients).

Hoffman and colleagues and Park and coworkers reported a 38 per cent mortality rate in a series in which they operated on all neonates with similarly serious hindbrain dysfunction.[20, 54] Ten years later, Vandertop, from the same institution, reported a series of 17 infants decompressed with a 12 per cent mortality, using the same indications for surgery.[66] In the 1992 series of Pollack and colleagues, 13 infants were decompressed; this series had a 23 per cent mortality.[56] The author's data indicate that many children who would have been operated on according to the aforementioned criteria survive well without surgery. The natural history of hindbrain dysfunction in the neonate appears to be one of gradual improvement over time in those children who survive the acute problems. For that reason, the author believes it is best to temporize as much as possible in these newborn children and to operate only when no other course is possible.

HYDROCEPHALUS

In Laurence's 1964 study of the natural history of myelomeningocele, hydrocephalus was evident clinically in 73 per cent of the children.[24] Shunting was attempted in 53 of 407 patients (13 per cent) but probably was not effective in any case. Eight of the 53 children (15 per cent) had arrest of the hydrocephalus.

In the author's study of an initial group of 100 children, 80 per cent showed clinical evidence of hydrocephalus requiring shunting.[36] In 20 per cent, shunting was not performed. However, in this group, not all children were evaluated radiologically. In a second group of 100 children, routine ultrasound studies of the head detected ventricular dilatation in 95 per cent. Shunts were required in 90 per cent of the 100 children. In a third group of almost 100 patients, a pattern similar to that of the second group has emerged. Thus, it would appear that approximately 10 per cent of patients with a myelomeningocele do not require shunt diversion of cerebrospinal fluid. The criteria used for deciding to place the initial shunt were (1) rapid, progressive enlargement of ventricular size or head circumference; (2) stridor, apnea, or gastroesophageal reflux attributed to hindbrain dysfunction from Chiari II malformation; (3) continued leakage of cerebrospinal fluid at the closure site; (4) evidence of developmental delay; and (5) cosmetically unpleasant head shape.

Shunt revisions were required in 52 per cent of the patients by 6 years of age.[36] No attempt was made to perform elective shunt lengthening as the child grew. Instead, adequate length was placed in the peritoneal cavity at the initial insertion. Almost half (48 per cent) of all the children reached the sixth year of life without any shunt revision. Another one third of the children

had only one or two revisions by the sixth year. The remaining 20 per cent required between three and nine revisions.

In the entire series of 285 patients, 264 (93 per cent) developed ventricular enlargement. Of the 264 with enlarged ventricles, 245 (93 per cent) had shunts performed. Thus, 86 per cent of the entire group received shunts. The size of the ventricles varied after shunting: 40 per cent showed slit ventricles, 20 per cent had ventricles of normal size, and 40 per cent had enlarged ventricles. The intelligence quotient did not correlate with ventricular size, except in the extreme case, ventricles were 4+ dilated after shunting (<1 cm of cortical mantle).[62] Only 14 per cent of those with 4+ ventricles, but 70 per cent of all other surviving children, have intelligence quotients higher than 80. The shunt revision rate in children with slit ventricles has been twice that of the other groups combined.

INFECTION

In Laurence's study, intracranial infection was the most common cause of death.[24] Analysis of that study reveals that most children became infected by way of the unrepaired myelomeningocele. In the author's experience, the incidence of ventriculitis is affected by the speed with which the myelomeningocele is repaired: it has been 7 per cent in those repaired within 48 hours of birth and 37 per cent in those repaired after 48 hours.[36] However, some studies have not shown any increase in neurological defects caused by delay in closing the back, although delay did cause a significant increase in the mortality rate.[6]

Since it has become routine practice to close the myelomeningocele within 48 hours and to use antibiotics to control infection, the incidence of infection of the central nervous system has declined. The overall incidence of shunt infection in the first group of 100 patients in the author's series was 12 per cent at 8 to 12 years of follow-up.[36]

INTELLIGENCE QUOTIENT

In Laurence's study, half the children who survived with moderate to severe hydrocephalus had intelligence quotients higher than 85.[24] Several children were well above average. In the past decade, a number of studies have reported a significant reduction in the quotient in cases in which the myelomeningocele was associated with hydrocephalus severe enough to require a shunt. Soare and Raimondi evaluated 173 unselected children with myelomeningocele.[61] The mean intelligence quotient of those with myelomeningocele alone was 102. The mean level of children with myelomeningocele and hydrocephalus was 87, a significant difference. Put differently, 97 per cent of those with myelomeningocele alone had quotients higher than 80, whereas only 63 per cent of those with myelomeningocele and hydrocephalus were above 80. Allowing for the heterogeneity of patient populations, differences in treatment regimens, and variations in the tests used to evaluate intelligence quotient, the intelligence level can be expected from these results to be significantly lower if the myelomeningocele is associated with hydrocephalus. However, infection was an uncontrolled variable that may have affected the findings.

In 1974, Hunt and Holmes reported that infection of the central nervous system dramatically lowered the intelligence quotients of patients with shunts and hydrocephalus compared with those of patients who required no shunt or who remained infection-free despite shunting.[21] Therefore, the author and his associates made a complete survey of 167 of the original 173 patients in the Soare-Raimondi study to determine the age at onset and the duration of any infection, the causative organism, and the severity of the process as judged by protein level, glucose level, and cell count in the cerebrospinal fluid.[35] The patients were separated into three groups: (1) those without shunts, (2) those with shunts without infection, and (3) those with shunts with infection. Only patients with shunts suffered infection of the central nervous system. As previously reported, the mean intelligence quotient of those not requiring a shunt was 102.[35] The mean quotient of those patients who did receive shunts but remained free of infection was 95. This level is not significantly different from that of the group without shunts. Those children who received shunts and then developed an infection had a mean intelligence quotient of only 73, which is significantly different from the results in the other two groups. Put another way, of those who did not require a shunt, 87 per cent had intelligence quotients higher than 80, whereas, of those with shunts who developed infections of the central nervous system, only 31 per cent had quotients higher than 80. The data therefore indicate that hydrocephalus alone is not a significant limiting factor in the ultimate intellectual growth of the child, but infection of the central nervous system is. Control of shunt infection must be a major concern for all physicians treating patients with myelomeningocele.

In the author's series, children from the first and second groups of 100 are now old enough for reliable intelligence testing. A total of 73 per cent of the survivors of the first group have intelligence quotients higher than 80.[36] In comparison, 80 per cent of survivors in Lorber's series of selected patients showed quotients higher than 80, a significant difference.[26] However, it is essential to take into account the difference in mortality rates between the two series. In Lorber's series, only 29 of 100 children survived with quotients higher than 80, whereas, in the author's series, 62 of 100 children survived with levels higher than 80—more than twice as many. Expressed another way, application of Lorber's selection criteria meant that for every surviving child with an intelligence quotient higher than 80, one child with a potential to be above 80 was left untreated and subsequently died.

Intelligence quotient is not the sole predictor of performance. Studies have demonstrated that as many as one half of children with myelomeningocele have some learning disability.[1] The severity of the learning disabil-

ity in the author's first two groups has yet to be determined. Some evidence indicates that most of the children have attention deficit disorders and that many respond to Ritalin, with marked improvement in school performance, especially in the area of mathematics.

The impact of the shunt procedure and subsequent control of hydrocephalus on the child's ultimate intelligence is difficult to determine. Laurence's paper shows that half of survivors with untreated, moderate to severe hydrocephalus have average or above-average intelligence.[24] Treatment of the hydrocephalus increases patient survival, protects vision, and may preserve intelligence in the remaining half of children who are destined to be retarded. The results suggest that it is more important to prevent progression of the hydrocephalus than to achieve a specific ventricular size. It is also evident that complications of the shunt procedure inflict retardation on a number of children. Shunt infection can reduce intelligence. Early aggressive shunting can produce slit ventricles and create difficulty in maintaining a functioning shunt in this population. Alternatively, delay in shunting until after the cranial sutures close and the intracranial volume becomes fixed increases the risk of subdural hematoma after shunting.

Routine assessment of the child's intellectual function is valuable not only in projecting future competitiveness but also as a baseline for shunt function. The author has seen a number of children with subtle shunt malfunctions that were discovered on medical psychological evaluation.

URINARY CONTINENCE

Before 1975, many children with myelomeningocele underwent a series of urinary diversion procedures in an effort to minimize the loss of renal function from infection.[23] The consequences of these procedures and the odor of urine made these children social pariahs. Since 1975, introduction of clean intermittent catheterization and advanced pharmacotherapy has permitted these children to develop "social" continence of urine.[23] That is, they can avoid incontinence in social situations and can behave like other children by maintaining a schedule of self-catheterization (or parent-performed catheterization) in the bathroom. These children do not have normal neuromuscular control of urination, but they can have normal social behavior.

In the author's series, almost 85 per cent of the 6- to 10-year-old population have been able to achieve such social continence of urine.[36] By adolescence, 75 per cent of the young adults have been able to perform their own catheterization program. Many of these children have a chronic low-grade cystitis, and the long-term effect of this infection on bladder mucosa is worrisome.[34] Urinary diversions are now rare. More than 100 patients from our total clinic population have undergone reimplantation procedures ("undiversions") during the last 10 years. A small number of selected children have been treated with artificial sphincters. As a result, these children no longer exude the objectionable order of urine. They are accepted by their peers, and they are placed in regular schools in the mainstream of education.

MOTOR AND SENSORY FUNCTION

Most children with myelomeningocele are born with a neurological deficit. In the author's series, 37 per cent of patients with myelomeningocele showed significant motor recovery shortly after surgical closure of the back. This motor improvement provided active function across a joint that was previously nonfunctional and persisted throughout the follow-up period. In the author's experience, delay in closing the myelomeningocele of more than 72 hours after birth decreases motor function in a small percentage of children. Other studies have not documented any increase in the degree of neurological deficit in patients who survive delayed closure.[28]

COMMUNITY AMBULATION AND SCHOOLING

Patients are designated community ambulators if they can move about the community without resorting to wheelchairs. Because of their motor deficits, many patients require reciprocal braces, canes, and walkers to assist them in maintaining the erect posture necessary for becoming community ambulators. However, as these children become older, the increase in their body weight may exceed the increase in their motor strength, leading to greater difficulties in walking. Many ultimately become wheelchair-bound.

As adults, most myelomeningocele patients with thoracic-level function require the use of wheelchairs to be mobile. In spite of this, the author does not agree with placing these children into a wheelchair immediately. Rather, they are started in the erect position and then "graduated" into wheelchairs if necessary. Electing to use a wheelchair must not be seen as failure. Rather, the children choose to use the wheelchair in order to conserve energy for other activities of daily living. That these patients are able to move about the community and accomplish their business is socially more important than whether they do so by brace or by wheelchair.

Complete ambulation data are available on 80 of 85 survivors from the first group of 100 patients with myelomeningocele. Ambulation was precluded in 13 children with severe central nervous system involvement in the form of significant mental retardation, hypotonia, or both. These children are unlikely to be competitive and independent. In the children without such severe involvement, the community ambulation rate is 89 per cent after 8 to 12 years of follow-up. This community ambulation group represents 75 per cent of all surviving children and 60 per cent of the original group of 100. Community ambulation was achieved by 100 per cent of those patients with sacral and lower lumbar myelomeningoceles and by 63 per cent of those

with higher lesions. Use of the reciprocating brace has markedly increased the number of children with thoracic-level function who ambulate. However, after 13 to 17 years of follow-up, the ambulation rate has fallen to 53 per cent. This decrease was expected and, again, is not regarded as failure. It is certainly more energy-efficient to use a wheelchair as the child without motor function below the waist grows into a young adult.

COMPETITIVE INDIVIDUALS

Children with intelligence quotients of 80 or higher will probably be able to compete successfully in society as adults and can become self-supporting citizens. Individuals with quotients lower than 70 are unlikely to be competitive. The author's data indicate that approximately 10 per cent of unselected children with a myelomeningocele will be unable to function independently as adults.[34] Mental retardation, hindbrain dysfunction, and hypotonia are the most common causes of inability to function independently.

Attempts to assess the independence of the adult patient population have only now been undertaken. Of 71 adult patients living in the Chicago area, 80 per cent live with relatives, but 82 per cent are independent in activities of daily living. Thirty per cent are attending or have finished college, but only 32 per cent are employed full-time. Preliminary returns from a national questionnaire show high rates of employment and ambulation.[10] However, in this preliminary data, only one third of those responding had hydrocephalus. This skewing reflects the fact that, in the past, the least affected individuals survived best. Those individuals with the most severe problems have died or have been lost to follow-up.

Late Complications

It was long assumed that gradual deterioration in neurological function was the natural history for children with myelomeningocele. This assumption has been proved wrong. It is now clear that neurological deterioration should not occur, at least into adulthood, provided that late complications of myelomeningocele are sought and treated diligently.

It is too soon to state with certainty what the outcome will be for children treated now, because it will take further observations to determine the long-term effects of such things as clean intermittent catheterization on the urethral mucosa, the effects of repeated trauma to joints that lack sensation, and the life expectancy of a patient with a shunt. The number of independent adults who have reached middle age is not sufficient to produce a clear picture of the probable outcome and complications that will be faced by the children treated now. However, the major late complications in patients with myelomeningocele include the Chiari II malformation, tethering by scarring of the spinal cord to the closure, and hydromyelia—all leading to scoliosis, spasticity, and loss of function.

CHIARI II MALFORMATION

In a few patients, the hindbrain dysfunction associated with the Chiari II malformation (Fig. 33–13) continues to present problems through childhood and into adolescence and early adulthood.[12, 18, 22, 53] Pain at the base of the skull and neck posteriorly, nystagmus, weakness in the upper extremities, lower cranial nerve symptoms, and hypotonia or spasticity are common features of this problem. Early recognition and treatment can preserve function and occasionally can prevent sudden death.[63] Posterior cervical decompression is much more likely to be effective in correcting symptoms in this age group than in newborns.

Late progressive scoliosis and spasticity insidiously rob a number of children of function. This scoliosis develops proximal to the level of the myelomeningocele and is not associated with vertebral anomalies. The role that the Chiari II malformation and cervical compression plays in this late deterioration is not clear. Hall and colleagues demonstrated that the central canal communicates with the ventricular system in hydromyelia, and they advocated the establishment of a functioning ventricular shunt to manage the hydromyelia.[15, 16] A shunt malfunction is the first problem to be ruled out, and this evaluation certainly must be done before cervical decompression is attempted. Resolution of the neurological deterioration with cervical decompressive laminectomy and plugging of the obex has been reported.[41, 53, 54] This procedure is based on the hydrodynamic theory proposed by Morgagni

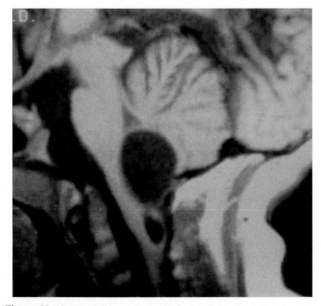

Figure 33–13

Magnetic resonance image of an adolescent with a Chiari II malformation and syringobulbia. The child's hindbrain symptoms markedly improved after cervical decompression and fenestration of the cyst.

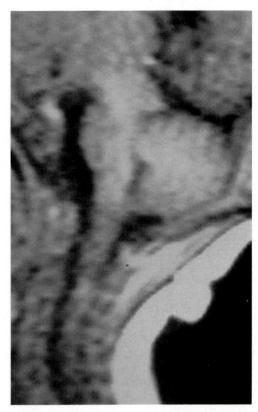

Figure 33–14

The figure shows a magnetic resonance image of an infant with apnea. Notice the minimal findings of a Chiari II malformation; this was confirmed at surgery. The child remained apneic after decompression.

and modified by Gardner.[14, 42, 53] In Park's series, the condition of 8 of 12 children improved after cervical decompression and plugging of the obex, and the condition of the other 4 remained unchanged.[54]

Although Park stated that "hydromyelia and compression of the brain stem are solely or concurrently responsible,"[53] and Hoffman felt that "although investigations . . . will show the malformation, they are not essential" and that "myelography is unnecessary because all of these infants have the malformation,"[18] magnetic resonance imaging findings may not correlate well with the clinical manifestations. Many children with progressive scoliosis, spasticity, or both have little evidence of hindbrain compression and no hydromyelia. One unfortunate child in our series is quadriparetic and ventilator-dependent but has almost no evidence of a Chiari II malformation or hydromyelia (Fig. 33–14). The author also has seen segmental hydromyelia and syringomyelia and, occasionally, holocord hydromyelia in which the central canal does not appear to communicate with the ventricular system. In these cases, the origin of the fluid and the hydrodynamics of the lesion are difficult to explain.

If scoliosis fails to respond to a shunt revision, a cervical decompression may be performed if there is magnetic resonance imaging evidence of hindbrain compression and hydromyelia. The author's results have been mixed but best in children with evidence of hindbrain dysfunction, upper extremity involvement, or both.

HYDROMYELIA

Hydromyelia signifies dilatation of the central canal of the spinal cord (Fig. 33–15), just as hydrocephalus signifies dilatation of the ventricles of the brain. In patients with myelomeningocele, cerebrospinal fluid has been shown to pass from the ventricles to the central canal through the iter of the central canal at the level of the obex. Hydromyelia therefore may be the consequence of untreated or inadequately treated hydrocephalus.[15, 16]

The most common symptoms of hydromyelia are rapidly progressive scoliosis, weakness of the upper extremities, spasticity, and an ascending motor loss in the lower extremities. In patients with myelomeningocele, the incidence of hydromyelia has been reported to vary from 50 to 80 per cent.[5, 27] This wide variation probably reflects the degree to which hydrocephalus was controlled, the difficulty in making the diagnosis accurately before the availability of neuroimaging, and the diligence with which the diagnosis was sought. In the author's series, computed tomography and magnetic resonance imaging demonstrated the presence of hydromyelia in 40 per cent of the cases studied.

Several methods are available to investigate the

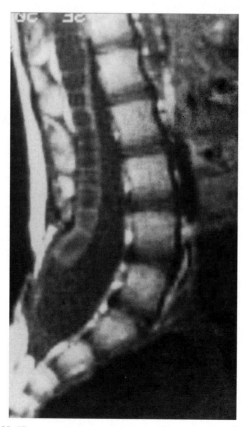

Figure 33–15

This magnetic resonance image shows severe hydromyelia and a tethered spinal cord.

causes of late deterioration of spinal cord function.[44, 45, 47–49] For the head, computed tomography scanning will probably be replaced by magnetic resonance imaging.[46] In patients with symptomatic hydromyelia, even if the head scan is unchanged from previous examinations, it must be determined that the shunt is actually working properly before other forms of therapy are undertaken. The author has had several cases in which the shunt was revised despite an unchanged computed tomography scan and which resulted in dramatic improvement or stabilization of the scoliotic curve.

Kyphoscoliosis has been reported to be present in 90 per cent of patients with myelomeningocele.[55, 60] It is most often progressive in patients with retethering of the cord by scar. Therefore, kyphoscoliosis should be viewed as a symptom of an underlying problem. Aggressive treatment of tethered cord and hydromyelia may be able to reduce the incidence of kyphoscoliosis to less than 20 per cent. Aggressive treatment of hydromyelia in children with a myelomeningocele who are experiencing the onset of scoliosis at levels rostral to the myelomeningocele may improve or stabilize the curve in 80 per cent of the patients.

If hydromyelia persists despite a functioning shunt, and if hindbrain compression is present by magnetic resonance imaging, posterior cervical decompression is indicated. The author prefers posterior cervical decompression to opening of the fourth ventricle. Venes and associates have advocated placing a catheter into the fourth ventricle at the time of decompression to bypass the central canal of the spinal cord; 10 of 14 patients showed improvement after this procedure.[67] If this procedure fails or in the absence of clinical or neuroimaging evidence of hindbrain compression, a shunt from the central canal to the pleural cavity may be placed with a flushing device over a rib.

In a child with a thoracic-level myelomeningocele, it is difficult to know whether the kyphosis is treatable and whether the progression of kyphosis can be arrested. Because the laminae are widely everted in spina bifida, the paraspinal muscles that develop along the laminae come to lie in an abnormal position lateral to—or even ventral to—the spinal canal. As a result, the spinal extensor muscles come to serve as spinal flexors. They no longer oppose the pull of the psoas but augment it. This abnormal, unstable relationship almost always leads to progressive "jack-knife" kyphosis requiring spinal fusion. Reigel has suggested that early kyphectomy and untethering of the spinal cord can slow or even arrest this process.[57]

RETETHERING OF THE SPINAL CORD

Limitation of movement of the distal end of the spinal cord can produce a variety of symptoms referable to deterioration of spinal cord function. This fixation, or tethering, of the end of the spinal cord allows intermittent "bow-stringing" of the spinal cord between the normal cephalic attachment and the point of the tether. Yamada and colleagues have supplied data that support the concept that the spinal cord stretches under tension, that the distal cord vasculature is attenuated by this stretching, and that the distal spinal cord consequently suffers intermittent ischemia that results in myelomalacia.[70] The author believes that the middle and upper levels of the spinal cord are compressed anteriorly against the apices of the curved vertebral column and deteriorate from chronic cord compression.

The most common symptoms of cord tethering in patients with myelomeningocele are subtle atrophy, pain, progressive orthopedic foot deformities, ascending motor loss, spasticity, and scoliosis.[19, 38, 57] Commonly, the pain radiates into the legs, especially with exercise. Pain, sensory loss, and motor loss usually do not follow dermatomal patterns. The children may exhibit lordosis and a bent-knee posture on standing.[57] In children previously doing well, hip dislocation may be the first sign of neurological deterioration. Bladder and bowel dysfunction or a change in catheterization pattern may signal an urgent situation requiring immediate attention.

In addition to these signs of cord tethering, patients with myelomeningocele often exhibit subtle changes in muscle tone, usually spasticity and functional muscle loss.[39] These changes are often insidious and can be picked up only by a scheduled routine of close follow-up observation. Routine muscle function examinations have proved very useful for early detection of this problem. Other investigators have reported that routine testing of somatosensory evoked potentials reliably detects early spinal cord deterioration.[57]

The incidence of retethering is probably related to the type of initial repair that is performed. Tight closure that restricts the underlying neural elements is a serious hazard to the child, because of the risks of immediate ischemic cord damage and later retethering of the spinal cord. Loose, or patulous, closure provides a generous fluid compartment in which the spinal cord may float away from the surgical scar. In addition, if it is possible to roll the neural placode into a tube by use of pia-to-pia suturing, one can sequester the raw tissue of the neural placode deep to the glistening pia of the "remade" cord and reduce the raw surface most likely to scar to a vertical mid-dorsal suture line (Fig. 33–16). Both factors help reduce the incidence of rescarring.[59]

Of 153 patients with retethering of the cord, 38 per cent had associated hydromyelia, and 16 per cent had an inclusion dermoid tumor, or epidermoid tumor. Fifty per cent of the children presented with progressive scoliosis; 51 per cent had motor loss; 40 per cent had spasticity.[17] Pain was the principal symptom in two children. After release, 53 per cent had improvement in their scoliosis, 14 per cent were stable, and 33 per cent progressed (Fig. 33–17).[17] Sixty-four per cent had improvement, or decrease, in their spasticity, whereas 36 per cent remained stable. Bladder and bowel function improved in 25 per cent, and pain was relieved in 100 per cent of the patients. Motor improvement was noted in 57 per cent; however, the condition of three children worsened. One of these children was significantly weaker in his legs after release but had a marked improvement in his scoliosis.

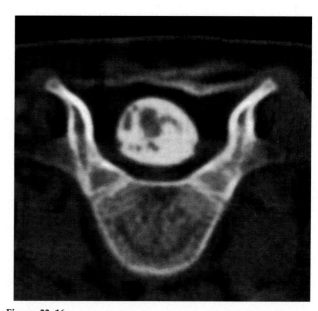

Figure 33–16

A computed tomography myelogram demonstrates the reconstructed neural tube floating in spinal fluid. Notice the widely everted lamina.

OTHER CAUSES

A shunt malfunction often is the cause of hydromyelia or hindbrain compression. The author has seen several children with progressive weakness of the lower extremities who recovered after a shunt revision. Subtle shunt malfunction can mimic any of the conditions and cause all the signs of deterioration mentioned previously. Therefore, it is essential to establish first that the shunt is functioning properly. Other treatable causes of late deterioration in neurological function include syringobulbia, inclusion dermoid tumors or epidermoid tumors (Fig. 33–18), arachnoid cysts (Fig. 33–19), undetected thick filum terminale, and diastematomyelia.

Syringobulbia presents clinically in the same manner as late manifestations of the Chiari II malformation. Although syringobulbia has not been reported in other series,[5, 59] the author has seen three cases. Magnetic resonance imaging demonstrates the lesion well (see Fig. 33–13), and intraoperative ultrasound localizes the cavity within the brain stem.[59] Syringobulbia has been managed with laser fenestration and by placing a small tube from the cavity to the subarachnoid space. Dramatic, almost immediate, improvement has occurred in the children managed by this method.

Arachnoid cysts produce symptoms very similar to those of a tethered cord. Magnetic resonance imaging is less effective in identifying the lesion than is the minimyelogram. After the cyst has been identified, its outer membrane is totally or partially removed, and the cavity is communicated with the subarachnoid space (see Fig. 33–19*A*, *B*).

Diastematomyelia and a thick filum terminale are the result of incomplete evaluation of the child at the time of the initial repair of the myelomeningocele. Again, the symptoms are those of a tethered cord. Plain

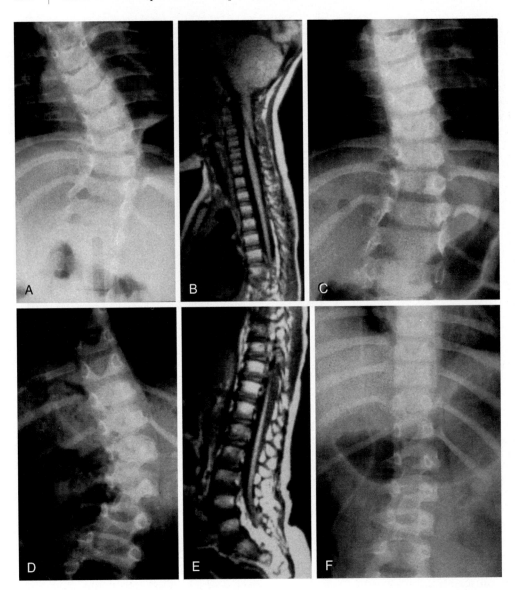

Figure 33–17
Composite spine films of two children with scoliosis and tethered cord. *A and D.* Preoperative views. *C and F.* Postoperative views. *B and E.* Magnetic resonance images show the absence of hydromyelia. Notice the postoperative improvement in the curve.

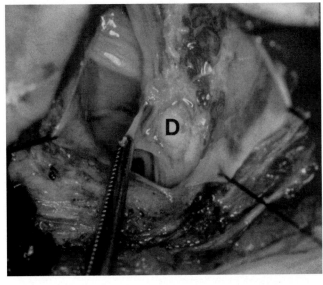

Figure 33–18
An operative photograph of an inclusion dermoid (D) which was found and removed at the time of untethering of the spinal cord.

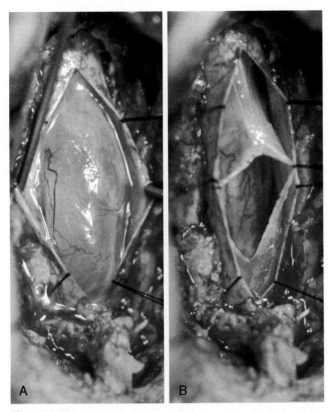

Figure 33–19

A. An arachnoid cyst posterior to the thoracic spinal cord is shown. *B.* After the arachnoid cyst was opened, the flattened spinal cord was seen anteriorly.

spine radiography usually suggests the presence of a diastematomyelia. Computed tomography with myelography or magnetic resonance imaging should delineate both of these problems.[49] The treatment is the same as in either of these lesions in the absence of a myelomeningocele. In addition, it is usually necessary to untether the distal spinal cord at the closure site.

The signs and symptoms of an inclusion dermoid tumor or epidermoid tumor are difficult to separate from those of a tethered cord because the two are almost invariable associated.

A not infrequent problem is that neither the Chiari II malformation nor a tethered cord can be excluded—or both are contributing to the problem. In these cases, the author has performed cervical decompressions and untethered the spinal cord during the same operation. If the child's condition precludes a double procedure, a cervical decompression is done first.

In summary, late deterioration is not uncommon in children with myelodysplasia. Most, possibly all, of this deterioration is preventable or correctable; it is not simply the natural history of this disease. Regularly scheduled evaluations of intellectual, musculoskeletal, and urinary systems are essential. If the observer is familiar with the signs and the symptoms of the various causes of deterioration and utilizes ultrasound, myelography, and neuroimaging techniques, the most probable cause can be identified, and a treatment plan can be outlined.

REFERENCES

1. Agnes, P., and McLone, D. G.: Learning disabilities in children with a myelomeningocele. Personal communication, 1987.
2. Ames, M., and Schut, L.: Diagnosis and treatment: Results of treatment of 171 consecutive myelomeningoceles—1962 to 1968. Pediatrics, 50:466, 1972.
3. Barson, A. J.: The vertebral level of termination of the spinal cord during normal and abnormal development. J. Anat. 106:489, 1970.
4. Caldarelli, M., Di Rocco, E., and McLone, D. G.: Chiari II malformation: Clinical manifestations and indications for decompression. In McLaurin, R., ed.: Proceedings of the Second Symposium on Spina Bifida. New York, Praeger Publishing, 1986, pp. 174–181.
5. Cameron, A. H.: The Arnold-Chiari and other neuro-anatomical malformations associated with spina bifida. J. Pathol. Bacteriol. 73:195, 1957.
6. Charney, E., Weller, S. C., Sutton, L. N., et al.: Management of the newborn with myelomeningocele: Time for a decision-making process. Pediatrics, 75:58, 1985.
7. Dandy, W. E.: Extirpation of the choroid plexus of the lateral ventricles in communicating hydrocephalus. Ann. Surg., 68:569, 1918.
8. Dandy, W. E., and Blackfan, K. D.: International hydrocephalus: An experimental, clinical and pathological study. Am. J. Dis. Child., 8:406, 1914.
9. DeRuysch, F., and Morgagni, G. B.: Considerations generales et observations particulaires sur le spina bifida. J. Med., 27:162, 1806.
10. Dias, L.: Personal communication.
11. Emery, J. L., and Lendon, R. G.: The local cord lesion in neurospinal dysraphism (meningomyelocele). J. Pathol., 110:83, 1973.
12. Fernbach, S. K., and McLone, D. G.: Derangement of swallowing in children with myelomeningocele. Pediatr. Radiol., 15:311, 1985.
13. Gardner, W. J.: Myelomeningocele, the result of rupture of the embryonic neural tube. Cleve. Clin. Q., 27:88, 1960.
14. Gardner, W. J.: Hydrodynamic mechanisms of syringomyelia: Its relationship to myelocele. J. Neurol. Neurosurg. Psychiatry, 28:247, 1965.
15. Hall, P. V., Campbell, R. L., and Kalsbeck, J. E.: Meningomyelocele and progressive hydromyelia: Progressive paresia in myelodysplasia. J. Neurosurg., 43:457, 1975.
16. Hall, P. V., Lindseth, R. E., Campbell, R. L., et al.: Myelodysplasia and developmental scoliosis: A manifestation of syringomyelia. Spine, 1:48, 1956.
17. Herman, J. M., McLone, D. G., Storrs, B. B., et al.: Analysis of 153 patients with myelomeningocele or spinal lipoma reoperated upon for a tethered cord. Pediatr. Neurosurg., 19:243–249, 1993.
18. Hoffman, H. J., Hendrick, E. B., and Humphreys, R. P.: Manifestations and management of Arnold-Chiari malformations in patients with myelomeningocele. Child's Brain, 1:255, 1975.
19. Hoffman, H. J., Hendrick, E. B., and Humphreys, R. P.: The tethered spinal cord: Its protean manifestations, diagnosis and surgical correction. Child's Brain, 2:145, 1976.
20. Hoffman, H. J., Park, T. S., Hendrick, E. B., et al.: Manifestazioni e trattamento della malformazione di Arnold-Chiari nel bambino con mielomeningocele. In DiRocco, M., and Caldarelli, M., eds.: Mielomeningocele. Rome, Casa del Libro Editrice, 1983, pp. 251–260.
21. Hunt, G. M., and Holmes, A. E.: Some factors relating to intelligence in treated hydrocephalic children. Am. J. Dis. Child., 127:664, 1974.
22. Ishak, B., McLone, D. G., and Seleny, F.: Autonomic dysfunction associated with Arnold-Chiari malformation. Child's Brain, 7:146, 1981.
23. Kaplan, W. E.: Management of the urinary tract in myelomeningocele. Probl. Urology, 2:121–131, 1988.
24. Laurence, K. M.: The natural history of spina bifida cystica: Detailed analysis of 407 cases. Arch. Dis. Child., 39:41, 1964.
25. Lorber, J.: Results of treatment of myelomeningocele: An analysis of 524 unselected cases, with special reference to possible selection for treatment. Dev. Med. Child Neurol., 13:279, 1971.
26. Lorber, J., and Salfield, S.: Results of selective treatment of spina bifida cystica. Arch. Dis. Child., 56:822, 1981.

27. MacKenzie, N. G., and Emery, J. L.: Deformities of the cervical cord in children with neurospinal dysraphism. Dev. Med. Child Neurol., 13:58, 1972.

28. McLone, D. G.: Technique for closure of myelomeningocele. Child's Brain, 6:67, 1980.

29. McLone, D. G.: Results of treatment of children born with a myelomeningocele. Clin. Neurosurg., 30:407, 1983.

30. McLone, D. G.: The handicapped newborn: Diagnosis, prognosis and outcome—the neonatal view. Issues Law Med., 1:15-24, 1986.

31. McLone, D. G.: Arguments against selection. Clin. Neurosurg., 34:359, 1986.

32. McLone, D. G.: Treatment of myelomeningocele: Arguments against selection. In Little, J. R., ed.: Clinical Neurosurgery. Vol. 33. Baltimore, Williams & Wilkins, 1986, pp. 359–370.

33. McLone, D. G.: Spina bifida today: Problems adults face. Semin. Neurol., 9:169, 1989.

34. McLone, D. G.: Continuing concepts in the management of spina bifida. Pediatr. Neurosurg., 18:254, 1992.

35. McLone, D. G., Czyzewski, D., Raimondi, A., et al.: Central nervous system infections as a limiting factor in the intelligence of children with myelomeningocele. Pediatrics, 70:338, 1982.

36. McLone, D. G., Dias, L., Kaplan, W. E., et al.: Concepts in the management of spina bifida. In Humphreys, R. P., ed.: Concepts in Pediatric Neurosurgery. 5th ed. Basel, S. Karger, 1985, pp. 14–28.

37. McLone, D. G., and Knepper, P. A.: On the role of complex carbohydrates and neurulation. Pediatr. Neurosurg., 12:2, 1986.

38. McLone, D. G., and Naidich, T. P.: Spinal dysraphism: Experimental and clinical. In Holtzman, R. N. N., and Stein, B. M., eds.: The Tethered Spine. New York, Thieme-Stratton, 1985, pp. 14–28.

39. McLone, D. G., and Naidich, T. P.: Myelodysplasia and tethered spinal cord. In Tachdjian, M. O., ed.: Pediatric Orthopedics. New York, Praeger Publishing, 1986, pp. 164–173.

40. McLone, D. G., and Naidich, T. P.: Myelomeningocele: Outcome and late complications. In McLaurin, R. L., Schut, L., Venes, J., et al., eds.: Pediatric Neurosurgery, Philadelphia, W. B. Saunders, 1989, pp. 53–70.

41. Milhorat, T. H.: Hydrocephalus: Historical notes, etiology and clinical diagnosis. In McLaurin, R. L., ed.: Pediatric Neurosurgery. New York, Grune & Stratton, 1982, p. 200.

42. Morgagni, G. B.: The Seats and Causes of Disease Investigated by Anatomy. London, R. Miller & J. Cadell, 1969.

43. Morton, M.: Spina bifida aperta: Treatment by injection. Br. Med. J. 1:381, 1875.

44. Naidich, T. P., Harwood-Nash, D. C., and McLone, D. G.: Radiology of spinal dysraphism. Clin. Neurosurg., 30:341, 1983.

45. Naidich, T. P., Maravilla, K., and McLone, D. G.: The Chiari II malformation. In McLaurin, R. L., ed.: Proceedings of the Second Symposium on Spina Bifida. New York, Praeger Publishing, 1986, pp. 164–173.

46. Naidich, T. P., and McLone, D. G.: The investigation of hydrocephalus by computed tomography. In Little, J. R., ed.: Clinical Neurosurgery. Baltimore, Williams & Wilkins, 1984, pp. 527–539.

47. Naidich, T. P., and McLone, D. G.: Myelocele and myelomeningocele. In McLaurin, R. L., ed.: Proceedings of the Second Symposium on Spina Bifida. New York, Praeger Publishing, 1986, pp. 119–128.

48. Naidich, T. P., McLone, D. G., and Fulling, K. H.: The Chiari II malformation: Part 4. The hindbrain deformity. Neuroradiology, 25:179, 1983.

49. Naidich, T. P., McLone, D. G., and Harwood-Nash, D.: Dysraphism. In Newton, T. H., and Potts, D. G., eds.: Modern Neuroradiology. Vol. 1. Computed Tomography of the Spine and Spinal Cord. San Francisco/New York, Clavadel Press, 1982, pp. 299–355.

50. Nulsen, F. E., and Spitz, E. B.: Treatment of hydrocephalus by direct heart shunt from ventricle to jugular vein. Surg. Forum, 2:399, 1952.

51. Osaka, K., Matsumoto, S., and Tanimura, T.: Myeloschisis in early human embryos. Child's Brain, 4:347, 1978.

52. Padget, D. H.: Spina bifida and embryonic neuroschisis—a causal relationship: Definition of postnatal confirmations of a bifid spine. Johns Hopkins Med. J., 128:233, 1968.

53. Park, T. S., Cail, W. S., Maggio, W. M., et al.: Progressive spasticity and scoliosis in children with myelomeningocele. J. Neurosurg., 62:367, 1985.

54. Park, T. S., Hoffman, H. J., Hendrick, E. B., et al.: Experience with surgical decompression of the Arnold-Chiari malformation in young infants with myelomeningocele. Neurosurgery, 12:147, 1983.

55. Piggott, H.: The natural history of scoliosis in myelodysplasia. J. Bone Joint. Surg. Br., 62:54, 1980.

56. Pollack, I. F., Pang, D., Albright, A. L., et al.: Outcome following hindbrain decompression of symptomatic Chiari malformations in children previously treated with myelomeningocele closure and shunts. J. Neurosurg., 77:881, 1992.

57. Reigel, D. H.: Tethered spinal cord. In Humphreys, R. P., ed.: Concepts in Pediatric Neurosurgery. Vol. 4. Basel, S. Karger, 1983, pp. 142–164.

58. Reigel, D. H., and McLone, D. G.: Myelomeningocele: Operative treatment and results. In Marlin, A. E., ed.: Concepts in Pediatric Neurosurgery. Vol. 8. Basel, S. Karger, 1988, pp. 41–50.

59. Reigel, D. H., and McLone, D. G.: Spina bifida. In Mustarde, J. C., and Jackson, I. T., eds.: Plastic Surgery in Infancy and Childhood. London, Churchill Livingston, 1988, pp. 477–485.

60. Shurtleff, D. B., Goiney, R., Gordon, L. H., et al.: Myelodysplasia: The natural history of kyphosis and scoliosis. A preliminary report. Dev. Med. Child Neurol., 18:126, 1976.

61. Soare, P. L., and Raimondi, A. J.: Intellectual and perceptual motor characteristics of treated myelomeningocele children. Am. J. Dis. Child., 131:199, 1977.

62. Storrs, B. B., and McLone, D. G.: Ventricular size and intelligence in myelodysplastic children. In Marlin, A. E., ed.: Concepts in Pediatric Neurosurgery. Vol. 8. Basel, S. Karger, 1988, pp. 51–66.

63. Tomita, T., and McLone, D. G.: Acute respiratory arrest: A complication of malfunction of the shunt in children with myelomeningocele and Arnold-Chiari malformation: A report of three cases. Am. J. Dis. Child., 137:142, 1983.

64. Trowbridge, A.: Three cases of spina bifida, successfully treated. Boston Med. Surg. J., 1:753, 1828.

65. Tulpius, N.: Obs Med Lib III Cap XXIX XXX 1641:229

66. Vandertop, W. P., Apio, A., Hoffman, H. J., et al.: Surgical decompression for symptomatic Chiari II malformation in neonates with myelomeningocele. J. Neurosurg., 77:541–544, 1992.

67. Venes, J. L., Black, K. L., and Latack, J. T.: Preoperative evaluation and surgical management of the Arnold-Chiari II malformation. J. Neurosurg., 64:363, 1986.

68. Vesalius, A.: DeCorporis Humani Fabrica. Basileau, Joannis Oporini, 1543.

69. Warkany, J., Wilson, J. G., and Geiger, J. F.: Myeloschisis and myelomeningocele produced experimentally in the rat. J. Comp. Neurol., 109:34, 1958.

70. Yamada, S., Schreider, S., Ashwal, S., et al.: Pathophysiologic mechanisms in the tethered spinal cord syndrome. In Holtzman, R. N. N., and Stein, B. M., eds.: The Tethered Spine. New York, Thieme-Stratton, Inc., 1985.

CHAPTER 34

Lipomyelomeningocele and Myelocystocele

Within the spectrum of spinal dysraphism are many skin-covered malformations associated with spina bifida occulta. Occurring once in each 4,000 births, lipomyelomeningocele is a subcutaneous lipoma of the lumbosacral region connected by a fibrous stalk traversing a bone defect to an intradural and intramedullary, fatty mass. At most medical centers, lipomyelomeningocele is the most common malformation leading to spinal cord tethering; the frequency ranges from 8 to 25 per cent of myelomeningoceles.[4, 16, 42] Myelocystocele is a rare lesion characterized by a cystic terminal dilatation of the central spinal canal into a meningocele. Either lesion may be suspected on physical examination, and the patient is usually neurologically intact at birth. Magnetic resonance imaging facilitates diagnosis of these lesions because it provides multiplanar visualization and greater sensitivity to associated malformations than does contrast-enhanced computed tomography.

The repair techniques for these malformations are based on embryonic development and anatomy. Surgical repair is recommended at the time of diagnosis because spinal cord tethering, with sudden or progressive neurological deterioration, is possible at any age. The optimal management of children with either malformation requires close cooperation between the pediatric neurosurgeon and the specialists involved with treating congenital defects. This chapter reviews the embryology, clinical presentation, radiology, and surgical management of lipomyelomeningoceles and myelocystoceles.

Embryology

Three complex and dynamic migrations of embryonic tissue initiate central nervous system development.[21] From gestational days 18 through 27, the neural tube is formed by *primary neurulation*. Closure of the neural groove begins in the future hindbrain region and progresses to close, first, the rostral neuropore and then the caudal neuropore, which later corresponds to the S2 level of the spinal cord. There is tight adherence between the superficial cutaneous ectoderm and neuroectoderm until neural tube closure is complete. During dysjunction, these two layers separate, allowing dorsolateral migration of mesoderm. Caudal to the posterior neuropore, beneath intact cutaneous ectoderm, is the primitive streak cell mass that extends into the embryonic tail fold. The primitive streak lies in close proximity to the developing hindgut and mesonephros. During *secondary neurulation*, or *canalization*, this cell mass acquires neuronal features and fuses with the more rostral neural tube. *Regression* of the caudal cell mass begins before canalization is complete. The distal neural lumen involutes and narrows, forming the filum terminale and the cauda equina.

Lipomyelomeningocele formation may reflect focal premature dysjunction.[27] Focal separation of neural ectoderm from cutaneous ectoderm allows migration of periaxial mesoderm into the developing neural tube, leading to dorsal lipomyeloschisis. Intramedullary fat remains continuous with subcutaneous adipose tissue along a fibrous stalk. The mesoderm primarily matures as fat, although tissues of mixed embryonic origin may be found within lipomyelomeningoceles, including bone, cartilage, blood vessels, renal epithelium, and gastric mucosa.[1, 7, 45] The role of energy transfer among membrane-bound glycosaminoglycans in premature dysjunction has been investigated by McLone and associates.[25, 26]

Myelocystocele formation probably reflects interruption of secondary neurulation and regression. These processes involve changes within the caudal cell mass during the fourth and fifth weeks of gestation. Simultaneously with distal neural development, the hindgut, cloacal membrane, and primitive perineum are formed.

P. M. Kanev • M. S. Berger

The caudal cell mass and the developing genitourinary system are closely approximated, and myelocystocele is frequently associated with cloacal exstrophy and anal stenosis.[18-20]

McLone and Naidich have speculated that distorted circulation of the cerebrospinal fluid within the distal neural tube forces terminal ventricle dilation.[23] A trumpet-like conus distorts the dorsal mesenchyme, resulting in spina bifida and formation of meningocele. Terminal cord enlargement allows contact of the distended conus with subcutaneous adipose tissue and impairs cephalad cord migration, leading to tethering.

Clinical Presentation

A midline or eccentric lumbosacral soft tissue mass is present in almost all newborn children with lipomyelomeningocele. The intergluteal fold is commonly obscured and distorted by a myelocystocele, but it is preserved with a lipomyelomeningocele (Fig. 34–1). Cutaneous defects can include meningocele manqué, dimples, and hemangiomas (Table 34–1); anal stenosis and other genitourinary malformations are common (Table 34–2). Cloacal or bladder exstrophy is associated with many myelocystoceles. Among 571 patients reported with lipomyelomeningocele, the overall female-to-male predominance was 1.33 to 1.[2, 10-13, 16, 37]

Scoliosis, varus or valgus foot deformities, and muscle mass asymmetry may be detected on clinical examination, and associated spinal malformations may include sacral dysgenesis (see Table 34–2). Most children have intact neurological function at birth; orthopedic deformities, motor or sensory deficits, and bladder paralysis are progressive with increasing patient age (Fig. 34–2). Asymmetrical weakness with patchy sensory loss is a common presentation accompanying both lipomyelomeningocele and myelocystocele. Detection of bladder paralysis in children younger than 2 to 3 years of age is unreliable except by urodynamics, ultrasound examination, and dynamic, contrast-enhanced studies of bladder emptying.[2] Forty-two per cent of 197 patients with lipomyelomeningocele cared for at Children's Memorial Hospital in Chicago were found to have a neurogenic bladder on presentation.[12] Foster and colleagues recorded abnormal urodynamic studies in 42 per cent of 12 patients younger than 18 months of age with lipomyelomeningocele. Despite normal voiding patterns, cystometrography confirmed flaccid bladder musculature in six of these patients and normal function in five.[8] Nineteen patients older than 18 months of age were studied by this group, and only four had normal bladder function. In another series of patients reported by Atala and colleagues, abnormal urodynamics were recorded in each of six older patients with lipomyelomeningocele.[2] Paralysis of bowel and bladder is complete when motor or sensory deficits are detected on neurological examination.[2, 16]

Older patients present with tethered spinal cord symptoms that include pain, scoliosis, gait and posture deformity, and progressive neurogenic bladder. Low

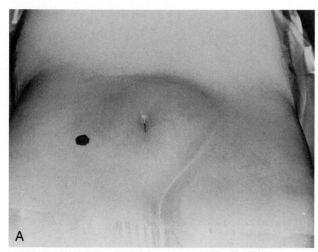
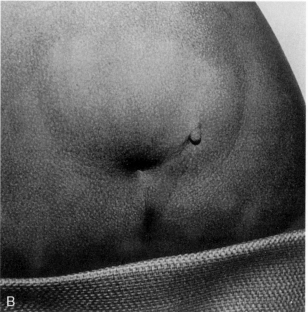

Figure 34–1

A. Infant with a lumbosacral lipomyelomeningocele. The intergluteal crease is preserved, and there is a small hemangioma and skin dimple. *B.* Infant with a sacral myelocystocele and associated skin tag and dimple obscuring the intergluteal fold.

back and radicular pain have been described, and Lhermitte's sign has occurred during sexual intercourse, jogging, labor and delivery, gynecological examination, weight lifting, and local percussive impact on the lower spine.[42] Insidious loss and sudden deterioration of neurological function can occur at any age into adulthood.[22, 23, 37] The causes of neurological deterioration include stretching injury and vascular compromise of spinal cord tethering, compression from expansion of intramedullary lipoma with weight gain, and local trauma.

Radiological and Preoperative Studies

Conventional radiography of the lumbosacral spine almost always gives abnormal results. Plain films dem-

Table 34–1

CUTANEOUS MANIFESTATIONS AMONG 614 PATIENTS WITH LIPOMYELOMENINGOCELE

	Chicago (n = 197)	Toronto (n = 97)	Seattle (n = 80)	Paris (n = 73)	Philadelphia (n = 43)	Osaka (n = 38)	Boston (n = 35)	San Francisco (n = 31)	New York (n = 20)	Total (n = 614)
Soft tissue mass	108	97	80	60	31	32	35	25	18	486
Skin dimples	38	26	14	22		19	10	—	6	135
Hemangiomas	35	24	9	17	4	6	7	—	1	103
Hair patches	9	1	11	6	5	2	1	—	5	40
Skin tags	6	5	6	6	5	2	1	—	—	31
Atretic or denuded skin patches	7	1	—	2	—	8	—	—	—	18
Dermal sinus	9	—	—	5	—	—	—	—	—	14
Hyperpigmentation	7	—	—	—	—	—	—	—	7	14
Hypopigmentation	—	3	3	—	—	—	—	—	2	8

Data from Atala et al.,[2] Foster et al.,[8] Hakuba et al.,[10] Harrison et al.,[11] Harvey et al.,[12] Hoffman et al.,[13] Kanev et al.,[16] Pierre-Kahn et al.,[37] and Sutton et al.[43]

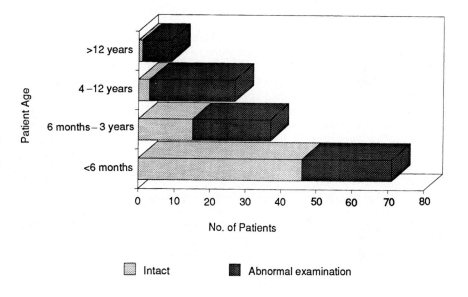

Figure 34–2

Preoperative neurological function in 144 children with lipomyelomeningocele as a function of patient age. (Data from references 13 and 16.)

Table 34–2

ASSOCIATED ANOMALIES AND MALFORMATIONS AMONG 578 PATIENTS WITH LIPOMYELOMENINGOCELE

	Chicago (n = 197)	Toronto (n = 97)	Seattle (n = 80)	Paris (n = 73)	Philadelphia (n = 43)	Osaka (n = 38)	San Francisco (n = 31)	New York (n = 20)	Total (n = 578)
Foot deformity	6	4	4	3	—	—	11	5	33
Scoliosis	12	1	7	—	—	—	1	—	21
Sacral dysgenesis	16	—	4	—	—	—	—	—	20
Hydromyelia	—	3	2	7	6	—	—	2	19
Anal displacement or stenosis	14	1	2	1	—	—	—	—	18
Leg length discrepancy	—	4	—	6	—	—	—	—	10
Skin ulceration	—	—	9	—	—	—	—	—	9
Diastematomyelia	—	3	1	1	1	1	—	—	7
Dermoid or epidermoid cyst	—	3	—	2	—	—	—	1	6
Cloacal exstrophy	—	—	—	—	5	—	—	—	5
Split spinal cord	—	3	—	—	—	1	—	—	1

Data from Atala et al.,[2] Hakuba et al.,[10] Harrison et al.,[11] Harvey et al.,[12] Hoffman et al.,[13] Kanev et al.,[16] Pierre-Kahn et al.,[37] and Sutton et al.[43]

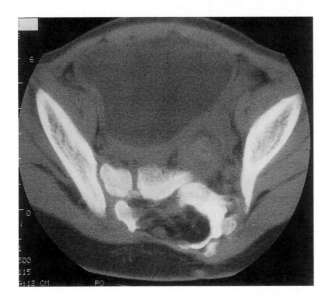

Figure 34–3

Axial metrizamide-enhanced computed tomography of a transitional lipomyelomeningocele in a 4-year-old female. There is an eccentric lobulated intradural mass and left sacral dysgenesis.

onstrate spina bifida with a widened canal and associated sacral dysgenesis, anomalous bone, hemivertebrae, and diastematomyelia. Because of immature calcification in children younger than 18 months of age, the usefulness of plain radiography may be limited. Ultrasound readily demonstrates the two-compartment cysts of a myelocystocele, and diminished cord pulsation confirms spinal cord tethering with both lipomyelomeningocele and myelocystocele.[31]

Finely sectioned axial computed tomography with sagittal reconstructions after intrathecal administration of contrast material defines the precise relations of bony landmarks to neural tissue and the nerve roots and demonstrates cord and meningocele kinking by fibrous bands (Fig. 34–3).[30, 32] Magnetic resonance imaging has become the study of choice for visualization of the multiplanar anatomical relations of myelocysto-

celes and lipomyelomeningoceles. The lipoma signal is high attenuation on T1-weighted views and gives diminished signal intensity on T2-weighted sequencing. Attachment anatomy is most accurately defined with sagittal T1-weighted images (Fig. 34–4), and associated hydromyelia, diastematomyelia, or stalk inclusion cysts (Fig. 34–5) are readily displayed. Peacock and Murovic demonstrated the usefulness of magnetic resonance imaging in visualization of the paired cystic compartments and related lipoma and bony malformations of a myelocystocele (Fig. 34–6).[35]

Bladder function is comprehensively assessed by urodynamics and dynamic contrast voiding studies. Renal and bladder ultrasound examination defines the anatomy of the kidney and collecting systems and confirms hydroureter or hydronephrosis. Surveillance urine cultures should be monitored regularly. Electro-

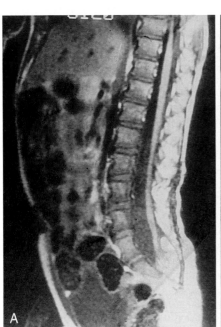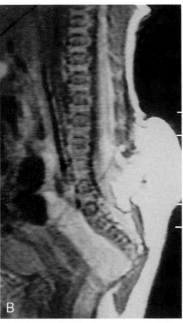

Figure 34–4

A. Sagittal T1-weighted magnetic resonance image of a transitional lipomyelomeningocele. The lipoma attaches cephalad to the dorsal spinal cord, and fat arising from the conus fills the distal thecal cul-de-sac. *B.* Sagittal T1-weighted magnetic resonance image of a 4-month-old girl with a dorsal lipomyelomeningocele. The lipoma stalk attaches to the dorsal spinal cord along a broad interface.

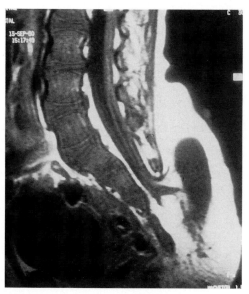

Figure 34–5

Sagittal T1-weighted magnetic resonance image of 4-year-old girl with dorsal lipomyelomeningocele that had a 5-cm inclusion cyst within the lipoma stalk.

dura is deficient laterally and anterolaterally, and stalk adherence to the dura is more tenuous than with dorsal attachment. The more complex transitional lipomyelomeningocele combines elements of dorsal and caudal lipoma attachment.

The authors have encountered a single case of Hakuba type I lipomyelomeningocele associated with bony diastematomyelia and a thickened filum terminale; stalk attachment was dorsal, and the bony spur divided the cord between the conus and the stalk. Division of adhesions and release of cord tethering is most difficult with types I, II, and variant III-a attachment anatomy.

Caudal lipomyelomeningoceles are encountered within the sacral spinal canal, and dorsal variants can be found at any lumbosacral level. The most common attachment is transitional; it occurs broadly from lumbar to lumbosacral regions. There is no correlation between lipoma size, location, or attachment anatomy and neurological function.[16, 17, 39] Lipid metabolism is identical to that of normal subcutaneous adipose tissue, and malignant transformation of a lipoma to liposarcoma or malignant teratoma is very rare.[9, 12, 29]

myography supplements routine muscle strength examination by physicians and physical therapists. Changes in urodynamic studies and denervation potentials or fibrillations may be the earliest evidence of neurological injury and progressive cord tethering.

Intracranial malformation or hydrocephalus is rare in patients with lipomyelomeningocele or myelocystocele. Magnetic resonance imaging of the brain has demonstrated the Chiari I malformation in several patients and a Chiari II malformation accompanying a cervicothoracic myelocystocele in a single child.[28, 30, 37]

Anatomical Classification

Three classifications of lipomyelomeningocele attachment were originally described by Chapman.[5, 6] The dorsal variant directly attaches to the dorsal surface of the caudally displaced spinal cord (Fig. 34–7). Dura, lipoma stalk, and arachnoid are tightly fused along a broad spinal interface. Sensory nerve roots enter the dorsolateral surface of the cord just lateral to this interface, and motor roots emerge more ventrally.

Hakuba and colleagues defined a classification scheme with four types and six subtypes of lipomyelomeningoceles (Table 34–3).[10] Neural elements remain within the spinal canal in type III (intraspinal) malformations. Subtype III-b is equivalent to a dorsal lipomyelomeningocele, and attachment by a narrow lipoma stalk through a small dural defect is seen in subtype III-c.

Caudal lipomyelomeningocele emerges from the conus medullaris and engulfs the cauda equina, filling the capacious distal thecal cul-de-sac. Functional and aberrant nerve roots traverse the lipoma mass. The

Surgical Treatment

Ethical considerations have prevented a randomized prospective study of the efficacy of repair of lipomyelo-

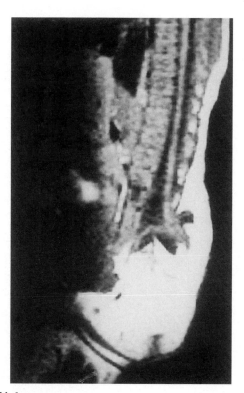

Figure 34–6

Sagittal T1-weighted magnetic resonance image of a sacral myelocystocele showing a terminal myelocystocele inserting into subcutaneous lipoma. The meningocele is dorsal and superior to the expanded spinal cord.

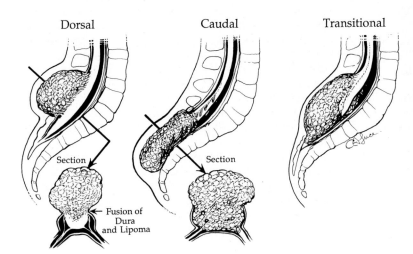

Figure 34–7

Lipomyelomeningocele anatomical classification. *Dorsal.* Lipoma stalk attaches to the dorsal dysraphic spinal cord and extends a variable intramedullary distance. *Caudal.* Lipoma arises from the conus medullaris and fills the terminal thecal sac; nerve roots may traverse the lipoma mass. *Transitional.* Lipomyelomeningocele combines dorsal attachment with nerve roots coursing anterolateral from stalk-cord interface and caudal lipoma origin. (Adapted from Chapman, P. H.: Congenital intraspinal lipomas: Anatomic considerations and surgical treatment. Child's Brain, *9:*37–47, 1982. Reprinted by permission of S. Karger AG, Basel.)

Table 34–3
CLASSIFICATION OF LIPOMYELOMENINGOCELES

Hakuba Type	Subtype	Description	Chapman Designation
I		Anomalous lipoma with associated spinal malformations, i.e., diastematomyelia	
II		Extraspinal lipoma—the spinal cord protrudes from the spinal canal via spina bifida	
	II-a	Kyphotic variant: the protruded cord curves and returns intraspinal	
	II-b	The conus protrudes extraspinal and fuses in a caudal attachment with the subcutaneous lipoma	
	II-c	The conus and distal thecal sac protrude extraspinal with broad caudal fusion with the subcutaneous lipoma	
III		Intraspinal variant: the cord remains within the spinal canal	
	III-a	The conus fuses with the subcutaneous lipoma through a caudal dural defect—roots are found in the lipoma dorsal to the line of attachment	Similar to caudal variant
	III-b	Lipoma attachment to the dorsal cord—roots are anterolateral to line of fusion	Identical to dorsal variant
	III-c	There is a fibrofatty stalk attachment to the conus	
IV		Epidural lipoma is attached to conus by a narrow fibrous band	

meningocele and myelocystocele. At the time of lipo-myelomeningocele diagnosis, approximately two thirds of children younger than 6 months of age are intact, whereas only a limited number of patients older than 4 years of age retain normal neurological and bladder function. Intact neurological function deteriorates in a negative logarithmic relation to increasing patient age, which implies that deficits will eventually develop in all patients (Fig. 34–8). From these observations, it can be assumed that the natural history of each malformation is progressive and results in irretrievable loss of neurological function with age.

Advocates of surgery recommend repair and release of cord tethering in advance of bladder paralysis and function loss. The most persuasive data that surgery is superior to conservative management show that, in most series, patients with normal bladder function on long-term follow-up invariably underwent surgery at an early age, in advance of neurological deterioration. Given the limited surgical risk of nerve injury, prophylactic repair appears justified, and predictable function loss can be avoided.[8, 16] The goals of surgery for either malformation are release of cord tethering, preservation of neural elements, lipoma debulking, and watertight dural reconstruction and skin closure. Surgery should be performed at the time lipomyelomeningocele is diagnosed; in newborns, repair is delayed until the child is 1 to 2 months of age.

SURGICAL TECHNIQUE FOR LIPOMYELOMENINGOCELE

After induction of general anesthesia and Foley catheter placement, the child is positioned prone with lateral padded rolls supporting the chest and abdomen. In children younger than 1 year of age, the arms are best supported alongside the trunk; in older patients, elevation of the arms above the shoulder positions the surgeon closer to the patient. Betadine scrub solution is used to prepare the skin from the intergluteal fold to well above the superficial lipoma mass.

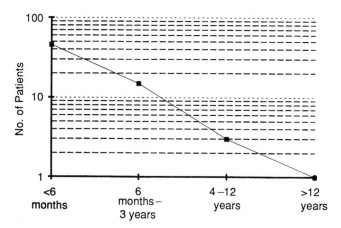

Figure 34–8

Logarithmic relation between patient age and intact neurological function at the time of diagnosis of lipomyelomeningocele in 65 children. (Data from references 13 and 16.)

The authors recommend a midline skin incision made from above to below the lipoma mass, although some groups use a curved incision.[10, 11, 40] To protect their vascular supply, skin flaps at least 1 cm in thickness are developed, and the dome of the lipoma is exposed. Subcutaneous tissue cephalad to the lipoma is divided with electrocautery until intact lumbosacral fascia is encountered. The cephalad pole of the fatty mass is gently elevated until the fascia defect and lipoma stalk are apparent; the caudal pole may blend into superficial fibers of the gluteal muscles, obscuring the plane of dissection. The lipoma stalk is defined circumferentially. To facilitate further exposure, the authors divide the stalk flush at the fascia, using a carbon dioxide laser or monopolar cautery.

The paraspinal muscles are dissected in a subperiosteal fashion from the first intact spinous process and the lamina cephalad to the stalk. Thick, fibrous epidural bands that notch the spinal cord and dura are frequently encountered, and they are sharply divided. The dura is opened with a No. 11 scalpel. Although it is displaced caudad, spinal cord anatomy at this level is normal. Loop or microscope magnification allows identification of dorsal nerve roots as they traverse the subarachnoid space. There may be dural or pial fat infiltration. The arachnoid is maintained intact and dissected free from the lateral dura with microsurgical techniques. A Woodson elevator or dental instrument passes easily in this plane.

As the stalk of a dorsal lipomyelomeningocele is approached, the lipoma, arachnoid, dorsal cord, and dura are tightly adherent just medial to the dorsal root entry zone. In the type II (extraspinal) Hakuba variant, the path of sensory roots may be quite variable because of cord rotation or dorsal displacement of the spinal cord and lipoma from within the canal (Fig. 34–9). These fused elements are divided with sharp microdissection until the lateral spinal cord is free of dural adhesion and cord mobility is confirmed. Intradural dissection must continue below the caudal stalk attachment to inspect for a thickened filum terminale.

For a caudal lipomyelomeningocele, lateral adhesions along the caudally-displaced spinal cord are divided until the conus and lipoma mass are encountered. Further dissection into the capacious thecal cul-de-sac becomes difficult because the lipoma-dura interface is tenuous and dura is deficient laterally and anterolaterally. Nerve roots traverse the lipoma mass and are best identified as they exit the neural foramina. At a level below the lowest roots, the lipoma stalk is divided to release cord tethering.

Dissection of a transitional lipomyelomeningocele begins above the conus and, by means of the techniques already described for dorsal attachment and dissection within the distal cul-de-sac, proceeds as a caudal variant.

The carbon dioxide surgical laser, adjusted for 10 to 15 mW pulse or continuous output, is ideal for lipoma resection. Vaporization minimizes neural tissue manipulation, and photocoagulation achieves excellent hemostasis of the small to medium-sized blood vessels common within the stalk and lipoma mass. The Cavi-

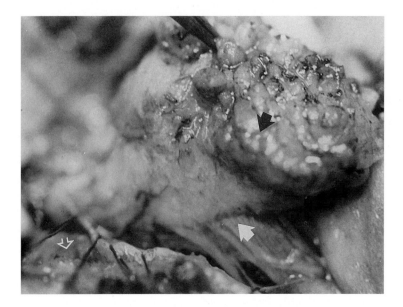

Figure 34–9

Operative photograph of dorsal lipomyelomeningocele arising from the lumbosacral spinal cord. There was extraspinal cord protrusion, although the nerve roots returned to the spinal canal. The lipoma stalk is divided flush with lumbosacral muscle fascia *(black arrow)*. The dura is dissected free from adherence along the lipoma-cord interface *(open arrow)*. Nerve roots of the cauda equina return to the distal thecal sac *(white arrow)*. The dorsal roots entry zone lies lateral to the attachment of dura, lipoma stalk, and spinal cord.

tron ultrasonic aspirator may also aid resection of the lipoma or stalk. Its usefulness is limited if the lipoma mass or stalk contains extensive fibrous tissue, bone, or cartilaginous material. A dorsal stalk attachment is sectioned just above the lipoma-cord interface. Intramedullary lipoma is encountered to a variable degree, and judicious laser resection is justified to debulk the expanded spinal cord. There is a fibrous interface between the lipoma and neural tissue, but it is tenuous and indistinct; aggressive laser vaporization within the cord can produce neurological deficits and must be avoided. With a caudal or transitional variant, the laser is used after section of the lipoma stalk below the last-exiting roots to debulk the lipoma within the terminal thecal sac. The debulking must proceed with great care because functional roots along with aberrant roots and fibrous bands traverse the lipoma. Electrical stimulation and functional monitoring during lipoma vaporization can minimize the risk of nerve root injury. Aberrant nerve roots within the lipoma mass may be sectioned if no response to electrical stimulation is encountered.[5, 7]

There are many techniques for monitoring lumbar and sacral root function, including peripheral nerve compound action or somatosensory evoked potential recording, electromyography monitoring of the anal sphincter and of the muscles, and rectal or bladder manometry.* The last technique involves pressure recording through a double-lumen Foley catheter during bladder or external sphincter contraction. Pressure changes are very rapid in response to stimulation and allow surgical maneuvers to be modified. The fact that electrophysiological monitoring has often prevented injury of functional nerve tissue that otherwise would be sectioned is the most compelling argument for its use.

It is not possible to fully untether the spinal cord in all cases of lipomyelomeningocele, although this situation is unusual in the author's experience. If the

spinal cord is rotated, nerve roots are shortened and angulated, limiting settling of the conus within the enlarged terminal thecal sac. Other limitations that may be encountered include sacral dysgenesis, conjoined nerve roots, and kyphotic cord displacement.[3, 10, 30]

As recommended by McLone and colleagues, the authors routinely suture the pia-arachnoid and reconstitute a tubular spinal cord and conus.[28] Intact circumferential pia may deter repeat cord tethering, and it minimizes contact of the subarachnoid space with fat droplets and charred debris after laser vaporization. Closure may also minimize inflammatory chemical meningitis. To decrease retethering, Sakamoto and colleagues recommend manipulating the conus into the center of the spinal canal and placing 8–0 or 9–0 stay sutures from the ventrolateral pia to the ventral dura. Bone grafts of rib or iliac crest, fashioned to resemble lamina, are used to reconstruct the dorsal elements at bifid vertebral levels. Central tack-up sutures secured to the reconstructed arch tent the dura away from the conus to maximize the subarachnoid space.[41]

Another maneuver that is critical to minimize repeat tethering is redundant dural closure. Redundant closure assures a wide contact of cerebrospinal fluid around the lower spinal cord to limit adhesions between neural tissue and the dura. In all cases, the authors incorporate cadaveric dura patch grafts closed with running 4–0 absorbable sutures. Muscle fascia is reapproximated with interrupted sutures in a watertight manner. Stalk defects that cannot be closed primarily should be augmented with cadaveric dura or fascia patches. Zide and co-workers have described a technique of lateral fascia-releasing incisions for midline closure of large defects, and they report no leaks of cerebrospinal fluid in their patients.[46, 47] If a large soft tissue defect is present after removal of the lipoma, "dead space" can be minimized by anchoring subcutaneous sutures directly to the lumbosacral fascia. A vertical mattress-suture skin closure may add another barrier against leaks of cerebrospinal fluid.

---

*See references 14, 15, 33, 34, 36, and 38.

Table 34–4
SURGICAL COMPLICATIONS AFTER REPAIR OF LIPOMYELOMENINGOCELE IN 562 PATIENTS

Patient Series	No. of Patients Who Underwent Surgery	Cerebrospinal Fluid Leak	Wound Infection	Wound Breakdown	Postoperative Neurological Deficits	Perioperative Mortality	Meningitis
Chicago	197	23	8	8	1	—	—
Toronto	97	3	—	—	—	—	—
Seattle	80	2	14	7	3	—	1
Paris	64	26	—	—	2	—	—
Osaka	38	—	—	—	2	2	—
Boston	35	—	—	—	1	—	—
San Francisco	31	3	4	—	—	—	—
New York	20	—	—	—	—	—	—
Total	562	57	26	15	9	2	1

Data from Atala et al.,[2] Foster et al.,[8] Hakuba et al.,[10] Harrison et al.,[11] Harvey et al.,[12] Hoffman et al.,[13] Kanev et al.,[16] and Pierre-Kahn et al.[37]

MYELOCYSTOCELE REPAIR

After the patient is positioned supine, a midline incision is made, and subperiosteal muscle dissection exposes the first intact lamina. After laminectomy, fibrous epidural bands are divided; the normal dura is opened, and the incision is carried into the meningocele. The spinal cord and roots can be visualized within the subarachnoid space as they course back toward the spinal canal. There is a trumpet-like enlargement of the conus that flares into the subcutaneous fat. Dissection through this lipoma exposes the terminal cyst in direct communication with a hydrosyringomyelia of the central canal. Below the origin of the third sacral nerve roots, the lipoma and edges of the myelocystocele are excised, untethering the spinal cord. After retubularization of the edges of the terminal cyst, dural flaps are mobilized and closed with a running absorbable suture; usually, there is sufficient dura and patch grafting is unnecessary. Midline wound closure proceeds in layers by techniques similar to those described for lipomyelomeningocele.

Complications of Surgery

Neurosurgeons during the 1960's believed that lipomyelomeningocele resections in young children carried excessive risk of nerve injury and recommended surgery limited only to debulking of the subcutaneous lipoma mass.[24, 44] Advancements in understanding of the embryology and anatomy of complex spinal dysraphism have led to the development of more aggressive surgical procedures. At the same time, surgical complications have steadily diminished with improvements in pediatric anesthesia, laser resection, the operating microscope, and electrophysiological monitoring.

Lipoma resection and release of cord tethering can be accomplished with very limited neurological risk, regardless of patient age. A review of published reports shows that postoperative deficits were encountered in only 9 of 562 patients (Table 34–4). Three children cared for at the Children's Medical Center in Seattle who had intact neurological function on preoperative examination sustained unilateral S1 root injury; lipoma attachment in each case was transitional, with kyphotic cord displacement and rotation.[16] In another series of patients reported by Harvey and colleagues, a similar injury occurred in one patient.[12] The risk of acquired postoperative bladder paralysis is less than 1 per cent. Cerebrospinal fluid leaks were the most common postoperative complication reported. These ranged from self-limiting subcutaneous collections to chronic fistulas requiring re-exploration and dural repair. The incidence of wound dehiscence or infection was 7 per cent; extensive resection of subcutaneous lipoma thins the overlying skin flaps and promotes ischemia, necrosis, and impaired wound healing. Only two patient deaths occurred in 562 cases.

Long-Term Outcome

Ninety-five per cent of 153 neurologically intact children who underwent surgery retained normal bladder function on long-term follow-up that ranged from 6 months to more than 20 years (Table 34–5).[12, 13, 16, 37] Only five of these patients (3.3 per cent) experienced

Table 34–5
LONG-TERM POSTOPERATIVE FOLLOW-UP AMONG 153 PATIENTS WITH LIPOMYELOMENINGOCELE WHO HAD INTACT PREOPERATIVE NEUROLOGICAL FUNCTION

	No. of Children with Preoperative Intact Neurological and Bladder Function	No. of Children with Normal Postoperative Neurological and Bladder Function on Long-Term Follow-Up
Chicago	61	60
Seattle	38	38
Toronto	27	22
Paris	27	25
Totals	153	145
		95%

Data from Harvey et al.,[12] Hoffman et al.,[13] Kanev et al.,[16] and Pierre-Kahn et al.[37]

Table 34–6

LONG-TERM FOLLOW-UP OF 273 PATIENTS WITH LIPOMYELOMENINGOCELE WHO HAD PREOPERATIVE MOTOR AND SENSORY DEFICITS

Patient Series	No. of Children with Preoperative Motor, Sensory, or Bladder Deficits	No. of Children with Improved Postoperative Motor and Sensory Examination	No. of Children with Stable Postoperative Motor and Sensory Examination
Chicago	145	65	78
Toronto	35	9	21
Seattle	42	42	0
Paris	37	14	23
Boston	14	10	4
Totals	273	140	126
		51%	46%

Data from Harvey et al.,[12] Hoffman et al.,[13] Kanev et al.,[16] and Pierre-Kahn et al.[37]

late deterioration and required reoperation for release of tethering. Among 273 children with preoperative motor or sensory deficits, improvement in neurological function was recorded in half (Table 34–6).[12, 13, 16, 37] In a population of 80 patients cared for at Seattle Children's Hospital, children with preoperative function at the L4 or L5 level improved to S1 or S2 over 12 to 18 months after surgery. There was improved ambulation and perineal sensation among children with preoperative sacral level function; however, there was no recovery of complete bladder paralysis in any patient.[16] The recovery of continence among patients with preoperative bladder dysfunction was 13 per cent (Table 34–7).[12, 13, 16, 37] Curvature improved in 6 of 13 patients with scoliosis, but no significant changes in orthopedic foot deformities were encountered.[12, 13, 16]

Late deterioration can occur at any time after initial surgical repair into adulthood. The symptoms of repeat cord tethering included progressive scoliosis curvature, radicular or low back pain, foot ulceration, and reduced continence. Any child with late changes in neurological function should promptly be studied with magnetic resonance imaging to investigate treatable causes, including syrinx formation, diastematomyelia, growth of residual lipoma tissue, and retethering. The overall incidence of retethering after primary repair in 403 patients was 15 per cent (Table 34–8).[12, 13, 16, 37] The statistically significant risk factors that predict retethering include initial surgery on a patient older than 1 year of age and the presence of a preoperative neurological deficit.[12] Retethering was not increased among patients experiencing cerebrospinal fluid leaks, wound infections, or other postoperative complications.

Bladder and bowel paralysis is the most significant complication of lipomyelomeningocele or myelocystocele. Among 42 children with bladder paralysis followed at Children's Medical Center in Seattle, at least one urinary tract infection occurred each year, and 16 patients required hospitalizations for pyelonephritis.[16] Clean intermittent bladder catheterization, antibiotic prophylaxis, and urinary acidification are critical to minimize kidney injury from chronic infection. Despite these measures, some children have required additional surgery, including construction of ileal conduits, bladder augmentation, or renal transplantation. Bowel management includes diet control, enemas, and digital stimulation.

Almost all children with lipomyelomeningocele or myelocystocele have normal intelligence and school performance. More than 95 per cent of patients are ambulatory, with limited requirements for bracing or wheelchair assistance.

Table 34–7

RECOVERY OF CONTINENCE AMONG 260 PATIENTS WITH LIPOMYELOMENINGOCELE WHO HAD PREOPERATIVE UROLOGICAL DYSFUNCTION

Patient Series	No. with Preoperative Urological Abnormality	No. Improved and Continent After Operation
Chicago	115	21
Toronto	35	5
Seattle	42	0
Paris	35	3
San Francisco	22	4
Boston	11	1
Totals	260	34
		13%

Data from Harvey et al.,[12] Hoffman et al.,[13] Kanev et al.,[16] and Pierre-Kahn et al.[37]

Table 34–8

LATE DETERIORATION FROM RETETHERING AMONG 403 PATIENTS WITH LIPOMYELOMENINGOCELE

Patient Series	No. of Patients	No. of Patients with Late Deterioration from Retethering
Chicago	197	36
Toronto	62	10
Seattle	80	11
Paris	64	3
Totals	403	60
		15%

Data from Harvey et al.[12] Hoffman et al.,[13] Kanev et al.,[16] and Pierre-Kahn et al.[37]

Conclusions

The evaluation of a child with a lumbosacral mass or cutaneous stigmata of occult spinal dysraphism is one of the most common reasons for referral to a pediatric neurosurgeon. A high index of suspicion must be maintained despite normal examination results, and a screening magnetic resonance imaging is warranted. Conservative management of lipomyelomeningocele or myelocystocele is no longer justified. Predictable neurological deterioration and loss of bladder function can be avoided by early surgery in the intact child. Late deterioration and retethering is reduced in children who are operated on when they are younger than 1 year of age, and there is limited risk of nerve injury at any age. Surgery should be performed at the time of diagnosis, and long-term care should be managed within a multidisciplinary program for congenital defects. Surgery that is accomplished before the appearance of deficits maintains normal neurological function so that children can develop unencumbered by motor paralysis or incontinence. For the pediatric neurosurgeon, there is little that could be more satisfying.

REFERENCES

1. Alston, S. R., Fuller, G. N., Boyko, O. B., et al.: Ectopic renal tissue in a lumbosacral lipoma: Pathologic and radiologic findings. Pediatr. Neurosci., 15:100–103, 1989.
2. Atala, A., Bauer, S. B., Dyro, F. M., et al.: Bladder functional changes resulting from lipomyelomeningocele repair. J. Urol., 148:592–594, 1992.
3. Barolat, G., Schaeffer, D., and Zeme, S.: Recurrent spinal cord tethering by sacral nerve root following lipomyelomeningocele surgery [Case report]. J. Neurosurg., 75:143–145, 1991.
4. Bruce, D. A., and Schut, L.: Spinal lipomas in infancy and childhood. Child's Brain, 5:192–203, 1979.
5. Chapman, P. H.: Congenital intraspinal lipomas: Anatomic considerations and surgical treatment. Child's Brain, 9:37–47, 1982.
6. Chapman, P. H., and Beyerl, B.: The tethered spinal cord, with particular reference to spinal lipoma and diastematomyelia. In Hoffman, H. J., and Epstein, F., eds.: Disorders of the Developing Nervous System. Boston, Blackwell Scientific, 1986, pp. 109–131.
7. Chapman, P. H., and Davis, K. R.: Surgical treatment of spinal lipomas in childhood. In Raimondi, A. J., ed.: Concepts in Pediatric Neurosurgery. Vol. 3. Basel, Karger, 1983, pp. 178–190.
8. Foster, L. S., Kogan, B. A., Cogen, P. H., et al.: Bladder function in patients with lipomyelomeningocele. J. Urol., 143:984–986, 1990.
9. Giudicelli, Y., Pecquery, R., Agli, B., et al.: Lipoprotein lipase and hormone-sensitive activities in human subcutaneous lipomas: Comparison with normal subcutaneous adipose tissue. Clin. Sci. Med., 50:315–318, 1976.
10. Hakuba, A., Fujitani, K., Hoda, K., et al.: Lumbo-sacral lipoma, the timing of the operation and morphological classification. Neuro-orthopedics, 2:34–42, 1986.
11. Harrison, M. J., Mitnick, R. J., Rosenbluth, B. R., et al.: Leptomyelolipoma: Analysis of 20 cases. J. Neurosurg., 73:360–367, 1990.
12. Harvey, C. F., Dias, M. S., and McLone, D. G.: Spinal cord lipomas 1971–1991: A twenty year experience [Abstract]. Pediatric Section Meeting, American Association of Neurologic Surgeons, Vancouver, B. C., 1992.
13. Hoffman, H. J., Taecholarn, C., Hendrick, E. B., et al.: Management of lipomyelomeningoceles: Experience at the Hospital for Sick Children, Toronto. J. Neurosurg., 62:1–8, 1985.
14. Ikeda, K., Kubota, T., Kashihara, K., et al.: Anorectal pressure monitoring during surgery on sacral lipomyelomeningocele. J. Neurosurg., 64:155–156, 1986.
15. James, H. E., Mulcahy, J. J., Walsh, J. W., et al.: Use of anal sphincter electromyography during operations on the conus medullaris and sacral nerve roots. Neurosurgery, 4:521–523, 1979.
16. Kanev, P. M., Lemire, R. J., Loeser, J. D., et al.: Management and long term follow-up review of children with lipomyelomeningocele, 1952–1987. J. Neurosurg., 73:48–52, 1990.
17. Lassman, L. P., and James, C. C.: Lumbosacral lipomas: Critical survey of 26 cases submitted to laminectomy. J. Neurol. Neurosurg. Psychiatry, 30:174–181, 1967.
18. Lemire, R. J., and Beckwith, J. B.: Pathogenesis of congenital tumors and malformations of the sacrococcygeal region. Teratology, 25:201–213, 1982.
19. Lemire, R. J., and Beckwith, J. B.: The spectrum of neural tube defects of the caudal spine in infants. In Arima, M., Suzuki, Y., and Yabuuchi, H., eds.: The Developing Brain and Its Disorders. Tokyo, University of Tokyo Press, 1984, pp. 29–42.
20. Lemire, R. J., Graham, C. B., and Beckwith, J. B.: Skin-covered sacrococcygeal masses in infants and children. J. Pediatr., 79:948–954, 1971.
21. Lemire, R. J., Loeser, J. D., Leech, R. W., et al.: Normal and Abnormal Development of the Human Nervous System. New York, Harper & Row, 1975, pp. 1–421.
22. Loeser, J. D., and Lewin, R. J.: Lumbosacral lipoma in the adult [Case report]. J. Neurosurg., 29:405–409, 1968.
23. Lunardi, P., Missori, P., Ferrante, L., et al.: Long-term results of surgical treatment of spinal lipomas: Report of 18 cases. Acta Neurochir. (Wien), 104:64–68, 1990.
24. Matson, D. D.: Neurosurgery of Infancy and Childhood. 2nd ed. Springfield, Charles C. Thomas, 1969, p. 46.
25. McLone, D. G., and Knepper, P. A.: Role of complex carbohydrates and neurulation. Pediatr. Neurosci., 12:2–9, 1985–1986.
26. McLone, D. G., and Naidich, T. P.: Spinal dysraphism: Experimental and clinical. In Holzmann, R. N., and Stein, B. M., eds.: The Tethered Spinal Cord. New York, Thieme-Stratton, 1985, pp. 3–13.
27. McLone, D. G., and Naidich, T. P.: The tethered spinal cord. In McLaurin, R. L., Schut, L., Venes, J. L., et al., eds.: Pediatric Neurosurgery, 2nd ed. Philadelphia, W. B. Saunders, 1989, pp. 71–96.
28. McLone, D. G., Mutluer, S., and Naidich, T. P.: Lipomyelomeningocele of the conus medullaris. In Raimondi, A. J., ed.: Concepts in Pediatric Neurosurgery. Vol. 3. Basel, Karger, 1983, pp. 170–177.
29. Mickle, J. P., and McLennan, J. E.: Malignant teratoma arising within a lipomyelomeningocele [Case report]. J. Neurosurg., 43:761–763, 1975.
30. Naidich, T. P., McLone, D. G., and Mutluer, S.: A new understanding of dorsal dysraphism with lipoma (lipomyeloschisis): Radiologic evaluation and surgical correction. A.J.R., 140:1065–1078, 1983.
31. Naidich, T. P., Radkowski, M., and Britton, J.: Real-time sonographic display of caudal spinal anomalies. In Naidich, T. P., and Quencher, R., eds.: Clinical Neurosonography: Ultrasound of the Central Nervous System. Berlin, Springer-Verlag, 1986, pp. 146–161.
32. Oakes, W. J.: Management of spinal cord lipomas and lipomyelomeningoceles. In Wilkins, R., and Rengachary, S., eds.: Neurosurgery Update II: Vascular, Spinal, Pediatric and Functional Neurosurgery. New York, McGraw-Hill, 1991, pp. 345–352.
33. Pang, D.: Use of an anal sphincter monitor for identification of sacral nerve roots and conus. In Holzmann, R. N. N., and Stein, B. M., eds.: The Tethered Spinal Cord. New York, Thieme-Stratton, 1985, pp. 3–13.
34. Pang, D., and Casey, K.: Use of an anal sphincter pressure monitor during operations on the sacral spinal cord and nerve roots. Neurosurgery, 13:562–568, 1983.
35. Peacock, W. J., and Murovic, J. A.: Magnetic resonance imaging of myelocystoceles: Report of two cases. J. Neurosurg., 70:804–807, 1989.
36. Phillips, L. H., and Park, T. S.: Electrophysiological monitoring during lipomyelomeningocele resection. Muscle Nerve, 13:127–132, 1990.
37. Pierre-Kahn, A., Lacombe, J., Pichon, J., et al.: Intraspinal lipomas with spina bifida: Prognosis and treatment in 73 cases. J. Neurosurg., 65:756–761, 1986.

38. Reigel, D. H.: Tethered spinal cord. *In* Humpreys, R., ed.: Concepts in Pediatric Neurosurgery. Vol. 4. Basel, Karger, 1983, pp. 142–163.

39. Rogers, H. M., Long, D. M., Chou, S. N., et al.: Lipomas of the spinal cord and cauda equina. J. Neurosurg., *34*:349–354, 1971.

40. Rosenbloom, B. R., Harrison, M. J., and Rothman, A. S.: Lumbosacral lipomas. Contemp. Neurosurg., *10*:1–8, 1988.

41. Sakamoto, H., Hakuba, A., Fujitani, K., et al.: Surgical treatment of the retethered spinal cord after repair of lipomyelomeningocele. J. Neurosurg., *74*:709–714, 1991.

42. Schut, L., Bruce, D. A., and Sutton, L. N.: The management of the child with a lipomyelomeningocele. Clin. Neurosurg., *30*:446–476, 1983.

43. Sutton, L. N., Duhaime, A. C., and Schut, L.: Lipomyelomeningocele. *In* Park, T. S., ed.: Contemporary Issues in Neurological Surgery: Spinal Dysraphism. Oxford, Blackwell Scientific, 1992, pp. 59–73.

44. Till, K.: Spinal dysraphism: A study of congenital malformations of the lower back. J. Bone Joint Surg. [Br.], *51*:415–422, 1969.

45. Walsh, J. W., and Markesbery, W. R.: Histological features of congenital lipomas of the lower spinal cord. J. Neurosurg., *52*:564–569, 1980.

46. Zide, B. M.: How to reduce the morbidity of wound closure following extensive and complicated laminectomy and tethered cord surgery. Pediatr. Neurosurg., *18*:157–166, 1992.

47. Zide, B. M., Epstein, F. J., and Wisoff, J.: Optimal wound closure after tethered cord correction [Technical note]. J. Neurosurg., *74*:673–676, 1991.

CHAPTER 35

Occult Spinal Dysraphism

Occult spinal dysraphism denotes a group of various skin-covered congenital anomalies characterized by incomplete fusion and deformation of neural elements, meninges, vertebral bone, and skin. It contrasts to open spinal dysraphism (e.g., myelomeningocele) mainly by the presence of intact skin coverage over the anomalous spinal and intraspinal structures. The number of patients with occult spinal dysraphism treated in many pediatric centers exceeds that of patients with open spinal dysraphism. Included in occult spinal dysraphism are lipomyelomeningocele, spinal lipoma, meningocele, myelocystocele, caudal regression syndrome, craniovertebral anomalies, tethered spinal cord, diastematomyelia, neurenteric cyst, and dermal sinus. Despite their remarkable pathological complexics, many of these lesions were traditionally difficult to diagnose in patients. Neuroimaging techniques, however, allow in vivo delineation of abnormalities in exquisite detail, thus rendering early intervention possible. In this chapter, five occult dysraphic lesions requiring neurosurgical treatment are discussed: tethered spinal cord syndrome, diastematomyelia, neurenteric cyst, spinal dermal sinus, and spinal meningocele. Other lesions are discussed elsewhere in this book.

Tethered Spinal Cord Syndrome

The tethered spinal cord syndrome consists of the abnormally low conus medullaris tethered by thickened filum terminale and associated neurological impairment. A few reports in the 1950's indicated a possible association of the abnormally thick filum terminale with progressive neurological deficits after improvement of neurological symptoms was observed following sectioning of the filum.[20, 37] The anomaly, however, was not considered a distinct form of spinal dysra-

phism, and persistent skepticism about its existence as a separate syndrome continued until the 1970's, when radiography correlates of the tethered spinal cord were demonstrated by the newly developed contrast and air myelography.[3, 28, 32, 35, 68] In the 1970's and 1980's, computed tomography and magnetic resonance imaging have added a new dimension to understanding the tethered cord syndrome by visualizing other forms of spinal dysraphism in which a thick filum is not associated with the tethered spinal cord. There is little doubt among neurosurgeons about the relation of the tethered spinal cord with thick filum or the need for surgical intervention.

As alluded to earlier, the tethered spinal cord occurs as part of more serious problems in various forms of spinal dysraphism (e.g., myelomeningocele, lipomyelomeningocele, lipoma of the filum, diastematomyelia, and dermal sinus). Since individual forms of spinal dysraphism accompanying cord tethering are covered in preceding chapters, the focus in this chapter is on the tethered cord due to abnormally thick filum.

EMBRYOLOGY

By the 8th week of gestation, the embryonic spinal cord extends down to the caudal end of the spinal canal (Fig. 35–1).[26] At this stage of embryogenesis, the fibrous filum terminale begins to appear, which represents involuted spinal cord caudal to the second coccygeal segment after retrogressive dedifferentiation. Thereafter, the spinal cord and vertebrae grow longitudinally, with the vertebral column growing faster than the spinal cord. This disparate longitudinal growth rate results in an ascent of the spinal cord in relation to the vertebral level. The rate of ascent of the spinal cord is at its maximum between the 8th and 18th weeks, decreases during later gestation, and is minimal after the 25th week (Fig. 35–2).[7] At birth, the conus medullaris

T. S. Park • P. M. Kanev • M. M. Henegar • B. A. Kaufman

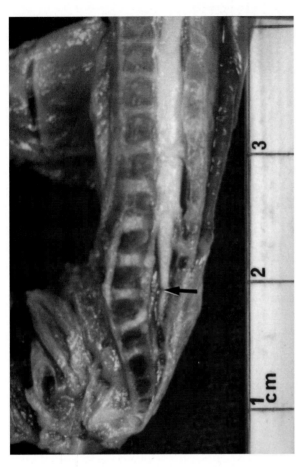

Figure 35–1

Sagittal section of a fetus with crown-rump length of 9.6 cm shows the spinal cord extending to the bottom of the dural sac. (From Hawass, N. D., El-Badawi, M. G., Fatani, J. A., et al.: Myelographic study of the spinal cord ascent during fetal development. A. J. N. R. *8*:691–695, 1987, © by American Society of Neuroradiology. Reprinted by permission.)

Figure 35–2

Vertebral level of spinal cord termination at different gestational ages. S, sacral; L, lumbar. The numbers 1 through 5 refer to the level of the vertebral body. (From Hawass, N. D., El-Badawi, M. G., Fatani, J. A., et al.: Myelographic study of the spinal cord ascent during fetal development. A. J. N. R. *8*:691–695, 1987, © by American Society of Neuroradiology. Reprinted by permission.)

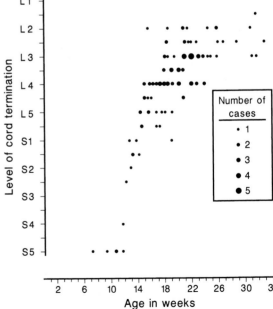

is opposite the T12 to L3 vertebral bodies, and no significant change in location of the conus relative to the vertebral level occurs, although some claim that there is further ascent of the spinal cord during the first 2 months of life.[60, 72] In parallel with this development of the spinal cord, the filum increases in thickness due to continuous intrinsic growth.[66] Thus, if the conus is anchored to a nonresilient thick filum between the 8th and 25th weeks of gestation, normal ascent of the cord would be inhibited, with the resultant low position of the conus.

PATHOGENESIS

Yamada and his colleagues expanded knowledge of pathogenesis of the tethered cord in a series of studies of adult cats subjected to mechanical traction of the distal spinal cord.[75-77] Noticeable elongation of the cat spinal cord and filum was demonstrated during application of weight traction, and once the weight traction was removed, the spinal cord and filum returned to normal shape and length.[67] A finding of particular importance was that the weight-induced stretching of the spinal cord was most pronounced below the attachment of the caudalmost dentate ligament, minimal in the thoracic cord, and absent in the cervical cord.[62, 67] The anatomical distortion of the spinal cord by traction was subsequently shown to accompany significant reduction of spinal cord blood flow and evoked potential activities.[38, 59, 76, 77] At a subcellular level, the cord tethering was associated with reduced mitochondrial oxidation of cytochrome a, a_3 during a hypoxic challenge, and untethering procedures reversed the metabolic disturbances, an observation made in humans as well as in animals.[76] Thus, convincing evidence exists that the tethered spinal cord causes anatomical and metabolic disturbances, which are reversed by early elimination of the tethering.

CLINICAL PRESENTATION

No significant sexual predilection has been observed in the incidence of tethered spinal cord syndrome. Almost half of patients show cutaneous stigmata.[28, 32, 35, 68] A hairy patch in the midline lumbosacral area is common (Fig. 35-3A), and a hemangioma or dimple may also be noted. The onset of symptoms occurs with spurts of linear growth between the ages of 5 and 15 years, but infants and children younger than 5 can manifest symptoms. In children, unusual exercise requiring spinal flexion may precipitate the onset of symptoms, but precipitant factors are uncommon.

The presenting symptoms and signs are neurological, orthopedic, or urological. Motor weakness is the most common presenting feature (76 per cent). Typically, the weakness is progressive, often associated with muscle wasting and a smaller leg on the affected side. Absent or hyperactive ankle jerk and Babinski's sign may be present. Because of these clinical presentations, patients sometimes have been labeled as having cerebral palsy or peroneal muscular atrophy. Detectable sensory loss is relatively uncommon. Trophic ulcerations, although described in earlier reports, are very uncommon, owing to early correct diagnosis. Pain is the initial presentation in 42 per cent of patients. It is located in the lumbosacral region, often radiates into one or both legs, and is aggravated by spinal flexion. Patients have difficulty in bending and touching their toes. Progressive scoliosis may result from the pain.

The orthopedic deformities include pes cavovarus with the smaller foot on the affected side, gait disturbance, and scoliosis. The predominance of orthopedic problems previously led to corrective orthopedic operations on the foot, which usually failed to correct the deformity. The primary urological problem, present in 35 per cent of patients, is a disturbance of bladder or bowel function or of both.[28] Urinary frequency, incomplete voiding, and enuresis are the manifestations of bladder involvement.[17, 19] Both orthopedic and urological symptoms are slowly progressive, culminating in irreversible damage.

The tight filum may cause development of neurological deterioration in adults after an entirely asymptomatic childhood. Likewise, symptoms are manifest in adulthood when the tethered spinal cord is part of a larger dysraphic condition. Pang and Wilberger noted that in adults circumstances precipitating the onset of neurological deterioration are often identifiable.[55] Some of their patients were engaged in body movements or posture that may subject the conus to stretching (i.e., childbirth in the lithotomy positions, straight leg-raising exercise in ballet practice, and forward bending in vehicular accident). Also, lumbar spondylosis or a herniated disc with crowding of intraspinal contents was present in some patients in whom symptoms were manifest after heavy lifting. In regard to clinical presentation, unlike children, adults often present with pain (78 per cent) and sensorimotor deficits (65 per cent); foot deformity of new onset and scoliosis are rare; and disturbance of bladder and bowel functions is as common as in children.

RADIOLOGICAL INVESTIGATION

Plain spine radiographs almost invariably demonstrate spina bifida occulta of L4, L5, or S1 vertebrae. Since spina bifida was present in all of their 86 children studied, Hendrick and colleagues suggested that normal spine radiographs nearly exclude the diagnosis.[51] However, the cord tethering may also occur in the absence of spina bifida, particularly in patients with a lipoma within the filum.[47] Although myelography with computed tomography and magnetic resonance imaging equally well define the tethered cord, magnetic resonance imaging is the radiological investigation of choice because of its noninvasiveness and superior resolution (see Fig. 35-3B). Current magnetic resonance imaging criteria of the cord tethering due to the tight filum are termination of the conus below the L3 vertebral body and the filum thicker than 2 mm. The location of the conus is determined by axial magnetic reso-

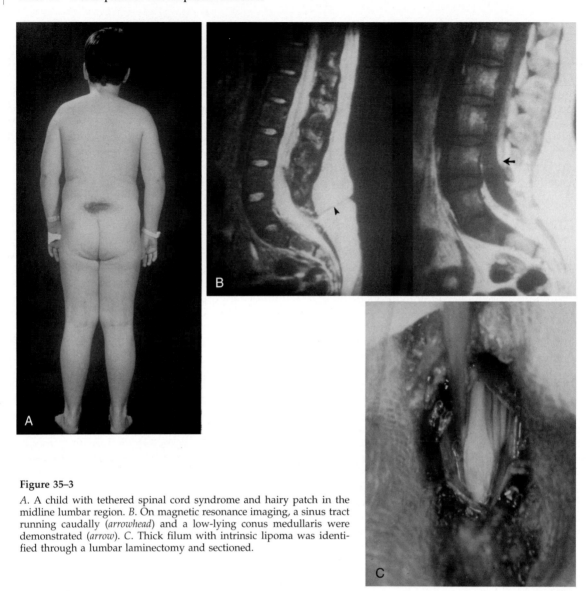

Figure 35–3

A. A child with tethered spinal cord syndrome and hairy patch in the midline lumbar region. *B.* On magnetic resonance imaging, a sinus tract running caudally (*arrowhead*) and a low-lying conus medullaris were demonstrated (*arrow*). *C.* Thick filum with intrinsic lipoma was identified through a lumbar laminectomy and sectioned.

nance imaging. On a sagittal image, the conus is seen to taper caudally and merge with the filum. When the filum is thickened, accurate localization of the conus may be difficult. Another point of caution is that in infants, magnetic resonance imaging does not delineate the thickened filum because of its small diameter compared with that of adults. In patients with demonstrated low-lying conus, the presence of fat within the filum renders cord tethering likely.[47]

TREATMENT

Operative Procedure. The purpose of spinal exploration in any patient with occult spinal dysraphism is to prevent later neurological deterioration. When the thickened filum and low-lying conus are demonstrated, surgical release of the tethered cord is justified even in the absence of neurological impairments. Laminectomy is carried out in the lumbosacral area. An extradural fibrous band that tethers the spinal cord and is rarely

encountered is divided. After the dura is opened, the taut, thickened filum is recognizable. It is advisable to examine the filum with the operating microscope for intrinsic lipoma or cystic dilation. In general, the appearance of the filum and adjacent nerve roots is readily differentiated, but when the differentiation is unclear, electrical stimulation of the presumed filum and monitoring of anal sphincter pressure or electromyography of the lower limb muscles may be helpful.[53] One should be aware, however, that current spread along the filum to the conus may result in visible responses on electromyography that could confuse surgeons. Once the filum is identified clearly (see Fig. 35–3C), a portion is separated from the roots, and particularly thin sacral roots are coagulated and divided. To avoid artifacts on postoperative magnetic resonance imaging, no metal clip is used. After sectioning, the proximal end of the filum is often seen to migrate cephalad as much as 2 cm before it nestles in the spinal canal. In patients in whom the spinal cord extends down to the bottom of the dural sac, no definable filum is present, and the spinal cord is bound to the end of the dural sac. In these patients, release of the tethered cord can be accomplished only by freeing the conus from the dura.

Outcome. Reports in the literature as well as clinical experience clearly point to significant benefits of releasing the tethered cord associated with a tight filum. The operation not only prevents the onset of neurological symptoms and signs but also halts or even reverses deterioration in some patients who present with neurological impairments.[28, 32, 68, 75] Reviewing a series of 86 children with symptomatic tight filum, Hendrick and associates noted no worsening in any of the patients, and all patients either improved or became stable postoperatively.[43] This has been the experience of other authors as well.[68, 75] Sectioning of the filum was most successful in patients with pain, because the back pain always completely subsides. These patients typically become much more mobile, being able to flex the back and touch their toes, which they could not do preoperatively. In regard to motor weakness, the outcome is modest; in the series of Hendrick and associates, the weak muscles detected in 65 patients returned to normal in 26, improved in 21, and remained unchanged in 18 patients.[43] A significant return of motor strength is followed by diminution in foot deformities and gait disturbance. Sensory deficits in the lower limbs reportedly resolved in all patients. Similarly, scoliosis was stabilized or improved in all patients so that some were able to cancel the proposed spinal fusion. The excellent outcome of scoliosis in this particular series is related to the lack of major vertebral anomalies in association with thickened filum, unlike other dysraphic conditions. Untethering of the conus resulted in resolution of symptoms of neurogenic bladder in most cases; 23 of 27 patients with such symptoms improved. These authors describe an adolescent who had lost a kidney as a result of neurogenic bladder and vesicourethral reflux and who resumed normal bladder function within 8 months after sectioning of the tight filum.

Diastematomyelia

Diastematomyelia is characterized by a longitudinal split of the spinal cord at one or more vertebral levels sometimes associated with a fibrous, bony, or cartilaginous spur dividing the spinal cord. The term "diastematomyelia," first coined by Ollivier in 1837, was derived from the Greek *diastema* meaning "cleft" and *myelos* meaning "spinal cord." This uncommon dysraphic lesion could rarely be diagnosed ante mortem before 1950 and was most often discovered serendipitously only on postmortem examinations.[45] At the Mayo Clinic from 1935 through 1967, only 10 cases were diagnosed during life and treated surgically.[16] Clinical awareness of the lesion was aroused by a few reports in 1950, and the subsequent advent of sophisticated myelography and computed tomography allowed in vivo diagnosis of the bony abnormalities associated with diastematomyelia. Magnetic resonance imaging has added further understanding of the lesion by disclosing diastematomyelia without a septum contained within a single dural tube and delineating syringomyelia above or below the split of the spinal cord. With an increasing number of cases discovered by the new imaging techniques, details of the clinical features of diastematomyelia have come to light.

Diplomyelia refers to a complete duplication of the spinal cord, each of which lies within the truly duplicated spinal canal. Each spinal cord has two dorsal horns and two ventral horns, which give rise to two dorsal and two ventral roots at each segment.[33, 51] Diplomyelia occurs only in association with true duplication of the spinal canal and in a nonviable fetus.[43, 51]

EMBRYOLOGY

The embryogenesis of this complex form of occult spinal dysraphism is not fully understood. Although lacking in concrete evidence, various theories have been advanced to explain the embryogenesis of diastematomyelia, an extensive review of which is available.[54] Briefly, the proposed theories focus on three different embryological abnormalities: (1) abnormal neurulation, (2) split notochord, and (3) accessory neurenteric canal.[8, 10, 21, 29, 54] The abnormal neurulation theory assumes that when the lateral extremes of the neural plate approach the midline dorsally to fuse and form the neural fold, they overconverge by continuous growth ventrally and ultimately fuse with the ventral portion of the plate on each side of the midline. As a result, two neural tubes are formed. If the space between the two cords is narrow, the intervening mesenchyme develops into pial membrane, but if the space is wide, more mesenchyme fills the space to develop the arachnoid-dural sheath and septum.[29] Gardner applied his hydrodynamic theory to suggest that overdistention of the central canal invokes a primary defect in neural tube formation.[47] The theory of a split notochord as the basic abnormality is proposed by Bentley and Smith.[26] Through the gap between the split notochord, a diverticulum herniates from the yolk sac and adheres to the dorsal ectoderm of skin anlage. Double neural plates thus result, and the subsequent neurulation forms the double spinal cords. Each hemicord induces the development of neural arch and midline bone septum, as the dorsal diverticulum involutes and develops into the various midline mesodermal products. Bremer suggested an accessory neurenteric canal as the primary embryological error for diastematomyelia.[60] Normally, a neurenteric canal, which appears for a short time in the region of the future coccyx, runs from the yolk sac cavity through the primitive pit (Henson's node) to the amniotic cavity. In cases of diastematomyelia, the accessory neurenteric canal is formed cephalad to the coccyx to split the notochord and neural plate for a varying distance from the primitive pit. Pang and colleagues modified the concept of Bremer by postulating that the accessory neurenteric canal might begin as an ectoendodermal adhesion in the midline, that endomesodermal elements grow in the midline to form endomesenchymal fistula, and that the neuroectoderm is bisected to produce split neural plates.[54] According to them, the septum in diastematomyelia arises from the midline mesenchyme.

PATHOLOGY

Pathological abnormalities in diastematomyelia are complex, involving in a variety of patterns the spinal cord, enwrapping meninges, median septum within the cleft, all elements of the vertebra, subcutaneous tissue, and skin. The advent of radiological imaging techniques made possible an understanding of complex pathology in diastematomyelia.

Meninges and Septum. With the wide use of computed tomography myelography in the 1970's, it became clear that diastematomyelia occurs either with or without an associated septum splitting the dural sac. The finding that was inconsistent with prior understanding was first reported by Scotti and associates; in a series of 21 patients examined by computed tomography myelography, they found classic diastematomyelia with a septum in only 6 patients, and other forms of diastematomyelia in the remaining 15 patients.[13] In 40 to 50 per cent of patients with diastematomyelia, a septum is seen to split the spinal cord as well as the dural sac. In this form of diastematomyelia, the two hemicords lie in two separate dura-arachnoid sheaths that merge into each other to reconstitute a single dura-arachnoid tube below and above the cleft.[25, 52, 64] The pial membrane covers the surface of each of the hemicords.[14] The medial walls of the duplicated dural sac form a dural sleeve that completely encircles the septum. The cleft splitting the dural sac is always longer than the cleft in the spinal cord. In the other 50 to 60 per cent of patients, diastematomyelia has no septum but has two split hemicords lying within a single arachnoid-dural sac (Fig. 35–4). As in the former form, the pial membrane envelops each hemicord in a separate pial sheath.

In virtually all patients with diastematomyelia and duplicated dural sacs, a fibrous partition or an osseous or osseocartilaginous spur traverses the dural cleft between and outside the medial walls of the duplicated dural sacs. The bone or cartilage spur is typically oriented sagittally; points forward, upward, or downward; and attaches to the vertebral body and lamina. The spur nearly always lies in the midsagittal plane of the vertebral body and divides the spinal canal into two approximately equal compartments. In the majority of cases, the broadest attachment of bone spur is dorsal at the lamina and the ventral attachment to the vertebral body is narrow, which makes it easier to remove the spur from the vertebral body than from the lamina. Rarely, however, the spur may be off the midline, arising from the pedicle.[64] The lamina to which the bone attaches is often markedly hypertrophic.

Both forms of diastematomyelia are associated with fibrous bands tethering the cord. According to James and Lassman, fibrous bands represent the atrophied aberrant dorsal roots, and single or multiple bands connect the spinal cord with the extradural neural arch or dura inside the dural sac.[64] Sometimes, the bands are between the hemicords and attach to the medial aspect of the hemicord, appearing as commissural bands. Not all fibrous bands are depicted by computed tomography or magnetic resonance imaging, but a common occurrence of fibrous bands in diastematomyelia was indicated by Pang, who found it in all of 18 patients surgically explored for treatment of diastematomyelia.[52] James and Lassman noted such bands in 8 of 11 surgically treated patients.[64]

Cleft in Spinal Cord and Hemicord. Whether or not diastematomyelia has an associated median septum splitting the dural sac, a cleft is present in the spinal cord and adjacent hemicords. The cleft in the spinal cord typically runs sagittally and extends through the spinal cord to form the two hemicords. The cleft extends for varying distances from 1 to as many as 10 vertebral segments.[64] The location of the cleft is exclusively lumbar in 47 per cent of patients, thoracolumbar in 27 per cent, exclusively thoracic in 23 per cent, and sacral or cervical in 1.5 per cent. Another cleft can be seen at more than one level with an intervening reunited cord in fewer than 1 per cent, as can multiple spurs within the same cleft.[25] The two hemicords reunite to reconstitute the single cord above and below the cleft in 91 per cent.[30] When the cleft begins in the lumbar region and extends caudally, it may split the conus, filum, and even the cauda equina.

The two hemicords are smaller than the cord above and below the point of reunion. The hemicords are of nearly equal size in 70 per cent of patients and noticeably asymmetrical in 30 per cent.[51] Each hemicord contains a dorsal and ventral horn, albeit in a disorganized form, which give rise to dorsal and ventral roots from the lateral aspect of each hemicord.[14, 29] Paramedian dorsal root may be identified near the septum, but paramedian ventral root is never present.[52] The central canal, when remaining patent rostral to the cleft, extends down to each hemicord and reunites below the cleft.[29, 51] Hydromyelia demonstrable on magnetic resonance imaging is found above or below the cleft in approximately 25 per cent of diastematomyelias.[63]

The type of splitting is not closely related to neurological symptoms and signs. Asymmetrical splitting may be associated with bilateral lower limb involvement, and the neurological deficit in the lower limb may be seen on the side of the larger rather than the smaller hemicord.[64] This suggests that intrinsic myelodysplasia is partly accountable for the pathogenesis of neurological deficits.

Vertebral Anomalies. Some form of dysraphic vertebral anomalies is always present in diastematomyelia, and the anomalies involve all elements of the vertebra.[25, 30, 52] Common anomalies of the vertebral body include hemivertebral hypoplasia or agenesis, partial or complete splitting of the bodies in the sagittal plane, a widened body with reduced thickness in the sagittal plane, a midline sagittal tract within the body, and narrowing of the intervertebral space and complete fusion of multiple segments. Anomalies of the vertebral bodies may involve multiple contiguous segments, or

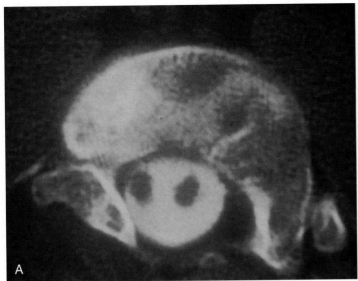

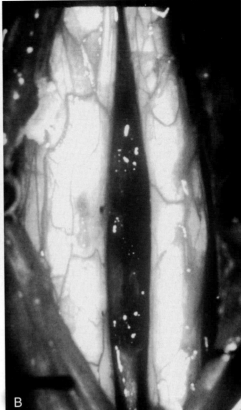

Figure 35–4

A. Contrast medium–enhanced computed tomography myelography showing diastematomyelia without median septum. Two hemicords are widely separated and enclosed by a single dural tube. *B.* Operative photograph showing a wide cleft in the spinal cord and hemicords.

a few segments may be skipped to involve more levels. In general, the severity of scoliosis correlates with the severity of the vertebral anomalies. Pang noted that severe vertebral anomalies were identified in 89 per cent of diastematomyelia patients with a median septum and in 33 per cent of diastematomyelia patients without a septum.[52]

Anomalies of the posterior vertebral elements are also common. In the neural arch, bifid lamina, a hypertrophic spinous process at the level of the diastematomyelia spur, and vertical fusion of laminae of two or more segments are seen. Anomalies of the pedicles are widening of the interpediculate distance, flattening of pedicles, and fusion of multiple segments of pedicles. Similar to the vertebral body anomalies, the incidence of the posterior element anomalies depends on the presence of the median septum; neural arch anomalies were seen in 84 per cent of diastematomyelias with a septum and in only 11 per cent of diastematomyelias without a septum.[52]

Other Congenital Anomalies. Of great significance is a high incidence of the abnormal placement of the conus medullaris in diastematomyelia, reported as 83 per cent.[25] The filum also may be thickened, exerting traction on the conus. Other associated anomalies include meningocele, myelomeningocele, lipomyelomeningocele, teratoma, and dermal sinus.

PATHOGENESIS

Although the mechanisms for neurological deterioration in diastematomyelia are not completely under-

stood, the pathogenesis is probably multifactorial, and several factors have been implicated. Herren and Edwards suggested direct pressure on the spinal cord from the septum and bone spur, a view supported by the fact that the hemicord often deviates away from the midline around the bone spur.[54] When the spur is large or scoliosis is severe, the deviation of the spinal cord becomes pronounced. Thus, in such a case the hemicord on the convex side of scoliosis may be under pressure from the median septum and spur. Tethering of the cord by the septum, a fibrous band, and a tight filum is also possible. Since ascent of the conus in relation to the vertebral column is minimal after birth, as noted in the discussion of tethered spinal cord syndrome, traction of the spinal cord with growth spurts is unlikely in patients with diastematomyelia. Rather, significant spinal cord traction is probably due to relative immobility of the spinal cord and repeat flexion-extension of the spine during vigorous physical activities.[68] Indeed, Russell and associates, reviewing 45 reported adult cases of symptomatic diastematomyelia, found the onset of neurological deterioration to follow flexion-extension injuries, strenuous exercise, and falls onto the back or buttocks in 9 cases.[71] Additional pathogenetic factors are syringomyelia and intrinsic myelodysplasia associated with diastematomyelia.[63, 64]

CLINICAL PRESENTATION

Diastematomyelia is three times more common in females than in males.[5, 23, 34, 39] The age at presentation ranges from 10 days to 76 years, with an average age of 4.3 to 6.5 years.[34, 39, 61] Most authors deny a hereditary influence because only a few case reports of familial diastematomyelia have been made.[39] In both children and adults, diastematomyelia is completely asymptomatic and is discovered as an incidental finding. Clinical manifestations of diastematomyelia are generally similar to those of other forms of occult spinal dysraphism, with presenting complaints being cutaneous abnormalities, orthopedic deformities, and neurological dysfunction. Cutaneous abnormalities are seen in as many as 71 per cent of patients, the most frequent abnormality being a hairy patch and the less frequent being nevus, dimple, meningocele, and lipoma.[36] Orthopedic syndromes include scoliosis and lower limb deformities. Scoliosis is due to associated vertebral anomalies and neurological dysfunction and tends to progress with growth spurts. Patients who have scoliosis without associated cutaneous abnormalities are often presumed to have congenital scoliosis. Thus, in such a series of patients, diastematomyelia was found to underlie scoliosis in 5 per cent.[73] Lower limb deformities include cavovarus foot, clawed toes, asymmetry in foot size and leg length, and trophic ulcerations. The neurological syndrome includes back and leg pain, muscle wasting and weakness in the leg, sensory loss, and disturbances of bladder and bowel control. Straight-leg raising may be restricted by sciatic pain, ankle and knee reflexes may be either diminished or brisk, and Babinski's response may be elicited.

Clinical onset of diastematomyelia is quite uncommon in adults, but it appears from the literature that adults predominantly present with pain and sensorimotor deficits and children present with skin lesions and foot deformities as well as sensorimotor deficits.[23, 34, 39, 52, 61] As noted earlier, in many adult patients, recognizable specific events (e.g., a blow to the back or excessive flexion-extension of back) precede the onset of neurological deterioration. In comparing diastematomyelia with and without a septum, Pang found no significant difference in the pattern and incidence of clinical manifestations between the two forms.[52]

RADIOLOGICAL INVESTIGATION

With new imaging techniques, it is possible to ascertain in exquisite detail the pathology of diastematomyelia. The purpose of investigation should be to visualize all abnormalities of the vertebra, spinal cord, median septum, and filum terminale. In the past, contrast-enhanced computed tomography myelography was the choice of investigation, but this invasive technique has largely been replaced by magnetic resonance imaging of the spine.[25] Plain spine radiographs taken before magnetic resonance imaging can help localize the site of diastematomyelia and concomitant vertebral anomalies. In patients with diastematomyelia with septum, computed tomography with three-dimensional reconstruction may be necessary to fully understand the anatomy of the bony septum and adjacent anomalies of the vertebral column (Fig. 35–5). Besides computed

tomography and magnetic resonance imaging, ultrasound has been shown to detect spinal dysraphism, and in the future, the technique may permit prenatal detection of diastematomyelia.[40]

TREATMENT

Although diastematomyelia sometimes remains completely asymptomatic, the lesion in the great majority of cases appears to produce neurological deficits.[23, 61] Guthkelch noted that of 17 children who had diastematomyelia with a septum and were initially treated conservatively 14 developed neurological symptoms later, whereas of 22 patients who received prophylactic surgery as soon as the diagnosis was established, only 1 showed deterioration (i.e., progression in scoliosis).[24] Thus, Guthkelch advocated early surgical intervention for all pediatric patients with diastematomyelia as a prophylactic measure against future neurological damage, an approach endorsed by the authors of this chapter and others.[34, 36, 39, 44] Diastematomyelia with a single dural tube was regarded as a nonsurgical lesion, but Pang advocated exploration of the cleft in the spinal cord to release the hemicord from tethering intrathecal fibrous bands.[51] In adult patients who have no symptoms despite diagnosed diastematomyelia, conservative management is appropriate.[23, 61]

Operative Procedures. When diastematomyelia is concurrent with meningocele and dermal sinus that appear more threatening clinically, the concurrent lesions should be treated first. The aim of surgery for diastematomyelia is to untether and decompress the spinal cord by removal of the median septum and adjacent dural sleeve, division of the fibrous band and thick filum tethering the cord, and reconstitution of the defect in the dorsal dural sac. The operation is performed with one of the variety of surgical techniques detailed by Meacham.[48] The patient is placed in the prone position and prepared for somatosensory evoked potential monitoring. The spinous process and lamina are exposed, with care taken to avoid inadvertent opening of the dural sac through a bifid lamina, which is often present at the level of the septum. From this point on, particularly in infants and young children, the operation proceeds with the aid of an operating microscope. Laminectomy is carried out one or two segments above and below the site of the lesion to expose the normal dural sac. The septum and surrounding dural sleeves are inspected. The lamina and spinous process at the level of the septum are often hypertrophic. Removal of the lamina begins laterally near the pedicle and continues medially toward the septum (Fig. 35–6A). The broadest attachment of the septum is most frequently dorsal, and the lamina is removed completely around a dorsal end of the septum. When fibrous bands attached to the neural arch are found, they are divided. The bony septum is freed from the dural sleeve and removed with a rongeur or a high-speed microdrill. The ventral septum is often narrow and attaches to the vertebral body via a fibrous or cartilaginous septum, enabling surgeons to avulse

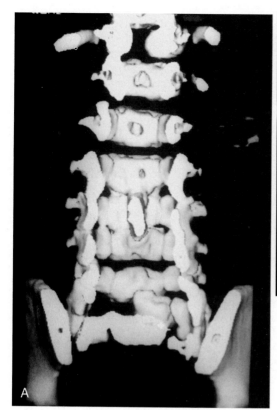

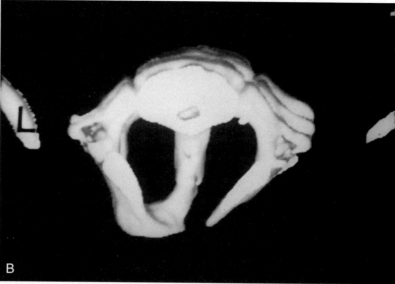

Figure 35–5

Computed tomography with three-dimensional reconstruction in an infant shows (*A*) bony septum attached to blocked lumbar vertebrae at L3–L4 ventrally and (*B*) partially hypertrophic and bifid lamina dorsally.

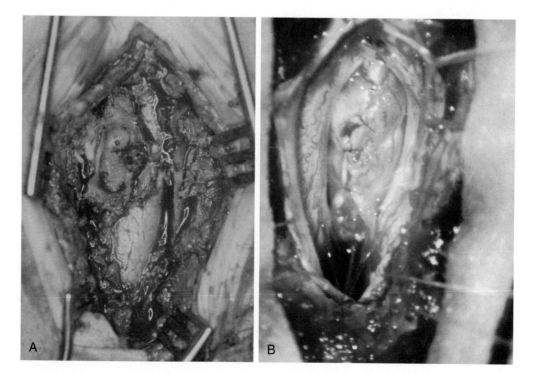

Figure 35–6

A. Operative photograph depicting bony septum and split dural sac. *B*. After resection of the bony septum and dural sleeve, hemicords were seen on each side. Note that there are no nerve roots between the hemicords. In this case, closure of the ventral dural defect was deemed safe and was performed.

the septum from the vertebral body. Excessive lateral movement of the bony septum between the dural sleeves may damage the hemicord. When the ventral attachment is broad and osseous, the septum is burred away down to the dorsal surface of the vertebral body. A brisk venous bleeding from the epidural vein is common as the ventral bony septum is removed. Once removal of the bony septum is finished, the dural sleeve is resected (see Fig. 35–6B) and any adhesions between the dura and hemicord are released. A complete resection of the dural sleeve is necessary to prevent regrowth of the bony septum. In cases in which the filum is seen in the operative field and cord tethering is suspected, the filum is divided. The dura is closed dorsally. A defect in the ventral dura, even if it is left open, does not cause a cerebrospinal fluid leak postoperatively. In cases of diastematomyelia with a single dural sac, the operation is much more straightforward: the cleft in the spinal cord is exposed, any bands or adhesions on the hemicord are released, and the dura is closed watertight.

Outcome. The reported outcome of surgery for diastematomyelia is in general excellent. As indicated by Guthkelch and others, prophylactic surgery on asymptomatic patients nearly always prevents development of neurological deterioration.[24, 34, 52] Furthermore, in patients with neurological deficits, surgery offers a good chance of diminishing the deficits. Kennedy, who reviewed 60 cases reported in the literature with sufficient details regarding the surgical outcome, noted neurological improvement in 73 per cent, no change in condition in 14 per cent, and worsening in 13 per cent.[30] Similar results were also described by others.[23, 61] The stable neurological condition achieved after the operation is likely to be sustained; in 21 patients surgically treated and followed for as many as 28 years (average follow-up, 13.7 years) Gower and co-workers reported improvement in 14 per cent, stable neurological condition 67 per cent, and worsening in 19 per cent.[75]

Neurenteric Cyst

Neurenteric cysts are rare malformations that lead to spinal cord compression or tethering. Embryologically, these cysts are derived from endoderm that is fused with the developing notochord during the third week of gestation. Although common near the cervicothoracic junction, they may be encountered anywhere from the cerebellopontine angle to the coccyx. In contrast to many congenital malformations of spinal dysraphism, clinical symptoms of neurenteric cysts may not be seen until the fourth or fifth decade of life. Magnetic resonance imaging has increased the diagnostic sensitivity for neurenteric cysts and facilitates surgical planning.

EMBRYOLOGY

Beginning on gestational day 15, gastrulation initiates the complex tissue migration that converts the early bilaminar embryo into three layers. The primitive streak begins as a thickening of the superficial ectoderm, which deepens rostrally to form Hensen's node or the primitive knot. Groove formation along the length of the primitive streak further deepens at Hensen's node to direct surface cell interposition between the ectoderm and endoderm to form paraxial mesoderm. Further surface cell migration cephalad between the mantles of paraxial mesoderm and the endoderm forms the notochordal process. Extension of the notochord is limited by the prochordal plate and caudad by the cloacal membrane.

The notochord begins as a solid core of cells, but cavitation extending from the primitive pit forms the notochordal canal. During intercalation, the notochordal process fuses with the ventral endoderm, opening this canal into the yolk sac. On gestation day 17 the neurenteric canal of Kovalevsky penetrates from Hensen's node through each cell layer, communicating the amniotic cavity to the inner yolk sac. This transient channel is closed during excalation with infolding of the notochordal plate in a cranial-to-caudal direction. The endoderm is reconstituted as a continuous cell layer, and the notochord becomes a solid core of tissue that induces formation of the neural plate and the vertebral bodies. With continued embryo growth, Hensen's node and the primitive streak are displaced caudad toward the sacrococcygeal region.[10] The superficial ectoderm is destined to form spinal cord and skin, whereas endoderm ultimately matures into the gastrointestinal and respiratory tracts. A remnant of the notochord persists as the nucleus pulposus of the disc space.

Several hypotheses concern the embryonic origin of neurenteric cysts. Common to all theories is that the cyst arises from a disorder of notochord formation. Incomplete excalation maintains the neurenteric canal with sagittal splitting of the notochord, explaining the common relationship of neurenteric cysts and diastematomyelia.[42] A dorsal intestinal fistula formation extends from the intestinal tract to the skin through a vertebral body defect, diplomyelia, and posterior spina bifida. In extreme cases, splitting of the spine, imperforate anus, and intestinal prolapse may occur.[57] Bremer has proposed ectopic or accessory neurenteric canals to explain dorsal fistula at locations cephalad to the coccyx.[60]

Partial obliteration of the neurenteric canal with incomplete variance of enteric fistula explains the spectrum of neurenteric cysts encountered clinically. Persistence of the anterior communication from the yolk sac into the developing spinal canal would maintain mucosa-lined tracts from the mediastinum or abdominal cavity through vertebral body defects.[2] Intradural, extramedullary cysts with or without spina bifida would develop from dorsal remnants of the neurenteric canal.[41] Focal segments of the neurenteric canal may persist, explaining anterior medullary or cerebellopontine angle cysts without accompanying vertebral or skull bone malformation.[15]

Other embryogenic theories include focal adhesions between the endoderm and ectoderm within the primitive streak. In this case, notochord development would be shifted, with disorganized induction of the spinal cord and vertebral bodies.[15, 49] Adhesions would prevent normal notochord invagination, interrupting mesoderm migration and development and leading to bladder exstrophy.[31] Visceral anomalies include enteric cysts, diverticula, adhesions, and fistulas.[1]

CLINICAL PRESENTATION

Neurenteric cysts present at any age from newborn to the fifth decade; there is a three-to-two male predominance. The malformations of the split notochord syndrome have been diagnosed prenatally by ultrasound and are apparent at birth; the complex association of intestinal protrusion, cloacal/bladder exstrophy, and renal dysgenesis may be fatal.[31, 57] Mediastinal and intra-abdominal cysts are usually symptomatic during the first decade of life; symptoms may include abdominal distention, dyspnea, hoarseness, and chronic pulmonary infection with partial bronchus obstruction. Children frequently present to a pediatric surgeon for evaluation of an abdominal mass or imperforate anus.[2]

The presentation of intraspinal cysts is more common during adulthood. The symptoms of spinal cord or nerve root compression may mimic other space-occupying lesions of the spinal canal, including disc herniation. Pain is the most common symptom and localizes to the spinal level of the malformation. When a long history of episodic paresis and dysesthesia is elicited, multiple sclerosis is considered in the differential diagnosis. Bacterial meningitis can occur when neurenteric cysts are accompanied by dorsal sinus tracts, whereas inflammation of the cerebrospinal fluid from contact with cyst contents is unusual. Fourth ventricular or cerebellopontine angle cysts may present as symptoms of increased intracranial pressure from ventricular obstruction and hydrocephalus.

In Agnoli and associates' review of 32 published cases of neurenteric cysts, the average patient age was 24 years and males outnumbered females 2.3 to 1.[20] The most common cyst location was cervical intradural extramedullary, followed by masses at the level of the conus medullaris. An intramedullary mass was encountered in only four cases. Neurological examination in each case revealed spastic paresis.

RADIOLOGICAL INVESTIGATION

Plain radiographs of the spine demonstrate spina bifida; a widened or split spinal canal; vertebral body defects, including block or hemivertebrae; vertebral bifurcation; and diastematomyelia. When the condition is accompanied by a mediastinal or intestinal enteric cyst, chest or abdominal radiographs reveal displacement of the bowel or a shift of the mediastinal contents. Fine-section axial computed tomography after intrathecal administration of contrast medium shows intradural extramedullary cysts and the spectrum of bone malformations. Magnetic resonance imaging has be-

come the study of choice for evaluating neurenteric cysts (Fig. 35–7).[11, 12, 49] The lobulated intradural extramedullary cysts are isointense or slightly hyperintense on T1-weighted images and slightly hyperintense with T2-weighted sequencing. The cyst wall does not enhance after gadolinium injection. Communication between mediastinal or intestinal cysts through a vertebral body defect into the spinal canal can be demonstrated with computed tomography or magnetic resonance imaging.

TREATMENT

Operative Procedure. Despite the ventral location of neurenteric cysts, a laminectomy is the surgical approach of choice. A wide posterior decompression directly exposes cysts located dorsal to the spinal cord. Exposure of thoracic cysts may require a costotransversectomy. The cyst is needle-punctured, and mucinous, viscous fluid is drained; rarely, calcification in the cyst wall is seen.[1, 15, 49] With collapse of the cyst, the walls are dissected free of the spinal cord with microsurgical techniques. Section of the denticulate ligaments affords access to cysts located ventral to the cord. Intraoperative ultrasound is a useful adjunct for localization of anterior or intramedullary cysts and guides the extent of resection. Access to cysts within the cerebellopontine angle or fourth ventricle is through midline or retromastoid posterior fossa craniectomy. Anterior dural defects are plugged with muscle or directly sutured.

The cyst is composed of a thick fibrous capsule lined by epithelium varying from cuboidal to columnar and pseudostratified; regions of ciliated epithelium are common. Periodic acid–Schiff staining highlights glycogen and mucinous deposits. A positive reaction may be observed on carcinoembryonic antigen immunohistochemical staining, and electron microscopy demonstrates microvilli and junctional complexes.[49]

Outcome. The prognosis after cord decompression in patients is excellent, and nearly all patients have diminished weakness and pain or recovery of neurological function.[1] Associated malformations in children with neurenteric cysts may be life-threatening or require long-term follow-up with multiple specialists. Although cyst recurrence is extremely unusual, periodical repeat magnetic resonance imaging is warranted with incomplete resection.

Spinal Dermal Sinus

Congenital spinal dermal sinus is an innocuous-appearing form of spinal dysraphism that can nevertheless produce significant morbidity if not managed in an appropriate fashion. Walker and Bucy introduced the term "congenital spinal dermal sinus" in 1934, although this entity was previously described by Verebely in 1913 and Moise in 1926.[50, 58, 65] The skin manifestation of a dermal sinus always consists of a hairline

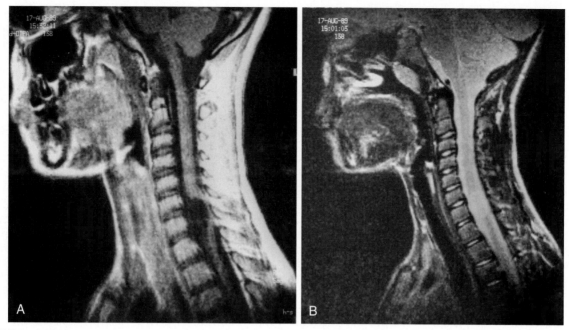

Figure 35–7

Neurenteric cyst typically situated ventral to the spinal cord appears hyperintense on both the T1-weighted (*A*) and the T2-weighted (*B*) magnetic resonance images. (Courtesy of Benjamin Lee, M.D., St. Louis Children's Hospital.)

ostium in the midline neuraxis. This skin defect represents the superficial stoma of an epithelium-lined tract that may extend into the intraspinal neural elements and provides an avenue for ingress of bacteria, leading to recurrent bacterial meningitis. In addition, epidermoid or dermoid cysts may accompany a dermal sinus.

PATHOLOGY

The appearance of the ostium of a dermal sinus is variable, and the stoma may be obscured by a hairy patch or skin nevus (Fig. 35–8A).[13, 74] The sinus tract itself is composed of a stratified squamous epithelial tube encased in dermal tissue. Repeated infections can disrupt this histological pattern.[13] In 6 to 7 per cent of the cases, the tract reportedly terminates dorsal to the spinal elements; in 10 to 20 per cent, it terminates in the extradural space, and 58 to 60 per cent of dermal sinuses terminate in the intradural space.[18] Approximately half of dermal sinuses display inclusion tumors along their course, which are epidermoid (see Fig. 35–8B), dermoid, or teratoma.[4] Dermoid and epidermoid tumors account for 83 per cent and 13 per cent of these tumors, respectively.[4, 9] Teratoma is rare and derives from each layer of the trilaminar embryo; it displays an age-related propensity toward malignant degeneration. Many thoracic dermal sinuses terminate in a mass of neuroglial tissue.[18, 74] A dermal sinus may be part of another spinal dysraphism (e.g., diastematomyelia, lipomyelomeningocele, tethered cord, or myelomeningocele).[4, 18]

CLINICAL PRESENTATION

The incidence of dermal sinus appears to be approximately 1 in 2,500 live births.[46, 58] French reported 13

per cent of dermal sinuses as occurring below the sacrococcygeal junction, 35 per cent in the lumbosacral junction, 41 per cent in the lumbar region, 10 per cent in the thoracic region, and 1 per cent in the cervical region.[17] However, dermal sinuses reported below the sacrococcygeal junction would have been sacrococcygeal dimples, which are seen in 2 to 4 per cent of newborns and almost invariably have no connection with intraspinal structures.[65]

About 75 per cent of patients present with symptoms attributable to the involvement of the central nervous system. Meningitis is the cause of presentation in 36 to 40 per cent of cases. Meningitis that is secondary to infection with multiple organisms and recurs despite successful antibiotic treatments should raise the suspicion of a dermal sinus. *Escherichia coli* and *Staphylococcus aureus* are the most frequently isolated pathogens. Almost half of the cases of meningitis from spinal dermal sinus are due to gram-negative organisms.[18, 74] *S. aureus* is the most common pathogen in meningitis from intracranial dermal sinuses.

Many inclusion tumors associated with dermal sinuses are asymptomatic, and some epidermoids and dermoids are discovered in evaluation of cord or cauda equina compression. The slow growth rate of these benign tumors results in late presentation after months or years of waxing and waning symptoms of neurological compromise. Thus, neurological deficits secondary to a tumor lead to a diagnosis of dermal sinus in approximately 47 per cent of patients older than 6 years of age but only 14 per cent of patients younger than 5 years of age. Nineteen per cent of patients displayed evidence of both tumor and infection; patients with infected inclusion tumors may exhibit rapid neurological worsening.[18, 22] Some patients may present with complaints of drainage of purulent material from

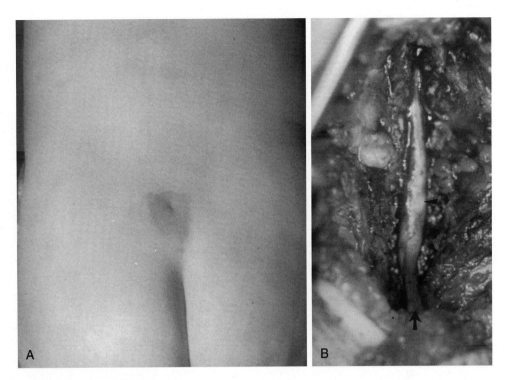

Figure 35–8

A. A skin dimple and nevus in the midline lumbar region of an infant. *B.* The dimple was connected to an extradural epidermoid tumor (*arrow*) by a sinus tract running cephalad (*arrowhead*).

the sinus tract. Although this drainage may represent a localized and superficial process, it may precede the onset of meningitis or intradural abscess.[4, 18, 69, 74]

Dermal sinus in the cervical region may track through the foramen magnum and enter the posterior fossa.[74] More important is that the cervical dermal sinus may accompany a posterior fossa dermoid or epidermoid tumor (Fig. 35–9).

Dermal sinuses in the sacrococcygeal region are often difficult to differentiate from pilonidal sinuses. Most authors consider pilonidal sinuses an acquired lesion of local inflammation and granulomatous response secondary to aberrant intracutaneous hair growth.[4, 13] Others, however, maintain that pilonidal sinuses are congenital lesions involving secondary infection of dermal sinuses or dermal rests of cells.[27, 56] Definitive classification may be difficult; however, the presence of intraspinal extension of the lesion should be ruled out.

DIAGNOSIS

All dermal sinuses located above the sacrococcygeal junction require thorough evaluation, including radiological investigation. In general, a sacrococcygeal dimple requires no investigation other than physical examination. Attempts to determine the nature of the tract by insertion of a probe into the ostium, which was frequently done previously, is discouraged, owing to a very low chance that it will yield diagnostic information and because of the significant risk of introducing bacteria into the intradural space. Likewise, contrast medium should not be injected into the tract for diagnostic purposes. Plain spine radiographs may reveal associated dysraphic changes.[74] In infants, ultrasound can be used to define not only the subcutaneous sinus

tract but also associated intraspinal dermoids and epidermoids.[65] In the past, contrast computed tomography myelography was widely employed, but this diagnostic modality has been replaced by magnetic resonance imaging.[6] Magnetic resonance imaging accurately depicts the extraspinal portion of the sinus tract and intramedullary tumors as well as allowing visualization of the cord for signs of cord tethering. Standard spin-echo magnetic resonance imaging sequences, however, do not reliably delineate an extramedullary tumor or the intraspinal extension of the sinus tract.[6] Consequently, in some patients, computed tomography myelography or ultrasound may be needed for complete preoperative evaluation.

SURGICAL TREATMENT

Given the high risk of infection and the significant morbidity associated with meningitis or infected inclusion tumors, all dermal sinuses located rostral to the sacrococcygeal region should be excised without undue delay irrespective of findings obtained on radiological studies.[13, 74] Excision should be complete, including removal of all intraspinal portions. Appropriate surgical intervention therefore requires provision for intradural and rostral extension of the resection bed.

Most authors agree with preoperative and postoperative prophylactic antibiotic treatment. Any sinus drainage should be cultured before initiation of antibiotic treatment. Recent meningitis and other overt infections mandate aggressive antibiotic therapy.[18, 74] Surgery should be delayed until overt infection is cleared unless urgent decompression is required. Morbidity from resection of a dermal sinus is low.

Preparations are made to extend the laminectomy

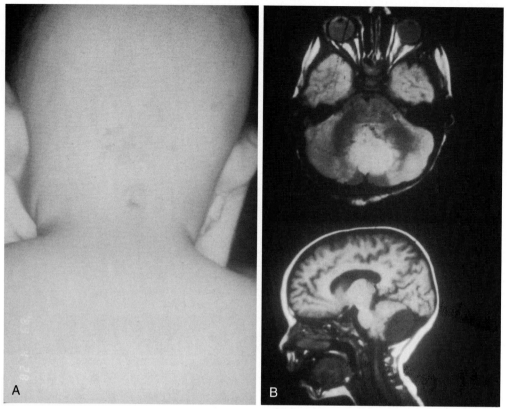

Figure 35–9

A child with a skin dimple and surrounding nevus in the cervical region (*A*) had a cerebellar dermoid tumor seen on magnetic resonance imaging (*B*).

rostrally. A skin incision is made around the ostium of the dermal sinus, and the sinus tract extending below the skin and passing through the dysraphic lamina or interlaminar space is preserved. The lamina involved by the sinus tract is removed, and then extradural elements are inspected. Sometimes, the sinus tract ends in dura without intradural extension (Fig. 35–10), and this needs to be confirmed by a dural opening. Epider-

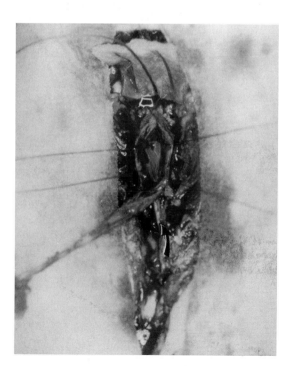

Figure 35–10

A skin dimple over the lower sacrum was attached to the bottom of the dural sac in an infant who presented with bouts of gram-negative meningitis. The filum terminale passes the dural sac and attaches to the lower sacrum (*arrow*).

moid may be present exclusively in the extradural space. The sinus tract extending intradurally may be connected to the filum and may result in thickened filum. In such cases, a tethered cord is often demonstrated by preoperative magnetic resonance imaging, and only a sectioning of the thickened filum is needed. If intradural inclusion tumors have been confirmed by magnetic resonance imaging, the laminectomy is extended to expose and remove the entire tumor. The tumor may be adherent to the filum and nerve roots in patients with prior meningitis, but in general it is easily freed from the neural elements. Multiple inclusion tumors with intervening normal cauda equina may be present. The importance of total removal of dermoid or epidermoid tumors at the first operation cannot be overemphasized, since infected tumors cause recurrent meningitis and total removal of recurrent tumors is nearly impossible. After tumor removal, the dura is closed in a watertight fashion.

Spinal Meningocele

POSTERIOR MENINGOCELE

A spinal meningocele is an unusual herniation of meninges through a defect of the posterior spinal arch. The most common location for these soft, noncompressible cutaneous lesions is lumbar or lumbosacral. Meningoceles are covered by full or partial thickness, and adjacent cutaneous defects may include meningocele manque, dimples, or hemangiomas. In contrast to myelocystocele, lipomyelomeningocele, or sacrococcygeal teratoma, transillumination is brilliant. There is a slight female predominance, and many children have normal neurological function. Spinal cord tethering is rare with simple meningocele but common when an associated dysraphic malformation such as a spinal lipoma, diastematomyelia, or thickened filum terminale is present. Patients with spinal meningocele rarely have hydrocephalus or Chiari malformation.

The anatomy of the spinal cord within the spinal canal is normal, and the cord rests on its ventral surface. Nerve roots of the cauda equina may, however, float within the cerebrospinal fluid sac. Plain spine films demonstrate a widened spinal canal limited to the level of the defect. Magnetic resonance imaging is the imaging technique of choice, as it accurately demonstrates normal intraspinal anatomy or associated bony or spinal malformations.

Meningocele repair is recommended at the time of diagnosis in infancy to prevent sac injury, cerebrospinal fluid leak, or infection. The child is positioned prone upon lateral padded rolls. A midline skin incision is made above or below the cutaneous lesion, and normal paraspinal muscle fascia is identified. The neck of the sac and the fascia defect are then circumferentially dissected, and the skin incision is extended for full exposure. The paraspinal muscles are then elevated lateral from the sac, allowing careful opening into the subarachnoid space. Using loupe or microscopy magni-

fication, an intradural exploration is completed, with careful inspection for entrapped nerve roots. The dura is closed with a running monofilament suture, and the muscle fascia defect is reapproximated. Skin closure is performed in two layers.

ANTERIOR SACRAL MENINGOCELE

An anterior sacral meningocele is a cystic meningeal herniation that passes ventrally through a bony sacral defect. In contrast to simple meningoceles, no cutaneous evidence of a sacral meningocele is observed; the coccygeal or sacral defect may be palpable during rectal examination. There is a nine-to-one female-to-male predominance, and initial diagnosis following pelvic ultrasound during pregnancy is very common. Presenting symptoms include chronic constipation, abdominal mass or fullness, recurrent urinary obstruction, and dysmenorrhea. Nearly all patients have normal results on neurological examination.

Plain spine films reveal the scimitar sign, a sickle-shaped bony sacral defect. Ultrasound demonstrates a fluid-filled mass separate from adjacent pelvic organs. Computed tomography myelography most accurately demonstrates the relationship of the sac and the communication from the spinal subarachnoid space. Magnetic resonance imaging demonstrates the relationships of the meningocele with the pelvic organs in three dimensions and may reveal associated malformations, including pelvic teratoma or hamartoma, spinal lipoma, or dermoid inclusion cysts.

Cyst aspiration or drainage should never be attempted by any route because of the risks of meningitis and death. There is a high mortality rate at labor from pelvic obstruction, infection, or cyst rupture. When this meningocele is diagnosed during pregnancy, elective delivery of the child by cesarean section on maturity of fetal pulmonary indices is recommended. Elective surgical management requires sacral laminectomy and intradural exploration to expose the anterior communication with the meningocele; it is rare that nerve roots herniate into the sac. The walls of the meningocele collapse after aspiration of cerebrospinal fluid from the sac. The defect is closed with a primary suture repair or obliterated with a fascia graft. Autologous fibrin glue may be useful to help secure a watertight closure. A transabdominal surgical approach is necessary when a solid-tissue mass lies within the meningocele sac. Postoperative ultrasound or magnetic resonance imaging is recommended to monitor any persistent cerebrospinal fluid within the meningocele sac.

REFERENCES

1. Agnoli, A. L., Laun, A., and Schonmayr, R.: Enterogenous intraspinal cysts. J. Neurosurg., 61:834–840, 1984.
2. Alrabeeah, A., Gillis, D. A., Giacomantonio, M., et al.: Neurenteric cysts: A spectrum. J. Pediatr. Surg., 23:752–754, 1988.
3. Anderson, F. M.: Occult spinal dysraphism: Diagnosis and management. J. Pediatr., 73:163–177, 1968.

4. Bale, P. M.: Sacrococcygeal developmental abnormalities and tumors in children. Perspect. Pediatr. Pathol., *1*:9–56, 1984.

5. Banna, M.: Syringomyelia in association with posterior fossa cysts. A. J. N. R., *9*:867–873, 1988.

6. Barkovich, A. J., Edwards, M. S., and Cogen, P. H.: MR evaluation of sinal dermal sinus tracts in children. A. J. N. R., *12*:123–129, 1991.

7. Barson, A. J.: The vertebral level of termination of the spinal cord during normal and abnormal development. J. Anat., *106*:489–497, 1970.

8. Bentley, J. F., and Smith, J. R.: Developmental posterior enteric remnants and spinal malformations. Arch. Dis. Child., *35*:76–86, 1960.

9. Black, S. P., and German, W. J.: Four congenital tumors found at operation within the vertebral canal: With observations on their incidence. J. Neurosurg., *7*:49–61, 1950.

10. Bremer, J. L.: Dorsal intestinal fistula; accessory neurenteric canal; diastematomyelia. Arch. Pathol., *54*:132–138, 1952.

11. Brooks, B. S., Duvall, E. R., el Gammal, T., et al.: Neuroimaging features of neurenteric cysts: Analysis of nine cases and review of the literature. A. J. N. R., *14*:735–746, 1993.

12. Brunberg, J. A., Latchaw, R. E., Kanal, E., et al.: Magnetic resonance imaging of spinal dysraphism. Radiol. Clin. North Am., *26*:181–205, 1986.

13. Cheek, W. R., and Laurent, J. P.: Dermal sinus tracts. Concepts Pediatr. Neurosurg., *6*:63–75, 1985.

14. Cohen, J., and Sledge, C. B.: Diastematomyelia. Am. J. Dis. Child., *100*:257–263, 1960.

15. D'Almeida, A. C., and Stewart, D. H.: Neurenteric cyst: Case report and literature review. Neurosurgery, *8*:596–599, 1981.

16. Dale, A. J.: Diastematomyelia. Arch. Neurol., *20*:309–317, 1969.

17. Flanigan, R. C., Russell, D. P., and Walsh, J. W.: Urologic aspects of tethered cord. Urology, *33*:80–82, 1989.

18. French, B. N.: Midline fusion defects and defects of formation. *In* Youmans, J. R., ed.: Neurological Surgery. 3rd ed. Philadelphia, W. B. Saunders, 1990, pp. 1081–1235.

19. Fukui, J., and Kakizaki, T.: Urodynamic evaluation of tethered cord syndrome including tight filum terminale. Urology, *16*:539–552, 1980.

20. Garceau, G. J.: The filum terminale syndrome (the cord-traction syndrome). J. Bone Joint Surg., *35*:711–716, 1953.

21. Gardner, W. J.: Diastematomyelia and the Klippel-Feil syndrome. Cleve. Clin. Q., *31*:19–44, 1964.

22. Gindi, S. E., and Fairburn, B.: Case reports and technical notes: Intramedullary spinal abscess as a complication of a congenital dermal sinus: Case report. J. Neurosurg., *30*:494–497, 1969.

23. Gower, D. J., Del Curling, O., Kelly, D. L., et al.: Diastematomyelia: A 40-year experience. Pediatr. Neurosci., *14*:90–96, 1988.

24. Guthkelch, A. N.: Diastematomyelia with median septum. Brain, *97*:729–742, 1974.

25. Harwood-Nash, D. C., and McHugh, K.: Diastematomyelia in 172 children: The impact of modern neuroradiology. Pediatr. Neurosurg., *16*:247–251, 1990.

26. Hawass, N. D., El-Badawi, M. G., Fatani, J. A., et al.: Myelographic study of the spinal cord ascent during fetal development. A. J. N. R., *8*:691–695, 1987.

27. Haworth, J. C., and Zachary, R. B.: Congenital dermal sinuses in children: Their relation to pilonidal sinuses. Lancet, *2*:10–14, 1955.

28. Hendrick, E. B., Hoffman, H. J., and Humphreys, R. P.: The tethered spinal cord. Clin. Neurosurg., *30*:457–463, 1983.

29. Herren, R. Y., and Edwards, J. E.: Diplomyelia (duplication of the spinal cord). Arch. Pathol., *30*:1203–1214, 1940.

30. Hilal, S. K., Marton, D., and Pollack, E.: Diastematomyelia in children. Radiology, *112*:609–621, 1974.

31. Hoffman, C. H., Dietrich, R. B., Pais, M. J., et al.: The split notochord syndrome with dorsal enteric fistula. A. J. N. R., *14*:622–627, 1993.

32. Hoffman, H. J., Hendrick, E. B., and Humphreys, R. P.: The tethered spinal cord: Its protean manifestations, diagnosis, and surgical correction. Childs Brain, *2*:145–155, 1976.

33. Hori, A., Fischer, G., Dietrich-Schott, B., et al.: Dimyelia, diplomyelia, and diastematomyelia. Clin. Neuropathol., *1*:23–30, 1982.

34. Humphreys, R. P., Hendrick, E. B., and Hoffman, H. J.: Diastematomyelia. Clin. Neurosurg., *30*:436–456, 1983.

35. James, C. C., and Lassman, L. P.: Spinal dysraphism: The diagnosis and treatment of progressive lesions in spina bifida occulta. J. Bone Joint Surg. [Br.], *44*:828–840, 1962.

36. James, C. C., and Lassman, L. P.: Diastematomyelia: A critical survey of 24 cases submitted to laminectomy. Arch. Dis. Child., *39*:125–130, 1964.

37. Jones, P. H.: Tight filum terminale. Arch. Surg., *73*:556–566, 1956.

38. Kang, J. K., and Kim, M. C.: Effects of tethering on regional spinal cord blood flow and sensory-evoked potentials in growing cats. Childs Nerv. Syst., *3*:35–39, 1987.

39. Kennedy, P. R.: New data on diastematomyelia. J. Neurosurg., *51*:355–361, 1979.

40. Korsvik, H. E., and Keller, M. S.: Sonography of occult dysraphism in neonates and infants with MR imaging correlation. Radiographics, *12*:297–306, 1992.

41. Macdonald, R. L., Schwartz, M. L., and Lewis, A. J.: Neurenteric cyst located dorsal to the cervical spine: Case report. Neurosurgery, *28*:583–588, 1991.

42. Mann, K. S., Khosla, V. K., Gulati, D. R., et al.: Spinal neurenteric cyst: Association with vertebral anomalies, diastematomyelia, dorsal fistula, and lipoma. Surg. Neurol., *21*:358–362, 1984.

43. Mathern, G. W., and Peacock, W. J.: Diastematomyelia. *In* Park, T. S., ed.: Contemporary Issues in Neurological Surgery: Spinal Dysraphism. Oxford, Blackwell Scientific, 1992, pp. 91–103.

44. Matson, D. D.: Neurosurgery of Infancy and Childhood. Springfield, Charles C Thomas, 1969, pp. 84–95.

45. Matson, D. D., Woods, R. P., Campbell, J. B., et al.: Diastematomyelia (congenital clefts of the spinal cord): Diagnosis and surgical treatment. Pediatrics, *6*:98–112, 1950.

46. McIntosh, R., Merritt, K., Richards, M. R., et al.: The incidence of congenital malformations: A study of 5,964 pregnancies. Pediatrics, *14*:505–521, 1954.

47. McLendon, R. E., Oakes, W. J., Heinz, E. R., et al.: Adipose tissue in the filum terminale: A computed tomographic finding that may indicate tethering of the spinal cord. Neurosurgery, *22*:873–876, 1988.

48. Meacham, W. F.: Surgical treatment of diastematomyelia. J. Neurosurg., *27*:78–85, 1967.

49. Miyagi, K., Mukawa, J., Merkaru, S., et al.: Enterogenous cyst in the cervical spinal canal: Case report. J. Neurosurg., *68*:292–296, 1988.

50. Moise, T. S.: *Staphylococcus* meningitis secondary to a congenital sacral sinus: With remarks on the pathogenesis of sacrococcygeal fistula. Surg. Gynecol. Obstet., *42*:394–397, 1926.

51. Naidich, T. P., and Harwood-Nash, D. C.: Diastematomyelia: Hemicord and meningeal sheaths; single and double arachnoid and dural tubes. A. J. N. R., *4*:633–636, 1983.

52. Pang, D.: Split cord malformation: II. Clinical syndrome. Neurosurgery, *31*:481–500, 1992.

53. Pang, D., and Casey, K.: Use of an anal sphincter pressure monitor during operations on the sacral spinal cord and nerve roots. Neurosurgery, *13*:562–568, 1983.

54. Pang, D., Dias, M. S., and Ahab-Barmada, M.: Split cord malformation: I. A unified theory of embryogenesis for double spinal cord malformations. Neurosurgery, *31*:451–480, 1992.

55. Pang, D., and Wilberger, J. E.: Tethered cord syndrome in adults. J. Neurosurg., *57*:32–47, 1982.

56. Patey, D. H., and Scarff, R. W.: Pathology of postanal pilonidal sinus: Its bearing on treatment. Lancet, *2*:484–486, 1946.

57. Pathak, V. B., Singh, S., and Wakhu, A. K.: Double split of notochord with massive prolapse of the gut. J. Pediatr. Surg., *23*:1039–1004, 1988.

58. Powell, K. R., Cherry, J. D., Hougen, T. J., et al.: A prospective search for congenital dermal abnormalities of the craniospinal axis. J. Pediatr., *87*:744–750, 1975.

59. Purtzer, T. J., Yamada, S., and Tani, S.: Metabolic and histologic studies of chronic model of tethered cord. Surg. Forum, *36*:512–514, 1985.

60. Reimann, A. F., and Anson, B. J.: Vertebral level of termination of the spinal cord with report of a case of sacral cord. Anat. Rec., *88*:127–138, 1944.

61. Russell, N. A., Benoit, B. G., and Joaquin, A. J.: Diastematomyelia in adults [Abstract]. Pediatr. Neurosurg., *16*:252–257, 1990.

62. Sarwar, M., Crelin, E. S., Kier, E. L., et al.: Experimental cord stretchability and the tethered cord syndrome. A. J. N. R., *4*:641–643, 1983.

63. Schlesinger, A. E., Naidich, T. P., and Quencer, R. M.: Concurrent hydromyelia and diastematomyelia. A. J. N. R., 7:473–477, 1986.
64. Scotti, G., Musgrave, M. A., Harwood-Nash, D. C., et al.: Diastematomyelia in children: Metrizamide and CT metrizamide myelography. A. J. R., 135:1225–1232, 1980.
65. Storrs, B. B., and Walker, M. L.: Sacral dermal sinus: Occult sacral masses discovered by routine ultrasound. Concepts Pediatr. Neurosurg., 7:172–178, 1987.
66. Streeter, G. L.: Factors involved in the formation of the filum terminale. Am. J. Anat., 25:1–11, 1919.
67. Tani, S., Yamada, S., and Knighton, R. S.: Extensibility of the lumbar and sacral cord. J. Neurosurg., 66:116–123, 1987.
68. Till, K.: Spinal dysraphism: A study of congenital malformations of the lower back. J. Bone Joint Surg. [Br.], 51:415–422, 1969.
69. Venger, B., Laurent, J. P., Cheek, W. R., et al.: Congenital thoracic dermal sinus tracts. Concepts Pediatr. Neurosurg., 9:161–172, 1989.
70. Verebely, T. V.: Ein Foll von intraverteholer Dermoidzyte. Virchows Arch. Pathol. Anat., 213:541–544, 1913.

71. Walker, A. E., and Bucy, P. C.: Congenital dermal sinuses: A source of spinal meningeal infection and subdural abscesses. Brain, 57:401–421, 1934.
72. Wilson, D. A., and Prince, J. R.: MR imaging determination of the location of the normal conus medullaris throughout childhood. A. J. N. R., 10:258–262, 1989.
73. Wilson, D. A., and Prince, J. R.: MR imaging determination of the location of the normal conus medullaris throughout childhood. A. J. N. R., 10:259–262, 1989.
74. Wright, R. L.: Congenital dermal sinuses. Progr. Neurol. Surg., 4:175–191, 1971.
75. Yamada, S.: Tethered spinal cord: Pathophysiology and management. In Park, T. S., ed.: Spinal Dysraphism. Oxford, Blackwell Scientific, 1992, pp. 74–90.
76. Yamada, S., Zinke, D. E., and Sanders, D.: Pathophysiology of "tethered cord syndrome." J. Neurosurg., 54:494–503, 1981.
77. Yamada, S., Knierim, D., Yonekura, M., et al.: Tethered cord syndrome. J. Am. Paraplegia Soc., 6(3):58–61, 1983.

Hydrocephalus in Childhood

Enclosed in a bony structure that is noncompliant over a short period of time, the central nervous system can be divided into three components: the parenchyma, fluids, and the vascular system.

The cerebral parenchyma is composed of both neural and glial cells. Although it is incompressible, the parenchymal volume can increase through cellular multiplication or can decrease through cellular destruction due to various mechanisms.

The vascular system is the only system open to the "outside" via the carotid and vertebral arteries and the jugular veins. It is compressible and therefore susceptible to rapid changes in volume.

The fluids of the central nervous system are of two types: cerebrospinal fluid and extracellular fluid. Both originate from the vascular system, both are resorbed in the vascular system. The two circulations maintain a constant relation through the ependymal wall and the perivascular spaces.[236]

In this environment, hydrocephalus is defined as a hydrodynamic disorder of the cerebrospinal fluid that leads to an increase in the volume occupied by this fluid in the central nervous system.*

In addition to hydrocephalus, conditions such as cerebral atrophy and focal destructive lesions also lead to an abnormal increase in fluid volume. In these conditions, a loss of cerebral tissue leaves vacant space that is passively filled with cerebrospinal fluid. Such situations are not the result of a hydrodynamic disorder and therefore are not classified as hydrocephalus, even if etymologically they indeed are.

The incidence of hydrocephalus is not exactly known, and it most probably varies according to the health care situation in each country. The incidence of 3 cases per 1,000 live births, which is generally reported, concerns only congenital hydrocephalus cases and does not reflect the incidence of acquired cerebrospinal fluid hydrodynamic disturbances. Based on the commercial data available, there are about 80,000 to 100,000 shunts implanted each year in the developed countries. Little information is available for the other countries; it is probable that in these countries many patients still do not receive treatment. The incidence of human hydrocephalus presents a bimodal curve, with one peak in infancy, related to the various forms of congenital malformations, and another peak during the adult years, mostly related to so-called normal-pressure hydrocephalus. Adult hydrocephalus represents approximately 40 per cent of the total cases of hydrocephalus. In children, the revision rate for a valve is 1.5 to 2.5, that is, a child will need an average of 1.5 to 2.5 additional valves to replace or to add to the first valve implanted. Taking these figures into account, the number of "new" hydrocephalic patients in the pediatric population treated each year could be estimated at 15,000 to 25,000. These figures remained stable or slightly decreased in the 1980's; a more pronounced reduction seems to be appearing in this decade.

Physiology

Under normal conditions, cerebrospinal fluid is produced mainly by a process of ultrafiltration at the level of the nontight junction of the capillary endothelial wall of the choroid plexus.* The resulting fluid is secreted into the ventricles by the choroidal epithelium. Sodium-potassium adenosine triphosphatase in the apical membrane of the choroidal epithelial cell plays a key role in cerebrospinal fluid formation.[219, 289, 306] The choroid plexus forms a true blood-fluid barrier; even

---

*See references 18, 73, 84, 130, 265, and 266.

*See references 29, 181, 187, 218, and 238.

C. Sainte-Rose

under extreme conditions sodium, potassium, calcium, and chloride concentrations remain constant in the cerebrospinal fluid.[156, 181] The fluid secretion rate, investigated in different species, appears to be continuous and stable under normal conditions. This rate of secretion is proportional to the weight of the choroid plexus. In most adult mammals, the choroid plexus constitutes approximately 0.25 per cent of brain weight, which represents 2 to 3 g of choroid plexus in humans. The secretion rate is approximately 21 mL per hour in childhood and adulthood.* There are no specific data concerning the neonatal period.[316] In this age group, the choroid plexus is relatively bigger than it is later in life. In addition to producing cerebrospinal fluid, the choroid plexus is responsible for the active transportation of folates, vitamin C, vitamin B₆, and deoxyribonucleosides.[281] It also plays an important role in cerebrospinal fluid purification, both by active resorption mechanisms (i.e., inorganic ions, drugs, or neuromediator metabolites) and by the passive transportation of metabolic wastes and macromolecules.[156] The cerebrospinal fluid secretion rate is not influenced by acute variations of intracranial pressure within normal physiological limits, but chronic increases in pressure, such as those that occur in hydrocephalus, apparently reduce cerebrospinal fluid formation and may result in atrophy of the choroid plexus. Since cerebrospinal fluid formation is an active phenomenon, it is modified by drugs that have an effect on pertinent metabolic processes. However, the predominant type of sodium-potassium adenosine triphosphatase in the choroid plexus seems to differ from that of other tissues and is much less sensitive to cardiac glycoside inhibition, at least at clinically tolerable doses.[316] Experimental inhibition of carbonic anhydrase by acetazolamide reduces cerebrospinal fluid production by about 50 per cent.[76, 180] Furosemide is also able to achieve the same results; however, the underlying mechanism remains unclear.[42, 243] In addition, although both furosemide and acetazolamide independently reduce cerebrospinal fluid formation by about 50 per cent, the combination of these two agents reduces production by 75 per cent.[42]

Other areas of the central nervous system are apparently also involved in cerebrospinal fluid production.[189] It is generally accepted that the major source of this extrachoroidal fluid formation is the extracellular fluid by way of the ependyma. Under normal circumstances, the percentage of the secretion produced by the choroid plexus is about 80 per cent.[181] From its ventricular origin, cerebrospinal fluid flows to its absorption sites. As shown by cine-magnetic-resonance studies, it is a complex bidirectional phenomenon comprising anterograde and retrograde flows. This pulsatile flow is dependent on the cardiac pulse and the subsequent central nervous system displacement.

Most of the cerebrospinal fluid is resorbed at the level of the cranial venous sinuses. This resorption, or more exactly the flow of cerebrospinal fluid into the venous blood, is a passive phenomenon that obeys the pressure gradient existing between the subarachnoid

space and the sinus. The resorption rate is linear above a pressure threshold that is equal to the venous sinus pressure (approximately 5 cm H_2O in an adult in the supine position). The passage of cerebrospinal fluid into the venous blood occurs at the level of arachnoid villi mainly located along the large cranial venous sinuses. The exact mechanism of this passage is still debated. Two apparently opposing views of cerebrospinal fluid absorption (process of filtration across a membrane, and direct fluid flow through arachnoid villi) have been reconciled by the hypothesis of a vacuolar transport system.[8, 273, 299, 300, 329] Noteworthy is the fact that the arachnoid villi are not mature at birth; they continue to develop during the first few months of life. It is probable that the cerebrospinal fluid resorption capacities develop in parallel.

Alternative routes of cerebrospinal fluid resorption exist, in addition to arachnoid granulations. For instance, considerable evidence from animal studies suggests that lymphatic resorption is substantial.[181] This resorption was found to occur principally via the lymphatics of the cranial and spinal nerves. At present, the role of these alternative routes in humans, under normal or pathological conditions, is not clear.[181, 188] There is also some clinical evidence for a potential role of the central canal of the spinal cord in cerebrospinal fluid resorption, at least in children.

Intracranial pressure, defined as cerebrospinal fluid hydrostatic pressure, results from the active secretion of cerebrospinal fluid and the resistances that oppose its flow and passive resorption in the venous system. Intracranial pressure represents the equilibrium point where cerebrospinal fluid resorption equals cerebrospinal fluid secretion (Fig. 36–1). Intracranial pressure is directly related to venous sinus pressure and passively follows its variations.[215, 244] This correlation explains intracranial pressure variations related to postural changes from a "positive" value in a supine position to a subatmospheric value when standing.[174, 175] In the

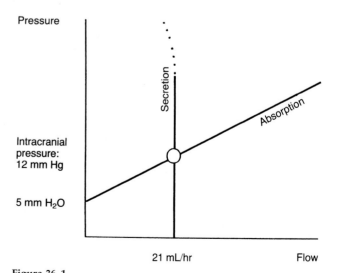

Figure 36–1

Diagram of cerebrospinal fluid secretion and absorption. Normal intracranial pressure is established at the pressure level where the absorption rate is equal to the secretion rate.

---

*See references 39, 70, 88, 172, 181, 239, and 316.

recumbent child and adult at rest, the normal basal intracranial pressure is around 12 ± 2 cm H_2O. In the newborn and during infancy, intracranial pressure values are lower. Values commonly reported in the literature are 2 to 4 cm H_2O for neonates.[318] This pressure increases and stabilizes around adult values as the skull ossifies and the sutures and fontanelles close.

Pathophysiology

From the preceding text, it is easy to understand that, in theory, hydrocephalus can result from three mechanisms: overproduction of cerebrospinal fluid, increased resistance to cerebrospinal fluid flow, and increased venous sinus pressure.

The consequence of all three mechanisms is an increase in cerebrospinal fluid pressure in order to maintain balanced secretion and resorption rates.[18] The mechanisms responsible for ventricular dilatation are not fully understood. However, ventricular enlargement cannot be considered as a simple accumulation of fluid due to an imbalance between production and absorption. The mechanisms of this enlargement are complex and probably come into play at different times during the development of hydrocephalus. Ventricular dilatation may result from (1) a compression of the cerebrovascular system, which is displaceable; (2) a redistribution of cerebrospinal fluid or extracellular fluid, or both, in the central nervous system; (3) a modification of the mechanical properties of the brain (increase in brain elasticity, alterations in the viscoelastic properties of brain, alteration of "brain turgor"); (4) the effect of the cerebrospinal fluid pulse pressure, which is still debated (some studies emphasize its importance as a causative factor in hydrocephalus, others suggest that it could be a contributory factor to ventricular expansion); (5) loss of brain substance, which in the long run contributes to the dilatation of the ventricles; and (6) in younger patients, an increase in skull volume due to the application of abnormal forces on functional cranial sutures. At this age, this additional volume is a major factor in the increase in cerebrospinal fluid.[292]

Once the hydrocephalic process has been initiated, secondary events may occur to further compromise the cerebrospinal fluid circulation and resorption. The possible role of an enhanced pulse pressure has been cited. A secondary elevation in sagittal venous sinus pressure that occurs with hydrocephalus from other causes may exacerbate an already existing absorption problem. In laboratory animals with communicating hydrocephalus, secondary occlusion of the aqueduct of Sylvius has been demonstrated. It has been suggested that this mechanism may occur with hydrocephalus associated with myelodysplasia and even with childhood hydrocephalus of other etiologies.[109]

Overproduction of cerebrospinal fluid (Fig. 36–2A) is almost exclusively due to choroid plexus tumors (papilloma or carcinoma).[92, 178, 190, 319] Overproduction, by itself, leads to an increase in intracranial pressure to

keep fluid secretion and resorption in balance and thus results in ventricular enlargement.[231] It should be stressed, however, that in patients having choroid plexus tumors, other factors (compression of the fluid pathways, fibrosis of the subarachnoid pathways or arachnoid villi resulting from microhemorrhages) can also contribute to increased cerebrospinal fluid outflow resistance, as is suggested by the frequent persistence of the hydrocephalic condition after tumor resection. There have been a few reports of cerebrospinal fluid overproduction in the absence of choroid plexus tumors. Finally, cerebrospinal fluid overproduction has been implicated as the causative agent in cases of hydrocephalus accompanying hypervitaminosis A.

An obstacle to cerebrospinal fluid flow (see Fig. 36–2B) is at the origin of most cases of hydrocephalus. The increased resistance caused by the obstacle leads to a proportional increase in cerebrospinal fluid pressure to keep resorption balanced. Hydrocephalus is usually classified according to the location of the blockage: whether it is in the ventricles or downstream from the ventricles, where it may be noncommunicating or communicating, respectively. The site of the ventricular dilatation depends on the location of the blockage, which explains why hydrocephalus can also be described as biventricular, triventricular, or quadriventricular. The blockage can result from various pathologies: (1) malformations causing local narrowing of the cerebrospinal fluid pathways (e.g., aqueductal stenosis, Chiari malformation); (2) mass lesions leading to an intrinsic or extrinsic compression of the cerebrospinal fluid pathways (e.g., intraventricular tumor, paraventricular tumor, arachnoid cyst, hematoma); and (3) inflammatory processes (e.g., infections, hemorrhages) and diseases, such as mucopolysaccharidoses, inducing ependymal reactions, leptomeningeal fibrosis, and obliteration of arachnoid villi.

Increases in venous sinus pressure (see Fig. 36–2C) have a double consequence: (1) an increase in cortical venous pressure, leading to a larger intracranial vascular volume, and (2) an increase in intracranial pressure up to the level required to maintain cerebrospinal fluid flow against an abnormally high venous sinus pressure. The clinical consequences of this venous hypertension depend on skull compliance. If the cranial sutures are closed, the ventricular dilatation is counteracted by the concomitant increase in vascular volume. In this case, the raised venous pressure translates into the clinical picture of pseudotumor cerebri. Conversely, if the skull is compliant, abnormally increased intracranial pressure leads to expansion of the cranium and, therefore, to an increase in fluid volume. This increase in venous sinus pressure can be of organic origin (sinus, jugular, or superior vena cava thrombosis, tumor invading the sinus, achondroplasia) or functional origin (high-flow arteriovenous malformation).[191, 237, 244]

The degree of increased resistance of the cerebrospinal fluid flow, and the speed with which the hydrodynamic disturbance develops, influence the clinical picture. All the intermediate levels between a case of acute intracranial hypertension and a chronic picture of cerebral dysfunction may be observed.

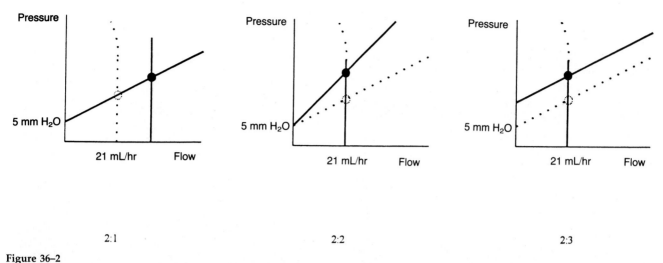

Figure 36–2

Overproduction of cerebrospinal fluid (A), increase in resistance to cerebrospinal fluid flow (B), and increase in venous sinus pressure (C) lead to an increase in intracranial pressure to maintain the balance between absorption and secretion.

Pathology

Dilatation of the ventricular cavities is associated with ependymal alterations, a thin, stretched cortical mantle, and altered cerebral vascularization. As previously stated, the type of ventricular dilatation depends on the location of the blockage. Some characteristics are related to age. It seems that the mechanical properties of the immature cerebral parenchyma may favor the elective dilatation of the posterior part of the lateral ventricles. Two mechanisms have been proposed to explain this phenomenon: higher compliance of the posterior skull before fusion of the cranial sutures, and lesser distensibility of the anterior ventricular system surrounded by the compact gray matter structure of the basal ganglia.

The thinning and stretching of the cortical mantle are the consequences of the dilatation of the ventricular cavities. The pathological features depend on the extent of the disease. In the acute phase, there exists an edema of the white matter around the ventricles, and relatively few neuronal lesions are present. At a later stage, the edema disappears and is replaced by fibrosis, and a process of axonal degeneration (demyelination) responsible for cerebral atrophy and focal loss of the neuronal population.[49, 77, 106, 320, 321] The ventricular ependyma is particularly vulnerable. In the acute phase, a cellular flattening and loss of cilia are observed; at a later stage, dramatic disruption of the ependymal membrane occurs. Finally, the ependymal membrane is largely destroyed, and the ventricular surface is recovered by a substitute glial tissue.[17] It has been recently demonstrated that neurons of the cerebral cortex are also affected, with decreases in their synaptic connections and dendritic richness.[179] These alterations are usually well correlated with the patient's clinical status. The reconstitution of the cerebral cortical mantle after shunting results not in the restoration of lost elements, but rather in the formation of glial scar.[240, 241] Concurrent with parenchymal injury, alterations in the vascular system are observed, consisting of a depletion of the capillary bed, which regenerates itself after treatment of the hydrocephalus.

Biochemical changes have been reported to result from the hydrocephalic process. These studies were motivated by the search for a potential prognostic marker of brain damage. For instance, there is an increase in the protein content of cerebrospinal fluid as well as specific alteration of its electrophoretic pattern in various hydrocephalic conditions.[50, 51, 276] Also, concentrations of fatty acids, xanthine, hypoxanthine, and ganglioside GM_1 were found to be of some interest as prognostic factors.[28, 108, 204, 264]

Etiology

PRENATAL CAUSES

Prenatal causes are responsible for congenital hydrocephalus that arises in utero and manifests itself either in utero or after birth.[2] They can be of malformative (sporadic developmental anomalies or genetically determined malformations), infectious, or vascular orgin. In a significant number of patients the etiology remains unknown; these cases of hydrocephalus are said to be idiopathic.

Stenoses of the Aqueduct of Sylvius Due To Malformation. These stenoses are responsible for approximately 10 per cent of all cases of hydrocephalus in newborns.[16] Their incidence is 0.5 to 1 case per 1,000 births, with a risk of recurrence in siblings of 1 to 4 per cent according to the different studies.[147] These stenoses are of nontumoral origin. Three types have been described: (1) aqueductal gliosis representing an overgrowth of fibrillary glia that constricts the lumen; (2) forking of the aqueduct, in which it is replaced by several canaliculi, sometimes obstructed; and (3) aqueduct obstruction by a thin ependymal septum generally

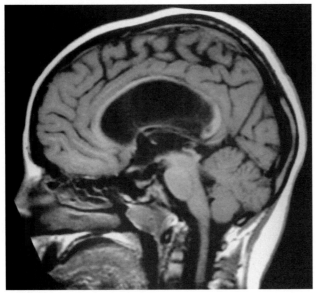

Figure 36–3

Aqueduct stenosis due to malformation seen on a midsagittal plane of a T1-weighted magnetic resonance image in a 15-year-old girl examined because of delayed puberty.

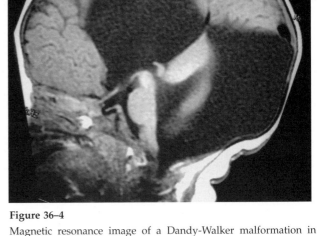

Figure 36–4

Magnetic resonance image of a Dandy-Walker malformation in a newborn. Hydrocephalus and agenesis of the corpus callosum are associated, in this case, with the posterior fossa cyst.

located in its caudal end.[242, 268] With the exception of Bickers-Adams syndrome, aqueductal stenosis is usually sporadic and rarely hereditary. The stenosis can be associated with other malformations (e.g., Arnold-Chiari malformation, occipital encephalocele).

Despite its congenital origin, the alteration of cerebrospinal fluid dynamics can remain compensated and undiagnosed for several years. Frequently, it is in retrospect that episodes of headaches in the patient's history, slightly increased head circumference, or subtle motor problems are recognized during investigation of a late acute decompensation of the hydrocephalic process or because of endocrine disorders (Fig. 36–3).

Dandy-Walker Malformation. This malformation affects 2 to 4 per cent of newborns with hydrocephalus. Of unknown etiology, Dandy-Walker malformation includes a cystic expansion of the fourth ventricle and hypoplasia of the cerebellar vermis (Fig. 36–4).[48, 107, 131] Hydrocephalus is generally explained by an inadequate communication between the dilated fourth ventricle (Dandy-Walker cyst) and the subarachnoid spaces.[290, 291] Hydrocephalus may be present at birth, but in 80 per cent of cases it develops within the first 3 months.[137] Associated brain and systemic malformations are numerous (agenesis of the corpus callosum, cleft palate, ocular anomalies, cardiac anomalies). Among facial anomalies, facial angiomas are found in 10 per cent of cases. The association of facial and cardiac anomalies favors the hypothesis that the onset of the malformation occurs between the time of formation and that of migration of the neural crest cells.[137] This malformation is often responsible for a characteristic deformation of the head, which is expanded posteriorly.

Arnold-Chiari Malformation (Type II). Although Arnold-Chiari malformation type II is composed of a complex constellation of central nervous system abnormalities, there are two characteristic malformations in the posterior fossa. The brain stem is elongated and malformed, and the cerebellar tonsils are elongated and extend into the cervical spinal canal (Fig. 36–5).[107, 109, 192] These malformations obliterate the posterior fossa cisterns and compromise the outlets of the fourth ventricle. Arnold-Chiari malformation is present in virtually all patients with a myelomeningocele, although

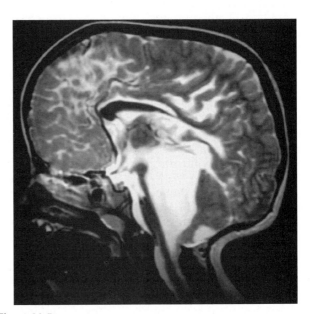

Figure 36–5

Arnold-Chiari type II malformation is an entity much more complex than simple ectopia of the cerebellar tonsils. An example of a magnetic resonance image of a child with myelomeningocele, Arnold-Chiari type II malformation, and postshunt trapped fourth ventricle, showing a dramatic change in the posterior fossa anatomy.

not all develop an active hydrocephalus that requires shunting (80 per cent).[308] The hydrocephalus is typically overt within the first month of life and is frequently exacerbated by the surgical closure of the spinal defect. The pathogenesis of the ventricular enlargement is probably related to an increase in cerebrospinal fluid outflow resistance at the level of the fourth ventricle and its outlet foramina. Associated primary or secondary aqueductal stenosis is frequently reported.

Other Rare Malformations. Other rare malformations include agenesis of the foramen of Monro, agenesis of the cerebrospinal fluid resorption sites, and a number of complex malformation syndromes without chromosome abnormalities.[7, 59, 110]

In Utero Infections. In utero infections can induce hydrocephalus when they involve the central nervous system. In addition to the impairment of cerebrospinal fluid flow, these infections are often responsible for parenchymal damage that largely influences the infant's ultimate developmental prognosis. Among the diseases that affect fetuses, special mention should be made of congenital toxoplasmosis that causes secondary aqueductal stenosis, affects the subarachnoid spaces, and causes parenchymal damage. These lesions may develop during the second trimester of pregnancy. Viral infections have also been implicated in the occurrence of congenital hydrocephalus. For instance, cytomegalovirus infection may induce a basal arachnoiditis leading to impairment of cerebrospinal fluid flow. As with toxoplasmosis, associated cerebral tissue loss can be extensive and can contribute to the ventricular enlargement.

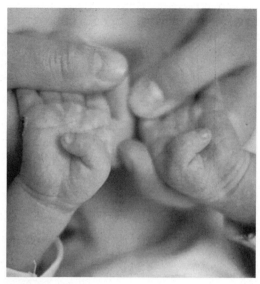

Figure 36–7

Typical thumb deformity in Bickers-Adams syndrome.

Hydrocephalus Associated with Destructive Cerebral Lesions of Ischemic Origin. Some rare cases of hydrocephalus are associated with cerebral lesions of ischemic origin (Fig. 36–6).

Rare Genetic or Family Hydrocephalus. X-linked hydrocephalus (Bickers-Adams syndrome) is a well-defined, recessively transmitted disorder that accounts for roughly 7 per cent of cases of hydrocephalus in males.[32, 105, 287] The condition is characterized by stenosis of the aqueduct of Sylvius and severe mental retardation.[304] About half of affected children have an adduction-flexion deformity of the thumb (Fig. 36–7). This syndrome can also exist without hydrocephalus. Cases of familial hydrocephalus striking both sexes are rare and could be transmitted recessively. In the lissencephaly of the Walker type, the recessive hereditary transmission is debated. The condition could result from an intrauterine viral infection transmitted by the mother to the fetus. Hydrocephalus may be present in cases of major chromosome aberrations affecting chromosome 8, 9, 13, 15, 18, or 21, or minor aberrations (1q25-qtr duplication).[150, 271]

POSTNATAL CAUSES

Postnatal causes are the most frequent.

Mass Lesions

Mass lesions are responsible for about 20 per cent of all cases of hydrocephalus in children. Exceptionally, the lesion can be a choroid plexus tumor whose pathogenic mechanism originated earlier (Fig. 36–8).

Generally, the expansive process causes an increased resistance to cerebrospinal fluid flow (Fig. 36–9). The nature of the process can vary; it is tumoral in many cases. However, any mass lesion can create an obstacle to cerebrospinal fluid flow (e.g., arachnoid cyst, ab-

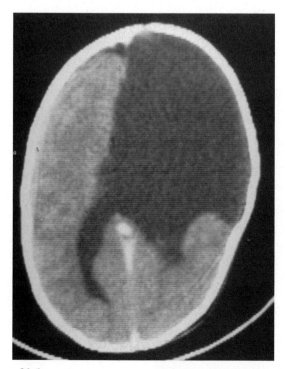

Figure 36–6

Computed tomogram of a case of congenital hydrocephalus probably due to a prenatal ischemic disorder.

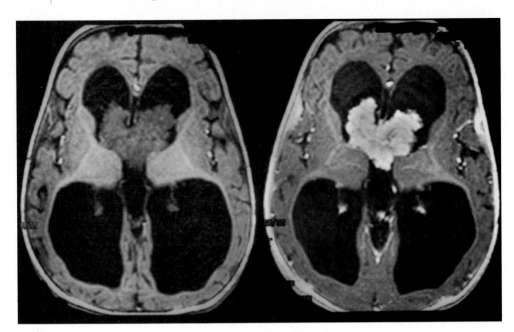

Figure 36–8

Choroid plexus papilloma in a 3-year-old boy suffering from intracranial hypertension.

scess, hematoma). In childhood, the most frequent location of these tumors is the posterior fossa (astrocytomas, medulloblastomas, ependymomas, dorsally exophytic brain stem tumors).[5, 95, 286] Other rare tumors are usually accompanied by hydrocephalus: tumors of the pineal region; gliomas in the mesencephalic region close to the aqueduct of Sylvius; and tumors below or in the third ventricle, particularly frequent in children (e.g., craniopharyngioma, hypothalamic glioma, optic glioma).[166, 217, 250] Some of these tumors can be responsible for arachnoid metastases. Intracranial spread and proliferation of tumor cells through the subarachnoid pathways is another potential cause of tumoral hydrocephalus. Despite their supposed congenital origin, colloid cysts of the third ventricle are rarely diagnosed in children.[170]

Arachnoid cysts and neuroepithelial cysts constitute the second most frequent type of mass lesion able to compromise cerebrospinal fluid flow (Fig. 36–10). They are most often encountered in the suprasellar region, the foramen magnum, and the posterior fossa, where it is important that they be distinguished from Dandy-Walker malformations (Fig. 36–11).[131] The location of the cyst largely determines the clinical picture. Posterior fossa and foramen magnum cysts tend to manifest themselves earlier than suprasellar cysts, the diagnosis of which can be very delayed. Aneurysm of the vein of Galen is very often accompanied by hydrocephalus. The pathogenesis of this hydrocephalus is debated. In a number of patients, there is unquestionably an extrinsic compression of the aqueduct of Sylvius; in other patients, the increase in venous pressure created by the

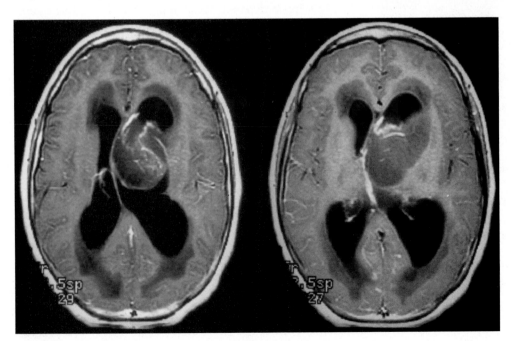

Figure 36–9

The developmental pattern of ventricular enlargement associated with tumors is related to the location of the tumor along the cerebrospinal fluid pathways. In this example, a benign astrocytic thalamic lesion was responsible for biventricular hydrocephalus.

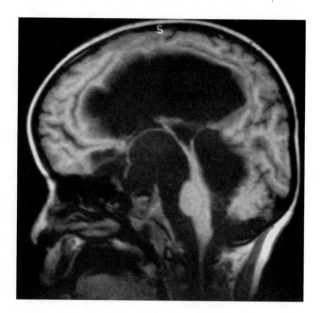

Figure 36–10

Two cysts, above and below the cerebral peduncle, were responsible for a case of severe hydrocephalus caused by aqueductal stenosis in this 2-year-old boy.

vascular shunt may be the origin of the ventricular dilatation (Fig. 36–12). In support of the venous origin theory, there have been reports of stabilization of the ventricular enlargement in some patients cured of their arteriovenous malformation.

Finally, a spinal tumor can be associated with hydrocephalus. The pathogenesis of this unexceptional entity is still debated. There are at least three possible pathological explanations of this association: a subarachnoid spreading of the spinal lesion (observed even with benign tumor); an alteration of the cerebrospinal fluid outflow of the fourth ventricle by the rostral expansion of a tumor involving the cervicomedullary junction; and subarachnoid fibrosis resulting from repeated contamination of the cerebrospinal fluid by blood byproducts (fibrin coming from the tumor or from a tumoral cyst?).

Hemorrhage

The causes of the hemorrhage may vary (prematurity, head injury, rupture of a vascular malformation), as may the effects it has on the cerebrospinal fluid hydrodynamics.[31, 207, 297] At an acute stage of the hemorrhage, transformation of fibrinogen into fibrin and clots generated by the bleeding create mechanical obstacles to cerebrospinal fluid flow in the narrowest parts of its pathways (aqueduct of Sylvius, basal cisterns, subarachnoid spaces, arachnoid villi); increased cerebrospinal fluid viscosity following bleeding is insufficient to induce hydrocephalus (Fig. 36–13).[93] At a chronic stage, leptomeningeal fibrosis develops in a percentage of the cases, leading to a permanently increased resistance to cerebrospinal fluid flow. This two-step evolution must be taken into account in planning treatment,

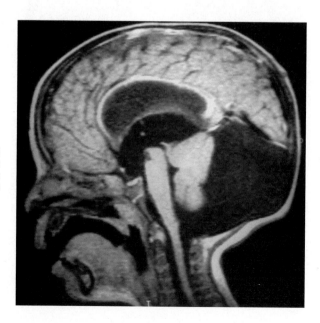

Figure 36–11

The differential diagnosis of Dandy-Walker malformation (see Fig. 36–4) and arachnoid cyst of the posterior fossa can be difficult even with magnetic resonance imaging. An asymmetry of the cystic formation and visualization of the cerebellar vermis on the midsagittal slice of a magnetic resonance image, as in this case, point toward an arachnoid cyst.

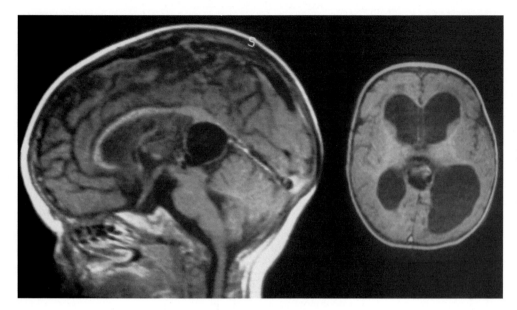

Figure 36–12

Hydrocephalus associated with vein of Galen malformation may be of venous origin or may be related to aqueductal stenosis. Both etiologies have been demonstrated.

because not all of these patients develop permanent hydrocephalus. There is a correlation between the extent of the bleeding and the risk of hydrocephalus at all stages.

Intraventricular hemorrhage in preterm infants is usually due to ventricular contamination by a hemorrhage occurring in the germinal matrix at the level of the caudate nucleus.[9, 136, 208, 209] It is usually reported that one third of premature infants weighing less than 1,500

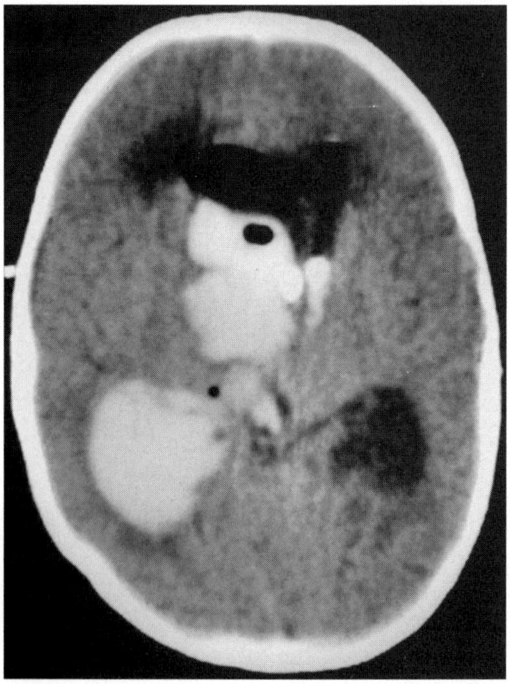

Figure 36–13

In the acute phase of an intraventricular hemorrhage, hydrocephalus is related to the mechanical obstacle created by the clot in the cerebrospinal fluid circulation. The goal of the treatment is to prevent the occurrence of chronic alterations in the subarachnoid spaces and arachnoid villi.

g or born before 32 weeks of gestation will develop periventricular-intraventricular hemorrhage.[44, 45] Progressive hydrocephalus may occur in those patients with the most severe bleeds. Despite significant progress in the management of these patients, some still require shunting.[213]

Meningitis

All bacterial meningitis can degenerate into hydrocephalus by inducing leptomeningeal fibrosis or inducing inflammatory aqueductal stenosis. Gram-negative central nervous system infection in neonates is of particular interest because of its association with cerebrospinal fluid contamination and brain tissue contamination. These patients will frequently develop a multiloculated hydrocephalus resulting in devastating brain damage (Fig. 36–14).[160] Tuberculous meningitis is almost always accompanied by a ventricular dilatation that generally evolves chronically and is due to arachnoiditis of the basal cisterns.[305, 310] With respect to geographical considerations, cysticercosis is one of the major causes of hydrocephalus; in these cases impairment of cerebrospinal fluid outflow can be due to an obstacle within the ventricles (parasitic cyst) or impairment of the subarachnoid spaces.[78, 159, 254, 278]

Hydrocephalus of Venous Origin

As previously cited, increased venous sinus pressure may result in hydrocephalus only as long as the skull is compliant. The increase in venous pressure is secondary to an anatomical or functional blockage. Examples of anatomical blockages are achondroplasia, in which the venous drainage is frequently impaired at the level of the cranial base; some craniostenoses; tumors compressing or invading the venous sinuses; and sinus, bijugular, or vena cava thrombosis (Fig. 36–15).[125, 216, 244, 326] Functional impairment of the venous

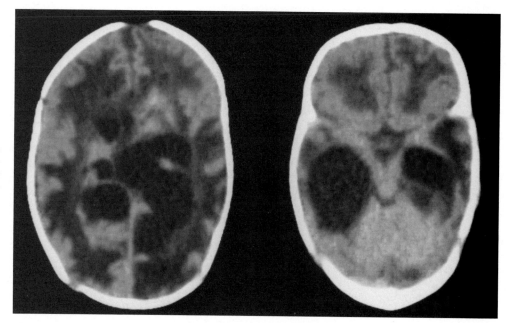

Figure 36–14

Gram-negative infection of the central nervous system in neonates can lead to very severe multiloculated hydrocephalus, as in this case.

sinus outflow is generally due to high-flow arteriovenous malformations.

Iatrogenic Hydrocephalus

Iatrogenic hydrocephalus is extremely rare.

Acute or chronic hypervitaminosis A has been reported to be a possible cause of hydrocephalus. The mechanism would be an increased secretion of cerebrospinal fluid or an increased permeability of the blood-brain barrier.

Idiopathic Hydrocephalus

In a significant number of cases, the etiology of hydrocephalus remains uncertain or unknown. The same causes previously listed may have gone undiagnosed, for example, a small bleed or improperly treated meningitis.[124]

Clinical Aspects

SIGNS AND SYMPTOMS

Clinical symptoms vary with the age of the patient and the circumstances of diagnosis.

During infancy, abnormally rapid head growth is the most common sign of hydrocephalus. It is always present in chronic hydrocephalus occurring before the age of 2 years, be it of prenatal or postnatal origin.

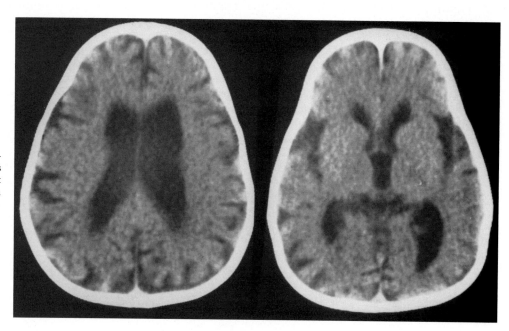

Figure 36–15

In hydrocephalus of venous origin, dilatation of the ventricles is associated with an enlargement of the subarachnoid spaces, as in this patient with achondroplasia.

Macrocrania is often a revealing sign. It can be defined as a head circumference higher than two standard deviations above normal, or the 98th percentile of the age class. Its extent varies according to the duration of evolution, the age at onset, and the progression of the hydrocephalus. More than macrocrania, a discontinuity in the slope of the head circumference growth curve should alert the physician.[193]

Macrocrania may be accompanied by four other signs of intracranial hypertension. First, excessive tension of the anterior fontanelle can be observed in infants. The anterior fontanelle is normally flat or slightly concave in an infant held erect (when he or she is not crying). Second, a disjunction of the sutures can be seen or palpated. Third, the scalp is thin and shiny with veins plainly visible. Fourth, among ocular signs, the setting-sun eye phenemenon is, in infants, characteristic of intracranial hypertension due to hydrocephalus.[52] Both ocular globes are deviated downward, and the upper lids are retracted. This phenomenon is somewhat reminiscent of the Parinaud syndrome and most likely represents dysfunction of the tectal region. Esotropia, due to sixth nerve and, occasionally, partial third nerve palsy, may be encountered; these oculomotor manifestations disturb binocular vision and carry the potential risk of amblyopia in infants. Papilledema is not frequent, but a funduscopic examination may reveal retinal venous engorgement or even early signs of optical atrophy. Signs of acute intracranial hypertension are more frequent in children than in infants as a result of skull rigidity. The symptoms include headaches, vomiting, alteration of consciousness, oculomotor disorders, and signs of brain stem dysfunction in the most advanced cases (posterior cerebellar fits linked to a tonsillar herniation, bradycardia, and respiratory arrhythmia). In the newborn, acute intracranial hypertension is revealed by a bulging, tensed fontanelle, with a cranial volume that may be only slightly enlarged. In all cases, signs of intracranial hypertension represent a neurosurgical emergency requiring neuroradiological examination to ensure that the diagnosis is correct.

Chronic intracranial hypertension presents especially marked symptoms in children. Because infants have distensible skulls, this hypertension manifests mainly as progressive abnormal head growth, accompanied, sooner or later, by an alteration in the development of intelligence, affecting verbal capabilities more than nonverbal ones. Once the sutures have closed, the most common symptoms include headaches, at first sporadic, then getting progressively worse, sometimes accompanied by typically early-morning abdominal pains, with nausea and vomiting. In addition to these two essential symptoms, changes in behavior and a decline in school performance as well as sometimes memory loss may be seen. At a later stage, the clinical picture may also comprise failed mental functioning with drowsiness. Chronic intracranial hypertension may delay the diagnosis, allowing significant brain damage to occur.

Sometimes patients first present with other neurological symptoms, which are more frequently observed in patients seen for macrocrania or intracranial hypertension.[58] A spasticity affecting generally the inferior limbs is interpreted as the consequence of a pyramidal tract stretched around dilated lateral ventricles. Usually discrete or subtle, this spasticity can be more severe and induce gait disturbance. Abnormal movements (e.g., bobble-head doll syndrome) are rare.

Endocrine disorders are uncommon and rarely revealing. They are thought to be linked to the distraction of the hypothalamus and pituary stalk by a dilated third ventricle.[13] They are often seen in cases of aqueductal stenosis. These disorders can lead to growth retardation, obesity, and precocious or delayed onset of puberty.[85]

DIAGNOSIS

The diagnosis of hydrocephalus is based on three types of data: historical data, physical examination, and clinical work-up.

History

It is essential to be aware of and to identify any entity known to be associated with hydrocephalus. Hydrocephalus is expected when certain conditions are identified ahead of the disease onset, as is the case with myelomeningoceles, which are always associated with an Arnold-Chiari type II malformation. It is also the case with some acquired causes, such as ventricular hemorrhage of the premature baby, bacterial meningitis, achondroplasia, and mucopolysaccharidoses.

Clinical Data

Hydrocephalus is suspected in cases of macrocrania; a disruption in the head circumference growth curve is always pathological and should alert the physician to investigate. Nonpathological big heads do exist, as does the notion of familial macrocrania. Neuroradiological examinations generally show unusually inflated subarachnoid spaces with slightly dilated ventricles. These particular cases, sometimes grouped under the designation "external hydrocephalus," could result from a delayed maturity of the cerebrospinal fluid resorption sites.[54] In any case, this condition constitutes a quite benign deviation from the normal spontaneous evolution, with no tendency to aggravation. This benign type of macrocrania usually remains on the same percentile along the head circumference growth curve, albeit at +2 to +4 standard deviations (Fig. 36–16). Generally, the dilatation of the subarachnoid spaces decreases after the cranial vault has ossified.[161]

The rapid cranial growth of the premature infant may be accompanied by a disjunction of the sutures and thus mimic hydrocephalus.[41, 270] There are other causes of macrocrania associated with intracranial hypertension in the child, such as chronic subdural hematomas (Fig. 36–17).

In real life, the most important problem is the clinical identification of the abnormal head and the subsequent

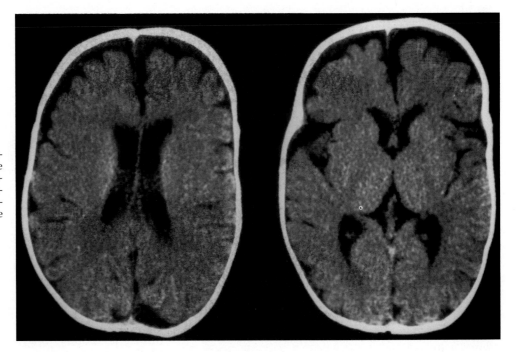

Figure 36–16

"External hydrocephalus" is a benign condition, observed in male infants and requiring no treatment. It may be difficult to differentiate from true subdural cerebrospinal fluid collections (see Fig. 36–17).

need for neuroradiological investigations enabling differentiation between hydrocephalus and conditions with similar presentations.

Neuroradiological Examinations

As long as the anterior fontanelle is largely permeable, transfontanellar ultrasound offers a simple, innocuous way of visualizing the ventricular dilatation.[27, 53, 133] This examination enables the detection of an "expected" hydrocephalus before its first clinical manifestation. Transfontanellar ultrasound has considerably helped the diagnosis and management of intrauterine hydrocephalus.[66, 132] However, this examination is in many cases insufficient to ensure the etiological diagnosis.

Computed tomography illustrates the ventricular dilatation, its topography, and the concurrent dilatation of the subarachnoid spaces.[4] The evolution of the disease can be appreciated by showing signs of fluid passage through the ependymal wall. This egression of fluid from the ventricles appears as a periventricular lucency that predominates at the levels of the frontal and occipital horns. This examination, easily conducted, can reveal the existence and the nature of an obstacle to cerebrospinal fluid flow. It facilitates the follow-up of treatment and the detection of secondary complications. It must be pointed out, however, that the total number of computed tomography scans through the ocular globes should be limited because of the underlying risk of cataract formation.

Magnetic resonance imaging is the examination of

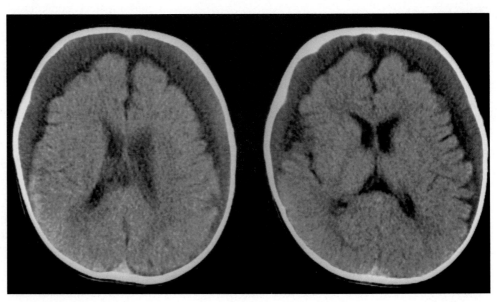

Figure 36–17

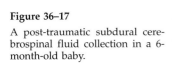

A post-traumatic subdural cerebrospinal fluid collection in a 6-month-old baby.

choice if elective scheduling is compatible with the need for a quick diagnosis. The duration of the scan necessitates immobilization or general anesthesia for noncompliant and younger patients. The presence of a metallic prosthesis may hamper the interpretation of the examination through artifact or, in the case of magnetic material, contraindicate use of the modality. Compared with computed tomography, magnetic resonance imaging offers a better morphological definition of the ventricles and of some causal lesions. It enables a pathophysiological approach to understanding the hydrodynamic disorder through the analysis of the cerebrospinal fluid flow, and the volumes of the different intracranial components.

Chronic intracranial pressure monitoring can be useful under certain circumstances.[1] In infants, the monitoring is done transcutaneously, through the anterior fontanelle, with fontanelle pressure sensors. In children, intracranial pressure monitoring is an invasive technique. The study of intracranial pressure variations requires long-term recordings, particularly at night during REM (rapid-eye-movement) sleep, which allows a finer analysis than does a baseline pressure study.[83]

The study of cerebral blood flow by Doppler ultrasound enables the calculation of a flow resistance index, which is high in cases of hydrocephalus. Some authors have reported a significant positive correlation between the ventricular dilatation and the resistance index at the level of the anterior cerebral artery in progressive hydrocephalus, as well as in normal-pressure hydrocephalus. The increased resistance index that implies a fall in cerebral diastolic blood flow is attributed to the compression or suppression, or both, of the vessels under the effect of the ventricular dilatation.

Other procedures such as lumbar puncture and angiography are sometimes useful in the etiological diagnosis.

Treatment

The situation today is such that probably no two neurosurgeons agree on what is the best approach to treating a particular hydrocephalic patient. The development of implantable shunt devices was, indeed, a major step forward in the treatment of this pathological condition.[196, 197] However, to quote McLaurin, it can be said that "the history of the evolution of ventricular shunting for hydrocephalus is largely a history to prevent the complications of shunting."[185] This fight against shunt complications and commercial competition led to a wide array of available devices.* In addition, alternative treatments other than shunts exist, but their indications are not well defined, nor are these techniques well known everywhere.[140] This confusing situation is the result of a lack of reliable scientific data supporting different therapeutic approaches, and

---

*See references 145, 177, 221, 222, 245, 278, and 327.

frequent lack of interest for a neurosurgical problem usually considered as minor. It could be worthwhile, however, for neurosurgeons to agree on some simple guidelines: (1) since a shunt insertion represents a lifetime commitment to an imperfect device, all attempts should be made to avoid it; (2) shunt selection should be based, as much as possible, on scientific data; and (3) good surgical technique is the best guarantee of fewer shunt complications.

Since alteration of cerebrospinal fluid hydrodynamics can occur under variable conditions, there are several therapeutic possibilities that must be discussed for each particular case.

TEMPORARY TREATMENT

Medical treatment tries to limit the evolution of hydrocephalus by decreasing the fluid secretion of the choroid plexus (acetazolamide, 100 mg per kg per day; furosemide, 1 mg per kg per day) or by increasing its resorption (isosorbide). Such treatment always constitutes a temporary treatment either before a more definitive therapeutic strategy is initiated or, in some specific cases, while the patient is observed for the spontaneous resolution of the hydrodynamic alteration.[272] Medical treatment is not effective in the long-term treatment of chronic hydrocephalus, and it may induce metabolic consequences.

External drainage of cerebrospinal fluid is performed through a ventricular catheter connected to an external drainage bag. It constitutes a temporary solution for patients whose hydrocephalus is potentially transitory or who have an ongoing infection.[210] The limits of this type of treatment lie in the risk of cerebrospinal fluid contamination and the need to maintain the patient under close monitoring. Similar to this method, repeated cerebrospinal fluid taps performed with subcutaneous ventricular access devices enable control of ventricular enlargement.

These methods of temporary control of ventricular dilatation can be helpful in particular circumstances and must be considered. For example, in posthemorrhage hydrocephalus, treatment of the acute phase of ventricular enlargement using a temporary method of drainage (i.e., external ventricular drainage, ventricular access devices) or medical treatment saves a significant number of patients from a permanent shunt.[14, 99, 122, 155, 176] In addition, these methods allow clearing of debris or clots from the cerebrospinal fluid for patients who will receive a shunt.

ALTERNATIVES TO SHUNTING

Alternatives to shunting exist mainly in the treatment of hydrocephalus when there is an obstacle within the ventricles, including the outlets of the fourth ventricle (e.g., aqueductal stenosis, posterior fossa tumor, arachnoid cysts). These treatments must be considered first, even if they are less straightforward than is simple shunt insertion. The restoration of a normal or close to normal cerebrospinal fluid circulation will

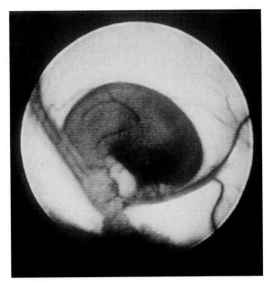

Figure 36–18

Endoscopic view of the right foramen of Monro in a 10-year-old female with hydrocephalus due to a pineal tumor (see color section in this volume).

always be better than any artificial drainage. In some cases, however, these treatments are not sufficient. Their results must be carefully assessed, and if they are suboptimal, the surgeon should not rule out a shunt.

Etiological Treatment

Treatment of the underlying etiology is the best therapeutic strategy for hydrocephalus. It may consist of controlling a case of vitamin A intoxication, radical resection of a mass lesion that is hindering flow, rapid clearance of the blood in cerebrospinal fluid, or correcting a malformation. Although in some cases the need for temporary symptomatic treatment prior to treatment of the etiology has to be discussed, the treatment of an apparent causal lesion does not always re-establish normal fluid flow. This outcome most probably occurs because the etiology is multifactorial or because of the appearance of secondary alterations of fluid flow. For example, the most common brain tumors in childhood are located in the posterior fossa and are responsible for varying degrees of ventricular enlargement in the majority of cases. Ideally, tumor removal should cure hydrocephalus; it does indeed happen in a large number of cases, as many as 80 per cent. However, some patients, particularly the youngest, still need to have shunts inserted after tumor surgery, probably because of postsurgical leptomeningeal fibrosis. It may also be necessary, under very specific conditions (to gain time), to control the intracranial hypertension prior to tumor surgery, even if the old habit of routinely inserting a shunt in these patients prior to tumor removal is no longer valid. Routine preoperative shunting may induce shunt dependency in patients who will no longer be hydrocephalic after re-establishment of normal cerebrospinal fluid circulation. A second promising example is the use of thrombolytic

agents in cases of posthemorrhage hydrocephalus. Urokinase instilled in the ventricles via a ventricular access device seems to be able to reduce the incidence of permanent hydrocephalus and to mitigate the need for shunt placement.[148, 205, 251, 269]

Membrane Fenestration

In cases of aqueduct stenosis or, more generally, alteration of cerebrospinal fluid flow in the posterior fossa (including posterior fossa tumors), fenestration of the floor of the third ventricle establishes an alternative route for cerebrospinal fluid flow toward the subarachnoid spaces.[140, 158, 252] In addition to restoration of a pseudophysiological cerebrospinal fluid circulation, third ventriculostomy re-establishes a uniform hydrostatic pressure regimen in the whole central nervous system, preventing the development of a pressure gradient on the vulnerable midline structures.[157] Magnetic resonance imaging and, particularly, cine-phase contrast studies have greatly improved the diagnosis of this type of hydrocephalus, illustrating the aqueduct stenosis and its etiology but also giving semiquantitative information on the cerebrospinal fluid flow alteration. At present, perforation of the floor of the third ventricle to bypass the blocked aqueduct is most effectively performed endoscopically.[248] A rigid or flexible neuroendoscope is introduced into the lateral ventricle through a coronal burr hole 2 to 3 cm from the midline. The foramen of Monro is located through identification of the choroid plexus and the septal and thalamostriate veins (Fig. 36–18; see color section in this volume). The endoscope is then passed into the third ventricle. Landmarks in the third ventricle are, posterior to anterior, the mamillary bodies, the dome of the division of the basilar artery (often visible through the attenuated floor), the dorsum sellae, and the infundibular recess (Fig. 36–19; see color section in this volume). An orifice

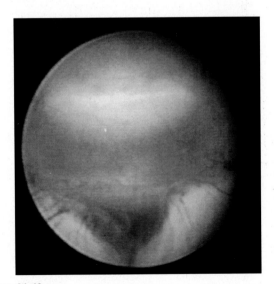

Figure 36–19

Landmarks on the floor of the third ventricle can be more or less obvious, depending on the degree of attenuation. Visualization and "palpation" of the posterior clinoid recesses is the safest way of avoiding arterial injury (see color section in this volume).

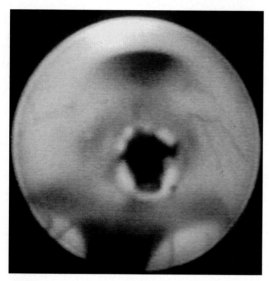

Figure 36–20

The risk of secondary obliteration of the hole in the floor of the third ventricle is almost nil because of the amplitude of the pulsatile flow at this level (see color section in this volume).

is created in front of the division of the basilar artery, putting into communication the third ventricle and the prepeduncular cistern (Fig. 36–20; see color section in this volume). Several methods, namely, laser, monopolar wire coagulator, radiofrequency, and balloon catheter, may be used to perforate the ventricle floor.[135] For safety reasons, the author prefers to make an initial microperforation using a coagulation wire or a contact laser. This hole is then dilated with a balloon catheter. One must be aware that the decrease in ventricle size after an efficient third ventriculostomy is less signifi-

cant than that after shunting. Evidence of flow at the level of the ventriculostomy orifice illustrated by phase-contrast magnetic resonance imaging (Fig. 36–21) and normalization of the clinical symptoms are more important in evaluating the benefits of treatment than is the decrease in ventricle size.

When arachnoid cysts impair the cerebrospinal fluid circulation, they too can be treated with endoscopic fenestration in many cases. It is necessary, however, to establish communication not only between the cyst and the nearest ventricle but also between the cyst and the subarachnoid spaces. In other words, the proximal and distal walls of the cyst must be perforated. Cysts located in the suprasellar region, the foramen magnum, or the posterior fossa or within the ventricles are potential indications for this method of treatment.

At present, about 25 per cent of patients with hydrocephalus can be cured without shunt placement (aqueduct stenosis, 10 per cent; tumors, 10 per cent; cyst, 5 per cent). It is probable that in the near future more shunts can be avoided (through the use of thrombolytic agents or extension of endoscopic procedures).

SHUNTS

Despite the interest in alternative treatments, the majority of patients still need to have shunts inserted.[86] The aim of shunting is to establish a communication between the cerebrospinal fluid (ventricular or lumbar) and a drainage cavity (e.g., peritoneum, right atrium, pleura). The choice of the cavities to drain from and to varies with each individual case. The peritoneal cavity is a preferred drainage site in children, because it enables the implantation of an important length of drain-

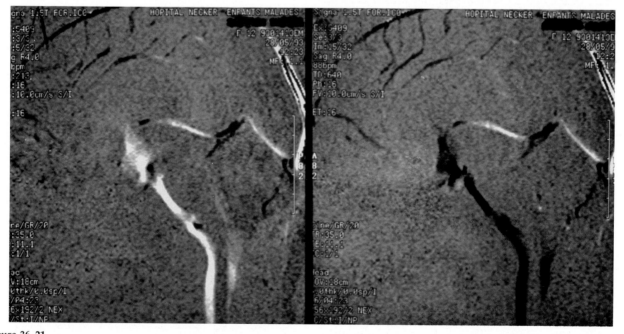

Figure 36–21

Cine-phase-contrast magnetic resonance imaging allows visualization and quantification of the flow at the level of the third ventriculostomy orifice.

age catheter to allow for growth, and it predisposes to less severe infectious complications than does the right atrium.[146, 234, 302, 324] Other drainage sites (e.g., pleura, gallbladder) can be helpful in very specific circumstances, even if they carry a high risk of shunt complications.[30, 141, 307, 322] The cerebrospinal fluid is usually drained from the ventricles; however, in the case of communicating hydrocephalus it may be drained from the lumbar subarachnoid spaces.* In addition to its specific complications, lumbar drainage has recently been implicated in causing tonsillar herniations, at least in children.† Until more is known, this modality is recommended only as a last resort. The perfect shunt does not exist; however, a wide number of available devices and judicious selection can allow an acceptable compromise in most cases. In fact, the selection of a shunt seems very often more subjective than scientific. Shunt selection by a particular surgeon is often influenced by historical precedent, anecdotal experience, marketing techniques, and financial considerations, as well as scientific principle. In addition, while shunts may differ significantly in their profile and mechanism, from the hydrodynamic standpoint they can be classified in only two or three categories. Prior to selecting and inserting a shunt system, the surgeon must consider several factors.[95, 96, 229, 255] The choice of shunt profile for preventing the occurrence of skin problems can be influenced by the age, weight, skin thickness, and head size of the patient. The choice of hydrodynamic properties of the system can be influenced by the size of the ventricles, the patient's stature, the patient's status (e.g., vegetative, normal), the pathogenesis of the hydrocephalus, and the evolutionary course of the disease. Surgical placement can be influenced by anatomical considerations and the potential for contamination (e.g., internal lines, gastrostomy, tracheotomy, laparotomy, artificial bladder). The status of the cerebrospinal fluid (e.g., debris from a recent hemorrhage) may require postponing shunt insertion. Anatomical considerations, such as loculated ventricles, must lead one to consider endoscopic surgery first; there is rarely an indication for using more than one shunt system.

Equipment

A shunt assembly is composed of three basic elements: proximal tubing, a valve system, and distal tubing. In addition, several components can be added to the shunt line. Since the large number of available devices are mainly the result of commercial competition, it is interesting to evaluate them in an attempt to determine their strengths and weaknesses.

Basic Components

All shunts are basically made from the same components, that is, silicone elastomer with or without barium impregnation, polycarbonate, polyethylene, polysulfone, and various metals. At present, pure silicone

appears to be the most appropriate material to achieve biocompatibility. There have been several reports, however, implicating silicone as a causative agent for host reactions and suggesting the need for a more biologically inert material.[113, 115, 288, 289] Several available valve systems incorporate metallic components or even magnets, which can produce artifact on magnetic resonance imaging.

Ventricular Catheters

Size. It appears that so-called small or ultrasmall catheters were designed to be less traumatic in infants. Since no hard data exist comparing the risks of neurological consequences (epilepsy), catheter obstruction, and skin problems to catheter diameters, the author reserves comment on the validity of various catheter diameters (except for commercial purposes).[72, 167]

Stiffness. Catheter stiffness is a function of the grade of the silicone, on one hand, and the thickness of the tubing (external diameter − internal diameter), on the other hand. This parameter is a compromise between two risks (for straight ventricular catheters). The catheter must be soft enough to prevent injury to the ventricular wall, with its subsequent migration into the brain parenchyma, and yet must be firm enought to be kink resistant and retain its straight shape.

Length. The length of ventricular catheters is directly related to the surgical technique.

Shape. Because of their elasticity, straight catheters have the advantage, when used alone, without a right-angle device, and inserted via an occipital route, to go naturally up in the ventricles, away from the choroid plexus. Preshaped right-angle catheters, or straight catheters used with a right-angle sleeve, have the advantage of staying where they are placed at the time of shunt insertion.

Tip (Flanged or Not Flanged). Flanged catheters of various design were proposed either to prevent obstruction by the choroid plexus or to prevent debris from going into the system at the time of shunt insertion.[127] They do not achieve these goals. What's more, these devices seem to favor firm choroid plexus attachment to the ventricular catheter.

Extracranial-Intracranial Transition Zone (Burr Hole Reservoir, Right-Angle Connector, Right-Angle Clip)

Preshaped Catheters. The simplest way of passing through the burr hole is to use a preshaped right-angle ventricular catheter. Because of their predetermined length, however, it is necessary to keep in stock several different catheters to match the needs of each particular case.

Straight Catheters. They can be precisely trimmed to the desired length for each case. At the burr hole site, this type of catheter either can be bent (the risk of kinking with the existing material being minimum) or can be maintained at a right angle with some addi-

---

*See references 15, 62, 138, 151, 153, 261, 283, and 284.
†See references 63, 64, 164, 184, 263, and 285.

tional device. The right-angle clips can erode the skin when they are made of hard plastic.

Burr Hole Reservoir. A straight ventricular catheter can be connected to a reservoir that fits in the burr hole. Both catheter and reservoir must be a one-component device, thus avoiding potential disconnection that can result in loss of the catheter in the ventricle. In addition, insertion of a burr hole reservoir requires a larger incision in order to avoid placing the device directly under the scar.

Right-Angle Connectors (Metal or Plastic). This device requires a ligature under the skull, with the aforementioned risk of a lost intracranial catheter; it should be avoided.

Reservoir (Shape, Size, Location, and Tap)

A reservoir provides easy access to the system for fluid sampling, patency testing, and direct intracranial pressure monitoring, but these advantages must be balanced against the risk of contamination related to tapping the shunt and the risk of mechanical complications associated with the reservoir.[194, 296] Antibiotics can be infused through the reservoir, but most shunt infections require removal of the entire contaminated shunt as definitive treatment. If a reservoir is deemed necessary, it must have certain characteristics. It must be tough enough to sustain needle perforations and yet be soft enough not to cause skin erosion. The reservoir must be of a profile compatible with pediatric use; however, it must also be capable of being palpated under the skin of an adult. This device can be located at the burr hole level, in line with the valve proximal to it, or integrated into the valve system. In any case, the reservoir increases the total volume of the valve system and requires a larger subcutaneous dissection for it to be properly inserted compared with a valve without a reservoir.

Valve (Location, Profile, and Pressure-Flow Characteristics)

Location. Except for distal-slit valves, which must be avoided because of their almost unique tendency to cause distal obstruction, all the valves are located proximal in the shunt system.[246, 247, 280] The surgeon decides how far from the burr hole site the valve is placed. One must remember that the valve is a point of inherent fixation in the system and can lead to fracture, disruption, or migration of the tubing if it is located too far from the other site of fixation, the burr hole. To prevent skin erosion it has been suggested that some larger devices should be placed at the neck and even at the prethoracic level. This location is of concern, at least in children, because of the potential for growth between these two points of fixation.

Profile. The valve must be of a size appropriate for use in infants. But, why do we have pediatric and adult models? Hopefully, a child will grow, and cerebrospinal fluid physiology is not that different in adults and children. The shape of the valve seems more important. Some devices with a cylindrical shape can

migrate easily under the skin if they are not properly secured by a nonabsorbable ligature.

Pumping Device. With present day technology, there is no need to pump a shunt to enhance flow. In addition, with the availability of computed tomography, magnetic resonance imaging, and ultrasound, a pumping device is comparatively unreliable for assessing shunt function.

Hydrodynamic Characteristics. From the hydrodynamic standpoint, there are three generations of valves: (1) pressure-regulating valves (externally adjustable or not), (2) siphon-resistive devices, and (3) a flow-regulating system. With the exception of the third group, most valves act as pressure regulators.[226, 280] A one-way valve mechanism, calibrated at a certain opening pressure, tries to maintain a constant pressure across the valve (differential pressure) regardless of the drainage flow. Several mechanisms can be used to achieve this (i.e., ball-in-cone valve, silicone rubber diaphragm valve, duckbill valve, silicone rubber slit valve). Although they differ in their mechanical construction, they all achieve the same result: when the differential pressure across the valve increases, the valve opens, and cerebrospinal fluid flows freely. An ideal pressure regulator would give a horizontal pressure-flow curve. In real life, there exist functional imperfections responsible for some alterations in the pressure-flow curve (Fig. 36–22). Each valve comes in different pressure ranges. The denominations and spectra of these pressure ranges vary with each manufacturer; typically: low pressure, less than 40 mm H_2O; medium pressure, 40 to 80 mm H_2O; high pressure, greater than 80 mm H_2O. By definition, the drainage flow of these valves is very sensitive to variations in differential pressure. The wide range of pressure induced by postural changes, rapid-eye-movement (REM) sleep, and effort is known to generate an overdrainage several times higher than cerebrospinal fluid secretion.[56, 57, 325, 328] Two complementing factors enable these pressure-regulating systems to effectively treat hydrocephalus: the choice of an opening pressure that provides an acceptable balance between overdrainage and underdrainage;

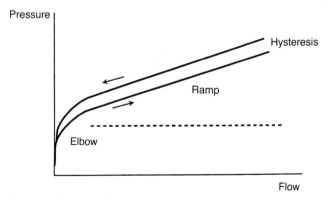

Figure 36–22

The perfect pressure-regulating mechanism maintains a constant differential pressure regardless of the flow rate (*horizontal line* on the pressure-flow graph). The actual mechanisms used in construction of hydrocephalus valves must overcome several functional realities, that is, "elbow," ramp, and hysteresis.

and the resilience of the human body. However, several complications (slit ventricles, pericerebral effusions, craniostenosis, cranioencephalic disproportion, ventricular exclusion, ventricular catheter obstructions) are directly or indirectly linked to the inadequacy of the cerebrospinal fluid drainage observed with these shunts. To try to remedy these drawbacks, several alternatives have been proposed over the past 15 years: valves with externally adjustable opening pressures, siphon-resistive devices, and a flow-regulating system.

Valves with Externally Adjustable Opening Pressures. These valves (programmable Medos valve* and Sophy valve†) are derived from conventional systems. They allow for fine-tuning in vivo of the balance between underdrainage and overdrainage, but the hydrodynamic characteristics of these shunts are the same as those of standard valves.[177] The adjustable function is obtained with the use of magnets built into the valve mechanism.

Siphon-Resistive Devices. These devices (Antisiphon device‡ and Siphon control device, Delta valve§) react to the hydrostatic pressure that appears when the patient leaves the recumbent position, to increase the opening pressure of the system proportionally to the vertical distance between the two ends of the distal tubing.[103, 120, 145, 221] In theory, a shunt system with a siphon-resistive device would react only to proximal pressure variations upstream (intracranial pressure + the hydrostatic pressure between the ventricles and the device).[297] This system tends to maintain a constant positive intracranial pressure, even when the person is standing. In addition, proper function of this device is contingent on atmospheric pressure, which is not always the case in the scar tissue that develops around the device.[74, 75, 89, 182, 183]

Flow-Regulating System. This system (Orbis-Sigma valve‖), contrary to a pressure regulator, tries to maintain a constant flow at different pressures.[245] This flow-regulating function is achieved by increasing the valve resistance as the differential pressure increases. The pressure-flow curve of a perfect flow regulator would be a straight vertical line, which is not exactly the case in real life (Fig. 36–23). The flow regulation of the existing system is set close to the cerebrospinal fluid secretion rate (18 to 30 mL per hour). These characteristics allow the device to limit the overdrainage phenomenon, with interesting clinical results.[71, 249] A certain residual overdrainage, however, can still be observed in patients who have retained some physiological cerebrospinal fluid resorption capacity. In addition, the very significant flow restriction built into the system requires that specific precautions be taken at the time of shunt insertion (clean cerebrospinal fluid, no leak of cerebrospinal fluid around the ventricular catheter).

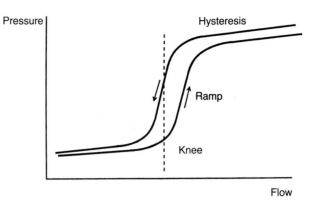

Figure 36–23

Contrary to pressure regulation, flow regulation tries to maintain a constant flow through the valve, regardless of the differential pressure. The ideal pressure-flow curve is a straight vertical. The actual mechanism demonstrates some functional restrictions, that is, "knee," ramp, hysteresis.

Distal Tubing (Size, Length, and Types of Ends)

Although not proven scientifically, a pure platinum-cured silicone outer wall seems less prone to promoting calcification than does barium-impregnated tubing. As previously stated, there is no rationale for distal-slit–ended catheters (with valve function or not). To the author's knowledge, the length of the tubing introduced into the peritoneal cavity is an exceptionally rare cause of problems. Thus, at least 25 cm has to be inserted to allow for growth and to avoid lengthening procedures without adverse sequelae.

Miscellaneous Accessories

The existing accessories, which can be added to the shunt system, have induced numerous shunt complications, without any proof of their effectiveness or usefulness. A Millipore (micropore) filter invariably induces shunt obstruction, an on-off device can lead to accidental arrest of flow, and telemetric pressure sensors are not convenient at the present time.[56, 67]

Connections of the Different Elements (One-Piece, Two-Piece, Three-Piece, and Multipiece Systems)*

Any connection is a weak point in a shunt system and carries several risks. Disconnection can occur in cases of improper ligature. Fracture can result from the different physical properties of the two materials. Migration or fracture can take place because when the connection is located on the distal tubing, it creates a point fixation. For these reasons it is safer to avoid the use of connectors distal to the valve and to select a system in which the distal tubing is joined with the valve. What happens at the proximal end of the valve system is more questionable. On one hand, disconnection at this level is quite rare and is influenced

---

*Codman & Sturleff, Inc., Randolph, Massachusetts.
†Sophysa S.A., Besançon, France.
‡American V. Mueller, Chicago, Illinois.
§PS Medical, Santa Barbara, California.
‖Cordis Corp., Miami, Florida.

---

*See reference 126.

essentially by the surgical technique; on the other hand, a one-piece system requires an external stylet for catheter introduction. This device is more traumatic to the brain and the dura, leading to a higher risk of cerebrospinal fluid leak around the ventricular catheter. In addition, clots and debris entering the catheter at the time of insertion flow directly into the system and increase the risk of shunt obstruction.

Surgical Technique

Even if the perfect shunt existed, it would rapidly be rendered useless by inappropriate surgical technique. The purpose of this section is not to legislate on shunt surgery but to describe the operation as the author performs it. This is to serve only as a model to demonstrate general surgical principles that apply to the insertion of most available shunts. Only ventriculoperitoneal and ventriculoatrial insertion will be described. General concerns, such as the role of the people in the operating room, the timing of shunt surgery, and the number of procedures per day, have been recently analyzed and correlated with occurrence of shunt infection. These measures could be applied to any type of shunt surgery.

Preoperative Preparation. Unless the operation is an emergency, the preparation of the patient begins the night before surgery. One scrub of the abdomen and the scalp is performed using a slow-release iodine soap solution. This scrub is repeated in the morning just prior to surgery. The hair is not shaved. If deemed necessary, clipping is performed by the surgeon himself.

Anesthesia. Prior to induction of anesthesia, it is important to verify that there are available at least two sets of the equipment that the surgeon intends to insert. The patient will be operated on while under general anesthesia with orotracheal intubation. The electrodes for electrocardiography must not be placed on the anterior chest wall that will be included in the surgical field in the case of a ventriculoperitoneal shunt. The bladder is emptied by manual suprapubic pressure in anesthetized children or by straight catheterization if there is any suspicion of a full bladder. A single perioperative dose of antibiotics is administered at the induction of anesthesia. The author prefers the administration of cefotaxime, 100 mg per kg, and fosfomycin, 100 mg per kg.

Positioning of the Patient. Positioning of the patient is a critical stage. It is important that the line joining the cranial incision and the abdominal one is linear. This avoids extra skin incisions at the neck or the thoracic level. The patient is placed in the prone position, the head is rotated to the contralateral side, and the neck is hyperextended with a shoulder roll.

Prepping and Draping. The hair is clipped over the skin incision. The operative field is widely and meticulously prepped with a slow-release iodine solution. A 4-cm-wide strip of skin is draped from the burr hole site to the umbilicus in the case of ventriculoperitoneal shunt insertion, or to the nipple for a ventriculoatrial shunt.

Skin Incision. The skin incision must be small; a 2- to 3-cm linear incision is enough to insert any of the available shunt systems. Gentle retraction permits placement of the burr hole at an adequate distance from the incision site. The classic half-moon flap (of any size) is unnecessary and serves only to compromise vascularization, predisposing to the occurrence of skin problems.

Burr Hole Placement. The ideal placement for the burr hole is controversial and is still a matter of discussion among neurosurgeons. The choice between the frontal and the occipital burr hole sites is essentially a function of institutional preferences, surgeon's conviction, and ventricular configuration. The author generally prefers the relative simplicity of a posterior burr hole placement, except when the anterior horns are the most dilated portion of the ventricular system. A frontal burr hole is positioned on the coronal suture in line with the medial canthus. A posterior burr hole is positioned on the lambdoid suture in line with the lateral canthus and the apex of the ear. It must be remembered that in some pathological conditions, such as Dandy-Walker malformation or large arachnoid cysts of the posterior fossa, the transverse sinus can be displaced in a much higher position; in these patients, preoperative identification of the transverse sinus by magnetic resonance imaging is required.

The size of the burr hole depends on the configuration of the shunt, and the thickness of the calvaria. If a free ventricular catheter is used, a burr hole needs only to be large enough (4 mm) to allow punctiform coagulation of the dura. However, in children, with thick calvaria and small ventricles, the burr hole must be large enough to allow modifications of the ventricular track. Also a larger diameter may be necessary if a burr hole reservoir is used. In infants with distended sutures, trephination can be frequently achieved simply with electrocautery.

Subgaleal Dissection. The creation of a small subgaleal pocket to allow easy placement of the valve and appropriate skin closure is of primary importance. When subgaleal dissection is too small, excessive traction on the distal catheter, or multiple manipulations of the valve, may be required, which predispose the system to injury. If the pocket is made too large, there is the potential for subcutaneous hematomas, collections of cerebrospinal fluid, or shunt migration. The author prefers to create a small subgaleal pocket with scissors. In a single movement, the scissors are introduced closed to the desired distance from the incision and pulled out opened. Repetition of the same movement increases the risk of contamination by organisms from the edges of the incision.

Shunt Passing

Ventriculoperitoneal Shunt Insertion. The stiffness and the length of the shunt tunneler are adapted to the patient. The author uses two different types of tunneler, a very malleable 45-cm-long tunneler in patients younger than 1 year of age, and a stiffer 65-cm-long tunneler for others. It is of primary importance to introduce the shunt passer into the previously created pocket. Care should be taken at the level of the neck and clavicle, to avoid vascular injuries or pleural perforation. One hand is pushing on the tunneler not too far from the scalp incision while the direction is controlled with the other hand through the skin covered with an adhesive plastic sheet. The track of the shunt passer must never become too superficial. This precaution reduces the risks of skin perforation and possibly the risk of delayed tubing calcification. When the tip of the tunneler arrives in the periumbilical region, it is delivered through a stab incision. Under certain circumstances it may be impossible to rotate the head for adequate positioning of the patient (e.g., upper spine fusion, cranioskeletal anomalies), or it may be too risky to place the shunt anteriorly (e.g., tracheotomy, jugular central line). In these cases, the shunt can be placed posteriorly. It is not recommended to use this route as a first choice, because the mechanical demands on the tubing are greater in this position, leading to a higher risk of calcification, fracture, or disconnection.

Ventriculoatrial Shunt Insertion. In the case of ventriculoatrial shunt insertion, tunneling is stopped at the midneck level, on the anterior edge of the sternocleidomastoid muscle. It is only at this time, and not before, that the surgeon opens the sterile blister containing the shunt. Many surgeons recommend soaking the shunt in an antiseptic solution (e.g., bacitracin). Some surgeons try to check the hydrodynamic characteristics of the valve in the operating room prior to insertion. What can be adequately tested is only the patency of the system, and these manipulations are probably the cause of some shunt contaminations. The distal tubing is then connected to the tunneler and pulled through, leaving it in place under the skin. Many surgeons recommend passing the shunt tunneler in a distal to proximal direction. The author, however, does not recommend this method, because he finds it difficult to maintain a subgaleal plane at the scalp level.

Opening of the Dura. The dura opening is performed blindly with coagulation using a monopolar or a bipolar cautery. The opening must be smaller than the outer diameter of the ventricular catheter, to ensure a tight dural catheter seal, especially in newborns with large ventricular dilatation and a thin cortical mantle. This is essential to reduce the risk of cerebrospinal fluid leakage around the catheter. A larger coagulation of the dura or a cruciform incision, as described by several authors, does not give any advantage over the aforementioned technique and increases the risk of subcutaneous cerebrospinal fluid leaks.

Ventricular Catheter Placement. The controversy over the ideal placement of the ventricular catheter tip is too complex to be discussed here. However, some concepts must be emphasized. It seems more appropriate to locate the tip of the ventricular catheter in the most dilated part of the ventricle for two main reasons: (1) such placement reduces the risk of malposition; and (2) the portion of the ventricle that is most dilated preoperatively will probably remain so after shunting, reducing the risk of the catheter's coming into contact with the choroid plexus and ventricle walls. The catheter, stiffened by its stylet, is introduced into the brain, through the punctiform coagulation site, and aimed toward the appropriate position. The surgeon realizes that the ventricle has been entered because of the kinesthetic sensation resulting from perforation of the ependyma and because cerebrospinal fluid will start to drip out the distal end of the catheter. At this time the stylet must be removed and the catheter gently advanced into the ventricle with a smooth forceps. It is useful to calculate the appropriate length of the catheter on computed tomography or plain x-ray films prior to surgery. A fiberoptic endoscope, if available, can be advantageously used in place of the classic stylet, allowing direct visualization.

Cleaning the Shunt System and Checking Its Function. Before connecting the catheter to the valve, 2 to 3 mL of cerebrospinal fluid is drained for routine cerebrospinal fluid sampling (culture and cell count) and to allow clearing of clots and debris. After connecting the catheter to the valve, some cerebrospinal fluid is gently aspirated from the distal end, and the absence of residual debris in the valve is checked. The valve is then inserted under the scalp by smoothly pulling the distal catheter with one hand while the other hand is controlling, through the skin, its progression in the subgaleal pocket. At this stage it is mandatory to verify that the shunt is functional. Cerebrospinal fluid must flow from the distal end of the tubing prior to its insertion in the drainage cavity. Shunt function may be encouraged by lowering slightly its distal end to increase the differential pressure applied to the drainage system.

Distal Insertion. In the case of a ventriculoperitoneal shunt, the author prefers to introduce the distal catheter into the peritoneal cavity by trocar puncture.[171] This technique is not advised in the case of previous abdominal surgery, where there is a risk of intraabdominal adhesions. In these cases, a minilaparotomy or the use of an endoscopic trochar is safest. In the case of a ventriculoatrial shunt, a percutaneous method is preferred in older patients.[298] The jugular vein is tapped and catheterized with a lead wire, and the needle replaced with a peel-away introducer. Under fluoroscopy, the appropriate length of catheter is determined (this length is approximately equal to the distance between the neck incision and the nipple minus 2 cm). The catheter is then trimmed to the appropriate length and introduced via the peel-away introducer.

Skin Closure. The only acceptable definition for skin closure is that it must be perfect. If the scalp incision is of the appropriate length, a two-layer closure with three to four stitches is enough. The wound is then protected with a loose adhesive surgical dressing.

As already stated, what has been described is only an example of surgical procedure for shunt insertion. There are probably many other possibilities. What is important, however, is that surgeons be convinced that shunt surgery is the major cause of shunt complications. They must be able to justify their choices at each step of the procedure.

Postoperative Management

The immediate postoperative period is critical. Special attention must be paid in two respects: (1) prevention of skin problems leading to shunt contamination, and (2) assessment of shunt function and detection of early shunt complications. The best way of avoiding skin problems is to perform perfect skin closure. In addition, any pressure over the valve system, even for a short period, must be avoided. This is of particular interest in the youngest or debilitated patients. Parents and nurses must be aware of the mechanisms of these complications, their risks, and their prevention. For most of the available shunts, no special positioning is required after shunting. However, some surgeons used to leave patients treated with a standard shunt in a recumbent position for 1 or 2 days after surgery, to minimize the risk of development of subdural cerebrospinal fluid collections. Conversely, when a high-resistance device is used in patients who are not able to function normally (infants, comatose patients), it can be worthwhile to artificially increase the pressure differential across the valve by positioning the patient semisitting. This maneuver increases the flow through the shunt and helps reduce the risk of cerebrospinal fluid leaking around the ventricular catheter and accumulating in the subcutaneous tissue.

Following a plain x-ray film of the inserted material and clinical evidence of normal function, the patient can be discharged from the hospital after a few days. The parents or the patient himself, if old enough, must be provided with all pertinent information about the shunt and shunt surgery. A follow-up examination is scheduled at 3 months after surgery, with computed tomography or magnetic resonance imaging performed.

Shunt Revision

The causes of shunt revision are so numerous that it is impossible to describe all the possible situations. However, some guidelines have to be kept in mind to avoid potentially serious complications.

It is mandatory to identify and correct the cause of the first failure. It is interesting to note that in most of the reported series occurrence of a shunt complication is highly correlated with occurrence of a subsequent one of the same type. For instance, a simple reconnection of a calcified distal tubing disconnected from the valve will inevitably result in another disconnection or fracture if the distal tubing is not entirely replaced.

In the case of very small ventricles, replacement of the ventricular catheter can be a frightening experience. It is essential to prevent cerebrospinal fluid leakage, which can further decrease the size of this already small ventricle. Good exposure of the catheter at the burr hole level is crucial. The obstructed catheter is removed and immediately replaced with a new one without its stylet. The new catheter is gently pushed through the pre-established tract in the ventricles using smooth forceps. Multiple taps, which carry the risk of bleeding, should be avoided. A safer alternative is to use an aid, such as a fiberoptic endoscope, a catheter stylet, ultrasound, a digitizer, or stereotactic insertion, if the new catheter does not pass easily on the first attempt.

When one is faced with an occluded or stuck ventricular catheter, there is a risk of major hemorrhage if the attached catheter is simply avulsed. It is often possible to pass a coagulation wire (used for endoscopic procedures) along the length of the adherent tubing. Frequently this maneuver allows a sufficient degree of retraction of the invading choroid plexus to withdraw the catheter easily and safely.

Disruption of tubings, evidenced on plain x-ray film, in a patient free from signs and symptoms does not usually mean arrested hydrocephalus. The fibrous sheath that develops around the silicone tube in its subcutaneous tract is capable, at least for a time, of acting as a conduit for cerebrospinal fluid. Removal of the shunt can lead to life-threatening complications.

In any case, the function of the system must be checked prior to insertion of the distal tubing in the drainage cavity.

SHUNT COMPLICATIONS

Shunt complications are numerous. They can be categorized into three groups: (1) infection; (2) mechanical failure; and (3) functional failure, resulting from an inadequate flow rate of a normally functioning shunt. Shunt infections put patients at increased risk for intellectual impairment, development of loculated ventricles, and even death.[142, 188, 313] Noninfectious shunt complications result in a low but real percentage of death or neurological impairment and require revision and an additional surgery with all its risks.* Finally, from an economical point of view, each malfunction doubles the cost of the treatment. In trying to reduce the rate of shunt complications, it is necessary to define and understand the causes of these problems; they often arise from multifactorial etiologies. One must never lose sight of the fact that any choice among the numerous possibilities that exist in the treatment of hydrocephalus is usually the result of a compromise between two or more risk factors. The shunt characteristics, including configuration, hydrodynamic properties, and material, are compromises among ease of insertion, risk of disconnection, risk of early or late obstruction, expense, and ease of manufacture. As far as the patient is concerned, one often compromises adequate profile and pressure-flow characteristics at the time of surgery and later on in life. As far as the surgeon is concerned, compromise exists as well at many stages in patient management.

Shunt Infection

In some cases, shunt infection remains remarkably difficult to establish. A simple working definition is the following: unequivocal evidence of infection of the shunt equipment, the overlying wound, the cerebrospinal fluid, or the distal drainage site related to the shunt. Unequivocal evidence of shunt infection requires demonstration of the organism(s) on Gram stain or culture

---

*See references 202, 214, 246, 247, 253, and 262.

from material in, on, or around the shunt, or from fluid withdrawn from the shunt. Most shunt infections appear within the first 2 months after surgery. The most common organisms infecting shunts during this period are staphylococci: approximately 40 per cent of shunt infections are caused by *Staphylococcus epidermidis*, and 20 per cent by *S. aureus*.* Other species isolated from infected shunts include the Coryneforms, streptococci, enterococci, aerobic gram-negative rods, and yeasts.[24] Because the most common organisms are part of the skin flora, and shunt infection usually occurs during the postoperative period, endogenous spread from the patient or surgical staff would be the logical route of infection. Various studies have, indeed, shown this to be the case.[20, 61, 267] Late shunt infections usually demonstrate a very different bacteriological profile, involving predominantly gram-negative bacilli. There is usually an attributable cause of infection, including bowel perforation, skin necrosis, exophytic tube calcifications, laparotomy, and *Haemophilus influenzae* meningitis.[267]

To understand the issues surrounding the prevention and treatment of shunt infections, it is important to examine the detailed mechanisms by which shunt systems become colonized with microorganisms. The implanted shunt is almost immediately coated with a glycoproteinaceous conditioning film, derived from serum and extracellular matrix proteins, providing potential receptor sites for bacterial or tissue adhesion.[117, 309] The shunt material's surface properties determine the sequence and layering of the deposited proteins. It is at this stage that there is competition for shunt surface adhesion between the host tissue cells and whatever bacteria may exist in the vicinity. This competition for adhesion has been termed the "race for surface."[117] The relative success of either the bacteria or the host cell in this race determines, in large part, the ultimate clinical scenario associated with the implanted shunt. If tissue cells are the first to adhere to and integrate with the shunt surface, this eukaryotic cell surface provides resistance to any further colonization attempts by bacteria. Tissue integration with the shunt surface, however, is limited to the portion of the shunt that lies within the subcutaneous tissue and generally does not occur on the distal portion that lies within the peritoneal cavity. It is during this crucial stage of surface adhesion that maintaining a sterile shunt system is of paramount importance. Bacterial adhesion is a complicated process that involves both physical and chemical interactions.[117] As it approaches the shunt surface, the bacterium, like any particle, acts under the influence of Van der Waals forces and attractive hydrophobic interaction between its surface and that of the shunt. Such forces may place the bacterium close enough to the shunt surface to allow for irreversible adhesion. This irreversible binding occurs as the result of interaction between specific fibrinal adhesions or bacterial exopolysaccharides, or both, and the conditioning film receptor on the shunt surface.[19] Initially, cell division within the bacterial microcolonies and,

later, recruitment and aggregation of bacteria from the surrounding environment produce a continuous biofilm on the shunt surface. This biofilm is composed of bacteria, either singly or in microcolonies, all embedded in an anionic matrix of exopolymers and trapped molecules.[68] Eventually the shunt infection becomes clinically detectable, although it may take as long as several months to manifest. The existence of bacteria in the form of a biofilm is one of the most important properties of bacterial colonization of biomaterials. This mode of growth has been shown to be associated with an appreciable measure of protection against many common antibacterial agents, including antibodies, white cells, surfactants, and antibiotics. The protective effects of the biofilm provide an explanation for the relative lack of success associated with the treatment of shunt infections by the exclusive use of systemic and/or intraventricular antibiotics.[82, 154] Aggressive antimicrobial chemotherapy may clear the acute inflammation, but the organisms within the surface biofilm will only be reduced in number and will rarely be eradicated. The biofilm mode of growth may explain the various clinical scenarios that are commonly associated with the different infecting organisms.[25] Organisms that lack the ability to adhere to the shunt surface, such as *S. aureus*, are more likely to be associated with a wound infection of the surrounding tissue that secondarily infects the shunt. Those organisms that can produce extracellular slime, however, particularly *S. epidermidis*, possess an enhanced ability to bind to the shunt material. Therefore, they are able to form a biofilm on the luminal shunt surface and then present as true shunt colonization, not as a wound infection.

Risk Factors for Shunt Infection

Despite the information available on the pathogenesis of shunt infection, few factors have been clearly identified as risk factors. Young age has represented a higher risk in a number of studies.[10, 128, 232] This may be related to relative immaturity of the immune system, the vulnerability of thin skin, or other factors. Poor skin condition or other concurrent sites of infection have been shown to increase the risk of shunt infection. Other factors may also promote infection, such as the duration of the operation and the presence of cerebrospinal fluid leak or drainage. The experience of the surgeon may influence infection rate, as it may interact with the previously mentioned factors.

Clinical Features

The clinical features depend on the site of infection. Wound infections are usually manifested as fever, reddening of the incision site or shunt tract, and, with progression of the infection, discharge of pus from the incision. In chronic wound infections, the shunt may actually become exposed as the wound breaks down. Any leakage of cerebrospinal fluid from the incision because of an improperly placed or malfunctioning shunt also often results in contamination and subsequent infection. Meningitis manifests as fever, head-

---

*See references 23, 36, 220, 232, 267, and 313.

ache or irritability, and often some neck stiffness, if not nuchal rigidity. Peritonitis is less common; the patient typically presents with fever, anorexia or vomiting, and abdominal tenderness. The severity of the symptoms depends, to some extent, on the infecting organism. Patients infected with *S. epidermidis* may look remarkably well and may have intermittent fever or irritability only. They may also present, particularly at the beginning, with signs of a typical shunt obstruction without fever or leukocytosis.[313] Patients with infected abdominal pseudocysts may present with a mass only. Historically, patients with ventriculoatrial shunts may manifest shunt nephritis or cor pulmonale, in addition to presenting with signs of a septicemia.[234, 282] Shunts have been demonstrated to be impervious to bacterial migration across the shunt wall, so spread occurs along the inside or the outside of the shunt.[121] Although the possibility of retrograde bacterial movements up the lumen of the shunt has been disputed, clear evidence of infectious spread from the peritoneal cavity to the brain has been reported.[22, 114] In terms of differential diagnoses, all patients with suspected shunt infection should have a thorough history and physical examination to rule out other possible sources of infection. This is particularly important in children, in whom any of the common childhood febrile illnesses, such as otitis media, or urinary tract infection (particularly in patients with myelomeningocele) can resemble a shunt infection.

Diagnostic Tests

Routine blood work frequently reveals a polymorphonuclear leukocytosis. Blood, urine, sputum, and wound sites should be cultured if they are clinically suspected. Plain x-ray film examination of the shunt system can verify its integrity, the presence of possible perforated abdominal viscus, and whether there are any extraneous pieces of shunt equipment from previous revisions that may or may not be contaminated. Computed tomography or magnetic resonance imaging of the head, displaying the size and configuration of the ventricles, not only helps determine whether the shunt is obstructed but also may influence decisions to remove the infected shunt and to insert an external ventricular drain. Placing such a drainage system in a patient with an infected functional shunt and slit ventricles may be quite difficult. Abdominal ultrasound should be performed in any patient with abdominal pain or tenderness or a mass. Cerebrospinal fluid, obtained via lumbar puncture or reservoir aspiration, examined for cell count, stained with Gram stain, and cultured, will confirm the diagnosis of shunt infection and quickly give an index of the probable infecting organism. It has been reported that shunt aspiration provides a diagnostic yield of approximately 95 per cent. The author suggests that lumbar puncture, even if it is truly less efficient, may be sufficient for a correct diagnosis in these infected patients. In addition, almost all recent series put the risk of shunt infection at less than 3 per cent. The author feels that when these two considerations are balanced against the potential com-

plications associated with reservoirs (disconnection, skin erosion, subcutaneous fluid accumulation), their routine use can be discussed. Sustained elevation of serum levels of C-reactive protein following shunt insertion is also strongly correlated with the presence of shunt infection.[25] Cerebrospinal eosinophilia (defined as more than 7 per cent of the total cereobrospinal white cell count) also correlates with shunt infection.[303] At the time of surgery, ventricular cerebrospinal fluid should be resampled. All hardware removed should be sent to the microbiology laboratory for culture. The manner in which the shunt material is handled is important in preventing contamination at the time of removal by the wound edges.[23]

Treatment of Shunt Infection

The number of combinations and permutations in the treatment of shunt infection is almost as great as the variety of shunt equipment and techniques of shunt placement.[55, 257, 317] The main treatment options encompass whether the shunt hardware is removed, whether interval external drainage is established, and whether intraventricular antibiotics are administered. There are three general treatment options. First is treatment with antibiotics alone. This type of therapy carries the lowest cure rate and the highest morbidity and mortality rates.[104] Given the production of a biolayer by the most common infecting organisms and their accompanying resistance to antibiotics, it seems logical that any treatment short of removal of the shunt hardware would be less than successful. There are some important exceptions. Organisms that cause meningitis in the general population and infect patients with shunts can usually be treated with antibiotics alone if they are discovered at the time of shunt insertion. *Haemophilus influenzae* infection, meningococcal meningitis, and even gonococcal meningitis in the presence of a shunt have been successfully treated with antibiotics alone.[168, 169, 211, 212, 233] Although not well documented in the literature, patients presenting with pneumococcal meningitis can also be successfully treated with antibiotics alone. Inherent in this form of treatment is the assumption that the cerebrospinal fluid will be resampled to verify sterilization. Failure of the fluid to clear within 48 to 72 hours should prompt removal of the shunt equipment.

The second general treatment option is shunt removal, with immediate replacement. This type of treatment carries a high cure rate. It is an attractive option, as it saves the patient from having to undergo a subsequent surgical procedure. There is no guarantee, however, that the cerebrospinal fluid is sterile at the time of immediate reinsertion (usually at an alternative site). The author prefers to wait a few days, treating the patient with antibiotics alone, for verified fluid sterilization prior to removing the contaminated system and replacing the shunt.

The third treatment option is shunt removal combined with antibiotic treatment given at intervals, usually with external ventricular drainage. This type of treatment carries the highest cure rate and the lowest mortality rate; however, it is burdensome in terms of surgical procedure for the patient.[313] At least two operations are necessary, and these involve two or three surgical sites: the original incision, a new external drainage location, and possibly a new shunt site. External ventricular drainage largely restricts the patient to bed, carries the risk of dislodgment (particularly in children), and can lead to recontamination of the cerebrospinal fluid by either the same or a different organism. An external drain can also become obstructed or can overdrain, leading to subdural fluid collections. It may be difficult to insert an external drain in patients with small ventricles, in which case externalization of the peritoneal catheter may be the only option to establish interval drainage.

Prevention of Shunt Infection

Given the considerable morbidity, let alone the financial cost, of shunt infections, prevention is the leading consideration for the future. Preoperative skin preparation with iodine-based agents tends to remove transient skin flora and to reduce but not eliminate resident flora that remain viable in the portals of sweat and sebaceous glands and hair follicles.[20] Shaving with a razor more than a few hours before surgery has been clearly related to an increased incidence of infection.[152, 263] A recent study concluded that forgoing shaving did not increase the risk of any neurosurgical procedure, including shunts.[323] While adhesive drapes prevent the shunt from coming into contact with exposed skin, they do not appear to lower the bacterial density of wounds or the postoperative infection rate.[223] Adhesive drapes may also permit accumulation of sweat under the drapes, leading to spillage and contamination of the incision.[21]

Perhaps nothing has aroused as much controversy in the quest for reduced shunt infection as the use of prophylactic antibiotics. A number of randomized controlled trials comparing the effects of antibiotic prophylaxis have been reported.* Only one study detected a significant reduction in infection with the use of antibiotics, but the infection rate was very high (23 per cent).[36] All the trials suffered from the lack of a sufficient number of patients to detect a statistical difference, if one existed. To get around this problem, the trials were combined and a meta-analysis performed that demonstrated a significant decline in infection rates with the use of prophylactic antibiotics.[129, 165] All the centers selected for this study, however, had a baseline infection rate greater than 15 per cent. Since most centers are now reporting very low infection rates (<3 per cent) with the use of prophylactic antibiotics, and as there is evidence by meta-analysis that these drugs are efficacious, it seems reasonable to use them. For this therapy to be effective, there must be adequate tissue levels of the antibiotics at the time of incision.[128] The overall duration of antibiotic administration should be a relatively short period (usually 24 hours), because there is no evidence of benefit from prolonged administration and to prevent superinfection and the

development of resistant organisms.[43] It is best to use relatively narrow-spectrum drugs that are effective against the most likely infecting organism (i.e., staphylococci).

Silastic is relatively biocompatible and thus induces minimal inflammation of the host tissue, thereby enhancing early tissue colonization of the surface and maintaining local tissue resistance.[38] Silastic does, however, contain surface imperfections that can harbor bacterial colonies.[121] Smoother surfaces, or electrically charged surfaces, may prove to be more resistant to colonization.[24]

Mechanical Shunt Failure

Definition of mechanical shunt failure is not easy. The literature is sometimes quite confusing, for two main reasons. The first is the debate surrounding what constitutes a shunt failure. While problems directly related to the shunt itself (e.g., proximal obstruction of the ventricular catheter) are universally acknowledged as shunt complications, problems related to imperfect shunt function (e.g., slit ventricles, subdural cerebrospinal fluid collection, postural headache) are sometimes more difficult to interpret.[102, 195] Finally, some shunts are inserted with deliberate plans to revise them (i.e., lengthen or upgrade the valve) at some point in the future. While these revisions are carried out in an elective and planned fashion, the author still maintains that as far as the patient is concerned, they represent complications. In terms of imperfect shunt function, any problem related to the treatment of hydrocephalus that requires a subsequent operation seems a reasonable definition of a shunt complication. The second reason for uncertainty regarding the definition of mechanical shunt failure is that noninfectious shunt complications result from a variety of causes, each with a different relative time of onset. While an improperly tied connector manifests itself very quickly, problems such as degeneration and fracture of the tubing may take many years. For this reason, it is necessary to have sufficient follow-up to detect the shunt failures that occur late after surgery. It is also necessary to use appropriate statistical analysis (life-table analysis) to adequately assess the probability of each type of shunt failure at various times after surgery.

Mechanical shunt complications can be classified in several different ways. They can be categorized by function into two groups: underdrainage and overdrainage. They can also be grouped according to a particular component of the device: complications at the level of the ventricular catheter, valve system, connectors, and so forth. Finally, these complications can also be classified according to their mechanisms, such as improper placement of the ventricular catheter, improper placement of the distal tubing in the drainage cavity, overdissection of the subcutaneous tissue, migration of the shunt system, clots in the ventricle, debris entering the valve at the time of shunt insertion, and occlusion of the catheter by choroid plexus. Actually, it seems most logical to use these three different classifications all together: the first one giving the net

---

*See references 21, 26, 36, 37, 87, 128, 199, 228, 256, 314, and 315.

effect for the patient, the second giving the site of the complication, and the third identifying the mechanism of that complication. Finally, it is possible to relate these complications to the etiology (surgical technique, patient management, or the device itself). This allows better identification and understanding of the interactions between these factors (collectively or individually) and shunt malfunction. The acquisition of these data is mandatory to optimize the present treatment of hydrocephalus and to define areas for future progress.

Mechanical shunt complications were previously believed to be time-related events. This is understandable when one looks at the survival rates of different series of shunted patients (Fig. 36–24). The risk of shunt failure is maximal during the first few months after surgery, ranging from 20 to 40 per cent at 1-year follow-up. Later on, after this critical period, the risk varies between 0 and 5 per cent per year for these series of patients treated with different types of valves. The mean survival time for a shunt was about 5 years in series of patients treated with standard valves. An analysis of the time of occurrence of each type of complication and their distribution over time shows some significant differences; some types of shunt failure tend to occur soon after surgery, and others later. For some failures the "at-risk" period is quite short, whereas other failures are distributed throughout the life of the system. For a particular type of shunt failure, the causative factors are frequently not the same over time. For example, the ventricular catheter can be occluded soon after surgery by debris, or later by the choroid plexus. It is also probable that these factors are not the same in children and adults. Although several observations and, occasionally, specific procedural recommendations can be made to aid in avoiding mechanical shunt complications, what frequently emerges is the enormous complexity of interrelated factors. Attempts to avoid one set of predisposing factors often lead to increased exposure to others. The management of these complications, when they occur, requires careful analysis so that other unexpected problems do not ensue.[96, 116, 134]

Occlusions

Shunt occlusions represent about one half of all shunt complications in the pediatric population. The risk of shunt obstruction varies over the course of follow-up. The risk is highest in the immediate postoperative period. The role of debris or clots in the cerebrospinal fluid and a possible misplacement of the proximal tubing are probably predominant in early

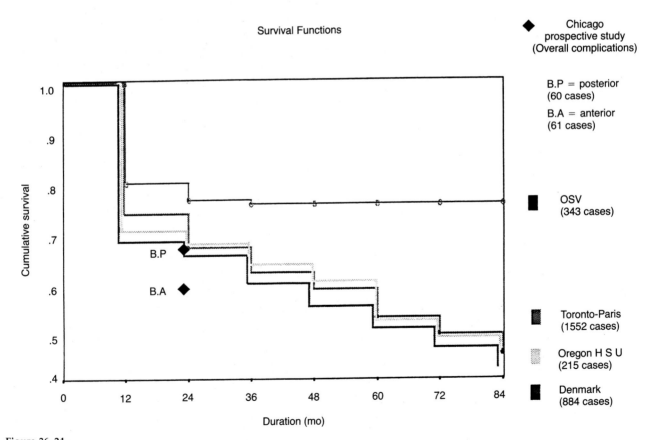

Figure 36–24

As demonstrated in all the reported series from different sources (prospective and retrospective), analyzed with life-table methods, the actuarial probability of occurrence of shunt mechanical complications is maximal during the first few months after surgery and similar between the series.[33, 214, 247, 249] These complications seem to be related mainly to surgical factors during that period. Later on, only two types of complications (proximal obstruction related to chronic overdrainage, and fracture related to the material) are mostly observed. It is interesting to note that limitation of the overdrainage phenomenon, as achieved with the Orbis-Sigma valve (OSV series), is able to reduce the risk of shunt complications by a factor of 2 at 5-year follow-up (50 versus 25 per cent).

occlusions, whereas choroid plexus, ependymal reaction, or immune reactions are predominant in producing delayed occlusion. Although there has been extensive discussion in the literature about delayed occlusions, in fact about one fourth of these occlusions occur soon after insertion. A shunt can be occluded at three different levels: the entry point (proximal occlusion), the valve system (valve obstruction), and the distal end (distal catheter occlusion). While factors influencing these occlusions are still being investigated, it is interesting to note that early occlusions are related more often to patient management and surgical technique. Late occlusions, however, are related mostly to the materials used and the hydrodynamic properties of the system. Nevertheless, an analysis of the potential causes of these types of shunt failure still needs to be made.

Proximal Occlusions. Ideally, an inert catheter floating in a pristine cavity filled with pure water has no reason to ever become obstructed. Silicone catheters, however, are not entirely inert, and cerebrospinal fluid may contain various debris or tissue. In addition, the cavity can become contracted to the point of putting the catheter and the wall of the cavity in apposition, or the choroid plexus can be swept along by the current into the proximal catheter. This type of complication may be related to various factors.

Contents of Cerebrospinal Fluid. Blood or cellular debris has a propensity to block the small lumina and distal holes of ventricular catheters. A period of temporary external drainage appears to be the solution to this problem.

Location of Catheter Tip. Catheter location is probably one of the most ancient controversies in the treatment of hydrocephalus.[6, 23] This debate is centered around standard teaching, which dictates that the choroid plexus is the agent most responsible for proximal catheter obstruction. Conventional wisdom states that the ventricular catheter must be placed in front of the foramen of Monro to avoid the choroid plexus. A ventricular catheter inserted in the frontal horn via an occipital route, however, can be drawn backward onto the choroid plexus by head growth. Alternatively, collapse of the ventricles may cause the catheter to migrate into the surrounding brain. Moreover, there are several other tissues besides choroid plexus that may obstruct the catheter. These include ependymal cells, glial tissue, connective tissue, and leptomeninges.[34, 66, 111, 112, 259] The results of the reported series are controversial.[6, 32] Actually, it is probable that there is no ideal place to locate the tip of the ventricular catheter; probably the least risky location is the one that remains the largest after drainage. This site varies from one patient to another. Not all parts of the ventricular system are distended to the same degree. In children, particularly those with congenital anomalies, the occipital horns remain dilated, and catheter tips located there may have a lower risk of obstruction.[227] It has also been suggested that ventricular catheters should be placed using visual assistance (e.g., endoscopy, radiography, ultrasound).[312] While such placement avoids insertion in the temporal horn or intraparenchymal

placement, these methods bring their own risks of morbidity which have not been fully evaluated at present.

Ventricle Size. The size of the ventricle is an important factor in delayed proximal catheter occlusion. Slitlike ventricles occurring after shunting are common in patients treated with standard pressure-regulating devices, and this condition can be found in as many as 40 per cent of patients at 3-year follow-up (Fig. 36–25). Sooner or later, the risk of proximal occlusion in this situation is almost inevitable. The occurrence of slit ventricles is related to the patient's age at the time of shunt insertion (potential of brain growth), the existence of brain atrophy prior to shunting, brain compliance (probably related to the evolution of the disease), and the hydrodynamic properties of the shunt. Although all available shunts overdrain to some degree, some newly developed shunts, which limit overdrainage, have been recently reported to demonstrate a decreased incidence of slitlike ventricles.

Valve Obstructions. The second component at risk for obstruction is the valve system itself. Rarely, an occlusion may be due to defective manufacturing of the device, which mandates a patency check at the time of insertion. Depending on the type, shunt valves have critical areas of flow restriction and dead space that are predisposed to accumulation of debris and tissue colonization. Systems that limit overdrainage (mentioned previously) require severe flow restriction in the valve system and could have adverse consequences, with an increased risk of valve obstruction. From a theoretical point of view, there is a risk of valve obstruction under three different conditions. First, at the time of shunt insertion there is always a risk of contamination of the valve with clot, parenchymal tis-

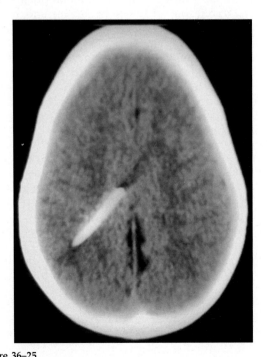

Figure 36–25

Slit ventricles are highly correlated with the occurrence of delayed proximal obstruction regardless of the location of the tip of the ventricular catheter.

sue, or other debris from the ventricular catheter. Second, bacterial proliferation in a shunt system can first present as a valve occlusion. Third, late valve obstruction, in addition to the possibility of debris or clot accumulation, raises the question of a cellular immune reaction, as suggested in well-documented cases of sterile shunt malfunctions.[113] In other words, valve obstruction can result from an active phenomenon (bacterial proliferation, development of an immune reaction) or a passive phenomenon (accumulation of debris of various origins). Valve obstruction can be at least partially prevented by improving valve design (avoiding dead spaces) and by careful surgical technique (minimizing the introduction of debris or clots into the system at the time of shunt insertion).

Distal Obstructions. The risk of distal occlusion varies according to the site of drainage and the design of the material.[3] Distal-slit catheters (the slits may or may not function as valves) carry a higher risk of occlusion. There is dead space beneath the slits that favors the progressive accumulation of debris, leading to plugging of the catheter. This tissue is composed of granuloma-like nodules of relatively acellular fibrin clumps surrounded by a large number of macrophages, a few mesothelial cells, lymphocytes, and fibroblasts. Some of the macrophages form multinucleated giant cells. The risk of this type of obstruction does not exist with open-ended distal tubing. Relative obstructions are due to lowering of the absorptive capacity of the peritoneal cavity (ascites or abdominal pseudocyst). Most of these phenomena have a clear origin (peritoneal infections, tumor seeding, mucopolysaccharidosis). In some cases, however, despite extensive investigation the cause of the malabsorption remains unclear (immune reaction?). In ventriculoatrial shunts, the tip of the drainage catheter may migrate out of the right atrium and become occluded with thrombus. Peritoneal catheters are free from this risk.

In summary, shunts occlude for a variety of reasons and under various circumstances. Ideally, occlusions could be prevented by draining pure cerebrospinal fluid from a noncollapsed part of the ventricles. This goal is difficult to attain; however, it is possible to define some guidelines:

1. Attempt to shunt the cleanest cerebrospinal fluid, which may mean using alternative methods such as external ventricular drainage or a transitory ventricular access port in patients with evidence of debris in the cerebrospinal fluid at the time of diagnosis.

2. Choose a nonflanged ventricular catheter and an open distal tubing.

3. Position the tip of the ventricular catheter in the place that is expected to remain the most dilated after drainage.

4. Choose a shunt with the appropriate flow-pressure characteristics, to limit the phenomenon of chronic overdrainage and to reduce the risk of catheter obstruction from ventricular collapse.

5. Check that the system, particularly the valve, is free from debris or clots and that it is flowing normally prior to inserting the distal end in the drainage cavity.

Disconnection and Fracture

The second most frequent cause of shunt failure in pediatric series is shunt fracture or disconnection. These complications can be observed throughout the follow-up period. Factors that can predispose to these types of complications include the design of the shunt; the construction material; and the surgical technique. There are strong interactions between these factors and factors related to the patients themselves. For example, younger patients have more potential for growth and therefore a greater risk of shunt fracture or disconnection. As a patient grows, the shunt must be free to move under the skin. Any point of fixation, creating tension in the material, can lead to fracture. Also, host reaction to foreign material results in degradation and calcification (the degree is specific to the host and the type of silicone), leading to shunt failure.[90, 115]

Surgical Technique. A loose ligature or absorbable suture at connector sites will lead to disconnection when stress is applied to the shunt system. Rough manipulation, particularly with metal instruments, can result in small erosions or even full-thickness tears in the tubing, leading to shunt fracture later on. As already stated, it is important not to place a connector too far distal from the valve in the subcutaneous tissue; this will lead to recurrent fracture or migration.

Design of the Shunt. The risk of disconnection exists mainly at points of connection in the shunt system. One-piece shunts avoid this problem. However, although the use of a one-piece system decreases the risk of fracture, it increases the risk of occlusion at the time of shunt insertion. It must be stressed that all connections have to be outside of the cranial cavity. Any connection at or deeper than the burr hole level can end in the loss of the ventricular catheter at the time of shunt revision.

Material. It has been demonstrated that the association of materials with different physical properties (e.g., steel, silicone) in tubing results in breakdown of the silicone (e.g., metal spring peritoneal catheters). Hard nylon connectors erode the Silastic tubing under the continual stresses associated with movement. It has also been demonstrated that even pure silicone catheters progressively deteriorate after implantation, altering the mechanical properties of the material. Host reactions against the subcutaneously implanted silicone induce calcification deposits on the outer wall of the catheter, creating points of fixation in the subcutaneous tissues (Fig. 36–26).[90, 115] Because of children's growth, these fixations stretch the tubing and can induce a fracture, a disconnection (if there are any connectors), or a narrowing of the lumen (increasing the resistance of the system). Calcifications, which may take years to develop, most commonly occur at the neck and thoracic level. They rarely develop in fatty tissue or the abdominal cavity, and they are never seen in the cerebrospinal fluid. There has been some recent speculation that barium-impregnated tubing or peroxide-cured silicone, or both, promote calcification, leading manufacturers to produce catheters with an outer wall of pure platinum-cured silicone.

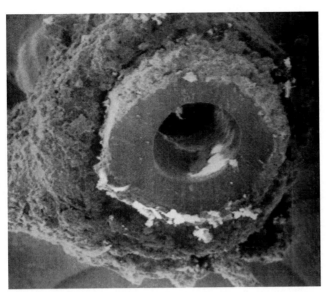

Figure 36–26

The unsolved problem of distal catheter calcification in its subcutaneous tract prevents free movement of the tube under the skin and is responsible for a large number of delayed fractures or migrations of the system in children.

In summary, a distal tubing, coated with pure silicone and joined to the valve system, and proper ligatures to connect the ventricular catheter to the valve seem, at present, the best that can be done to reduce these types of complications. Research and development in tubing materials, however, is required to better understand and thus avoid calcifications and their sequelae.

Migration

There are important similarities between shunt migrations and fractures. Actually, in many cases, a shunt that is not able to migrate (because of the valve shape, fixation of the valve in the subcutaneous tissue, or fixation at the burr hole) will fracture later on (Fig. 36–27). To migrate, a shunt needs to be under traction (traction = point of fixation + patient growth) and to be able to move in the subcutaneous tissue (improperly fixed tube-shaped valve). These two requirements indicate the two potential causes of this type of complication. It appears that the critical issues in preventing shunt migration are proper valve fixation (adequate suturing and proper pocket dissection) and attention to valve shape.

Improper Placement

The shunt can be improperly placed at the level of the ventricles or at the level of the drainage cavity. The frequency of these types of complications remains unacceptably high.

Ventricular Level. Today, for various reasons, placement of the ventricular catheter will probably remain a "blind" procedure in most cases. A well-trained neurosurgeon is the best guarantee in preventing this type

of complication.[206] In particularly difficult circumstances (slit or loculated ventricles), additional methods of localization (endoscopy, ultrasound, tripod, stereotactic) can be helpful.[274] In the future, fiberoptic stylets and computerized placement of shunts will probably become cost effective and practical enough to justify routine use.

Peritoneal Level. Trocar or no trocar? While this question stimulates controversy among neurosurgeons, one must admit that there are no reported differences between these two techniques. The answer to the question seems to be one of common sense. It is dangerous to tap a peritoneal cavity in the case of previous abdominal surgery; otherwise, it is faster and as safe to use a trocar. Once again, it is more a question of the skill and experience of the surgeon. In the near future it is probable that a trocar allowing visualization (endoscopic trocar) will solve the problem.

Right Atrial Level. Electrocardiography or fluoroscopy is usually utilized to correctly position the tip of the catheter in the right atrium.[46, 235]

Skin Problems and Subcutaneous Cerebrospinal Fluid Effusion

Skin Problems. As with other types of shunt complications, skin problems are usually the result of an interaction among the patient, the surgical technique, and the materials. Problems can present at the scar level because of improper surgery or as necrosis of the

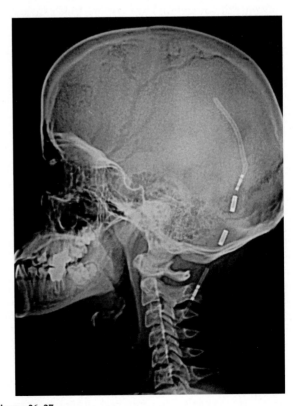

Figure 36–27

Migration and fracture are very similar in their etiologies. It can be said that when a point of fixation under the skin exists in a growing child, a shunt that is not able to migrate will fracture later on.

skin over the shunt due to pressure. These types of complications carry a major risk of shunt contamination, and all attempts must be made to prevent their occurrence.

Patient. Careful evaluation of the local risk factors (e.g., erosion, previous scar, skin thickness) prior to surgery, choosing the least "aggressive" shunt material, and taking special surgical care of patients in the high-risk group can help minimize potential complications. Long-term compression of the skin over the shunt (e.g., tight bandage) must be avoided. Proper in-hospital management and education of family members are mandatory in bed-ridden patients (young or comatose).

Surgery. Ideally, the valve system must be placed in a pocket of appropriate size under the galea, through a small skin incision.

Shunt Design. Large valve size, sharp edges, and hard plastic can lead to the occurrence of skin injury and necrosis. At connectors, the use of large-caliber wire with a big knot is injurious to the skin. The knot must be turned down into the subcutaneous tissue.

Subcutaneous Fluid Collections. Subcutaneous accumulation of cerebrospinal fluid is usually due to shunt obstruction. Under certain conditions, however, this type of complication can be observed with a well-functioning shunt: when resistance around the ventricular catheter is less than the shunt resistance or when the skin can be easily hydrodissected (infants, overdissection). The use of a high- or variable-resistance valve, large ventricles (thin cortex at insertion site), a large opening in the dura, overdissection, and the patient's age (loose skin in infants) are factors that can lead to this type of complication even if the shunt is functioning normally. Once the fluid has started to collect, it is difficult to stop because the movement of the shunt into the pouch of cerebrospinal fluid will facilitate the leak. This problem is avoided by keeping the dural opening small, by minimizing trauma to the brain, and by adjusting patient positioning immediately after surgery (to artificially increase drainage long enough to allow proper healing). If the goal is to drain these patients and to prevent the occurrence of secondary chronic overdrainage complications (e.g., slit ventricles, craniostenosis) with one surgery, some kind of compromise (i.e., patient positioning) has to be accepted. In contradistinction, some surgeons recommend treating infants with an initial low-resistance, low opening-pressure shunt, and then scheduling a shunt replacement when they are older. The author finds this type of management questionable for two reasons. First, if this second operation is not done, there is increased probability of chronic overdrainage complications. Second, the patient is exposed to the potential risks of two operations.

Overdrainage

Overdrainage is a constant problem with existing valves.[98] For example, the potential drainage capacity of a "low-resistance medium-pressure" valve is well over 200 mL per hour for a 25 cm H_2O differential pressure, whereas cerebrospinal fluid production is only around 21 mL per hour. Any increase in the differential pressure across the system, above the opening pressure of the valve, may cause overdrainage. This point is frequently reached during daily life (e.g., postural changes, rapid-eye-movement sleep, physical efforts). This risk of overdrainage can be minimized by increasing the opening pressure of the valve, by adding a siphon-resistive device to the system, or by using a flow-regulating device. Even if these devices represent progress, none of these solutions are able to provide a drainage flow rate exactly meeting the requirements of each particular case. In addition, these systems carry their own risks of malfunction. The adverse consequences of an overdrainage phenomenon are emphasized by the intraventricular location of the drainage site. In nature, the cerebrospinal fluid flows from the ventricles to the subarachnoid spaces, while in a shunted patient the point of lower pressure corresponds to the drainage site. This overdrainage phenomenon is directly responsible for several complications, namely, orthostatic hypotension, subdural cerebrospinal fluid collections, slit-ventricle syndrome, craniosynostosis, and loculation of the ventricles.* As the overdrainage phenomenon is related in part to postural changes and patient height, this risk is highest in the oldest patients. Altogether, this complication represents fewer than 10 per cent of shunt failures in pediatric series, and about 30 per cent in adult series. Besides these classic complications, overdrainage is also highly correlated with the occurrence of obstruction of the ventricular catheter due to the slit-ventricle effect previously mentioned.

Subdural Cerebrospinal Fluid Collections. The risk of subdural cerebrospinal fluid collection is related to (1) the drainage capacity of the shunt (valve opening pressure, valve resistance, differential pressure across the shunt), and (2) the size of the ventricles and the compliance of the brain. Most patients with shunts demonstrate enlargement of their subarachnoid spaces, which is actually an indirect sign of a well-functioning shunt. In some cases, disruption of the arachnoid, or the stretched subarachnoid vessels, can lead to hygroma or a true subdural hematoma, respectively. These complications occur spontaneously in most cases, but they can be elicited by minor head trauma or a previous injury of the arachnoid (e.g., ventricular tap, intracranial pressure sensor). At present, the best way of preventing this type of complication is with the judicious use of a valid shunt alternative (third ventriculostomy) or an overdrainage-limiting device. Not all subdural cerebrospinal fluid collections require treatment; for instance, hygromas in symptom-free patients can resolve spontaneously. In other cases, limiting the drainage by increasing the valve opening pressure or by using a flow-rate–limiting system can be successful. Finally, insertion of a subdural drain that functions at a pressure lower than that of the ventricular system (tubing without interposition of a valve) solves the problem in most cases by restoring a pres-

---

*See references 12, 94, 97, 101, 102, and 118.

sure gradient between the ventricles and the subarachnoid space.[144]

Slit-Ventricle Syndrome. There are numerous definitions of this syndrome in the literature, probably because it represents a mixture of different types of shunt complications.[149, 162, 200, 201] Strictly speaking, it is a syndrome of transient intracranial hypertension occurring in patients with a fully patent shunt and slit ventricles.[94, 97] In these patients, a dramatic decrease in the volume of the cranial cerebrospinal fluid compartment leads to loss of the cerebrospinal fluid's buffering reserve for volumetric modifications of the other two compartments (brain parenchyma and blood). In this condition, any alteration in the fragile equilibrium (e.g., fever, minimal head trauma, rapid-eye-movement sleep), usually of no consequence, results in severe intracranial hypertension. The possible solutions to this problem are overdrainage limitation or cranial expansion, or both.

Craniostenosis. Craniostenosis is frequently observed in the pediatric patient who has had a shunt implanted. The phenomenon is due to a chronic low intracranial pressure level, below physiological values, and is rarely, by itself, an indication for reoperation. More often, premature closing of the cranial vault sutures, and chronic overdrainage of the cerebrospinal fluid and brain growth (in infants), contribute to the development of cranioencephalic disproportion and slit ventricles.[139] Patients who require cranial expansion generally present with cranioencephalic disproportion. Subtemporal decompression is no longer utilized; cranioplasty techniques currently employed in craniofacial surgery are preferred.[143] In a couple of cases, in patients with a very thick cranial vault, the author has split the tables of the skull, which may provide enough additional cranial volume.

Loculation of the Ventricles. Loculated ventricles in hydrocephalic patients are usually observed after an inflammatory process, such as meningitis or hemorrhage.[4, 160] In some cases, however, the excessive drainage of cerebrospinal fluid, by itself, seems to be able to induce a loculation in the ventricular system.[101, 173, 200] It is probable that in some cases, tethering and obstruction can develop at the sites of maximal restriction in the cerebrospinal fluid pathway (foramen of Monro or aqueduct of Sylvius). This loculation of the ventricular system can require several drainage sites for the condition to be adequately treated. To prevent generation of a pressure gradient in the central nervous system, one should connect the ventricular catheters to the same valve, instead of using several different shunt systems. When possible, the most satisfactory solution is to re-establish communication within the ventricles by neuroendoscopy; however, one must keep in mind that endoscopic surgery generates debris in the ventricles, which can lead to obstruction of the existing shunt system.

Orthostatic Hypotension. Clinical symptoms of orthostatic hypotension (headaches, nausea) are frequently observed in older patients after shunt insertion.[102] Usually, these symptoms disappear after a short period of time, as patients adapt themselves to the new hydrodynamic conditions. In some cases, however, it is necessary to upgrade the opening pressure of the valve or to use a more resistant shunt.

Unclear Etiologies

From time to time, patients with shunts undergo a second operation for unclear reasons; subtle symptoms (mild deterioration, lowering of mental capacity, episodic headaches) and a constellation of subjective factors can result in surgery. The shunt is generally found to be patent and, depending on the customs of different institutions, can be either changed entirely or re-placed in the drainage cavity after being shortened by a few centimeters. Some of these cases are recognized later on as an early stage of contamination; some are probably related to a partial obstruction of the drainage system; and in some the etiology still remains unclear. In this last group, the patient probably had suspicious symptoms too easily and too frequently attributed to shunt malfunction. In other words, patients with shunts can demonstrate symptoms and signs such as headaches, nausea, vomiting, mental deterioration, and seizures that are not related to improper function of the shunt. Instead of performing needless surgery, it could be worthwhile to enlist the use of further studies in unclear cases.

For inherent technical reasons, it is probable that a "shunt forever" is an impossible dream, but delaying the occurrence of shunt malfunction for as long as possible is a realistic goal. Although some problems, such as deterioration of the silicone tubing, remain to be solved, several causes of shunt malfunction can be avoided. While shunt failures are inevitable, they are in large part quite preventable. At present, it seems that the surgeon has an important role to play in this challenge, as surgery is a major cause of shunt complications. Major progress in the treatment of hydrocephalus will have been achieved when every neurosurgeon is convinced that shunt surgery is as important as any other type of neurosurgery and requires the same efforts.

Outcome

Historically, the prognosis for hydrocephalus has been poor, with a high mortality rate (up to 80 per cent).[100, 330] Shunts, and improvement in general medical care, have significantly changed the overall outcome figures over the past three decades. Thanks to the progress made, the prognosis of children with hydrocephalus today depends more on the prognosis of the causative lesion than on the hydrocephalus itself.[79, 81] The outlook for the individual with hydrocephalus is quite variable and depends on a complex interplay of factors, including diagnostic category, patient age, associated abnormalities, and other complications (e.g., epilepsy, supratentorial malformations). For example, a history of brain injury, such as trauma, hemorrhage, and infection, may adversely affect the prognosis for cognitive function.[47, 163, 258] Treatment also has a risk of further complication, which can compromise intellectual function.[40, 186] However, efforts have been made to define prognostic factors related to hydrocephalus itself, as opposed to its associated cause.[224, 275, 294, 301] The pathophysiological effects of hydrocephalus itself are poorly understood. The most commonly reported finding is an uneven development of cognitive function in childhood, with verbal intelligence higher than nonverbal. Potential alterations of motor and visual function related to enlargement of the ventricles can be expected to have an ultimate impact on nonverbal intelligence.* The "site of alteration" of the cerebrospinal fluid circulation has been reported to influence intellectual outcome and, more specifically, nonverbal intelligence in some studies, but such a relationship is contradicted in others.[69] Prenatal hydrocephalus is generally considered to have a more severe prognosis, with only one third of the patients having an intelligence quotient above 80.[60, 293] The thickness of the cortical mantle, assessed preoperatively, has been reported to correlate with prognosis.[331] However, since the degree of reduction of ventricle size varies with the treatment modality (e.g., third ventriculostomy versus standard shunt), postoperative cortical mantle thickness is a poor prognostic indicator. Finally, treatments have resulted in functional recovery without a real understanding of anatomical correlation. In other words, the goal of normalization of radiological images by whatever means is probably too simplistic to be accepted.[119]

REFERENCES

1. Abbott, R., Epstein, F. J., and Wisoff, J. H.: Chronic headache associated with a functioning shunt: Usefulness of pressure monitoring. Neurosurgery, 28:72, 1991.
2. Adams, C., Johnston, W. P., and Nevin, N. C.: Family study of congenital hydrocephalus. Dev. Med. Child Neurol., 24:493, 1982.
3. Agha, M. D., Amendola, M. A., Shirazi, K. K., et al.: Abdominal complications of ventriculoperitoneal shunts with emphasis on the role of imaging methods. Surg. Gynecol. Obstet., 156:473, 1983.
4. Albanese, V., Tomasello, F., Sampaolo, S., et al.: Neuroradiological findings in multiloculated hydrocephalus. Acta Neurochir. (Wien), 60:297, 1982.
5. Albright, L., and Reigel, D. H.: Management of hydrocephalus secondary to posterior fossa tumors. J. Neurosurg., 46:52, 1977.
6. Albright, A. L., Haines, S. J., and Taylor, F. H.: Function of parietal and frontal shunts in childhood hydrocephalus. J. Neurosurg., 69:883, 1988.
7. Aleksic, S., Budzilovich, G., Creco, M. A., et al.: Intracranial lipomas, hydrocephalus, and other CNS anomalies in oculoauriculo-vertebral dysplasia (Goldenhar-Gorlin syndrome). Child's Brain, 11:285, 1984.
8. Alksne, J. F., and Lovings, E. T.: Functional ultrastructure of the arachnoid villus. Arch. Neurol., 27:371, 1972.
9. Allan, W. C., Holt, P. J., Sawyer, L. R., et al.: Ventricular dilation after neonatal periventricular-intraventricular hemorrhage: Natural history and therapeutic implications. Am. J. Dis. Child., 136:589, 1982.
10. Ammirati, M., and Raimondi, A. J.: Cerebrospinal fluid shunt infections in children: A study on the relationship between the

11. Anderson, E. M., and Plewis, I.: Impairment of a motor skill in children with spina bifida cystica and hydrocephalus: An exploratory study. Br. J. Psychol., 68:61, 1977.
12. Andersson, H.: Craniosynostosis as a complication after operation for hydrocephalus. Acta Paediatr. Scand., 55:192, 1966.
13. Antoniou, A. G., and Emery, J. L.: The infundibulum of the hypophysis in hydrocephalus. Z. Kinderchir. Grenzgeb., 28:321, 1979.
14. Anwar, M., Kadam, S., Hiatt, I. M., et al.: Serial lumbar punctures in prevention of posthemorrhagic hydrocephalus in preterm infants. J. Pediatr., 107:446, 1985.
15. Aoki, N.: Lumboperitoneal shunt: Clinical applications, complications, and comparison with ventriculoperitoneal shunt. Neurosurgery, 26:998, 1990.
16. Avman, N., Gokalp, H. Z., Arasil, E., et al.: Symptomatology, evaluation, and treatment of aqueductal stenosis. Neurol. Res., 6:194, 1984.
17. Bannister, C. M., and Mundy, J. E.: Some scanning electron microscopic observations of the ependymal surface of the ventricles of hydrocephalic Hy3 mice and a human infant. Acta Neurochir. (Wien), 46:159, 1979.
18. Barlow, C. F.: CSF dynamics in hydrocephalus, with special attention to external hydrocephalus. Brain Dev., 6:119, 1984.
19. Bayston, R., and Penny, S. R.: Excessive production of mucoid substance by Staphylococcus SIIA: A possible factor in colonisation of Holter shunts. Dev. Med. Child Neurol. 14(Suppl. 27):25, 1972.
20. Bayston, R., and Lari, J.: A study of the sources of infection in colonised shunts. Dev. Med. Child Neurol., 16(Suppl. 32):17, 1974.
21. Bayston, R.: Antibiotic prophylaxis in shunt surgery. Dev. Med. Child Neurol., 17(Suppl. 35):99, 1975.
22. Bayston, R., and Spitz, L.: The role of retrograde movement of bacteria in ventriculo-atrial shunt colonisation. Z. Kinderchir., 25:352, 1978.
23. Bayston, R., Leung, T. S. M., Wilkins, B. M., et al.: Bacteriological examination of removed cerebrospinal fluid shunts. J. Clin. Pathol., 36:987, 1983.
24. Bayston, R., Grove, N., Siegel, J., et al.: Prevention of hydrocephalus shunt catheter colonisation in vitro by impregnation with antimicrobials. J. Neurol. Neurosurg. Psychiatry, 52:605, 1989.
25. Bayston, R.: Hydrocephalus Shunt Infections. London, Chapman & Hall, 1989, pp. 12–57.
26. Bayston, R.: A prospective randomised controlled trial of antimicrobial prophylaxis in hydrocephalus shunt surgery. Z. Kinderchir., 45(Suppl. I):5, 1990.
27. Bejar, R., Curbelo, V., Coen, R. W., et al.: Diagnosis and follow-up of intraventricular and intracerebral hemorrhages by ultrasound studies of the infant's brain through the fontanelles and the sutures. Pediatrics, 66:661, 1980.
28. Bejar, R., Saugstad, O. D., James, H., et al.: Increased hypoxanthine concentrations in cerebrospinal fluid of infants with hydrocephalus. J. Pediatr., 103:44, 1983.
29. Bering, E. A.: Circulation of the cerebrospinal fluid: Demonstration of the choroid plexuses as the generator of the force for flow of fluid and ventricular enlargement. J. Neurosurg., 19:409, 1962.
30. Bernstein, R. A., and Hsueh, W.: Ventriculocholecystic shunt: A mortality report. Surg. Neurol., 23:31, 1985.
31. Beyerl, B., and Black, P.: Posttraumatic hydrocephalus. Neurosurgery, 15:257, 1984.
32. Bickers, D. S., and Adams, R. D.: Hereditary stenosis of the aqueduct of Sylvius. J. Neuropathol., 8:104, 1959.
33. Bierbrauer, K. S., Storrs, B. B., McLone, D. G., et al.: A prospective, randomized study of shunt function and infections as a function of shunt placement. Pediatr. Neurosurg., 16:287, 1990/91.
34. Bigio, M. R. D., and Bruni, E.: Reaction of rabbit lateral periventricular tissue to shunt tubing implants. J. Neurosurg., 64:932, 1986.
35. Blakemore, C.: Effects of visual experience on the developing brain. Mod. Probl. Paediatr., 13:229, 1974.
36. Blomstedt, G. C.: Results of trimethoprim-sulfamethoxazole prophylaxis in ventriculostomy and shunting procedures. J. Neurosurg., 62:694, 1985.

---

*See references 11, 35, 80, 91, 123, and 332.

37. Blum, J., Schwartz, M., and Voth, D.: Antibiotic single-dose prophylaxis of shunt infections. Neurosurg. Rev., 12:239, 1989.
38. Borges, L. F.: Cerebrospinal fluid shunts interfere with host defenses. Neurosurgery, 10:55, 1982.
39. Boulard, G., Ravussin, P., and Gúerin, J.: A new way to monitor external ventricular drainage. Neurosurgery, 30:636, 1992.
40. Boynton, B. R., Boynton, C. A., Merritt, T. A., et al.: Ventriculoperitoneal shunts in low birth weight infants with intracranial hemorrhage: Neurodevelopmental outcome. Neurosurgery, 18:141, 1986.
41. Bridgers, S. L., and Ment, L. R.: Absence of hydrocephalus despite disproportionately increasing head size after the neonatal period in preterm infants with known intraventricular hemorrhage. Child's Brain, 8:423, 1981.
42. Buhrley, L. E., and Reed, D. J.: The effect of furosemide on sodium-22 uptake into cerebrospinal fluid and brain. Exp. Brain Res., 14:503, 1972.
43. Burke, J. F.: The effective period of preventive antibiotic action in experimental incisions and dermal lesions. Surgery, 50:161, 1961.
44. Burstein, J., Papile, L. A., and Burstein, R.: Intraventricular hemorrhage and hydrocephalus in premature newborns: A prospective study with CT. A.J.R., 132:631, 1979.
45. Camfield, P. R., Camfield, C. S., Allen, A. C., et al.: Progressive hydrocephalus in infants with birth weights less than 1,500 g. Arch. Neurol., 38:653, 1981.
46. Cantu, R. C., Mark, V. H., and Austen, W. G.: Accurate placement of the distal end of a ventriculoatrial shunt catheter using vascular pressure changes. J. Neurosurg., 27:584, 1967.
47. Cardoso, E. R., and Galbraith, S.: Posttraumatic hydrocephalus: A retrospective review. Surg. Neurol., 23:261, 1985.
48. Carmel, P. W., Antunes, J. L., Hilal, S. K., et al.: A Dandy-Walker syndrome: Clinico-pathological features and re-evaluation of modes of treatment. Surg. Neurol., 8:132, 1980.
49. Castejon, O. J.: Transmission electron microscope study of human hydrocephalic cerebral cortex. J. Submicrosc. Cytol. Pathol. 26:29, 1994.
50. Cerda, M., and Bassauri, L.: Isoelectric focusing of cerebrospinal fluid proteins in children with nontumoral hydrocephalus: A preliminary report. Child's Brain, 6:140, 1980.
51. Cerda, M., Vielma, J., Martinez, C., et al.: Poly-acrylamide gel electrophoresis of cerebrospinal fluid proteins in children with nontumoral hydrocephalus. Child's Brain, 6:140, 1980.
52. Cernerud, L.: The setting-sun eye phenomenon in infancy. Dev. Med. Child Neurol., 17:447, 1975.
53. Chambers, S. E., Hendry, G. M., and Wild, S. R.: Real-time ultrasound scanning of the head in neonates and infants, including a correlation between ultrasound and computed tomography. Pediatr. Radiol., 15:4, 1985.
54. Chapman, P. H.: External hydrocephalus. In Humphreys, R. P., ed.: Concepts in Pediatric Neurosurgery. Vol. 4. New York, Karger, 1983, pp. 102–118.
55. Chapman, P. H., and Borges, L. F.: Shunt infections: Prevention and treatment. Clin. Neurosurg., 32:652, 1984.
56. Chapman, P. H., Griebel, R., Cosman, E. R., et al.: Telemetric ICP measurement in normal and shunted, hydrocephalic patients. In Chapman, P. H., ed.: Concepts in Pediatric Neurosurgery. Vol. 6. New York, Karger, 1985, pp. 115–132.
57. Chapman, P. H., Cosman, E. R., and Arnold, M. A.: The relationship between ventricular fluid pressure and body position in normal subjects and subjects with shunts: A telemetric study. Neurosurgery, 26:181, 1990.
58. Chattha, A. S., and Delong, G. R.: Sylvian aqueduct syndrome as a sign of acute obstructive hydrocephalus in children. J. Neurol. Neurosurg. Psychiatry, 38:288, 1975.
59. Chemke, J., Czernobilsky, B., Mundel, G., et al.: A familial syndrome of central nervous system and ocular malformations. Clin. Genet., 7:1, 1975.
60. Chervenak, F. A., Duncan, C., Ment, L. R., et al.: Outcome of fetal ventriculomegaly. Lancet, 2:179, 1984.
61. Choux, M., Genitori, L., Lang, D., et al.: Shunt implantation: Reducing the incidence of shunt infection. J. Neurosurg., 77:875, 1992.
62. Chuang, S., Hochhauser, L., Fitz, C., et al.: Lumbo-peritoneal shunt malfunction: A new, reliable CT sign. Acta Neuroradiol., 10(Suppl. 369):645, 1986.
63. Chumas, P. D., Armstrong, D. C., Drake, J. M., et al.: Tonsillar herniation: The rule rather than the exception after lumboperitoneal shunting in the pediatric population. J. Neurosurg., 78:568, 1993.
64. Chumas, P. D., Kulkarni, A. V., Drake, J. M., et al.: Lumboperitoneal shunting: A retrospective study in the pediatric population. Neurosurgery, 32:376, 1993.
65. Cochrane, D. D., and Myles, T.: Management of intrauterine hydrocephalus. J. Neurosurg., 57:590, 1982.
66. Collins, P., Hockley, A. D., and Woollam, D. H. M.: Surface ultrastructure of tissues occluding ventricular catheters. J. Neurosurg., 48:609, 1978.
67. Cosman, E. R., Zervas, N. T., Chapman, P. H., et al.: A telemetric pressure sensor for ventricular shunt systems. Surg. Neurol., 11:287, 1979.
68. Costerton, J. W., Cheng, K. J., Geesey, G. G., et al.: Bacterial biofilms in nature and disease. Annu. Rev. Microbiol., 41:435, 1987.
69. Cull, C., and Wyke, M. A.: Memory function of children with spina bifida and shunted hydrocephalus. Dev. Med. Child Neurol., 26:177, 1984.
70. Cutler, R. W. P., Page, L., Galicich, J., et al.: Formation and absorption of cerebrospinal fluid in man. Brain, 92:707, 1968.
71. Czosnyka, M., Maksymowicz, W., Batorski, L., et al.: Comparison between classic-differential and automatic shunt functioning on the basis of infusion tests. Acta Neurochir. (Wien), 106:1, 1990.
72. Dan, N. G., and Wade, M. J.: The incidence of epilepsy after ventricular shunting procedures. J. Neurosurg., 65:19, 1986.
73. Dandy, W. E., and Blackfan, K. D.: Internal hydrocephalus: An experimental, clinical, and pathological study. Am. J. Dis. Child., 8:406, 1914.
74. Da Silva, M. C., and Drake, J. M.: Effect of subcutaneous implantation of anti-siphon devices on CSF shunt function. Pediatr. Neurosurg., 16:197, 1990/91.
75. Da Silva, M. C., and Drake, J. M.: Complications of CSF shunt anti-siphon devices. Pediatr. Neurosurg., 17:304, 1991/92.
76. Davson, H., and Segal, M. B.: The effects of some inhibitors and accelerators of sodium transport on the turnover of ^{22}Na in the cerebrospinal fluid and the brain. J. Physiol. (Lond.), 209:131, 1970.
77. Del Bigio, M. R., Bruni, J. E., and Fewer, H. D.: Human neonatal hydrocephalus: An electron microscopic study of the periventricular tissue. J. Neurosurg., 63:56, 1985.
78. Del Brutto, O. H., and Sotelo, J.: Neurocysticercosis: An update. Rev. Infect. Dis., 10:1075, 1988.
79. Dennis, M., Fitz, C. R., Netley, C. T., et al.: The intelligence of hydrocephalic children. Arch. Neurol., 38:607, 1981.
80. De Vlieger, M., Sadikoglu, S., Van Eijndhoven, J. H., et al.: Visual evoked potentials, auditory evoked potentials, and EEG in shunted hydrocephalic children. Neuropediatrics, 12:55, 1981.
81. Dennis, M., Fitz, C. R., Netley, C. T., et al.: The intelligence of hydrocephalic children. Arch. Neurol., 38:607, 1981.
82. Diaz-Mitoma, F., Harding, G. K. M., Hoban, D. J., et al.: Clinical significance of a test for slime production in ventriculoperitoneal shunt infections caused by coagulase-negative staphylococci. J. Infect. Dis., 156:555, 1987.
83. DiRocco, C., McLone, D. G., Shimoji, T., et al.: Continuous intraventricular cerebrospinal fluid pressure recording in hydrocephalic children during wakefulness and sleep. J. Neurosurg., 42:683, 1975.
84. DiRocco, C., Caldarelli, M., Maira, C., et al.: The study of cerebrospinal fluid dynamics in apparently "arrested" hydrocephalus in children. Child's Brain, 3:359, 1977.
85. DiRocco, C., Iannelli, A., Borrelli, P., et al.: Surgically treatable growth retardation due to non-neoplastic pituitary-hypothalamic dysfunction. Child's Brain, 11:353, 1984.
86. DiRocco, C.: The Treatment of Infantile Hydrocephalus. Vol. 2. Boca Raton, FL, CRC Press, 1987, pp. 155–168.
87. Djindjian, M., Fevrier, M. J., Otterbein, G., et al.: Oxacillin prophylaxis in cerebrospinal fluid shunt procedures: Results of a randomized open study in 60 hydrocephalic patients. Surg. Neurol., 25:178, 1986.
88. Drake, J. M., Sainte-Rose, C., Da Silva, M. C., et al.: Cerebrospinal fluid flow dynamics in children with external ventricular drains. Neurosurgery, 28:242, 1991.

89. Drake, J. M., Da Silva, M. C., and Rutka, J. T.: Functional obstruction of an anti-siphon device by raised tissue capsule pressure. Neurosurgery, 32:137, 1993.

90. Echizenya, K., Satoh, M., and Mural, H.: Mineralization and biodegradation of CSF shunting systems. J. Neurosurg., 67:584, 1987.

91. Ehle, A., and Sklar, F.: Visual evoked potentials in infants with hydrocephalus. Neurology, 29:1541, 1979.

92. Eisenberg, H. M., McComb, J. G., and Lorenzo, A. V.: Cerebrospinal fluid overproduction and hydrocephalus associated with choroid plexus papilloma. J. Neurosurg., 40:381, 1974.

93. Ellington, E., and Margolis, G.: Block of arachnoid villus by subarachnoid hemorrhage. J. Neurosurg., 30:651, 1969.

94. Epstein, F., Marlin, A. E., and Wald, A.: Chronic headache in the shunt-dependent adolescent with nearly normal ventricular volume: Diagnosis and treatment. Neurosurgery, 3:351, 1978.

95. Epstein, F., and Murali, R.: Pediatric posterior fossa tumors: Hazards of the "preoperative" shunt. Neurosurgery, 3:348, 1978.

96. Epstein, F.: How to keep shunts functioning, or "The Impossible Dream." Clin. Neurosurg., 32:608, 1984.

97. Epstein, F.: Increased intracranial pressure in hydrocephalic children with functioning shunts: A complication of shunt dependency. In Shapiro, K., Marmarou, A., and Portnoy, H., eds.: Hydrocephalus. New York, Raven Press, 1984, pp. 315–321.

98. Faulhauer, K., and Schmitz, P.: Overdrainage phenomena in shunt-treated hydrocephalus. Acta Neurochir. (Wien), 45:89, 1978.

99. Fleischer, A. C., Bundy, A. L., Hutchinson, A. A., et al.: Sonographic depiction of changes in ventricular size associated with repeated ventricular aspirations. J. Ultrasound Med., 2:499, 1983.

100. Foltz, E. L., and Shurtleff, D. B.: Five-year comparative study of hydrocephalus in children with and without operation (113 cases). J. Neurosurg., 20:1064, 1963.

101. Foltz, E. L., and Shurtleff, D. B.: Conversion of communicating hydrocephalus to stenosis or occlusion of the aqueduct during ventricular shunt. J. Neurosurg., 24:520, 1966.

102. Foltz, E. L., and Blanks, J. P.: Symptomatic low intracranial pressure in shunted hydrocephalus. J. Neurosurg., 68:401, 1988.

103. Fox, J. L., Portnoy, H. D., and Shulte, R. R.: Cerebrospinal fluid shunts: An experimental evaluation of flow rates and pressure values in the anti-siphon valve. Surg. Neurol., 1:299, 1973.

104. Frame, P. T., and McLaurin, R. L.: Treatment of CSF shunt infections with intrashunt plus oral antibiotic therapy. J. Neurosurg., 60:354, 1984.

105. Friedman, J. M., and Santos-Ramos, R.: Natural history of X-linked aqueductal stenosis in the second and third trimesters of pregnancy. Am. J. Obstet. Gynecol., 150:104, 1984.

106. Gadsdon, D. R., Variend, S., and Emery, J. L.: Myelination of the corpus callosum: II. The effect of relief of hydrocephalus upon the processes of myelination. Z. Kinderchir., 28:314, 1979.

107. Gardner, E., O'Rahilly, R., and Prolo, D.: The Dandy-Walker and Arnold-Chiari malformations: Clinical, developmental, and teratological considerations. Arch. Neurol., 32:393, 1975.

108. Gerosa, M. A., and Carteri, A.: Cerebrospinal fluid levels of cyclic nucleotides in non-neoplastic hydrocephalus: Preliminary report. Child's Brain, 6:45, 1980.

109. Gilbert, J. N., Jones, K. L., Rorke, L. B., et al.: Central nervous system anomalies associated with meningomyelocele, hydrocephalus, and the Arnold-Chiari malformation: Reappraisal of theories regarding the pathogenesis of posterior neural tube closure defects. Neurosurgery, 18:559, 1986.

110. Gilles, F. H., and Davidson, R. I.: Communicating hydrocephalus associated with deficient dysplastic parasagittal arachnoidal granulations. J. Neurosurg., 35:421, 1971.

111. Giuffrè, R.: Choroidal and ependymal reactions. J. Neurosurg. Sci., 20:123, 1976.

112. Go, K., Ebels, E., and Van Woerden, H.: Experiences with recurring ventricular catheter obstructions. Clin. Neurol. Neurosurg., 83:47, 1981.

113. Gower, D. J., Lewis, J. C., and Kelly, D. L.: Sterile shunt malfunction: A scanning electron microscopic perspective. J. Neurosurg., 62:1079, 1984.

114. Gower, D. J., Horton, D., and Pollay, M.: Shunt-related brain abscess and ascending shunt infection. J. Child Neurol., 5:318, 1990.

115. Griebel, R. W., Hoffman, H. J., and Becker, L.: Calcium deposit on CSF shunts: Clinical observations and ultrastructural analysis. Child's Nerv. Syst., 3:180, 1982.

116. Griebel, R., Khan, M., and Tan, L.: CSF shunt complications: An analysis of contributory factors. Child's Nerv. Syst., 1:77, 1985.

117. Gristina, A. G.: Biomaterial-centered infection: Microbial adhesion versus tissue integration. Science, 237:1588, 1987.

118. Gruber, R.: The problem of chronic overdrainage of the ventriculo-peritoneal shunt in congenital hydrocephalus. Z. Kinderchir., 31:362, 1980.

119. Gruber, R.: Should "normalization" of the ventricles be the goal of hydrocephalus therapy? Z. Kinderchir., 38(Suppl. 2):80, 1983.

120. Gruber, R., Jenny, P., and Herzog, B.: Experiences with the anti-siphon device (ASD) in shunt therapy of pediatric hydrocephalus. J. Neurosurg., 61:156, 1984.

121. Guevara, J. A., Zuccaro, G., Trevisan, A., et al.: Bacterial adhesion to cerebrospinal fluid shunts. J. Neurosurg., 67:438, 1987.

122. Gurtner, P., Bass, T., Gudeman, S. K., et al.: Surgical management of posthemorrhagic hydrocephalus in 22 low-birth-weight infants. Child's Nerv. Syst., 8:198, 1992.

123. Guthkelch, A., Sclabassi, R. J., Hirsch, R. P., et al.: Visual evoked potentials in hydrocephalus: Relationship to head size, shunting, and mental development. Neurosurgery, 14:283, 1984.

124. Gutierrez, Y., Friede, R. L., and Kaliney, W. J.: Agenesis of arachnoid granulations and its relationship to communicating hydrocephalus. J. Neurosurg., 43:553, 1975.

125. Haar, F. L., and Miller, C. A.: Hydrocephalus resulting from superior vena cava thrombosis in an infant: Case report. J. Neurosurg., 42:597, 1975.

126. Haase, J., Bang, F., and Tange, M.: Danish experience with the one-piece shunt: A long-term follow-up. Child's Nerv. Syst., 3:93, 1987.

127. Haase, J., and Weeth, R.: Multiflanged ventricular catheter for hydrocephalus shunts. Acta Neurochir. (Wien), 33:213, 1976.

128. Haines, S. J., and Taylor, F.: Prophylactic methicillin for shunt operations: Effect on incidence of shunt malfunction and infection. Child's Brain, 9:10, 1982.

129. Haines, S. J.: Do antibiotics prevent shunt infections? A meta-analysis [Abstract]. Pediatric Section of the American Association of Neurological Surgeons. 1991.

130. Hakim, S., Venegas, J. G., and Burton, J. D.: The physics of the cranial cavity, hydrocephalus and normal pressure hydrocephalus: Mechanical interpretation and mathematical model. Surg. Neurol., 5:187, 1976.

131. Haller, J. S., Wompert, S. M., Rabe, E. F., et al.: Cystic lesions of the posterior fossa in infants: A comparison of the clinical, radiological, and pathological findings in Dandy-Walker syndrome and extra-axial cysts. Neurology, 21:494, 1971.

132. Hanigan, W. C., Gibson, J., Kleopoulox, N. J., et al.: Medical imaging of fetal ventriculomegaly. J. Neurosurg., 64:575, 1986.

133. Harmat, G., Paraicz, E., and Szenasy, J.: Ultrasound control of progressive hydrocephalus in infancy. Child's Brain, 11:230, 1984.

134. Hayden, P. W., Shurtleff, D. B., and Stuntz, T. J.: A longitudinal study of shunt function in 360 patients with hydrocephalus. Dev. Med. Child Neurol., 25:334, 1983.

135. Heilman, C. B., and Cohen, A. R.: Endoscopic ventricular fenestration using a "saline torch." J. Neurosurg., 74:224, 1991.

136. Hill, A., and Rozdilsky, B.: Congenital hydrocephalus secondary to intra-uterine germinal matrix/intraventricular haemorrhage. Dev. Med. Child Neurol., 26:524, 1984.

137. Hirsch, J. F., Pierre-Kahn, A., Renier, D., et al.: The Dandy-Walker malformation: A review of 40 cases. J. Neurosurg., 61:515, 1984.

138. Hoffman, H. J., Hendrick, E. B., and Humphreys, R. P.: New lumboperitoneal shunt for communicating hydrocephalus: Technical note. J. Neurosurg., 44:258, 1976.

139. Hoffman, H. J., and Tucker, W. S.: Cephalocranial disproportion: A complication of the treatment of hydrocephalus in children. Child's Brain, 2:167, 1976.

140. Hoffman, H. J., Harwood-Nash, D., Gilday, D. L., et al.: Percutaneous third ventriculostomy in the management of noncommunicating hydrocephalus. In Epstein, F., Hoffman, H. J., and Raimondi, A. J., eds.: Concepts in Pediatric Neurosurgery. Vol. 1. New York, Karger, 1981, pp. 87–106.

141. Hoffman, H. J., Hendrick, E. B., and Humphreys, R. P.: Experience with ventriculo-pleural shunts. Child's Brain, 10:404, 1983.

142. Hoffman, H. J., Soloniuk, D., Humphreys, R. P., et al.: A concerted effort to prevent shunt infection. In Matsumoto, S., and Tamaki, N., eds.: Hydrocephalus: Pathogenesis and Treatment. New York, Springer-Verlag, 1991, pp. 510–514.

143. Holness, R. O., Hoffman, H. J., and Hendrick, E. B.: Subtemporal decompression for the slit-ventricle syndrome after shunting in hydrocephalic children. Child's Brain, 55:137, 1979.

144. Hoppe-Hirsch, E., Sainte-Rose, C., and Renier, D.: Pericerebral collections after shunting. Child's Nerv. Syst., 3:97, 1987.

145. Horton, D., and Pollay, M.: Fluid flow performance of a new siphon-control device for ventricular shunts. J. Neurosurg., 72:926, 1990.

146. Hougen, T. J., Emmanoulides, G. C., and Moss, A. J.: Pulmonary valvular dysfunction in children with ventriculovenous shunts for hydrocephalus: A previously unreported complication. Pediatrics, 55:836, 1975.

147. Howard, F. M., Till, K., and Carter, C. O.: A family study of hydrocephalus resulting from aqueduct stenosis. J. Med. Genet., 78:252, 1981.

148. Hudgins, R. J., Boydston, W. R., Hudgins, P. A., et al.: Treatment of intraventricular hemorrhage in the premature infant with urokinase. Pediatr. Neurosurg., 20:190, 1994.

149. Hyde-Rowan, M. D., Rekate, H. L., and Nulsen, F. E.: Reexpansion of previously collapsed ventricles: The slit ventricle syndrome. J. Neurosurg., 556:536, 1982.

150. Ishida, A., Sawaishi, Y., Goto, A., et al.: Two siblings with partial trisomy 15 and monosomy 21 associated with central nervous system anomalies. Tohoku J. Exp. Med., 171:277, 1993.

151. Ishiwata, Y., Yamashita, T., Ide, K., et al.: A new technique for percutaneous study of lumboperitoneal shunt patency. J. Neurosurg., 68:152, 1988.

152. Jackson, D. W., Pollock, A. V., and Tindal, D. S.: The value of a plastic adhesive drape in the prevention of wound infection. Br. J. Surg., 58:340, 1971.

153. James, H. E., and Tibbs, P. A.: Diverse clinical applications of percutaneous lumboperitoneal shunts. Neurosurgery, 8:39, 1981.

154. James, H. E., Wilson, H. D., Connor, J. D., et al.: Intraventricular cerebrospinal fluid antibiotic concentrations in patients with intraventricular infections. Neurosurgery, 10:50, 1982.

155. James, H. E., Bejar, R., Meritt, A., et al.: Management of hydrocephalus secondary to intracranial hemorrhage in the high-risk newborn. Neurosurgery, 14:612, 1984.

156. Johanson, C. E.: Potential for pharmacologic manipulation of the blood–cerebrospinal fluid barrier. In Neuwelt, E. A., ed.: Implications of the Blood-Brain Barrier and Its Manipulation. Vol. 1. New York, Plenum Press, 1989.

157. Johnson, D. L., Fitz, C., McCullough, D. C., et al.: Perimesencephalic cistern obliteration: A CT sign of life-threatening shunt failure. J. Neurosurg., 64:386, 1986.

158. Jones, R. F. C., Stening, W. A., and Brydon, M.: Endoscopic third ventriculostomy. Neurosurgery, 26:86, 1990.

159. Joubert, J.: Cysticercal meningitis: A pernicious form of neurocysticercosis which responds poorly to praziquantel. S. Afr. Med. J., 77:528, 1990.

160. Kalsbeck, J. E., DeSousa, A. L., Kleiman, M. B., et al.: Compartmentalization of the cerebral ventricles as a sequela of neonatal meningitis. J. Neurosurg., 52:547, 1980.

161. Kendall, B., and Holland, I.: Benign communicating hydrocephalus in children. Neuroradiology, 21:93, 1981.

162. Kiekens, R., Mortier, W., Pothmann, R., et al.: The slit-ventricle syndrome after shunting in hydrocephalic children. Neuropediatrics, 13:190, 1982.

163. Krishnamoorthy, K. S., Kuehnle, K. J., Todres, I. D., et al.: Neurodevelopmental outcome of survivors with posthemorrhagic hydrocephalus following grade II neonatal intraventricular hemorrhage. Ann. Neurol., 15:201, 1984.

164. Kushner, J., Alexander, E., Davis, C. H., et al.: Kyphoscoliosis following lumbar subarachnoid shunts. J. Neurosurg., 34:783, 1971.

165. Langley, J. M., LeBlanc, J. C., Drake, J. M., et al.: Efficacy of antimicrobial prophylaxis in cerebrospinal fluid shunt placement: A meta-analysis. Clin. Infect. Dis., 17:98, 1993.

166. Lee, B. C. P.: Magnetic resonance imaging of periaqueductal lesions. Clin. Radiol., 38:527, 1987.

167. Leggate, J. L., Baxter, P., Minns, R. A., et al.: Epilepsy following ventricular shunt placement. J. Neurosurg., 68:318, 1988.

168. Leggiadro, R. J., Atluru, V. L., and Katz, S. P.: Meningococcal meningitis associated with cerebrospinal fluid shunts. Pediatr. Infect. Dis., 3:489, 1984.

169. Lerman, S. J.: Haemophilus influenzae infections of cerebrospinal fluid shunts: Report of two cases. J. Neurosurg., 54:261, 1981.

170. Loch Macdonalds, R., Humphreys, R. P., Rutka, J. T., et al.: Colloid cysts in children. Pediatr. Neurosurg., 20:169, 1994.

171. Lockhart, C., Selman, W., Rodziewicz, G., et al.: Percutaneous insertion of peritoneal shunt catheters with use of the Verres needle. J. Neurosurg., 60:444, 1984.

172. Lorenzo, A. V., Page, L. K., and Watters, G. V.: Relationship between cerebrospinal fluid formation, absorption, and pressure in human hydrocephalus. Brain, 93:679, 1970.

173. Lourie, H., Shende, M. C., Krawchenko, J., et al.: Trapped fourth ventricle as delayed complication of ventricular shunting: Report of two unusual cases. Neurosurgery, 7:279, 1980.

174. Magnaes, B.: Body position and cerebrospinal fluid pressure: Part 1. Clinical studies on the effect of rapid postural changes. J. Neurosurg., 44:687, 1976.

175. Magnaes, B.: Body position and cerebrospinal fluid pressure: Part 2. Clinical studies on orthostatic pressure and the hydrostatic indifferent point. J. Neurosurg., 44:698, 1976.

176. Marlin, A. E., Rivera, S., and Gaskill, S. J.: Treatment of posthemorrhagic ventriculomegaly in the preterm infant: Use of the subcutaneous ventricular reservoir. Concepts Pediatr. Neurosurg., 8:15, 1988.

177. Matsumae, M., Sato, O., Itoh, K., et al.: Quantification of cerebrospinal fluid shunt flow rates: Assessment of the programmable pressure valve. Child's Nerv. Syst., 5:356, 1989.

178. Matsushima, T.: Choroid plexus papillomas and human choroid plexus: A light and electron microscopic study. J. Neurosurg., 59:1054, 1983.

179. McAllister, J. P., Maugans, T. A., Shah, V. M., et al.: Neuronal effects of experimentally induced hydrocephalus in newborn rats. J. Neurosurg., 63:776, 1985.

180. McCarthy, K. D., and Reed, D. J.: The effect of acetazolamide and furosemide on cerebrospinal fluid production and choroid plexus carbonic anhydrase activity. J. Pharmacol. Exp. Ther. 189:194, 1974.

181. McComb, J. G.: Review article: Recent research into the nature of cerebrospinal fluid formation and absorption. J. Neurosurg., 59:369, 1983.

182. McCullough, D. C., and Wells, M.: Complications with antisiphon devices in hydrocephalics with ventriculoperitoneal shunts. In American Society for Pediatric Neurosurgery, ed.: Concepts in Pediatric Neurosurgery. Vol. 2. New York, Karger, 1982, pp. 63–75.

183. McCullough, D. C.: Symptomatic progressive ventriculomegaly in hydrocephalics with patent shunts and anti-siphon devices. Neurosurgery, 19:617, 1986.

184. McIvor, J., Krajbich, J. I., and Hoffman, H. J.: Orthopaedic complications of lumboperitoneal shunts. J. Pediatr. Orthop., 8:687, 1988.

185. McLaurin, R. L.: Shunt complications. In Section of Pediatric Neurosurgery of the AANS: Pediatric Neurosurgery: Surgery of the Developing Nervous System. New York, Grune & Stratton, 1982, pp. 243–253.

186. McLone, D. G., Czyzewski, D., Raimondi, A. J., et al.: Central nervous system infections as a limiting factor in the intelligence of children with myelomeningocele. Pediatrics, 70:338, 1982.

187. Milhorat, T. H.: Choroid plexus and cerebrospinal fluid production. Science, 166:1514, 1969.

188. Milhorat, T. H., Mosher, M. B., Hammock, M. K., et al.: Evidence for choroid plexus absorption in hydrocephalus. N. Engl. J. Med., 283:286, 1970.

189. Milhorat, T. H.: The third circulation revisited. J. Neurosurg., 42:628, 1975.

190. Milhorat, T. H., Hammock, M. K., Davis, D. A., et al.: Choroid plexus papilloma: I. Proof of cerebrospinal fluid overproduction. Child's Brain, 2:273, 1976.

191. Mueller, S. M., Bell, W., Cornell, S., et al.: Achondroplasia and hydrocephalus: A computerized tomographic, roentgenographic, and psychometric study. Neurology, 27:430, 1977.

192. Naidich, T. P., McLone, D. G., and Fulling, K. H.: The Chiari II malformation: Part IV. The hindbrain deformity. Neuroradiology, 25:179, 1983.

193. Nellhaus, G.: Head circumference from birth to eighteen years: Practical composite international and interracial graphs. Pediatrics, 41:106, 1968.

194. Noetzel, M. J., and Baker, R. P.: Shunt fluid examination: Risks and benefits in the evaluation of shunt malfunction and infection. J. Neurosurg., 61:328, 1984.

195. Nowak, T. P., and James, H. E.: Migraine headaches in hydrocephalic children: A diagnosis dilemma. Child's Nerv. Syst., 5:310, 1989.

196. Nulsen, F. E., and Becker, D. P.: Control of hydrocephalus by valve-regulated shunt. J. Neurosurg., 26:362, 1967.

197. Nulsen, F. E., and Spitz, E. B.: Treatment of hydrocephalus by direct shunt from ventricle to jugular vein. Surg. Forum, 2:399, 1951.

198. O'Brien, M., Parent, A., and Davis, B.: Management of ventricular shunt infections. Child's Brain, 5:304, 1979.

199. Odio, C., Mohs, E., Sklar, F. H., et al.: Adverse reactions to vancomycin used as prophylaxis for CSF shunt procedures. Am. J. Dis. Child., 138:17, 1984.

200. Oi, S., and Matsumoto, S.: Morphological findings of post shunt slit-ventricle in experimental canine hydrocephalus: Aspects of causative factors of isolated ventricles and slit-ventricle syndrome. Child's Nerv. Syst., 2:179, 1986.

201. Oi, S., and Matsumoto, S.: Infantile hydrocephalus and slit-ventricle syndrome in early infancy. Child's Nerv. Syst., 3:145, 1987.

202. Olsen, L., and Frykberg, T.: Complications in the treatment of hydrocephalus in children. Acta Paediatr. Scand., 72:385, 1983.

203. Onodera, Y., and Ito, H.: Fatty acid in cerebrospinal fluid of congenital hydrocephalus. Child's Brain, 3:101, 1977.

204. Onodera, Y., Kawaguchi, T., and Itoh, H.: Fatty acid of cerebrospinal fluid in arrested hydrocephalus. Child's Brain, 9:95, 1982.

205. Pang, D., Sclabassi, R. J., and Horton, J. A.: Lysis of intraventricular clot with urokinase in a canine model: 2. In vivo safety study of intraventricular urokinase. Neurosurgery, 19:547, 1986.

206. Pang, D., and Grabb, P. A.: Accurate placement of coronal ventricular catheter using stereotactic coordinate-guided freehand passage. J. Neurosurg., 80:750, 1994.

207. Paoletti, P., Pezzotta, S., and Spanu, G.: Diagnosis and treatment of post-traumatic hydrocephalus. J. Neurosurg. Sci., 27:171, 1983.

208. Papile, L. A., Burstein, J., Burstein, R., et al.: Incidence and evolution of the subependymal and intraventricular hemorrhage: A study of infants with birth weights less than 1.500 gm. J. Pediatr., 92:529, 1978.

209. Papile, L. A., Burstein, J., Burstein, R., et al.: Posthemorrhagic hydrocephalus in low-birth-weight infants: Treatment by serial lumbar punctures. J. Pediatr., 97:273, 1980.

210. Papo, I., Caruselli, G., and Luongo, A.: External ventricular drainage in the management of posterior fossa tumors in children and adolescents. Neurosurgery, 10:13, 1982.

211. Patriarca, P. A., and Lauer, B. A.: Ventriculoperitoneal shunt–associated infection due to Haemophilus influenzae. Pediatrics, 65:1007, 1980.

212. Petrak, R. M., Pottage, J. C., Harris, A. A., et al.: Haemophilus influenzae meningitis in the presence of a cerebrospinal fluid shunt. Neurosurgery, 18:79, 1986.

213. Pezzota, S., Locatelli, D., and Bonfanti, N.: Shunt in high-risk newborns. Child's Nerv. Syst., 3:114, 1987.

214. Piatt, J. H., and Carlson, C. V.: A search for determinants of cerebrospinal fluid shunt survival: Retrospective analysis of 14-year institutional experience. Pediatr. Neurosurg., 19:233, 1993.

215. Pierre-Kahn, A., Gabersek, V., and Hirsch, J. F.: Intracranial pressure and rapid eye movement sleep in hydrocephalus. Child's Brain, 2:156, 1976.

216. Pierre-Kahn, A., Hirsch, J. F., Renier, D., et al.: Hydrocephalus and achondroplasia: A study of 25 observations. Child's Brain, 7:205, 1980.

217. Pollack, I. E., Pang, D., and Albright, A. L.: The long-term outcome in children with late-onset aqueductal stenosis resulting from benign intrinsic tectal tumors. J. Neurosurg., 80:681, 1994.

218. Pollay, M.: Formation of cerebrospinal fluid: Relation of studies of isolated choroid plexus to the standing gradient hypothesis. Neurosurgery, 42:665, 1975.

219. Pollay, M., Hisey, B., Reynolds, E., et al.: Choroid plexus Na$^+$/K$^+$-activated adenosine triphosphatase and cerebrospinal fluid formation. Neurosurgery, 17:768, 1985.

220. Pople, I. K., Bayston, R., and Hayward, R. D.: Infection of cerebrospinal fluid shunts in infants: A study of etiological factors. J. Neurosurg., 77:29, 1992.

221. Portnoy, H. D., Schulte, R. R., Fox, J. L., et al.: Anti-siphon and reversible occlusion valves for shunting in hydrocephalus and preventing postshunt subdural hematomas. J. Neurosurg., 38:729, 1973.

222. Post, E. M.: Currently available shunt systems: A review. Neurosurgery, 16:257, 1985.

223. Raahave, D.: Effect of plastic skin and wound drapes on the density of bacteria in operation wounds. Br. J. Surg., 63:421, 1976.

224. Raimondi, A. J., and Soare, P.: Intellectual development in shunted hydrocephalic children. Am. J. Dis. Child., 227:664, 1974.

225. Raimondi, A. J., Robinson, J. S., and Kuwamura, K.: Complications of ventriculo-peritoneal shunting and a critical comparison of the three-piece and one-piece systems. Child's Brain, 3:321, 1977.

226. Rayport, M., and Reiss, J.: Hydrodynamic properties of certain shunt assemblies for the treatment of hydrocephalus: Part 1. Report of a case of communicating hydrocephalus with increased cerebrospinal fluid production treated by duplication of shunting device. Part 2. Pressure-flow characteristics of the Spitz-Holter, Pudenz-Heyer, and Cordis-Hakim shunt systems. J. Neurosurg., 30:455, 1969.

227. Reeder, J. D., Kaude, J. V., and Setzer, E. S.: The occipital horn of the lateral ventricles in premature infants: An ultrasonographic study. Eur. J. Radiol., 3:148, 1983.

228. Reider, M. J., Frewen, T. C., and Del Maestro, R. F.: The effects of cephalothin prophylaxis in postoperative ventriculoperitoneal shunt infections. Can. Med. Assoc. J., 136:935, 1987.

229. Rekate, H. L.: To shunt or not to shunt: Hydrocephalus and dysraphism. Clin. Neurosurg., 332:593, 1984.

230. Rekate, H. L., Erwood, S., Brodkey, J. A., et al.: Etiology of ventriculomegaly in choroid plexus papilloma. Pediatr. Neurosci., 12:196, 1985/86.

231. Rekate, H. L.: Classification of slit-ventricle syndromes using intracranial pressure monitoring. Pediatr. Neurosurg., 19:15, 1993.

232. Renier, D., Lacombe, J., Pierre-Kahn, A., et al.: Factors causing acute shunt infection: Computer analysis of 1174 operations. J. Neurosurg., 61:1072, 1984.

233. Rennels, M. B., and Wald, E. R.: Treatment of Haemophilus influenzae type b meningitis in children with cerebrospinal fluid shunts. J. Pediatr., 97:424, 1980.

234. Roa, P. S., Molthan, M. E., and Lipow, H. W.: Cor pulmonale as a complication of ventriculoatrial shunts: Case report. J. Neurosurg., 333:221, 1970.

235. Robertson, J. T., Schick, R. W., Morgan, F., et al.: Accurate placement of ventriculo-atrial shunt for hydrocephalus under electrocardiographic control. J. Neurosurg., 18:255, 1961.

236. Rosenberg, G. A., Kyner, W. T., and Estrada, E.: Bulk flow of brain interstitial fluid under normal and hyperosomolar conditions. Am. J. Physiol., 238:F42, 1980.

237. Rosman, N. P., and Shands, K. N.: Hydrocephalus caused by increased intracranial venous pressure: A clinicopathological study. Ann. Neurol., 3:445, 1978.

238. Rougemont, J., de, Ames, A., III, Nesbett, F. B., et al.: Fluid formed by choroid plexus: A technique for its collection and a comparison of its electrolyte composition with serum and cisternal fluids. J. Neurophysiol., 23:485, 1960.

239. Rubin, R. C., Henderson, E. S., Ommaya, A. K., et al.: The production of cerebrospinal fluid in man and its modification by acetazolamide. J. Neurosurg., 25:430, 1966.

240. Rubin, R., Hochwald, G. M., Tiell, M., et al.: Reconstitution of the cerebral cortical mantle in shunt-corrected hydrocephalus. Dev. Med. Child Neurol., 17(Suppl. 35):151, 1975.

241. Rubin, R. C., Hochwald, G. M., Tiell, M., et al.: Hydrocephalus:

III. Reconstruction of the cerebral cortical mantle following ventricular shunting. Surg. Neurol., 5:179, 1976.

242. Russell, D. S.: Observations on the Pathology of Hydrocephalus (Special Report Series Medical Research Council, No. 265). London, HM Stationery Office, 1949.

243. Sahar, A., and Tsipstein, E.: Effects of mannitol and furosemide on the rate of formation of cerebrospinal fluid. Exp. Neurol., 60:584, 1978.

244. Sainte-Rose, C., Lacombe, J., Pierre-Kahn, A., et al.: Intracranial venous sinus hypertension: Cause or consequence of hydrocephalus in infants? J. Neurosurg., 60:727, 1984.

245. Sainte-Rose, C., Hooven, M. D., and Hirsch, J. F.: A new approach in the treatment of hydrocephalus. J. Neurosurg., 66:213, 1987.

246. Sainte-Rose, C., Hoffman, H. J., and Hirsch, J. F.: Shunt failure. In Marlin, A. E., eds.: Concepts in Pediatric Neurosurgery. Vol. 9. Basel, Karger, 1989, p. 7.

247. Sainte-Rose, C., Piatt, J. H., Renier, D., et al.: Mechanical complications in shunts. Pediatr. Neurosurg., 17:2, 1991/92.

248. Sainte-Rose, C.: Third ventriculostomy. In Manwaring, K. H., and Crone, K. R., eds.: Neuroendoscopy. Vol. 1. New York, Mary Ann Liebert Publisher, 1992, pp. 47–62.

249. Sainte-Rose, C.: Shunt obstruction: A preventable complication? Pediatr. Neurosurg., 19:156, 1993.

250. Sanford, R. A., Bebin, J., and Smith, R. W.: Pencil gliomas of the aqueduct of Sylvius: Report of two cases. J. Neurosurg., 57:690, 1982.

251. San Frutos, M. A., Fernandez-Pavon, A., Perez Higueras, A., et al.: Local urokinase for the treatment of ventriculitis complications. Acta Paediatr. Scand., 75:497, 1986.

252. Sayers, M. P., and Kosnick, E. J.: Percutaneous third ventriculostomy: Experience and technique. Child's Brain, 2:24, 1976.

253. Sayers, L. N., Moosy, J., and Guthkelch, N.: Malfunctioning ventriculoperitoneal shunts. J. Neurosurg., 56:511, 1982.

254. Scharf, D.: Neurocysticercosis: Two hundred thirty-eight cases from a California hospital. Arch. Neurol., 45:777, 1988.

255. Schick, R. W., and Matson, D. D.: What is arrested hydrocephalus? J. Pediatr., 558:791, 1961.

256. Schmidt, K., Gjerris, F., Osgaard, O., et al.: Antibiotic prophylaxis in cerebral fluid shunting: A prospective randomized trial in 152 hydrocephalic patients. Neurosurgery, 17:1, 1985.

257. Schurtleff, D. B., Foltz, E. L., Weeks, R. D., et al.: Therapy of Staphylococcus epidermidis: Infections associated with cerebrospinal fluid shunts. Pediatrics, 53:55, 1974.

258. Scott, D. T., Ment, L. R., Ehrenkranz, R. A., et al.: Evidence for late developmental deficit in very low birth weight infants surviving intraventricular hemorrhage. Child's Brain, 11:261, 1984.

259. Sekhar, L. N., Moossy, J., and Guthkelch, A. N.: Malfunctioning ventriculoperitoneal shunts: Clinical and pathological features. J. Neurosurg., 56:411, 1982.

260. Selman, W. R., Spetzler, R. F., Wilson, C. B., et al.: Percutaneous lumboperitoneal shunt: Review of 130 cases. Neurosurgery, 6:255, 1980.

261. Selman, W. R., and Spetzler, R. F.: New lumboperitoneal shunt catheter. Surg. Neurol., 21:58, 1984.

262. Serlo, W., Fernell, E., Heikkinen, E., et al.: Functions and complications of shunts in different etiologies of childhood hydrocephalus. Child's Nerv. Syst., 6:92, 1990.

263. Seropian, R., and Reynolds, B. M.: Wound infections after preoperative depilatory versus razor preparation. Am. J. Surg., 121:251, 1971.

264. Shapiro, K., Ginns, E., and Braden, K.: GM_1 ganglioside concentration in the cerebrospinal fluid of hydrocephalic infants and children. Z. Kinderchir., 334:419, 1981.

265. Shapiro, K., Fried, A., and Marinarou, A.: Biomechanical and hydrodynamic characterization of the hydrocephalic infant. J. Neurosurg., 63:69, 1985.

266. Shapiro, K., and Fried, A.: Pressure-volume relationships in shunt-dependent childhood hydrocephalus: The zone of pressure instability in children with acute deterioration. J. Neurosurg., 64:390, 1986.

267. Shapiro, S., Boaz, J., Kleiman, M., et al.: Origin of organisms infecting ventricular shunts. Neurosurgery, 22:868, 1988.

268. Shellshear, I., and Emery, J. L.: Gliosis and aqueductule formation in the aqueduct of Sylvius. Dev. Med. Child Neurol., (Suppl. 37):22, 1976.

269. Shen, P. H., Matsuoka, Y., Kawajiri, K., et al.: Treatment of intraventricular hemorrhage using urokinase. Neurol. Med. Chir. (Tokyo), 30:329, 1990.

270. Sher, P. K., and Brown, S. B.: A longitudinal study of head growth in pre-term infants: II. Differentiation between "catch-up" head growth and early infantile hydrocephalus. Dev. Med. Child Neurol., 17:711, 1987.

271. Sheridan, M., Chaseling, R., and Johnston, I. H.: Hydrocephalus, lumbal canal stenosis and Maroteaux-Lamy syndrome (mucopolysaccharidosis type 6): Case report. J. Neurosurg. Sci., 36:215, 1992.

272. Shinnar, S., Gammon, K., Bergman, E. W., et al.: Management of hydrocephalus in infancy: Use of acetazolamide and furosemide to avoid cerebrospinal fluid shunts. J. Pediatr., 107:31, 1985.

273. Shinya, K., Tetsumori, Y., Toshihiko, K., et al.: A light and electron microscopy and immunohistochemical study of human arachnoid villi. J. Neurosurg., 69:429, 1988.

274. Shkolnik, A., and McLone, D. C.: Intraoperative real-time ultrasonic guidance of ventricular shunt placement in infants. Radiology, 141:515, 1981.

275. Shurtleff, D. B., Foltz, E. L., and Loeser, J. D.: Hydrocephalus: A definition of its progression and relationship to intellectual function, diagnosis, and complications. Am. J. Dis. Child., 125:688, 1973.

276. Silva, C. A., and Sá, M.: Electrophoretic pattern of cerebrospinal fluid proteins in non-neoplastic infantile hydrocephalus. Acta Neurol. Scand., 57:317, 1978.

277. Slabaugh, R. D., Smith, J. A., Lemons, J., et al.: Neonatal intracranial hemorrhage and complicating hydrocephalus. JCU 12:261, 1984.

278. Sotelo, J., and Marin, C.: Hydrocephalus secondary to cysticercotic arachnoiditis: A long-term follow-up review of 92 cases. J. Neurosurg., 66:686, 1987.

279. Sotelo, J.: A new ventriculoperitoneal shunt for treatment of hydrocephalus: Experimental results. Revue Europeanne de Biotechnologie Medicale, 15:257, 1993.

280. Sparrow, O. C.: Laboratory performances of single-piece ventriculoperitoneal shunts with distal slit-valve control. J. Neurosurg., 70:496, 1989.

281. Spector, R.: Vitamin homeostasis in the central nervous system. N. Engl. J. Med., 296:1393, 1977.

282. Sperling, D. R., Patrick, J. R., Anderson, F. M., et al.: Cor pulmonale secondary to ventriculo-auriculostomy. Am. J. Dis. Child., 107:308, 1964.

283. Spetzler, R., Wilson, C., and Grollmus, J.: Percutaneous lumboperitoneal shunt. J. Neurosurg., 43:770, 1975.

284. Spetzler, R. F., Wilson, C. B., and Grollmus, J. M.: Percutaneous lumboperitoneal shunt: Technical note. J. Neurosurg., 43:770, 1975.

285. Steel H. H., and Adams, D. J.: Hyperlordosis caused by the lumboperitoneal shunt procedure for hydrocephalus. J. Bone Joint Surg., 54:1537, 1972.

286. Stein, B. M., Fraser, R. A. R., and Tenner, M. S.: Normal pressure hydrocephalus: Complication of posterior fossa surgery in children. Pediatrics, 49:50, 1972.

287. Strain, L., Gosden, C. M., Brock, D. J. H., et al.: Genetic heterogeneity in X-linked hydrocephalus: Linkage to markers within Xq27.3. Am. J. Hum. Genet., 54:236, 1994.

288. Sugar, O., and Bailey, O. T.: Subcutaneous reaction to silicone in ventriculoperitoneal shunts: Long-term results. J. Neurosurg., 41:367, 1974.

289. Sweadner, K. J., and Gilkeson, R. C.: Two isozymes of the Na,K-ATPase have distinct antigenic determinants. J. Biol. Chem., 260:9016, 1985.

290. Taggart, J. K., and Walker, A. E.: Congenital atresia of the foramens of Luschka and Magendie. Arch Neurol Psychiatry, 48:583, 1942.

291. Tal, Y., Freigang, B., Dunn, H. G., et al.: Dandy-Walker syndrome: Analysis of 21 cases. Dev. Med. Child Neurol., 22:189, 1980.

292. Tamaki, N., Yamashita, H., Kimura, M., et al.: Changes in the components and content of biological water in the brain of experimental hydrocephalic rabbits. J. Neurosurg., 73:274, 1990.

293. Tardieu, M., Evrard, P., and Lyon, G.: Progressive expanding congenital porencephalies: A treatable cause of progressive encephalopathy. Pediatrics, 68:198, 1981.

294. Tew, B., and Laurence, K. M.: The effects of hydrocephalus on intelligence, visual perception, and school attainment. Dev. Med. Child Neurol., (Suppl. 35):129, 1975.

295. Tew, B., and Laurence, K.: The clinical and psychological characteristics of children with the "cocktail party" syndrome. Z. Kinderchir. Grenzgeb., 28:360, 1979.

296. Thomas, G. G., and Cudmore, R. E.: The advantages of a ventriculostomy reservoir with the Holter valve system. J. Pediatr. Surg., 11:63, 1976.

297. Tokoro, K., and Chiba, Y.: Optimum position of the antisiphon device. Neurosurgery, 27:332, 1990.

298. Tomita, T.: Placement of a ventriculoatrial shunt using external jugular catheterization: Technical note. Neurosurgery, 14:74, 1984.

299. Tripathi, B. S., and Tripathi, R. C.: Vacuolar transcellular channels as a drainage pathway for cerebrospinal fluid. J. Physiol., 239:195, 1974.

300. Tripathi, R. C.: Ultrastructure of the arachnoid mater in relation to outflow of cerebrospinal fluid: A New concept. Lancet, 2:8, 1973.

301. Tromp, C. N., Van Den Burg, W., Jansen, A., et al.: Nature and severity of hydrocephalus and its relation to later intellectual function. Z. Kinderchir. Grenzgeb., 28:354, 1979.

302. Tsingoglou, S., and Eckstein, H. B.: Pericardial tamponade by Holter ventriculoatrial shunts. J. Neurosurg., 36:695, 1971.

303. Tung, H., Raffel, C., and McComb, J. G.: Ventricular cerebrospinal fluid eosinophilia in children with ventriculoperitoneal shunts. J. Neurosurg., 75:541, 1991.

304. Turner, G., Turner, B., and Collins, E.: X-linked mental retardation without physical abnormality: Renpenning's syndrome. Dev. Med. Child Neurol., 13:71, 1971.

305. Upadhyaya, P., Bhargava, S., Sundaram, K. R., et al.: Hydrocephalus caused by tuberculous meningitis: Clinical picture, CT findings, and results of shunt surgery. Z. Kinderchir., 38(Suppl. 2):76, 1983.

306. Vates, T. S., Bonring, S. L., Oppelt, W. W.: Na-K activated adenosine triphosphatase formation of cerebrospinal fluid in the cat. Am. J. Physiol., 206:1165, 1964.

307. Venes, J. L., and Shaw, R. K.: Ventriculo-pleural shunting in the management of hydrocephalus. Child's Brain, 55:45, 1979.

308. Venes, J. L., Black, K. L., and Latack, J. T.: Preoperative evaluation and surgical management of the Arnold-Chiari II malformation. J. Neurosurg., 64:363, 1986.

309. Vercelloti, G. M., McCarthy, J. B., Lindholm, P., et al.: Extracellular matrix proteins (fibronectin, laminin and type IV collagen) bind and aggregate bacteria. Am. J. Pathol., 120:13, 21, 1985.

310. Visudhiphan, P., and Chiemchanya, S.: Hydrocephalus in tuberculous meningitis in children: Treatment with acetazolamide and repeated lumbar puncture. J. Pediatr., 95:657, 1979.

311. Volpe, J. J.: Neonatal intraventricular hemorrhage. N. Engl. J. Med., 303:886, 1981.

312. Vries, J. K.: Endoscopy as an adjunct to shunting for hydrocephalus. Surg. Neurol., 13:69, 1980.

313. Walters, B. C., Hoffman, H. J., Hendrick, E. B., et al.: Cerebrospinal fluid shunt infections: Influences on initial management and subsequent outcome. J. Neurosurg., 60:1014, 1984.

314. Walters, B. C., Goumnerova, L., Hoffman, H. J., et al.: A randomized controlled trial of perioperative rifampin/trimethoprim in cerebrospinal fluid shunt surgery. Child's Nerv. Syst., 8:253, 1992.

315. Wang, E. E. L., Prover, C. G., Hendrick, E. B., et al.: Prophylactic sulfamethoxazole and trimethoprim in ventriculoperitoneal shunt surgery: A double-blind, randomized, placebo-controlled trial. J.A.M.A., 251:1174, 1984.

316. Welch, K.: The principle of physiology of the cerebrospinal fluid in relation to hydrocephalus, including normal-pressure hydrocephalus. In Friedlander, W. J., ed.: Current Reviews: Advances in Neurology. Vol. 13. New York, Raven Press, 1975, pp. 247–332.

317. Welch, K.: The prevention of shunt infection. Z. Kinderchir., 22:465, 1977.

318. Welch, K.: The intracranial pressure in infants. J. Neurosurg., 52:693, 1980.

319. Welch, K., Strand, R., Bresnan, M., et al.: Congenital hydrocephalus due to villous hypertrophy of the telencephalic choroid plexuses: Case report. J. Neurosurg., 59:172, 1983.

320. Weller, R. O., and Shulman, K.: Infantile hydrocephalus: Clinical, histological, and ultrastructural study of brain damage. J. Neurosurg., 36:255, 1972.

321. Weller, R. O., and Williams, B. N.: Cerebral biopsy and assessment of brain damage in hydrocephalus. Arch. Dis. Child., 550:763, 1975.

322. West, C. G. H.: Ventriculovesical shunt: Technical note. J. Neurosurg., 553:858, 1980.

323. Winston, K. R.: Hair and neurosurgery. Neurosurgery, 2:320, 1992.

324. Wyatt, R. J., Walsh, J. W., and Holland, N. H.: Shunt nephritis: Role of the complement system in its pathogenesis and management. J. Neurosurg., 55:99, 1981.

325. Yamada, H., Tajima, M., and Nagaya, M.: Effects of respiratory movements on cerebrospinal fluid dynamics in hydrocephalus infants with shunts. J. Neurosurg., 42:194, 1975.

326. Yamada, H., Nakamura, S., Tajima, M., et al.: Neurological manifestations of pediatric achondroplasia. J. Neurosurg., 54:49, 1981.

327. Yamada, H.: A flow-regulating device to control differential pressure in CSF shunt systems: Technical note. J. Neurosurg., 57:570, 1982.

328. Yamada, S., Ducker, T. B., and Perot, P. L.: Dynamic changes of cerebrospinal fluid in upright and recumbent shunted experimental animals. Child's Brain, 1:187, 1975.

329. Yamashima, T.: Ultrastructural study of the final cerebrospinal fluid pathway in human arachnoid villi. Brain Res., 384:68, 1988.

330. Yashon, D., Jane, J. A., and Sugar, O.: The course of severe untreated infantile hydrocephalus: Prognostic significance of the cerebral mantle. J. Neurosurg., 23:509, 1965.

331. Young, H., Nulsen, F., Weiss, M., et al.: The relationship of intelligence and cerebral mantle in treated infantile hydrocephalus. Pediatrics, 52:38, 1973.

332. Zeiner, E. H. K., Prigatano, C. P., Pollay, M., et al.: Ocular motility, visual acuity and dysfunction of neuropsychological impairment in children with shunted uncomplicated hydrocephalus. Child's Nerv. Syst., 2:115, 1985.

Hydrocephalus in Adults

Adult hydrocephalus is a relatively common problem that may be difficult to treat satisfactorily because of uncertainty in diagnosis and complexity of shunt placement. It can present with high cerebrospinal fluid pressure and headache, vomiting, coma, and death or with low pressure and a gradual slowing of intellectual and motor activity. Three issues usually face the neurosurgeon in its management: whether to insert a shunt at all, how to make sure that the shunt is at the appropriate pressure, and how to avoid the complications of shunting. This chapter discusses the classification, etiology, clinical pattern, differential diagnosis, treatment, and outcome of adult hydrocephalus in both its high-pressure and normal-pressure forms.

Classification

Hydrocephalus can be broadly defined as an excess of cerebrospinal fluid in the head. This is usually in the ventricular system, although in external hydrocephalus in children, fluid accumulates in the subarachnoid space. "Hydrocephalus" implies an alteration in cerebrospinal fluid dynamics as a cause of increased ventricular volume; "ventriculomegaly" is a more general term that covers ventricular enlargement from whatever cause, including atrophy.

A number of adjectives are used to describe hydrocephalus. "Internal" hydrocephalus indicates ventricular enlargement; "external" hydrocephalus refers to the enlargement of subarachnoid spaces over the cortical surface. In "communicating" hydrocephalus, the ventricular system is in communication with the subarachnoid space of the brain and spinal cord; in the "noncommunicating" form, there is a block either within the ventricular system or in its outlets to the subarachnoid space, so that the ventricles and subarachnoid space are discontinuous. "Obstructive" hydrocephalus describes an obstruction to the flow of cerebrospinal fluid; most hydrocephalus is obstructive in that a blockage to flow is the cause, rather than an overproduction of fluid.

The time course of the hydrocephalus is described by the terms "acute," "subacute," and "chronic." Acute hydrocephalus usually occurs over days, subacute over weeks, and chronic over months and years. The terms "symptomatic" and "asymptomatic" describe the clinical findings that accompany the hydrocephalus: symptomatic patients have complaints and findings attributable to their hydrocephalus, and asymptomatic patients do not. This distinction may be obscured because some symptoms are very subtle and some cannot easily be differentiated from those of the coexisting neurological disorder. "Arrested" hydrocephalus suggests that whatever factors have led to ventricular enlargement in the past are no longer active. "Ex vacuo" hydrocephalus implies that ventricular enlargement is the result of primary cortical atrophy.

In this chapter, hydrocephalus is discussed in its high-pressure and normal-pressure forms. Either can have acute or chronic onset, although acute onset of symptoms of normal-pressure hydrocephalus is unusual.

High-Pressure Hydrocephalus

High-pressure and normal-pressure hydrocephalus are located on a continuum, with somewhat artificial divisions by symptomatology. A process that obstructs cerebrospinal fluid pathways within the ventricular system or over the convexities may lead to either form of hydrocephalus. The difference between high-pressure and normal-pressure hydrocephalus appears to be the severity of obstruction and the ability of the brain to adapt to whatever lesion caused ventricular enlargement. The same causes can produce either form.

P. McL. Black

ETIOLOGY

Table 37–1 lists the causes of hydrocephalus found by Katzman in a series of adult patients.[69] Virtually all high-pressure hydrocephalus in adults is caused by obstruction to the flow of cerebrospinal fluid through the ventricular system and subarachnoid pathways, with an increase in mean and pulsatile pressures in the ventricular system and subsequent ventricular dilatation.[84] Symptoms may be the result of increased intracranial pressure and diminished cerebral blood flow; unchecked, they can lead to foramen magnum herniation and death.

The causes of hydrocephalus can be found anywhere along the cerebrospinal fluid pathways. Many of them are neoplastic. In the lateral ventricles, these include choroid plexus papilloma, ependymoma, subependymal giant cell astrocytoma, glioma, metastatic tumor, and meningioma. Obstruction of the third ventricle can be caused by intraventricular masses, such as colloid cyst, astrocytoma, ependymoma, choroid plexus papilloma, meningioma, or parasitic cyst; compression of the posterior aspect of the ventricle by a pineal region tumor or cyst; and compression from the suprasellar region by a craniopharyngioma, pituitary adenoma, ectopic pinealoma, hypothalamic or optic nerve glioma, chordoma, hamartoma, tuberculum sellae meningioma, or metastatic tumor.

Intrinsic tumors in the aqueduct are rare, but they do occur, and pontine gliomas may narrow the aqueduct secondarily. The most common cause of aqueductal narrowing, however, is congenital aqueductal stenosis, which may not be symptomatic until adult life.[5] Obstruction occurring within the fourth ventricle may result from ependymoma, medulloblastoma, choroid plexus papilloma, subependymoma, epidermoid, or parasitic cyst. Extrinsic compression of the fourth ventricle and aqueduct can be found with medulloblastomas, tumors of the cerebellar hemisphere (e.g., astrocytoma, hemangioblastoma, metastasis), or lesions of the cerebellopontine angle, including vestibular schwannomas, meningiomas, and epidermoids.

Primary obstruction in the subarachnoid pathways is most often seen after subarachnoid hemorrhage caused by aneurysmal rupture, but it can occur after head trauma.[9, 11, 40] Other causes include meningitis, meningeal carcinomatosis, and any mass that obliterates the subarachnoid space over all or part of the convexity, including hemisphere tumors (especially meningiomas), gliomatosis, subdural hematomas, and arachnoid cysts.

CLINICAL PRESENTATION

High-pressure hydrocephalus accompanies subarachnoid hemorrhage and meningitis regularly enough that it should be anticipated in any patient with either of these conditions. It may follow the original event by several weeks. Patients with specific causes of hydrocephalus may have symptoms of hydrocephalus without localizing symptoms; these include headache, nausea, ataxia, and disturbances in vision. The headache tends initially to be bifrontal, is usually more severe in the morning because cerebrospinal fluid is drained less in the recumbent position, and may be relieved by sitting up. As the symptoms progress, the headache may awaken the patient at night and become generalized and continuous. Neck pain may develop and is of concern because it may indicate protrusion of the cerebellar tonsils into the foramen magnum.

Nausea and vomiting are usually associated with headache. Unlike nausea from vestibular disease, the nausea caused by hydrocephalus is not exacerbated by particular head movements. Abdominal pain is also unusual. Vomiting characteristically occurs early in the morning, when the headache is most severe.

Ataxia is truncal, with an unsteady and broad-based gait. Limb ataxia may be present if a mass in the cerebellar hemisphere is the cause of the hydrocephalus.

Disturbances of vision may include loss of acuity, diplopia from abducens nerve weakness, or inability to look up. Episodic "graying out" of vision is a sign of serious optic nerve compromise by increased intracranial pressure and should be treated emergently.

On examination, papilledema is an important sign of increased intracranial pressure. Abducens nerve weakness is not localizing but indicates pressure elevation. Failure of upward gaze and of accommodation indicates pressure on the tectal plate. Truncal ataxia may accompany hydrocephalus by itself or may be a sign of a vermian cerebellar lesion. Other focal signs may indicate the presence of a specific lesion.

DIAGNOSTIC TESTS

Computed tomography is the usual initial diagnostic test in evaluating a patient with symptoms of high-pressure hydrocephalus. It should be done both with and without intravenous contrast agents; in this way, ventricular enlargement can be identified, and the underlying cause may also be established (Fig. 37–1). Magnetic resonance imaging is an even more useful test in imaging hydrocephalus and identifying its cause

Table 37–1
ETIOLOGY OF HYDROCEPHALUS IN ADULT PATIENTS

Cause	No. of Patients	Percentage
Subarachnoid hemorrhage	315	34
Idiopathic	314	34
Head injury	102	11
Tumors	54	6
Prior operation	43	5
Aqueduct stenosis	34	3
Meningitis	34	3
Others	39	4

Modified from Katzman, R.: Low pressure hydrocephalus. *In* Wells, C. E., ed.: Dementia. Philadelphia, F. A. Davis, 1977. Used by permission.

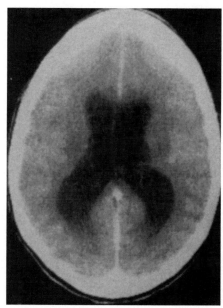

Figure 37–1

Computed tomography in a typical patient with hydrocephalus and increased cerebrospinal fluid pressure. There is loss of the sulcal pattern and a tight appearance to the brain.

(Fig. 37–2). It may demonstrate a low-grade tumor more accurately than computed tomography; furthermore, assessment of the flow of cerebrospinal fluid is possible with magnetic resonance imaging and may help establish physiologically significant hydrocephalus.[22]

Lumbar puncture can be dangerous in a patient with hydrocephalus and symptoms of increased intracranial pressure and should be deferred until after computed tomography is performed. Lumbar puncture in a patient with an intracranial mass may lead to tonsillar impaction and central herniation.

Angiography is used today only to evaluate apparently vascular lesions seen on computed tomography or magnetic resonance imaging. Ventriculography and pneumoencephalography are of historical interest only. Cerebral blood flow testing, positron emission tomography, single photon emission computed tomography (SPECT),[132] visual evoked responses, and cerebrospinal fluid biochemical tests are of research interest only (see discussion below).

MANAGEMENT

Shunting is the definitive therapy for high-pressure hydrocephalus, as discussed below. In the acute state, intravenous mannitol, 1 g per kg as a bolus, may prevent death from herniation, but a ventricular catheter should be inserted as quickly as possible, as discussed in the next paragraph. In the subacute state, corticosteroids may diminish cerebrospinal fluid pressure enough to get a patient ready for semielective surgery.

Emergent ventriculostomy may be necessary if ob-

tundation or loss of vision is a component of the high-pressure hydrocephalus syndrome at presentation. Ventriculostomy can be done in the emergency room or in the intensive care unit if there is not enough time to go to the operating room. The most convenient site is a frontal point 10 cm behind the nasion and 3 cm to the right of the midline. After scalp shaving and careful antiseptic preparation, and with strict aseptic technique, the skin is infiltrated with a local anesthetic with epinephrine and incised 2 cm in a linear incision. A twist drill hole is made through the skull. The dura is opened, and a ventriculostomy catheter is inserted into the right frontal horn. The most reliable landmarks for directing the catheter are the medial canthus of the right eye and a point midway between the lateral margin of the orbit and the tragus. The catheter should be tunneled subgaleally for several centimeters before exiting from the skin and should then be connected to a closed-system drainage bag. Many centers use prophylactic methicillin or other penicillinase-resistant antibiotics intravenously during the period of ventricular drainage. Use of a tunneled catheter greatly reduces the risk of infection; the catheter can be kept in place for at least 5 days without infection.

If the hydrocephalus is less acute, the major management decision is whether to use a shunt as the primary treatment or to attempt to remove the underlying cause. This is especially true for patients with intraventricular tumors and for elderly patients with obstructive tumors, such as vestibular schwannomas. With improved micro-operative techniques, direct removal of the mass itself is increasingly advocated. If this is selected as the primary therapy, however, there is still a possibility that shunting will be required at a later date.

Some surgeons advocate routine preoperative shunting before removal of a mass lesion that obstructs the flow of cerebrospinal fluid. One cooperative study suggested that centers that use routine preoperative shunting have overall results similar to those of institutions that do not use this therapeutic plan.[86] Shunting with a midline cerebellar mass present may allow upward herniation through the tentorial notch. Furthermore, the shunt may spread malignant cells to the peritoneum if the primary process is a malignant tumor. Use of an inline filter helps prevent spread of malignant cells but may lead to later shunt malfunction. If a shunt is not placed preoperatively or intraoperatively, the patient must be watched closely during the immediate postoperative period for the development of hydrocephalus.

In proceeding with surgery in a patient with hydrocephalus, it is often helpful as the first step to tap the ventricle, perhaps leaving a catheter in place during the procedure. For cerebral masses, this can be done through a frontal burr hole; for posterior fossa masses, through a parieto-occipital one. Postoperatively, the burr hole site should be left for later urgent ventricular cannulation. Some surgeons leave a ventricular cannula in place, either attached to a reservoir subcutaneously or as an open drain, for 24 to 48 hours.

The techniques of shunt placement and their complications for both high-pressure and normal-pressure hy-

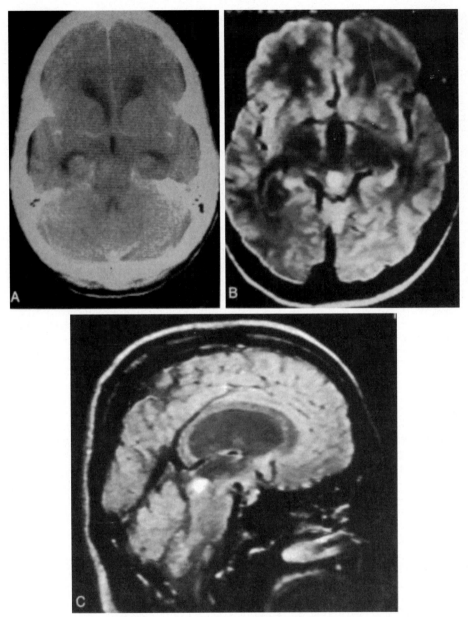

Figure 37–2

The usefulness of magnetic resonance imaging in assessing hydrocephalus of uncertain cause. *A.* Computed tomography section of a patient with hydrocephalus and a suggestion of a posterior third ventricular mass. *B.* The transaxial section of the magnetic resonance image displays a region of high signal in the brain stem more distinctly. *C.* Sagittal magnetic resonance imaging of the same lesion; the appearance is typical of a brain stem glioma.

drocephalus are discussed in the last section of this chapter. In general, shunting is a satisfactory method of managing high-pressure hydrocephalus. A high-pressure valve is usually satisfactory.

Normal-Pressure Hydrocephalus

Normal-pressure hydrocephalus is a condition characterized by normal cerebrospinal fluid pressure but enlarged ventricles. If it follows an event such as subarachnoid hemorrhage, its diagnosis is not problematic. If it occurs without a known previous cause, however,

it may be difficult to distinguish from Alzheimer's disease or other conditions with normal cerebrospinal fluid pressure and ventricular enlargement. A number of tests have been proposed to diagnose normal-pressure hydrocephalus in these circumstances. The most satisfactory criterion, however, remains the clinical presentation, that is, a syndrome of gait disturbance, slowing of thought and actions, dementia, and urinary incontinence.[10, 69, 98, 100, 105]

ETIOLOGY

Normal-pressure hydrocephalus can be divided into two large groups—that of known cause and that termed "idiopathic." The conditions that typically precede the syndrome are the same as those listed in Table 37–1; they all have a tendency to cause low-grade scarring or obstruction of the ventricular system and subarachnoid pathways around the base of the brain and convexities. The most common causes of normal-pressure hydrocephalus are aneurysm rupture and head trauma; trauma produces ventricular enlargement both by subarachnoid hemorrhage and by loss of tissue substance.[9, 11, 40] Brain tumors are a second cause; hydrocephalus depends in part on the size and location of the tumor, with posterior fossa tumors being especially prone to producing hydrocephalus. Paget's disease of bone is an unusual cause of obstruction of cerebrospinal fluid flow because of bony compression at the base of the brain.[81] Familial occurrence of normal-pressure hydrocephalus has been noted.[102] Marginal aqueductal stenosis may be a more common cause of this disorder than was previously thought. Meningeal inflammations such as tuberculous meningitis have a high incidence of delayed hydrocephalus. Finally, neurosurgery of any kind can cause hydrocephalus by releasing blood into the subarachnoid space.

PATHOPHYSIOLOGY

Cases with known cause are relatively easy to understand: there is increased resistance to the flow of cerebrospinal fluid within the ventricular system or subarachnoid spaces. This increased resistance is probably in the cerebrospinal fluid pathways around the brain and not in the arachnoid villi; an obstruction within arachnoid villi leads to pseudotumor cerebri rather than hydrocephalus if the sutures have closed.[12]

The pathophysiology of the idiopathic form is obscure. The mechanism of ventricular enlargement has not been fully explained, but there are at least three theories. Fishman and Hoff and Barber proposed that a transmantle gradient is established by a cerebrospinal fluid obstruction that provides a driving force for ventricular enlargement.[40, 59] Conner and co-workers have demonstrated that such a gradient occurs in cats with kaolin-produced experimental hydrocephalus, and Epstein has further analyzed the intracranial gradients that accompany hydrocephalus.[30, 37] There is evidence that relative aqueductal stenosis may be partially responsible for hydrocephalus after experimental subarachnoid hemorrhage.[15]

A second potential mechanism is increased pulse pressure within the ventricular system. DiRocco and colleagues have demonstrated that this mechanism is capable of increasing ventricular size in lambs without increasing the mean cerebrospinal fluid pressure.[33]

A third hypothesis grew out of the work of Salomon Hakim and his son Carlos.[51, 55] They consider that under normal circumstances, the brain acts like a sponge of viscoelastic material with a significant ability to "give" because of the venous capillaries, extracellular space, and lipids and proteins in the cerebral white matter. The pressure that controls the degree to which fluid may be displaced and the extent to which brain

parenchyma may be compressed is the gradient between the intraventricular cerebrospinal fluid pressure and the venous blood, that is, the effective cerebrospinal fluid pressure. For these authors, the gradient between cerebrospinal fluid pressure and venous pressure is the driving force for hydrocephalus. The normal effective cerebrospinal fluid pressure is lower than the bioelastic limit of the parenchyma; therefore, the pressure produces only a stress distribution within the cerebral tissue and does not squeeze out any liquid. Hydrocephalus is triggered by an initial increase in intraventricular pressure above venous pressure, raising the effective cerebrospinal fluid pressure, producing additional stress, and shifting fluid out of the cells. The periventricular region receives the greatest stress, and as this area yields, the ventricles enlarge. Figure 37–3 illustrates the relation between ventricle and parenchyma according to this last theory.

There is little pathological or physiological support in humans for these theories. In a few well-studied human cases of idiopathic normal-pressure hydrocephalus, scarring of the subarachnoid space has been demonstrated around the base of the brain.[32, 107] This is by no means a uniform finding at autopsy, however; in many cases, there is no evidence of obstruction of the cerebrospinal fluid pathway.[23] Similarly, the attempt to demonstrate cerebrospinal fluid dynamic abnormalities has produced confusing results. Some infusion studies have indicated that patients with normal-pressure hydrocephalus of unknown cause have increased resistance to cerebrospinal fluid outflow, but others are inconclusive on this matter.[74] The difficulty in using present methodology to measure compliance and resistance of the system accurately is a major problem. Specific studies are discussed in the section on deciding whether to do a shunt.

Assuming that there is increased resistance to cerebrospinal fluid flow at some level in the pathway, there are several explanations for the fact that the pressure does not seem to be elevated. Several investigators have suggested that patients with normal-pressure hydrocephalus have intermittently elevated cerebrospinal fluid pressure that may not be manifested on a single lumbar puncture but require long-term pressure monitoring.[122-124] Hakim and Adams have suggested that there is an initial rise in cerebrospinal fluid pressure that leads to ventricular enlargement and that this enlargement is maintained despite normal pressure because of Laplace's law. Although the pressure is normal, the enlarged ventricular area reflects increased force on the ventricular wall.[54] More recent studies suggest that attention must be directed increasingly to the parenchyma as well as to the cerebrospinal fluid in normal-pressure hydrocephalus.[12] Sklar and co-workers have demonstrated changes in brain elasticity, for example, which may be central to the development of ventricular enlargement despite normal pressures.[116]

A quite different approach to normal-pressure hydrocephalus than the study of cerebrospinal fluid physiology is implicit in the examination of cerebrospinal fluid peptides and other chemicals in this condition. Wikkelso and colleagues found that levels of somato-

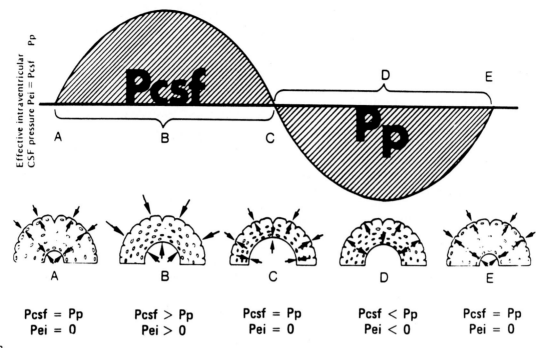

Figure 37–3

The development, maintenance, and resolution of hydrocephalus in the model proposed by Hakim. The model uses a gradient between cerebrospinal fluid and parenchymal pressure to explain the development and maintenance of hydrocephalus. In condition *A*, with normal ventricular size, there is a balance between pressures; in *B* an excessive cerebrospinal fluid pressure leads to progressive ventricular dilatation; and in *C* there is a steady state reached because of plastic deformation of the brain parenchyma. *D* and *E* show resolution of this situation with a shunt. Pcsf = intraventricular cerebrospinal fluid pressure; P_P = intraparenchymal venous pressure; Pei = effective differential cerebrospinal fluid pressure; Pei = Pcsf − P_P. (From Hakim, C.: The physics and physiopathology of the hydraulic complex of the central nervous system: The mechanics of hydrocephalus and normal pressure hydrocephalus. Unpublished dissertation, Cambridge, Massachusetts Institute of Technology, 1985. Used by permission.)

statin and peptide YY were decreased in patients with normal-pressure hydrocephalus and that delta-sleep–inducing peptide, vasoactive intestinal polypeptide, and somatostatin levels increased substantially after shunt placement.[135] Glial fibrillary acidic protein has been reported to be elevated in patients with normal-pressure hydrocephalus, and there are changes in cerebrospinal fluid vasopressin and brain-specific protein D_2.[3, 117, 118] This is a relatively underexplored area in this disease.

CLINICAL DIAGNOSIS

The diagnosis of normal-pressure hydrocephalus is still best made by clinical symptoms.[14, 23, 38, 103, 129] The chief feature is gait disturbance; the other two major components are memory loss, usually for recent events, and urinary incontinence. Slowing of thought and actions is also characteristic.

The syndrome is progressive, but the tempo of its evolution is highly variable. Symptoms may fluctuate. In some cases, the syndrome may develop months or years after the appearance of the etiological factor. Headache is not present. Aggressive behavior, seizures, and Parkinson-like symptoms have also been described in the presentation.[99, 101, 125]

On examination, extraocular movements are full; focal signs such as weakness or sensory loss are not present unless there has been brain damage related to the disease process that has caused the hydrocephalus. Difficulty in walking invariably occurs, and limb movements may be slow; muscle strength is usually normal. A Babinski response may be found in one or both feet, and reflexes may be somewhat increased. Sucking and grasping reflexes appear in the late stages. There is no sensory loss. Aphasia, visual field deficits, and parietal sensory findings are not features of normal-pressure hydrocephalus.

Disturbance of Gait. Gait disorder, usually the first symptom, may precede the other problems by months or even years. In some patients, the changes in gait and mentation occur at about the same time, whereas difficulty in walking occasionally follows other symptoms.

The gait problem varies from mild imbalance to an inability to walk or even stand.[27] There is often a history of falling. The major problem appears to be organizing a smooth gait.[38] Computerized gait evaluations have revealed characteristic short steps with difficulty in raising the legs, associated with almost continuous activity in antigravity muscles.[71] A motor abnormality may be present in the arms as well as the legs.[119]

Examination shows the steps to be shortened and the base widened. Balance is lost when turning. The patient is unable to perform tandem walking and sways during the Romberg test with eyes open or closed. Cerebellar ataxia is not present. Computed tomography correlations have suggested that large ventricles and gait disorder often appear together.[39, 72, 121] This gait syndrome may be more general in the elderly, however, rather than being specific for hydrocephalus.[36]

Disturbance of Mentation. The disorder in mentation can vary substantially from patient to patient. An impairment of recent memory is most characteristic; it may range from an inability to retain a fact for even a minute to a slight limitation revealed only by detailed testing.[38] The patient often appears to be "slowing up." Spontaneity and initiative are decreased, and interest in conversation, reading, writing, hobbies, and recreational activities declines. The family may report unconcern, apathy, lethargy, or the appearance of being withdrawn. Tasks are performed more slowly; attention and concentration are impaired. This complex of abnormalities has been termed the "abulic trait" by Fisher.[38]

The Wechsler-Bellevue test usually shows that verbal performance is relatively preserved but nonverbal performance (drawing, copying, arranging blocks, puzzle assembly, digit symbols, and picture-story arrangement) is more greatly impaired. Dyscalculia is usually present. As symptoms progress, the patient's responses become slower, to the point at which there may be no response to questions. If there is a response, it may be brief and only a partial answer. Voluntary movements are slow and delayed. In a few advanced cases, agitation and more complex disturbances in mental function may appear. Aberrant behavior, delusions, hallucinations, paranoia, and irrational speech are not usually part of the clinical picture. In an occasional patient, the presenting picture may be slowing of motor activity with rigidity and tremor that leads to the diagnosis of parkinsonism.

Incontinence. Urinary incontinence develops in some patients as a sense of urgency, but in most it is of the frontal lobe type, in which appropriate awareness of the need to urinate is diminished or lacking. Fecal incontinence is rare.

DIAGNOSTIC TESTS

Computed Tomography. Computed tomography is the most often used imaging test in the evaluation of a patient suspected of having normal-pressure hydrocephalus.[65, 66] This test gives an accurate assessment of the size of the ventricles, the extent of cortical atrophy, and the presence of localized pathological changes that may account for the hydrocephalic syndrome. Ideally, computed tomography in normal-pressure hydrocephalus shows marked enlargement of the ventricles but little or no evidence of atrophy; however, improvement has been noted in patients with significant cortical atrophy as well. Periventricular low absorption is an important finding in some patients.[17] Postoperatively, ventricular size can be easily measured, and the presence of subdural hematoma or hygroma can be evaluated. The use of computed tomog-

raphy to predict shunt response is discussed later in this chapter.

Magnetic Resonance Imaging. Magnetic resonance imaging is as important as computed tomography in the evaluation of adult hydrocephalus. With it, the ventricles can be imaged in the sagittal and frontal planes as well as in the transaxial plane used in computed tomography. Ventricular volumes can also be displayed and measured (Fig. 37–4; see color section in this volume).[29, 45] Subtle changes caused by microinfarcts in the parenchyma can be established, and, perhaps more important, flowing cerebrospinal fluid can be differentiated from stagnant cerebrospinal fluid. Continuing data suggest that the flow seen in the cerebral aqueduct is more prominent in normal-pressure hydrocephalus.[22, 82] Volumetric distinctions can also be made between normal-pressure and high-pressure hydrocephalus.[29] Normal-pressure hydrocephalus has an increased ventricular volume with normal subarachnoid volume; high-pressure hydrocephalus has an increased ventricular volume and diminished subarachnoid volume. Alzheimer's disease has increased ventricular and subarachnoid volumes.[45] Periventricular diminished signal on magnetic resonance imaging is not as useful as periventricular low density on com-

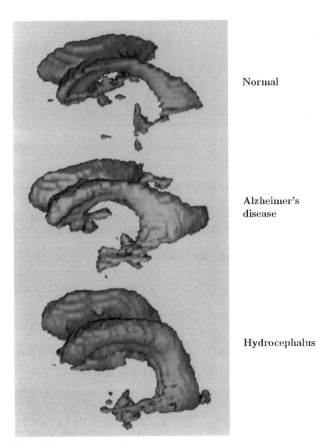

Normal

Alzheimer's disease

Hydrocephalus

Figure 37–4

Three-dimensional reconstruction of the ventricular system in a normal patient (*top*), a patient with Alzheimer's disease (*middle*), and a patient with idiopathic normal-pressure hydrocephalus (*bottom*) (see color section in this volume). (Courtesy of Ron Kikinis, John Martin, and Mitsunori Matsumae, Surgical Planning Laboratory, Brigham and Women's Hospital, Boston.)

puted tomography for establishing that hydrocephalus is active.

Lumbar Puncture. The measurement of cerebrospinal fluid pressure with the patient in the lateral recumbent position in the resting state usually reveals a pressure of less than 180 mm H_2O in normal-pressure hydrocephalus. Protein and sugar levels are normal unless altered by the disease process that has caused the hydrocephalus, and the cell count should also be normal. An improvement after draining of cerebrospinal fluid by lumbar puncture suggests that a shunt would be helpful; Haan and Thomeer suggested that temporary lumbar drainage be used as a predictive test.[49]

Isotope Cisternography. In this test, a radiolabeled isotope is injected into the lumbar subarachnoid space, and its passage into the brain and ventricles is visualized.[41, 57, 68, 136] The most commonly used isotope in the past was [131]iodine-labeled human serum albumin (RISA); currently, indium-labeled diethylenetriamine pentaacetic acid (DTPA) is the agent of choice. A dose of 500 mCi is injected into the lumbar subarachnoid space, and scans are done at 4, 24, 48, and 72 hours.

Three different flow patterns have been described: (1) the normal pattern, with flow over the convexities and not into the ventricles; (2) a pattern suggestive of idiopathic normal-pressure hydrocephalus, with ventricular entry and stasis within the ventricles for 72 hours but no ascent over the convexities; and (3) a "mixed" pattern, with variable ventricular entry and flow around the convexities.[68] Most patients are in the "mixed" category, with both ventricular entry and early convexity ascent. The relation of the findings to the response to shunting is so variable that this test is not usually helpful in the definitive evaluation of patients with normal-pressure hydrocephalus.[129]

Other Tests. Skull films are usually normal and show no evidence of chronic increased intracranial pressure. Studies of cerebrospinal fluid dynamics are discussed later. The measurement of transport of radioactive indicators from the cerebrospinal fluid to the plasma as an index of delay in absorption has been suggested, but correlation with the results of shunting has not been made. No consistent distinctive pattern of altered cerebral blood flow has been found, although diminished frontal flow bilaterally is a common finding.[83] Visual evoked potentials have little proven usefulness.[2]

Normal-Pressure Hydrocephalus with Known Etiology

Subarachnoid Hemorrhage. Some enlargement of the ventricular system has been reported in 67 per cent of patients after subarachnoid hemorrhage[11]; one report noted acute hydrocephalus in 40 per cent.[80] Initially, there may be a temporary increase in cerebrospinal fluid pressure, but in most cases the symptoms of hydrocephalus develop after the pressure has returned to a normal level. Frequently, the onset is delayed for one to several weeks after the hemorrhage. Rapid delayed deterioration may occur as long as 3 weeks after the hemorrhage.

In the acute stage, it may be difficult to differentiate the clinical signs of hydrocephalus from those of spasm or bleeding, and computed tomography plus arteriography may be necessary. In the chronic stage, the differential diagnosis is not as difficult. Dementia with severe impairment of memory and slowness of thought and movement may be the most prominent symptoms.

Hydrocephalus without symptoms should be monitored by regular computed tomography studies. If the ventricular size is increasing over several months, shunting should be considered. Within the first 2 weeks of hemorrhage, serial lumbar punctures or ventriculostomy may allow the patient to get through a period of high pressure without having to undergo operation. In most series, shunting is eventually required for 10 to 15 per cent of patients with symptoms of subarachnoid hemorrhage; the response to placement of a shunt is good in 80 per cent of cases.[11, 40]

Trauma. The natural history of patients who develop large ventricles after head trauma has not been fully studied.[9] In many cases, it is difficult to differentiate the direct effects of the brain injury from those secondary to obstruction of cerebrospinal fluid flow.[79] The mechanism for development of hydrocephalus is thought to be scarring and obstruction of the basal cisterns as the result of subarachnoid hemorrhage. Rarely, there may be obstruction of a major venous sinus or a block in the third ventricle or the aqueduct, and in some cases primary cortical tissue loss is an important contributing factor. As with spontaneous subarachnoid hemorrhage, symptoms may be associated with mildly elevated or normal cerebrospinal fluid pressure. The onset of disturbance of mentation or a disorder of gait may be delayed for several weeks or even months after the trauma. In these circumstances, improvement after insertion of a shunt can be striking. However, in patients in whom enlarged ventricles are associated with failure to recover fully after a serious head injury, the results are variable, probably because of underlying brain damage.

Meningitis. On rare occasions, obliteration of the subarachnoid space develops after meningitis. Symptoms of normal-pressure hydrocephalus may be noted early in the illness, or they may not be manifested for several months. A shunt is indicated if spontaneous recovery does not occur. In most cases of bacterial meningitis, ventriculostomy should be used until the cerebrospinal fluid is sterile before permanent shunt placement. For tuberculosis or fungal meningitis, concern about spreading organisms should not prevent shunt replacement.

Intracranial Tumors. Enlarged ventricles associated with partial obstruction of the cerebrospinal fluid pathways by a brain tumor may produce symptoms of normal-pressure hydrocephalus. As with high-pressure hydrocephalus, judgment is necessary about whether to place a shunt first or to remove the primary lesion. If there is no urgency and the lesion will have to be removed in any case, its removal should be done first.

Postoperative. Several days or weeks after intracranial operation, particularly after a posterior fossa exploration, symptoms of normal-pressure hydrocephalus may develop. Computed tomography shows enlarged ventricles. If the symptoms do not improve spontaneously over a short period of time, a shunt is indicated.

Aqueduct Stenosis. Symptoms related to hydrocephalus secondary to aqueduct stenosis may not occur until adult life.[5] The majority of patients present with symptoms and signs of increased intracranial pressure, but the syndrome of normal-pressure hydrocephalus may also be seen. The ventricular system may be very large.

Patients with this problem are often young and have symptoms of intermittent headache as well as mental slowing. With an implanted telesensor, it may be possible to monitor cerebrospinal fluid pressure in these patients for a period before deciding to shunt; however, shunting should be done if there is evidence of elevated intracranial pressure or intellectual or motor decline. Sagittal magnetic resonance imaging of the brain stem and aqueduct is useful to exclude a pontine glioma as a cause of stenosis. It is possible that third ventriculoscopy done by endoscopy can avoid a shunt in these patients.

Idiopathic Normal-Pressure Hydrocephalus

Idiopathic normal-pressure hydrocephalus is an intriguing syndrome that has generated more publications than its incidence would suggest. It has been given a number of names, including occult hydrocephalus, hydrocephalic dementia, low-pressure hydrocephalus, Hakim's syndrome, Hakim-Adams syndrome, and ventricular enlargement and gait abnormality.[24, 40, 69, 78]

In the history of this disorder, Salomon Hakim suggested in 1964 that ventriculomegaly may be a cause of dementia and gait disturbance without an antecedent neurological event.[52] He and Adams were able to find several cases that led to further publications.[1] Early enthusiastic reports of shunt success were followed by later studies with varying results.* The efficacy of shunt placement has been increasingly questioned by some authors.[44, 88, 130] One example is an interinstitutional study from Amsterdam that showed, among 166 patients, a marked improvement in only 15 per cent, and a shunt morbidity of 28 per cent.[130]

Depending on the criteria for success, however, the contemporary literature reports an overall improvement rate of about 60 to 74 per cent in idiopathic normal-pressure hydrocephalus patients with shunts and a marked improvement rate in about 50 per cent.† Larsson and colleagues, for example, found that 73 per cent of 74 patients improved after shunt surgery.[77] Despite the varying responses to shunt placement, this syndrome remains an important treatable cause of gait disorder and of dementia in selected patients.‡

The differential diagnosis in idiopathic normal-pressure hydrocephalus includes Alzheimer's disease, Parkinson's disease, depression, and multi-infarct dementia. Alzheimer's disease is usually characterized by memory loss out of proportion to the gait disorder (at least in the early stages); this is the most important differential feature. In Alzheimer's disease, cortical deficits such as aphasia and frontal lobe release signs may be part of the clinical presentation; they are rare in normal-pressure hydrocephalus. The definitive diagnosis may be possible only by biopsy, however. The tremor and rigidity of Parkinson's disease help differentiate it from idiopathic normal-pressure hydrocephalus, as does the lack of incontinence. However, the two conditions may coexist. Depression may cause memory loss and a slow, shuffling gait; again, incontinence is not usually a feature, and the patient should fulfill diagnostic criteria for depression. Multi-infarct dementia may sometimes be differentiated by the presence of multiple low-absorption regions on computed tomography or magnetic resonance imaging.

The major treatment in idiopathic normal-pressure hydrocephalus is placement of a shunt. In considering whether to insert a shunt, two types of findings can be distinguished: those that seem irrelevant to the decision and those that seem to have prognostic value.

Findings That Can Probably Be Ignored in the Decision to Shunt in Idiopathic Normal-Pressure Hydrocephalus

Evidence of Cerebrovascular Disease. Evidence of atherosclerotic brain disease on computed tomography or magnetic resonance imaging does not prevent a good outcome from shunting.[35, 50, 95] Many patients with clinical normal-pressure hydrocephalus of unknown cause have cerebrovascular disease, including deep white-matter infarction. Koto and co-workers reported a greater likelihood of improvement after shunting in patients with hypertension and focal ischemic signs than in their nonhypertensive counterparts.[75] Casmiro and colleagues found that hypertension, ischemic heart disease, ischemic changes on electrocardiography, low cholesterol levels, and diabetes were correlated with the development of symptomatic idiopathic normal-pressure hydrocephalus.[24]

Atrophy on Computed Tomography. Early reports suggested that atrophy implied a poor shunt response. However, data from Salmon's work, from Vasilouthis, from the Mayo Clinic, and from the author's institution all support the view that improvement can occur if atrophy is present, although the chances of improvement are somewhat better if there is no atrophy.*

Normal or Mixed Cisternographic Pattern. Initial reports were enthusiastic about the use of radionuclide cisternography as a predictive test for shunting in idiopathic normal-pressure hydrocephalus.[57, 108, 127] However, there appears to be less reliance on this technique in more recent reports. The author has found that a pattern typical of normal-pressure hydrocephalus was helpful in predicting a good shunt response but that a normal or mixed pattern could also be associated with

---

*See references 4, 6, 7, 8, 13, 48, 91, 96, 104, 110, 123, 127, and 128.
†See references 8, 15, 17, 19, 23, 46, 48, 60, 78, 89, 120, and 131.
‡See references 14, 17, 46, 70, 78, and 98.

*See references 4, 14, 78, 103, 109, 110, and 111.

a good response.[14] Borgesen and colleagues suggested that a normal indium-DTPA pattern predicted normal conductance of cerebrospinal fluid and therefore made shunting ill-advised; however, they did not specify whether shunts failed to improve the conditions of patients treated by these principles.[21] Vanneste and colleagues used a multicenter study to demonstrate that cisternography did not improve predictive power.[129] Metrizamide computed tomography cisternography has been suggested as a replacement for indium cisternography in elucidating cerebrospinal fluid dynamics; however, its role remains to be defined.[34]

Altered Cerebral Blood Flow Measurements. Some investigators have suggested a characteristic pattern of cerebral blood flow in patients with normal-pressure hydrocephalus.[83, 89, 90] Others have found that no distinctive pattern of blood flow characterizes patients with idiopathic normal-pressure hydrocephalus.[64, 126] Blood flow measurements may identify shunt nonresponders early in the postoperative period, because patients with normal-pressure hydrocephalus have an increase in blood flow after shunting.[47, 83, 89, 90]

One report suggests that positron emission tomography shows a pattern of global hypometabolism in normal-pressure hydrocephalus and one of frontotemporal hypometabolism in dementia caused by Alzheimer's disease, but this requires further study.[67]

Findings That Favor a Decision to Shunt

Significant Gait Disturbance. Cerebrospinal fluid shunting was initially considered most important as a treatment for memory loss; however, it now appears that the presence of a gait disturbance is the major element in predicting shunt success. There appears to be a general relationship between large ventricles and gait disturbance.[39, 72, 121] There is also a definite relationship between gait disturbance and success of shunting. Fisher found that gait disturbance preceded impaired mentation in 12 of 16 patients who responded to a shunt; 9 of 11 patients who did not respond to a shunt had little or no gait disturbance.[38] Jacobs and colleagues reported that none of their patients who were able to walk without difficulty had improvement after shunting.[66] Laws and Mokri emphasized the importance of gait difficulty, and their group has reported a 74 per cent success rate when difficulty in walking was a major criterion for shunting.[78, 103] Vassilouthis used gait disturbance as an essential criterion to obtain an 87.5 per cent success rate after shunting.[131] Graff-Radford and colleagues found that gait disturbance preceding other symptoms implied a good shunt response.[46]

The author's experience has been that gait disturbance is the finding most likely to respond dramatically to shunting, although it is not always necessary to have gait difficulty as the primary or predominant syndrome to achieve shunt success.

Altered Cerebrospinal Fluid Dynamics with Increased Cerebrospinal Fluid Outflow Resistance. There is a substantial literature on cerebrospinal fluid physiology in idiopathic normal-pressure hydrocepha-

lus.* If 180 mm H_2O is taken as the upper limit of normal pressure, some patients with normal pressures on a single determination will have high pressures at some time over a 24-hour period. Using epidural pressure recording, Symon's group has identified a subgroup of patients with idiopathic normal-pressure hydrocephalus associated with pressure peaks greater than 20 mm Hg or recurrent B-wave activity.[122–124] Symon and Hinzpeter reported that these patients have a higher improvement rate with shunting than do patients with entirely normal pressure traces.[123] Similar evidence of intermittently elevated pressures has been found with ventricular pressure recording. Crockard and colleagues divided patients with hydrocephalus into those with intermittent elevations of intracranial pressure and those without such elevations.[31] They found that ventricular size was the same in both groups but that there was more sulcal atrophy in patients without elevated intracranial pressure. They did not comment on shunt outcome.

Hartmann and Alberti used overnight recording to select patients for shunting but did not place shunts in patients who had normal traces.[56] Chawla and associates monitored intracranial pressure by either a subdural transducer or a ventricular catheter in 12 patients; they found that 7 patients with flat recordings did not improve but 5 patients with B waves did.[28] However, these latter 5 patients all had lumbar puncture pressures above 15 mm Hg, making them not true examples of normal-pressure hydrocephalus. Borgesen and colleagues reported that 13 of 14 patients with B waves more than 50 per cent of the time on an intraventricular overnight recording improved with shunting.[18–20] Foltz and Aine suggested that the pattern of the cerebrospinal fluid pulse wave rather than the mean pressure measurement is the critical feature of analysis in hydrocephalus.[42] They believed that the pulse pressure and systolic waveform established the diagnosis of hydrocephalus in 10 patients with idiopathic normal-pressure hydrocephalus; however, correlation was not made with outcome.

The situation with regard to lumbar infusion testing is more complicated than that with overnight recording.[36, 61] The infusion test, described as a method of assessing resistance to cerebrospinal fluid absorption, has been used to demonstrate impaired absorption in normal-pressure hydrocephalus.[61, 72] It has little relation to computed tomography patterns.[73] Moreover, it has not been consistently useful as a predictive test for shunting. Kosteljanetz found that outflow resistance measurements did not help predict shunt result.[74] This may be a result of testing artifact or of misinterpretation of results. Alternatively, it may be that constant-rate infusion misrepresents some important features of cerebrospinal fluid physiology. Similarly, pressure volume testing by means of a single lumbar puncture may not be completely accurate.

To avoid the problem of a constant-rate infusion technique, Sklar and colleagues have developed a servocontrol system that quickly reaches and maintains a

---

*See references 17–21, 26, 30, 56, 61, 73, 74, 76, 85, and 94.

given cerebrospinal fluid pressure.[115] It is therefore a constant-pressure system requiring only one lumbar puncture. However, its efficacy in predicting shunt outcome has not been tested in large numbers of patients.

Because of the difficulties with lumbar infusion testing, Borgeson, Gjerris, Sorensen and associates have used lumboventricular perfusion to predict shunt outcome.[17-21] This technique uses infusion through a lumbar catheter with a ventricular catheter for outflow and infusion pressure set by the height of the ventricular outflow. Absorption volume is calculated and plotted against pressure; the slope of the resulting regression line is the conductance to outflow of cerebrospinal fluid in milliliters per minute per mm Hg. What is being measured is the ease with which fluid is removed from the cerebrospinal fluid space by absorptive mechanisms. Borgesen and Gjerris reported on the results of lumboventricular perfusion in 80 patients with normal-pressure hydrocephalus, 40 of whom had the idiopathic variety. Using a criterion for shunting that required conductance to be less than 0.12 mL per minute per mm Hg, they found that 21 (70 per cent) of 31 patients with idiopathic normal-pressure hydrocephalus had a good response to shunting; if the cutoff had been 0.8 mL per minute per mm Hg, all patients would have responded.[19] Later reports have confirmed these results.[20, 21]

These authors found that outflow conductance measurements did not correlate with lumbar infusion results, suggesting that lumbar infusion itself may not provide accurate predictive data. Although lumboventricular perfusion appears to be a useful predictive test, it is limited by the need for a ventricular catheter. However, at the present time it appears to be the most satisfactory test of cerebrospinal fluid dynamics for prediction of shunt outcome.

Improvement After Lumbar Puncture. Lumbar puncture in a patient with a persistent dural defect can be regarded as a kind of temporary fistula that lowers the cerebrospinal fluid pressure; it is therefore reasonable to consider this as a therapeutic trial of cerebrospinal fluid diversion. Bret and colleagues, Fisher, and Wikkelso and associates all found that improvement in gait after lumbar puncture was a reliable indicator of shunt success.[23, 38, 133]

Computed Tomography with Periventricular Low Absorption. Mori and co-workers noted that periventricular low absorption on computed tomography was an indication of increased likelihood of shunt success in patients with hydrocephalus.[92] This finding has been shown to result from increased periventricular water in experimental hydrocephalus and appears to be caused by similar phenomena in human patients.[58, 93] Borgesen and Gjerris reported that all 16 patients with periventricular lucency improved; this finding appears to be a useful predictor of shunt success.[19]

Computed Tomography with Small Sulci. Other computed tomography findings are less clearly helpful in predicting shunt response. The previous section has discussed the fact that large sulci do not preclude an effect from shunting. Small sulci in combination with large ventricles, however, are associated with a high likelihood of improvement after shunting. In Borgesen's series, 16 patients with this finding all had a good shunt response.[19] Benzel and colleagues found that the absence of gyral atrophy and sylvian fissure enlargement in association with the typical clinical syndrome predicted a good shunt response.[8] Other computed tomography features associated with a good shunt response are enlarged third ventricle and temporal horns.[134]

Cerebrospinal Fluid Flow Void in the Aqueduct. Bradley and colleagues reviewed 20 patients with idiopathic normal-pressure hydrocephalus to assess which responded to shunt placement and found that the magnitude of the cerebrospinal fluid flow void predicted shunt response accurately.[22]

Subcortical Low Flow on Positron Emission Tomography or Single Photon Emission Computed Tomography. Waldemar and colleagues reported diminished subcortical flow in normal-pressure hydrocephalus patients who improved after shunt placement.[135]

The choice of shunt placement often requires clinical judgment of the most experienced kind, and neurosurgical consultation with a senior surgeon may be helpful. Figure 37–5 presents a summary of decision-making for patients with idiopathic normal-pressure hydrocephalus and incorporates some of these data.

Shunt Operations

The definitive treatment of symptomatic hydrocephalus is usually placement of a shunt to drain cerebrospinal fluid from the ventricle to a body vein or cavity. The basic shunt procedures and their complications are presented in this section.

TECHNIQUE

Ventriculoperitoneal shunting is the easiest and most widely used technique for shunt placement in adults (Fig. 37–6); ventriculovenous (ventriculoatrial) shunting is also acceptable (Fig. 37–7).[63, 97] Lumboperitoneal shunting is acceptable in communicating hydrocephalus but carries the risk of tonsillar herniation and acquired Arnold-Chiari malformation.

Any of the currently available valve systems may be used; it is important in selecting a valve to have a reliable opening pressure on cerebrospinal fluid testing. There are three types of valve: the slit valve, which is the most common and uses the pressure required to open a slit between two deformable pieces of plastic as its pressure regulator; the spring valve, which uses the resilience of a spring; and the flow-controlled valve, which relies on the narrow diameter of the tubing to provide resistance. There are also adjustable valve systems on the market (see later).

Larsson and colleagues used a high-pressure valve in 13 patients and found that clinical improvement occurred within the first 3 months after shunting and

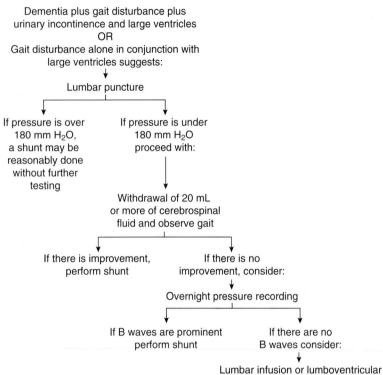

Figure 37–5

Paradigm for decision-making in idiopathic normal-pressure hydrocephalus. Each result indicates further procedures or tests to be considered.

did not increase as the valve pressure was lowered below the initial high setting (170 mm H_2O). The mean intracranial pressure did not decrease at the initial high-pressure setting and yet did go on to decrease with lower valve pressures.[77] At the other extreme, McQuarrie and colleagues believed that a low-pressure system was the optimum one for effective shunt placement.[87] Schmitt and Spring found that all 21 of the patients they treated with a Sophy adjustable valve improved at pressures set between 130 and 170 mm H_2O, compared with improvement in only 7 of 15 patients treated with conventional valves with either high or medium pressures.[112] Sindou and colleagues found that 36 per cent of patients required adjustment of valve pressure when the Sophy system was available to them, suggesting that adjustment of pressure is an important potential adjunct to successful shunting.[114] The Medos valve, which can vary the pressure from 30 to 200 mm H_2O in 10-mm increments, allows precise setting of valve pressures and is currently in clinical trial. It allows the surgeon to modify the pressure noninvasively through an externally applied magnetic coil and has been useful in treating chronic subdural hygromas after shunting, slit-ventricle syndrome, and traditional cases of normal-pressure hydrocephalus.[16]

For shunt implantation in the usual case, the right scalp, neck, anterior chest, and abdomen are shaved and isolated with Steri-Drapes after general anesthesia has been induced. Prophylactic intravenous antibiotics are given. The skin is prepared, and incision sites are marked out.

In the scalp, either a frontal or a parieto-occipital site may be used. The frontal burr hole is best placed 10 cm from the nasion and 2.5 cm to the right of the midline. Usually, it is best to seat the valve and peritoneal tubing subgaleally before inserting the ventricular catheter. It is important to test the valve by filling it with sterile saline or water and testing the run-off and closing pressure, holding the distal end horizontal. The shunt assembly is then attached to the ventricular catheter, and confirmation of good flow from the peritoneal tubing is made. It is helpful to mark the direction of catheter insertion before drapes are placed; appropriate landmarks are the inner canthus of the right eye in the mediolateral plane and a point midway between the lateral orbital rim and the tragus in the anteroposterior plane. Aiming more posteriorly (e.g., at the tragus) puts the catheter in the third ventricle. For occipital burr hole placement, a point 6 cm above the inion and 3 cm to the right of the midline is chosen. In this approach, the catheter is inserted to aim 1 cm above the nasion. The skin flap in either case is made as a small curvilinear incision situated so that shunt tubing does not cross under it.

After burr hole placement and coagulation of the dura, the ventricle is sounded with a No. 19 ventricular needle or shunt catheter. For frontal cannulation, 6 cm of catheter is left below the dura in final position. Initially, an additional 1 cm may be necessary to obtain good flow; the catheter should then be drawn back to 6 cm. In the occipital region, 11 cm of catheter is usual, although the distance can be estimated on the scalp as the distance to the lateral orbit.

There are a number of possible incisions for insertion of the peritoneal catheter. A subcostal muscle-splitting incision in the right upper quadrant is a relatively easy

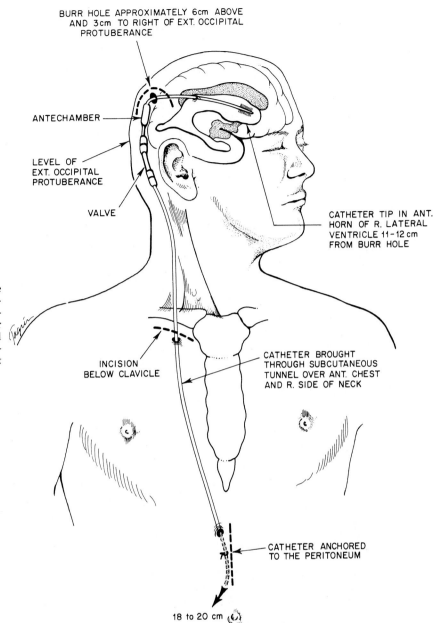

BURR HOLE APPROXIMATELY 6cm ABOVE AND 3cm TO RIGHT OF EXT. OCCIPITAL PROTUBERANCE

ANTECHAMBER

LEVEL OF EXT. OCCIPITAL PROTUBERANCE

VALVE

CATHETER TIP IN ANT. HORN OF R. LATERAL VENTRICLE 11–12 cm FROM BURR HOLE

INCISION BELOW CLAVICLE

CATHETER BROUGHT THROUGH SUBCUTANEOUS TUNNEL OVER ANT. CHEST AND R. SIDE OF NECK

CATHETER ANCHORED TO THE PERITONEUM

18 to 20 cm

Figure 37–6

Placement of ventriculoperitoneal shunt in the adult by means of an occipital burr hole. Usually a midline incision is made above the umbilicus. The peritoneal catheter is inserted for a distance of at least 18 to 20 cm. It is anchored at the peritoneum and placed in a subcutaneous tunnel over the anterior chest and the right side of the neck.

technique. An alternative is a midline incision through the rectus fascia; in this approach, differentiating properitoneal fat from omentum may not be easy, and care should be taken to be certain that the peritoneal cavity is entered. Confirmation of peritoneal entry can be made by visualizing the bowel or liver. The peritoneal tubing is inserted for a distance of 20 to 30 cm. The peritoneum and fascia should be closed separately and firmly. A suture is tied around the catheter and anchored to the fascia.

If a venous shunt is used, an oblique incision is made over the upper portion of the anterior border of the sternocleidomastoid muscle (see Fig. 37–7). The common facial vein is identified and ligated, and the cardiac catheter is inserted through this vein and into the jugular vein for a distance of 20 to 25 cm. The catheter is filled with a radiopaque substance, and a radiograph is taken to verify that the tip of the catheter is positioned at the level of the sixth thoracic vertebra. If the catheter is already radiopaque, dye is not needed.[63]

For ventriculopleural shunting, an incision is made between the second and the third ribs lateral to the midclavicular plane, and the tubing is inserted after puncture of the parietal pleura. A chest film should be obtained in the first postoperative week.

Accessories may help ensure successful shunt placement. An implanted telesensor device may allow postoperative noninvasive monitoring of cerebrospinal fluid pressure.[26] An antisiphon device stops flow at atmospheric pressure; some surgeons believe that it is helpful to prevent negative pressures and subsequent subdural hygroma or hematoma formation. An on-off device allows the shunt to be turned off; it is important

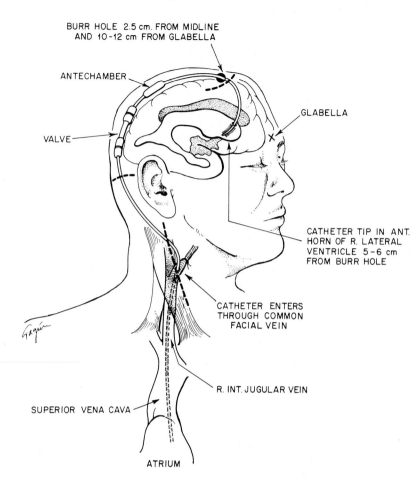

BURR HOLE 2.5 cm. FROM MIDLINE
AND 10-12 cm FROM GLABELLA

ANTECHAMBER

GLABELLA

VALVE

CATHETER TIP IN ANT.
HORN OF R. LATERAL
VENTRICLE 5-6 cm
FROM BURR HOLE

CATHETER ENTERS
THROUGH COMMON
FACIAL VEIN

R. INT. JUGULAR VEIN

SUPERIOR VENA CAVA

ATRIUM

Figure 37–7

Placement of ventriculovenous shunt in the adult by means of a frontal burr hole. The burr hole is usually on the right side and is placed behind the anterior hairline, 10 to 12 cm from the glabella and 2.5 to 3.0 cm from the midline. The landmarks for insertion are the inner canthus of the eye in the frontal plane and a point just in front of the external auditory meatus in the lateral plane. The catheter should lie at a depth of 5 to 6 cm from the external table of the skull. The neck incision is made in a skin crease and centered over the upper portion of the sternocleidomastoid muscle. Usually the catheter can be inserted through the common facial vein. The position of the distal end of the catheter is checked by radiography; it should be at the level of the sixth or seventh thoracic vertebra.

to be able to see it in x-ray profile to know whether it is on or off. In-line filters can be used if there are abnormal cells in the cerebrospinal fluid; these filters may be useful in preventing tumor spread into the abdomen but can be expected to occlude.

POSTOPERATIVE COMPLICATIONS

Major complications after shunting for high-pressure hydrocephalus are infrequent; the most common are shunt malfunction and infection. In normal-pressure hydrocephalus, complications are considerably more common, perhaps because of the age of patients and the complexity of accurate diagnosis. The incidence of reported complications is as high as 35 per cent; in Bret and Chazal's series, there were subdural collections in 16.8 per cent of patients, shunt malfunction in 10.6 per cent, sepsis in 4 per cent, and seizures in 4 per cent.[23] Puca and colleagues found a 28.65 per cent incidence of shunt revision, most often from distal malposition, obstruction, or infection.[106]

Overdrainage. Overdrainage occurred in one of seven cases in the series reported by Sindou and colleagues; it may be construed either as mismatching of valve pressure to the patient's ventricular system or as siphoning.[43, 53, 114] It can result in a low-pressure syndrome and, ultimately, in chronic subdural hematoma or hygroma formation. Chapman and Fox and their colleagues have analyzed the effect of shunting on intracranial pressure in the upright position, emphasiz-

ing the degree to which siphoning occurs in most shunt systems; this is presumably an important factor in the low-pressure syndrome and in formation of subdural collections.[25, 43]

Subdural Hygromas. Subdural hygromas are a major potential problem in shunt placement for normal-pressure hydrocephalus. They often present as apparently asymptomatic lesions in a patient who may not be responsive to shunt placement, and the clinical issue is whether to drain them. The author's policy is to watch them expectantly with computed tomography in 1 month unless they are producing mass effect or symptoms; if they are enlarging, it is necessary to drain them and either tie off the shunt for 1 to 3 months, revise it to a higher-pressure valve, or insert an antisiphon device. Tearing of bridging veins may cause them to become subdural hematomas, which, with repeated small bleeding episodes, can enlarge. Illingworth found a substantial incidence of subdural hematomas in his series.[62]

Low-Pressure Syndrome. Low-pressure syndrome can be as debilitating as hydrocephalus; it is characterized by headache worse on sitting up and by nausea; particularly characteristic is pain at the base of the neck. Revision to a higher-pressure valve, a valve adjustment if the patient has a variable-pressure valve, or insertion of an antisiphon device is a reasonable option for treatment, but the syndrome usually does not resolve spontaneously.

Underdrainage. Underdrainage results in failure of the ventricles to diminish in size as the patient remains symptomatic. It may be difficult to establish that this is the cause of failure of improvement; Sindou and colleagues found that the shunt pressure was lowered 20 times in 69 patients with normal-pressure hydrocephalus using a variable-pressure valve.[114] This indicates how often valve adjustment could be helpful if there were a ready mechanism for carrying this out.

Matching of shunt pressure to the patient's needs is not an easy matter. Although the changes in ventricular size that occur after shunting do not always correlate with the clinical results, the possibility of varying the valve pressure according to the patient's needs is an attractive one.[113]

Shunt Malfunction. Shunt malfunction may occur more often than is suspected in normal-pressure hydrocephalus. Larsson and colleagues, for example, found a 31 per cent incidence.[77]

Valve pumping is not a reliable indicator of shunt function. If shunt malfunction is suspected from increasing symptoms, the first step is to repeat the computed tomography study. The ventricles usually begin to diminish in size within a week in high-pressure hydrocephalus; in that condition, continued enlargement suggests shunt malfunction. In normal-pressure hydrocephalus, the ventricles may remain large despite good shunt function. A lumbar puncture should be performed to establish whether the system is functioning at the pressure for which the valve was engineered. Puncture of the shunt reservoir tests the shunt but carries the risk of subsequent infection. If the reservoir is punctured, inability to withdraw cerebrospinal fluid suggests ventricular catheter obstruction. The next step is to revise the catheter operatively, because attempting to flush it may dangerously increase partially decompensated intracranial pressure. If there is ready withdrawal of cerebrospinal fluid, shunt tubing b̶t̶ the ventricular catheter and the reservoir sh compressed very firmly, and run-off into the pe catheter should be evaluated. In this case, att irrigation is worthwhile, with the tubing into th tricle compressed if possible.

Ventricular catheter malfunction may be diffi diagnose, especially if the catheter is only part cluded. In that case, the cerebrospinal fluid pre on shunt tap may seem normal; however, a poor waveform and poor catheter flow are indicativ malfunction. Operative revision is indicated. V malfunction may occur from a change in characteri of the plastic or obstruction by debris. It can best diagnosed by exploration of the shunt and disc nection in the operating room. Peritoneal catheter struction may be caused by omentum, by debris, or infection. Cultures of cerebrospinal fluid are importa to obtain if there is peritoneal catheter obstruction b cause of the possibility of low-grade infection as cause of peritoneal malabsorption. Like valve malfunction, peritoneal catheter dysfunction can be diagnosed with certainty only through surgery.

Seizures. Seizures are an infrequent complication of shunt placement, occurring in about 5 per cent of patients. Occipital catheter placement may be associated with a lesser chance of seizure disorder than is frontal placement. The author does not use prophylactic anticonvulsants.

Intracerebral Hemorrhage. Intracerebral hemorrhage is an uncommon complication of catheter placement, with a 1 per cent incidence. Care in directing the catheter is an important step in the prevention of intracerebral hemorrhage, so multiple passes should be avoided. The most important determination is where the burr hole is in relation to midline and sutures.

Shunt Infection. Infection of a shunt is often indolent in adults, as it is in children. Peritoneal catheter malfunction is a common manifestation, and cerebrospinal fluid cultures from the shunt tubing should be obtained during revision of a shunt for peritoneal malfunction. Although some authors have suggested that infection can be treated with antibiotics alone, the best course is to remove the entire shunt system. External ventriculostomy may be needed until the infection resolves (usually in about 1 week).

Medical Problems. A number of medical problems may occur in patients with idiopathic normal-pressure hydrocephalus because of their age. The author's experience, however, has been that contemporary anesthesia techniques have not made age a contraindication if the patient is likely to be helped by shunt placement.

REFERENCES

1. Adams, R. D., Fisher, C. M., Hakim, S., et al.: Symptomatic occult hydrocephalus with "normal" cerebrospinal fluid pressure: A treatable syndrome. N. Engl. J. Med., 273:117–126, 1965.
2. Alani, S. M.: Pattern-reversal visual evoked potentials in patients with hydrocephalus. J. Neurosurg., 62:234–237, 1985.
3. Albechtsen, M., Sorenson F., et al.: High cerebrospinal ... illary acidic protein in ... phalus. J. Neurol. Sci.,
... eatment of parenchy- ... triculo-atrial shunting ... 78–482, 1967. ... on-neoplastic stenosis ... and adult life. Surg.
... s with low-pressure ... uid diversion with ...), 27:11–15, 1972. ... Surgical indications ... tive analysis of the ... results of surgical ...)76.
... : Communicating ... after ventricular ...), 1990. ... hydrocephalus.
... rocephalus: Re- ... g., 53:371–377, 1980. ... us and vasospasm following sub- ... ...emorrhage from ruptured intracranial aneurysms. Neurosurgery, 18:12–16, 1986.
12. Black, P. McL., and Conner, E. S.: Chronic increased intracranial pressure. In Asbury, A. K., McKhann, G. M., and McDonald, W. I., eds.: Diseases of the Nervous System. Philadelphia, W. B. Saunders, 1986.
13. Black, P. McL., and Sweet, W. H.: Normal-pressure hydrocephalus, idiopathic type: Selection of patients for shunting proce-

dures. *In* Little, J., ed.: Advances in Neurosurgery: Lumbar Disc, Adult Hydrocephalus. Baltimore, Williams & Wilkins, 1985, pp. 106–110.

14. Black, P. McL., Ojemann, R. G., and Tzouras, A.: Cerebrospinal fluid shunts for dementia, gait disturbance, and incontinence. Clin. Neurosurg., 32:632–656, 1985.

15. Black, P. McL., Tzouras, A., and Foley, L.: Cerebrospinal fluid dynamics and hydrocephalus after experimental subarachnoid hemorrhage. Neurosurgery, 17:55–62, 1985.

16. Black, P. McL., Hakim, R., and Olsen-Bailey, N.: The use of the Codman-Medos Programmable Hakim Valve in the management of patients with hydrocephalus: Illustrative cases. Neurosurgery, 34:1110–1113, 1994.

17. Borgesen, S. E., and Gjerris, F.: The predictive value of conductance to outflow of cerebrospinal fluid in normal-pressure hydrocephalus. Brain, 105:65–86, 1982.

18. Borgesen, S. E., Gjerris, F., and Sorensen, S. C.: The resistance to cerebrospinal fluid absorption in humans: A method of evaluation by lumboventricular perfusion, with particular reference to normal-pressure hydrocephalus. Acta Neurol. Scand., 57:88–96, 1978.

19. Borgesen, S. E., Gjerris, F., and Sorensen, S. C.: Intracranial pressure and conductance to outflow of cerebrospinal fluid in normal-pressure hydrocephalus. J. Neurosurg., 50:489–493, 1979.

20. Borgesen, S. E., Gjerris, F., and Sorensen, S. C.: Cerebrospinal fluid conductance and compliance of the craniospinal space in normal-pressure hydrocephalus. J. Neurosurg., 51:521–525, 1979.

21. Borgesen, S. E., Westergard, L., and Gjerris, F.: Isotope cisternography and conductance to outflow of cerebrospinal fluid in normal-pressure hydrocephalus. Acta Neurochir. (Wien), 57:67–73, 1981.

22. Bradley, W. C., Whittemore, A. R., Kortman, K. E., et al.: Marked cerebrospinal fluid void: Indicator of successful shunt in patients with suspected normal-pressure hydrocephalus. Radiology, 178:459–466, 1991.

23. Bret, P., and Chazal, J.: L'Hydrocéphalie chronique de l'adulte. Neurochirurgie, 36(Suppl. 1):1–159, 1990.

24. Casmiro, M., D'Alessandro, R., Cacciatore, F. M., et al.: Risk factors for the syndrome of ventricular enlargement with gait apraxia (idiopathic normal-pressure hydrocephalus): A case-control study. J. Neurol. Neurosurg. Psychiatry, 52:847–852, 1989.

25. Chapman, P. H., Cosman, E. R., and Arnold, M. A.: The relationship between ventricular fluid pressure and body position in normal subjects and subjects with shunts: A telemetric study. Neurosurgery, 26:181–189, 1990.

26. Chapman, P. H., Cosman, E. R., Zervas, N. T., et al.: A telemetric pressure sensor for ventricular shunt systems. Surg. Neurol., 11:287–294, 1979.

27. Chawla, J. C., and Woodward, J.: Motor disorder in "normal-pressure hydrocephalus." Br. Med. J., 1:485–486, 1972.

28. Chawla, J. C., Hulme, A., and Cooper, R.: Intracranial pressure in patients with dementia and communicating hydrocephalus. J. Neurosurg., 40:376–380, 1974.

29. Condon, B., Patterson, J., Wyper, D., et al.: Use of magnetic resonance imaging to measure intracranial cerebrospinal fluid volume. Lancet, 1:1355–1357, 1986.

30. Connor, E. S., Black, P. McL., and Foley, L.: Experimental normal-pressure hydrocephalus is accompanied by increased transmantle pressure. J. Neurosurg., 61:322–328, 1984.

31. Crockard, H. A., Hanlon, K., Duda, E. E., et al.: Hydrocephalus as a cause of dementia: Evaluation by computerized tomography and intracranial pressure monitoring. J. Neurol. Neurosurg. Psychiatry, 40:736–740, 1977.

32. DeLand, F. H., James, A. E., Jr., Ladd, D. J., et al.: Normal-pressure hydrocephalus: A histologic study. Am. J. Clin. Pathol., 58:58–63, 1972.

33. DiRocco, C., Petterossi, V. C., Caldarelli, M., et al.: Communicating hydrocephalus induced by mechanically increased amplitude of the intraventricular cerebrospinal fluid pressure: Experimental studies. Exp. Neurol., 59:40–52, 1978.

34. Drayer, B. P., and Rosenbaum, A. E.: Dynamics of cerebrospinal fluid system as defined by cranial computed tomography. *In* Wood, J. H., ed.: Neurobiology of Cerebrospinal Fluid. Vol. 1. New York, Plenum Press, 1980.

35. Earnest, M. P., Fahn, S., Karp, J. H., et al.: Normal-pressure hydrocephalus and hypertensive cerebrovascular disease. Arch. Neurol., 31:262–266, 1974.

36. Elble, R. J., Hughes, L., and Higgins, C.: The syndrome of senile gait. J. Neurol., 23:71–75, 1992.

37. Epstein, C. M.: The distribution of intracranial forces in acute and chronic hydrocephalus. J. Neurol. Sci., 21:171–180, 1974.

38. Fisher, C. M.: The clinical picture in occult hydrocephalus. Clin. Neurosurg., 24:270–284, 1977.

39. Fisher, C. M.: Hydrocephalus as a cause of disturbance of gait in the elderly. Neurology, 32:1358–1363, 1982.

40. Fishman, R. A.: Occult hydrocephalus [Letter]. N. Engl. J. Med., 27:466–467, 1966.

41. Fleming, I. F. R., Shepard, R. H., and Turner, V.: Cerebrospinal fluid scanning in the evaluation of hydrocephalus: A clinical review of 100 patients. *In* Cisternography and Hydrocephalus: A Symposium. Springfield, IL, Charles C Thomas, 1972.

42. Foltz, E. L., and Aine, C.: Diagnosis of hydrocephalus by cerebrospinal fluid pulse-wave analysis: A clinical study. Surg. Neurol., 15:283–293, 1980.

43. Fox, J. L., McCullough, D. C., and Green, R. C.: Effect of cerebrospinal fluid shunts on intracranial pressure and on cerebrospinal fluid dynamics—a new technique of pressure management: Results and concepts—a concept of hydrocephalus. J. Neurol. Neurosurg. Psychiatry, 36:302–312, 1973.

44. Friedland, R. P.: "Normal"-pressure hydrocephalus and the saga of the treatable dementias [Clinical conference]. J.A.M.A., 262:2577–2581, 1989.

45. Gleason, P. L., Black, P. McL., and Matsumae, M.: The neurobiology of normal-pressure hydrocephalus. Neurosurg. Clin. North Am., 4(4):667–675, 1993.

46. Graff-Radford, N. R., and Godersky, J. C.: Normal-pressure hydrocephalus: Onset of gait abnormality before dementia predicts good surgical outcome. Ann. Neurol., 43:940–942, 1980.

47. Grubb, R. L., Raichle, M. E., Gado, M. H., et al.: Cerebral blood flow, oxygen utilization, and blood volume in dementia. Neurology, 27:905–910, 1977.

48. Guidetti, B., and Gagliardi, F. M.: Normal-pressure hydrocephalus. Acta Neurochir. (Wien), 27:1–9, 1972.

49. Haan, J., and Thomeer, R. T. W. M.: Predictive value of temporary external lumbar drainage in normal-pressure hydrocephalus. Neurosurgery, 22:388–391, 1988.

50. Haidri, N. H., and Modi, S. M.: Normal-pressure hydrocephalus and hypertensive cerebrovascular disease. Dis. Nerv. Syst., 38:918–921, 1977.

51. Hakim, C.: The physics and physiopathology of the hydraulic complex of the central nervous system: The mechanics of hydrocephalus and normal-pressure hydrocephalus. Unpublished dissertation. Cambridge, Massachusetts Institute of Technology, 1985.

52. Hakim, S.: Some observations on cerebrospinal fluid pressure hydrocephalic syndrome in adults with "normal" cerebrospinal fluid pressure: Recognition of a new syndrome. [English translation]. Bogota, Columbia, Javeriana University School of Medicine, 1964.

53. Hakim, S.: Hydraulic and mechanical mis-matching of valve shunts used in treatment of hydrocephalus: The need for a servo-valve shunt. Dev. Med. Child Neurol., 15:646–653, 1973.

54. Hakim, S., and Adams, R. D.: The special clinical problem of symptomatic hydrocephalus with normal cerebrospinal fluid pressure: Observations on cerebrospinal fluid pressure; observations on cerebrospinal fluid hydrodynamics. J. Neurol. Sci., 2:307–327, 1965.

55. Hakim, S., Venegas, J. G., and Burton, J. D.: The physics of the cranial cavity, hydrocephalus, and normal-pressure hydrocephalus: Mechanical interpretation and mathematical model. Surg. Neurol., 5:187–210, 1976.

56. Hartman, A., and Alberti, E.: Differentiation of communicating hydrocephalus and presenile dementia by continuous recording of cerebrospinal fluid pressure. J. Neurol. Neurosurg. Psychiatry, 40:630–640, 1977.

57. Heinz, E. R., David, D. O., and Karp, H. R.: Abnormal isotope cisternography in symptomatic occult hydrocephalus: A correla-

tive isotopic-neuro-radiological study in 130 subjects. Radiology, 95:109–120, 1970.

58. Hirtasuka, H., Tabata, H., Tsuruoka, S., et al.: Evaluation of periventricular hypodensity in experimental hydrocephalus by metrizamide computed tomographic ventriculography. J. Neurosurg., 56:235–240, 1982.

59. Hoff, J., and Barber, R.: Transcerebral mantle pressure in normal-pressure hydrocephalus. Arch. Neurol., 31:101–105, 1974.

60. Hughes, C. P., Siegel, B. A., Coxe, W. S., et al.: Adult idiopathic communicating hydrocephalus with and without shunting. J. Neurol. Neurosurg. Psychiatry, 41:961–971, 1978.

61. Hussey, F., Schanzer, B., and Katzman, R.: A simple constant fusion manometric test for measurement of cerebrospinal fluid absorption: II. Clinical studies. Neurology, 20:665–680, 1970.

62. Illingworth, R. D.: Subdural hematoma after treatment of chronic hydrocephalus by ventriculo-caval shunts. J. Neurol. Neurosurg. Psychiatry, 33:95–99, 1970.

63. Illingworth, R. D., Logue, V., Symon, L., et al.: The ventriculo-caval shunt in the treatment of adult hydrocephalus: Results and complications in 101 patients. J. Neurosurg., 35:681–685, 1971.

64. Ingvar, D. H., and Gustafson, L.: Regional cerebral blood flow in organic dementia with early onset. Acta Neurol. Scand., 46(Suppl. 43):42–73, 1971.

65. Jacobs, L., and Kinkel, W.: Computerized axial transverse tomography in normal-pressure hydrocephalus. Neurology, 26:501–507, 1976.

66. Jacobs, L., Conti, D., and Kinkel, W. R.: "Normal"-pressure hydrocephalus: Relationships of clinical and radiographic findings to improvement following shunt surgery. J.A.M.A. 235:510–512, 1976.

67. Jagust, W. L., Freidland, R. P., and Budinger, T. F.: Positron emission tomography with ^{18}F-fluorodeoxyglucose differentiates normal-pressure hydrocephalus from Alzheimer dementia. J. Neurol. Neurosurg. Psychiatry, 48:1091–1096, 1985.

68. James, A. E., Jr., DeLand, F. H., Hodges, F. J., III, et al.: Normal-pressure hydrocephalus: Role of cisternography in diagnosis. J.A.M.A., 213:1615–1622, 1970.

69. Katzman, R.: Low-pressure hydrocephalus. In Wells, C. E., ed.: Dementia. Philadelphia, F. A. Davis, 1977.

70. Kaye, J. A., Grady, C., Haxby, J. V., et al.: Plasticity in the aging brain: Reversibility of anatomic, metabolic, and cognitive deficits in normal-pressure hydrocephalus following shunt surgery. Arch. Neurol., 47:1226–1341, 1990.

71. Knutsson, E., and Lying-Tunnel, U.: Gait apraxia in normal-pressure hydrocephalus: Patterns of movement and muscle activation. Neurology, 35:155–160, 1985.

72. Koller, W. C., Glatt, S. C., and Wilson, R. S.: Senile gait: Correlation with computed tomographic scans. Ann. Neurol., 12:87, 1982.

73. Kosteljanitz, M., and Ingstrup, H. M.: Normal-pressure hydrocephalus: Correlation between computed tomography and measurements of cerebrospinal fluid dynamics. Acta Neurochir. (Wien), 77:8–13, 1985.

74. Kosteljanitz, M., Nehen, A. M., and Kaaland, J.: Cerebrospinal fluid outflow resistance measurements in the selection of patients for shunt surgery in the normal-pressure hydrocephalus syndrome: A controlled trial. Acta Neurochir. (Wien), 104:48–53, 1990.

75. Koto, A., Rosenberg, G., Zingesser, L. H., et al.: Syndrome of normal-pressure hydrocephalus: Possible relation to hypertensive and arteriosclerotic vasculopathy. J. Neurol. Neurosurg. Psychiatry, 40:73–79, 1977.

76. Lamas, E., and Lobato, R. O.: Intraventricular pressure and cerebrospinal fluid dynamics in chronic adult hydrocephalus. Surg. Neurol., 12:287–295, 1977.

77. Larsson, A., Wikkelso, C., Bilting, M., et al.: Clinical parameters in 74 consecutive patients shunt-operated for normal-pressure hydrocephalus. Acta Neurol. Scand., 84:475–482, 1991.

78. Laws, E. R., Jr., and Mokri, B.: Occult hydrocephalus: Results of shunting correlated with diagnostic tests. Clin. Neurosurg., 24:316–333, 1977.

79. Lewin, W.: Preliminary observations on external hydrocephalus after severe head injury. Br. J. Surg., 55:747–751, 1969.

80. Longstreth, W. T. J. R., Nelson, L. M., Koepsell, T. D., et al.: Clinical course of spontaneous subarachnoid hemorrhage: A population-based study in King County, Washington. Neurology, 43:712–718, 1993.

81. Martin, B. J., Roberts, M. A., and Turner, J. W.: Normal-pressure hydrocephalus and Paget's disease of bone. Gerontology, 31:397–402, 1985.

82. Mascalchi, M., Arnetoli, G., Inzitari, D., et al.: Cine-MR imaging of aqueductal CSF flow in normal-pressure hydrocephalus syndrome before and after CSF shunt. Acta Radiol., 34:586–592, 1973.

83. Mathew, N. T., Meyer, J. S., Hartman, A., et al.: Abnormal cerebrospinal fluid–blood flow dynamics: Implications in diagnosis, treatment, and prognosis in normal-pressure hydrocephalus. Arch. Neurol., 32:657–664, 1975.

84. McComb, J. G.: Recent research into the nature of cerebrospinal fluid formation and absorption. J. Neurosurg., 59:369–383, 1983.

85. McCullough, D. C., and Fox, J. L.: Negative intracranial pressure in adults with shunts and its relationship to the production of subdural hematoma. J. Neurosurg., 40:372–375, 1974.

86. McLaurin, R. L.: On the use of precraniotomy shunting in the management of posterior fossa tumors in children: A cooperative study. Concepts Pediatr. Neurosurg., 6:1–5, 1985.

87. McQuarrie, I. G., Saint-Louis, L., and Scherer, P. B.: Treatment of normal-pressure hydrocephalus with low versus medium pressure cerebrospinal fluid shunt. Neurosurgery, 15:484–488, 1984.

88. Messert, B., and Wannamaker, B. B.: Reappraisal of the adult occult hydrocephalus syndrome. Neurology, 24:224–231, 1974.

89. Meyer, J. S., Kitagaura, Y., Tanabashi, N., et al.: Evaluation of treatment of normal-pressure hydrocephalus. J. Neurosurg., 62:513–521, 1985.

90. Meyer, J. S., Kitagaura, Y., Tanabashi, N., et al.: Pathogenesis of normal-pressure hydrocephalus: Preliminary observations. Surg. Neurol., 23:121–133, 1985.

91. Michelson, W. J., Schlesinger, E. B., and Bailey, S.: Factors involved in surgical management of normal-pressure hydrocephalus. Acta Radiol. Diagn., 13:570–574, 1972.

92. Mori, K., Murata, T., Nakano, Y., et al.: Periventricular lucency in hydrocephalus on computerized tomography. Surg. Neurol., 8:337–340, 1977.

93. Mosely, I. F., and Radu, W. E.: Factors influencing the development of periventricular lucencies in patients with raised intracranial pressure. Neuroradiology, 17:65–69, 1979.

94. Nelson, J. R., and Goodman, S. J.: An evaluation of the cerebrospinal fluid infusion test for hydrocephalus. Neurology, 21:1037–1053, 1971.

95. Noda, S., Fujita, K., Kusunoki, T., et al.: Hypertensive vasculopathy as a causative factor of normal-pressure hydrocephalus: A clinical analysis. No Shinkei Geka, 9:1033–1039, 1981.

96. Nornes, H., Rootwelt, I. S., and Sjaastad, O.: Normal-pressure hydrocephalus. Eur. Neurol., 1:261–274, 1973.

97. Ojemann, R. G.: Initial experience with the Hakim valve for ventriculovenous shunting: Technical note. J. Neurosurg., 28:283–287, 1968.

98. Ojemann, R. G.: Normal-pressure hydrocephalus. Clin. Neurosurg., 18:337–370, 1971.

99. Ojemann, R. G.: Normal-pressure hydrocephalus. In Critchley, M., O'Leary, J. L., and Jennett, B., eds.: Scientific Foundations of Neurology. Philadelphia, F. A. Davis, 1972, pp. 302–308.

100. Ojemann, R. G., and Black, P. McL.: Evaluation of the patient with dementia and treatment of normal-pressure hydrocephalus. In Wilkins, R. H., and Rangachary, S. S., eds.: Neurosurgery. New York, McGraw-Hill, 1984, pp. 312–321.

101. Ojemann, R. G., Fisher, C. M., Adams, R. D., et al.: Further experience with the syndrome of "normal"-pressure hydrocephalus. J. Neurosurg., 31:279–294, 1969.

102. Penry, R. K., Berger, A., and Gorss, E.: Familial occurrence of normal-pressure hydrocephalus. Arch. Neurol., 41:335–337, 1984.

103. Petersen, R. C., Mokri, B., and Laws, E. R., Jr.: Response to shunting procedure in idiopathic normal-pressure hydrocephalus. Ann. Neurol., 12:99, 1982.

104. Philippon, J., Ancri, D., and Pertuiset, B.: Hydrocephalie a pression normal (enregistrement de la pression etude radiologique, transit isotopique). Rev. Neurol. (Paris), 125:347–358, 1971.

105. Pickard, J. D.: Adult communicating hydrocephalus. Br. J. Hosp. Med., 27:35–44, 1982.

106. Puca, A., Anile, C., Maira, G., et al.: Cerebrospinal fluid shunting for hydrocephalus in the adult: Factors related to shunt revision. Neurosurgery, 29:822–826, 1991.

107. Ribadeau-Dumas, J. L., Ricou, P., Verdure, L., et al.: Etude anatomique d'un cas d'hydrocephalie a pression normale. Neurochirurgie, 22:138–145, 1976.

108. Rossi, G. F., Galli, G., DiRocco, C., et al.: Normotensive hydrocephalus: The relations of pneumoencephalography and isotope cisternography to the results of surgical treatment. Acta Neurochir. (Wien), 30:69–83, 1974.

109. Salmon, J. H.: Senile dementia: Ventriculo-atrial shunt for symptomatic treatment. Geriatrics, 24:67–72, 1969.

110. Salmon, J. H.: Adult hydrocephalus: Evaluation of shunt therapy in 80 patients. J. Neurosurg., 37:423–428, 1972.

111. Salmon, J. H., and Armitage, T. L.: Surgical treatment of hydrocephalus ex-vacuo: Ventriculo-atrial shunt for degenerative brain disease. Neurology, 18:1223–1226, 1968.

112. Schmitt, J., and Spring, A.: Die Therapie des Normaldruck Hydrocephalus mit dem transcutan magnetisch versteelbaren Ventil. Neurochirurgia (Stuttgart), 33(Suppl. 1):23–26, 1990.

113. Shenkin, H. A., Greenberg, J. O., and Grossman, C. B.: Ventricular size after shunting for idiopathic normal-pressure hydrocephalus. J. Neurol. Neurosurg. Psychiatry, 38:833–837, 1975.

114. Sindou, M., Guyotat-Pelissou, I., Chidiac, A., et al.: Transcutaneous pressure adjustable valve for the treatment of hydrocephalus and arachnoid cysts in adults: Experiences with 75 cases. Acta Neurochir. (Wien), 121:135–139, 1993.

115. Sklar, F. H., Beyer, C. W., Jr., Ramanathas, M., et al.: Servocontrolled lumbar infusions: A clinical tool for the determination of cerebrospinal fluid dynamics as a function of pressure. Neurosurgery, 3:170–175, 1978.

116. Sklar, F. H., Diche, J. T., Beyer, C. W., et al.: Brain elasticity changes with ventriculomegaly. J. Neurosurg., 53:173–179, 1980.

117. Sorensen, P. S., Gjerris, F., Ibsaur, S., et al.: Low cerebrospinal fluid concentration of brain-specific protein D_2 in patients with normal-pressure hydrocephalus. J. Neurol. Sci., 62:59–65, 1983.

118. Sorensen, P. S., Hammer, M., Vorstrup, S., et al.: Cerebrospinal fluid and plasma vasopressin concentration in dementia. J. Neurol. Neurosurg. Psychiatry, 46:911–916, 1983.

119. Spelberg-Sorensen, R., Jansen, E. L., and Gjerris, F.: Motor disturbance in normal-pressure hydrocephalus: Special reference to stance and gait. Arch. Neurol., 43:34–38, 1986.

120. Stein, S. C., and Langfitt, T. W.: Normal-pressure hydrocephalus: Predicting the results of cerebrospinal fluid shunting. J. Neurosurg., 41:463–470, 1974.

121. Sudarski, L., and Ronthal, M.: Gait disorders among elderly patients. Arch. Neurol., 40:740–743, 1983.

122. Symon, L., and Dorsch, N. W. C.: Use of long-term intracranial pressure measurement to assess hydrocephalic patients prior to shunt surgery. J. Neurosurg., 42:258–273, 1975.

123. Symon, L., and Hinzpeter, T.: The enigma of normal-pressure hydrocephalus: Tests to select patients for surgery and to predict shunt function. Clin. Neurosurg., 24:285–315, 1977.

124. Symon, L., Dorsch, N. W. C., and Stephens, R. J.: Pressure waves in so-called low-pressure hydrocephalus. Lancet, 2:1291–1292, 1972.

125. Sypert, G. W., Leffman, H., and Ojemann, G. A.: Occult normal-pressure hydrocephalus manifested by Parkinsonism-dementia complex. Neurology, 23:234–238, 1973.

126. Tamaki, N., Kusunoki, T., Wakabayashi, T., et al.: Cerebral hemodynamics in normal-pressure hydrocephalus: Evaluation by ^{133}Xe inhalation and dynamic computed tomographic study. J. Neurosurg., 61:510–515, 1984.

127. Tator, C. H., and Murray, S. A.: A clinical, pneumoencephalographic and radio-isotope study of normal-pressure communicating hydrocephalus. Can. Med. Assoc. J., 105:573–579, 1971.

128. Udvarhely, G. B., Wood, J. H., James, A. E., Jr., et al.: Results and complications in 55 shunted patients with normal-pressure hydrocephalus. Surg. Neurol., 3:271–275, 1975.

129. Vanneste, J., Augustijn, P., Davies, F. Z., et al.: Normal-pressure hydrocephalus: Is cisternography useful in selecting patients for a shunt? Arch. Neurol., 49:366–370, 1992.

130. Vanneste, J., Augustijn, P., Dirven, C., et al.: Shunting normal-pressure hydrocephalus: Do the benefits outweigh the risks? A multicenter study and literature review. Neurology, 42:54–59, 1992.

131. Vassilouthis, J.: The syndrome of normal-pressure hydrocephalus. J. Neurosurg., 61:501–509, 1984.

132. Waldemar, G., Schmidt, J. F., Delecluse, F., et al.: High-resolution SPECT with [^{99m}Tc]-d, 1-HMPAO in normal-pressure hydrocephalus before and after shunt operation. J. Neurol. Neurosurg. Psychiatry, 56:655–664, 1993.

133. Wikkelso, C., Andersson, H., and Blomstrand, C.: The clinical effect of lumbar puncture in normal-pressure hydrocephalus. J. Neurol. Neurosurg. Psychiatry, 45:64–69, 1982.

134. Wikkelso, C., Andersson, H., Blomstrand, C., et al.: Computed tomography of the brain in the diagnosis of and prognosis in normal-pressure hydrocephalus. Neuroradiology, 31:160–165, 1989.

135. Wikkelso, C., Ekman, R., Westergren, I. K., et al.: Neuropeptides in cerebrospinal fluid in normal-pressure hydrocephalus and dementia. Eur. Neurol., 31:88–93, 1991.

136. Wolinsky, J. S., Barnes, B. D., and Margolis, M. T.: Diagnostic tests in normal-pressure hydrocephalus. Neurology, 23:706–713, 1973.

CHAPTER 38

Infections of Cerebrospinal Shunts

The infection of cerebrospinal fluid shunts is a common complication that has tainted the considerable success attained in treating hydrocephalus. Hydrocephalus of a variety of causes affects 1 in 1,000 children.[49] If untreated, 50 to 60 per cent of children with hydrocephalus die, and the majority of the remainder have retardation or suffer from the disfigurement of macrocephaly.[49, 74] The initial difficulties and flaws in shunt design encountered during the 1940's and 1950's have been overcome, and shunts have become the mainstay of treatment for these patients. Most children with hydrocephalus now survive to adulthood and lead normal, productive lives. Infections are the second most common problem interfering with this successful outcome (Fig. 38–1). Patients whose shunts have become infected have been shown to have double the mortality and threefold number of shunt-related operations as do patients with shunts who do not sustain a shunt infection.[111, 125, 128] The mortality from shunt infection–related ventriculitis is between 30 and 40 per cent.[27, 83, 90] Furthermore, shunt infections account for the greatest morbidity associated with cerebrospinal fluid infection in the pediatric patients.[123] Some reports indicate that, even when infections are successfully treated, long-term morbidity includes seizures, cognitive deficiencies, and psychomotor retardation.[27, 85, 127]

Many studies of shunt infections have been characterized by methodological flaws, and, although important progress has been made, the prevention of shunt infection remains largely an unsolved problem. The basic mechanisms of pathogenesis are incompletely understood, although what has been learned has yielded important and useful strategies for intervention in the prevention and treatment of shunt infection. Controversy abounds over the best methods of infection prevention and treatment. Clinically, however, there is little doubt that shunt infections are difficult to treat and require prolonged hospitalization and additional invasive procedures for the patient with a shunt.

TERMINOLOGY

Shunt infections can be broadly classified into "internal" and "external" infections. Although this terminology is somewhat antiquated, it is useful in defining two different clinical syndromes that arise as a result of shunt infection. Internal infection refers to an infection of the luminal surface of the shunt catheter, the valve, or the reservoir (or any combination of these). These are the so-called "true" shunt infections that are associated with increased morbidity and mortality because of the frequency of associated ventriculitis. The clinical syndrome is dependent on the severity of the infection, the infecting organism, and the type of shunt. By contrast, external shunt infection refers to an infection of the adluminal surface of the shunt and the subcutaneous tract through which it passes. Typically, these are clinically manifest as foreign body infections and tend to be more self-limited and associated with lower morbidity because the cerebrospinal fluid is not involved. Often, an associated lesion in the skin appears adjacent to the shunt tract and presages the occurrence of external infection.

EPIDEMIOLOGY AND RISK FACTORS

Reported rates of infection range from 2 to 39 per cent; however, a trend toward somewhat lower rates has been observed, such that most recent series report a 5 to 10 per cent infection rate.[51, 70, 100, 102, 131] The exact reason for the improvement over the past 20 years is not known, although an attractive hypothesis includes

Jeffrey P. Blount's research is supported by the Peyton Society and NIH in-training grant 1-T32-NSO7361.

J. P. Blount • S. J. Haines

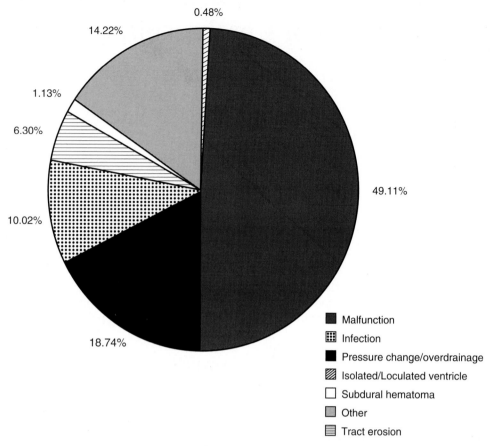

Figure 38–1

Indication for shunt revision for a series of 619 shunt revisions performed at the University of Minnesota Hospital and Clinic/Variety Club Children's Hospital. Data are based on a retrospective review of 989 cerebrospinal fluid diversion procedures performed on 450 patients seen at the University of Minnesota between June 1, 1982, and June 1, 1992. There were 370 first shunts placed and 619 revisions or adaptations.

closer attention to surgical technique, improved prophylactic antibiotics, and a trend toward an increase in the number of shunt surgeries being performed at large specialized centers that accumulate considerable experience with the placement and revision of shunts.

An important consideration in any discussion of infection rate concerns the determination of what individuals constitute the numerator and denominator.[43] For example, the numerator may represent the number of infected patients or infected shunts, whereas the denominator can reflect the total number of patients, the total number of shunts placed, or the total number of procedures.[43] Markedly different results can be produced, and the surgeon must be careful to understand the relevant terminology when making comparisons.

The highest incidence of wound infection is found in the youngest patients.[27, 96, 114, 125] Pople and co-workers found that patients who received shunts at an age of less than 6 months experienced a 15.7 per cent rate of infection, whereas those who received shunts at an age of 6 months or more showed a 5.6 per cent rate of infection.[95] Likewise, George and associates demonstrated a 13.6 per cent rate of infection for patients younger than 4 years of age. This rate was decreased to 6.8 per cent for patients between the ages of 4 and 61 years.[51] Interestingly, they found that the rate of

infection was also elevated in patients older than 61 years of age (16.7 per cent).[51] Initially, the proposed reason for a higher rate of infection in the young was immunological immaturity. Renier and colleagues have observed that the period between the first 2 and 6 months of life, which corresponds with a period of lowered serum immunoglobulin (IgG) levels, is when neonates are particularly susceptible to shunt infection.[102] Pople and co-workers counter this claim with the observation that levels of maternal antibody are high in the neonate, and they further attest to cases of shunt infection in which serum levels of antibody specific for the infecting organism were high.[95] They claim instead that qualitative and quantitative differences in the microbial flora of the neonate account for the elevated risk of infection.[95] Aerobic *Staphylococcus* species and *Propionibacterium acnes* are found in greater density on the face and head in childhood than in adulthood.[26] It has also been observed that there is a greater density of both aerobic staphylococci and anaerobic diphtheroids on the head and neck than on the trunk or limbs.[26] D'Angio and co-workers demonstrated a high incidence of a single biotype of *Staphylococcus epidermidis* on neonates in an intensive care setting and concluded that hospitalized neonates frequently become rapidly colonized by a single highly resistant strain.[36]

Shapiro and associates also noted a greater incidence of infection in younger patients, although they did not attribute this to skin flora.[114] Only 20 per cent of the shunt infections in their series of 413 patients were caused by the same strains of bacteria as those cultured from the skin preoperatively. The relationship between the cause of hydrocephalus and the subsequent risk of shunt infection is less clear. Some authors have suggested that patients with spinal dysraphism show greater rates of shunt infection.[62, 82] McCullough and colleagues report that the infection rate in patients with spina bifida was twice that for those with hydrocephalus from other causes, but they note that this difference was not statistically significant.[82] Several other studies have shown no correlation between infection rates and the cause of hydrocephalus.[51, 70, 114, 129]

The correlation between the rate of infection and whether a shunt is an initial shunt or revision is also controversial. Renier and colleagues claim a statistically significant reduction in the rate of infection between primary shunt insertion (8.4 per cent), revisions for obstruction (5 per cent), and revisions following removal for infection (17.5 per cent).[102] Other investigators have also noted higher rates of infection for shunt revisions.[51] By contrast, many authors have observed no significant differences.[42, 125]

Similarly, the correlation with the type of shunt is controversial. In an early report, Little and Rhoton showed that 24 per cent of patients with ventriculoatrial shunts became infected, whereas only 11 per cent of patients with ventriculoperitoneal shunts became infected.[77] Ignelzi and Kirsch also demonstrated a similar trend.[65] However, as pointed out by Fan-Havard and Nahata, these investigators failed to control for the larger number of patients undergoing ventriculoatrial shunt placement than ventriculoperitoneal placement.[43] Significant differences are not realized when the incidence of infection is compared. Studies by several other groups have demonstrated no difference in rates of infection between the types of shunts.[51, 70, 111]

Several other factors have been suggested as risk factors for shunt infection (Table 38–1). Of particular note is poor skin condition or skin infection, which has been found to be highly associated with shunt infection in several studies.[95, 102] One study demonstrated that patients with dermatitis or eschar on the scalp showed an infection rate of 13 per cent, whereas those without these lesions had a 3.8 per cent incidence of infection.[102]

Anatomy and Physiology

PATHOPHYSIOLOGY

The fundamental pathophysiological mechanisms involved in cerebrospinal fluid shunt infection can be broadly categorized into bacterial mechanisms and host-shunt–related mechanisms.

Bacterial Mechanisms

Mechanisms of Bacterial Adhesion

The adherence of microorganisms to foreign bodies or tissue substratum is a complex process that is dependent on the interaction of multiple sets of opposing forces. The principal factors involved in the initial attachment of bacteria include the basic physicochemical forces of the molecules, specific bacteria-mediated attachment functions, and host-derived proteoglycan films that coat the foreign body and function as receptors for bacteria.[34, 38] Irreversible adhesion is dependent on synthetic biochemical reactions that are time-dependent and organism-specific.[53]

The molecular structure of all particles confers certain electrochemical forces to the particles. The electrostatic forces vary, depending on the composition of the particles, but most bacterial cells are negatively charged.[38] Substrata and polymers are also normally negatively charged; however, this can be altered by pH or tissue damage that results from surgery, trauma, or infection.[38, 53] Initial adherence requires that the repulsion of like-charged surfaces must be overcome. Electromagnetic forces generated by atomic and molecular vibrations of similar frequencies between molecules are termed "Van der Waals forces."[53] Their degree of attraction or repulsion is in part determined by the distance between the objects. At the secondary minimum (a distance of approximately 10 nm), the force is

Table 38–1
RISK FACTORS FOR SHUNT INFECTION

Factor	References
Young age	51, 96, 102
Infection, disruption, or poor condition of skin	43, 90, 95, 102
Concomitant systemic infection at time of shunting	30, 102
Postoperative wound dehiscence	102
Prolonged operating time	46
Limited surgeon experience with cerebrospinal fluid shunts	30, 91, 123
Cause of hydrocephalus (myelomeningocele > others)	51, 62, 70, 82, 114, 129
Shunt revision (versus initial shunt)	51, 102, 125
Ventriculoatrial versus ventriculoperitoneal shunt	51, 65, 70, 77, 111
Shunt surgery done late in day	30, 123
Increased number of people in operating room	58
Ventricular catheter revision	102

attractive but becomes increasingly repulsive as particles are brought closer together until the primary minimum is reached; at this point, the force becomes attractive once again (Fig. 38–2).[53]

Hydrophobic forces are considerably stronger than Van der Waals forces and act over distances of 10 to 20 nm.[98] These forces arise from the change in free energy resulting from the direct interaction of particles of differing hydrophobicity. Hydrophobic properties of polymers are important determinants of the binding affinity of the coagulase-negative staphylococci.[53] Adhesins (or lectins) are bacterial cell surface markers that bind to specific receptors on substrate surfaces, increasing the binding affinity of the bacteria.[38, 98] Often, adhesins are located on the distal end of fimbriae, which are filamentous structures that extend from the bacterial cell surface and function primarily in cell adhesion.[38]

When a foreign body is implanted, it is rapidly covered with a film of soluble connective tissue containing fibronectin, fibrinogen, or collagen, or other proteins.[53, 98] Glycoprotein coverings may play an important role in bacterial adhesion because some contain distinct binding sites for bacteria. For example, fibronectin binds *S. epidermidis* and *S. aureus* at specific binding sites.[53] Such proteins may modulate the binding capacity of microorganisms.[98]

Once irreversible binding has occurred, a metabolic microclimate termed the "microzone" may form at the interface of the bacteria and colonized surface. Within the microzone, host factors that are antagonistic to bacterial proliferation are excluded, and bacterial aggregation and proliferation occur.[53] An important event within the microzone is the sequestration of iron within the microzone via the exclusion of host proteins that normally lower iron concentrations below levels needed by pathogenic bacteria.[53] Bacterial aggregation may then continue until the colonized surface area reaches its carrying maximum, at which time aggregation factors decrease and colonies become subject to shear forces and demonstrate dispersion.[53] The cycle then may repeat itself as individual bacterial colonies encounter additional foreign material and as colonization continues to spread.

Bacteriology of Shunt Infection

An understanding of bacterial mechanisms in shunt infections arises from an understanding of the bacteriology of shunt infection. Shunt infections are dominated by organisms of low virulence. *S. epidermidis* (formerly *S. albus*) is the most common pathogen and accounts for 50 to 75 per cent of shunt infections in virtually all series (Table 38–2).* The next most frequently encountered organisms include *S. aureus*, the gram-negative bacilli, and the anaerobic diphtheroids (e.g., *P. acnes*).[43, 49, 70, 90] Some of these organisms demonstrate unique features that appear to facilitate the colonization and subsequent infection of a shunt.

The initial event in any foreign body infection is exposure of the foreign body to the infecting organism, with the subsequent colonization of the foreign body. Two early observations provided initial insight into one mechanism by which bacteria gain access to an

*See references 47, 49, 65, 70, 84, 90, and 111.

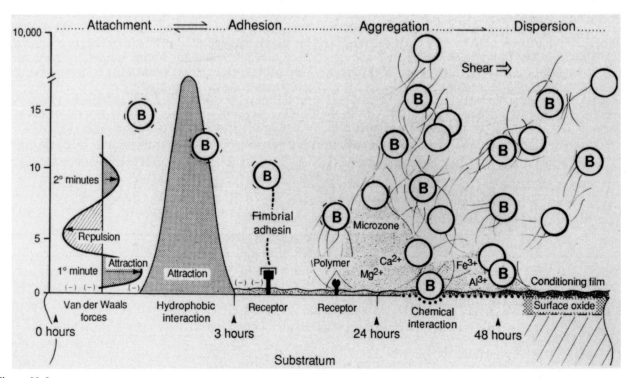

Figure 38–2

Molecular sequences in bacterial adhesion to foreign body. (From Gristina, A. G.: Biomaterial-centered infection: Microbial adhesion versus tissue integration. Science, 237:1588–1595, 1987. Copyright 1987 by the AAAS. Reprinted by permission.)

Table 38–2

COMMON ORGANISMS IN SHUNT INFECTION*

Pathogen	Percentage of Total Infections	References
Staphylococcus epidermidis	89	65
	55–62	47, 70, 86, 111, 114
	39–48	91, 102, 127
Staphylococcus aureus	20–28	47, 91, 102, 111, 127
Propionibacterium acnes (includes diphtheroids and *Corynebacterium* species)	55	101
	14	47
	5	114
	4	86
	1	111
Gram-negative bacilli	44	127
	15–22	47, 86, 91, 102, 114
Streptococci	4–12	47, 102, 111, 127
Candida species	3	47

*Referenced studies are published primary retrospective clinical cerebrospinal fluid shunt series that quantify bacteriological profile.

implanted shunt. First, it was noted that *S. epidermidis* and other skin commensals make up a great percentage of shunt infections.[61, 62] It was further noted that 70 per cent of shunt infections occur within 2 months of implantation.[49, 51, 70, 111] This suggested that skin commensal organisms were colonizing and infecting the shunt following their introduction into the wound at the time of surgery. Bayston and Lari demonstrated that organisms isolated from shunt infections were often present on the skin surface, nose, or ears of the patient before surgery.[14] Fifty-eight per cent of the wounds sampled before final closing were found to contain organisms that were earlier cultured from the skin.[14] These observations were later extended when it was shown that bacterial density on the skin adjacent to the wound significantly correlated with the incidence of infection.[95]

The mechanisms by which bacteria gain access to shunts are outlined in Table 38–3 and discussed later in this chapter. Other common skin commensal organisms that are found in shunt infections include *P. acnes, S. aureus,* and the streptococci (*Streptococcus pyogenes, S. viridans, S. pneumoniae*).

S. epidermidis is particularly well adapted for shunt colonization and infection. In early serological studies, Holt identified a subclass of these bacteria that were particularly prevalent in shunt infection.[61] An early classification scheme of aerobic cocci was proposed by Baird-Parker.[6] This scheme enabled the division of the staphylococci into 6 categories (from SI to SVI) on the basis of results of tests for the presence of coagulase, phosphatase, and acetoin production, as well as the aerobic production of acid from mannitol, lactose, and L-arabinoside. It soon became evident that Baird-Parker group SII was disproportionately represented in infected shunts.[61] This prompted further analysis and subdivision of this group. Holt subdivided Baird-Par-

ker class SII into subgroups on the basis of the in vitro capabilities of the organisms.[61] Further evaluation of infected shunts revealed that subgroup IIA was the most commonly isolated staphylococci from infected shunts.[61]

The Baird-Parker classification system was subsequently replaced; however, the isolation of this subclass prompted studies into the properties of the SIIA subgroup of staphylococci. Several authors found that staphylococci of the IIA subgroup had the capability of synthesizing and secreting a glycolipid mucoid substance that was termed "slime" (Fig. 38–3).[33, 111] The frequency with which slime was seen with class IIA staphylococci and the incidence of class IIA staphylococcal infection of shunts raised the question of the pathophysiological role of slime.

Studies from infected intravascular catheters also demonstrated the capability of subgroup IIA staphylococci to synthesize slime.[33] Christiansen and co-workers found that 63 per cent of strains of *S. epidermidis* that infected intravascular devices were associated with slime production.[33] This contrasted with 37 per cent of randomly collected skin isolates and blood culture contaminates. This difference was statistically significant ($P < .05$). Further studies have indicated a general predilection of slime-producing *S. epidermidis* in infections of implanted biomaterials that are made of polymers.[31, 32]

An important finding emerged from these studies. Several lines of data support a primary role of this glycolipid substance in the pathogenesis of coagulase-negative staphylococcal shunt infections.[15] The chemical structure of slime is not completely understood; however, it is apparent that it consists of a complex variety of neutral, acidic, and amino sugars.[78] Ludwicka and associates have reported that slime is 40 per cent carbohydrate and 27 per cent protein by weight.[78] Slime differs from a true bacterial capsule in that it is loosely bound to multiple cells in a cluster, whereas a capsule tightly surrounds a single cell.[78, 93]

The evolutionary advantage of slime production is unknown. Coagulase-negative staphylococci normally

Table 38–3

MECHANISMS OF BACTERIAL ACCESS TO CEREBROSPINAL FLUID SHUNTS

Colonization
Primary
Introduction of skin-dwelling commensal organisms to the surgical wound at the time of shunt implantation
Secondary
Introduction of skin-dwelling commensal organisms through skin lesion or during invasive surgical procedure
Hematogenous Spread
Blood-borne microorganisms seed the shunt apparatus and initiate infection; of particular importance in ventriculoatrial shunts in which distal tip may be seeded following an episode of transient bacteremia
Retrograde Transmission
From distal infection, with retrograde ascension of infection; may occur with bowel penetration; may cause ascending gram-negative infection

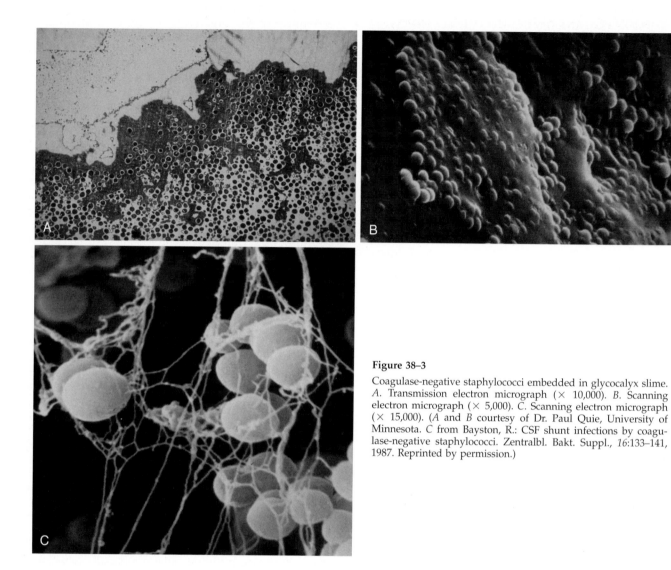

Figure 38–3

Coagulase-negative staphylococci embedded in glycocalyx slime. *A.* Transmission electron micrograph (× 10,000). *B.* Scanning electron micrograph (× 5,000). *C.* Scanning electron micrograph (× 15,000). (*A* and *B* courtesy of Dr. Paul Quie, University of Minnesota. *C* from Bayston, R.: CSF shunt infections by coagulase-negative staphylococci. Zentralbl. Bakt. Suppl., *16*:133–141, 1987. Reprinted by permission.)

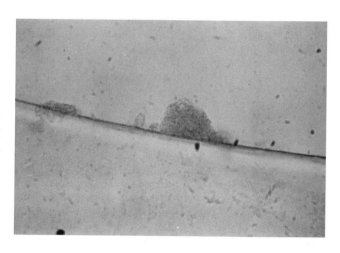

Figure 38–4

Microcolonies of coagulase-negative staphylococci are adherent to a colonized shunt. Note the adhesion of the microcolonies to the luminal surface. (From Bayston, R.: CSF shunt infections by coagulase-negative staphylococci. Zentralbl. Bakt. Suppl., *16*:133–141, 1987. Reprinted by permission.)

colonize the skin and mucous membranes of humans and animals. Slime production may facilitate colonization of surfaces by enabling organisms to adhere together in large cell clusters and carry out substance exchange between cells.[94]

The introduction of a plastic or polymer substance presents a novel environment for colonization (Fig. 38–4). Although its exact pathophysiological role is unknown, slime appears to have several important functions in the colonization of plastic surfaces. First, it facilitates the growth of the organism on smooth surfaces via an unknown mechanism.[33] Although this was initially thought to be due to an adhesive function, it later became evident that the primary forces involved in cell adhesion to surfaces were surface charges, hydrophobic/hydrophilic interactions, Van der Waals forces, and fimbrial adhesion.[53] Bacterial adherence to plastics in vitro correlates well with the production of infections.[5] Some authors have speculated that the production of slime may increase the hydrophobicity of the organism and thus promote association with an inert surface.[94] Although some adhesive properties have not been excluded, it is now thought that surface determinants on the cell membrane are primary in providing adherence to a polymer surface.[78, 93]

Second, slime matrix acts as a mechanical barrier that may protect the bacteria from host defense mechanisms or systemic antibiotics. This barrier may be very thick. Studies of infected intravascular devices have demonstrated staphylococci embedded beneath a matrix up to 160 μm in thickness.[94] Peters and colleagues have demonstrated that nafcillin-sensitive coagulase-negative staphylococci become resistant to oxacillin when grown in vitro on a polymer surface, and they have hypothesized that the barrier effect of the slime matrix may play an important role in the development of this resistance.[93] These results suggest that staphylococci are more resistant to antibiotics when grown on polymeric or plastic foreign surfaces.[5] A clinical corollary of this observation is that standard minimum inhibitory concentration values for a given antibiotic against a strain of coagulase-negative staphylococci may not be accurate for a foreign body–related infection. In related studies, these authors found a greater than 15-fold increase in the minimal inhibitory concentration for multiple antibiotics to S. epidermidis when grown in a medium that promoted slime formation as compared with bacteria grown in a slime-inhibiting medium.[94] Collectively, these and other studies suggest that slime plays an important role in protecting bacteria from antibiotics.

Staphylococcal slime has also been shown to have a variety of effects on the host immune system. The barrier effect that is important in protecting the bacteria from antibiotics also shields them from endogenous bactericidal compounds such as lysozyme, an endogenous enzyme that is lytic to bacteria and is found in the cerebrospinal fluid of 8 per cent of patients. In addition, a variety of effects on granulocytes, mononuclear cells, and lymphocytes have been demonstrated in vitro.[52, 68] Johnson and co-workers have suggested that staphylococcal slime alters polymorphonuclear

neutrophil function without affecting the viability of the neutrophils.[68] These investigators demonstrated that staphylococcal slime decreases chemotaxis and bacterial uptake by neutrophils and that in its presence superoxide generation, adherence, and degranulation are increased.[68] A direct effect on lymphocytes has also been demonstrated. Gray and associates have shown that slime inhibits the lymphoproliferative response to several standardized mitogens in vitro.[52] It also induces an alteration of cell surface antigens with a consequent inversion of the ratio of T helper (CD4) and T suppressor (CD8) cells.[52] The level of natural killer cell activity also appears to be decreased by staphylococcal slime.[52] Whether these events are seen in vivo is unknown, yet a bacteria-induced immunosuppressive effect is consistent with the indolent, refractory nature of coagulase-negative staphylococcal shunt infection.

Some authors have correlated symptoms with the slime-producing capability of the infecting organism. Fever was higher and shunt obstruction and abdominal pain occurred significantly more frequently when the infection was due to a slime-producing organism.[37]

Mechanisms of shunt infection are not as well studied for other microorganisms as as they are for the coagulase-negative staphylococci. Barrett has identified surface proteins, which he has named "protein A" and "clumping factor," in certain strains of S. aureus.[7] Preliminary evidence suggests that they may play a role in the organism's ability to bind to plastic shunt polymer.

A small but significant percentage of shunt infections arise from gram-negative organisms. Although these infections are less common, they are of great importance clinically because they have traditionally been associated with high morbidity and mortality rates. Sells and colleagues reported that gram-negative infections constituted only 20 of 217 infections in a retrospective 10-year review.[113] However, they found high morbidity and mortality rates in 18 of 20 patients for whom follow-up data were available. Thirty-nine per cent died from ventriculitis, 22 per cent sustained definite central nervous system damage, 17 per cent were mentally retarded, and 22 per cent showed no residual sequelae.[113]

A large review of gram-negative shunt infections has suggested that patients with these infections can be successfully treated with prompt shunt removal, external ventricular drainage, and intravenous administration of ceftriaxone.[120] These authors consider ceftriaxone the agent of choice because of its ability to penetrate the blood-brain barrier. Intraventricular administration of antibiotics is recommended when the cerebrospinal fluid glucose level is less than 10 mg per dL. When patients were treated appropriately, no mortality and a low (13 per cent) incidence of central nervous system damage following gram-negative shunt infection were observed.[120]

The hematogenous spread of bacteria may be particularly important in patients with ventriculoatrial shunts. The distal catheter tip may be vulnerable to seeding with bacteria during transient bacteremic episodes. This mechanism is hypothesized to account for the higher rate of infections in those with ventriculoatrial shunts, although little firm evidence supports this widely held contention.

Bacteria may also gain access to an implanted shunt from an ascending infection following abdominal sepsis or shunt perforation of the bowel.[49, 84, 120] Several case reports have demonstrated the onset of gram-negative shunt infections following other localized gram-negative infections (bowel perforations, abdominal catastrophes, meningitides) that occurred temporally distant from the time of surgery and in which the blood cultures were positive for gram-negative organisms.[64, 123] In other reports, bowel penetration has not produced clinical infection and only came to attention when the shunt catheter protruded from the anus.[105, 112] Ascending infection is an infrequently observed mechanism, although gram-negative pathogens overwhelmingly predominate in retrograde shunt infection.[64]

As greater attention has been devoted to anaerobic organisms, progressively more evidence has accumulated to suggest that they are important pathogens in shunt infection.[20, 26, 42] *P. acnes* is a pleomorphic gram-positive rod that is found in high concentration on human skin. Rekate and co-workers found that *P. acnes* was the most common cause of shunt infection in a large metropolitan center.[101] The detection of *P. acnes* may prove elusive for several reasons. First, anaerobic cultures must be sent for analysis and observed for a prolonged period (7 to 10 days) before anaerobic infection can be excluded.[20, 26, 42, 101] The organism is a fastidious anaerobe that may fail to grow unless cultured and transported under anaerobic conditions.[20, 101] Second, the clinical presentation of *P. acnes* infection varies greatly. *P. acnes* shunt infections commonly present as a shunt malfunction, but the clinical spectrum ranges from asymptomatic colonization to fulminant meningitis and midbrain encephalitis. Finally, *P. acnes* is normally found in high concentration on the human skin and is, therefore, frequently considered a contaminant. Designating a *P. acnes* culture a contaminant is potentially hazardous because the occurrence of shunt infection with *Propionibacterium* after previous positive culture results had been disregarded has been demonstrated.[26] The intervening history was often marked by repeated episodes of shunt failures and replacements. The authors believe that any positive culture result for *P. acnes* mandates a second culture, which, if also yielding a positive result, should prompt therapy for shunt infection. Despite its indolent course and varied presentation, untreated *P. acnes* shunt infection may progress to cause neurological deterioration, midbrain encephalitis, or death.[20, 26]

Host-Shunt–Related Mechanisms

Guevara and associates studied the mechanisms of bacterial adhesion to cerebrospinal fluid shunts with the use of electron microscopy and identified topographical irregularities along the surface of the catheter that were selectively colonized by infecting microorganisms.[54] These irregularities appeared to shelter and hide bacteria within the walls of the shunt (Fig. 38–5).[54] Assays of bacterial adherence strength demonstrated

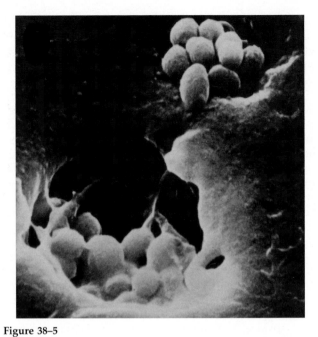

Figure 38–5

Scanning electron micrograph demonstrating colonies of *Staphylococcus aureus* embedded within the inner surface of a shunt catheter (× 10,670). Infecting organisms may selectively colonize imperfections in the shunt catheter surface and gain protection from host bactericidal mechanisms and antibiotics. (From Guevara, J. C., Zuccaro, G., Trevisan, A., et al.: Bacterial adherence to CSF shunts. J. Neurosurg., 67:438–445, 1987. Photograph courtesy of Dr. Claudio DeNoya.)

that cells of *Klebsiella pneumoniae* retained adherence to the internal shunt walls despite rates of flow up to 200 times greater than those normally demonstrated in vivo.[54] Further, studies utilizing intrashunt antibiotics have failed to eradicate bacterial colonization of the shunt despite the maintenance of antibiotic levels at 200-fold the minimal inhibitory concentration of the colonizing organism.[13, 115] These observations support the concept that microscopic irregularities in the catheter may protect colonizing microorganisms from the bactericidal effects of antibiotics and the clearance effect of the cerebrospinal fluid.

Pioneering studies by Borges suggested that the shunt itself may interfere with the host immune response to a shunt infection.[23] In an in vitro model of shunt infection, Borges demonstrated that the ability of leukocytes to phagocytose bacteria was decreased in the presence of a shunt.[23] Leukocytes were also noted to be unable to adhere well to a shunt catheter. This would impair the immune response because neutrophilic migration to the site of infection is dependent on surface adherence. It was also observed that neutrophils in the immediate proximity of the shunt showed a high rate of exocytosis of myeloperoxidase, which is an important component of the intracellular microbicidal system.[23]

Natural History

The natural history of shunt infection has never been completely studied. Untreated ventriculoperitoneal shunt infection may lead to ventriculitis or obstruction, with the attendant hazards of increased intracranial pressure. Chronic low-grade shunt infection can be associated with intellectual, psychological, and neurological deficits.[27, 85, 113, 127] Untreated ventriculoatrial shunt infections can be associated with such serious complications as glomerulonephritis, pulmonary emboli, cor pulmonale, thrombosis of the superior vena cava, pulmonary hypertension, cardiac tamponade, pleural effusion, atrial or ventricular perforation, and endocarditis.*

Diagnosis

CLINICAL PRESENTATION

The clinical presentation of shunt infection can be highly varied and is dependent on the location of the infection, the infecting organism, and the age of the patient. Internal or true shunt infections range from incidentally discovered asymptomatic infections to fulminant life-threatening ventriculitis. In the neonate, the signs and symptoms of shunt infection include alterations of feeding, irritability, vomiting, fever, lethargy, somnolence, and bulging fontanelle.[27, 43, 49] In the older child or adult, nonspecific signs often predominate. Headache, fever, vomiting, meningismus, obstructive symptoms, and abdominal pain may all be signs of shunt infection. Although meningismus may be present in severe shunt infections, its absence should not be taken as evidence against the diagnosis of shunt infection.[43, 49] Retrospective studies have suggested that it is present in only about a one third of documented shunt infections.[111, 127]

A large retrospective study by Walters and colleagues suggests that a commonly overlooked presentation of shunt infection is shunt obstruction.[127] Only half of the patients who presented with obstructive symptoms who were later found to have a shunt infection were initially considered to have an infected shunt.

As the understanding of the mechanisms and causes of shunt infection has grown, it has become evident that a high index of suspicion is necessary in the diagnosis of shunt infection. This is particularly true in the evaluation of neonates and of those with infections arising from anaerobic organisms. The clinical manifestations of shunt infection in a neonate may be subtle and difficult to detect. Seemingly unrelated events, such as poor feeding or failure to thrive, may be the first harbinger of infection. Likewise, infections with anaerobic organisms may be more indolent and present with less striking symptoms than those with more typical aerobic pathogens.

The timing of shunt infections is also characteristic. Seventy per cent of all shunt infections occur within the first 2 months after shunt placement, and 80 per cent occur within the first 6 months.[49, 51, 70, 111] Most external shunt infections occur in the immediate postoperative period.[43, 49]

The patient with shunt infection may present with abdominal signs; these may range from the presence of a painless, localized fluid collection to an acute abdomen.[50, 55, 64, 103] The presence of a localized abdominal fluid collection, or pseudocyst, is highly suggestive of infection in any patient with a ventriculoperitoneal shunt.[50, 55] Hahn and co-workers found active infection in 36 per cent and a recent history of shunt infection in 62 per cent of patients who had abdominal pseudocysts.[55] Edwards has commented that 80 per cent of patients in combined series of patients with pseudocyst had infected shunts.[50] Rarely, patients with shunt infection may present with signs of an acute abdomen.[64, 103] These patients can usually be treated with catheter externalization and antibiotics if shunt infection is the source of their abdominal problem. Therefore, it is essential to obtain cerebrospinal fluid from the shunt of any patient who presents with an acute abdomen. Failure to recognize the diagnosis of shunt infection may cause significant delays in the institution of appropriate treatment or may subject the patient to unnecessary abdominal surgical procedures.[64, 103]

Clinical signs of ventriculoatrial shunt infection include fever and, rarely, manifestations of shunt nephritis.[46, 99, 121] Shunt nephritis was first described by Black and associates in 1965 and occurs when bacteremia resulting from shunt infection gives rise to antibody deposition in the renal glomeruli.[21] Subsequent deposition and activation of complement induces a glomerulopathy that is clinically manifest by hematuria, anemia, hepatosplenomegaly, nephrotic syndrome, and, in some cases, an associated purpuric rash.[99, 121] Serum studies reveal an increase in IgG and IgM concentrations, erythrocyte sedimentation rate, and white blood cell counts but a decrease in circulating complement precursor (C3) levels.[64] Renal biopsy typically reveals lobular glomerulonephritis with mesangial cell proliferation and capillary basement membrane thickening. Electron microscopy has confirmed the presence of mesangial deposits in 77 per cent of patients and subendothelial deposits in 73 per cent, and immunofluorescent studies have revealed that deposits most commonly consist of immunoglobulin and complement precursors (C3).[121] Glomerulonephritis occurs only in a small percentage of patients with recurrent ventriculoatrial shunt infection but can cause chronic renal failure or death.[99, 121] Shunt nephritis is now rare because of the prevalence of ventriculoperitoneal shunts and of a greater awareness of this diagnosis among physicians caring for children with shunts.

External shunt infections are local infections of the adluminal side of the catheter and of the subcutaneous tract in which it is placed. They are clinically manifest by erythema, tenderness, and induration over the shunt catheter tract. These features may progress to breakdown of the tract, with the resultant exposure of the catheter. Often, these infections are precipitated in neonates by fluid tracking along the side of the catheter (Fig. 38–6). Cerebrospinal fluid may leak from the incision site and result in colonization and external infection. As the

---

*See references 4, 19, 46, 85, 99, and 121.

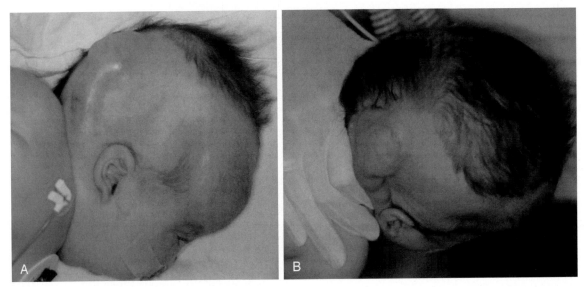

Figure 38–6

A and B. Subcutaneous cerebrospinal fluid collecting along the shunt tract may leak through the incision and significantly increase the likelihood of external shunt infection. (Courtesy of Dr. James Rutka, Hospital for Sick Children, Toronto, Ontario, Canada.)

cerebrospinal fluid is often not infected in external shunt infections, meningeal and obstructive symptoms are often absent, and signs of local infection predominate. A clinical corollary to this is that tapping of the shunt when external infection is suspected may serve to introduce bacteria into an otherwise sterile space.

INVESTIGATIONS FOR DIAGNOSING SHUNT INFECTION

Because the symptoms of shunt infection are nonspecific, it is essential that cerebrospinal fluid culture be performed for any patient suspected of harboring a shunt infection (an exception to this may occur when an external infection is suspected; see later in this chapter). However, it is often advisable to have a pediatrician inspect the child carefully for any other signs of infection that can be diagnosed noninvasively (e.g., otitis media, pharyngitis) before a shunt tap is undertaken. Many infections present with nonspecific symptoms in pediatric patients, and those patients with shunts are as susceptible to those infections as are their counterparts who do not have shunts. This fact notwithstanding, the neurosurgeon still must bear the primary responsibility for ensuring that a patient does not harbor a shunt infection: he or she should continue to follow any patient with a shunt in whom the possibility of shunt infection exists until another source of infection has been identified, treatment instituted, and clinical improvement noted. A shunt tap should be performed in any shunted patient in whom the possibility of shunt infection is suspected and in whom no other source of infection can be identified. Shunt aspiration is safe, is effective in providing useful information about the status of a given shunt, and is associated with a minimally increased risk of secondary (tap-related) shunt infection.[86, 89] Conversely, tapping a shunt in the presence of another documented infection is inadvisable and contraindicated because it may serve to introduce infection into an otherwise sterile shunt system.

The rate of return of a positive result on culture of a shunt tap sample is significantly increased when antibiotic treatment is not initiated until after the tapping is completed.[86, 123] One study found that shunt fluid aspiration yielded a positive culture result in 95 per cent of patients who were not receiving antibiotic therapy.[86] All cerebrospinal fluid should undergo glucose and protein determination, complete blood cell count, and culture for aerobic and anaerobic microorganisms.

If the clinical presentation suggests the presence of an external shunt infection with associated erythema, tenderness, swelling, and induration along the catheter tract, then the clinician may forego a shunt tap, as these infections involve the shunt tract rather than the cerebrospinal fluid. Consequently, cerebrospinal fluid cultures are less likely to yield positive results, and thus the risk of introducing infection into the shunt is increased. Sampling only the perishunt effusion may be useful in this circumstance. If it is possible to sample the cerebrospinal fluid at a site remote from the tract infection, it is advisable to do so in order to ensure that the sample is sterile. Appropriate treatment of an external shunt infection includes removal of the shunt and institution of antibiotic therapy.

Findings on cerebrospinal fluid analysis that are consistent with shunt infection include hypoglycorrhachia, elevation of protein level, and pleocytosis.[43, 49, 70, 111] Often, the glucose level is only minimally decreased.[49] The degree of pleocytosis has been shown to correlate with the incidence of positive culture results in several studies.[43, 132] Yogev and Davis found that culture results were positive in 89 per cent of patients in whom the cerebrospinal fluid had a white blood cell count greater than 100 per mm^3, whereas positive culture results were observed in only 47 per cent of patients who had a count of less than 20 per mm³.[132] The serum white blood cell count has little diagnostic value in ventriculoperitoneal shunt infection. One survey found that one quarter of patients with ventriculoperitoneal shunt infections have peripheral white blood cell counts of less than 10,000 per mm³, and only one third of patients with shunt infections have counts of greater than 20,000 per mm³. By contrast, blood studies are very important in suspected ventriculoatrial shunt infection. The peripheral white blood cell count is often elevated and blood culture results are positive in 80 per cent of cases of infected ventriculoatrial shunts.[46, 121] The rate of return of positive blood culture results can be increased if the reservoir of the shunt is pumped before the blood sample is collected.[123]

Gram staining of cerebrospinal fluid from infected shunts is useful for several reasons. First, it may demonstrate organisms that fail to grow in culture because of the institution of antibiotic therapy before shunt tapping. Bayston and co-workers identified 2 cases out of 23 in which organisms that had failed to grow in culture owing to the presence of antibiotics were observable on microscopy.[19] Furthermore, Gram staining results may allow preliminary identification of the infecting organism and thus may facilitate antibiotic selection. Certain organisms require prolonged incubation time in culture (e.g., *P. acnes*).[20, 26, 101] If such an organism is identified on Gram staining, it allows the closer targeting antibiotic therapy and mandates prolonged observation of culture results.

Positive results on cerebrospinal fluid culture are the sine qua non of shunt infection.[71] Establishing the diagnosis of shunt infection is not difficult if the patient is febrile, the inflammatory response is pronounced, the glucose level is diminished, and Gram stain and culture results are positive. However, more commonly, the symptoms are nonspecific, the cerebrospinal fluid results are minimally to mildly abnormal, and the results of Gram staining are negative. Furthermore, the most common organisms in shunt infections are common skin commensals that sometimes make interpretation of positive culture results for skin flora difficult. For this reason, Venes has suggested that a positive diagnosis of shunt infection can be made when the culture results are positive and the cerebrospinal fluid white blood cell count is less than 10 per mm³ with a shift to the left.[123] Others have suggested that the diagnosis requires that two or more culture specimens obtained from the shunt reservoir yield the same bacterial species, that the Gram staining be consistent with the organism cultured, or that signs of surgical wound infection be present.[133] The authors think that these criteria are too rigid when an infection is clinically suggested and the organism is a *Staphylococcus* species. In these circumstances, a single positive culture result should prompt treatment. If infection is not clinically suspected or if an unusual organism is cultured, a repeat culture is required for the diagnosis.

Some authors have advocated the use of serum C-reactive protein as a marker of shunt infection. C-reactive protein is an acute-phase reactant (immune globulin) found in serum following nonspecific tissue damage or destruction.[12] It is not found in the absence of a pathological process, nor is it specific to any given source. Consequently, it is limited in its specificity but may serve as a useful marker of nonspecific inflammation or in discerning infection from noninfectious obstruction.[12]

Another serological test for determining shunt infection is the assay for an antibody to a common antigen shared by most pathogenic strains of coagulase-negative staphylococci. Bayston has found that children whose shunts were shown to be colonized with *S. epidermidis* demonstrated consistently higher antibody titers than those whose shunts were not colonized.[11] Normal titers rise throughout childhood and into adolescence to a range of 380 to 1,200.[13] Bayston states that levels greater than 1,200 are uncommon in the absence of infection but advocates that baseline levels should be obtained and followed in patients with shunts.[11] A sharp increase in titers is highly associated with infection and may predate symptomatic infection.[13] Others have found that these assays are lacking in sensitivity and specificity or are too cumbersome for routine clinical use.[43, 49]

The role of fungi in shunt infection must also not be overlooked. Fungal cultures are indicated if the results of bacterial cultures of the cerebrospinal fluid are repeatedly negative in the patient with pleocytosis and symptoms of shunt malfunction or infection.[49]

Prophylaxis and Treatment

PROPHYLAXIS

The prevention of shunt infection has received considerable attention in the neurosurgical literature and yet remains controversial. Current efforts in prophylaxis are centered on two interventions: the use of prophylactic preoperative and perioperative antibiotics, and the local prevention of contamination of the shunt from the skin and operative environment.

Use of Prophylactic Antibiotics

The early studies of Burke demonstrated a benefit from prophylactic antibiotic use in general surgery and defined the temporal relationship between the surgical incision and the administration of antibiotic.[25] Maximal prophylactic benefit was attained when the antibiotic was administered before wound inoculation. Early trials featured a course of prolonged antibiotic use throughout the perioperative period, but it was soon recognized that this often encouraged the overgrowth of resistant organisms and resulted in more serious clinical infection. Treatment paradigms then shifted to short courses of the preoperative administration of range-narrow antibiotics that were targeted at the most frequent pathogens for a given procedure.[25, 56] Since that time, selected trials in vascular, orthopedic, and gynecological surgery have demonstrated some benefit to the prophylactic use of antibiotics, although the majority of studies have suffered from methodological flaws.[28, 40, 41] There is now conclusive evidence that perioperative systemic antibiotic prophylaxis reduces wound infection rates in clean neurosurgical operations.[57] Multiple published trials examine the effect of prophylactic antibiotics in shunt surgery.* These trials are outlined in Table 38–4. However, no definitive prospective randomized clinical trial has yet been performed. A multicenter randomized prospective trial was recently abandoned in the United Kingdom owing to the failure to enroll sufficient numbers of patients in a period of time short enough for statistical significance to be achieved.[17] Other prospective trials have been reported. Haines and Taylor were the first to report a prospective, double-blind, randomized trial addressing the efficacy of prophylactic antibiotics in the prevention of shunt infection.[58] Seventy-four children undergoing shunt surgery were randomly assigned to receive either methicillin or a placebo. The incidence of infection

*See references 1, 17, 22, 39, 58, 66, 82, 100, 110, 126, and 129.

was followed for 6 months. No statistically significant difference in the rate of infection was noted between the two groups; however, the methicillin-treated patients demonstrated a significantly ($P < .05$) decreased incidence of late (2 to 6 months) complications when compared with those in the placebo-treated group.[58] Wang and associates noted a similar incidence of infection between a group given a placebo (7.7 per cent) and one treated with trimethoprim-sulfamethoxazole (7.2 per cent) in a double-blind, randomized, placebo-controlled study of 120 patients undergoing shunt surgery.[129] Likewise, Walters and colleagues could not demonstrate a statistically significant difference between patients treated with trimethoprim and rifampin and those given a placebo.[126] Blomstedt reported a statistically significant reduction in infection rate in patients who received perioperative trimethoprim-sulfamethoxazole when compared with those who were given a placebo.[22] Although the study design was a double-blind, randomized prospective trial, several methodological problems occurred. The total patient

Table 38–4

EFFICACY OF PROPHYLACTIC ANTIBIOTICS IN SHUNT SURGERY*

Author(s) (Year)	Reference	Treatment Group	No. of Patients	Incidence of Infection (Per Cent)	Comments
Bayston (1975)	10	Placebo	78	2.6	No reduction in wound contamination with prophylactic antibiotics
		Cloxacillin	34	0	
		Gentamicin	20	0	
McCullough et al. (1980)	82	No antibiotic (prior to 1974)	257	8.9	Sequential study, nonrandomized
		Methicillin (after 1974)	435	5.2	
Ajir et al. (1981)	1	Placebo	60	23.3	Single-dose treatment; difference with/ without antibiotics significant
		No antibiotic (shunt placement)	73	5.5	For revision ($P < .05$); no staphylococcal infections in methicillin-treated group
		Methicillin (shunt placement)	34	8.8	
		No antibiotic (shunt revision)	32	12.5	
		Methicillin (shunt revision)	32	0	
Haines et al. (1982)	58	Placebo	39	12.8	Randomized, double-blind trial; differences between treatment and control not statistically significant for early infection; significant reduction in late infections with antibiotics
		Methicillin	35	5.7	
Wang et al. (1984)	129	Placebo	65	7.7	Double-blind randomized placebo-controlled study; no statistically significant difference between groups
		Trimethoprim-sulfamethoxazole	55	7.3	
Schmidt et al. (1985)	110	Placebo	73	5.5	Study not blinded; no support for prophylactic antibiotics obtained
		Methicillin/erythromycin	79	8.9	
Blomstedt (1985)	22	Placebo	60	23.3	Double-blind randomized controlled study; statistically significant differences support prophylaxis
		Trimethoprim-sulfamethoxazole	62	6.5	
Djindjian et al. (1986)	39	Placebo	78	20	
		Oxacillin	30	3.3	
Reider et al. (1987)	100	Placebo	31	9.7	Randomized double-blind placebo-controlled trial; meta-analysis did not reach statistical significance for series selected
		Cephalothin	32	6.3	
Walters et al. (1992)	126	Rifampin/trimethoprim	130	12	Differences not statistically significant
		Placebo	113	19.5	

*Series included are controlled prospective trials referenced in *Index Medicus* and are restricted to operations for cerebrospinal fluid diversion. Allocation to treatment and control groups was performed at random.

population was only 122, patients younger than 12 years of age were excluded from the study, and an unusually high baseline incidence of infection (29 per cent) was observed.[22] In a nonblinded prospective trial, Schmidt and co-workers found no support for the use of prophylactic antibiotics.[110] Seventy-nine patients were treated with preoperatively administered methicillin and erythromycin, and 73 were given a placebo. Rates of infection did not differ significantly.[110] Also, Bayston noted no difference between patients treated prophylactically with gentamicin or with cloxacillin when compared with those receiving a placebo in a prospective randomized trial that was not blinded.[11]

The majority of studies of the efficacy of antibiotic prophylaxis in shunt surgery are retrospective.* The results of these studies are mixed. Salmon observed a decrease in the infection rate from 19 to 3 per cent following the initiation of antibiotic prophylaxis.[108] Ajir and colleagues found a significant ($P < .05$) reduction in infections associated with shunt revisions following the initiation of prophylactic antibiotic therapy.[1] No change in infection rate was noted for primary shunt insertion with prophylactic antibiotic use. Gardner and Gordon retrospectively reviewed 200 cases of shunt placement or revision and concluded that technical factors and surgical experience were more important in the prevention of shunt infection than was the use of prophylactic antibiotics.[48] Collectively, these studies provide no conclusive evidence about the use of prophylactic antibiotics.

The combined data of many reported series may be evaluated with the statistical method of meta-analysis. Meta-analysis "critically reviews and statistically combines the results of previous research."[107] Haines and Walters have performed meta-analysis on nine randomized series of shunt infections and concluded that prophylactic antibiotics are useful in reducing the incidence of infection by about 50 per cent.[59] The effect of prophylactic antibiotics appears to be strongly related to the baseline rate of infection in that all benefit of prophylactic antibiotics is lost when the baseline rate of infection is less than 5 per cent. These findings were suggested in earlier studies in which statistically significant improvements in the rate of infection with prophylactic antibiotics correlated with higher baseline rates of infection. Langley and associates have performed meta-analysis on a series of 12 neurosurgical series of shunt infections. They also concluded that the perioperative use of antibiotics significantly reduces the rate of subsequent shunt infection.[73]

Prevention of Wound Colonization

As a greater understanding of the microbiology of shunt infection has evolved, more attention has been devoted to the local environment and to the prevention of colonization of the shunt. The timing of shunt infection strongly suggests that the most common means of inoculation of the catheter is bacterial colonization at the time of shunt placement.[14] As described earlier, the shunt environment offers a unique environment for bacteria, an environment to which certain organisms seem particularly well adapted. Other findings have supported the critical relationship between the skin flora found adjacent to the wound and the subsequent occurrence of shunt infection. Several investigators have found that organisms isolated from shunt infections were often present on the surface of the skin adjacent to the wound before surgery.[43, 49, 90, 95, 111] Pople and co-workers reported that the bacterial density on the skin adjacent to the surgical wound correlated with the incidence of shunt infection.[95] Klingman studied the bacteriology of the scalp and found significant numbers of gram-positive cocci in the infundibulum of the hair follicle (the uppermost portion of the follicle at its opening to the skin surface).[72] Although topically applied iodine is lethal to surface bacteria, it may fail to reach all of the resident flora lying deep in the hair follicles.[14] Forrest and Cooper have demonstrated the re-emergence of skin bacteria as soon as 10 minutes after the surgical scrub and suggest that this represents a real risk for colonization of the shunt.[46] Venes notes that an essential part of the protocol that enabled a significant decrease in the rate of shunt infection included exclusion of the skin area from the operative field and "strict avoidance of contact between shunt tubing and the patient's skin."[123] Others have also reported significant reductions in the rate of shunt infection when protocols that emphasized fastidious attention to technique and the avoidance of shunt contact with the skin were initiated.[29, 30, 97]

The preoperative use of shampoos with bactericidal agents may be employed to reduce the bacterial density of the scalp before shunt surgery. Although the efficacy of this method of prophylaxis has not been investigated with a prospective randomized trial, chlorhexidine shampoos have been found to reduce skin flora and have been associated with reductions in the rate of infection in vascular and abdominal surgery.[24] A single report in neurosurgical patients has shown a reduction in postoperative scalp flora density in those who underwent preoperative skin preparation compared with those who did not.[75] Given the importance of local bacteria in shunt colonization, the efficacy of preoperative shampoos in reducing skin bacterial density, and the minimal toxicity associated with the use of these agents, it appears reasonable to recommend the prophylactic use of bactericidal shampoos as part of the overall program of infection prophylaxis.

Some surgeons have attempted to isolate completely the surgical site from the operative environment with the use of a surgical isolator.[60, 102] The isolator is a clear plastic enclosure that separates the wound from the operative environment. Hirsch and co-workers reported a reduction in the rate of shunt infection from 19.7 to 7.4 per cent following the initiation of the use of a surgical isolator.[60] However, this series was sequential, and other investigators found no effect on the incidence of shunt infection when a surgical isolator was used. Airborne bacteria are, however, considered important by many investigators.[91, 102, 117, 119] Choux demonstrated an exponential increase in the number

---

*See references 1, 10, 39, 48, 49, 66, 67, 108, 126, and 129.

of airborne microorganisms over the course of an operating day. This is the rationale for performing shunt surgery early in the day, as is practiced at some large pediatric neurosurgical centers.

A promising experimental method for preventing the bacterial colonization of implanted shunts involves the impregnation of catheters with antibiotics.[18] Bayston and associates have impregnated Silastic catheters with rifampin, trimethoprim, spiramycin, clindamycin, and diethanolamine and have shown that the processed catheters demonstrated antimicrobial activity in vitro. Clindamycin and rifampin were the most effective and prevented colonization at the catheters' tips despite the presentation of three separate challenge doses of S. epidermidis.[18] Further testing is needed to determine the safety and in vivo efficacy of this promising approach.

TREATMENT OF ESTABLISHED INFECTION

The treatment of shunt infection has long been a subject of controversy centering on the need for removal of the infected shunt. Although there is little disagreement that an infected shunt system that is also dysfunctional warrants prompt removal, the appropriate management of an infected shunt that is functioning properly has generated considerable disagreement.

Medical Treatment

Serious complications may accompany the removal of intraventricular shunt catheters. Fatal intraventricular hemorrhage may occur when a shunt catheter is withdrawn (Fig. 38–7). Strands of choroid plexus may become embedded in the tip of the ventricular catheter and may be torn on its removal. Although intraventricular endoscopy may reduce the likelihood of this complication, any removal of an intraventricular shunt catheter involves some risk of hemorrhage. Shunt removal may also put the shunt-dependent patient at risk for an increase in intracranial pressure. External drainage devices may facilitate the management of elevated intracranial pressure but can also lead to superinfection and other complications. Furthermore, recannulating the ventricle may be difficult if a patient has slitlike ventricles, and the removal of ventriculoatrial shunts is typically associated with the loss of the vein for replacement. Concerns for these complications prompted some investigators to attempt the eradication of shunt infections with intravenous and intraventricular antibiotics without removal of the infected shunt.[83, 122, 127] In general, the use of systemic antibiotics without concomitant application of intrashunt antibiotics has failed to eliminate reliably shunt infection. Several authors have, however, reported successful eradication of shunt infections with the use of intrashunt and systemic antibiotics without shunt removal.[44, 83, 122, 127] McLaurin demonstrated the successful treatment of 9 of 22 shunt infections with intravenous and intra-

ventricular antibiotics.[83] Likewise, Mates and colleagues and Bayston and Rickwood separately reported an 87.5 per cent and a 90 per cent rate of eradication of infection that developed within 2 weeks of shunting with the use of intrashunt and systemic antibiotics.[16, 80] The proponents of this approach emphasize the importance of fastidious attention to cerebrospinal fluid antibiotic levels, of repeated culture, and of the preparedness to remove catheters if clinical improvement is not observed. A careful review of clinical series of patients treated medically for shunt infection reveals that the majority required shunt replacement or manipulation during the course of their treatment. This observation coupled with generally better rates of cure with surgical treatment has promoted a trend toward the surgical treatment of shunt infections at most centers.

Surgical Treatment

Several studies support removal of infected shunts as the most effective means of treating shunt infection (Table 38–5).[91, 116, 117, 125] The review of Walters and colleagues of 222 patients over a 20-year period revealed that those patients who were treated with antibiotics alone demonstrated a 14 per cent rate of cure and a 36 per cent mortality rate.[127] By contrast, the group of patients treated with removal of their shunts and the administration of antibiotics demonstrated a 59 per cent rate of cure and an 18 per cent mortality rate from shunt infection. Furthermore, more than half of the patients who received only antibiotics died, and their deaths were found to be related to the infection itself and not to the underlying disease.[127] James and coworkers prospectively evaluated 30 patients with shunt infections.[66] They found that removal of the shunt, the use of antibiotics, and the delayed replacement of the shunt resulted in a 100 per cent rate of cure. If the shunt was immediately replaced, the cure rate was 90 per cent. By contrast, treatment with antibiotics without shunt removal resulted in a 30 per cent rate of infection eradication.[66]

The extent of shunt removal and its correlation with outcome from infection has received little attention in the neurosurgical literature. No study to date has specifically addressed differences in outcome whether the entire shunt or just the distal end is externalized and subsequently revised. Clearly, the appropriate course of action is dictated by the specifics of the individual situation. However, given the propensity of certain species of pathogenic microbes to invade a shunt (see earlier) and evade immune surveillance, it would seem logical to replace as much of the shunt system as possible at the time of revision for infection. Similarly, the appropriate end point for treatment before shunt revision following infection has received little attention. Venes advocates leaving the shunt externalized and maintaining antibiotic therapy until either three successive negative results on cerebrospinal fluid cultures are obtained or the fever has disappeared for at least 24 hours.[123]

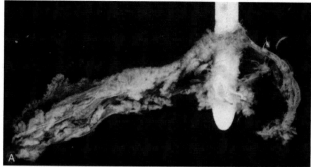

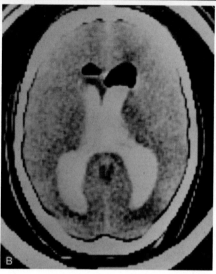

Figure 38–7

Fatal intraventricular hemorrhage may accompany the removal of shunts that have been in place for a prolonged period; however, the removal of any catheter is associated with some risk of hemorrhage.

Treatment Plan

The approach to the patient with an infected shunt is outlined in Figure 38–8. Treatment of shunt infection with antibiotics alone is reserved for those few cases in which unusual surgical circumstances exist. High surgical risk and a shortage of alternative shunt sites are two such indications for a trial of antibiotic therapy alone. However, the failure of antibiotics alone to clear infections in cerebrospinal fluid shunts is well documented. Furthermore, as outlined above, several unique characteristics of the bacteria-shunt environment serve to protect colonizing bacteria and promote infection. An understanding of these basic pathophysiological mechanisms should enable the clinician to predict the failure of infection eradication without removal of an infected shunt. Consequently, the authors strongly favor the removal of infected cerebrospinal fluid shunts and the institution of antibiotic therapy. The decision about the immediate replacement of infected shunts is dependent on whether there is evidence of ventriculitis and, at the authors' institution, is approached conservatively. External ventricular drainage is a necessary and useful adjunct to shunt removal in many patients because it enables removal of an infected shunt with constant control of intracranial pressure. Antibiotics may also be administered directly into the infected shunt with this approach. This direct administration ensures high drug concentrations in the cerebrospinal fluid and enables monitoring of intra-cranial pressure and antibiotic levels. When the infection is controlled (three consecutive negative culture results observed for the length of time required for the first culture to grow), the external ventricular drain is removed and a new shunt is placed in a different site. The principal risk of external ventricular drainage is superinfection with a more virulent nosocomial organism.[49]

Delayed replacement of an infected shunt involves complete removal of the infected foreign body, treatment with antibiotics, and the subsequent placement of a new shunt. This eliminates the need to place the new shunt into the previously infected tract and ventricle. However, the disadvantage of this approach is that the hydrocephalus is not treated during the interval between removal and replacement, which leaves the patient at risk for increased intracranial pressure. Delayed replacement may be a useful strategy in cases of communicating hydrocephalus.

The same approach is undertaken when an infection with anaerobic diphtheroids (*P. acnes*) is diagnosed. Although the pathophysiological mechanisms for these organisms are not as well understood as are those for the coagulase-negative staphylococci, the combined clinical literature demonstrates that shunt infections with *P. acnes* may progress to cause neurological deterioration and death.[20, 26] Owing to this, the authors advocate the complete removal of the infected shunt and the administration of antibiotics (penicillin G).

Shunt externalization and culture and Gram staining

Table 38–5
RESULTS OF DIFFERENT MODALITIES OF TREATING SHUNT INFECTION

Author	Total No. of Infections	Treatment Modality	Rate of Cure (Per Cent)	Comment/Conclusion
James et al.[66]	30	Shunt removal; external ventricular drainage with intravenous and intraventricular antibiotics	100	Randomized prospective trial; small size precludes statistical significance
Forward et al.[47]	34	Remove all components of shunt; systemic antibiotics	100	Retrospective study; small number of patients precludes statistical significance
		Partial removal of shunt; systemic antibiotics	53	Unacceptably high rate of failure with nonsurgical therapy
		No surgery; systemic antibiotics (oral and intravenous)	50	Higher effectiveness of antibiotics with intraventricular administration
Frame et al.[44]	12	Intravenous antibiotics and intrashunt methicillin	71 (with one course) 100 (with two courses)	Study supportive of nonsurgical treatment of shunt infection; small number of patients precludes statistical significance
Odio et al.[91]	59	No shunt removal; antibiotics alone	62	Relapses occurred only in cases in which the shunt was not removed; study is retrospective; significant differences in infection rates noted among the 5 neurosurgeons contributing to this study
		Immediate shunt removal, external ventricular drainage, intravenous antibiotics	92	
		Delayed shunt removal, external ventricular drainage, intravenous antibiotics	89	
Walters et al.[127]	267	Intravenous antibiotics	9	Surgical therapy results in higher cure rate; retrospective study; mortality lower when initial therapy is surgical
		Intravenous and intraventricular antibiotics	43	
		Shunt removal, immediate replacement, intravenous antibiotics	56	
		Shunt removal, external ventricular drainage, intravenous antibiotics, delayed replacement	58	
		Shunt removal, intravenous antibiotics, no replacement	52	

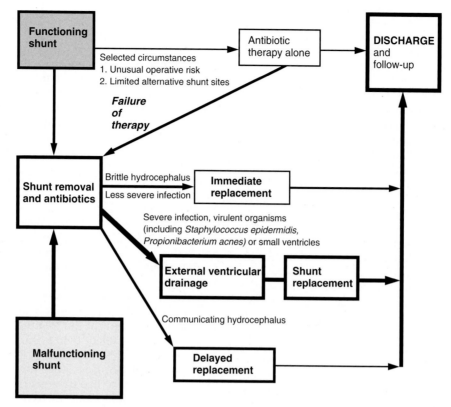

Figure 38–8

Algorithm for a recommended approach to the patient with shunt infection. Arrow thickness correlates with the frequency of approach. (Adapted and redrawn from Walters, B. C.: Cerebrospinal fluid shunt infection. Neurosurg. Clin. North Am., 3:387–401, 1992. Used by permission.)

of the cerebrospinal fluid are the first steps in the approach to the patient with a ventriculoperitoneal shunt who presents with abdominal signs. Once cerebrospinal fluid has been sent for analysis, antibiotic therapy is initiated. If the patient is stable, then a period of close, careful observation is undertaken for 4 to 6 hours. Reynolds and co-workers have demonstrated that the majority of patients with an acute abdomen as a result of ventriculoperitoneal shunt infection improve rapidly with shunt externalization and the institution of antibiotic therapy. If no improvement in the clinical condition is observed, then exploratory laparotomy is considered.

Initial Choice of Antibiotics

It is axiomatic in treating any infectious problem that the sensitivity results of the cultured organism direct the choice of antibiotics. However, at times, the clinical appearance is consistent with infection, but the Gram staining of the sample from the shunt tap does not reveal any bacteria. Often, several days in culture are required before a pathogen is definitively identified; a still greater time is required for sensitivity results to return. As a result, the initial choice of antibiotic therapy is usually empiric and is based on knowledge of the epidemiology and bacteriology of shunt infection, the sensitivity spectra and pharmacokinetics of various antibiotics, and the clinical characteristics of the pa-

tient. A low-grade fever with signs of intermittent obstruction may suggest an anaerobic infection, whereas high fevers and meningeal signs are indicative of gram-negative infection. However, clinical syndromes do not reliably predict the identity of the infecting organism. Consequently, initial empiric antibiotic coverage should be broad and potent. It must be re-emphasized that, except in extreme circumstances, no antibiotic therapy should be instituted until after cerebrospinal fluid is obtained for culture because the premature administration of antibiotics may adversely affect the capability of the infecting organism to grow in culture and, thus, may preclude its identification. Each hospital has its own individual patterns of infection and antibiotic sensitivity with which the neurosurgeon should become familiar.

Staphylococci are implicated in the overwhelming majority of shunt infections. Therefore, empiric therapy for virtually all shunt infections includes the use of antistaphylococcal agents. Vancomycin (in children, 45–60 mg per kg per day divided into 6- to 8-hour doses; in adults, 2 g per day divided in 6-hour doses) induces alterations in bacterial cell wall membranes by blocking a critical step of cell wall synthesis.[124] Few strains of staphylococci are resistant, although the penetration of vancomycin into the cerebrospinal fluid is poor in the absence of inflammation and is variable in its presence.[93, 124] Some authors have therefore suggested that vancomycin is ineffective for prophylaxis but may be useful in the treatment of cerebrospinal fluid shunt infection.[76] Leroux and co-workers demonstrated cerebrospinal fluid levels of 0.1 to 1.5 μg per mL after intravenous administration of vancomycin in the absence of inflammation.[76] Peak levels of 30 to 40 μg per mL are desirable, and levels greater than 50 μg per mL may be considered toxic.

Bactericidal cerebrospinal fluid levels of vancomycin may be ensured with intrathecal administration (5 to 20 mg).[93, 124] Rapid equal distribution of vancomycin within the fluid has been demonstrated following a single intrathecal dose in an experimental model of hydrocephalus.[63] Clinical experience has, however, shown great variability in the cerebrospinal fluid concentration of vancomycin following intrathecal administration. Although several reports show peak levels of 200 to 300 μg per mL following administration of a 20-mg dose, peaks as high as 600 μg per mL have been demonstrated after the intrathecal administration of a 10-mg dose.[3, 92] Levels in excess of 200 μg per mL may be associated with ototoxicity and nephrotoxicity.[3, 124] Leroux and co-workers demonstrated no correlation between cerebrospinal fluid levels and ventricular size, a patient's weight, meningeal inflammation, and serum levels.[76] The effect of hydrocephalus on the pharmacokinetics of intrathecally administered antibiotics is unknown, although some authors have hypothesized that clearance times are prolonged owing to the impairment of cerebrospinal fluid flow dynamics. Despite their widespread clinical use, the pharmacokinetics of intrathecal antibiotics are poorly understood, and no specific guidelines for dosages have been established. Intrathecally administered antibiotics must, therefore, be used judiciously because of the lack of controlled clinical trials documenting the safety and efficacy of this practice.[130]

The efficacy of vancomycin may also be increased with the concomitant administration of rifampin (20 mg/kg per day, not to exceed 600 mg per day, intravenously or perorally).[104] Rifampin is a useful adjunct because of its capacity to kill intracellular organisms, its good cerebrospinal fluid penetration, and its high level of activity against staphylococci.[104] Archer found rifampin to be the single most active agent against all isolates of *S. epidermidis* from infected valves or shunts.[2] Further, this drug shows excellent synergism with vancomycin and is well absorbed when given orally. Sippel and associates found that the cerebrospinal fluid levels of orally administered rifampin (25 mg per kg) exceeded the minimum inhibitory concentration for all strains of staphylococci tested by at least 1,000-fold on the second day of therapy.[118] Rifampin must be given concomitantly with another antimicrobial if the emergence of resistant strains is to be prevented.[104]

Teicoplanin is a new glycopeptide antibiotic that is closely related to vancomycin. It has demonstrated great efficacy against staphylococci. Like vancomycin, teicoplanin has poor central nervous system penetration, and intrathecal dosing has been recommended. It is not yet approved for usage in the United States; however, the European experience has demonstrated its efficacy in treating resistant shunt infection when it is given intrathecally (5 to 40 mg).[35]

Although the antistaphylococcal penicillins (nafcillin, methicillin) are highly effective against *S. aureus*, many strains of the coagulase-negative staphylococci are resistant. Archer found that 63 per cent of *S. epidermidis* strains were resistant to antistaphylococcal penicillins and cephalosporins.[2] Gardner and Gordon observed that infections caused by methicillin-resistant *S. epidermidis* usually fail to respond to other beta-lactam antibiotics regardless of reports of in vitro susceptibility.[48] Pediatric patients who are given methicillin, nafcillin, or oxacillin must be closely observed for hematological abnormalities (neutropenia and eosinophilia) and elevated liver function values.[27] Furthermore, there is considerable variability among individuals with respect to total clearance time and cerebrospinal fluid concentration following the administration of a standard dose.[69, 88]

Some authors have described trimethoprim-sulfamethoxazole (20 mg trimethoprim per kg per day) as a good initial agent in the treatment of shunt infection because of its excellent blood-brain barrier penetration, high rate of oral absorption, and low incidence of resistance in staphylococci.[89] Trimethoprim-sulfamethoxazole, like rifampin, has demonstrated the capability of eliminating bacteria within leukocytes and has demonstrated synergy with antistaphylococcal agents.[126] Trimethoprim-sulfa inhibits the level of dihydrofolic reductase of bacteria much more efficiently than the same enzyme in mammalian cells.[106] It should not be administered to patients younger than 2 months of age, and in the presence of renal failure, the dose must be reduced.[106]

In addition to antistaphylococcal agents, an agent with broad coverage is often added. Chloramphenicol (25 to 100 mg per kg per day, perorally or intravenously, divided into 6-hour doses) was formerly a primary choice in the treatment of ventriculitis because of its broad spectrum and excellent penetration into the central nervous system.[9] Peak serum chloramphenicol levels of between 10 to 25 μg per mL are recommended.[9] Chloramphenicol levels in the cerebrospinal fluid may be 30 per cent of plasma levels in noninflamed meninges and 45 to 90 per cent of these levels when the meninges are inflamed.[45] However, it lacks bactericidal activity within the central nervous system and may be associated with severe adverse effects. The most serious of these includes a dose-dependent irreversible aplastic anemia and the gray syndrome.[9] Because the severe toxicity is dose-dependent and interindividual variability in pharmacokinetics is considerable, careful serum monitoring is important when therapy with chloramphenicol is undertaken.

Ceftriaxone is a long-acting third-generation cephalosporin that has excellent cerebrospinal fluid penetration in the presence of inflammation and a broad range of antimicrobial efficacy.[8] Following intravenous administration of doses of 50 to 75 mg per kg, cerebrospinal fluid concentrations of 98 to 484 μg per mL were observed. This exceeded the minimal inhibitory concentration of the staphylococcal species tested and that of several gram-negative species (*Haemophilus influenzae, Escherichia coli, Neisseria meningitidis*) by several hundred- to a thousand-fold.[8] A recent prospective nonrandomized trial demonstrated the efficacy of ceftriaxone (50 mg per kg per day, intravenously, divided into 12-hour doses) in treating ventriculitis associated with shunt infection.[109] All nine patients treated with ceftriaxone were cured of infection. Organisms included *S. epidermidis, H. influenzae, Klebsiella* species, *E. coli,* and *Enterobacter* species.[109]

The clinical appearance of an acutely ill patient raises the suspicion of gram-negative shunt infection. The aminoglycoside antibiotics (gentamicin, tobramycin, amikacin) show high in vitro efficacy against gram-negative organisms but are limited by their poor capacity for crossing the blood-brain barrier.[130] Intrathecal aminoglycoside therapy has been used effectively in the treatment of life-threatening gram-negative shunt infection. The greatest experience has been gained with gentamicin in the treatment of gram-negative meningitides of infancy. Intrathecal doses of 0.5 to 8.0 mg have demonstrated efficacy against gram-negative organism–related ventriculitis when systemic therapy failed.[130] One study demonstrated increased mortality with the use of intraventricular gentamicin, although methodological factors may have significantly affected the outcome of this study.[81, 130] The considerable clinical experience with intrathecal gentamicin suggests that it is safe; however, reports of toxic manifestations include transient ototoxicity and seizures. Tobramycin and amikacin are useful substitutes when culture results indicate resistance to gentamicin.[130] Although the anaerobic diphtheroids (e.g., *P. acnes*) are widely sensitive to several antibiotics, including gentamicin, rifampin, clindamycin, and chloramphenicol, penicillin is the usual drug of choice. This is because of the universal sensitivity of *P. acnes* to penicillin, its good penetration of the blood-brain barrier, and the low incidence of toxicity associated with its use.[42, 79]

Microbicidal levels of antibiotics in the cerebrospinal fluid are a cornerstone of therapy for shunt infections. Because cerebrospinal fluid lacks both the opsonins and complement found in blood, bactericidal levels are essential. For difficult infections, it is highly recommended that bactericidal titers for the antibiotic being used against the identified organism strain be established. The sensitivity of the identified strain of pathogen should always be tested against the antibiotic employed. Optimal cerebrospinal fluid levels in the treatment of cerebrospinal fluid shunt infection should be at least 30 times the minimal inhibitory concentration levels.[130]

Summary and Conclusions

Cerebrospinal fluid shunt infections are important because they occur frequently and are associated with high rates of morbidity and mortality. Their pathogenesis is incompletely understood, but it is evident that certain strains of bacteria are particularly well adapted for the colonization and infection of shunts. The primary sources of shunt infection are skin commensals of low virulence that appear to be introduced at the time of shunt implantation. The anaerobic diphtheroids are important and common sources of shunt infection that are underidentified. Unfortunately, there is no known method for the elimination of shunt infection from neurosurgical practice. However, the incidence of shunt infection may be reduced through the meticulous intraoperative prevention of wound colonization and with the use of prophylactic antibiotics. Shunt infections vary significantly in their clinical presentation, and a high index of suspicion is essential for timely diagnosis. Treatment varies according to the clinical status of the patient, the functional status of the shunt, and the species of the infecting organism. Further studies are needed for better delineation of the pathophysiological mechanisms of shunt infection and so that new strategies of prevention and treatment can be developed, analyzed, and implemented.

Acknowledgments

The assistance provided by John A. Campbell in reviewing the University of Minnesota experience is gratefully acknowledged.

REFERENCES

1. Ajir, F., Levin, A. B., and Duff, T. A.: Effect of prophylactic methicillin on cerebrospinal fluid infection in children. Neurosurgery, 9:6–8, 1981.
2. Archer, G. L.: Antimicrobial susceptibility and selection of resistance among *Staphylococcus epidermidis* isolates recovered from patients with infection of indwelling foreign devices. Antimicrob. Agents Chemother., 14:353–359, 1978.
3. Arroyo, J. C., and Quindlen, E. A.: Accumulation of vancomycin after intraventricular infusions. South. Med. J., 76:1554, 1983.
4. Arze, R. S., Rashid, H., Morley, R., et al.: Shunt nephritis: Report of two cases and review of the literature. Clin. Nephrol., 19:48–53, 1983.
5. Ashkenazi, S.: Bacterial adherence to plastics. Lancet, 1:1075–1076, 1984.
6. Baird-Parker, A. C.: The classification of staphylococci and micrococci from world wide sources. J. Gen. Microbiol., 38:363–387, 1965.
7. Barrett, S. P.: Protein-mediated adhesion of *Staphylococcus aureus* to silicone implant polymer. J. Med. Microbiol., 20:249–253, 1985.
8. Barson, W. J., Miller, M. A., Brady, M. T., et al.: Prospective comparative trial of ceftriaxone vs. conventional therapy for treatment of bacterial meningitis in children. Pediatr. Infect. Dis., 4:362–368, 1985.
9. Bartlett, J. G.: Chloramphenicol. Med. Clin. North Am., 66:91–102, 1982.
10. Bayston, R.: Antibiotic prophylaxis in shunt surgery. Dev. Med. Child Neurol., 35(Suppl. 17):99–103, 1975.
11. Bayston, R.: Serological surveillance of children with CSF shunting devices. Dev. Med. Child Neurol., 17:104–110, 1975.
12. Bayston, R.: Serum C-reactive protein test in diagnosis of septic complications of cerebrospinal fluid shunts for hydrocephalus. Arch. Dis. Child., 54:545–548, 1979.
13. Bayston, R.: CSF shunt infections by coagulase-negative staphylococci. Zentralbl. Bakt. Suppl., 16:133–142, 1987.
14. Bayston, R., and Lari, J.: A study of the sources of infection in colonised shunts. Dev. Med. Child Neurol., 16:16–22, 1974.
15. Bayston, R., and Penny, S. R.: Excessive production of mucoid

substance in staphylococcus SIIA: A possible factor in colonisation of Holter shunts. Dev. Med. Child Neurol., *14*:25–28, 1972.

16. Bayston, R., and Rickwood, A. M. K.: Factors involved in the antibiotic treatment of cerebrospinal fluid shunt infection. Z. Kinderchir., *34*:339–345, 1981.

17. Bayston, R., Bannister, C., Boston, V., et al.: A prospective randomised controlled trial of antimicrobial prophylaxis in hydrocephalus shunt surgery. Z. Kinderchir., *45*(Suppl.):5–7, 1990.

18. Bayston, R., Grove, N., Siegal, J., et al.: Prevention of hydrocephalus shunt catheter colonization in vitro by impregnation with antimicrobials. J. Neurol. Neurosurg. Psychiatry, *52*:605–608, 1989.

19. Bayston, R., Leung, T. S., Wilkins, B. M., et al.: Bacteriological examination of removed cerebrospinal fluid shunts. J. Clin. Pathol., *36*:987–990, 1983.

20. Beeler, B. A., Crowder, J. G., Smith, J. W., et al.: *Propionibacterium acnes*: Pathogen in central nervous system shunt infection. Am. J. Med., *36*:987–990, 1976.

21. Black, J. A., Challacombe, D. N., and Ockenden, B. G.: Nephrotic syndrome associated with bacteremia after shunt operations for hydrocephalus. Lancet, *2*:921–922, 1965.

22. Blomstedt, G.: Results of trimethoprim-sulfamethoxazole prophylaxis in ventriculostomy and shunting procedures. J. Neurosurg., *62*:694–697, 1985.

23. Borges, L. F.: Cerebrospinal fluid shunts interfere with host defenses. Neurosurgery, *10*:55–59, 1982.

24. Brandberg, A., and Andersson, I.: Pre-operative whole-body disinfection by shower bath with chlorhexidine soap: Effect on transmission of bacteria from skin flora. *In* Maibach, H. I., and Alv, R., eds.: Skin Microbiology: Relevance to Clinical Infection. New York, Springer-Verlag, 1981, pp. 98–102.

25. Burke, J. F.: The effective period of preventative antibiotic action in experimental incisions and dermal lesions. Surgery, *50*:161–168, 1961.

26. Camarata, P. J., McGeachie, R. E., and Haines, S. J.: Dorsal midbrain encephalitis caused by *Propionibacterium acnes*: Report of two cases. J. Neurosurg., *72*:654–659, 1990.

27. Chapman, P. C., and Borges, L. F.: Shunt infections: Prevention and treatment. Clin. Neurosurg., *23*:652–664, 1984.

28. Chodak, G. W., and Plaut, M. E.: Use of systemic antibiotics for prophylaxis in surgery. Arch. Surg., *112*:326–334, 1977.

29. Choux, M.: Shunt implantation: Toward zero infection. Child's Nerv. Syst., *4*:181, 1988.

30. Choux, M., Genitori, L., Lang, D., et al.: Shunt implantation: Reducing the incidence of shunt infection. J. Neurosurg., *77*:875–880, 1992.

31. Christiansen, G. D., Baddour, L. M., and Simpson, W. A.: The role of adherence in the pathogenesis of coagulase-negative staphylococcal infections. Zentralbl. Bakt. Suppl., *16*:103–109, 1987.

32. Christiansen, G. D., Baddour, L. M., and Simpson, W. A.: Phenotypic variation of *Staphylococcus epidermidis* slime production in vitro and in vivo. Infect. Immunol., *55*:2870–2877, 1987.

33. Christiansen, G. D., Simpson, W. A., Bisno, A. L., et al.: Adherence of slime-producing strains of *Staphylococcus epidermidis* to smooth surfaces. Infect. Immunol., *37*:318–325, 1982.

34. Colleen, S., Herrstrom, P., Wieslander, A., et al.: Physico-chemical properties of *Staphylococcus epidermidis* and *Staphylococcus saprophyticus* as studied by aqueous polymer two-phase systems. Scand. J. Infect. Dis. Suppl., *24*:165–172, 1980.

35. Cruciani, M., Navarra, A., DiPerri, G., et al.: Evaluation of intraventricular teicoplanin for the treatment of neurosurgical shunt infections. Clin. Infect. Dis., *15*:285–289, 1992.

36. D'Angio, C. T., McGowan, K. L., Baumgart, S., et al.: Surface colonization with coagulase-negative staphylococci in premature neonates. J. Pediatr., *114*:1029–1034, 1989.

37. Diaz-Mitoma, F., Harding, G. K. M., Hoban, D. J., et al.: Clinical significance of a test for slime production in ventriculoperitoneal shunt infections caused by coagulase-negative staphylococci. J. Infect. Dis., *156*:555–560, 1987.

38. Dickinson, G. M., and Bisno, A. L.: Infections associated with indwelling devices: Infections related to extravascular devices. Antimicrob. Agents Chemother., *33*:602–605, 1989.

39. Djindjian, M., Fevrier, M. J., Otterbein, G., et al.: Oxacillin prophylaxis in cerebrospinal fluid shunt procedures: Results of a randomized open study in 60 hydrocephalic patients. Surg. Neurol., *25*:178–180, 1986.

40. Dor, P., and Klasterski, J.: Prophylactic antibiotics in oral pharyngeal and laryngeal surgery for cancer (a double-blind study). Laryngoscope, *83*:1992–1998, 1973.

41. Ericson, C., Lidgren, L., and Lindberg, L.: Cloxacillin in the prophylaxis of postoperative infection of the hip. J. Bone Joint Surg. [Am.], *55*:808–813, 1973.

42. Everett, E. D., Eickoff, T. C., and Simon, R. H.: Cerebrospinal fluid shunt infections with anaerobic diphtheroids (*Propionibacterium* species). J. Neurosurg., *44*:580–585, 1976.

43. Fan-Havard, P., and Nahata, M. C.: Treatment and prevention of infections of cerebrospinal fluid shunts. Clin. Pharm., *6*:866–868, 1987.

44. Frame, P. T., and McLaurin, R. L.: Treatment of CSF shunt infections with intrashunt plus oral antibiotic therapy. J. Neurosurg., *60*:354–360, 1984.

45. Friedman, C. A., Lovejoy, F. C., and Smith, A. L.: Chloramphenicol disposition in infants and children. Pediatrics, *95*:1071–1077, 1979.

46. Forrest, D. M., and Cooper, D. G. W.: Complications of ventriculo-atrial shunts: A review. J. Neurosurg., *29*:506–512, 1968.

47. Forward, K. R., Fewer, H. D., and Stiver, H. G.: Cerebrospinal fluid shunt infections. J. Neurosurg., *59*:389–393, 1983.

48. Gardner, B. D., and Gordon, D. S.: Postoperative infection in shunts for hydrocephalus: Are prophylactic antibiotics necessary? B.M.J., *284*:1914, 1982.

49. Gardner, P., Leipzig, T., and Phillips, P.: Infections of central nervous system shunts. Med. Clin. North Am., *69*:297–314, 1985.

50. Gaskill, S. J., and Marlin, A. E.: Pseudocysts of the abdomen associated with ventriculoperitoneal shunts: A report of twelve cases and a review of the literature. Pediatr. Neurosci., *15*:23–27, 1989.

51. George, R., Leibrock, L., and Epstein, M.: Long-term analysis of cerebrospinal fluid shunt infections: A 25-year experience. J. Neurosurg., *51*:804–811, 1979.

52. Gray, E. D., Oeters, G., Verstegen, M., et al.: Effect of extracellular slime substance from *Staphylococcus epidermidis* on the human cellular immune response. Lancet, *1*:365–367, 1984.

53. Gristina, A. C.: Biomaterial-centered infection: Microbial adhesion versus tissue integration. Science, *237*:1588–1595, 1987.

54. Guevara, J. A., Zuccaro, G., Trevisan, A., et al.: Bacterial adhesion to cerebrospinal fluid shunts. J. Neurosurg., *67*:438–445, 1987.

55. Hahn, Y. S., Engelhard, H., and McLone, D.: Abdominal CSF pseudocyst: Clinical features and surgical management. Pediatr. Neurosci., *12*:75–79, 1985.

56. Haines, S. J.: Systemic antibiotic prophylaxis in neurological surgery. Neurosurgery, *6*:355–361, 1980.

57. Haines, S. J.: Efficacy of antibiotic prophylaxis in clean neurosurgical operations. Neurosurgery, *24*:401–405, 1989.

58. Haines, S. J., and Taylor, F.: Prophylactic methicillin for shunt operations: Effects on incidence of shunt malfunction and infection. Child's Brain, *10*:10–22, 1982.

59. Haines, S. J., and Walters, B. C.: Antibiotic prophylaxis for CSF shunts: A meta-analysis. Neurosurgery, *34*:87–92, 1994.

60. Hirsch, J. F., Renier, E., and Pierre-Kahn, A.: Influence of the use of a surgical isolator on the rate of infection in the treatment of hydrocephalus. Child's Brain, *4*:137–150, 1978.

61. Holt, R.: The classification of staphylococci from colonized ventriculo-atrial shunts. J. Clin. Pathol., *22*:475–482, 1969.

62. Holt, R. J.: Bacteriological studies on colonised ventriculoatrial shunts. Dev. Med. Child Neurol., *12*:83–88, 1970.

63. Howard, M. A., Grady, M. S., Park, T. S., et al.: Pharmacokinetics of intraventricular vancomycin in hydrocephalic rats. Neurosurgery, *18*:725–728, 1986.

64. Hubschmann, O. R., and Countee, R. W.: Acute abdomen in children with infected ventriculoperitoneal shunts. Arch. Surg., *115*:305–307, 1980.

65. Ignelzi, R., and Kirsch, W. M.: Follow-up analysis of ventriculoperitoneal and ventriculoatrial shunts for hydrocephalus. J. Neurosurg., *42*:679–682, 1975.

66. James, H. E., Walsh, J. W., Wilson, H. D., et al.: Prospective randomized study of therapy in cerebrospinal fluid shunt infection. Neurosurgery, *7*:459–463, 1980.

67. James, H. E., Wilson, H. D., Connor, J. D., et al.: Intraventricular cerebrospinal fluid antibiotic concentrations in patients with intraventricular infections. Neurosurgery, 10:50–54, 1982.

68. Johnson, G. M., Regelmann, W. E., Gray, E. D., et al.: Staphylococcal slime and host defenses: Effects on polymorphonuclear granulocytes. Zentralbl. Bakt. Suppl., 16:33–43, 1987.

69. Kane, J. G., Parker, R. H., Jordan, G. W., et al.: Nafcillin concentration in cerebrospinal fluid during treatment of staphylococcal infections. Ann. Intern. Med., 87:309–311, 1977.

70. Keutcher, T. R., and Mealey, J.: Long-term results after ventriculoatrial and ventriculoperitoneal shunting for infantile hydrocephalus. J. Neurosurg., 50:179–186, 1979.

71. Klein, D. M.: Shunt infections. In Scott, M. S., ed.: Hydrocephalus. Concepts in Neurosurgery, Congress of Neurologic Surgeons (US). Vol. 3. Baltimore, Williams & Wilkins, 1990, pp. 87–97.

72. Klingman, A. M.: The bacteriology of the normal skin. In Maiback, H. I., and Hildick-Smith, G., eds.: Skin Bacteria and Their Role in Infection. New York, McGraw-Hill, 1965, pp. 13–35.

73. Langley, J. M., LeBlanc, J. C., Drake, J., et al.: Efficacy of antimicrobial prophylaxis in placement of cerebrospinal fluid shunts: Meta-analysis. Clin. Infect. Dis., 17:98–103, 1993.

74. Laurence, K. M., and Coats, S.: The natural history of hydrocephalus: Detailed analysis of 182 unoperated cases. Arch. Dis. Child., 37:345, 1962.

75. Leclair, J. M., Winston, K. R., Sullivan, B. F., et al.: Effect of preoperative shampoos with chlorhexidine or iodophor on emergence of resident scalp flora in neurosurgery. Infect. Control Hosp. Epidemiol., 9:8–12, 1988.

76. Leroux, P., Howard, M. A., and Winn, H. R.: Vancomycin pharmacokinetics in hydrocephalic shunt prophylaxis and relationship to ventricular volume. Surg. Neurol., 34:366–372, 1990.

77. Little, J. R., Rhoton, A. L., and Mellinger, J. F.: Comparison of ventriculoperitoneal and ventriculoatrial shunts for hydrocephalus in children. Mayo Clin. Proc., 47:397, 1972.

78. Ludwicka, A., Uhlenbruck, G., Peters, G., et al.: Investigation on extracellular slime substance produced by Staphylococcus epidermidis. Zentralbl. Bakt. Mikrobiol., 258:256–267, 1984.

79. Martin, W. J., Gardner, M., and Washington, J. A., II: In vitro antimicrobial susceptibility of anaerobic bacteria isolated from clinical specimens. Antimicrob. Agents Chemother., 1:148–158, 1972.

80. Mates, S., Glaser, J., and Shapiro, K.: Treatment of cerebrospinal fluid shunts with medical treatment alone. Neurosurgery, 11:781–782, 1982.

81. McCracken, G. H., and Mize, S. G.: A controlled study of intrathecal antibiotic therapy in gram-negative enteric meningitis of infancy. J. Pediatr., 89:66, 1976.

82. McCullough, D. C., Kane, J. G., Presper, J. H., et al.: Antibiotic prophylaxis in ventricular shunt surgery. Child's Brain, 7:182–189, 1980.

83. McLaurin, R. L.: Infected cerebrospinal fluid shunts. Surg. Neurol., 1:191–195, 1973.

84. McLaurin, R. L.: Treatment of infected ventricular shunts. Child's Brain, 1:306–310, 1975.

85. McLone, D. G., Czyzewski, D., Raimondi, A. J., et al.: Central nervous system infections as a limiting factor in the intelligence of children with myelomeningocele. Pediatrics, 70:338–342, 1982.

86. Myers, M. G., and Schoenbaum, S. C.: Shunt fluid aspiration: An adjunct in the diagnosis of cerebrospinal fluid shunt infection. Am. J. Dis. Child., 129:220–222, 1975.

87. Nahata, M. C., DeBolt, S. L., and Powell, D. A.: Adverse effects of methicillin, nafcillin and oxacillin in pediatric patients. Dev. Pharmacol. Ther., 4:117–123, 1982.

88. Nahata, M. C., Fan-Havard, P., Kosnick, E. J., et al.: Pharmacokinetics and cerebrospinal fluid concentration of nafcillin in pediatric patients undergoing cerebrospinal fluid shunt placement. Chemotherapy, 36:98–102, 1990.

89. Noetzel, M. J., and Baker, R. P.: Shunt fluid examination: Risks and benefits in the evaluation of shunt malfunction and infection. J. Neurosurg., 61:328–332, 1984.

90. O'Brien, M., Parent, A., and Davis, B.: Management of ventricular shunt infections. Child's Brain, 5:304–309, 1979.

91. Odio, C., McCracken, G. H., and Nelson, J.: CSF shunt infections in pediatrics. Am. J. Dis. Child., 138:1103–1108, 1984.

92. Pau, A. K., Smego, R. A., and Fisher, M. A.: Intraventricular vancomycin: Observations of tolerance and pharmacokinetics in two infants with ventricular shunt infections. Pediatr. Infect. Dis., 5:93–96, 1986.

93. Peters, G., Locci, R., and Pulverer, G.: Adherence and growth of coagulase-negative staphylococci on surfaces of intravenous catheters. J. Infect. Dis., 146:479–482, 1982.

94. Peters, G., Schumacher-Perdreau, F., Jansen, B., et al.: Biology of Staphylococcus epidermidis extracellular slime. Zentralbl. Bakt. Suppl., 16:15–32, 1987.

95. Pople, I. K., Bayston, R., and Hayward, R. D.: Infection of cerebrospinal fluid shunts in infants: A study of etiological factors. J. Neurosurg., 77:29–36, 1992.

96. Pople, I. K., Quinn, M. W., and Bayston, R.: Morbidity and outcome of shunted hydrocephalus. Z. Kinderchir., 45:29–31, 1990.

97. Puca, A., Anile, C., Maira, G., et al.: Cerebrospinal fluid shunting for hydrocephalus in the adult: Factors related to shunt revision. Neurosurgery, 29:822–826, 1991.

98. Quie, P. G., and Belani, K. K.: Coagulase-negative staphylococcal adherence and persistence. J. Infect. Dis., 156:543–547, 1987.

99. Rames, L., Wise, B., Goodman, J. R., et al.: Renal disease with Staphylococcus albus bacteremia: A complication of ventriculoatrial shunts. J.A.M.A, 212:1671–1677, 1970.

100. Reider, M. J., Frewen, T. C., Delmaestro, R. F., et al.: The effect of cephalothin prophylaxis on postoperative ventriculoperitoneal shunt infections. Can. Med. Assoc. J., 136:935–938, 1987.

101. Rekate, H. L., Ruch, T., and Nulsen, F. E.: Diphtheroid infections of cerebrospinal fluid shunts: The changing pattern of shunt infection in Cleveland. J. Neurosurg., 52:553–556, 1980.

102. Renier, D., Lacombe, J., Pierre-Kahn, A., et al.: Factors causing acute shunt infection: Computer analysis of 1,174 operations. J. Neurosurg., 61:1072–1078, 1984.

103. Reynolds, M., Sherman, J. O., and Mclone, D. G.: Ventriculoperitoneal shunt infection masquerading as an acute surgical abdomen. J. Pediatr. Surg., 18:951–953, 1983.

104. Ring, J. C., Cates, K. L., Belani, K. K., et al.: Rifampin for CSF shunt infections caused by coagulase-negative staphylococci. J. Pediatr., 95:317–319, 1979.

105. Rubin, R. C., Ghatak, N. R., and Visudhipan, P.: Asymptomatic perforated viscus and gram-negative ventriculitis as a complication of valve-regulated ventriculoperitoneal shunts. J. Neurosurg., 37:616–619, 1972.

106. Rubin, R. H., and Swartz, M. N.: Trimethoprim-sulfamethoxazole. N. Engl. J. Med., 303:426–431, 1980.

107. Sacks, H. S., Berrier, J., Reitman, D., et al.: Meta-analysis of randomized controlled trials. N. Engl. J. Med., 316:450–455, 1987.

108. Salmon, J. H.: Adult hydrocephalus, evaluation of therapy in 80 patients. J. Neurosurg., 37:423, 1972.

109. Schaad, U. B., and Stoeckel, K.: Single-dose pharmacokinetics of ceftriaxone in infants and young children. Antimicrob. Agents Chemother., 21:248–253, 1982.

110. Schmidt, K., Gjerris, F., Osgaard, O., et al.: Antibiotic prophylaxis in cerebrospinal fluid shunting: A prospective randomized trial in 152 hydrocephalic patients. Neurosurgery, 17:1–5, 1985.

111. Schoenbaum, S. C., Gardner, P., and Shillito, J.: Infections of cerebrospinal fluid shunts: Epidemiology, clinical manifestations and therapy. J. Infect. Dis., 131:543–552, 1975.

112. Schulhy, L. A., Worth, R. M., and Kalsbeck, J. E.: Bowel perforation due to peritoneal shunt. Surg. Neurol., 3:265–268, 1975.

113. Sells, C. J., Shurtleff, D. B., and Loeser, J. D.: Gram-negative cerebrospinal fluid shunt–associated infections. Pediatrics, 59:614–618, 1977.

114. Shapiro, S., Boaz, J., Kleiman, M., et al.: Origin of organisms infecting ventricular shunts. Neurosurgery, 22:868–871, 1988.

115. Sheth, N. K., Fransom, T. R., and Sohule, P. G.: Influence of bacterial adherence to intravascular catheters on in vitro antibiotic susceptibility. Lancet, 2:1266–1268, 1985.

116. Shurtleff, D. B., Stuntz, J. T., and Hayden, P. W.: Experience with 1,201 cerebrospinal fluid shunt procedures. Pediatr. Neurosci., 12:49–57, 1985.

117. Shurtleff, D. B., Foltz, E. L., Weeks, R. D., et al.: Therapy of Staphylococcus epidermidis: Infections associated with cerebrospinal fluid shunts. Pediatrics, 53:55–62, 1974.

118. Sippel, J. E., Mikhail, I. A., Girgis, N. I., et al.: Rifampin concentration in cerebrospinal fluid of patients with tuberculous meningitis. Am. Rev. Respir. Dis., *109*:579–580, 1974.

119. Spanu, G., Karussos, G., Adinolfi, D., et al.: An analysis of cerebrospinal fluid shunt infections in adults: A clinical experience of 12 years. Acta Neurochir., *80*:79–82, 1986.

120. Stamos, J. K., Kaufman, B. A., and Yogev, R.: Ventriculoperitoneal shunt infections with gram-negative bacteria. Neurosurgery, *33*:858–862, 1993.

121. Stickler, G. B., Shin, M. H., Burke, E. C., et al.: Diffuse glomerulonephritis associated with infected ventriculoatrial shunt. N. Engl. J. Med., *279*:1077–1082, 1968.

122. Tomaszek, D. E., and Powers, S. K.: Treatment of cerebrospinal fluid and syringosubarachnoid shunt infection with systemic and intrathecal antibiotics. Neurosurgery, *17*:327–328, 1985.

123. Venes, J. L.: Infections of CSF shunt and intracranial pressure monitoring devices. Infect. Dis. Clin. North Am., *3*:289–299, 1989.

124. Visconti, E. B., and Peter, G.: Vancomycin treatment of cerebrospinal fluid shunt infection. J. Neurosurg., *51*:245–246, 1979.

125. Walters, B. C.: Cerebrospinal fluid shunt infection. Neurosurg. Clin. North Am., *3*:387–401, 1992.

126. Walters, B. C., Goumnerova, L., Hoffman, H. J., et al.: A randomized controlled trial of perioperative rifampin/trimethoprim in cerebrospinal fluid shunt surgery. Child's Nerv. Syst., *8*:253–257, 1992.

127. Walters, B. C., Hoffman, H. J., Hendrick, E. B., et al.: Cerebrospinal fluid shunt infection. J. Neurosurg., *60*:1014–1021, 1984.

128. Walters, B. C., Hoffman, H. J., Hendrick, E. B., et al.: Decreased risk of infection in cerebrospinal fluid shunt surgery using prophylactic antibiotics: A case-control study. Z. Kinderchir., *40*:15–18, 1985.

129. Wang, E. L., Prober, C. G., Hendrick, B. E., et al.: Prophylactic sulfamethoxazole and trimethoprim in ventriculoperitoneal shunt surgery: A double-blind, randomized, placebo-controlled trial. J.A.M.A., *251*:1174–1177, 1984.

130. Wen, D. Y., Bottinni, A. G., Hall, W. A., et al.: The intraventricular use of antibiotics. Neurosurg. Clin. North Am., *3*:343–353, 1992.

131. Yogev, R.: Cerebrospinal fluid shunt infections: A personal view. Pediatr. Infect. Dis., *4*:113–118, 1985.

132. Yogev, R., and Davis, A. T.: Neurosurgical shunt infections: A review. Child's Brain, *6*:74–81, 1980.

133. Younger, J. J., Christiansen, G. D., Bartley, D. L., et al.: Coagulase-negative staphylococci isolated from cerebrospinal fluid shunts: Importance of slime production, species identification and shunt removal to clinical outcome. J. Infect. Dis., *156*:548–554, 1987.

Arachnoid Cysts

The definition "primary (or true) congenital arachnoid cyst" is applied to collections of fluid that develop within the arachnoid membrane because of splitting or duplication of this structure.[149] The definition is meant to differentiate congenital arachnoid cysts from the "secondary" or "false" arachnoid cysts that have been described in the past with a variety of names, such as "leptomeningeal cysts," "chronic cystic arachnoiditis," and "leptomeningitis chronica circumscripta adhaesiva seu cystica."[119] These cysts are, in fact, acquired accumulations of cerebrospinal fluid that result from postinflammatory loculation of the subarachnoid space in patients with head injury, intracranial infection, or hemorrhage; their lining membrane is characterized by the presence of inflammatory cells and hemosiderin deposits.[33, 137, 151, 167, 175]

Similarly, the presence of glial tissue and epithelial cells differentiates the less common glioependymal cysts, which may also develop (although rarely) within the subarachnoid space.[54, 122] As the term *cyst* defines a closed cavity of abnormal origin, arachnoid cysts should be differentiated from congenital or acquired focal dilations of the subarachnoid space that maintain free communications with the natural pathways of the cerebrospinal fluid circulation, such as dilated cisterns, arachnoid pouches, sacs, and diverticula, as well as the cavities that result from cavitation processes of the brain—namely, the porencephalic cavities and the cavities that occur secondary to vascular infarction.

Several aspects of congenital arachnoid cysts have not yet been clarified. First, their differentiation from other intrathecal cystic lesions may be difficult despite the relative ease of recognition presently allowed by the modern diagnostic tools of neuroimaging. Second, the surgical indications as well as the choice of the surgical modalities remain a matter of discussion in many instances, depending on the limited knowledge available on the physiopathogenetic mechanisms and natural history of this specific pathological entity. Further uncertainty is added by the relative unpredictability of the surgical outcome in a significant proportion of cases.

General Survey

According to the most credible physiopathogenetic interpretation, arachnoid cysts originate from a minor aberration in the development of the arachnoid mater that leads to a splitting or duplication of this membrane.[25, 44, 48, 150, 162] The malformative origin is supported by several observations, such as the similar distribution in adults and children (Table 39–1), the occasional occurrence in siblings, the relationship with the cisterns (and, in particular, with the sporadic occurrence in both sylvian cisterns), the presence of accompanying anomalies of the venous architecture (e.g., the absence of the sylvian vein), and association with other congenital anomalies, namely, agenesis of the corpus callosum and Marfan's syndrome.*

Unfortunately, the amount of knowledge regarding the specific developmental anomaly accounting for the formation of arachnoid cysts is very limited. However, it has been propounded that these cysts as well as the arachnoid diverticula could originate either from a defect in the condensation of the primitive mesenchyma, which forms the outer layer of the arachnoid membrane and the dura, or from abnormalities in the flow of the cerebrospinal fluid, which creates the subarachnoid space in the earliest phases of embryogenesis.[64, 116]

Arachnoid cysts are rare, although they may develop anywhere in the subarachnoid space along the cerebro-

---

*See references 24, 28, 35, 39, 58, and 70.

C. Di Rocco

Table 39–1

TOPOGRAPHIC DISTRIBUTION OF INTRACRANIAL ARACHNOID CYSTS

	General Population*		Pediatric Population†	
	No. of Cases	Per Cent	No. of Cases	Per Cent
Supratentorial	161	77	366	77
Sylvian fissure	103	50	162	34
Sellar region	18	9	73	15
Cerebral convexity	9	4	70	15
Interhemispherical fissure	10	5	36	8
Quadrigeminal plate	21	10	25	5
Infratentorial	47	23	112	23
Median	19	9	86	17.5
Cerebellar hemisphere	22	11	24	5
Retroclival	6	3	2	0.5
Total	208		478	

*Data from cases in the literature (1831–1980) collected by Rengachary and Watanabe.[135]
†Data from cases in the literature (1962–1991) collected by Di Rocco and Caldarelli.[39]

spinal axis (Table 39–2). Their reported incidence accounts for only 1 per cent of intracranial space–occupying lesions.[10, 25, 27, 44, 141] However, an apparent relative increase in frequency and a shift in age distribution toward the first years of life have been described in recent years, reflecting the impact of the wide application of computed tomography, magnetic resonance imaging, and ultrasonographic techniques.[39]

In many instances, the recognition of an arachnoid cyst is an incidental finding in asymptomatic subjects examined for head injury or, in infants, for an aspecific macrocrania suggesting an underlying hydrocephalus. The actual low incidence of arachnoid cysts is supported by the correlation between data obtained from the clinical experience (prior to the introduction of computed tomography, magnetic resonance imaging, and ultrasonography) and those obtained from autopsy observations. In 1960, for example, Nagoulitch and Per-

Table 39–2

ANATOMICAL CLASSIFICATION OF ARACHNOID CYSTS

Intracranial Cysts
  Extradural intradiploic cysts
    Supratentorial
    Infratentorial
  Intradural cysts
    Supratentorial
      Sylvian
      Sellar and suprasellar
      Cerebral convexity
      Interhemispherical
      Intraventricular
    Optic nerve
    Quadrigeminal plate
    Infratentorial
      Cerebellar hemisphere
      Midline vermian–cisterna magna
      Cerebellopontine angle
      Intraventricular
      Retroclival
Spinal Cysts
  Extradural cysts
  Intradural cysts

ovitch[114] estimated that only 0.7 per cent of their infant patients with intracranial space–occupying lesions harbored an arachnoid cyst. In the same year, Cassinari and co-workers[23] analyzed 3,706 subjects with an intracranial mass and found only 13 cases of arachnoid cysts—that is, 0.4 per cent. The same incidence (i.e., 0.4 per cent) was subsequently reported by Shuangshoti[159] and by Tamaki and co-workers.[166] On the other hand, in 1977, Shaw and Alvord[158] described only 5 arachnoid cysts in 5,000 human brain and spinal cord specimens (i.e., an incidence of 0.1 per cent). Later, Adam and co-workers[3] reported only 5 arachnoid cysts in 3,000 consecutive fetal and neonatal autopsies; their findings correspond to an incidence of 0.17 per cent. It should be stressed, however, that many arachnoid cysts may remain asymptomatic for several years or for an entire lifetime, depending on their size and location, so they may escape detection; similarly, the thin cyst wall may be easily torn when the brain and the spinal cord are removed in autopsy examinations, precluding correct recognition especially in cases of small lesions.

Arachnoid cysts are nearly always sporadic and single; males are involved in more than two thirds of the cases.[39, 60] The bilateral occurrence of more or less symmetrical cysts has been reported, although rarely, in normal as well as in neurologically impaired children. In the latter instance, especially in patients with bitemporal cysts, the differential diagnosis should be made with lesions resulting from perinatal hypoxia.[70, 142] The great majority of arachnoid cysts are detected in the first two decades of life; the largest proportion of infantile cases is currently recognized during the first 2 years.[39]

The natural history of arachnoid cysts is not well known. Some of these cysts are quiescent throughout life, some remain dormant for many years before showing clinical manifestations, and some even disappear spontaneously, although this last possibility is the exception.[16, 141]

In some cases, however, arachnoid cysts may become symptomatic as they progressively enlarge and interfere with adjacent neural structures or with cerebrospinal fluid circulation. Symptoms and signs include cranial enlargement, localized cranial bulging, clinical manifestations of increased intracranial pressure, epileptic seizures, psychomotor retardation, and focal neurological deficits. Hydrocephalus of either a communicating or an obstructive type is often present. In the elderly, syndromes of dementia with some similarities to those seen in normal-pressure hydrocephalus have also been described.[30, 40, 88]

Distinctive clinical pictures have been reported in relation to the specific localization of the cysts, such as endocrine disorders in patients with cysts in the region of the sella turcica, acute subdural hematomas following minor head injury in patients with cysts localized to the middle cranial fossa, and the so-called "bobble-head doll" syndrome, which is characterized by a to-and-fro bobbing of the head on the trunk first described in two children with cysts in the suprasellar region and in the anterior part of the third ventricle.[18]

The reason why arachnoid cysts actually expand has been the subject of debate for a long time. One hypothesis postulates the existence of an osmotic gradient between the cystic content and the cerebrospinal fluid; this explanation, however, is not supported by the characteristics of the fluid contained in the cysts, which is similar to normal cerebrospinal fluid.[46, 63]

The theories currently accepted to explain the progressive enlargement of arachnoid cysts postulate two principal mechanisms. According to the first theory, an arachnoid cyst may enlarge even when it does not communicate with the subarachnoid space (noncommunicating arachnoid cyst) because of fluid production by the cells that form its wall.[89] Morphological evidence supporting the secretory properties of the cells of the cyst wall has been suggested by the similarity of the cyst lining to the subdural neuroepithelium and to the neuroepithelial lining of arachnoid granulations (e.g., the presence in both of intercellular clefts, desmosomal intercellular junctions, pinocytotic vesicles, multivesicular bodies, lysosomal structures, and basal lamina) as well as by the presence of microvilli on the luminal surface.[45, 64] Enzyme ultracytochemical evidence of the secretory nature of arachnoid cysts has been provided by the demonstration of a structural organization consisting of sodium-potassium adenosine triphosphatases in the plasma membranes that line the cyst cavity and of alkaline phosphatase on the opposite plasma membranes, indicating fluid transport toward the lumen of the cavity.[63, 64]

The second theory (the "ball-valve" hypothesis) postulates the existence of an anatomical communication that acts as a functional one-way valve between the subarachnoid space and the cyst (communicating arachnoid cyst); this communication allows the cerebrospinal fluid to enter the cyst cavity.[160] The pressure gradient for the movement of cerebrospinal fluid into the arachnoid cyst would be ensured by transitory increases in cerebrospinal fluid pressure, especially those increases brought about by cerebral artery systolic oscillations or by pulsations transmitted through the veins.[153, 178] The one-way pulsatile movement of the cerebrospinal fluid into the cyst can be directly demonstrated by magnetic resonance imaging studies, although the mechanism is tenable only in cases in which the intracystic pressure does not exceed the amplitude of the pulse pressure of cerebrospinal fluid.

In recent years, the relationship between arachnoid cysts and normal cerebrospinal fluid pathways has been investigated almost exclusively with computed tomography after intrathecal injection of metrizamide (Fig. 39–1).[87, 94, 146] With this type of investigation, the typical cyst can be easily differentiated because of its low density observed immediately after contrast medium injection into the subarachnoid space. In some cases, however, a partial penetration of the contrast medium into the cyst cavity may be observed after 8 to 12 hours. The cyst content may continue to show an increased density even when the subarachnoid space is no longer enhanced by the metrizamide. In some cases, the cyst is not penetrated by the contrast medium even on delayed scans.[34, 69] Rarely, the contrast agent diffuses within the cyst and the subarachnoid space simultaneously.

According to some authors, rapidly filling cysts do not improve following treatment, whereas slowly filling or noncommunicating cysts behave like expanding lesions, which respond favorably to surgical treatment.[55, 59] It has also been hypothesized that the different morphofunctional patterns of arachnoid cysts might actually correspond to different evolutive stages of the same lesion, when a rapidly filling arachnoid pouch is transformed into a slowly filling or noncommunicating cyst because of the progressive obliteration of the anatomical communication with the subarachnoid space.[59]

The optimal therapy for patients with arachnoid cysts still remains a matter of discussion. Conservative management has been proposed for patients who do not have signs of increased intracranial pressure or of focal neurological deficits.[141] This attitude is supported by cases in which unexpected deterioration and even death occurred following surgical procedures for cyst exploration and excision.[64, 104] The abrupt displacement of brain structures following an excessively rapid decompression of the cyst or postoperative infections and hemorrhages account for these severe complications.[5, 178]

On the other hand, surgical treatment, even in asymptomatic patients, is favored on the basis of observations of intracranial bleeding associated with the presence of an arachnoid cyst that occurred after mild head injury. There is an obvious indication for surgical treatment in patients showing signs of intracranial hypertension that is due either to a progressive enlargement of the cyst or to an associated hydrocephalus or subdural hematoma. Also, surgical intervention should be considered for patients with focal neurological signs or seizure disorders that are possibly related to the presence of the cyst. The goal of surgical treatment is to eliminate the pressure exerted by the lesion, either directly (by excision of the cyst membrane or by opening of the cyst into the subarachnoid space or cerebral ventricles after craniotomy or endoscopic approach) or indirectly (by insertion of a diversionary device for the

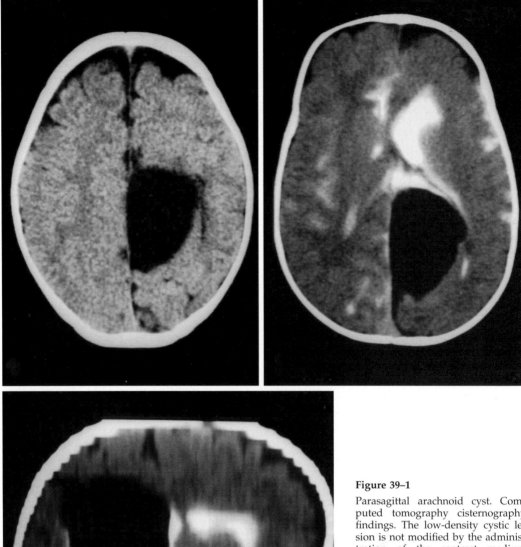

Figure 39–1

Parasagittal arachnoid cyst. Computed tomography cisternography findings. The low-density cystic lesion is not modified by the administration of the contrast medium within the cerebral ventricles and subarachnoid spaces.

shunting of the fluid from the cyst to the peritoneal cavity or, occasionally, to the venous bloodstream).

Total excision of the cyst membrane, which appears to be the most rational treatment in light of the secretory properties of the cyst wall, can unfortunately be accomplished only rarely because of the tight anatomical relationship between this structure and the underlying neural tissue. In some cases, however, extensive (although incomplete) removal of the cyst lining or opening of the cyst suffices to relieve clinical symptoms and is followed by a volumetric reduction of the cyst on postoperative computed tomography scans.

Failure of the operation and recurrence of the cyst after direct excision of its membrane have been re-ported to occur at a rate of approximately 25 per cent.[71, 110] This relatively high recurrence rate, which may result from an excessively limited excision of the cyst wall, from secondary obliteration of the artificial opening, or from insufficient absorption of cerebrospinal fluid within the subarachnoid space, has led some neurosurgeons to prefer shunting of the cyst fluid, a procedure that could eventually be combined with ventriculoperitoneal shunting for an associated hydrocephalus.[61, 163] The main advantages of a shunting procedure are its technical feasibility and its low morbidity and mortality rates, even in very young patients. Furthermore, such an operation is apt to ensure a more gradual reduction in volume of the cyst. Disadvantages include the well-known complications of cerebrospinal fluid shunts, such as mechanical complications and infections.[29]

Intracranial Arachnoid Cysts

Arachnoid cysts that develop within the intracranial compartment may range in size from a few centimeters in diameter to huge sacs that occupy half of the skull compartment and cause significant distortion and displacement of the underlying nervous structures. The typical location of intracranial cysts is intradural, with the possible exception of those arachnoid malformations that may be found in the diploë of the skull, in the orbit, in the epicranial space, or in the midline posterior parietal region at the level of the obelion[86, 174] (see Table 39–2). Only rarely do intracranial arachnoid cysts develop in sites anatomically unrelated to the cerebral cisterns, such as the optic nerve, the sulci of the cerebral convexity, and the cerebral ventricles.

The pathogenesis of the intraventricular arachnoid cysts is a matter of debate. For some authors, in fact, these cysts represent a kind of "internal" meningocele; for others, they derive from the arachnoid layer transported along with the vascular mesenchyme when it invaginates through the choroidal fissure.[50, 105, 117]

Most commonly, intracranial arachnoid cysts maintain an anatomical relationship with the cisterns and apparently originate from a maldevelopment process of these spaces. Indeed, the huge cysts of the cerebral convexity may also be considered extensions of the cisternal spaces of the sylvian or of the interhemispheric fissures. The sylvian cistern represents the most frequent localization, whereas the clival region is the rarest. Some age-related differences exist, such as the higher incidence of the suprasellar and cerebral convexity cysts found in children and the major frequency of the lateral localization of the infratentorial cysts detected in adults (see Table 39–1).

Since the intracranial arachnoid cysts manifest clinical signs and symptoms according to the site of their development, these lesions are usually classified on the basis of their topographical localization (Table 39–2). From a practical point of view, however, the intradiploic, the optic nerve, the intraventricular, and the retroclival arachnoid cysts are of relatively little interest because of their rare occurrence.[21] In contrast, the other subgroups fall into typical clinical patterns, and each requires a specific approach for establishing the surgical indication and selecting the surgical modality.

SUPRATENTORIAL ARACHNOID CYSTS

Sylvian Fissure Cysts

The sylvian fissure represents the most common location of supratentorial arachnoid cysts, accounting alone for about one half of adult and one third of pediatric cases (see Table 39–1). These cysts are frequently small or medium in size. However, they can increase to a large volume, opening the fissure and exposing the entire insula as well as the main trunk and branches of the middle cerebral artery (Fig. 39–2). As a result, the anterior superior surface of the temporal lobe may become severely compressed or may be underdeveloped in patients with huge lesions, a finding once incorrectly termed "temporal lobe

Figure 39–2

Sylvian fissure arachnoid cyst on computed tomography and magnetic resonance imaging examinations. The frontal and the temporal lobes are compressed and divaricated by the lesion. The subarachnoid space over the convexity of the homolateral cerebral hemisphere are barely recognizable. The lateral cerebral ventricle is slightly compressed and controlaterally deviated together with the midline structures.

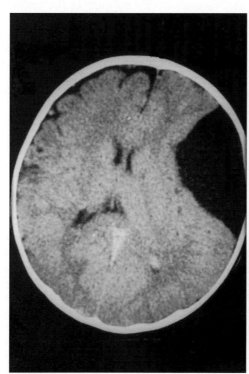
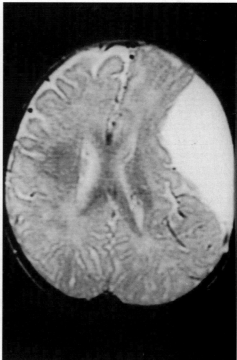

agenesis."[140, 157] The posterior inferior surface of the frontal lobe is also frequently involved by cysts that extend anteriorly and deeply toward the temporal fossa and the chiasmatic region (Fig. 39–3). Very rarely, these cysts develop bilaterally in both temporal regions.

Sylvian fissure cysts may manifest clinically at any age, but they become symptomatic more frequently in children and adolescents than in adults; in most series, infants and toddlers account for about one fourth of cases.[25] Males are approximately threefold more frequently affected than are females, and the left hemisphere is more commonly involved than is the right hemisphere.[57, 148] Headache, although seldom severe, is the most common presenting symptom. Mild proptosis is also a common complaint; controlateral motor weakness may be noted in advanced cases. In about 20 to 25 per cent of patients, arachnoid cysts of the sylvian fissure are revealed by focal or generalized seizures or by signs of increased intracranial pressure.

Mental impairment is rare, being found in only 10 per cent of cases; however, developmental delay is common in children with large lesions and is nearly constant and severe in subjects with bilateral cysts.[70] Facial pain has occasionally been described.[106] A localized bulging of the skull in the temporal region is a characteristic feature in one half of patients (see Fig. 39–3). In very young subjects, however, an asymmetrical macrocrania is more often observed. Skull anomalies are easily detected by standard x-ray examinations as well as by computed tomography of the skull, which demonstrates the outward bulging and thinning of the temporal squama and the elevation and anterior displacement of the lesser and greater wings of the sphenoid bone.[156, 160] On computed tomography scans, these cysts appear as well-defined lesions between the dura and the distorted brain, with the same density as cerebrospinal fluid and without contrast enhancement[11, 94] (see Fig. 39–3). The homolateral cerebral ventricle can be compressed or slightly displaced controlaterally; however, the cerebral ventricles usually are of normal size or only minimally dilated. Small and medium-sized lesions frequently show a biconvex or semicircular shape. With relatively large cysts, the sylvian fissure assumes a square configuration because of the compression of the adjacent frontal and temporal lobes and of the insula.[92]

When examined with metrizamide-enhanced computed tomography cisternography, sylvian fissure arachnoid cysts are characterized by different patterns of contrast medium penetration, which vary from the immediate filling and rapid clearance of the cyst cavity to the progressive accumulation of contrast medium and subsequent delayed clearance. According to Galassi and associates,[55, 56] a reverse relationship exists between middle fossa arachnoid cysts and the presence and ease of an anatomofunctional communication with the normal subarachnoid spaces. The authors differentiated three subgroups of increasing severity based on the computed tomography appearance and the cisternography findings. Type 1 cysts, which are the mildest form, are small, biconvex, or semicircular and are

confined to the anterior aspect of the temporal fossa. They are accompanied by negligible mass effect because of the free and rapid communication with the basal cisterns. Type 2 cysts, which are medium-sized and roughly triangular or quadrangular lesions with frequent but moderate mass effect, involve the anterior and middle portions of the temporal fossa and extend upward opening the sylvian fissure. These cysts fill with water-soluble contrast medium relatively late on computed tomography cisternography. Finally, type 3 cysts are large, roundish or oval lesions that occupy the middle cranial fossa almost entirely, effecting constant and severe compression of the adjacent nervous structures and eventually causing ventricular displacement and midline shift. The penetration of these cysts by contrast medium is absent or very much delayed because of the absent or functionally inadequate communication with normal cerebrospinal fluid pathways.

In the past, cerebral angiography contributed to the diagnosis by demonstrating specific dislocations of the main trunk and branches of the middle cerebral artery (in contrast with the hypoplasia of these vessels in the case of temporal lobe congenital dysplasia or acquired atrophia) as well as changes in the pattern of the temporal veins' drainage into the sphenoid sinus.[68, 148] Cerebral angiography has been replaced by magnetic resonance angiography (Fig. 39–4). When combined with surface anatomy scanning, magnetic resonance imaging may show the veins in relation to the cyst as maintaining their normal position near the inner face of the dura mater and may evidence, when present, the small abnormal arteries that run in some cases over the cyst wall. The demonstration of these abnormal arteries is particularly helpful in establishing surgical indication because these fragile vessels, which are draped over the outer membrane of the cyst and lack the support of the cerebral parenchyma (see Fig. 39–3), may easily be torn even in the event of minor head trauma. Indeed, although sylvian fissure arachnoid cysts may remain asymptomatic throughout a patient's life, they can show an acute increase in volume because of subdural or intracystic bleeding.[61, 98] Actually, a subdural hematoma is the most typical complication, occurring with relatively high frequency in association with these cysts and only rarely with cysts located in the other preferential intracranial sites.[13, 49]

Because of the unsatisfactory results of surgical methods that are limited to puncturing of the cyst through a burr hole, sylvian fissure arachnoid cysts are managed with essentially one of two main operative procedures: (1) excision of the cyst membranes, and (2) placement of a cystoperitoneal shunt. Sometimes, both procedures are combined in the same patient.

Resection of a cyst should be carried out through a frontotemporal craniotomy, with the complete exposure and, possibly, total removal of the outer membrane. The need to remove the inner membrane of the cyst is not universally accepted; in several cases, it has been possible to visualize the free movement of cerebrospinal fluid within the subarachnoid space underneath the membrane during the operation.[148] Direct excision of a cyst's linings, either the outer or both the

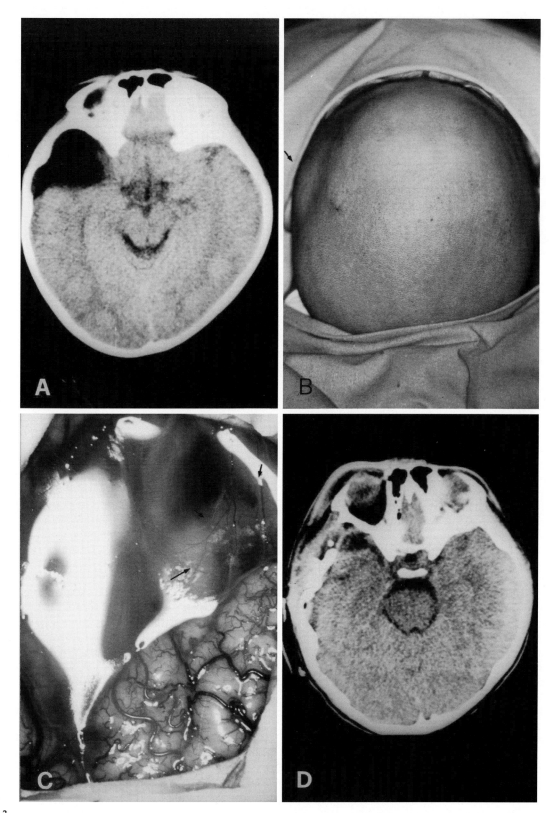

Figure 39–3

Sylvian fissure arachnoid cyst. Computed tomography demonstrates the lesion and its effect on the adjacent parenchymal and osseous structures. *A.* The greater sphenoid wing is anteriorly displaced. *B.* The bulging of the temporal bone *(arrow)* is apparent on physical inspection. *C.* The cyst wall with fine vessels *(arrows)* extends between the compressed temporal and frontal lobes. *D.* The re-expansion of the temporal pole is demonstrated by the postoperative computed tomography study.

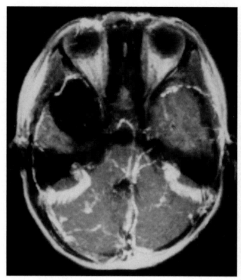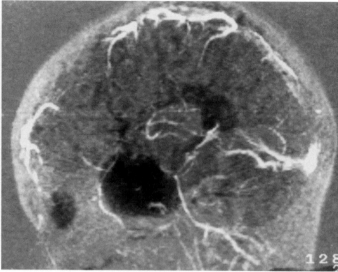

Figure 39–4

Axial and sagittal views of magnetic resonance imaging angiography superimposed on T1-weighted images of an arachnoid cyst of the sylvian fissure. Note the abnormal temporal venous pattern. (Courtesy of Dr. Y. Yamanouchi, Kansai University, Osaka, Japan.)

outer and the inner membranes, is often followed by reaccumulation of fluid after a variable period of time.[171] The recurrence rate diminishes when wide and multiple communications are made between the residual cyst cavity and the basal cisterns following opening of the arachnoid membrane at the incisura (Fig. 39–5). When this communication is inadequate, the cystic cavity may re-expand merely because of the accumulation of cerebrospinal fluid. In fact, the physiological direction of the cerebrospinal fluid circulation from the basal cisterns to the sylvian fissure may favor an imbalance between inflow and outflow of the fluid, with secondary accumulation within the cystic cavity.

A cystoperitoneal shunt alone offers a valid alternative to the direct operative approach by ensuring the outflow of fluid from the cyst and by decreasing the intracystic pressure, thus allowing the adjacent cerebral tissue to re-expand.[101] Some authors suggest combining the shunt procedure with the excision of the outer cyst membrane to prevent this membrane, which easily detaches from the dura mater after a shunt insertion, from plugging the shunt tube.[148] The possibility of episodes of intracranial hypertension following the shunting of a cyst has been pointed out; such episodes are apparently due to the same disturbances in cerebrospinal fluid dynamics that characterize pseudotumor cerebri syndromes.[102]

The treatment of asymptomatic arachnoid cysts of the sylvian fissure that are detected incidentally by computed tomography still remains very controversial, and a conservative attitude is often adopted, especially in patients with small lesions. A contribution to the surgical indication in asymptomatic patients may be provided by magnetic resonance imaging of those in whom the signal intensity of the cyst is greater than that of the cerebrospinal fluid, suggesting the presence of a previous, clinically unnoticed intracystic hemorrhage.

Sellar Region Cysts

Arachnoid cysts of the chiasmatic region are usually divided into two groups: (1) the suprasellar cysts that develop above the diaphragma sellae, and (2) the intrasellar cysts that are found within the sellar cavity. The latter are far less frequent than the former and are practically absent in children. Indeed, the mean age at clinical presentation for this type of lesion has been calculated to be around 42.2 years.[15]

On the other hand, the suprasellar variety may be regarded as a typical condition of pediatric patients. In 1982, for example, Hoffman and co-workers, reporting on a personal series of 8 cases and on 46 cases collected from the literature, found that about one sixth of the patients were infants younger than 1 year of age, one half were younger than 5 years of age, and only 13 per cent of the subjects were older than 20 years of age.[78] With the advent of computed tomography and ultrasonography, the mean age at diagnosis has become significantly lower, so that in our series of 15 children operated on in the last 10 years, the great majority of patients who were treated (78 per cent) were younger than 1 year of age. It is worth noting that in 2 of the 15 cases, the diagnosis was made in utero. A further consequence of the widespread use of the modern diagnostic techniques of neuroimaging is the relative increase in the incidence of sellar region cysts; in fact, these cysts, once regarded as rare, currently represent the second most common group among supratentorial intracranial arachnoid cysts.[66, 176] Affected males slightly outnumber females, with a male-to-female ratio of about one and one half to one.[125]

Intrasellar arachnoid cysts should not be confused with the so-called "empty sella" syndrome, which is secondary to an extension of the chiasmatic cistern into the sellar cavity because of either an abnormally large hiatus or of an excessively low attachment of the dia-

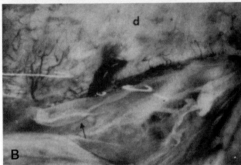

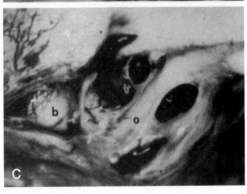

Figure 39–5

Operative findings in left sylvian fissure arachnoid cyst. *A* and *B*. After removal of the outer cyst membrane, the basal lining of the cyst *(arrows)* is detached from the dura (d) of the temporal cranial fossa. *C.* Additional openings are then made in the arachnoid close to the tentorial notch to improve fluid circulation. b, brain stem; o, oculomotor nerve.

phragma sellae below the level of the clinoid processes. Likewise, intrasellar arachnoid cysts should be differentiated from intrasellar diverticula of a normal arachnoid membrane that has herniated through the diaphragma sellae, allowing the progressive accumulation of cerebrospinal fluid within the sella turcica by means of a flap-valve mechanism. True intrasellar arachnoid cysts are thought to originate from a duplication of the arachnoid membrane from arachnoid remnants below the diaphragma sellae or, alternatively, from the arachnoid membrane that has herniated through the diaphragma sellae and lost its anatomical relationship with the intracranial subarachnoid space.[73, 139] In contrast to intrasellar arachnoid diverticula, contrast medium injected into the subarachnoid space very rarely enters intrasellar arachnoid cysts, even when the "hanging head" position is utilized during the examination. However, a pinhole communication of the cyst with the subarachnoid space has been demonstrated in some patients at surgery.[15, 79]

Intrasellar arachnoid cysts are usually located outside the pituitary gland at the level of the pars distalis or immediately below the dura mater. They develop within the sella turcica, compressing the hypophysis, inducing ballooning and posterior bowing of the sellar

contour, and displacing the diaphragma sellae upward. This last structure, however, remains intact even in the presence of a large suprasellar extension[14, 15] (Fig. 39–6). About one half of intrasellar arachnoid cysts are discovered incidentally in patients who were found to have anomalies of the sella turcica on x-ray examinations carried out after minor head trauma or because of endocrinological disturbances. Headache is the most common complaint. Magnified high-resolution computed tomography reconstruction of the sellar region in the coronal and sagittal planes is particularly helpful in establishing a diagnosis. Treatment consists mainly of transsphenoidal drainage of the lesion, followed by packing of the residual cavity with muscular tissue or dura substitution materials and by reconstruction of the floor of the sella turcica with nasal cartilage.

Usually, suprasellar arachnoid cysts expand in all directions; laterally, they can grow into one or both temporal fossae and posteriorly into the interpeduncular and prepontine cisterns, behind the clivus. When these lesions develop upward in the direction of the third ventricle, they gradually replace the space occupied by this structure, pushing its floor upward (Fig. 39–7). Hydrocephalus, which is commonly associated with this type of lesion, ensues when the foramina of

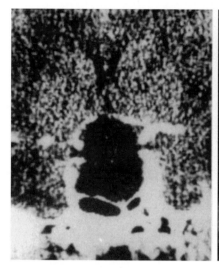
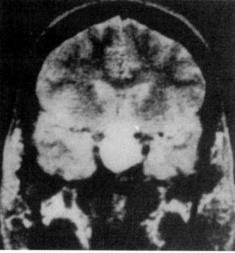

Figure 39–6

Intrasellar arachnoid cyst. Computed tomography and magnetic resonance imaging findings.

Monro or the basal cisterns, or both, are obstructed because of the cyst's enlargement.[116, 134]

A further impairment in cerebrospinal fluid circulation may be caused by the posterior dislocation of the midbrain, with secondary compression of the aqueduct of Sylvius (see Fig. 39–7). However, the obstructive nature of the ventricular dilation that accompanies suprasellar arachnoid cysts is questioned by some authors, who consider the possibility of a common maldevelopmental process accounting for both the formation of the arachnoid cyst and the hydrocephalus.[20] A significant proportion of suprasellar arachnoid cysts communicate with the subarachnoid space, and a ball-valve mechanism is presumed to account for their enlargement.[78] These cysts should be differentiated from di-

verticula of the arachnoid membrane of Liliequist, which develop upward and forward when the permeability of the membrane is altered by previous infection or by hemorrhage.[53] Besides the clinical manifestations of hydrocephalus, the symptoms of suprasellar arachnoid cysts include visual impairment and endocrine dysfunction.[113]

Most of the suprasellar arachnoid cysts that occur in children are found in subjects with enlarged heads, growth retardation, and possibly delayed psychomotor development.[42] In about one third of cases, the optic nerves and the chiasma may be stretched over the cyst wall, with variable resultant effects of visual impairment such as unilateral or bilateral decrease in visual acuity or bitemporal hemianopsia, or both. Endocrino-

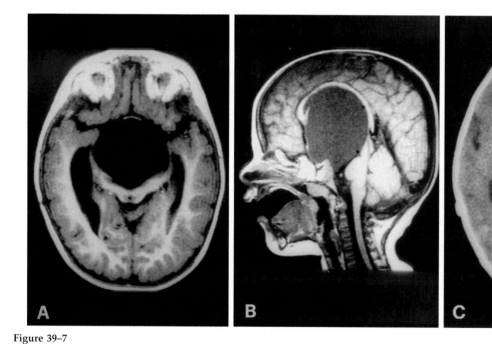
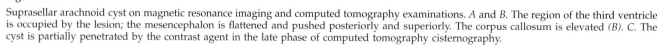

Figure 39–7

Suprasellar arachnoid cyst on magnetic resonance imaging and computed tomography examinations. A and B. The region of the third ventricle is occupied by the lesion; the mesencephalon is flattened and pushed posteriorly and superiorly. The corpus callosum is elevated (B). C. The cyst is partially penetrated by the contrast agent in the late phase of computed tomography cisternography.

logical disturbances are due to stretching and eventual disruption of the pituitary stalk and to compression of the inferomedial portions of the thalami, the tuber cinereum, and the mamillary bodies (Figs. 39–7 and 39–8). Growth retardation and isosexual precocious puberty represent the most common clinical manifestations of such endocrinopathy.[50, 129] However, in older children and adolescents, hypopituitarism is more frequently observed.[25, 42]

A typical but rare presentation is the so-called "bobble-head doll" syndrome.[6] The definition of the syndrome derives from the characteristic irregular and involuntary movements of the head, which occur in an anteroposterior direction two or three times per second and resemble those of dolls with a weighted head resting on a coiled spring.[18, 36] The to-and-fro bobbing of the head (and, in some cases, of the trunk) characterizes patients when they stand, whereas it is usually absent during sleep. The rhythmic movements can be interrupted voluntarily for only short periods of time. The syndrome, nearly always described in the pediatric age group, affects boys more frequently than girls, with a ratio of incidence of two to one.[83] Its pathogenesis is not well understood, although it has been attributed to the abnormal pressure exerted by the cyst on the third ventricle and on the dorsomedial nucleus of the thalamus.[147] Finally, in some patients, as in other patients with hydrocephalus, suprasellar arachnoid cysts may be clinically manifested by gait ataxia.[78] Computed tomography has currently replaced all the diagnostic tools previously utilized for the diagnosis, such as plain skull x-ray examination (J-shaped sella turcica), isotopic brain scanning (silent areas or areas of increased uptake), ventriculography (upward displacement of the floor of the third ventricle, and upward and backward displacement of the aqueduct), air encephalography (lack of visualization of the suprasellar portion of the chiasmatic cistern), and cerebral angiography (lateralization of the internal carotid arteries, elevation of the horizontal portions of the anterior cerebral arteries, enlargement of the circle of Willis, elevation and backward displacement of the internal cerebral veins, and elevation of the basal vein of Rosenthal).[84] The typical image of a suprasellar arachnoid

cyst on computed tomography scanning is a smooth, oval or round water-dense lesion in the region of the third ventricle, which, together with the superimposed frontal horns of the lateral cerebral ventricles, characteristically resembles the head of a rabbit in some patients[84, 113] (Fig. 39–7C). The differential diagnosis should be made with other possible cystic lesions of the region, such as Rathke's cleft cysts, cystic craniopharyngiomas, epidermoid cysts, and cystic gliomas, as well as with a dilated third ventricle.[87, 93] The differential diagnosis with a dilated third ventricle seen on computed tomography may be obtained with metrizamide-enhanced ventriculography. In patients in whom the aqueduct is not completely obstructed, the injection of metrizamide at the lumbar level may rapidly visualize the subarachnoid spaces and the ventricular system, outlining the negative image of the cyst. In the late stages of the examination (8 to 12 hours), a kind of inversion of the computed tomography image occurs as the contrast medium disappears from the subarachnoid space while the density of the fluid inside the lesion increases. After 24 hours, the contrast agent also disappears from inside the cystic cavity.[111, 146]

Magnetic resonance imaging is of great assistance in the recognition and differential diagnosis of suprasellar arachnoid cysts. Furthermore, the technique offers the advantage of multiplanar imaging. In particular, the sagittal images provide the best evaluation of the relationship between the cyst and the third ventricle that is necessary for planning the surgical treatment (see Fig. 39–7). During prenatal life, in the neonatal period, and during infancy, ultrasonography may further contribute to the diagnosis and the evaluation of the modification that is eventually to be induced by surgical treatment (Fig. 39–9).

At the time of this writing, there is no agreement on the best method for operative treatment of suprasellar arachnoid cysts. This is demonstrated by the availability of a variety of surgical options, from the simple bypass shunting of the cysts or the associate hydrocephalus, or both, to the resection of the cyst wall following craniotomy. The shunting of the associated hydrocephalus alone has been practically abandoned because in most patients the induced reduction in size

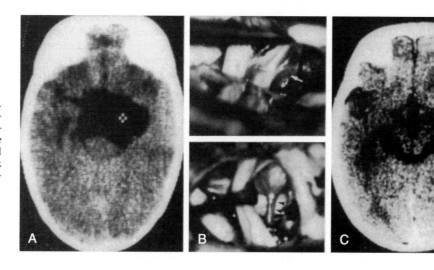

Figure 39–8
Suprasellar arachnoid cyst. *A.* Preoperative computed tomography scan. *B.* Intraoperative findings. Note the cyst displacing the optic nerves upward *(arrows)* and the hypoplastic pituitary stalk *(arrowheads). C.* Postoperative computed tomography scan.

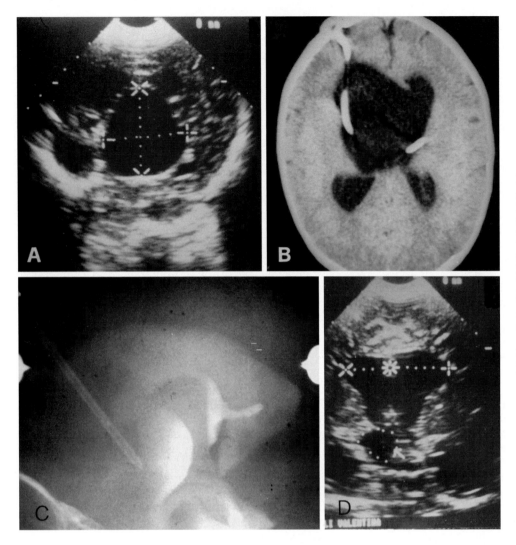

Figure 39–9

Suprasellar arachnoid cyst. *A.* Preoperative ultrasound examination demonstrates the cyst occupying the region of the third ventricle. *B.* A drainage catheter inserted percutaneously fails to penetrate the cyst wall, sliding over the cystic lesion and stopping within the opposite lateral ventricle. Stereotactic placement of a catheter draining from the cyst and from the lateral ventricle *(C)* is followed by the reduction in size of the cyst, as demonstrated by the postoperative ultrasound study *(D).*

of the cerebral ventricles does not modify the volume or the shape of the cyst itself, and in others it is even followed by the progressive enlargement of the lesion.[93, 125] In several instances, however, the shunting of the associated hydrocephalus is required after the excision of the cyst or the fenestration of its wall. In such cases, the persistence of the hydrocephalus may be the result of incomplete removal of the cyst membrane, with the persistence of a residual obstacle in cerebrospinal fluid circulation, or it may reflect a generalized defect in cerebrospinal fluid absorption, which cannot be cured by the simple elimination of the cyst.

The direct shunting of the cyst offers the great advantage of being a relatively safe surgical procedure in comparison with the more complex operations that require craniotomy.[72, 127] The operation, however, is accompanied by a surprisingly high percentage of failure owing to improper placement of the cranial catheter, which may easily slide over the elastic cyst membrane to accidentally penetrate the adjacent ventricular system (see Fig. 39–9), or because of the catheter's subsequent occlusion.[127, 132] Stereotactic techniques may facilitate the correct placement of the catheter into the cyst cavity or allow the simultaneous shunting of the lesion and the associated hydrocephalus by means of a cisto-

ventriculoperitoneal shunt[72] (see Fig. 39–9). Other authors have suggested that a separate tube be left in the residual cavity after the direct excision of the cyst membrane; this tube could be either connected to the ventricular system or joined to a pre-existing ventriculoperitoneal shunt by means of a Y-connector.[84]

The advantage of easier exposure of the cyst by prior insertion of a cerebrospinal fluid shunt device before the direct surgical management of the lesion has been stressed by some authors.[129] However, the direct excision, fenestration, or marsupialization of suprasellar arachnoid cysts by means of either a subfrontal, transventricular, transcallosal, or, less commonly, temporal approach is mainly favored because of the possibility of avoiding shunt dependency.[78, 129] In fact, percentages of subjects with suprasellar arachnoid cysts as high as 75 per cent have been reported to be cured by this type of treatment in the absence of an associated hydrocephalus.[127] Unfortunately, the recurrence of the lesion after marsupialization or fenestration procedures is quite common, especially in subjects with associated ventricular dilation. The cause of the complication has received two interpretations: (1) insufficient aggressiveness of the surgeon, and (2) the relative inability of the chiasmatic region to accommodate the diversion of fluid from inside the cyst.[38, 127] Hoffman and co-workers[78] have stressed the good results obtained with the use of a transcallosal approach to open the dome of the cyst into one of the lateral ventricles. The experience has been confirmed by Pierre-Kahn and co-workers,[125] who have adopted a procedure of percutaneous ventriculocistotomy performed under ventriculoscopic guidance. According to these authors, the intracranial pressure improved in their patients after the operation, despite the fact that in several instances the cyst was only partially reduced in size and that the cerebral ventricles remained larger than normal.

It should be noted that the symptoms of the bobble-head doll syndrome tend to persist even after surgical opening of a suprasellar arachnoid cyst in the majority of the patients; however, a few successful cases of the disappearance of the symptoms have been reported.[6, 178]

Cerebral Convexity Cysts

When confined to the surface of the cerebral hemispheres, arachnoid cysts may vary in size, from small lesions that compress the underlying brain and produce localized bulging of the skull, to huge lesions that extend over the hemisphere, dislocate the entire brain contralaterally, and cause asymmetrical cranial enlargement. These lesions differ from the arachnoid cysts localized in other intracranial regions because of their apparent lack of any anatomical relationship with a cisternal space. Also, their incidence is low,[25, 103] with females more frequently affected than males.

Arachnoid cysts overlying the cerebral cortex may be grossly subdivided into two main varieties that differ in their morphology, age distribution, and clinical manifestations; intermediate forms do exist but are rare. The first variety, *hemispherical cysts,* is represented by those huge fluid collections that extend over most or all of the surface of one cerebral hemisphere. The cerebral parenchyma and the lateral cerebral ventricle are compressed and contralaterally dislocated (Fig. 39–10). These cysts have been considered to be extreme extensions of sylvian fissure cysts, but they are not accompanied by any sign of temporal lobe aplasia and are characterized by a compressed rather than an enlarged sylvian fissure. In infants with macrocrania, the differential diagnosis of hemispherical arachnoid cysts

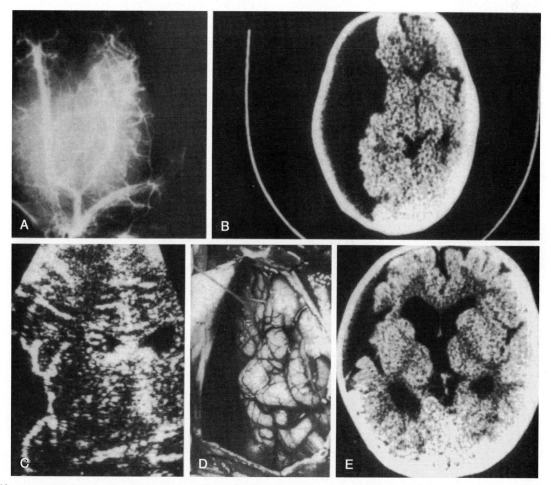

Figure 39–10

Left cerebral convexity arachnoid cyst. *A, B,* and *C.* Angiography, computed tomography, and ultrasonography findings. Note the mass effect of the cyst, the normal vascular supply of the underlying cerebral hemisphere, and the normal size of the lateral cerebral ventricles. *D.* After removal of the outer membrane of the cyst, its inner membrane is cautiously detached from the cerebral cortex. *E.* The postoperative computed tomography scan shows a partial re-expansion of the left cerebral hemisphere.

with unilateral subdural hygroma or chronic hematoma may be difficult clinically. However, infants with chronic subdural fluid collections are commonly symptomatic, although the clinical picture can be rather aspecific (failure to thrive, irritability, seizures, and psychomotor retardation). Computed tomography and magnetic resonance imaging allow differentiation of the two entities in nearly all cases. On computed tomography, the density of the hematoma, inferior or equal to that of the cerebral parenchyma because of the increased protein content, differs from the waterlike density of an arachnoid cyst. On magnetic resonance imaging, the high signal intensity of the hematoma on recovery sequences is characteristically different from the signal of cerebrospinal fluid and is similar to the signal of an arachnoid cyst. The flattening of the cerebral cortex in cases of chronic subdural hematoma, in contrast with the almost normal outline of this structure in cases of hemispherical arachnoid cyst, is the most typical differentiating feature on ultrasound examination (see Fig. 39–10).

The second variety, *focal cysts,* comprises small-sized lesions, the presence of which is usually suggested by a localized bulging of the skull (Fig. 39–11). The bone deformity suggests a long-standing process that probably began in early infancy; usually, it does not present any differential characteristic when compared with other osteolytic calvarial lesions. Even after the advent of computed tomography, the differential diagnosis with grade I cerebral gliomas can be difficult, especially when it is considered that both conditions may be clinically manifested by seizure disorder. Magnetic resonance imaging, however, does generally allow the correct diagnosis.

Clinical manifestations of cerebral convexity cysts vary in children and adults. In the pediatric group, a localized bulging of the skull without any accompanying signs of neurological dysfunction is the most frequent presenting sign of small or medium-sized lesions. Focal neurological signs are remarkably absent, even in children with large cysts, such as those that occupy the entire hemicranium. These patients surprisingly have only a cranial asymmetry, as the hemicranium harboring the cysts is obviously larger than the contralateral one. The characteristic cranial deformity, together with a normal findings on neurological examination, clearly differentiates children with cerebral convexity cysts from those with hemiaplasia cerebri caused by an arrest in the development of one carotid artery and its branches. In the case of hemispherical arachnoid cysts, cerebral angiography confirms the normal vascular supply to the brain and clearly demonstrates the mass effect of the lesion because of the contralateral displacement of the middle and anterior cerebral arteries together with the deep cerebral veins (see Fig. 39–10).

In adults, arachnoid cysts of the cerebral surface are often symptomatic and are manifested by signs of intracranial hypertension, epilepsy, and neurological deficits.[19, 62] These cysts can extend into underlying cerebral cortex, which may show secondary atrophic changes. Skull x-ray films are usually normal. Computed tomography scanning demonstrates rounded lesions with the same density as the cerebrospinal fluid but without the characteristic loculations typical of post-traumatic cysts.[144] Cerebral convexity cysts are generally treated following craniotomy that exposes the entire lesion as far as its point of contact with the normal cortex so as to ensure both the extensive excision of the outer cystic membrane and the ability to make an additional opening into the basal cisterns, if required (Fig. 39–12; see also Fig. 39–10).

Usually, it is not necessary to attempt removal of the medial cystic wall, which is intimately connected with the underlying cerebral cortex. In many subjects, the operation suffices to eliminate the lesion and allow the

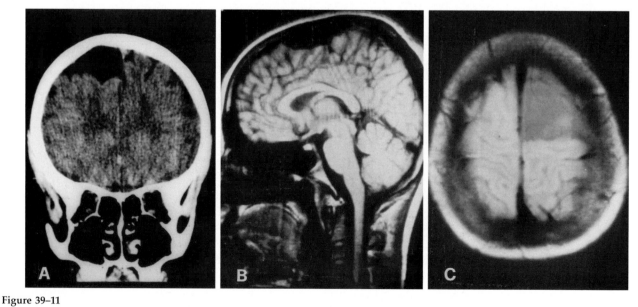

Figure 39–11

Cortical arachnoid cyst. *A.* Computed tomography demonstrates that the inner table of the skull is mildly deformed by the underlying cystic lesion. *B* and *C.* The mass effect of the cyst on the adjacent cerebral parenchyma is well evidenced by magnetic resonance imaging.

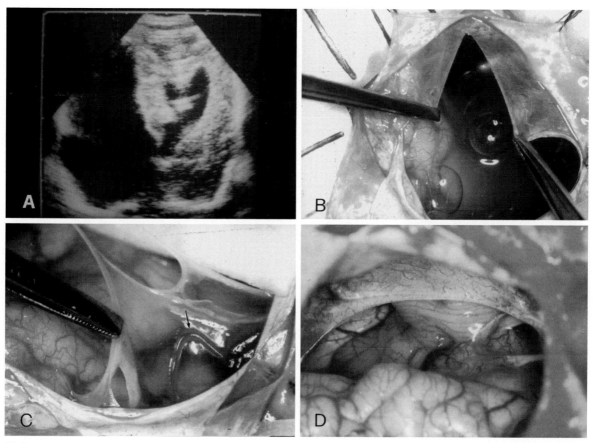

Figure 39–12

Hemispheric arachnoid cyst. Ultrasound preoperative examination *(A)* and intraoperative findings *(B, C,* and *D). C.* Note the abnormal vessel on the cyst lining *(arrow). D.* After cyst removal, the cerebellum and the brain stem as well as the fifth, sixth, seventh, and eighth cranial nerves are visualized.

local re-expansion of the cerebral parenchyma (see Fig. 39–10); however, in some subjects, especially in those with hemispheric arachnoid cyst, the circulation of the cerebrospinal fluid may remain relatively impaired despite the large excision of the cystic membrane and the multiple communications that can be made at the borders of the cyst (where the apparent reflexion or splitting of the arachnoid membrane has occurred). In such patients, reaccumulation of fluid over the cerebral hemisphere can be observed and favored in some cases by the incomplete re-expansion of the compressed cerebral parenchyma. The insertion of a shunt device from the residual cavity to the peritoneal cavity is believed to aid the re-expansion of the hemisphere and counteract the reaccumulation of fluid.

Interhemispherical Fissure Cysts

Arachnoid cysts that develop between the two hemispheres are defined by their anatomical relationship with the corpus callosum. In fact, the partial or complete agenesis of the corpus callosum is the only element that makes possible the classification of these cysts into two main varieties: (1) *interhemispherical cysts,* which are associated with a partial or complete agenesis of the corpus callosum (Fig. 39–13), and (2) *parasagittal cysts,* which are not accompanied by a defect in the

formation of the corpus callosum[120, 131] (Fig. 39–14; see also Fig. 39–1). It is unclear whether the occurrence of an interhemispherical cyst and the agenesis of the corpus callosum are causally related.[109, 126] Indeed, the hypothesis of a mechanical interference exerted by the cyst in the development of the midline commissure is contradicted by observations of patients in whom the complete agenesis of the corpus callosum is not accompanied by the formation of arachnoid cysts or is associated only with a lesion of minimal size.[135, 179] When the main interhemispherical commissure is partially developed, it determines the direction of growth of parasagittal cysts, allowing further subdivision into anterior, middle, and posterior varieties. The anterior cysts expand toward the cisterna laminae terminalis, and the posterior may reach the quadrigeminal cistern or develop around the splenium into the cavum veli interpositi. In some cases, the interhemispherical cysts expand into both the supratentorial and the infratentorial compartments, and they may occupy the cistern of the superior cerebellar vermis.

A very rare variety of interhemispherical arachnoid cyst that develops between the two folds of the dura forming the falx cerebri is the *interhemispherical intradural cyst.* It is believed to originate from the arachnoid that penetrates the dural sinuses at various places in the form of arachnoid villi.[76, 131] However, most authors

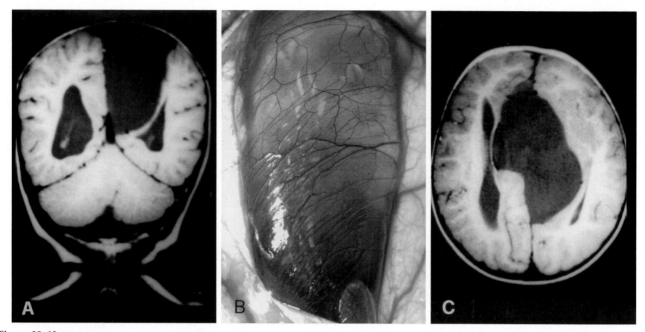

Figure 39–13

Interhemispherical arachnoid cyst. Magnetic resonance imaging *(A and C)* and intraoperative aspect *(B)*. The cyst lining, with its fine vessels, extends between the two cerebral hemispheres on both sides of the midline. The lateral cerebral ventricles are compressed and laterally dislocated *(A and C)*.

prefer to consider *epicranial arachnoid cysts,* which occur at the skull midline and usually in the parietal region, as a variant of meningoceles rather than as true interhemispherical cysts, even though these lesions are histologically arachnoid malformations.[86, 107]

The actual incidence of interhemispherical fissure cysts is not known, but these lesions are apparently rare; their relative incidence in all age groups and in pediatric patients is approximately 5 per cent and 8 per cent, respectively (see Table 39–1).

Despite the large dimensions that interhemispherical fissure cysts may reach in the course of time, their symptomatology can remain surprisingly poor.[27, 100] In many cases, in fact, the diagnosis is established incidentally. A spreading over of the medial side of the homolateral cerebral hemispheres, rather than a disruption of the fibers that normally pass the midline at the third month of fetal life, is thought to account for the absence or very low incidence of neurological deficits in patients with interhemispherical cysts and agenesis of the corpus callosum. In a large proportion of patients, macrocrania is the presenting sign; however, clinical manifestations of increased intracranial pressure are present in only about two thirds of cases.

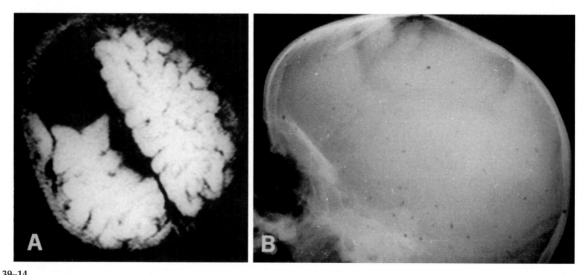

Figure 39–14

Parasagittal arachnoid cyst. *A.* Magnetic resonance imaging examination shows the cyst confined between the falx and the cerebral hemisphere. *B.* The erosion of the skull above the cystic lesion is evidenced by the skull x-ray film. Note the presence of a catheter draining from the cyst.

Localized bulging of the skull, although not so apparent and sharply radiologically defined as that of sylvian fissure arachnoid cysts, is the second most common finding (see Fig. 39–14). Hydrocephalus is mild or even absent in subjects with parasagittal cysts; on the other hand, ventricular dilation is relatively common in patients with interhemispherical cysts. In the latter instance, it is difficult to recognize the role exerted, respectively, by the cyst and by the maldevelopmental process of the commissura in the genesis of the altered cerebrospinal fluid dynamics.

Both varieties of arachnoid cyst occurring in the interhemispherical fissure present considerable difficulties for diagnosis, although the recognition of parasagittal cysts is facilitated by their unilaterality and by the absence of associated cerebral malformation (see Fig. 39–14). The preoperative differential diagnosis of parasagittal arachnoid cysts from other cystic lesions that may also develop along one side of the falx (e.g., glial, ependymal, choroid, and epithelial cysts) may be extremely difficult, even when computed tomography and magnetic resonance imaging are available. Coronal sections are particularly helpful in defining the wedge-shaped configuration of these lesions, which are sharply delimited on one side by the falx and are relatively more expanded toward the more compliant cerebral hemisphere and ventricle. Parasagittal arachnoid cysts are usually penetrated in a relatively short time by contrast medium injected into the cerebrospinal fluid spaces; however, the clearance of the agent from the cyst cavity is surprisingly slow. Among the various hypotheses propounded to explain the phenomenon, the most accepted theory postulates the presence of a unidirectional valvular communication with the subarachnoid space that allows the penetration of fluid but does not favor its clearance. The stasis of fluid within the cyst would be related to the characteristics of the cystic wall, which is rich in collagen fibers but lacking in elastic fibers.[135]

In cases of interhemispherical arachnoid cysts, the neurological findings alone may not suffice to differentiate these lesions from other midline cysts and from certain forms of agenesis of the corpus callosum, in particular type I-C prosencephaly.[37, 126] An associated midline cyst may be observed in about 25 per cent of patients with agenesis of the corpus callosum, and approximately 30 per cent of cases of holoprosencephaly are characterized by the presence of a dorsal cyst.[26] Some degree of elevation and "cystic" distention of the roof of the third ventricle (possibly simulating an interhemispherical cyst) may be detected in almost all malformations resulting in a defect of the corpus callosum. In such instances, the "cyst" is often indented at the midline by the free edge of the falx, bulging more or less symmetrically on both sides. As in most cases of interhemispherical arachnoid cysts, the falx is hypoplastic; the lesions are usually less indented, although they may assume a "batwing" appearance on coronal computed tomography or magnetic resonance imaging views. Hydrocephalus can be present in both conditions; however, in type I-C prosencephaly, the posterior part of the ventricular system is barely recognizable,

whereas in patients with arachnoid cysts the occipital horns of the lateral cerebral ventricles can be easily identified even though they are laterally displaced by the cystic lesion (see Fig. 39–13). A further distinguishing feature is the normal separation of the basal ganglia in the presence of an interhemispherical arachnoid cyst; this is in contrast to the varying degrees of fusion of the structures in prosencephaly.

Two main surgical options, which can be combined in some patients, are available for the treatment of interhemispherical fissure arachnoid cysts: (1) craniotomy with excision of the cystic lining, and (2) insertion of a cystoperitoneal shunt device. The removal of the cystic membrane has various results, ranging from adequate re-expansion of the cerebral parenchyma to the persistence of the midline cystic cavity (although reduced in size and freely communicating with the subarachnoid space). Both the direct excision of the cyst wall and the placement of the cystoperitoneal shunt usually allow the normalization of intracranial pressure in the vast majority of affected patients.

Quadrigeminal Plate Region Cysts

Arachnoid cysts developing in the region of the tentorial notch and the posterior end of the third ventricle may cause early neurological dysfunction as well as impaired cerebrospinal fluid dynamics because of the relatively restricted space available for the cysts' growth and their effect on important physiological functions of the adjacent neural structures. The direction of the expansion of these cysts may be lateral into the cisterna ambiens (Fig. 39–15), upward into the posterior part of the interhemispherical fissure, and downward into the cistern of the superior cerebellar vermis. When extremely large, arachnoid cysts of the quadrigeminal plate region may show both supratentorial and infratentorial extension (Fig. 39–16). Symptoms and findings include hydrocephalus secondary to compression of either the posterior part of the third ventricle or the aqueduct and to anomalies of pupillary reaction or eye movement due to compression of the quadrigeminal plate or stretching of the fourth cranial nerve. However, in patients with such cysts, impairment of upward conjugate gaze is considerably less frequent than in patients with tumors of the pineal region. Limb weakness and gait ataxia have occasionally been observed; bilateral deafness due to damage to the inferior colliculus is a rare finding.[75] In some patients, epilepsy is the main clinical manifestation.

Most of the arachnoid cysts of the quadrigeminal plate region described in the literature have been found in patients younger than 15 years of age, with a slightly higher incidence in girls than in boys.[75] Differentiation between arachnoid cysts of the quadrigeminal plate region and other congenital or acquired cystic lesions is often very difficult, especially in cases of cystic dilatation of the cisterna ambiens or complex cystic malformations with ependymal and glial elements contained in the cyst wall.[8, 67, 90] Differential diagnosis from dilated subarachnoid pouches of this region that result from postinflammatory loculation of the quadrigeminal cis-

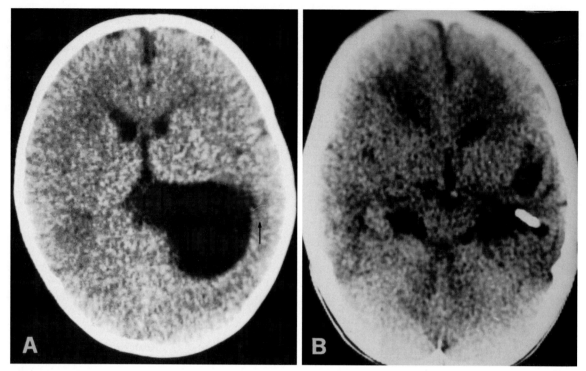

Figure 39–15

Quadrigeminal plate region arachnoid cyst. *A.* The lesion extends laterally, occupying the cisterna ambiens and dislocating the lateral cerebral ventricle *(arrow)*. *B.* Postoperative computed tomography demonstrates re-expansion of the brain following cystoperitoneal shunting treatment.

tern may be virtually impossible in the absence of reliable anamnestic findings. However, evidence of a posterior cranial fossa–occupying lesion allows easy differentiation of quadrigeminal plate region arachnoid cysts from subarachnoid pouches or dilated cisterns (the so-called cystlike "lesions of Kruyff"), which may be associated with a tumor of the posterior cranial fossa.[90] Quadrigeminal arachnoid cysts must also be differentiated from dilated suprapineal recesses of the third ventricle in cases of aqueductal stenosis and from atrial diverticula of the lateral cerebral ventricle caused by massive ventricular dilatation.[90, 115]

Magnetic resonance imaging and computed tomography provide the best diagnostic information by revealing the ovoid water-dense area posterior to the third ventricle (see Fig. 39–16). The relation of the cyst to the subarachnoid space can be defined by metrizamide-enhanced computed tomography cisternography. As is the case for arachnoid cysts situated elsewhere, penetration of the contrast medium into the cyst cavity and clearance of the contrast agent are usually delayed. Metrizamide often forms a "halo" in the subarachnoid space around the cyst, and this halo persists even when the agent has drained from other areas of the subarachnoid space.[75]

Treatment of arachnoid cysts of the quadrigeminal plate region is technically problematic because the region is not easily accessible. Establishing a shunt from the cyst or the lateral cerebral ventricle has not proved to be very satisfactory.[35, 129] Shunting associated with excision of the cyst lining may have a better rate of success.[69, 75]

The direct excision of the cyst membrane and the opening of the cyst into the subarachnoid space of the cisterna ambiens may be carried out by means of a supratentorial operation, with a low occipital craniotomy and transtentorial approach to the lesion, as well as by means of an infratentorial procedure, with incision or retraction of the cerebellum. To obtain a successful result, it is particularly important to establish a communication either between the cyst and the third ventricle through the posterior wall of the suprapineal recess or between the cyst and the fourth ventricle through the anterior medullary velum[75, 80] (see Fig. 39–16). Regardless of the surgical modality adopted, the rate at which cysts of the quadrigeminal plate region refill postoperatively and at which symptoms recur is considerably high.

INFRATENTORIAL ARACHNOID CYSTS

Posterior fossa arachnoid cysts are rather uncommon when compared with the more frequent supratentorial lesions (see Table 39–1). The estimated incidence of these lesions (approximately 25 per cent of all intracranial arachnoid cysts are infratentorial) may actually be even higher than their real incidence. In fact, their appearance between the 7th and 10th weeks of embryonic life temporally coincides with that of other cystic malformations of the posterior fossa with which these cysts are often confused—namely, the Dandy-Walker malformation and the Dandy-Walker variants. The ab-

Figure 39–16
Quadrigeminal plate region arachnoid cyst developing in both supratentorial and infratentorial compartments *(A and C).* The surgical treatment is followed by an obvious reduction in size of the lesion and by the disappearance of the associated hydrocephalus *(B and D).*

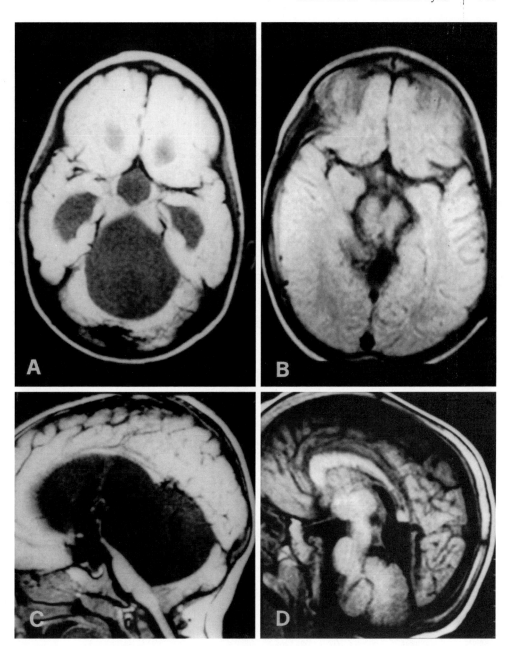

sence of vermian abnormalities is the main distinguishing feature of arachnoid cysts developing within the posterior cranial fossa, whereas the Dandy-Walker malformation and the Dandy-Walker variant are both characterized by the partial agenesis of the cerebellar vermis.[133] The absence of the foramen of Magendie is a further distinguishing feature of the Dandy-Walker malformation; in contrast, the communication between the fourth ventricle and the subarachnoid spaces is preserved in the Dandy-Walker variant.

The term *posterior fossa arachnoid cyst* should be reserved only for those cases in which the cyst does not communicate with the subarachnoid spaces and possibly exerts a compressive effect on the surrounding anatomical structures. This type of lesion is generated by a maldevelopmental process of the roof of the fourth ventricle. In this process, this structure fails to become entirely permeable and splits into two layers between

which the cerebrospinal fluid is "trapped" during embryonic life.[96] Morphologically similar but communicating with the perimedullary subarachnoid spaces are the cystic evaginations of the tela choroidea, which also occur without gross abnormalities of the cerebellar vermis.[133] This second type of cystic malformation of the posterior cranial fossa is often referred to as a "retrocerebellar arachnoid cyst" or a "cyst of the cisterna magna," even though it is correctly distinguished from a "true" arachnoid cyst by those authors who prefer different definitions, such as "Blake's pouch" or "subarachnoid pouch."[74, 177] The distinction is important when dealing with the incidence of posterior fossa arachnoid cysts, since retrocerebellar arachnoid pouches are common, and arachnoid cysts are relatively rare. However, with respect to physiopathogenic interpretation, the differentiation is considerably less important because the two entities are regarded as

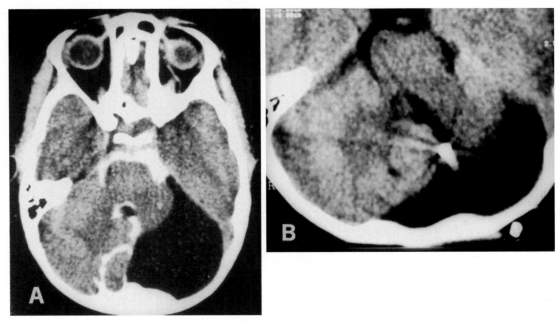

Figure 39–17

Lateral posterior fossa arachnoid cyst. *A.* Computed tomography cisternography demonstrates that the lesion does not communicate with the surrounding subarachnoid spaces. *B.* A moderate re-expansion of the cerebellum is noted after shunting of the cyst.

basically different aspects of the same nosographic entity.[58, 133]

In most patients, arachnoid cysts lie posteriorly within the posterior cranial fossa and have two main variants of anatomical distribution: (1) the midline posterior fossa arachnoid cyst, which pushes the vermis anteriorly while separating the two cerebral hemispheres (Fig. 39–17); and (2) the laterally located cyst, which overlays and compresses one cerebellar hemisphere (Fig. 39–18). A third, relatively common pattern

describes those cysts that develop within the cerebellopontine angle, displacing the cerebellum and brain stem contralaterally.[99, 112] Less commonly, arachnoid cysts of the posterior cranial fossa may extend to the level of the tentorial notch into the cisterna of the superior cerebellar vermis or into the internal auditory canal.[154, 169] Rare locations of these cysts, such as the retroclival space and the fourth ventricle, have also been described.[41, 88, 110] The incidence is slightly greater in males than in females. Posterior fossa arachnoid

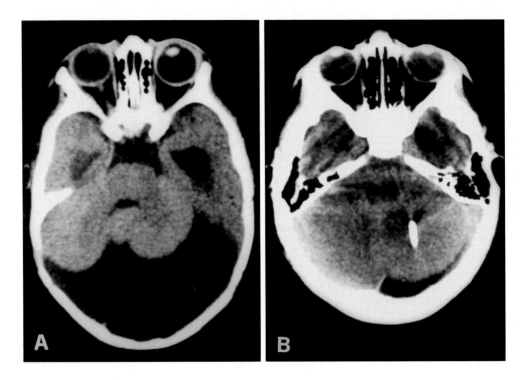

Figure 39–18

Posterior fossa arachnoid cyst. *A.* Preoperative computed tomography shows the thinning and bulging of the occipital squama. *B.* The shunting therapy is followed by cerebellar re-expansion and reduction in volume of the lesion. The occipital squama is obviously thickened.

cysts can cause symptoms at any age, but they tend to become symptomatic in a large proportion of patients during infancy and childhood.

Cerebellar Cysts

Macrocrania and signs and symptoms of increased intracranial pressure (in most instances because of the common association with hydrocephalus) are the most common clinical presentations of posterior fossa arachnoid cysts, especially when they occur in the pediatric population. Although hydrocephalus typically characterizes cysts localized at the midline (Fig. 39–19), ventricular dilation is also frequently associated with lesions that develop over the cerebellar hemispheres. In the latter instance, however, nystagmus and cerebellar signs may be important features of the clinical presentation. Unilateral or bilateral bulging of the occipital squama, although rare, can also be observed (see Fig. 39–19).

As for other types of intracranial arachnoid cysts, the active secretion of fluid by the cells of the cystic membrane or a ball-valve mechanism favoring the internal trapping of cerebrospinal fluid is believed to account for the progressive enlargement of these lesions.[12] Symptoms produced by expansion of a cerebellar arachnoid cyst differ in children and adults. In the first years of life, the main presenting signs and symptoms are macrocrania and various degrees of psychomotor retardation similar in every respect to those more commonly found in conventional hydrocephalus.[88, 112] In adults, the clinical picture is that of a slowly developing posterior fossa mass, the clinical course of which is often characterized by intermittent symptoms or is influenced by postural changes that suggest periodic volume fluctuations of the lesion.[58]

Although computed tomography and magnetic resonance imaging have made the diagnosis of cerebellar cysts relatively easy, some difficulties may still be encountered in differentiating these lesions from other cystic malformations or from anomalies of the subarachnoid spaces of the posterior cranial fossa—for example, "mega cisterna magna" and the so-called "Dandy-Walker cyst" (Fig. 39–20).[12] As originally defined, the term *mega cisterna magna* should be used to describe only those cases in which the enlargement of the retrocerebellar subarachnoid spaces depends on an associated hypoplasia of the cerebellar vermis, without any anomalies of the arachnoid membrane.[65] Some authors, however, use the term *mega cisterna magna* to describe a developmental defect resulting from a splitting of the falx cerebelli and the absence of the transverse arachnoid fold, which normally constitutes the upper limit of the cisterna magna.[133] This anatomical variant of the cisterna magna generally lacks clinical significance and does not require operative treatment because of its free communication with the cerebrospinal fluid pathways.[2, 65] In a few instances, however, the distinction between a retrocerebellar arachnoid cyst and a mega cisterna magna is difficult owing to the presence of signs such as enlargement of the posterior cranial fossa, thinning of the occipital bone, and hydrocephalus, which suggest a mass effect exerted by the accumulation of fluid within the abnormally large cisterna magna.[58, 143] The differentiation of midline retrocerebellar arachnoid cysts from the Dandy-Walker malformation is usually not particularly difficult. In contrast, differential diagnosis from the so-called Blake pouch, which usually communicates with the fourth ventricle and the perimedullary subarachnoid space, may be very difficult in cases in which the communication between the Blake pouch and the perimedullary subarachnoid space is lost.

Figure 39–19

Midline posterior fossa arachnoid cyst. The lesion occupies the entire posterior cranial fossa, pushing the cerebellar vermis anteriorly. *A.* The quadrigeminal plate is stretched and pushed upward so that it is barely recognizable on preoperative magnetic resonance imaging. *B.* This structure, as well as the cerebellar vermis, resumes its normal shape after shunting treatment of the cyst.

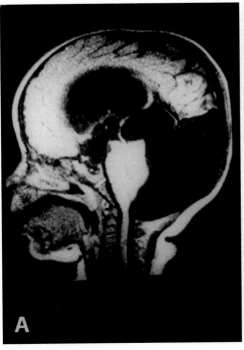
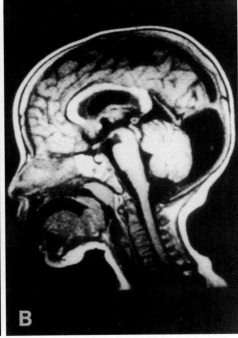

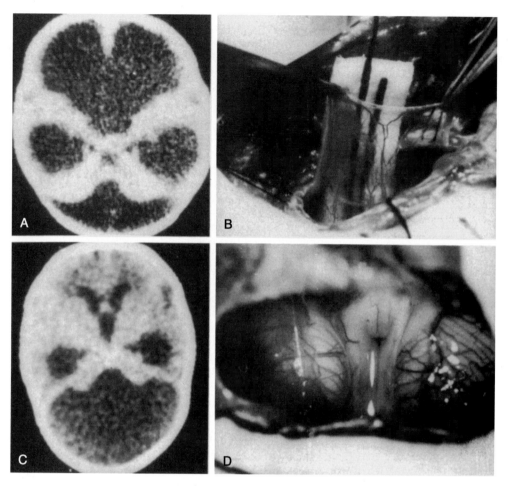

Figure 39–20

Computed tomography and operative findings in a child with a posterior arachnoid cyst (*A* and *B*) and a child with a Dandy-Walker cyst (*C* and *D*). Note the preserved cerebellar vermis in the patient with the posterior arachnoid cyst (*A*).

Cerebellar cysts become symptomatic because of the compression and distortion of the surrounding parenchymal structures and, in the large majority of cases, because of secondary hydrocephalus. Consequently, the surgical options include craniotomy with excision of the cyst membrane, shunting procedures of the cyst or the associated hydrocephalus (or both), and, finally, combination of the craniotomy and shunting operations. In the last instance, some clinicians prefer to shunt the cerebral ventricles or the residual cyst cavity after the craniotomy and resection of the cyst wall, whereas others favor the shunting therapy as the first surgical step prior to craniotomy.[103, 142, 155, 172]

In infants without hydrocephalus, the direct excision of the cyst membrane appears, at least theoretically, to be the most appropriate type of management. Indeed, in many cases, the operation is followed by the disappearance of the lesion and by cerebellar re-expansion. In some patients, however, the excision of the cyst wall is not sufficient to prevent the recurrence of the lesion; in others, it may be followed by the sudden appearance of unexpected postoperative hydrocephalus that is probably due to impairment of cerebrospinal fluid circulation or absorption within the peripheral subarachnoid spaces.[40, 112] Consequently, it is advisable to carry out careful preoperative assessment of cerebrospinal fluid dynamics, even in subjects in whom the cyst is not accompanied by an obvious hydrocephalus.[40, 103, 141]

Some authors consider the direct excision of the cyst lining to be the first-choice surgical option, even in patients with cerebellar arachnoid cysts associated with ventricular dilation.[58, 103] The policy is obviously based on the hypothesis that the associated hydrocephalus is secondary and obstructive. Other authors advocate the direct surgical approach, even in patients whose cysts appear to have some kind of communication with the neighboring cerebrospinal fluid spaces; this attitude is based on the assumption that a ball-valve mechanism or direct fluid secretion across the cyst wall contributes to the progressive enlargement of the lesion despite the anatomical communication with the surrounding subarachnoid space.[7, 146] Actually, the relationship between cerebellar cysts and the associated hydrocephalus cannot be explained on the basis of a mere obstruction of the cerebrospinal fluid circulation, as demonstrated by the relatively large number of patients who require cerebrospinal fluid shunting (either from the residual cyst cavity or from the cerebral ventricles) after an apparently successful excision of the cyst lining.[40, 112]

Some authors have proposed extrathecal shunting from a pathological cyst cavity as the only treatment to be performed.[100, 172] The advantage of this approach is essentially the simplicity of the operation; disadvantages include shunt malfunction, which has been reported with a frequency ranging from 10 to 26 per cent.[100, 103] This high percentage of failure places cerebellar cysts on a par with other cystic lesions of the posterior fossa, such as Dandy-Walker cysts and cysts associated with a rhombencephalon developmental anomaly, which also have a high incidence of occlusion of the cerebrospinal fluid shunting device, probably in relation to the limited amount of choroidal tissue available for cerebrospinal fluid production within the posterior cranial fossa to maintain the patency of the shunt device.[108]

Despite the wide range of surgical options and the divergent opinions on the best surgical approach, the great majority of patients who undergo surgery because of cerebellar arachnoid cysts benefit from such treatment. Nevertheless, some patients may continue to exhibit variable degrees of psychomotor retardation and focal neurological signs, even if the intracranial pressure has been fully normalized.

Cerebellopontine Angle Cysts

Congenital arachnoid cysts that develop from the arachnoid of the cerebellopontine angle are relatively rare in comparison with the more frequent cystic lesions of the region that result from inflammatory processes of the inner ear.[17, 145] In most cases, these congenital cysts are found in adulthood; males and females are equally affected.[99, 172] Symptoms include cochleovestibular dysfunction, cerebellar signs, and, less frequently, fifth and seventh cranial nerve deficits as well as pyramidal deficits.[77, 145] Papillary edema is often observed even in those patients without hydrocephalus; this finding has been explained by the possible impairment of the flow of cerebrospinal fluid within the basal cisterns.[144]

Rarely, arachnoid cysts in adults may remain confined within the internal auditory canal.[22, 154] This location has also been described in children, in whom the cyst induces a widening of the canal and facial palsy.[165, 169] Although in most patients the clinical history prior to diagnosis is relatively short, in some patients skull x-ray examination may show alteration of the temporal bone, which is indicative of a lesion that has been present for some time. Prior to the introduction of computed tomography, diagnosis was nearly always made during surgery for suspected acoustic neurinoma. Computed tomography and magnetic resonance imaging are currently the only diagnostic techniques with which an arachnoid cyst of the cerebellopontine angle can be correctly recognized.[22] The utility of computed tomography is, however, more limited in patients with cysts located within the internal auditory canal. Operative management involves excision of the lesion. However, although cerebellar and pyramidal deficits usually regress after surgery, cochleovestibular dysfunction improves only rarely.

Fourth Ventricle Cysts

The development of an arachnoid cyst within the fourth ventricle was first described in a child with a history of apparently arrested hydrocephalus.[41] Two further cases were subsequently reported in adults, both of whom presented with a clinical picture resembling that of normal-pressure hydrocephalus syndrome.[88, 170]

Differential diagnosis should be made with the so-called "encysted fourth ventricle." Following craniotomy, direct excision of the cyst membrane and shunting of the associated hydrocephalus have proved to be appropriate surgical management.

Intraspinal Arachnoid Cysts

Intraspinal arachnoid cysts originate from the arachnoid of the spinal cord, which extends to the sheaths of the spinal nerve roots. These cysts are relatively uncommon but must be differentiated from both other congenital intraspinal cystic lesions, such as neuroepithelial, neurenteric, and teratoid cysts, and from the acquired cystic cavities that result from postinflammatory adhesions within the subarachnoid space.[4, 51] Since the first observations of these cysts were made at the turn of the century, the cause and pathogenesis of intraspinal arachnoid cysts have been the subject of continuing debate.[152, 161] Their association with other congenital anomalies (i.e., diastematomyelia, or the abnormal fusion of vertebral bodies) and their occurrence in members of the same family or in patients with von Recklinghausen's disease have been cited as support for the congenital origin of these cysts.[1, 95] Three groups of authors have proposed different pathogenetic theories. The first group believes that intraspinal arachnoid cysts originate from an abnormal proliferation or distribution of the trabeculae that appear within the subarachnoid space during the early embryonic period.[168, 173] The abnormal arrangement of these trabeculae could lead to the formation of arachnoid diverticula in areas of lower resistance when they are under the effect of variations in cerebrospinal fluid pressure.[52, 164] Exclusion of these diverticula from the cerebrospinal fluid circulation and their subsequent development into cysts may gradually occur because of a valvular mechanism, or they may perhaps be precipitated by trauma.[9, 91]

A second group of authors considers intraspinal arachnoid cysts to be the result of a widening of the septum posticum, which divides the dorsal spinal subarachnoid space at the midline in the cervical and thoracic areas.[85, 124] This hypothesis would account for the frequent cervical and dorsal sites, as well as for posterior locations, of the spinal arachnoid cysts; however, it cannot explain cysts that are situated anterior to the spinal cord or close to the spinal roots. Finally, according to a third group's interpretation, spinal arachnoid cysts originate from a herniation of the arachnoid owing to a congenital defect of the dura mater.[47]

INTRADURAL ARACHNOID CYSTS

Intradural arachnoid cysts are commonly found in the thoracic segment posterior or posterolateral to the spinal cord; however, they may develop in the cervical and lumbar segments[118, 123] (Fig. 39–21). The occurrence of the lesion on the anterior or anterolateral aspect of the spinal cord is uncommon.[121] Intradural arachnoid cysts may be multiple and associated with extradural and perineural cysts.[169] Males and females are equally affected; cysts are usually diagnosed in the fifth decade of life, although younger persons can also be affected.[52]

The clinical presentation of intradural arachnoid cysts is quite variable, and no obvious relationship exists between the severity of signs and symptoms and the duration of the clinical history. Local or radicular pain, dysesthesia, motor deficit, and, in almost one half of all cases, bladder disturbances are the most frequent complaints, and they usually appear and evolve over a period of months or years. Pain is not characteristic, although in some instances pain similar to that associated with disc prolapse may be present.[130] In about one sixth of patients, the progression of symptoms is marked by transitory episodes of remission, which mimic those of demyelinating disease.[121, 130] In other patients, exacerbation of symptoms may occur with changes in posture and may be caused by fluctuations in cyst volume or by secondary stretching of the adjacent neural structures.[9] Only rarely is the presenting sign an anomaly of the spine such as scoliosis or kyphosis.[121] In most cases described in the literature, myelographic investigation performed in patients in both the prone and the supine positions has led to direct visualization of the cyst or has indirectly demonstrated the lesion by revealing a partial or complete intradural block. Plain x-ray films have usually not been helpful.[4] Magnetic resonance imaging and metrizamide-enhanced computed tomography myelography currently represent the diagnostic procedures of choice.

Macroscopically, intradural arachnoid cysts appear as translucent, round or oval cystic formations that vary in size (the size fluctuates with respiratory movements). In fewer than one third of cases, the cysts have a diverticular morphology. The coexistence of anomalous vessels on the dorsal aspect of the spinal cord is relatively common.[123] Occasionally, total excision of the cyst lining cannot be carried out because of adherence of the lesion to the spinal cord or nerve roots. In such cases, shunting of the cyst into the peritoneal cavity has been suggested, especially when a reaccumulation of fluid is demonstrated.[82]

Surgical treatment is followed by an immediate remission of symptoms in the majority of patients.

EXTRADURAL CYSTS

In most cases, extradural arachnoid cysts present as membranous diverticula connected by a narrow neck to a nerve root sleeve, usually at the entry of the root into the spinal subarachnoid space. More rarely, they are found on the posterior midline or in proximity to the point of fixation of the filum terminale. This characteristic topography seems to support the hypothesis that extradural arachnoid cysts develop through areas of lower resistance of the dura mater.[47] In fact, abnormal arachnoid proliferation and the occurrence of cystic cavities have been demonstrated with a relatively high frequency at the level of the lateral meningoradicular junctions.[138] Some of these cysts—that is, those located in the lumbar region and close to the attachment of the filum terminale—have also been likened by some authors to meningoceles and considered to result from defective closure of the posterior neuro-

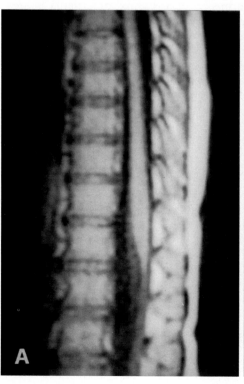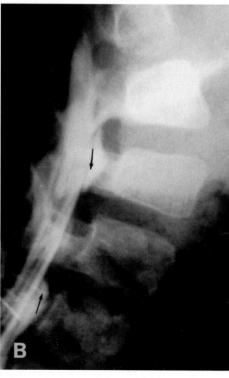

Figure 39–21

Intradural spinal arachnoid cyst. *A.* The magnetic resonance imaging examination shows the cyst pushing the conus and spinal roots backward. *B.* Myelography demonstrates the upper and inferior limits of the lesion *(arrows).* Note the scalloping of the corresponding vertebral body.

pore.[81] Extradural arachnoid cysts are rarely associated with intradural arachnoid cysts.[28]

The majority of extradural arachnoid cysts communicate with the subarachnoid space and are found in the inferior dorsal and dorsolumbar regions, usually in the retromedullary space.[32] Although also reported in children, these lesions are more frequently found in adolescents and young adults. Males and females are affected equally. Progressive limb weakness, associated in some patients with low thoracic pain or abdominal pain, usually dominates the clinical picture because of the frequent dorsal location of these cysts.[31, 32] It is worth noting that pain and sensorial disturbances may be considerably less important than the motor deficit or may even be lacking, despite the fact that extradural arachnoid cysts commonly lie on the posterior surface of the spinal cord. In some patients, the radicular pain may be due to an associated kyphoscoliosis rather than to the presence of the cyst itself. Sphincter disturbances are less common than they are in patients with intradural cysts. Extradural arachnnoid cysts may remain silent for a long time before they are diagnosed, as has been suggested by the frequency of concomitant vertebral deformities. In fact, kyphoscoliosis has been reported to occur in about one half of patients with the cysts along the dorsal spine. A plain x-ray study of the spine usually demonstrates any abnormalities, such as pedicular erosion with a widening of the interpedicular space, enlargement of the spinal canal, scalloping of the vertebrae, and signs of anterior vertebral epiphysitis reminiscent of Scheuermann's disease.[31] In rare instances, erosion of the sacral foramina may be due to arachnoid diverticula (incorrectly called "arachnoid root cysts"), which are usually observed along the lower lumbar and sacral roots during lumbar myelography. In most cases, diverticula have no clinical significance; however, in a few patients, they may be accompanied by radicular symptoms (Fig. 39–22).

Conventional myelography, metrizamide-enhanced computed tomography myelography, and magnetic resonance imaging currently appear to be the most appropriate diagnostic tools for the detection of extradural arachnoid cysts.[43]

Management consists of complete excision of the cyst. This procedure may occasionally be complicated by the adherence of the cyst membrane to the posterior surface of the dura mater or by extension of the membrane into the intervertebral foramina. Laminotomy rather than laminectomy is the preferred procedure because of the benign nature of the lesion and because of the need to spare the posterior vertebral arches in order to preserve spinal stability (especially in young patients or in patients with lesions extending over several spinal segments who may also have a kyphoscoliotic deformity).[28, 128]

REFERENCES

1. Aarabi, B., Pasternak, G., Hurko, O., et al: Familial intra-dural arachnoid cysts: Report of two cases. J. Neurosurg., 50:826–829, 1979.
2. Adam, R., and Greenberg, J. O.: The mega cisterna magna. J. Neurosurg., 48:190–192, 1978.
3. Adams, J. H., Corsellis, J. A. N., and Duchen, L. W., eds.: Greenfield's Neuropathology. 4th ed. London, E. Arnolds, 1984, pp. 426–427.
4. Agnoli, A. L., Schonmayr, R., and Laun, A.: Intraspinal arachnoid cysts. Acta Neurochir., 61:291–302, 1982.
5. Aicardi, J., and Bauman, F.: Supratentorial extracerebral cysts in infants and children. J. Neurol. Neurosurg. Psychiatry, 38:57–68, 1975.
6. Albright, L.: Treatment of bobble-head doll syndrome by trans-callosal cystectomy. Neurosurgery, 8:593–595, 1981.
7. Alker, G. F., Jr., Glasauer, F. E., and Leslie, E. V.: Radiology of a large cisterna magna cyst: A case report. Arch. Neurol., 36:376–379, 1979.
8. Alvord, E. C., Jr., and Marcuse, P. M.: Intracranial cerebellar meningo-encephalocele (posterior fossa cyst) causing hydrocephalus by compression at the incisura tentorii. J. Neuropathol. Exp. Neurol., 21:50–69, 1962.
9. Ambrosetto, C., Alvisi, C., and Ferraro, M.: Cisti leptomeningee spinali. Minerva Neuroch., 12:276–279, 1968.
10. Anderson, F. M., and Landing, B. H.: Cerebral arachnoid cysts in infants. J. Pediatr., 69:88–96, 1966.
11. Anderson, F. M., Segall, H. D., and Caton, W. L.: Use of computerized tomography scanning in supratentorial arachnoid cysts. J. Neurosurg., 50:337–338, 1979.
12. Archer, C. R., Darwish, H., and Smith, K., Jr.: Enlarged cisternae magnae and posterior fossa cysts simulating Dandy-Walker syndrome on computed tomography. Radiology, 127:681–686, 1978.
13. Auer, L. M., Gallhofer, B., Ladurner, G., et al.: Diagnosis and treatment of middle fossa arachnoid cysts and subdural hematomas. J. Neurosurg., 54:366–369, 1981.
14. Banna, M.: Arachnoid cysts in the hypophyseal area. Clin. Radiol., 25:323–326, 1974.
15. Baskin, D. S., and Wilson, C. B.: Transsphenoidal treatment of non-neoplastic intrasellar cysts. J. Neurosurg., 60:8–13, 1984.
16. Beltramello, A., and Mazza, C.: Spontaneous disappearance of a large middle fossa arachnoid cyst. Surg. Neurol., 24:181–183, 1985.
17. Bengochea, F. G., and Blanco, F. L.: Arachnoidal cysts of cerebellopontine angle. J. Neurosurg., 12:66–71, 1955.
18. Benton, J. W., Nellhaus, G., Huttenlocker, P. R., et al.: The bobble-head doll syndrome. Neurology, 16:725–729, 1966.
19. Bhandari, Y. S.: Non-communicating supratentorial subarachnoid cysts. J. Neurol. Neurosurg. Psychiatry, 35:763–768, 1972.
20. Binitie, O., Williams, B., and Case, C. P.: A suprasellar subarach-

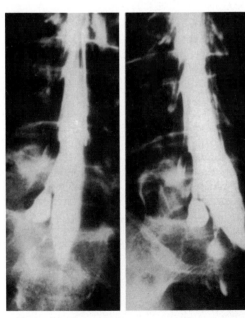

Figure 39–22
Arachnoid diverticula of the spinal nerve roots.

noid pouch: Aetiological considerations. J. Neurol. Neurosurg. Psychiatry, 47:1066–1074, 1984.

21. Bourekas, E. C., Raji, M. R., Dastur, K. J., et al.: Retroclival arachnoid cyst. A.J.N.R., 13:353–354, 1992.

22. Brooks, M. L., Mayer, D. P., Sataloff, R. T., et al.: Intracanalicular arachnoid cyst mimicking acoustic neuroma: CT and MRI. Comput. Med. Imaging Graph., 16:283–285, 1992.

23. Cassinari, V., Marossero, F., and Infuso, L.: Le cisti aracnoidali endocraniche. Riv. Neurol., 30:133–158, 1960.

24. Choux, M., Raybaud, C., Pinsard, N., et al.: Intracranial supratentorial cysts in children, excluding tumor and parasitic cysts. Child's Brain, 4:15–32, 1978.

25. Choux, M., and Yanez, A.: Arachnoid cyst. In Hoffman, H. J., and Epstein, F., eds.: Anomalies of the Developing Central Nervous System. Boston, Blackwell Scientific, 1987, pp. 175–189.

26. Chuan, G. S., and Harwood-Nash, D.: Tumors and cysts. In Naidich, T. P., and Quencer, R. M., eds.: Clinical Neurosonography. Berlin, Springer-Verlag, 1987, pp. 97–109.

27. Cilluffo, J. M., Onofrio, B. M., and Miller, R. H.: The diagnosis and surgical treatment of intracranial arachnoid cysts. Acta Neurochir., 67:215–229, 1983.

28. Cilluffo, J. M., Redmon, M. J., and Ebersol, M. J.: Idiopathic thoracic intradural and extradural arachnoid diverticula: Report of a case. Acta Neurochir., 65:199–206, 1982.

29. Ciricillo, S. F., Cogen, P. H., Harsh, G. R., et al.: Intracranial arachnoid cysts in children: A comparison of the effects of fenestration and shunting. J. Neurosurg., 74:230–235, 1991.

30. Clavel, M., Taborga, F. G., and Onzain, I.: Arachnoid cysts as a cause of dementia in the elderly. Acta Neurochir., 78:28–32, 1985.

31. Cloward, R. B.: Congenital spinal extradural cyst: Case report and review of literature. Ann. Surg., 168:851–864, 1968.

32. Combelles, G., Rousseaux, M., Dhellemmes, P., et al.: Kystes meninges extra-duraux rachidiens. Neurochirurgie, 29:13–19, 1983.

33. Craig, W.: Chronic cystic arachnoiditis. Am. J. Surg., 17:384–388, 1932.

34. Crisi, G., Calo, M., De Santis, M., et al.: Metrizamide-enhanced computed tomography of intracranial arachnoid cysts. J. Comput. Assist. Tomogr., 8:928–935, 1984.

35. Danzinger, J., and Boch, S.: Paracollicular arachnoid pouches. Am. J. Roentgenol. Radium Ther. Nucl. Med., 124:310–314, 1975.

36. Dell, S.: Further observations on the "bobble-headed doll syndrome." J. Neurol. Neurosurg. Psychiatry, 44:1046–1049, 1981.

37. Diebler, C., and Dulac, O.: Pediatric Neurology and Neuroradiology. Berlin, Springer-Verlag, 1987, pp. 67–68.

38. Di Rocco, C.: Surgical management of sellar and parasellar arachnoid cysts. Crit. Rev. Neurosurg., 1:353–360, 1991.

39. Di Rocco, C., Caldarelli, M., and Ceddia, A.: Incidence, anatomical distribution, and classification of arachnoidal cysts. In Raimondi, A. J., Choux, M., and Di Rocco, C., eds.: Intracranial Cyst Lesions. New York, Springer-Verlag, 1993, pp. 101–111.

40. Di Rocco, C., Caldarelli, M., and Di Trapani, G.: Infratentorial arachnoid cysts in children. Child's Brain, 8:119–133, 1981.

41. Di Rocco, C., Di Trapani, G., and Iannelli, A.: Arachnoid cyst of the fourth ventricle and "arrested" hydrocephalus. Surg. Neurol., 12:467–471, 1979.

42. Di Rocco, C., Iannelli, A., Borrelli, P., et al.: Surgically treatable growth retardation due to non-neoplastic pituitary-hypothalamic dysfunction. Child's Brain, 11:353–368, 1984.

43. Di Sclafani, A., and Canale, D. J.: Communicating spinal arachnoid cysts: Diagnosis by delayed metrizamide computed tomography. Surg. Neurol., 23:428–430, 1985.

44. Di Trapani, G., Di Rocco, C., Pizzolato, P., et al.: Arachnoid cysts in children: Ultrastructural findings of three cases. Ital. J. Neurol. Sci., 1:19–24, 1979.

45. Di Trapani, G., Di Rocco, C., Pocchiari, M., et al.: Arachnoid cysts in children: Ultrastructural findings. Acta Neuropathol. (Berl), 7(Suppl.):392–395, 1981.

46. Dyck, P., and Gruskin, P.: Supratentorial arachnoid cysts in adults: A discussion of two cases from a pathophysiologic and surgical perspective. Arch. Neurol., 34:276–279, 1977.

47. Elsberg, D. A., Dyke, O. G., and Brewer, E. D.: The symptoms and diagnosis of extradural cysts. Bull. Neurol. Inst. N. Y., 3:395–417, 1934.

48. Escourolle, R., Hauw, J. J., Hervé de Sigalony, J. P., et al.: Les kystes arachnoïdiens de l'adulte: Etude neuropathologique de 6 observations. Ann. Anat. Pathol., 19:257–274, 1974.

49. Eustace, S., Toland, J., and Stack, J.: CT and MRI of arachnoid cyst with complicating intracystic and subdural haemorrhage. J. Comput. Assist. Tomogr., 16:995–997, 1992.

50. Faris, A. A., Bale, G. F., and Cannon, B.: Arachnoid cyst of the third ventricle with precocious puberty. South Med. J., 64:1139–1142, 1971.

51. Fortuna, A., La Torre, E., and Ciappetta, P.: Arachnoid diverticula: A unitary approach to spinal cysts communicating with the subarachnoid space. Acta Neurochir., 39:259–268, 1977.

52. Fortuna, A., and Mercuri, S.: Intradural spinal cysts. Acta Neurochir., 68:289–314, 1983.

53. Fox, J. L., and Al-Mefty, O.: Suprasellar arachnoid cyst: An extension of the membrane of Liliequist. Neurosurgery, 7:615–618, 1980.

54. Friede, R. L., and Yasargil, M. G.: Supratentorial intracerebral epithelial (ependymal) cysts: review. Case reports and fine structure. J. Neurol. Neurosurg. Psychiatry, 40:127–137, 1977.

55. Galassi, E., and Gaist, G.: Dynamics of intracranial cyst formation and expansion. In Raimondi, A. J., Choux, M., and Di Rocco, C., eds.: Intracranial Cyst Lesions. New York, Springer-Verlag, 1993, pp. 53–88.

56. Galassi, E., Gaist, G., Giuliani, G., et al.: Arachnoid cysts of the middle cranial fossa: Experience with 77 cases treated surgically. Acta Neurochir., 42:201–207, 1988.

57. Galassi, E., Piazza, G., Gaist, G., et al.: Arachnoid cysts of the middle cranial fossa: A clinical and radiological study of 25 cases treated surgically. Surg. Neurol., 14:211–219, 1980.

58. Galassi, E., Tognetti, F., Frank, F., et al.: Infratentorial arachnoid cysts. J. Neurosurg., 63:210–217, 1985.

59. Galassi, E., Tognetti, F., Gaist, G., et al.: CT scan and metrizamide CT cisternography in arachnoid cysts of the middle cranial fossa: Classification and pathophysiological aspects. Surg. Neurol., 17:363–369, 1982.

60. Garcia-Bach, M., Isamat, F., and Vila, F.: Intracranial arachnoid cysts in adults. Acta Neurochir., 42:205–209, 1988.

61. Geissenger, J. D., Kohler, W. C., Robinson, B. W., et al.: Arachnoid cysts of the middle cranial fossa: Surgical consideration. Surg. Neurol., 10:27–33, 1978.

62. Ghatak, N. R., and Mushrush, G. J.: Supratentorial intra-arachnoid cyst: Case report. J. Neurosurg., 35:477–482, 1971.

63. Go, K. G.: Pathogenesis of arachnoid cysts in relation to the mechanism of cerebrospinal fluid absorption. In Raimondi, A. J., Choux, M., and Di Rocco, C., eds.: Intracranial Cyst Lesions. New York, Springer-Verlag, 1993, pp. 79–86.

64. Go, K. G., Houthoff, H. J., Blaauw, E. H., et al.: Arachnoid cysts of the sylvian fissure: Evidence of fluid secretion. J. Neurosurg., 60:803–813, 1984.

65. Gonsette, R., Potvliege, R., André-Balisaux, G., et al.: La méga grande citerne: Etude clinique, radiologique et anatomopathologique. Acta Neurol. Belg., 68:559–570, 1968.

66. Gonzales, C. A., Villarejo, F. J., Blazquez, M. G., et al.: Suprasellar arachnoid cysts in children. Acta Neurochir., 60:281–296, 1982.

67. Grollmus, J. M., Wilson, C. B., and Newton, T. H.: Paramesencephalic arachnoid cysts. Neurology, 26:128–134, 1976.

68. Hacher, H.: Abflusswege der Sylvischen Venegruppe. Radiologie, 12:383–387, 1968.

69. Handa, J., Nakano, H., and Aii, H.: CT cisternography with intracranial arachnoid cysts. Surg. Neurol., 8:451–454, 1977.

70. Handa, J., Okamoto, K., and Sato, M.: Arachnoid cyst of the middle cranial fossa: Report of bilateral cysts in siblings. Surg. Neurol., 16:127–130, 1981.

71. Harrison, M. J. G.: Cerebral arachnoid cysts in children. J. Neurol. Neurosurg. Psychiatry, 34:316–323, 1971.

72. Harsh, G. R. IV, Edwards, M. S. B., and Wilson, C. B.: Intracranial arachnoid cysts in children. J. Neurosurg., 64:835–842, 1986.

73. Harter, L. P., Silverberg, G. D., and Brant-Zawadzki, M.: Intrasellar arachnoid cyst: Case report. Neurosurgery, 7:387–390, 1980.

74. Harwood-Nash, D. C.: Neuroradiology in Infants and Children. St. Louis, C. V. Mosby, 1976, pp. 979–994.

75. Hayashi, T., Kuratomi, A., and Kuramoto, S.: Arachnoid cyst of the quadrigeminal cistern. Surg. Neurol., 14:267–273, 1980.

76. Haymaker, W., Foster, M. E., Jr.: Intracranial dural cysts, with report of case. J. Neurosurg., 1:211–218, 1944.
77. Higashi, S., Yamashita, J., Yamamoto, Y., et al.: Hemifacial spasm associated with a cerebellopontine angle arachnoid cyst in young adult. Surg. Neurol., 37:289–292, 1992.
78. Hoffman, H. J., Hendrick, E. B., Humphreys, R. P., et al.: Investigation and management of suprasellar arachnoid cysts. J. Neurosurg., 57:597–602, 1982.
79. Hornig, G. W., and Zervas, N. T.: Slit defect of the diaphragma sellae with valve effect: Observation of a "slit valve." Neurosurgery, 30:265–267, 1992.
80. Huckman, M. S., Davis, D. O., and Coxe, W. S.: Arachnoid cyst of the quadrigeminal plate. J. Neurosurg., 32:367–370, 1970.
81. Hyndman, O. R., and Gerber, W. F.: Spinal extra-dural cyst, congenital and acquired: Report of cases. J. Neurosurg., 3:474–486, 1946.
82. Jensen, F. O., Knudsen, V., and Troesen, S.: Recurrent intraspinal arachnoid cyst treated with a shunt procedure. Acta Neurochir., 39:127–129, 1977.
83. Jensen, H. P., Pendl, G., and Goerke, W.: Head bobbing in a patient with a cyst of the third ventricle. Child's Brain, 4:235–241, 1978.
84. Kasdon, D. L., Douglas, E. Z., and Brougham, M. F.: Suprasellar arachnoid cyst diagnosed preoperatively by computerized tomographic scanning. Surg. Neurol., 7:299–303, 1977.
85. Kim, J. H., Shucart, W. A., and Haimovici, H.: Symptomatic arachnoid diverticula. Arch. Neurol., 31:35–37, 1974.
86. Kirchner, S. G., and Long, W. R.: Epicranial arachnoid cyst. South. Med. J., 77:905–906, 1984.
87. Kishore, P. R. S., Krishna Rao, C. V. G., Williams, J. P., et al.: The limitation of computerized tomographic diagnosis of intracranial midline cysts. Surg. Neurol., 14:417–431, 1980.
88. Korosue, K., Tamaki, N., Fujiwara, K., et al.: Arachnoid cyst of the fourth ventricle manifesting normal pressure hydrocephalus. Neurosurgery, 12:108–110, 1983.
89. Krawchenko, J., and Collins, G. H.: Pathology of an arachnoid cyst. J. Neurosurg., 50:224–228, 1979.
90. Kruyff, E.: Paracollicular plate cysts. A.J.R., 95:899–916, 1965.
91. Kuhlendahl, A.: Spinale Arachnoidalzysten. Zentralbl. Neurochir., 19:198–204, 1959.
92. La Cour, F., Trevor, R., and Casey, M.: Arachnoid cysts and associated subdural hematoma. Arch. Neurol., 35:84–89, 1978.
93. Lee, B. C. P.: Intracranial cysts. Radiology, 130:667–674, 1979.
94. Leo, J. S., Pinto, R. S., Hulvat, G. F., et al.: Computed tomography of arachnoid cysts. Radiology, 130:675–680, 1979.
95. Lesbros, D., Guillaud, R., and Frerebeau, P.: Kyste arachnoidien intra-dural rachidien. Arch. Fr. Pediatr., 42:309–311, 1985.
96. Le Schey, W. H., Jr.: Posterior fossa arachnoid cysts. J. Maine Med. Assoc., 70:398–405, 1979.
97. Lesoin, F., Dhellemmes, P., Rousseaux, M., et al.: Arachnoid cysts and head injury. Acta Neurochir., 69:43–51, 1983.
98. Lisovoski, F., Danziger, N., Helias, A., et al.: Kyste arachnoïdien de la fosse temporal: Hématome sous-dural: Apport de l'IRM. Rev. Neurol. (Paris), 148:151–151, 1992.
99. Little, J. R., Gomez, M. R., and MacCarthy, C. S.: Infratentorial arachnoid cysts. J. Neurosurg., 39:380–386, 1973.
100. Locatelli, D., Bonfanti, N., Sfogliarini, R., et al.: Arachnoid cysts: Diagnosis and treatment. Child's Nerv. Syst., 3:121–124, 1987.
101. Lodrini, S., Lasio, G., Fornari, M., et al.: Treatment of supratentorial primary arachnoid cysts. Acta Neurochir., 76:105–110, 1985.
102. Maixner, V. J., Besser, M., and Johnston, I. H.: Pseudotumor syndrome in treated arachnoid cysts. Child's Nerv. Syst., 8:207–210, 1992.
103. Marino, V. M., Undjian, S., and Wetzka, P.: An evaluation of the surgical treatment of intracranial arachnoid cysts in children. Child's Nerv. Syst., 5:177–183, 1989.
104. Markakis, E., Heyer, R., Stoeppler, L., et al.: Die Aphasie der perisylvischen Region. Neurochirurgia, 22:211–220, 1970.
105. Martinez-Lage, J. F., Poza, M., Sola, J., et al.: Congenital arachnoid cyst of the lateral ventricles in children. Child's Nerv. Syst., 8:203–206, 1992.
106. Martuza, R. L., Ojemann, R. G., Shillito, J., Jr., et al.: Facial pain associated with a middle fossa arachnoid cyst. Neurosurgery, 8:712–716, 1981.
107. McLaurin, R. L.: Parietal encephaloceles. Neurology, 14:764–772, 1964.
108. McLone, D. G., Naidich, T. P., and Cunningham, T.: Posterior fossa cysts: Management and outcome. Concepts Pediatr. Neurosurg., 7:134–141, 1987.
109. Menezes, A. H., Bell, W. E., and Perret, G. E.: Arachnoid cysts in children. Arch. Neurol., 37:168–172, 1980.
110. Milhorat, T. H.: Pediatric Neurosurgery. Contemp. Neurol. Series, 16:192–197, 1978.
111. Mori, K.: Anomalies of the Central Nervous System. New York, Thieme Stratton, 1985, pp. 25–34.
112. Mori, K., Hayashi, T., and Handa, H.: Infratentorial retrocerebellar cysts. Surg. Neurol., 7:135–142, 1977.
113. Murali, R., and Epstein, F.: Diagnosis and treatment of suprasellar arachnoid cyst. J. Neurosurg., 50:515–518, 1979.
114. Nagoulitch, I., and Perovitch, M.: Les collections liquidiennes extra-cérebrales chez l'enfant. Lyon Chir., 56:726–739, 1960.
115. Naidich, T. P., McLone, D. G., Hahn, Y. S., et al.: Atrial diverticula in severe hydrocephalus. A.J.N.R., 3:257–266, 1982.
116. Naidich, T. P., McLone, D. G., and Radkowski, M. A.: Intracranial arachnoid cyst. Pediatr. Neurosci., 12:112–122, 1985–1986.
117. Nakase, H., Hisanaga, M., Hashimoto, S., et al.: Intraventricular arachnoid cyst: Report of two cases. J. Neurosurg., 68:482–486, 1988.
118. Okamura, M., and Sumita, I. C.: Cisto aracnoideo cervical cirurgico. Seara Med. Neurocir., 14:143–151, 1985.
119. Oliver, L. C.: Primary arachnoid cysts: Report of two cases. B. M. J., 1:1147–1149, 1958.
120. Osaka, K., and Matsumoto, S.: Hydrocephalus in neurosurgical practice. J. Neurosurg., 48:767–803, 1978.
121. Palmer, J. J.: Spinal arachnoid cysts: Report of six cases. J. Neurosurg., 41:728–735, 1974.
122. Patrick, B. S.: Ependymal cyst of the sylvian fissure. J. Neurosurg., 35:751–754, 1971.
123. Pau, A., Viale Sehrbundt, E., and Turtas, S.: Spinal intradural arachnoid cysts. Neurochirurgia, 25:19–21, 1982.
124. Perret, G., Green, D., and Keller, J.: Diagnosis and treatment of intradural arachnoid cysts of the thoracic spine. Radiology, 79:425–429, 1962.
125. Pierre-Kahn, A., Capelle, L., Brauner, R., et al.: Presentations and management of suprasellar arachnoid cysts. J. Neurosurg., 73:355–359, 1990.
126. Probst, F. P.: The Prosencephalies. Berlin, Springer-Verlag, 1979, pp. 107–115.
127. Raffel, C., and McComb, J. G.: To shunt or to fenestrate: Which is the best surgical treatment for arachnoid cysts in pediatric patients? Neurosurgery, 23:338–342, 1988.
128. Raimondi, A. J., Gutierrez, F. A., and Di Rocco, C.: Laminotomy and total reconstruction of the posterior spinal arch for spinal canal surgery in childhood. J. Neurosurg., 45:555–560, 1976.
129. Raimondi, A. J., Shimoji, T., and Gutierrez, F. A.: Suprasellar cysts: Surgical treatment and results. Child's Brain, 7:757–772, 1980.
130. Raja, I. A., and Hankinson, J.: Congenital spinal arachnoid cysts. J. Neurol., 33:105–110, 1970.
131. Rao, K. C. V. G., Gunadi, I. K., and Diaconis, J. N.: Interhemispheric intradural cyst. J. Comput. Assist. Tomogr., 6:1167–1171, 1982.
132. Rappaport, Z. H.: Suprasellar arachnoid cysts: Options in operative management. Acta Neurochir., 122:71–75, 1993.
133. Raybaud, C.: Cystic malformations of the posterior fossa: Abnormalities associated with the development of the roof of the fourth ventricle and adjacent meningeal structures. J. Neuroradiol., 9:103–133, 1982.
134. Rengachary, S. S.: Intracranial, arachnoid and ependymal cysts. In Wilkins, R. H., and Rengachary, S. S., eds.: Neurosurgery. New York, McGraw-Hill, 1985, pp. 2160–2172.
135. Rengachary, S. S.: Parasagittal arachnoid cyst: Case report. Neurosurgery, 9:70–75, 1981.
136. Rengachary, S. S., and Watanabe, I.: Ultrastructure and pathogenesis of intracranial arachnoid cysts. J. Neuropathol. Exp. Neurol., 40:61–83, 1981.
137. Rengachary, S. S., Watanabe, I., and Brackett, C. E.: Pathogenesis of intracranial arachnoid cysts. Surg. Neurol., 9:139–144, 1978.
138. Rexed, B.: Arachnoidal proliferation with cyst formation in hu-

man spinal nerve roots at their entry into the intervertebral foramina: Preliminary report. J. Neurosurg., 4:414–421, 1947.

139. Ring, B. A., and Waddington, M.: Primary arachnoid cyst of the sella turcica. Am. J. Radiol., 98:611–615, 1966.

140. Robinson, R. G.: The temporal lobe agenesis syndrome. Brain, 87:87–106, 1964.

141. Robinson, R. G.: Congenital cysts of the brain: Arachnoid malformations. Progr. Neurol. Surg., 4:133–174, 1971.

142. Rossitch, E., Jr., and Oakes, W. J.: Klüver-Bucy syndrome in a child with bilateral arachnoid cysts: Report of a case. Neurosurgery, 24:110–112, 1989.

143. Rousseaux, M., Dhellemmes, P., Clarisse, J., et al.: Les kystes et les pseudokystes arachnoïdiens sous, retro et supracérébelleux de l'adulte. Neurochirurgie, 28:245–253, 1982.

144. Rousseaux, M., Lesoin, F., Christiaens, J. L., et al.: Kystes arachnoïdiens plurilobés pariétaux de l'adulte: Deux observations. Neurochirurgie, 30:245–248, 1984.

145. Rousseaux, M., Lesoin, F., Petit, H., et al.: Les kystes arachnoïdiens de l'angle ponto-cérébelleux. Neurochirurgie, 30:119–124, 1984.

146. Ruscalleda, J., Guardia, E., dos Santos, F. M., et al.: Dynamic study of arachnoid cysts with metrizamide. Neuroradiology, 20:185–189, 1980.

147. Russo, R. H., and Kindt, G. W.: A neuroanatomical basis for the bobble-head syndrome. J. Neurol., 41:720–723, 1974.

148. Sato, K., Shimoji, T., Yaguchi, K., et al.: Middle fossa arachnoid cyst: Clinical, neuroradiological and surgical features. Child's Brain, 10:301–316, 1983.

149. Schachenmayr, W., and Friede, R. L.: Fine structure of arachnoid cysts. J. Neuropathol. Exp. Neurol., 38:434–446, 1978.

150. Schachenmayr, W., and Friede, R. L.: The origin of subdural neomembranes: I. Fine structure of the dura-arachnoid interface in man. Am. J. Pathol., 92:53–68, 1978.

151. Scherer, E.: Über Cystenbildung der weichen Hirnhäute im Liquorraum der Sylvischen Furche mit hochgradiger Deformierung des Gehirns. Ztschr. Ges. Neurol. Psychiat., 152:787–799, 1935.

152. Schlesinger, H.: Beitrage zur Klinik der Ruckenmarks und Wirbelsäulentumoren. Jena, G. Fischer, 1898, pp. 162–163.

153. Schreiber, M. S.: Primary congenital arachnoid cysts. Med. J. Aust., 2:802–803, 1959.

154. Schuknecht, H. F., and Gao, Y. Z.: Arachnoid cyst in the internal auditory canal. Ann. Otol. Rhinol. Laryngol., 92:535–541, 1983.

155. Serlo, W., Wendt, L. V., Heikkinen, E., et al.: Shunting procedures in the management of intracranial cerebrospinal cysts in infancy and childhood. Acta Neurochir., 76:111–116, 1985.

156. Seur, N. H., and Kooman, A.: Arachnoid cyst of the middle fossa with paradoxical changes of the bony structures. Neuroradiology, 12:177–183, 1976.

157. Shaw, C. M.: "Arachnoid cysts" of the sylvian fissure versus "temporal lobe agenesis" syndrome. Ann. Neurol., 5:483–485, 1979.

158. Shaw, C. M., and Alvord, E. C.: Congenital arachnoid cysts and their differential diagnosis. In Vihken, P. J., and Bruyn, G. W., eds.: Congenital Malformation of the Brain and Skull. Part II. Amsterdam, Elsevier North-Holland, 1977, pp. 75–135.

159. Shuangshoti, S.: Calcified congenital arachnoid cyst with heterotopic neuroglia in wall. J. Neurol. Neurosurg. Psychiatry, 41:88–94, 1978.

160. Smith, R. A., and Smith, W. A.: Arachnoid cysts of the middle cranial fossa: Surgical considerations. Surg. Neurol., 5:246–252, 1976.

161. Spiller, W. G., Musser, J. H., and Martin, E.: A case of intradural spinal cyst with operation and recovery, with a brief report of eleven cases of tumor of the spinal cord or spinal column. Trans. Coll. Physicians Philadelphia, 25:1–18, 1971.

162. Starkman, S. P., Brown, T. C., and Linell, E. A.: Cerebral arachnoid cysts. J. Neuropathol. Exp. Neurol., 17:484–500, 1958.

163. Stein, S. C.: Intracranial developmental cysts in children: Treatment by cistoperitoneal shunting. Neurosurgery, 8:647–650, 1981.

164. Strully, K. J.: Meningeal diverticula of sacral nerve roots (perineural cysts). J.A.M.A., 161:1147–1152, 1956.

165. Sumner, T. E., Benton, C., and Marshak, G.: Arachnoid cyst of the internal auditory canal producing facial paralysis in a three-year-old child. Pediatr. Radiol., 114:425–426, 1975.

166. Tamaki, N., Taomoto, K., Fujiwara, K., et al.: Temporal arachnoid cysts in children: Neurological and etiological considerations. Brain Nerve, 28:937–950, 1976.

167. Taveras, J. M., and Ransohoff, J.: Leptomeningeal cysts of the brain following trauma with erosion of the skull: A study of seven cases treated by surgery. J. Neurosurg., 10:233–241, 1953.

168. Teng, P., and Papatheodorou, C.: Spinal arachnoid diverticula. Br. J. Radiol., 39:249–254, 1966.

169. Thijissen, H. O. M., Marres, E. H. M., and Slooff, J. C.: Arachnoid cyst simulating intrameatal acoustic neuroma. Neuroradiology, 11:205–207, 1976.

170. Turgut, M., Ozcan, O. E., and Onol, B.: Case report and review of the literature: Arachnoid cyst of the fourth ventricle presenting as syndrome of normal pressure hydrocephalus. J. Neurosurg. Sci., 36:55–57, 1992.

171. Van der Meche, F. G. A., and Braakman, R.: Arachnoid cysts in the middle cranial fossa: Cause and treatment of progressive and non-progressive symptoms. J. Neurol. Neurosurg. Psychiatry, 46:1102–1107, 1983.

172. Vaquero, J., Carrillo, R., Cabezudo, J. M., et al.: Arachnoid cysts of the posterior fossa. Surg. Neurol., 16:117–121, 1981.

173. Verga, P.: Di alcune formazioni cistiche della dura madre spinale e della loro interpretazione patogenetica. La Speriment., 763:124–147, 1925.

174. Weinand, M. E., Rengachary, S. S., McGregor, D. H., et al.: Intradiploic arachnoid cysts: Report of two cases. J. Neurosurg., 70:954–958, 1980.

175. Weinman, D. F.: Arachnoid cysts in the sylvian fissure of the brain. J. Neurosurg., 22:185–187, 1965.

176. Wells, R. G., Sty, J. R., Young, L. W., et al.: Radiological case of the month. Am. J. Dis. Child., 142:1081–1082, 1988.

177. Williams, B.: Subarachnoid pouches of the posterior fossa with syringomyelia. Acta Neurochir., 47:187–217, 1979.

178. Williams, B., and Guthkelch, A. N.: Why do central arachnoid pouches expand? J. Neurol. Neurosurg. Psychiatry, 37:1085–1092, 1974.

179. Zingesser, L., Schechter, M., Gonatas, N., et al.: Agenesis of the corpus callosum associated with an inter-hemispheric arachnoid cyst. Br. J. Radiol., 37:905–909, 1964.

Craniosynostosis

lthough skull shape irregularity has been recognized since antiquity, the study of abnormal skull growth related to craniosynostosis had its scientific origin in the late 1700's. Sommerring noted that bone growth in the skull occurred primarily at suture lines and that when this growth site was prematurely bridged with bone an abnormal skull shape developed.[33] This was characterized by restriction of the skull's growth in a plane perpendicular to the plane of the fused suture. Similar observations were made by Otto in 1831 and Virchow in 1851.[18, 35] It was Virchow's widely publicized treatise on skull deformity that added impetus to the scientific study of abnormal skull form in craniosynostosis. He observed, as had earlier investigators, that skull growth occurred at suture lines in the skull and that when these suture lines were prematurely fused, skull deformity developed. Restriction of growth adjacent to the suture occurred, but compensatory growth occurred elsewhere in the skull to accommodate the growing brain. This understanding of normal and abnormal skull growth served as the basis for understanding skull abnormalities for the following 100 years (Fig. 40–1).

In the mid-20th century, however, the primary role of the cranial vault suture in the development of craniosynostosis skull deformities was questioned by van der Klaauw and Moss.[16, 34] Moss noted that surgeons operating on the skulls of children presumed to have craniosynostosis would occasionally find a patent cranial vault suture despite what appeared to be a typical craniosynostosis skull deformity (see Fig. 40–1).[2] Also, he recognized that there were some constant characteristic cranial base deformities associated with individual forms of craniosynostosis; and because the cranial base developed embryologically to maturity before the remainder of the cranial vault, he suggested that the cranial base abnormality was the site of primary pathological process and that the cranial vault suture abnormality (fusion) was *secondary* to the cranial base defor-

mity.[16] Testing this hypothesis in the laboratory, he removed a normal cranial vault suture and found that removal of the suture did not affect overall skull length.[15] This test indicated that the cranial vault suture, unlike the epiphysis of a long bone, does not serve as a growth site that pushes the bone ends apart with growth but is a passive recipient of growth influences.

The amount of bone deposited at the cranial vault suture is related to the strains that influence it. Brain enlargement, Moss believed, was the primary source of these tensile strains that caused the sutures to deposit bone.[17] This is known as the functional matrix theory, in which the functional enlargement or development of an organ system is the primary force in changing overall shape and determining final form. Even though brain enlargement may be the primary influence for skull enlargement, the role the vault suture plays in the development of the skull pathology associated with craniosynostosis must be determined by direct manipulation of growth at that suture.[15]

In 1979, Persson and colleagues reported that, in animals, selective restriction of an individual cranial vault suture's growth resulted in skull deformities that closely mimic the clinical condition of craniosynostosis involving the same cranial vault suture in humans.[31] Moreover, cranial base and even facial deformities develop *secondary* to the cranial vault suture restrictions.[1, 30] This observation indicates that cranial vault suture pathology may be primary in the development of craniosynostosis skull deformities leading to cranial base and facial deformity. Subsequently, Mooney and co-workers studied an animal model of congenital craniosynostosis in which cranial vault suture, vault, and cranial base abnormalities exist that closely resemble the findings of Babler and Persing on cranial suture restriction.[1, 10, 11] In addition, Opperman and colleagues' developmental studies demonstrate the very significant influence of mesenchymal tissues, in particular the

---

J. A. Persing • J. A. Jane

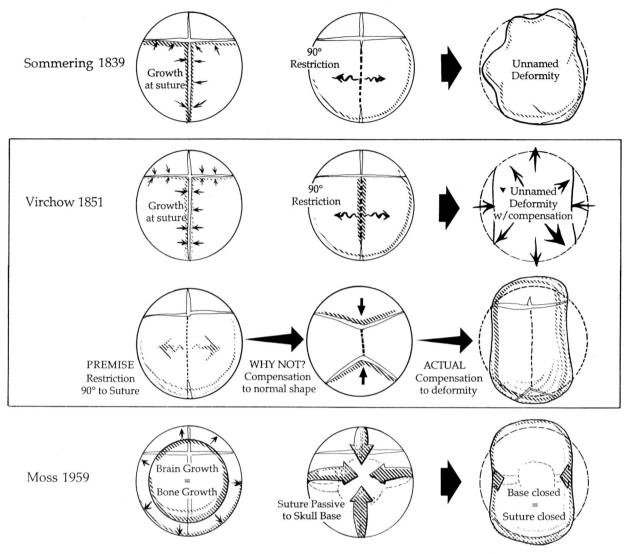

Figure 40–1

Earlier theories of cranial maldevelopment in craniosynostosis. Sommerring defines fusion of vault sutures with growth restrictions locally. Virchow describes fusion of vault sutures with local restriction of growth and more distant cranial vault compression. Moss describes functional matrix theory where skull base and brain growth dictate form.

dura and the periosteum at the suture, on the maintenance of patency of cranial vault sutures during development.[19, 20] Recognition of these factors in the development of the skull, especially matrix and cytokine influences such as transforming growth factor-beta and insulin-like growth factor II on overall skull development, are promising new areas for investigation since these factors are likely to play a role in the development of nonsyndromic craniosynostosis skull deformity.

Nonsyndromic and Syndromic Craniosynostosis

The incidence of craniosynostosis is approximately 1 in 10,000 live births. Most commonly affected is the sagittal suture, followed by the unilateral coronal, bilateral coronal, metopic, and lambdoid sutures.

Researchers have found further clinical evidence that cranial vault suture, not cranial base, pathology is of primary importance in developing skull shape pathology in nonsyndromic craniosynostosis. With surgical treatment of the cranial vault suture and bone but not the cranial base, preoperative and postoperative computed tomography shows that manipulation of the vault alone results in improvement of not only cranial vault but also cranial base pathology after surgery.[13] This indicates that removal of abnormal influence in the cranial vault suture may improve cranial base shape. Further analysis of skull growth after simple suture closure has revealed a predictable pattern based on certain rules. The ability to predict and understand the stereotypical deformity from observation of the vault suture suggests its primary role.[4, 7]

Additional studies are being done to further document skull growth changes by surgical manipulation, in particular by the use of mechanical devices to control or enhance growth influences.[4, 24] In the future, these devices may be used clinically to prolong corrective growth influences postoperatively.

Syndromic craniosynostosis is much less common and appears to be a more generalized disorder of mesenchymal development that may represent abnormalities in homeobox or *DOX* gene expression or both. Crouzon's syndrome occurs in 1 in 25,000 live births, and this bilateral coronal synostosis is frequently associated with exorbitism and midface hypoplasia. Apert's syndrome occurs in 1 in 100,000 live births; the features of brachycephaly due to coronal synostosis and midface hypoplasia are evident, but extremity syndactylies are also characteristic. There are more than 64 known craniofacial syndromes associated with craniosynostosis[3]; however, the cause of craniosynostosis is still unknown, although in some cases a genetic influence is undeniable. In the syndromic forms of craniosynostosis, autosomal dominant inheritance patterns are the general rule for the more commonly noted syndromes, such as Apert's, Crouzon's, and Pfeiffer's syndromes, whereas autosomal recessive inheritance (e.g., Carpenter's syndrome), characterized by abnormal skull shape deformities associated with polydactyly, is not commonly seen.

Diagnosis

Nonsyndromic craniosynostosis involving a single vault suture is ordinarily defined by observation of a typically deformed skull shape with radiographs serving as confirmatory evidence. The authors have developed a modification of the Virchow hypothesis on skull deformity to explain the skull shapes associated with individual forms of craniosynostosis.[4, 7] These patterns of skull abnormalities may be explained by invoking four tenets: (1) cranial vault bones directly adjacent to the prematurely fused vault suture act as a single bone plate, with reduced growth potential along all margins of that plate (Fig. 40–2A); (2) asymmetrical bone deposition occurs at vault sutures along the perimeter of the bone plate, with increased bone deposition occurring at the suture margin located farther away from the plate (see Fig. 40–2B); (3) the nonperimeter sutures in line with the fused suture deposit bone symmetrically at their sutural edges (see Fig. 40–2C); and (4) perimeter and sutures (in line) abutting the prematurely fused suture compensate to a greater degree than distant sutures (see Fig. 40–2D).

These basic rules allow for definition of cranial vault shape abnormality but do not determine etiology. This precise definition, however, is important, because skull deformity associated with craniosynostosis must be distinguished from skull deformity related to uterine molding; conditions such as plagiocephaly without craniosynostosis will improve with time and require no surgery, whereas craniosynostosis deformity will either maintain or increase skull deformity with time, indicating the need for surgery.

Operative Timing and Approaches

Experimental evidence demonstrates that improved skull form is achieved with an operation before the human equivalent of 6 months of age.[25] In clinical studies, more significant degrees of improvement were noted in patients younger than 6 months of age who underwent surgery than were observed in those patients who underwent surgery after 6 months of age. The cranial base deformities established in unilateral coronal synostosis were also corrected more successfully if surgery was performed early.[13]

The influence of surgical methods is not yet clearly defined; however, limited craniectomy procedures of few sutures appear to be beneficial in the very young patient with a mild deformity, whereas more comprehensive approaches to established skull deformity are more effective in the older child and in the child with more severe deformities at any age. Objective documentation of these approaches is not yet widespread, but Marsh and co-workers, comparing preoperative to postoperative skull shape and following a limited craniectomy procedure with a whole-vault cranioplasty approach for sagittal synostosis, showed that skull deformity was minimized with both the limited craniectomy and the more extensive cranioplasty procedure.[14] However, the skull shape returned to normal only in patients who underwent the more extensive cranioplasty procedure. Additional data are required to confirm initial impressions, but they are consistent with the hypothesis that early rapid growth of the brain allows the shape of the brain to shape the skull (Fig. 40–3).

Intracranial Pressure and Craniosynostosis

There has been long-standing concern about the restriction of brain growth in craniosynostosis due to cranial vault suture obliteration by bone; however, confusion has developed in assessing the risk of elevated pressure. This is in part related to an old practice of grouping patients with abnormal skull shapes together, including varied disorders such as poor brain development, microcephaly, and craniosynostosis. Now, imaging techniques can define vault synostosis, patency, and brain parenchyma abnormalities, and patients with microcephaly due to poor brain development can usually be distinguished from patients with skull deformity related to craniosynostosis.

Craniosynostosis, however, may result in increased intracranial pressure, which, in turn, may be associated with neurological dysfunction. Renier, in exhaustive studies, performed preoperative and postoperative recordings in patients with craniosynostosis.[32] Intracranial pressure elevation was defined as pressure greater than 15 mm Hg for more than 5 minutes in a nonanesthetized patient. Intracranial pressure elevation was particularly evident in patients with multiple suture

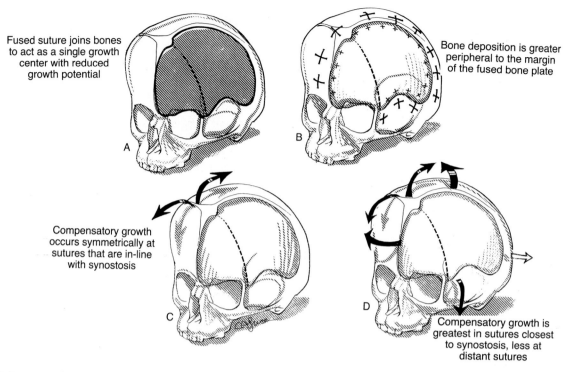

Figure 40–2

Observed characteristics of unilateral coronal synostosis. *A.* Fused left coronal suture *(dotted line)* joining frontal and parietal bone, which acts as a single growth center (bone plate) with reduced growth potential. *B.* The margin of the abutting sutures peripheral to the "fused bone plate" deposits a greater amount of bone at the suture *(large plus signs)* than at the margin of the suture adjacent to the fused bone plate *(small plus signs)*. *C.* Compensation for restricted skull growth occurs symmetrically at sutures that are "in line" with the fused suture. *D.* The greatest degree of compensation occurs in sutures closest to the fused suture *(black arrows)* and the least degree in sutures distant from the affected suture *(white arrow)*.

synostosis. In this study, 26 per cent of patients with bilateral coronal synostosis and 54 per cent of patients with bilateral coronal and metopic synostosis were shown to have elevated intracranial pressure. In single-suture stenosis, however, intracranial pressure elevation was much less frequently associated with cranial synostosis; 12 per cent of patients with unilateral coronal, 8 per cent with sagittal, and 6 per cent with metopic synostosis showed evidence of intracranial pressure elevation. The influence of this elevation on intelligence as measured by standard IQ tests showed a similar correlation: lower IQ scores were associated with greater frequency of intracranial elevation in craniosynostosis.

Operative Treatment

The technique of surgical reconstruction must be tailored to the type of synostosis present and also to

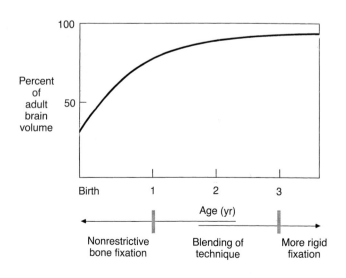

Figure 40–3

Brain growth as it relates to surgical technique of fixation of individual elements of bone during skull reconstruction. Note that nonrigid fixation methods are preferred during rapid phases of brain growth (e.g., in patients younger than 1 year of age), while patients older than 3 years are treated with more definitive fixation, since a high percentage of adult brain volume has already been achieved. Patients between 1 and 3 years of age receive a combination of fixation techniques.

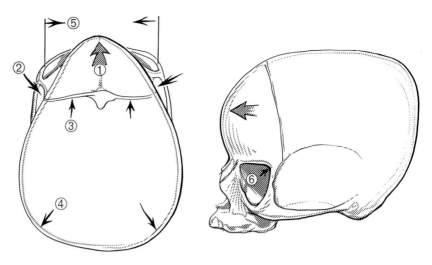

Figure 40–4

Features of the trigone-shaped skull of metopic synostosis: 1, ridging of the fused suture; 2, temporal narrowing; 3, patent coronal suture displaced anteriorly; 4, compensatory bulging of the parieto-occipital region, contributing to the pear-shaped appearance of skull; 5, narrowed bizygomatic dimension; and 6, posterior displacement of superolateral orbital rim.

the age of the patient. It is clear that reshaping bone in a child younger than 1 year of age is much more readily achieved without significant bone disruption than in the older child. The methods of fixation for reshaped skull segments should also be different for children who are very young to avoid induced abnormalities in brain development as a result of vault surgery and subsequent restriction of brain growth. Patients who are younger than 3 years old have a substantial amount of brain growth remaining, but because those older than 3 years old have already achieved approximately 85 to 90 per cent of their ultimate brain mass (see Fig. 40–3), the fixation techniques may be more rigid and inclusive in these children. In this chapter, the treatment of patients who are younger than 1 year old and those who are older than 3 years old is described, recognizing that patients between 1 and 3 years of age will require a blending of the techniques and approaches described for the other two time periods.

METOPIC SYNOSTOSIS

Metopic synostosis is characterized by metopic suture ridging, bilateral flattening of the frontal bones, anterior displacement of the coronal sutures, lateral flaring of the posterior parietal regions, hypotelorism, and flattening of the supraorbital ridges (Fig. 40–4). Viewed from above, the skull has a characteristic triangular shape known as trigonencephaly.

Operative Technique in the Child Younger Than 1 Year of Age

In children younger than 1 year of age, a zigzag variation on the coronal incision, sometimes called the stealth incision, may be used to minimize the visibility of incisional scalp alopecia (Fig. 40–5). Dissection of the anterior and posterior scalp flaps is conducted in the supraperiosteal plane, preferred because bleeding is reduced and the periosteal tissue left on the bone anchors individual bone fragments and maintains their alignment with subsequent remodeling.[23]

Incision of the periosteum approximately 1 cm above the supraorbital rim aids in subperiorbital dissection, to allow for bilateral orbital rim osteotomy and advancement (Fig. 40–6A). A bifrontal craniotomy is performed, and the posterior extent is located just anterior to the coronal suture. The orbital rims are reshaped to assume a more convex configuration, particularly in the supralateral orbital rim. No attempt is made to correct the hypotelorism that is evident on preoperative examination, since it is ordinarily relatively mild and does not constitute a significant long-term postoperative deformity.

Figure 40–5

Scalp incisions. *A*. Bicoronal skin incision. *B*. A zigzag coronal incision that provides greater access to anterior and posterior skull as well as more acceptable scar due to hair coverage. *C*. Reflection of anterior scalp flap with subperiosteal dissection in the supraorbital region.

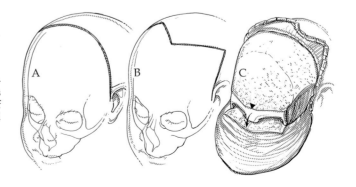

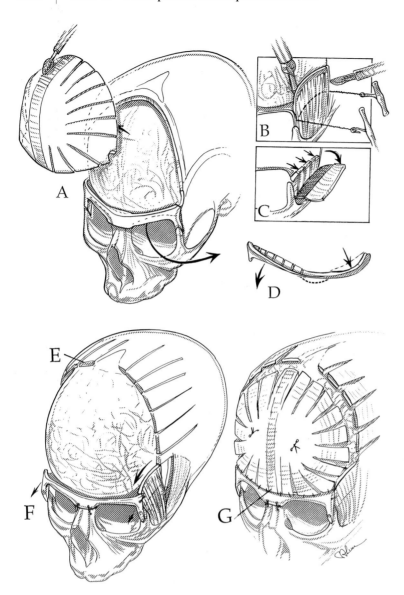

Figure 40–6

Early metopic synostosis. *A.* Bifrontal craniotomy is performed with burring of central ridge, peripheral radial osteotomy, and bilateral removal of visor. *B.* Composite vascularized temporalis squamous muscle flap is developed using Gigli saw and myotomy in the temporalis muscle. *C.* Composite flap is reflected laterally, and squamous temporal bone is split vertically into barrel staves and out- or infractured *(arrows)*. *D.* Supraorbital rim is recontoured with internal kerfs, and bending of rims is performed to achieve rounded contour. *E.* Anterior parietal bone undergoes parallel-oriented osteotomies to expand the parietal region laterally. *F.* Visor is reattached at nasion, and temporalis composite myo-osseous flap is advanced forward *(arrows)* to advanced orbital rims. *G.* Reshaped bifrontal bone is attached to supraorbital rim and underlying dura.

Additional reconstructive steps are taken in the temporal regions. Instead of dissecting the temporalis muscle from the infratemporal fossa, a composite resection of the squamous temporal bone and the overlying temporalis muscle is performed using a Gigli saw and a craniotome (see Fig. 40–6*B*). The remaining basal bone in the temporal region is split into vertical "staves" and fractured laterally, increasing the flare in the temporal region (see Fig. 40–6*C*) to counteract the concavity typically found in this region with metopic synostosis. The anterior parietal bone is divided with anteroposterior slats to increase the flare in the anterior parietal region. The bifrontal bone graft undergoes radial osteotomies, reshaping the bone to provide a less acutely angled midline shape and more prominence to the lateral superior frontal bone (see Fig. 40–6*B*). The midline frontal bone frequently requires shaping with a burr to reduce its prominence. The advanced supraorbital rim is affixed to the nasal bone and the anterior portion of the zygoma at the level of the frontal zygomatic suture. An oblique stair-step cut in the lateral zygomatic process of the frontal bone affords the necessary release and subsequent support for the advanced rim. A composite of temporalis muscle and squamous bone is attached laterally to the advanced supraorbital rims. At the coronal suture, the adjacent bone is removed, creating a neocoronal suture, to remove the bony restriction to expansion of the dura in this region after further anterior remodeling of the frontal bone. The scalp flap is then replaced.

A less radical procedure is used for less severe forms (Fig. 40–7)[5]; occasional simple burring down of a prominent metopic suture will suffice. If the lateral orbital rims do not seem to need advancement, then the temporalis muscle can be detached and reinserted in a more anterior position. Also, it is acceptable to remove the metopic suture down to the nasal suture along with the thickened medial orbital rim or frontal bone and reinsert on the frontal process of the zygoma along with the temporalis muscle.

Figure 40–7

Alternate treatment of mild metopic synostosis. *A.* Burring frontal midline prominence may be sufficient. *B.* Middle bifrontal craniotomy is performed, followed by removal of fused suture, midline dural plication, and removal of narrowed lateral frontal bone and abnormally thickened bone in the parasagittal region of the orbits. *C.* A new supraorbital rim is developed following the contouring of frontal bone graft and inferior displacement *(arrows)* to fill in bone defect removed by prior osteotomy. Temporalis muscle is advanced anteriorly.

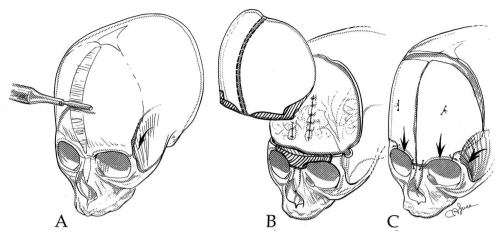

Operative Technique in the Child Older Than 3 Years of Age

In both the patient who is older than 3 years of age and the younger child, the same scalp and dissection plane is opted for and a bifrontal bone graft is elevated. In patients older than 3 years of age, the graft may be split vertically into anteroposterior slats, in which the intracranial surface of the bone undergoes "kerf" (weakening of the bone) to allow for remodeling (Fig. 40–8). The goal is to achieve a more round frontal form and less central V-shaped angularity. Supraorbital rims undergo the same form of elevation and advancement as in the younger child. The temporalis muscle and squamous portion of the temporal bone are elevated as a composite flap, advanced, and attached to the advanced superior orbital rim. The individual bone slats are reattached to the advanced superior orbital rim medially and laterally, with care taken to avoid significant bony defects, since osteogenesis in a more mature child is much less active than it is in a younger

child. In some instances, split calvarial bone grafting may be necessary to fill in bone gaps.

UNILATERAL CORONAL SYNOSTOSIS

Unilateral coronal synostosis is characterized by ridging of the prematurely fused half of the coronal suture, flattening of the ipsilateral frontal and parietal bones, bulging of the ipsilateral squamous portion of the temporal bone, and bulging of the contralateral frontal and parietal bones (Fig. 40–9). The nasal radix is deviated to the side of the fused suture, and the ear ipsilateral to the fused suture is displaced anteriorly compared with the contralateral ear. Confirmatory radiographic findings include the "harlequin" orbit deformity, characterized by elevation of the greater and lesser wings of the sphenoid ipsilateral to the fused coronal suture. Computed tomography of the cranial base demonstrates a shortened anterior cranial fossa and a narrowed sphenopetrosal angle ipsilateral to the fused coronal suture.

Figure 40–8

Mature bone remodeling for metopic synostosis. *A.* Bifrontal craniotomy is performed with elevation of bilateral supraorbital rims. *B.* Frontal bone is divided into slats with endocranial kerfs weakening the bone to allow bending *(arrow).* *C.* Remodeled bone is replaced on skull with temporalis composite myo-osseous flap and is advanced to prevent postoperative temporal hollowing. *D.* Split calvarial grafts are used to fill any significant bone deficits.

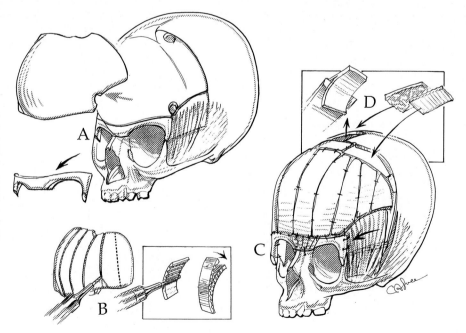

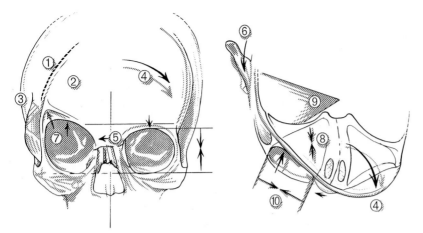

Figure 40–9

Unilateral coronal synostosis characteristics: 1, fused suture; 2, flattening of ipsilateral frontal bone; 3, bulging of right squamous temporal bone; 4, bulging of contralateral frontal bone; 5, nasal radix deviated to ipsilateral side; 6, ear ipsilateral to fused suture displaced anteriorly; 7, harlequin deformity, shown on radiograph, is superiorly displaced ipsilateral greater wing of sphenoid bone; 8, shortening of ipsilateral anterior cranial fossa; 9, narrowed ipsilateral sphenopetrosal angle; and 10, narrowing of ipsilateral mediolateral dimension of orbit.

Operative Technique in the Child Younger Than 1 Year of Age

The patient who is younger than 1 year old is placed in a supine position, and a zigzag coronal incision is carried out. The anterior scalp flap is dissected in the supraperiosteal plane to approximately 1 cm above the superior orbital rims. At this point, dissection is subperiosteal to define the orbital rims bilaterally. The mediolateral dimension of the orbital rim ipsilateral to the fused suture is measured and found to be narrower than it is contralaterally. The superoinferior dimension of the orbit contralateral to the fused suture is reduced compared with the rim ipsilateral to the fused suture.

A bifrontal craniotomy is performed, avoiding removal of the temporalis muscle from the underlying squamous temporal bone (Fig. 40–10). An orbital roof osteotomy, extending to the frontal zygomatic suture laterally to the midline, is carried out bilaterally to elevate and reshape the supraorbital rims. Contouring of the inner portion of the zygomatic process of the frontal bone is performed to equal the mediolateral dimension of the orbit on the contralateral side (Fig. 40–11). The superior orbital rim contralateral to the fused suture is shaped with a burr to achieve symmetry. A composite (the temporalis and squamous portion of the temporal bone) flap is elevated ipsilateral to the fused suture, and the basal coronal suture is resected to the frontal sphenoid suture.[29] The orbital rims are

contoured to achieve symmetry and to increase projection of this supralateral orbital rim ipsilateral to the fused half of the coronal suture. The orbital rims are secured with wire in the midline and sutured laterally at the frontal process of the zygoma. The nasal radix deviation is usually not corrected since it will be ameliorated with subsequent growth in the majority of patients. The temporalis-squamous temporal bone composite flap is attached to the advanced superior orbital rim ipsilateral to the previously fused suture. The frontal craniotomy bone is reshaped by radial osteotomy to increase projection in the flattened bone segment ipsilateral to the fused suture and to reduce projection of the bulging contralateral frontal bone. The bone is then affixed to the advanced supraorbital rims. For less severe conditions, particularly in younger children, similar techniques can give good results (Fig. 40–12).[9]

Operative Technique in the Child Older Than 3 Years of Age

The patient who is older than 3 years of age undergoes a coronal skin flap and periorbital dissection similar to that performed in the younger child (Fig. 40–13). A bifrontal bone graft is elevated, but instead of a bilateral orbital rim elevation a unilateral orbital rim elevation is performed ipsilateral to the fused coronal sutures. In the older child, the osteotomy extends infe-

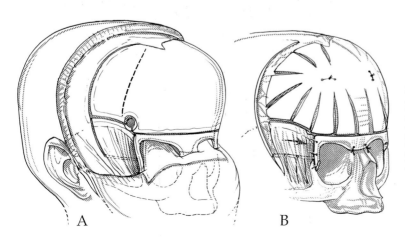

Figure 40–10

Early unilateral coronal synostosis. *A.* Bicoronal takedown and bifrontal craniotomy is done with burr hole placed superior to temporal crest. *B.* Bilateral supraorbital rim advancement and contouring is associated with composite advancement of myo-osseous flap (see also Fig. 40–6C).

A   B

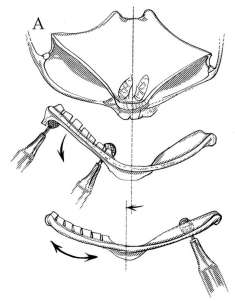

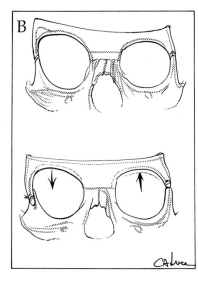

Figure 40–11

Anterior cranial fossa viewed from above in right-sided unilateral coronal synostosis. *A.* Superior orbital rim ipsilateral to fused suture is contoured by drill to equalize the mediolateral dimension of the orbit, bilaterally, and contour vertically oriented medial superior orbit ipsilateral to fused suture. Bone is advanced following weakening kerfs on orbital roof. *B.* Bilateral orbital rims are contoured and both advanced to equalize projection of orbital rims.

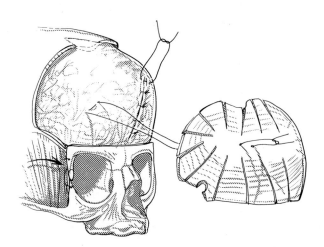

Figure 40–12

In simpler cases, treatment is directed to dural plication in the frontal region contralateral to the fused suture, contouring the frontal bone flap by radial osteotomy, and securing the flap to the dura and superior orbital rims. A simple advancement of the temporalis muscle is affixed to the advanced lateral orbital rim, which has been secured to the frontal process of the zygoma.

Figure 40–13

Mature bone remodeling techniques in unilateral coronal synostosis. *A.* Bifrontal osteotomy with myoosseous temporal bone flap outlined. *B.* Frontal bone divided into slats, and endocranial surface channeled with kerfs, contoured, and replaced. Superolateral orbital rim is advanced by C-shaped orbital osteotomy, and contralateral orbital rim and roof are equalized to height of fused suture by contouring.

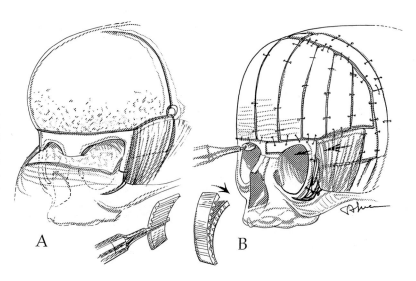

riorly into the body of the zygoma. The abnormal mediolateral dimension of the orbital rim (i.e., mediolateral shortening) ipsilateral to the fused suture is corrected by contouring the inner aspect of the zygomatic process of the frontal bone. The orbital rim to be advanced is now in the shape of a letter C.[12, 28, 37] Bone grafts are harvested from the parietal region to insert into the body of the zygoma, the anteriormost portion of which is now advanced in the orbital rim. The temporalis muscle composite flap is advanced, attaching the squamous portion of the temporal bone to the advanced orbital rim laterally. The bifrontal bone graft is split into slats approximately 1.5 cm wide, weakened on their undercranial surface by transversely oriented kerf channels, and then greenstick fractured to achieve the desired form. The individual slats are then attached to the superior orbital rim and to each other to achieve the final desired symmetry.

BILATERAL CORONAL SYNOSTOSIS

Bilateral coronal synostosis is characterized by ridging of the coronal suture, flattening of the caudal portion of the frontal bones and supraorbital ridges, and bulging of the cephalad portion of the frontal bones (Fig. 40–14). The occiput is flattened, and the squamous portion of the temporal bones is unusually prominent. The vertex of the skull is more anteriorly situated than normal. Radiographically, bilateral harlequin abnormalities are present in the orbits and basal computed tomography demonstrates shortened anterior cranial fossae and bilaterally narrowed sphenoid petrosal angles.

Operative Technique in the Child Younger Than 1 Year of Age

Because the abnormalities of coronal synostosis are situated both anteriorly and posteriorly within the skull, a different approach to intraoperative patient positioning is elected. The modified prone position, in which the anterior and posterior portions of the skull are exposed simultaneously, has proved optimal; however, to use this position certain precautions should be taken.[22] The presence of craniovertebral anomalies and the ability of the patient to tolerate this position must be assessed preoperatively. Cervical spine radiographs with flexion and extension lateral views and basal computed tomography are performed routinely to identify any patient who might be at risk for neurological injury. If anomalies such as the Arnold-Chiari malformation and instability of the cervical spine are identified, a two-stage approach with the patient alternately in a supine and then a prone position should be elected.

If no vertebral abnormalities exist, the patient's head is placed on a well-padded chin support (usually the combination of a bean bag and a well-cushioned anterior portion of a Philadelphia collar for stabilization).[21] After this, a coronal incision is performed and anterior and posterior supraperiosteal dissection is done (Fig. 40–15). The posterior limit is the foramen magnum, and the anterior limit is the lateral portion of the orbital rims at the level of the frontal zygomatic suture bilaterally. Frontal and parieto-occipital bone grafts are elevated, leaving bone over the vertex of the skull and two lateral struts of bone extending from the vertex to the base of the skull. Subperiosteal dissection is performed posteriorly in the occiput. Barrel stave osteotomies are performed in the occipital region,[27] with the individual bone segments fractured posteriorly to increase the potential space in the posterior skull later in surgery for the repositioned brain and dural envelope. The superior orbital rims are elevated bilaterally to the level of the frontal zygomatic suture, contoured, and fixed in the advanced position. The squamous portion of the temporal bone is elevated with the overlying temporalis muscle and advanced and attached to the superior orbital rims. The more basal temporal bone undergoes osteotomy and infracture to reduce the abnormal convexity in the region. An intracranial pressure monitor is placed in the right parietal bone, off the midline. The struts extending from the vertex of the skull in the parietal region to the basal temporal region are then divided, shifted posteriorly, and reduced in height (usually 1.0 to 1.5 cm) to change the position of the vertex of the skull, flatten the frontal contour, and reduce the height of the skull.

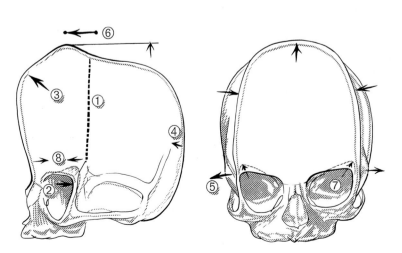

Figure 40–14

Features of bilateral coronal synostosis: 1, fused coronal suture; 2, recessed superior orbital rim; 3, prominent frontal bone; 4, flattening of occiput; 5, anteriorly displaced skull vertex; 6, shortened anterior cranial fossa; 7, harlequin deformity of greater wing of sphenoid; and 8, protrusion of squamous portion of temporal bone.

Figure 40–15

Early bilateral coronal synostosis technique. *A.* Osteotomies: 1, bifrontal craniotomy; 2, biparietal occipital craniotomy; 3, struts severed inferiorly, with bone removed *(shaded)* equal to anticipated height reduction; 4, barrel stave osteotomies in occiput, fractured posteriorly; 5, bilateral supraorbital rim elevation. *B.* Height reduction: 6, bilateral supraorbital rim advancement and fixation at nasion; 7, composite myoosseous temporalis flap advanced, fixed to rim; 8, intracranial pressure monitoring as height of skull is reduced; 9, height reduction achieved by slowly cinching wire struts; and 10, greater prominence achieved in parietal occiput. *C.* Completed remodeling of skull.

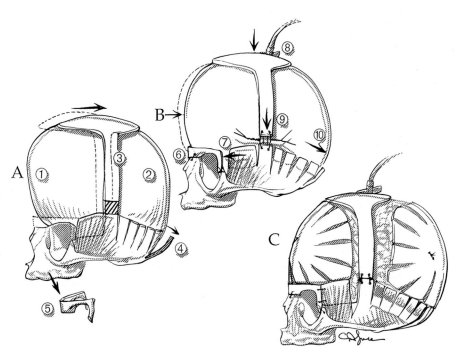

This height reduction accomplishes correction of the abnormal turret shape of the skull and encourages brain and dural shift to fill the space created in the occiput. This achieves the desired elongation of the anteroposterior axis of the skull. Reduction in the height of the skull is achieved slowly, monitoring intracranial pressure under the conditions of normotension and normocapnia. Intracranial pressure should only be elevated for brief periods, followed by rapid reduction to normal tension as the height of the skull is reduced. It is anticipated that reshaping the cranial vault will lead to temporary elevation in cranial pressure during the active dural remodeling process, but within a short period of time the removal of confining bone will reduce cranial pressure overall.

The bifrontal bone graft undergoes radial osteotomy reshaping to the desired effect and attachment to the superior orbital rim; however, the frontal bone is not attached to the anterior parietal region. A neocoronal suture bone defect approximately 1 cm wide is created at the site of the normal coronal suture. The posterior occipital bone is reshaped to achieve greater convexity, and a defect of approximately 1 cm is created between the reshaped bone graft and surrounding bone to allow for preferential expansion of the parieto-occipital region.

Operative Technique in the Child Older Than 3 Years of Age

In a child older than 3 years of age, a zigzag coronal incision and supraperiosteal dissection plane is carried out similar to the technique used for the younger child. After elevation of the bifrontal and parietal occipital bone grafts, barrel stave osteotomies are performed in the occipital region (Fig. 40–16). The orbital rims are elevated and advanced as a unit extending into the

frontal process of the zygoma. The two C-shaped rings of bone are advanced and stabilized. The squamous temporal bone and temporalis muscle are elevated as a composite and advanced to attach to the posterior border of the advanced orbital rim. The height of the skull is again reduced and the intracranial pressure is monitored as in the younger child; however, patients who are older than 3 years of age require a much more prolonged period of accommodation than the younger child, and less height reduction is ordinarily achieved. Correction of over 1 cm is unusual in the child older than 3 years of age, whereas 1.0 to 1.5 cm of correction is quite common in a child younger than 1 year of age.

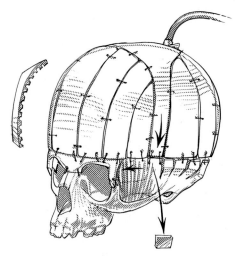

Figure 40–16

Bilateral coronal synostosis, mature bone techniques. Individual frontal and parietal bone divided into slats weakened by transversely oriented kerfs of the bone to allow bending of the skull. Height of the skull is reduced, equivalent to bone removed in parietal region.

The bifrontal and parietal occipital bone grafts are then remodeled by dividing the bone segments into vertical slats, weakened on the endocranial surface by kerfs, then reshaped with bone-molding instruments and microfracture. Individual bone slats are reapproximated frontally to the superior orbital rim and proceed posteriorly to the occiput.

SAGITTAL SYNOSTOSIS

Sagittal synostosis results in a skull shape that is characterized by biparietal narrowing, ridging of the sagittal suture, and bilateral bulging of the frontal or occipital regions or both (Fig. 40–17). Radiographically, fusion of the sagittal suture is evident. Individuality in surgical technique is necessary for addressing the most salient deformities. Usually, one of three varieties of sagittal synostosis predominates. These varieties are anterior compensation, posterior compensation, and "golf tee'" deformities. The anterior type can be treated with the standard π (pi) procedure with optional supplementary frontal craniotomy reshaping and dura plication.[8] The posterior variety needs a posterior π but this often also requires elevation of the parietal region. This is a variety of the golf-tee deformity, which may also be seen with frontal bossing and may need surgery via a modified prone position.

Operative Technique in the Child Younger Than 1 Year of Age

As in the child with bilateral coronal synostosis, a patient with complete sagittal synostosis frequently has simultaneous evidence of skull deformity in the anterior and posterior skull. For the most complete correction of these abnormalities, the patient is placed in the modified prone position;[22] however, before placing the child in this position, basal computed tomography and cervical spine radiography should be done to rule out cranial vertebral anomalies such as Arnold-Chiari type I malformation, cervical spine instability, or both. If anomalies are evident, a two-stage approach is more prudent.

If no cranial vertebral abnormalities exist, the patient's head is placed on a well-padded chin support and a zigzag coronal incision is carried out. The currently used procedure is a modification of a previously described π procedure (Fig. 40–18).[8, 36] Anterior and posterior scalp flaps are dissected in the supraperiosteal plane; and bifrontal, individual parietal, and occipital bone grafts are elevated. Since there are no significant orbital abnormalities evident in sagittal synostosis, no orbital dissection is performed. However, because of characteristic hollowing seen in this area, lateral barrel staves are carried out temporally through the squamous portion of the temporal bone and temporalis muscle. These bone segments are then outfractured to increase projection in this region. The skull is shortened anteriorly to posteriorly by first reshaping the occipital bone to a flatter plane and then attaching the reshaped bone posteriorly to the occiput. The paramedian parietal bone adjacent to the sagittal sinuses is elevated, the ridge contoured, and the bone attached posteriorly to the occipital bone. The bifrontal bone graft is ordinarily reshaped by radial osteotomy to correct abnormal convexity bilaterally in the supralateral frontal bones. To angulate the forehead posteriorly to resolve abnormal frontal prominence, a segment of the median parietal bone is removed, usually approximately 1.5 cm in length. When this is accomplished, an overlap of the lateral frontal bone is seen over the superior lateral orbital rim. A triangular wedge of bone is removed over this area to allow precise alignment with the superior orbital rim. The parietal bones are then re-

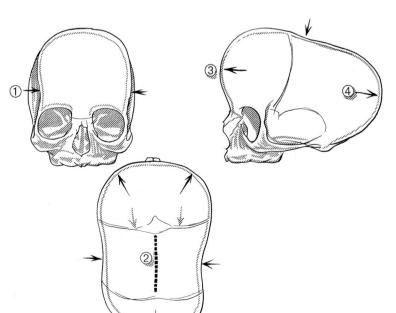

Figure 40–17

Sagittal synostosis characteristics: 1, bitemporal narrowing; 2, ridging of fused sagittal suture; 3, frontal bossing; and 4, occipital bossing.

Figure 40–18

Early sagittal synostosis, operative approach: 1, bifrontal craniotomy; 2, separate parietal craniotomies bilaterally; 3, biparietal occipital craniotomies; 4, lateral barrel stave osteotomies; 5, recontour of occiput and replacement of bone; 6, reduction in skull length by attachment of shortened midline bone; 7, contour of projecting sagittal ridge with reduction in length; 8, bifrontal bone graft has undergone radial osteotomy; 9, removal of infralateral frontal bone to allow posterior tilting of frontal bone on visor; and 10, parietal bone grafts attached to underlying dura.

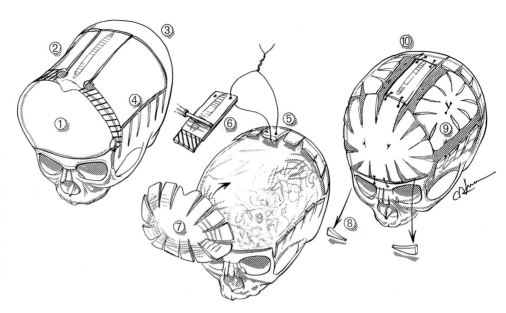

shaped with radial osteotomies to give a more convex form. Two paramedian neosagittal sutures are created by tailoring the remaining bone grafts so that there is a gap of approximately 1 cm between the midline bone and the parietal bone grafts. To allow relatively free lateral movement of the brain and bone in this region, the parietal bone grafts are sutured only to the underlying dura and not to adjacent bone, resulting in a more rounded skull form.

An alternative mode of treatment addresses the most salient deformity. Usually one of three varieties of sagittal synostosis predominates, and the surgical correction can be somewhat restricted. These varieties are anterior compensation (Fig. 40–19A), posterior compensation (see Fig. 40–19B), and golf tee deformity (see Fig. 40–19C). The anterior type can be treated by the standard π procedure employing optional supplementary frontal craniotomy with reshaping and dural plication (Fig. 40–20A and B).[36] The posterior variety needs a posterior π procedure, but this often also requires evaluation of the frontal region (see Fig. 40–20C and D). This is a variety of the golf tee deformity that may also be seen with frontal bossing and may need surgery with the patient in a modified prone position.

Operative Technique in the Child Older Than 3 Years of Age

The child with sagittal synostosis who is older than 3 years of age is placed in the modified prone position,

and anterior and posterior supraperiosteal scalp dissection, similar to Marchac's original procedure, is carried out as discussed for the younger child.[32] Serial bifrontal, bifrontoparietal, biparietal, and right occipital bone grafts are elevated (Fig. 40–21). The occiput convexity is flattened by radial osteotomy and greenstick fracture. However, the parietal bone is reshaped to a more convex form using kerfs on the endocranial surface of the bone and a series of controlled greenstick fractures. Bone grafts harvested from the occiput and anterior parietal region are inserted into the gaps created by lateral remodeling of the parietal bone in the temporal regions. The frontal bone graft is angulated posteriorly to achieve normal forehead contour. The bone overlapping the anterior parietal paramedian bone is resected in the form of a triangle. Barrel staves are performed in the temporal region, creating multiple composite flaps, and are fractured outward. The remodeled bone grafts are secured anterior to posterior and medial to lateral.

LAMBDOID SYNOSTOSIS

Children with lambdoid synostosis typically have flattening of the parietal occipital regions ipsilateral to the fused portion of the suture. If synostosis has occurred unilaterally, an asymmetrical occiput is seen, characterized by flattening of the occiput ipsilateral to the fused suture and contralateral bulging evident in

Figure 40–19

A. Fusion of anterior portion of sagittal suture with compensatory frontal bossing. B. Fusion of posterior sagittal suture with compensatory occipital bossing and bathrocephaly. C. Golf tee deformity: narrowing of posterior occiput with posterior sagittal fusion, resulting in frontal bulge compensation as viewed from above.

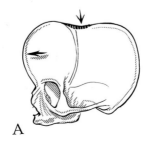
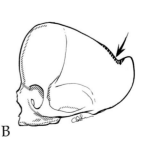
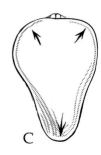

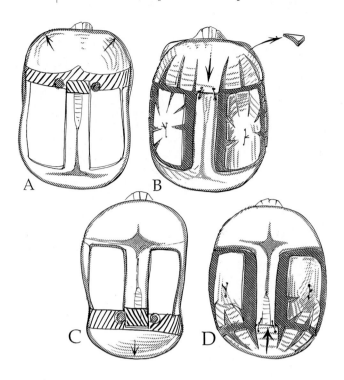

Figure 40–20

A and *B*. Primarily anterior sagittal fusion: *A*. Anterior π procedure: separate parietal craniotomies with removal of coronal suture. *B*. Remodeled bone sutured to dura after sagittal fixation and posterior tilt of frontal bone. *C* and *D*. Primarily posterior sagittal fusion: *C*. Posterior π procedure: occipital craniotomy, parietal craniotomies, and removal of lambdoid suture to allow forward movement of occiput. *D*. Remodeled bone returned as occiput is fixed to shortened sagittal strut.

the parietal occiput region (Fig. 40–22). If bilateral synostosis has occurred, then symmetrical flattening of the occiput is seen. If the synostosis is severe, skull deformities in the frontal region, which may include elevation of the vertex of the skull, are evident.

Operative Technique in the Child Younger Than 1 Year of Age

Individualization of surgical technique is required; however, most of the deformities can be satisfactorily corrected with placement of the patient in the prone position and surgical manipulations in the occipital bone.[26] If, however, vertex and frontal abnormalities exist, the patient should be placed in the modified prone position, similar to the position used for a patient with bilateral coronal synostosis. This discussion

will be restricted to patients having deformities in the parietal occiput.

A patient with occipital deformity is placed in the prone position, and a posteriorly "displaced" coronal incision is carried out (Fig. 40–23*A*). Dissection is performed in the supraperiosteal plane. A biparietal occipital bone graft is elevated in patients with unilateral synostosis or bilateral lambdoid synostosis, with care taken to avoid injury to the transverse sinus. Barrel stave osteotomies are performed in both unilateral and bilateral synostosis; in the bilateral lambdoid synostosis with bilateral posterior flattening evident, barrel staves are performed to increase bilateral occipital projection. In patients with unilateral lambdoid synostosis, the occiput is fractured posteriorly, unilaterally ipsilateral to the fused suture, and inwardly on the contralateral bulging side. The biparietal occipital bone

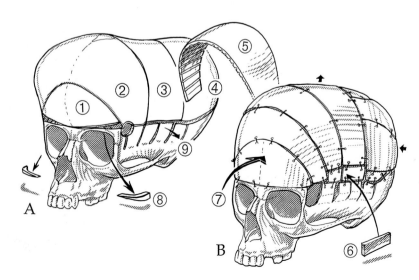

Figure 40–21

Serial bone grafts. *A*: 1, Bifrontal; 2, bifrontoparietal; 3, biparietal; 4, occipital; and 5, biparietal segment reformed with endocranial kerfs and greenstick fractures. *B*: 7, Bifrontal bone graft tilted posteriorly and upright, following removal of restraining triangle of frontal bone bilaterally (8).

Figure 40–22
Features of lambdoid synostosis. *A.* Unilateral lambdoid fusion: 1, unilateral fusion; 2, occipital flattening; and 3, ipsilateral to fusion: anteriorly displaced ear. *B* and *C.* Bilateral lambdoid fusion: 4, with bilateral occipital flattening; 5, prominence of frontal bone; and 6, elevation of skull vertex.

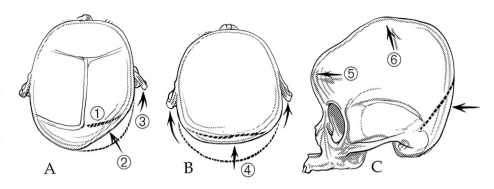

graft undergoes radial osteotomy and contouring to achieve symmetry (see Fig. 40–23*B*). In unilateral synostosis, the convex side is made flatter and the flatter side is made more convex with the use of greenstick fracture. In patients with bilateral lambdoid synostosis, a bilaterally convex occiput is achieved by similar methodology. The bone is then reattached to the dura and not to adjacent bone.

Operative Technique in the Child Older Than 3 Years of Age

In patients with this condition who are older than 3 years, a biparietal occipital bone graft is elevated and posterior barrel staves are performed in the basal occiput. In addition, a more anteriorly situated biparietal bone graft is harvested and used as a band to symmetrically re-form the occiput; the graft is attached more anteriorly with microplates and miniplates to the basal parietal bone. The more basal parietal occipital bone graft, which was deformed due to the synostosis, is placed in the more superior parietal region after contouring and reshaping.

CORRECTION OF "POSTERIOR" SYNOSTOSIS

Posterior deformities include unilateral and bilateral lambdoid synostosis with or without posterior sagittal

synostosis or squamosal synostosis. These are rare conditions, and the principal surgical difficulty lies in not being able to maintain the corrected posterior projection. Jane has been using a single-molded strip microplate attached just above the foramen magnum to correct this projection (Fig. 40–24). The dead space that is obtained is so large that Jane believes it is unlikely that significant inward migration would occur.

Operative Complications

Although surgical procedures for craniosynostosis are quite safe despite their extensive nature, complications may arise. Problems that may be associated with cranioplasty procedures are blood loss and associated air embolus.[6] Patients undergoing these operative procedures will lose blood at a slow rate from the cancellous portion of the bone, particularly if basal skull osteotomies are performed. Adequate preparation for blood replacement and monitoring for blood loss intraoperatively as well as in the immediate postoperative period is necessary. Because of low circulating blood volumes in very young patients, it is imperative that attention be paid to achieving good hemostasis intraoperatively and monitoring blood loss postoperatively. The most appropriate postoperative site is a highly skilled intensive care unit.

As a function of blood loss, with the patient in any position (supine, prone, or modified prone) osteotom-

Figure 40–23
Unilateral lambdoid technique. *A.* Biparieto-occipital bone flaps. *B.* Bifrontal asymmetry recontoured.

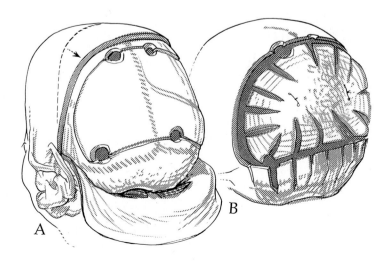

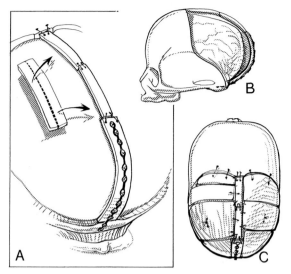

Figure 40–24

Treatment of rare posterior deformities. *A.* Greater convexity enhanced by microplate attachments to midline occipital bone supported by bone grafts. *B.* Microplate enhances retainment of occipital convexity. *C.* Increased occipital convexity and remodeled parietal and occipital bones.

ies in the bone may lead to air being incorporated into the vascular system. This possibility is anticipated by increasing circulating volume at the outset of surgery; by maintaining hypotension, but with high circulating volume, during osteotomies of the cranial bones; and by monitoring for the existence of air embolus with Doppler examination and carbon dioxide and nitrogen detection techniques.

Intracranial pressure elevation may occur in patients who undergo reduction of the height of the skull. This may be seen in the immediate perioperative period with the highest risk patients in the older than 1 year category, who have undergone reductions in skull height greater than 1.5 cm or who have had previous surgical procedures that have rendered the dura scarred and inelastic. Although this possibility is uncommon, it must be suspected in patients who are not rapidly returning to normal after surgery. In this instance, release of any cranial caudal restriction should be performed. Skull caps may be used postoperatively in this situation to gradually reduce the height of the skull without reliance on internal splints. It is cumbersome and less effective than the internal splints but may be safer in certain circumstances where internal splinting is not tolerated.

Philosophy of Treatment

For many years, the authors have advocated a more radical approach to the treatment of craniosynostosis. Early on, it was recognized that simple synostectomy was not enough and that more extensive procedures gave better results,[8] which led to a plea for bilateral procedures for unilateral synostosis.[9] The theoretical basis for this clinical approach was the observation that single-suture closure gave rise to a progressive series of compensations and that it is often the compensations that represent the principal deformity needing treatment.[7] Simple synostectomy may suffice for an early sagittal synostosis before frontal bossing or an occipital knob has occurred. An early unilateral coronal synostosis may not (but usually does) need a contralateral frontal correction to achieve an ideal result, but a bilateral coronal synostosis has a brachycephalic deformity that, in the authors' experience, cannot be corrected without extensive cranial remodeling. However, an individualized approach to each deformity is necessary as well. The surgical techniques shown in this chapter are not meant to be rigidly adhered to, but they should serve as a framework for treatment in particular patients.

REFERENCES

1. Babler, W. J., and Persing, J. A.: Experimental alteration of cranial suture growth: Effects on the neurocranium, basicranium and midface. *In* Dixon, A. P., and Samat, B. G., eds.: Factors and Mechanisms Influencing Bone Growth. New York, Alan R. Liss, 1982, pp. 333–345.
2. Bolk, L.: On the premature obliteration of sutures in the human skull. Am. J. Anat., *17*:495–523, 1915.
3. Cohen, M. M, Jr.: Craniosynostosis: Diagnosis, Evaluation, and Management. New York, Raven Press, 1986, pp. 1–606.
4. Delashaw, J. B., Persing, J. A., Broaddus, W. C., et al.: Rules for cranial vault growth. J. Neurosurg., *70*:159–165, 1989.
5. Delashaw, J. B., Persing, J. A., Park, T. S., et al.: Surgical approach for the correction of metopic synostosis. Neurosurgery, *19*:228–234, 1986.
6. Harris, M. M., Stratford, M. A., Rowe, R. W., et al.: Venous air embolism and cardiac arrest during craniectomy in a supine infant. Anesthesiology, *65*:547–550, 1986.
7. Jane, J. A., and Persing, J. A.: Neurosurgical treatment of craniosynostosis. *In* Cohen, M. M., ed.: Craniosynostosis: Diagnosis and Evaluation of Management. New York, Raven Press, 1986, pp. 249–320.
8. Jane, J. A., Edgerton, M. T., Futrell, J. W., et al.: Immediate correction of sagittal synostosis. J. Neurosurg., *49*:705–710, 1978.
9. Jane, J. A., Park, T. S., Zide, B. A., et al.: Alternative techniques in the treatment of unilateral coronal synostosis. J. Neurosurg., *61*:550–556, 1984.
10. Mooney, M. P., Losken, H. W., Siegel, M. I., et al.: Development of a strain of rabbits with congenital simple non-syndromic coronal suture synostosis: I. Breeding demographics, inheritance pattern, and craniofacial anomalies. Cleft Palate Craniofacial J., *31*:1–7, 1994.
11. Mooney, M. P., Losken, H. W., Siegel, M. I., et al.: Development of a strain of rabbits with congenital simple non-syndromic coronal suture synostosis: II. Somatic and craniofacial growth patterns. Cleft Palate Craniofacial J., *31*:8–16, 1994.
12. Marchac, D., and Renier, D.: Craniofacial Surgery for Craniosynostosis. Boston, Little, Brown, 1982.
13. Marsh, J., and Vannier, M. W.: Cranial base changes following surgical treatment of craniosynostosis. J. Neurosurg., *54*:601–606, 1981.
14. Marsh, J., Jenny, A., Galic, M., et al.: Surgical management of sagittal synostosis. *In* Persing, J., Edgerton, M., and Jane, J., eds.: Scientific Foundations and Surgical Treatment of Craniosynostosis. Baltimore, Williams & Wilkins, 1989, pp. 263–269.
15. Moss, M. L.: Growth of the calvaria in the rat: The determination of osseous morphology. Am. J. Anat., *94*:333–362, 1954.
16. Moss, M. L.: The pathogenesis of premature cranial synostosis in man. Acta Anat., *37*:351–370, 1959.
17. Moss, M. L.: Functional anatomy of cranial synostosis. Child's Brain, *1*:22–33, 1975.

18. Otto, A. W.: Lehrbuch der Pathologischen des Menschen und der Thiere. Berlin, Rucker, 1830.

19. Opperman, L. A., Sheen, R., Persing, J. A., et al.: In the absence of periosteum, transplanted fetal and neonatal rat coronal sutures resist osseous obliteration. J. Craniofacial Surg., 5:327–332, 1994.

20. Opperman, L. A., Sweeney, T. M., Redmon, J., et al.: Tissue interactions with underlying dura mater inhibit osseous obliteration of developing cranial sutures. J. Dev. Dynam., 198:312–322, 1993.

21. Park, T. S., Broaddus, W. C., Harris, M., et al.: Vacuum-stiffened bean bag for cranial remodeling procedures in the modified prone position. J. Neurosurg., 71:623–625, 1989.

22. Park, T. S., Haworth, C. S., Jane, J. A., et al.: Modified prone position for cranial remodeling procedures in children with craniofacial dysmorphism: A technical note. Neurosurgery, 16:212–214, 1985.

23. Persing, J. A., and Luce, C.: Remodeling techniques for immature and mature cranial vault bone: Technical note. J. Craniofacial Surg., 1:147–149, 1990.

24. Persing, J. A., Babler, W. F., Nagorsky, M. J., et al.: Skull expansion in experimental craniosynostosis. Plast. Reconstr. Surg., 78:594–603, 1986.

25. Persing, J. A., Babler, W. D., Winn, H. R., et al.: Age as a critical factor in the success of surgical correction of craniosynostosis. J. Neurosurg., 54:601–606, 1981.

26. Persing, J. A., Delashaw, J. B., Jane, J. A., et al.: Lambdoid synostosis: Surgical considerations. Plast. Reconstr. Surg., 81:852–860, 1988.

27. Persing, J. A., Edgerton, M. T., Park, T. S., et al.: Barrel stave osteotomy for correction of turribrachycephaly craniosynostosis deformity. Ann. Plast. Surg., 18:488–493, 1987.

28. Persing, J. A., Jane, J. A., Park, T. S., et al.: Floating C-shaped orbital osteotomy for orbital rim advancement in craniosynostosis: Preliminary report. J. Neurosurg., 72:22–26, 1990.

29. Persing, J. A., Mayer, P., Spinelli, H., et al.: Prevention of temporal hollowing following fronto-orbital advancement for craniosynostosis. J. Craniofacial Surg., 5:271–274, 1994.

30. Persing, J. A., Morgan, E. P., Cronin, A. J., et al.: Skull base expansion: Craniofacial effects. Plast. Reconstr. Surg., 87:1028–1033, 1991.

31. Persson, K. M., Roy, W. A., Persing, J. A., et al.: Craniofacial growth following experimental craniosynostosis and craniectomy in rabbits. J. Neurosurg., 50:187–197, 1979.

32. Renier, D.: Intracranial pressure in craniosynostosis: Pre- and postoperative recordings—correlation with functional results. *In* Persing, J., Edgerton, M., and Jane, J., eds.: Scientific Foundations and Surgical Treatment of Craniosynostosis. Baltimore, Williams & Wilkins, 1989, pp. 263–269.

33. Sommerring, S. T.: Vom Baue des Menschlichen. 2nd ed. Leipzig, Voss, 1839.

34. van der Klaauw, C. J.: Cerebral skull and facial skull. Arch. Neerl. Zool., 7:1–37, 1946.

35. Virchow, R.: Ueber den cretinismus, namentlich in Franken: Und euber pathologische Schadelformen. Verh. Phys. Med. Gesane Wurzburg, 2:230–271, 1851.

36. Vollmer, D. G., Jane, J. A., Park, T. S., et al.: Variants of sagittal synostosis: Strategies for correction. J. Neurosurg., 61:557–562, 1984.

37. Whitaker, L. A., Schut, L., and Kerr, L. P.: Early surgery for isolated craniofacial dysostosis: Improvement and possible prevention of increasing deformity. Plast. Reconstr. Surg., 60:575–581, 1977.

Congenital Craniofacial Malformations

This chapter considers craniofacial malformations that affect both the cranium and the face: first, facial clefts affecting the face and bone, and second, faciocraniosynostoses.

Facial Clefts

EMBRYOLOGY

The embryonic development of the face occurs very early, between the fourth and eight weeks of gestation.[22] The close relationship between the face and the brain is obvious when one observes that the midportion of the face develops immediately anterior to the forebrain by the differentiation of the broad midline frontonasal prominence (Fig. 41–1). Lateral to this midline prominence, paired elements appear, the nasal placodes and the maxillary process; they merge in the midline while the frontonasal prominence is displaced in a cephalic direction and narrows to form the bridge and root of the nose. Simultaneously, the tip of the nose is derived from the paired medial elements. The eyes are directly derived from the brain, and the optic vesicle starts as an outpouching of the forebrain that induces formation of a lens placode when it comes in contact with the surface ectoderm. The developing eyes, first positioned far laterally, move closer together as the frontonasal prominence narrows. The maxillary and mandibular processes also migrate and create the lower face (Fig. 41–2).

Clefts of the midline craniofacial structure occur when this delicate sequence of events is disrupted. If the frontonasal prominence remains in its embryonic position, the optic placodes cannot migrate toward the midline; this causes orbital hypertelorism, which is associated with various anomalies of the forehead and nose. On the other hand, arrested development of the frontonasal prominence produces major malformations such as cyclopia, ethmocephaly, and cebocephaly (Fig. 41–3). Hypotelorism represents to a milder degree the same anomaly. It is said that "the face predicts the brain," and the importance of the centrofacial anomaly appears to parallel the forebrain defect.[8]

ETIOLOGY

Because major facial clefts are rare, most of our knowledge of the pathogenesis of these malformations is based on studies of the formation of cleft lip and palate. From these investigations, four major categories of environmental factors have been identified: radiation, infection, maternal metabolic imbalances, and drugs and chemicals.[38] Radiation, infection, and maternal metabolic imbalances have not been reported to be responsible for craniofacial malformations. Drugs and chemicals such as tretinoin, thalidomide, corticosteroids, and even aspirin, with their increased use, are known to be responsible for malformations. Because the development of the face occurs so early in pregnancy, mothers may ingest various drugs while unaware of being pregnant.

The importance of heredity in the causation of craniofacial malformations is too difficult to clarify because of the limited number of cases. Nevertheless, the role of heredity is obvious in the more frequent clefts of lip, palate, and the lateral aspects of the orbit, as in Treacher Collins syndrome. Causal environmental and hereditary factors probably play varying roles in the formation of particular malformations.

CLASSIFICATION

Various systems of classification have been proposed for craniofacial clefts,[12, 37] but two of them are of special

D. Marchac • D. Renier

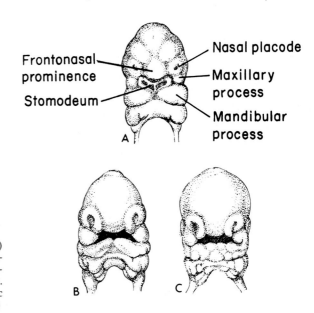

Figure 41–1

Embryonic development of the human face. *A.* Four-week embryo (3.5 mm) with designation of facial processes. *B.* Five-week embryo (6.5 mm). *C.* Six-week embryo (9 mm). *D.* Six-and-a-half-week embryo (12 mm). *E.* Seven-week embryo (19 mm). *F.* Eight-week embryo (28 mm) (After Patten.). (From Kawamoto, H.: Rare craniofacial clefts. *In* McCarthy, J., ed.: Plastic Surgery. Philadelphia, W. B. Saunders, 1990, p. 2924. Used by permission.)

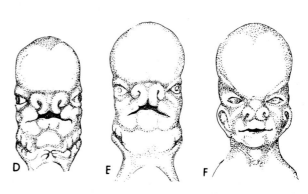

value when assessing craniofacial anomalies involving the neurosurgeon. These are the median facial clefts and the Tessier classification.

Median Facial Clefts

Median facial clefts can be divided into two categories: those presenting with a deficiency of tissue, with missing parts, and those without lack of tissue but presenting with a malformation, usually a widening.

Midline tissue deficiency malformations are almost always linked with a forebrain deficiency. The term arhinencephaly has been used, but *holoprosencephaly*, a term proposed by De Myer, Zeman, and Palmer, better reflects the lack of median tissues.[8] On the basis of this brain-facial linkage, and including some concepts of Cohen and associates, the holoprosencephalic malformations are divided into five types.[4]

Near-normal or excess tissue midline disorders do not, in contrast with the previous group, have a high

Figure 41–2

Contributions of the embryonic processes to the adult face. (From Kawamoto, H.: Rare craniofacial clefts. *In* McCarthy, J., ed.: Plastic Surgery. Philadelphia, W. B. Saunders, 1990, p. 2925.)

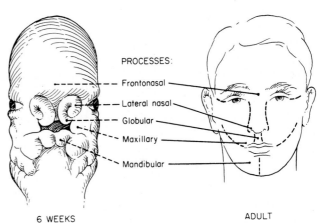

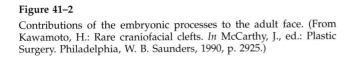

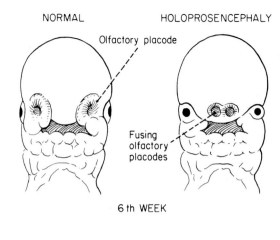

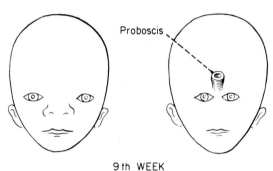

Figure 41–3

Embryonic face with developing holoprosencephaly. Because the development of the frontonasal process is inhibited, the olfactory and optic placodes assume a position closer to the midline. Formation of a proboscis is shown. It is postulated that cyclopia and ethmocephaly are formed by a similar mechanism, depending on the degree of convergence of the olfactory and optic placodes. (After Cohen and associates.) (From Kawamoto, H.: Rare craniofacial clefts. *In* McCarthy, J., ed.: Plastic Surgery. Philadelphia, W. B. Saunders, 1990, p. 2926.)

correlation between the facial anomalies and the underlying brain. The deformities can range from a notch in the upper lip and a widened nose to the most severe form of midline cleft (Fig. 41–4). The term *frontonasal dysplasia*, suggested by Sedano and associates for this group of anomalies, is used widely, especially among geneticists.[29] Frontonasal dysplasia and holoprosencephaly are at opposite ends in this system of classification of midline anomalies.

This system does not take into account all the asymmetrical and paramedian anomalies, and for easier comprehension and definition of treatment, the authors use the Tessier classification, which is based on clinical and operative experience.

Tessier Classification

In the Tessier classification, the orbit is regarded as the reference landmark, common to both the cranium and the face. The clefts, numbered from 0 to 14, rotate around the orbit, following constant lines through the skeleton and soft tissues (Fig. 41–5). Clefts can be mostly cranial if they run upward from the palpebral fissure or mostly facial if they run downward from the palpebral fissure. They are craniofacial if the upper and lower pathways are connected.[32]

The following combinations can be clinically observed: 0 and 14, 1 and 13, 2 and 12, 3 and 11, 4 and 10. This concept of time zones is very helpful when examining the patient and often permits finding the malformation along its entire length, above and below the orbit. The severity of the cleft is highly variable

and can range from a slight soft tissue indentation to a complete open cleft. The soft tissue and skeletal clefts are, on the whole, superposable, but description of the defect in relation to the skeletal cleft is more reliable because the skeletal landmarks are more consistent.

Unilateral and bilateral forms of the cleft are found in varying combinations. Three-dimensional computed tomography has greatly facilitated diagnosis.[7] Plastic models made from computed tomography images are also becoming available.

Some clefts, those affecting mostly the lateral aspect of the face, do not present any interest for the neurosurgeon. It is mostly central and paramedial clefts affecting the face and the cranium that are of interest because, in these cases, the cranium is the way of access for the surgical correction.

SURGICAL TREATMENT

Principles

Surgical treatment of facial clefts affecting the upper part of the face benefited greatly from the breakthrough made by Tessier to conceptually remove the separation existing between the face and the cranial base, between the territories of plastic and neurological surgery.[34] Tessier demonstrated that the frontocranial route was usable to get access to the nose and orbits and that frontocranial problems can be treated simultaneously

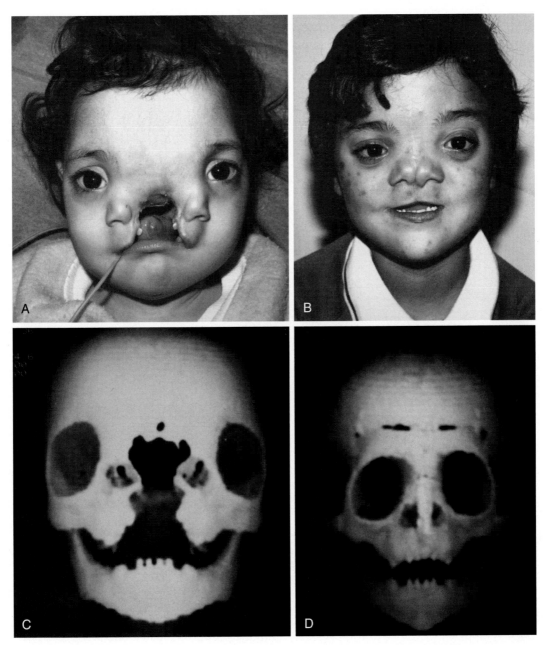

Figure 41–4
Major facial cleft 0–14 corrected by bipartition. *A.* An 8-month-old infant girl presenting with a wide cleft. The brain protrudes between the orbits and must be lifted before the mobilization. *B.* Patient at 4 years of age, before revision of the nasal dorsum and tip. *C* and *D.* Three-dimensional reconstructions before and after the bipartition procedure.

with facial problems. The fear of contamination from the facial cavities was so great among neurosurgeons in 1967 that, for their first case, Tessier and Guiot, his neurosurgical colleague, placed a dermal skin graft on top of the dura of the anterior cranial fossa after it had been elevated, sacrificing all the olfactory nerves. A few months later, they performed the combined craniofacial approach. By 1970, a one-stage procedure was considered safe. Converse had shown that the olfactory nerves could be preserved in most cases.[5] Preliminary disinfection of the nasal cavities, dissection of the mucosal domes and their immediate repair if opened, preservation or perfect repair of dura, changing of instru-

ments if passing through the facial cavities, and perioperative antibiotic therapy are all preventive means that help to avoid infection, osteitis, and meningitis.

The combined approach principally allows the surgeon to move the orbits and repair bony anomalies of the frontonasal complex. Orbital displacement is key to the treatment of major craniofacial clefts. The orbit can be moved on a horizontal, vertical, anterior, or posterior axis to correct all anomalies. It can be moved alone ("orbital shift") or in association with the lower part of the face ("bipartition"). The reconstruction of a missing orbital roof or part of the forehead, canthopexies, and correction of soft tissue problems can be per-

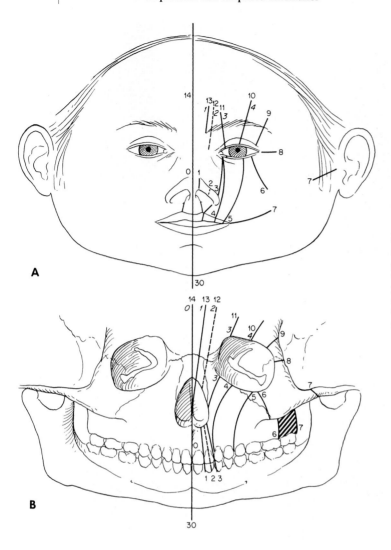

Figure 41–5

Classification of facial cranio-orbital clefts according to Tessier. *A.* Location of the clefts on the face. *B.* Skeletal pathways. The bony and soft tissue clefts coincide, and the orbit is the axis of rotation. This classification, based on clinical experience, is very helpful for analyzing the continuity of the cleft through the cranium, orbit, and midface. (Courtesy of Dr. P. Tessier, Paris.)

formed simultaneously. The age at operation is significant, especially if there is a cranial cleft.

Treatment of Symmetrical Orbital Hypertelorism

The two main aims of surgery for this condition are to bring the orbits closer together and to create a nose of normal appearance. The basic anatomical anomaly is an increase of the intraorbital distance, the nasal bones and glabellar region being much wider than usual. The enlarged portion of this medial part is removed, and, after mobilization of the orbits, the nasal skeleton is adjusted with the help of a bone graft if more dorsal projection is needed (Figs. 41–6 and 41–7).

The neurosurgical approach is fundamental because it allows access to the orbital roof and the central ethmoidosphenoidal area. Only in rare circumstances is it possible to move the lower three fourths of the orbits, leaving intact the roof and removing the excess width of the nose below the cribriform plate. This extracranial approach is possible only if the cribriform plate is very high and the deformity minimal. Raveh uses an inferior intracranial approach, cutting the orbital roof and the ethmoidal cells from below, without

a frontal craniectomy.[23] He claims to have good control of the dura and an improved postoperative period.

Like almost all craniofacial teams, the authors prefer to use the frontal approach to have a clear view of the anterior cranial fossa and to be able to repair the dura in the best possible manner, if necessary. In hypertelorism, anomalies of the midline often exist, and good exposure seems essential to control the dura.

Frontal Craniectomy. Frontal craniectomy allows access to the orbital roofs and medial area. The design of the frontal craniectomy must be carefully planned with the plastic craniofacial surgeon. The lower limit is of importance. Some surgeons, following Tessier's technique,[31] prefer to keep a piece of bone intact at the lower part of the forehead, between the frontal flap and the mobilized orbits. Because the supraorbital rim to be preserved is about 1 cm in height and the preserved frontal band also measures 1 cm, the lower limit of the frontal craniectomy must be at least 2 cm above the orbits. Many craniofacial surgeons, including the authors, do not preserve this horizontal band; the lower limit of the craniectomy with this approach is 1 cm above the orbits. This approach facilitates access to the anterior cranial fossa. An anteroposterior landmark and a stable point of fixation are fundamental. The

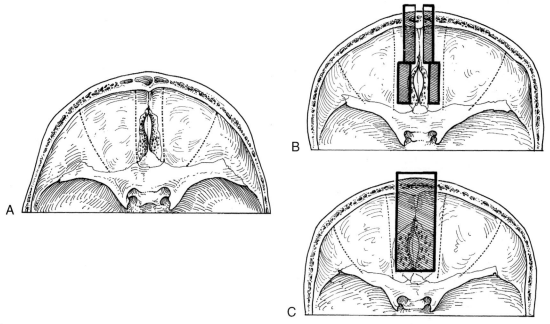

Figure 41-6

The anterior cranial base in hypertelorism. The main feature, in comparison with the normal (*A*), is the enlargement of the ethmoidal area, which pushes the orbits apart. *B*. After resection of the cranial base at the ethmoidal level, it is possible to bring the orbits closer together while preserving the groove of the olfactory nerves. *C*. In unfavorable cases, the olfactory groove is very wide, which necessitates sacrificing the central portion and crista galli, with subsequent loss of olfaction.

authors keep a low lateral spur of frontal bone to fulfill this purpose (Fig. 41-8). Therefore, the frontal craniectomy flap should take an upward angle at about the middle of the orbits.

Dural elevation of the frontal flap must be done with care because anomalies are frequently encountered—for example, a very deep groove for the longitudinal sinus or a thick or even bifid crista galli. After the frontal flap has been lifted up, careful elevation of the dura from the orbital roofs and from the edge of the great wing of the sphenoid bone and the adjacent part of the temporal fossa is performed. The difficult part is the central portion, around the cribriform plates. If the cribriform plate is normal or only moderately enlarged, the necessary resection to decrease the distance between the orbits is performed in the ethmoidal cells on each side of the cribriform plate. Sometimes, the cribriform plate is completely modified, the olfactory grooves being located very far apart, close to the medial wall of the orbits. In that case, sacrifice of the olfactory nerves is unavoidable during a medial resection (see Fig. 41-6).

Meticulous repair of the dura is mandatory after severance of the olfactory nerves. A periosteal patch is sometimes useful to reinforce the tightness. At this stage, the central resection is performed by the plastic craniofacial surgeon, who has previously dissected the nasal mucosal domes by going upward from below the nasal bones. The paranasal sections are performed vertically at a slightly divergent angle, and the transverse posterior section is then performed. It is usually made in front of the crista galli if the olfactory nerves are intact. In some cases, it is done posteriorly, removing almost all of the ethmoid bone. This medial resec-

tion is lifted en bloc and the nasal mucosal domes are exposed. If they are not intact, immediate suturing of the nasal mucosae is performed.

Next, the osteotomies are performed through the orbital roof, lateral orbital wall, and posterior medial wall. The lower osteotomies are different according to whether orbital shift or bipartition is being performed. The orbits are then brought together and contact is re-established in the midline. All the interposing elements must be removed, such as an enlarged superior nasal septum or residual ethmoidal cells posteriorly. Dura must be carefully protected during these maneuvers.

After the orbits are solidly fixed together in the midline by wires or miniplates, the neurosurgical portion of the procedure is almost completed. Tightness of the dura and absence of bleeding is checked in the anterior cranial fossa and temporal fossa, and the frontal bone flap is fitted back in place (Figs. 41-9 and 41-10).

Bone grafts are needed to close the gaps in the orbital walls and often to build up the nasal dorsum. These grafts are taken from the cranial vault. Sometimes, in adolescents and adults, it is possible to split the frontal bone flap and use the posterior aspect for bone grafts. More often, it is necessary to take bone grafts from the cranial vault, especially a straight, thick piece for the nose. It is convenient to take these bony pieces posterior to the frontal flap. In the authors' practice, bone dust from the burr holes and small residual bony fragments are mixed with fibrin glue and used to occlude the vault defects after the graft removals.

Even a significant displacement is well tolerated by the optic nerves. The optic nerve is not straight; it has a certain slackness that allows it to follow the displacement of the eyeball (see Fig. 41-7). To permit a

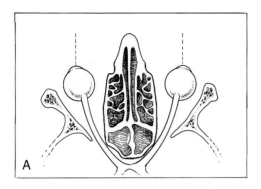

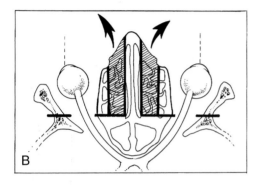

Figure 41–7

Correction of hypertelorism at the orbital level. *A.* Normal. *B.* The central, enlarged portion is narrowed by a central resection of the excess width of bone, either by a medial resection followed by a nasal bone graft or by a paramedial resection if the nose has a good projection and is symmetrical, as shown here. The lateral orbital walls are cut rather posteriorly to mobilize the ocular globe medially. *C.* After medial resection and mobilization of the orbits, the optic nerve is supple and long and easily allows ocular globe displacements.

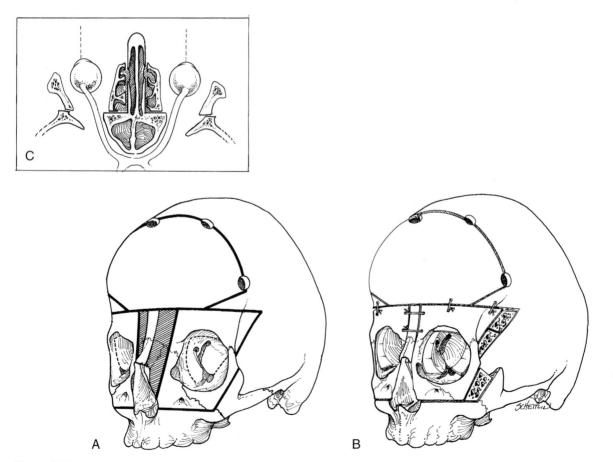

Figure 41–8

The orbital shift. *A.* A frontal flap gives access to the orbital roofs and to the vertical central area of the anterior cranial base. The medial resection is profound, and the orbital osteotomy is performed with a horizontal cut located below the infraorbital foramen. *B.* The orbits have been brought together. A bilateral frontal spur, which has been preserved during cutting of the frontal flap, allows solid fixation and precise repositioning. Bone grafts are placed in the gap created by the displacement and, if necessary, on the nose. It was advisable to keep the central part of the nose in the case illustrated in this drawing.

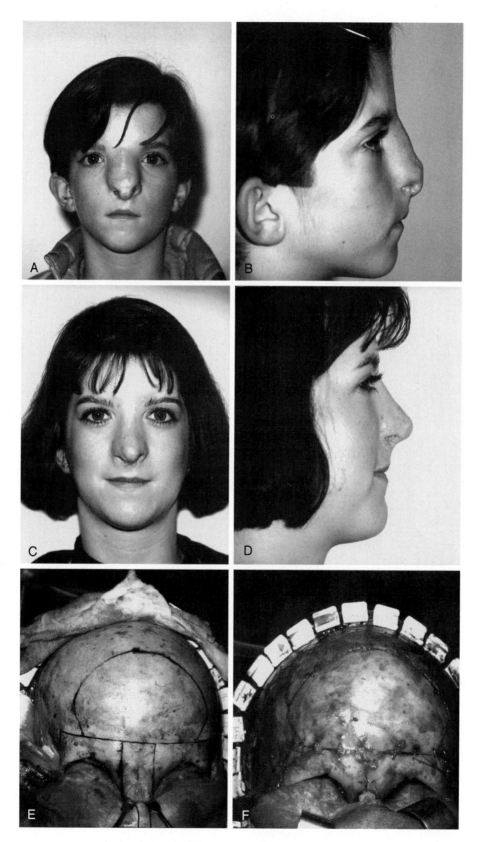

Figure 41–9

Hypertelorism with nasal clefts. *A* and *B.* An 8-year-old girl presented with a hypertelorism associated with nasal enlargement. *C* and *D.* Appearance is shown at 16 years of age, after orbital shift performed at 9 years of age and several operations on the nose. *E* and *F.* Operative views of this patient show the orbital displacement and frontal spurs.

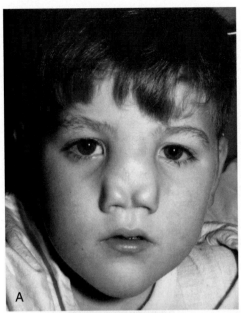

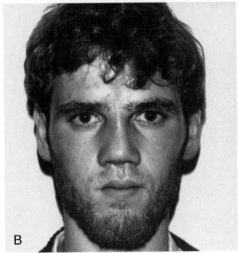

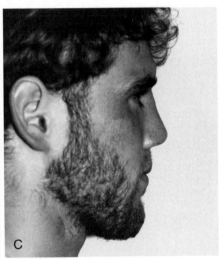

Figure 41–10

Hypertelorism and midline cleft. *A.* A 4-year-old boy presented with a midline cleft 0–14 with bifid nose and hypertelorism. *B* and *C.* Appearance at 17 years of age, after orbital shift at 5 years of age and complementary nasal bone graft at age 15.

good medial displacement of the eyeball, it is essential that the medial wall of the orbit also be displaced toward the midline. If the osteotomy is too anterior, there will be a step effect, limiting the displacement of the ocular globes.

Orbital Shift and Bipartition

There are two ways to mobilize the orbits when correcting an orbital hypertelorism. The classic approach, described by Tessier in 1967[34] consists of a mobilization of the orbits en bloc medially, the lower horizontal cuts being situated below the infraorbital rim, through the malar bones and maxillae.[30] Bipartition, proposed by van der Meulen and developed by Tessier, represents a mobilization of the two hemifaces.[33, 35, 36] Instead of cutting below the orbits, the surgeon makes the osteotomies through the zygomatic arch and the pterygomaxillary junction and medially through the palate. The medial resection must have an inverted "V" shape because there will be a movement of rotation, along with the narrowing on the midline.

This movement of rotation allows for widening of the maxillary arch and the nasal fossae and also for changing the axis of the orbits, which have a lateral slant (Fig. 41–11).

The choice between orbital shift and bipartition is linked to a series of factors:

The maxillary arch: if the maxillary arch is narrow and inverted, the incisors being higher than the molars, bipartition is the operation of choice because it widens the maxilla and improves the angle of the upper dentition. On the other hand, if the maxillary arch and occlusion are normal, it seems preferable to avoid an interpterygomaxillary disjunction.

The axis of the orbits: if the axis is normal, a horizontal mobilization is satisfactory; if they are laterally and downwardly oblique, bipartition corrects these anomalies.

The nasal fossae: if they are narrow, bipartition improves the airways.

Bipartition is the operation of choice in severe cases

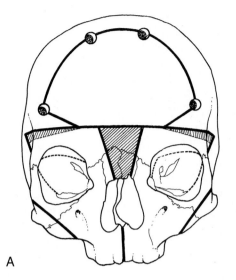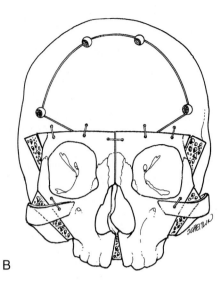

Figure 41–11
Correction of hypertelorism by facial bipartition. *A.* The orbits are mobilized with the maxilla, and the osteotomy performed involves the bone at the pterygomaxillary junction. A triangular resection is done on the midline, wider at the top. *B.* Rotation of the hemifaces is obtained with the narrowing, and the maxilla and nasal fossae become wider.

A   B

(Fig. 41–12; see Fig. 41–4), whereas orbital shift is indicated for more limited displacements. The bipartition principle can also sometimes be used to get access to a lesion of the cranial base. Some midline clefts are associated with an encephalocele of the ethmoidosphenoidal area, and, after midline splitting, easy access can be obtained to the encephalocele.

Asymmetrical Cases

Asymmetrical cases are more difficult to correct than symmetrical ones. Sometimes both orbits have to be moved in different ways; sometimes, only one of the orbits is involved in the planned displacement. The cranial base is also asymmetrical, and all the different distortions must be carefully evaluated by computed tomography and three-dimensional reconstructions. Paramedial clefts create a situation in which the affected orbit is displaced laterally and inferiorly to a variable degree. A frontal bony defect is often associated. The orbit may be of normal size but is sometimes of a reduced size (anophthalmia). Various anomalies of the maxillary and nasal portion of the face may also be associated.

After the anomaly has been understood and classified according to the Tessier system (see previous discussion), a plan of treatment is devised. The correction is fundamentally from top to bottom; that is, the frontal and orbital regions must be reconstructed first. In most cases, a bilateral asymmetrical correction is requested (Fig. 41–13).[16] The neurosurgical approach is by means of a frontal bone flap, its lower limit being carefully planned because of the variable movements of the supraorbital rim, often including elevation on one side and transversal movement only on the alternate side. In cases of paramedial clefts, the ethmoidal region is asymmetrical, and dural elevation should be performed with care. After the orbits are properly positioned, the frontal bone flap is adjusted and wired back.

Sometimes, only one orbit is displaced, usually inferiorly, with one globe located lower than the other, a condition termed *orbital dystopia*. In these situations, displacement of the entire orbit en bloc is the solution. Partial maneuvers such as elevation of the roof and placement of bone grafts on the floor usually produce disappointing results. The en bloc displacement of the orbit requires a frontal flap to gain access to the roof. This frontal flap can be unilateral and corresponds to the width of the orbital osteotomy. The frontal segment, removed to permit elevation of the supraorbital rim of the orbit, is utilized as a bone graft placed below the orbit to maintain the elevation and fill the bony gap created.

Soft Tissue Anomalies

Some craniofacial malformations involve only the skeleton—for example, mild symmetrical orbital hypertelorism, orbital dystopia, frontal or malar asymmetries, or malposition. Correction can be made through hidden approaches, such as bicoronal or vestibular incisions, and can leave almost invisible scars, as with the palpebral infraciliary approach.

Excess skin can adjust and retract. After correction of moderate hypertelorism, the excess skin of the glabellar region and dorsum of the nose retracts with the help of good undermining and a bone graft to lift the dorsum of the nose. Soft tissue correction must be considered in the initial plan of treatment, because the approach to the skeleton and the scalp incision can be influenced. For example, if a frontal skin flap is planned, the design of the coronal incision may have to be changed to avoid cutting through the future pedicle.

This section discusses mainly those facial clefts that associate soft tissue problems with skeletal anomalies. It is usually much easier to reconstruct the skeleton—to place the bones in good position—than to correct soft tissue deficiencies. All the resources of plastic surgery can rarely achieve a perfect contour with minimal scars. The authors briefly consider the main soft tissue problems encountered in major congenital craniofacial malformations.

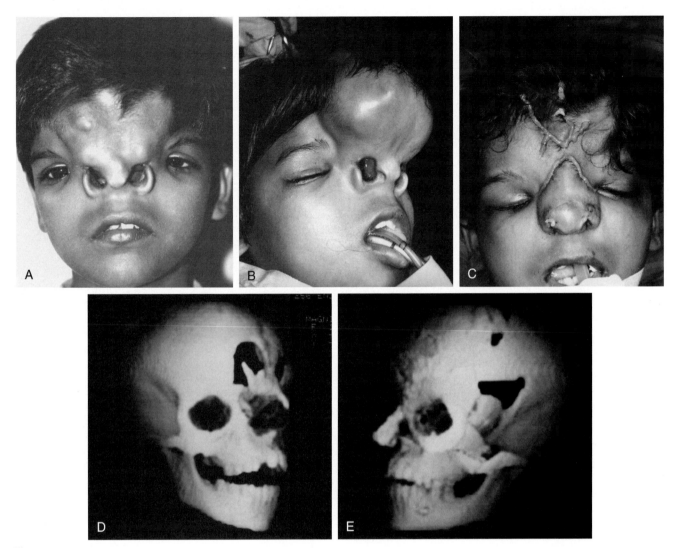

Figure 41–12

Nasal reconstruction combined with hypertelorism correction. *A.* This 8-year-old patient presented with a bilateral cleft 2, with enlarged nasal fossae located between the orbits, and absence of nasal dorsum. *B.* Expansion of the forehead skin is performed first to provide the amount of facial skin necessary to provide nasal reconstruction. *C.* The bipartition technique has been used to bring the orbits together. The retracted nostrils have been lowered and the frontal flap placed over the nose, which has been reconstructed with a bone graft. *D* and *E.* Three-dimensional reconstructions before and after correction.

Scalp and Eyebrows

Hairline distortion is frequently observed in cranio-facial clefts and reflects the continuity of the cleft at the scalp level. If a widow's peak of hair growing down onto the forehead has to be removed, it can be incorporated into a frontal skin resection that facilitates exposure. Eyebrows can be clefted or can be displaced. Differential repositioning of the forehead and scalp can correct the displacement of the eyebrows, usually by lowering them.

Nose

In symmetrical hypertelorism, presenting with an excess of skin at the level of the nasal dorsum, it is better to try to avoid the easy solution of a midline skin excision. Some of these scars do very well with time and become hardly visible, but others stretch, get pigmented, and remain very evident. It is therefore better to try skin retraction (discussed above).

If there is a cleft affecting the nose, it should be corrected at the time of the craniofacial surgery to utilize the wide undermining performed at the nose level. A cleft can be closed by reapproximation of tissue with plasties at the alar margins, but if there is a tissue deficiency, various nasal flaps should be considered. The excess skin existing on the upper part of the nose can be transferred to the lower part.

In some cases, the nose is very distorted and the shortage of skin is obvious from the start. The frontal area is the best zone from which to obtain the missing skin. Sometimes, correction of the hypertelorism creates an excess of skin tissue at the level of the forehead that can be used as a frontal flap. If the forehead skin is limited in surface, a preliminary frontal skin

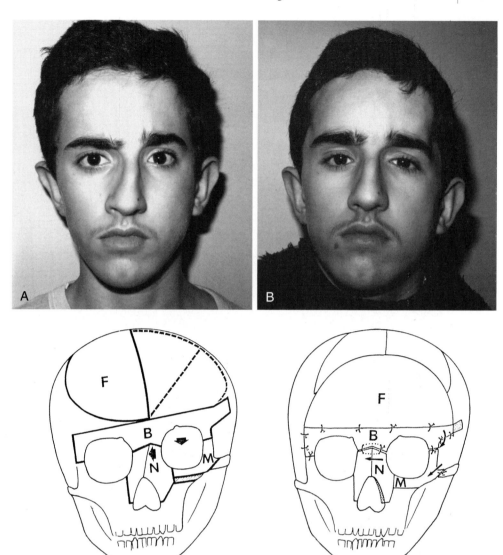

Figure 41–13

Orbital dystopia. *A.* This 13-year-old boy presented with a severe asymmetry secondary to an untreated left coronal synostosis. *B.* The same patient is shown after frontal, orbital, and nasal correction. *C* and *D.* The correction is obtained through frontal remodeling after elevation of the supraorbital bar, malar osteotomy, and perinasal mobilization. (*C* and *D* from Marchac, D., and Renier, D.: Craniofacial Surgery for Craniosynostosis. Boston, Little, Brown, & Co., 1982, p. 125.)

expansion may be necessary to provide the required amount (see Fig. 41–12). These nasal problems should be carefully considered beforehand because the usual bicoronal approach may have to be modified because of them.

Eyelids and Ocular Cavity

Clefts of the eyelids are located principally on the lower eyelid and are part of the midface reconstruction, as are oculonasal clefts. Regarding the craniofacial clefts discussed in this chapter, it is in the ocular cavity that problems are encountered.

If there is anophthalmia or microphthalmia, the bony orbit does not develop to its normal size. The preferred treatment is a progressive enlargement. Conformers are very difficult to place; intraorbital expanders are much more efficient and can produce an almost normal growth of the orbit. A prosthesis is fitted afterward. Nevertheless, this orbital expansion is difficult to execute and requires a very careful follow-up. If it fails or cannot be undertaken, the problem of a micro-orbit

must be faced. This orbit should first be placed in proper position, vertically and horizontally, in relation to the other orbit. It can then be surgically enlarged by expanding the whole circumference (Fig. 41–14). Access to the orbital roof is obtained with a localized frontal craniectomy, as for an orbital dystopia.[19]

Here also, the secondary soft tissue work of creating a good cavity capable of retaining an ocular prothesis and building up the short, retracted eyelids with auricular composite grafts is often more difficult and time-consuming than the skeletal work.

Faciocraniosynostoses

In addition to the risk of brain compression and cranial deformities observed in faciocraniosynostosis, facial involvement raises important problems, both functional (exorbitism, breathing impairment, swallowing and mastication difficulties) and morphological (facial retrusion, short nose, ocular malposition). The

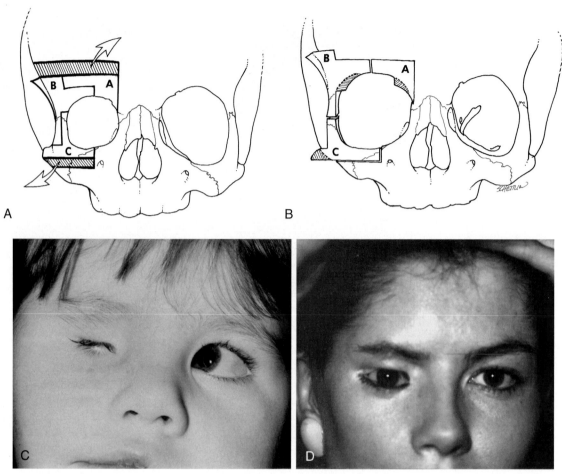

Figure 41–14

Correction of microphthalmic orbit. *A.* If early expansion was not performed or was unsuccessful, orbital enlargement can produce an orbit of sufficient size to create a cavity for the ocular prosthesis. After frontal flap elevation, the orbital rim is cut superiorly, laterally, and inferiorly to allow for enlargement. *B.* Appearance of the orbit after frontal and malar displacement and readjustment of the orbital rim is shown. *C.* A 4-year-old girl presented with a right microphthalmic orbit. *D.* The same patient is shown at 16 years of age, after orbit enlargement at 7 years of age, subsequent creation of an ocular cavity for a prosthesis, and composite grafts to the eyelids.

treatment of these patients must take into consideration all of these parameters, and close cooperation between the neurosurgeon and the plastic craniofacial surgeon is mandatory to determine a good plan of treatment and obtain optimal results.

DESCRIPTION AND CLASSIFICATION OF THE FACIOCRANIOSYNOSTOSES

Crouzon's Syndrome

Described by Crouzon in 1912, this syndrome involves only the face and cranium and is not associated with other anomalies elsewhere on limbs or trunk.[6] The fundamental factor is an underdeveloped midfacial mass that features exorbitism because of lack of depth of the orbits, inverted occlusion, and receding malar bones. The nose is short (Figs. 41–15 and 41–16). Cranially, a brachycephaly is usually present, but sometimes it may be a scaphocephaly or a cloverleaf skull.

The coronal and sagittal sutures are involved in almost all cases and are frequently associated with the lambdoid sutures. Usually, these sutural fusions do not exist at birth. The coronal and sagittal fusions appear at about 1 year of age, the lambdoid later in life. In some cases, the sagittal fusion appears first, presenting like a simple scaphocephaly, and the coronal fusion appears some months later. Commonly, the diagnosis of Crouzon's syndrome is difficult during the first year of life, even if the brachycephaly is obvious. It is often difficult to know whether the midface will be affected, even on radiological examination. Midface retrusion and exorbitism appear later in life.

In some cases, the diagnosis is evident at birth. In these cases, the malformation is usually severe, with marked frontofacial retrusion producing a severe exorbitism with a high risk of exposure keratitis or even luxation of the eyeballs. The retrusion of the maxillae is also severe, producing airway obstruction with obligatory mouth breathing (Fig. 41–17).

The relationship of the forehead and face is usually good in patients with Crouzon's syndrome. There is a

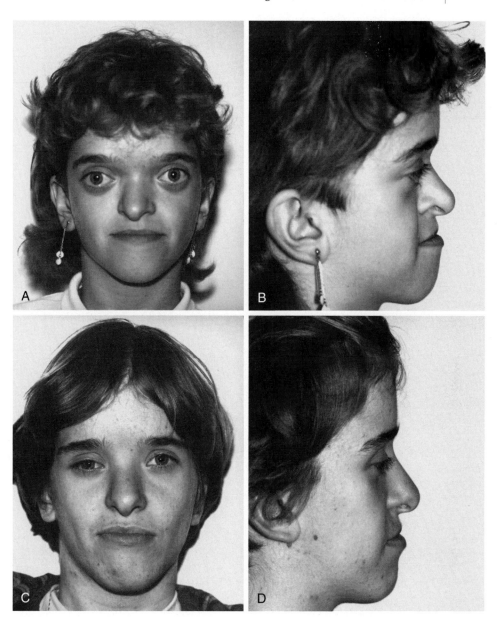

Figure 41–15
Facial advancement in a patient with Crouzon's syndrome. *A* and *B*. This patient, age 9 years, presented with a severe facial retrusion with exorbitism. She had a frontal advancement in infancy. *C* and *D*. The same patient is shown at 16 years of age, after the Le Fort III type of facial advancement.

backward horizontal displacement of all the frontofacial skeleton, as if it were held back by the synostosis.

Apert's Syndrome (Acrocephalosyndactyly)

First described by Apert in 1906, this syndrome is easy to recognize because of the associated syndactylies of the hands and feet.[1] These syndactylies are always severe and affect almost all the digits. They can range from a nearly complete fusion to fingers well-delineated but joined by skin[18] (Fig. 41–18).

The craniofacial involvement is also usually obvious at birth, with a brachycephaly, sometimes asymmetrical, associated with a facial retrusion of variable degree. Both coronal sutures are always fused, although some rare cases present without craniosynostosis (3 cases out of 64 in the authors' series). What distinguishes Apert's from Crouzon's syndrome is the exis-

tence of hypertelorism and open bite, the anterior part of the maxillary alveolar arch being higher than the posterior part. The face and forehead are also abnormally wide, and the anterior fontanelle is widely open during the first months of life.

Pfeiffer's Syndrome

Described by Pfeiffer in 1964, this syndrome is an association of faciocraniosynostosis and anomalies of hands and feet.[3] There is a brachycephaly by bicoronal synostosis (sometimes asymmetrical), a midface retrusion by maxillary hypoplasia, and a hypertelorism. Thumbs and great toes are broad with a varus deviation. Soft tissue syndactyly can be observed. As in Crouzon's and Apert's syndromes, some severe forms exist, with precocious marked frontofacial retrusion resulting in ocular and breathing problems. This condition is sometimes associated with a cloverleaf skull.

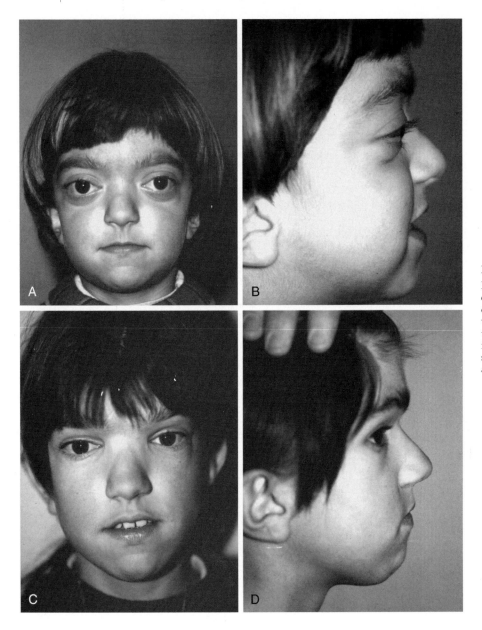

Figure 41–16

Frontofacial monobloc. *A* and *B.* A 7-year-old girl presented with Crouzon's syndrome. The exorbitism is significant as well as the dental retrusion, but the relationship between the forehead and nose is good. *C* and *D.* The same patient is shown 7 years after monobloc frontonasal advancement.

Saethre-Chotzen Syndrome

Described by Saethre in 1931 and Chotzen in 1932, this syndrome is characterized by the association of bicoronal synostosis, maxillary hypoplasia, ptosis, and ear anomalies.[3] The craniosynostosis is usually a brachycephaly or, in some cases, a plagiocephaly or even an oxycephaly (acrocephaly). The midface retrusion is most often mild. The ears have prominent antihelical crura. Some cases have soft tissue syndactyly in the hands.

Craniofrontonasal Dysplasia

In the group of craniofacial dysplasias (see discussion of median facial clefts), some cases present with a bicoronal craniosynostosis, featuring a subgroup called craniofrontonasal dysplasia. There is a brachycephaly, often marked, associated with the facial anomalies of frontonasal dysplasia, which include hypertelorism, broad nasal bridge, bifid nose, and, sometimes, soft tissue syndactyly.

ETIOLOGY

Although the majority of faciocraniosynostoses are sporadic, there is also evidence for a genetic origin, based on numerous observations of familial cases.[13, 14] Crouzon's syndrome occurs in 1 in 25,000 births, and the frequency of familial cases varies in the literature from 44 to 67 per cent.[3] The familial cases accounted for 26 per cent in the authors' series. In this series (Table 41–1), the rate of familial cases was lower in the precocious forms of Crouzon's syndrome than in the common type: 13 versus 29 per cent, respectively. The transmission is autosomal dominant. There is a great variability of expression, and both severe and mild forms can be observed in the same family. In fresh mutations (sporadic cases), the paternal age at conception is higher than the mean in the unaffected population.

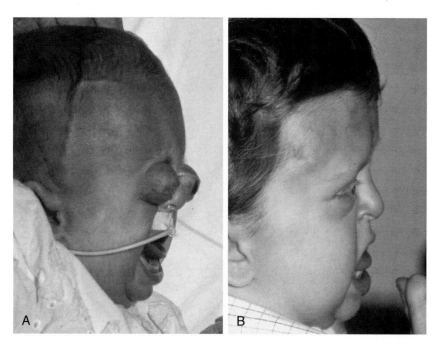

Figure 41–17

Early monobloc for severe exorbitism. *A.* This 2-month-old infant with Crouzon's syndrome has an exorbitism threatening his eyes. *B.* After early monobloc advancement at 3 years of age, the maxilla is still recessed but the exorbitism is corrected.

The incidence of Apert's syndrome is estimated to be between 1 in 100,000 and 1 in 160,000 births.[3] Most cases are sporadic; few affected patients have children because of the severity of the disease. However, a dominant transmission with complete penetrance has been reported in some cases. As in Crouzon's syndrome, the paternal age at conception is higher than average.

Pfeiffer's syndrome has an autosomal dominant transmission with complete penetrance and variable expression. In the authors' series, 41 per cent of the cases were familial.

Saethre-Chotzen syndrome has also an autosomal dominant transmission. The penetrance is incomplete, and the expression is variable. In the authors' series, 5 of the 9 cases were familial. This syndrome was localized on the short arm of chromosome 7 (7p22) by Brueton and colleagues in 1992.[2]

Females are much more affected by craniofrontonasal dysplasia than males, which is consistent with an X-linked inheritance. In the authors' series, 36 per cent of the cases were familial, and 91 per cent of the patients were females.

FUNCTIONAL ASPECTS

Intracranial Pressure

As in isolated craniosynostoses, the main problem of the faciocraniosynostoses is the risk of intracranial

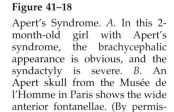

Figure 41–18

Apert's Syndrome. *A.* In this 2-month-old girl with Apert's syndrome, the brachycephalic appearance is obvious, and the syndactyly is severe. *B.* An Apert skull from the Musée de l'Homme in Paris shows the wide anterior fontanellae. (By permission of the Musée de l'Homme.)

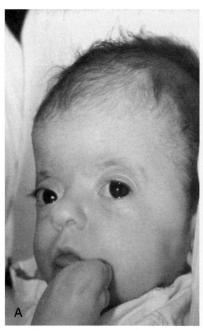

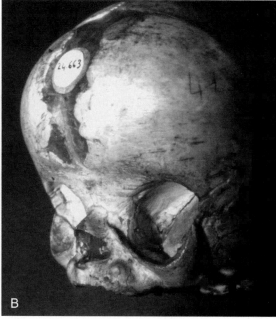

Table 41–1

DISTRIBUTION OF ISOLATED CRANIOSYNOSTOSIS AND CRANIOFACIAL SYNDROMES IN THE AUTHORS' SERIES (1976–1993)*

Type	No.	No. Operated
Scaphocephaly	511	343
Trigonocephaly	127	106
Pachycephaly	11	8
Plagiocephaly	177	173
Brachycephaly	84	78
Oxycephaly	120	81
Complex	77	69
Apert's syndrome	65	57
Crouzon's syndrome	66	59
Pfeiffer's syndrome	17	15
Saethre-Chotzen syndrome	9	9
Craniofrontonasal dysplasia	11	9
Other syndromes	24	17
TOTAL	1299	1024

*The syndromic craniosynostoses account for 14.8 per cent of the whole series.

hypertension and its possible mental or visual repercussions. The risk of intracranial hypertension varies according to the type of syndrome.[9, 10, 24, 27, 28] In the authors' series, intracranial pressure was recorded in 68 cases of faciocraniosynostosis. Intracranial hypertension was defined as a baseline pressure equal to or greater than 15 mm Hg. The frequency of intracranial hypertension was 62.5 per cent in Crouzon's syndrome, 45 per cent in Apert's syndrome, and 29 per cent in the others.

Without early treatment, intracranial hypertension can lead to optic atrophy and visual loss. This is observed mainly in Crouzon's syndrome. In the authors' series, papilledema was observed in 35 per cent and optic atrophy in 10 per cent of the Crouzon's cases. In the other syndromes, papilledema was observed in only 4 to 5 per cent, and no optic atrophy was observed.

In addition to the intracranial hypertension, some authors have implicated direct compression of the optic nerve in the optic canal. The authors have never observed this condition.

Mental Development

There is a great variability in mental level according to the different types of faciocraniosynostosis.[24–26] Comparing the scores before and after operation, three main factors appear as far as mental development is concerned. First, Apert's syndrome is much more serious than the other conditions, and this is equally true before and after surgical treatment (Table 41–2). Second, the result is better after early treatment (Table 41–3). Third, there is only a mild improvement in mental level after treatment, compared with the preoperative status. In other words, the main predictive factor is the preoperative mental level, which is best preserved by an early frontal release.

Brain Malformation

Faciocraniosynostoses are associated with brain malformations much more than are nonsyndromic isolated craniosynostoses. This is particularly true in Apert's syndrome. The nature and frequency of these malformations were studied by magnetic resonance imaging in the authors' series of children with Apert's and Crouzon's syndromes (Table 41–4). Only 14 patients with Apert's syndrome (25 per cent) had a normal brain on magnetic resonance imaging. In the whole series, 5 children with Apert's syndrome (7.7 per cent) and 19 children with Crouzon's syndrome (28.8 per cent) had to have shunts placed for hydrocephalus.

SURGICAL TREATMENT

Because faciocraniosynostoses are characterized essentially by backward displacement of the forehead and midface, both having to be moved forward, this condition can be treated by advancing the forehead and the face either separately or simultaneously.

Separate Frontal and Facial Advancement

Frontal Advancement

The main feature of faciocraniosynostosis (essentially Crouzon's and Apert's syndromes) is a recessed orbital bar, and it is treated like a brachycephaly (see Chapter 40). For an infant younger than 4 or 5 months of age, the authors perform a "floating forehead" type of advancement, the advanced forehead being fixed only to the root of the nose and to the lateral side of the orbits, with no connections to the posterior part of the cranial vault.[15, 16] The expanding brain is capable of pushing the advanced forehead forward.

Table 41–2

PREOPERATIVE AND POSTOPERATIVE MENTAL LEVEL ACCORDING TO THE TYPE OF FACIOCRANIOSYNOSTOSIS

Type	Preoperative		Postoperative	
	IQ > 90	Mean IQ	IQ > 90	Mean IQ
Apert's syndrome	6%	59	19%	65
Crouzon's syndrome	64%	88	72%	94
Saethre-Chotzen syndrome	40%	83	50%	93
Craniofrontonasal dysplasia	67%	93	71%	104
Other syndrome	56%	79	56%	79

Table 41–3

MENTAL RESULTS IN FACIOCRANIOSYNOSTOSIS ACCORDING TO AGE AT SURGERY

Type	Operated < 1 year			Operated > 1 year		
	N	*IQ > 90*	*Mean IQ*	*N*	*IQ > 90*	*Mean IQ*
Apert's syndrome	27	30%	71	15	0	54
Crouzon's syndrome	10	80%	95	19	68%	94
Other syndromes	17	71%	100	10	40%	78

If the patient is older than 4 to 5 months of age, the authors perform a horizontal tongue-in-groove advancement. The upper part of the forehead is remodeled according to each individual case, and a wide open fontanelle is closed by hinging two pieces of bone together. In the authors' experience, this frontal advancement in infants should be of 2 cm. At first, this creates an exaggerated frontal bulge, but it is the prerequisite for obtaining a satisfactory long-term result. The step-line effect can be attenuated by placing a small bone graft above the upper part of the nose.

Up until the child reaches 2 years of age, a wide bony defect can be left open on the vault after advancement because there will be rapid reossification. After 2 years of age, reossification becomes problematic, and defects must be closed. Bone splitting is rarely possible at this age. Bone fragments may be mixed with bone dust and fibrin glue to cover any existing defects.

The fixation of the advanced bony pieces in infants is done with wire and bone grafts. Only in rare instances is it necessary to use miniplates to stabilize the supraorbital bar after floating forehead advancement. In infants, miniplates are quickly embedded in the growing bone. Sometimes the miniplates protrude inside the cranium and the screws pierce the dura. Therefore, the authors strongly advise against their use in infants whenever stabilization can be achieved by other means.

Facial Advancement

Facial advancement is usually of the Le Fort III type. Le Fort described three main types of maxillary disjunction. Surgical facial advancement reproduces approximately the lines of fracture on the face. Tessier gave the names Le Fort I, II, and III to the facial osteotomies. Although Gillies was the first to perform a facial advancement in the late 1940's, Tessier was really the pioneer in craniofacial surgery.[11] He developed the Le Fort III type of advancement, his lines of osteotomy being deeper than those of Gillies and located behind the lacrymal apparatus.[30] The mobilized part includes the lower three fourths of the orbits, the nose, the malar bones, and the upper maxillae (Fig. 41–19).

A coronal approach allows the periosteal elevation around the orbits and at the root of the nose. The osteotomies are made with oscillating and reciprocating saws that cut through the root of the nose, medial wall, floor, and lateral wall of the orbit. A section is made on the orbital rim, usually at the level of the junction of the frontal and malar bones, then downward through the malar bone and the pterygomaxillary space. This interpterygomaxillary osteotomy is often difficult because the narrow groove is not easily detected. The maneuver is usually executed from above, especially in children, but can be done through an oral approach, especially in adolescents and adults, who have a thick bone at this level.

Progressive mobilization is done, fighting against the resisting muscles and mucosae. After the desired position is obtained, fixation is performed with the help of interposing bone grafts, wires, and miniplates placed between the zygomatic arch and the advanced malar bone. Intramaxillary fixation is used only in older children to ensure proper positioning and is removed after the miniplate fixation has been performed. Elastic tractions are placed after postoperative recovery to control occlusion.

The Le Fort II osteotomy mobilizes the nose and the

Table 41–4

ASSOCIATED BRAIN MALFORMATIONS IN A SERIES OF 55 CASES OF APERT'S SYNDROME AND 44 CASES OF CROUZON'S SYNDROME STUDIED BY MAGNETIC RESONANCE IMAGING

Area Involved or Syndrome	Abnormality	Apert's Syndrome	Crouzon's Syndrome
Corpus callosum	Hypoplasia	15	
	Aplasia	3	
Ventricles	Nonprogressive dilatation	21	12
	Hydrocephalus	5	15
Septum pellucidum	Cyst	13	
	Aplasia	15	
Chiari syndrome	Tonsillar herniation	1	25
	Tonsillar herniation plus syringomyelia		6

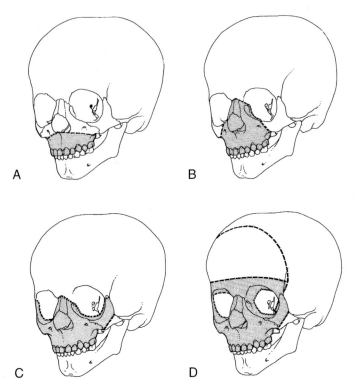

Figure 41–19

Facial advancements or osteotomies inspired by the classification of René Le Fort. *A.* Le Fort I mobilizes the dental part of the maxillae. *B.* Le Fort II advances the maxillae and the nose but leaves the malar bones and orbital rim in place. *C.* Le Fort III corresponds to a craniofacial disjunction and permits the advancement of the whole midface. *D.* In frontofacial monobloc, the totality of the orbits is advanced with the midface, and the forehead is advanced above, as necessary.

maxillae, leaving the malar bones in place, and does not modify the depth of the orbits. It is of limited indication in faciocraniosynostosis, in which an orbital deepening to correct the exorbitism is usually necessary.

The Le Fort I operation mobilizes only the upper maxillae, cutting horizontally slightly above the level of the floor of the nasal fossae. It permits advancing the dental portion of the maxillae and the nasal spine. In specific cases, intermediate osteotomies can be performed to mobilize to a variable degree some or all of the malar bones and the inferior orbital rim.

Simultaneous Frontal and Facial Advancement

In 1971 Tessier described the simultaneous advancement of the forehead and face in faciocraniosynostosis. He performed a Le Fort III osteotomy and, during the same session, frontal advancement and remodeling; the advanced frontal bandeau was fixed above the mobilized face.

Ortiz-Monasterio proposed in 1978 to perform a monobloc advancement in which the orbits and face are mobilized simultaneously and the upper part of the forehead is adjusted above, as required[21] (see Fig. 41–16). Good stability of the orbits and an absence of distortion of the junction between the nose and forehead are thus obtained. This technique allows for horizontal advancement only and can be used only in patients with Crouzon's syndrome who do not need nasal lengthening and have no open bite.

In patients with Apert's syndrome, a simultaneous narrowing of the face and correction of the hypertelor-

ism can be achieved by using the bipartition principle introduced by Van der Meulen and developed by Tessier.[33, 35, 36] The principle is to split the face down the middle, removing an inverted "V" of excess bone between the orbits and splitting the palate on the midline from the incisors backward. The two hemifaces can be moved, the orbits brought in closer together, and the upper maxillae widened (Fig. 41–20). Therefore, for patients with Apert's syndrome, a simultaneous frontofacial advancement and bipartition is performed. The bipartition can also be performed utilizing only a Le Fort III type of advancement (Fig. 41–21).

The open bite of the patient with Apert's syndrome cannot be corrected simultaneously with the facial correction; one merely obtains a correction of the inverted "V" deformation of the teeth. A Le Fort I osteotomy usually has to be done later.

The simultaneous frontofacial advancement is logical, permitting correction of the frontal and facial problems of faciocraniosynostosis in one operation. Its two major drawbacks are the magnitude of the operation and the risk of infection (meningitis or osteitis) from the communication between the anterior cranial base and the nasal cavities. It is possible to close this communication with the use of bone grafts and periostal flaps, but the risk of infection remains.

Indications

In infants, the authors perform a frontal advancement of the floating forehead type, up until the age of 5 months. In an older infant, a horizontal tongue-in-groove procedure is the operation of choice. A monobloc frontofacial advancement is performed only in cases of severe exorbitism[17, 20] (see Fig. 40–17).

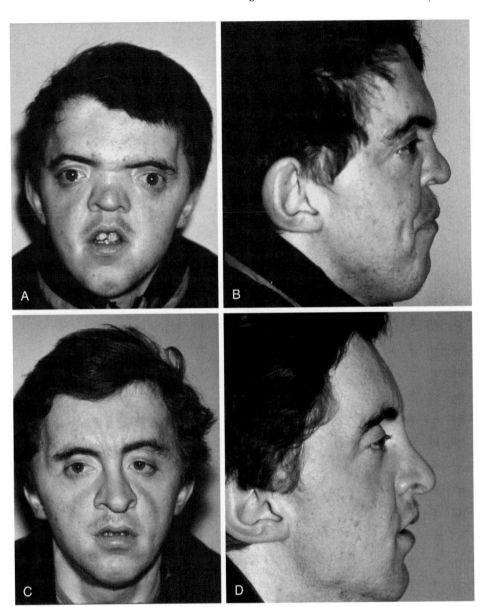

Figure 41–20

An adult with Apert's syndrome corrected by bipartition. *A* and *B*. This patient, age 19 years, had a previous frontal remodeling in childhood and presented with a major facial retrusion with hypertelorism. *C* and *D*. The same patient is shown after facial advancement with bipartition. The hypertelorism is corrected.

In children, if the forehead has been advanced earlier and is satisfactory, the authors postpone the facial advancement for as long as possible. The ideal is to wait until the eruption of final dentition, at about 11 or 12 years of age. If the facial retrusion is severe and creates functional (respiratory and masticatory) or psychological problems, the authors operate before school age, at about 5 years of age (see Fig. 41–21). The patient's parents are warned that a second advancement will be necessary after final dentition, usually a Le Fort I operation.

In unoperated patients, or if the forehead still recedes, a monobloc frontofacial advancement is considered in favorable cases. If the family prefers to avoid the infectious risks linked to the monobloc, a two-stage operation is performed—frontal advancement first, and facial advancement 6 to 9 months later.

It is often possible to further improve the appearance of the patient, when growth is almost completed, by frontal contouring, rhinoplasty, genioplasty, orthodontics, and, sometimes, orthognatic surgery (Fig. 41–22).

A new method of treatment of faciocraniosynostosis is under development called progressive distraction. It utilizes the Ilizarov principle of bony elongation. An appliance permitting a progressive advancement of the face or of the frontofacial complex is applied after mobilization or even after a simple corticotomy.

Endoscopy can be used to perform these bony sections without the need of a bicoronal approach. The operative and infectious risks should be eliminated by this progressive advancement technique.

Treatment of Associated Hydrocephalus

The association of craniosynostosis and hydrocephalus poses a difficult surgical problem. The treatment of the craniosynostosis is in conflict with the treatment of the hydrocephalus, because the former tends to enlarge skull volume, whereas the aim of the latter is to reduce the size of the cerebral ventricles and thus reduce the volume of the brain. Treating both problems at the

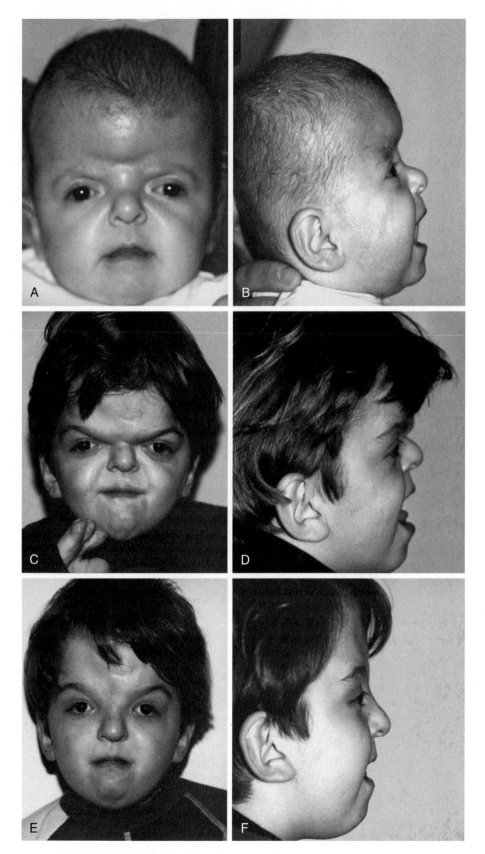

Figure 41–21

Two-step advancement in Apert's syndrome. *A* and *B*. An infant with Apert's syndrome, with the retruded supraorbital bar, just before floating forehead advancement. *C* and *D*. The same patient at 4 years of age is shown. The forehead is satisfactory, but the midface retrusion with hypertelorism is severe. *E* and *F*. The same patient is shown after facial advancement of the Le Fort III type combined with facial bipartition.

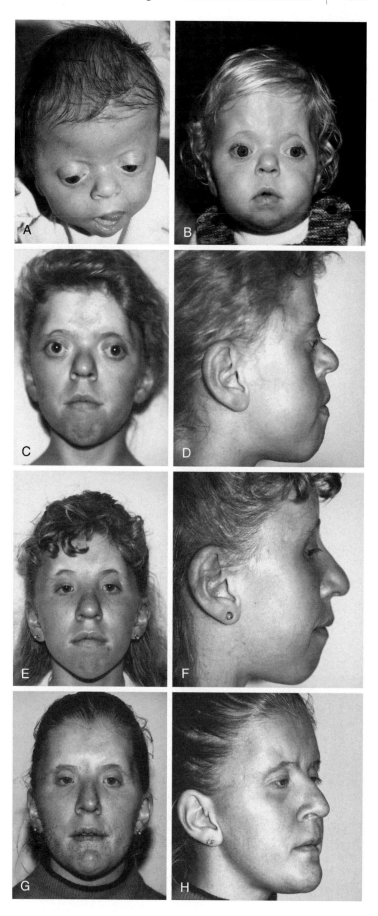

Figure 41–22

Secondary improvements in Apert's syndrome. *A.* A 6-month-old infant with Apert's syndrome with severe brachycephaly is shown. The same patient is shown after early frontal advancement and remodeling (*B*); at 11 years of age, with a severe facial retrusion (*C* and *D*); after facial advancement of the Le Fort III type (*E* and *F*); and at 16 years of age, after frontal contouring, rhinoplasty, and genioplasty (*G* and *H*). All three elements had to be improved to produce the final acceptable appearance.

same time produces a dead space between skull and brain that is not obliterated fast enough, the brain expansion being thwarted by the shunting of the cerebrospinal fluid. The question is to determine which must be treated first, craniosynostosis or hydrocephalus.

If the hydrocephalus is mild and slowly progressive, the craniosynostosis should be treated first. In this case, a shunt can be used to treat the hydrocephalus, if necessary, after the brain re-expansion has been completed. If the hydrocephalus is considerable or rapidly progressive, the shunt should be performed first. Then, the reduction in size of the ventricles is followed by computed tomography, and the craniosynostosis is treated after the size of the ventricles has decreased and is stable.

Craniofacial Surgery Is Teamwork

It is obvious from the congenital craniofacial malformations studied in this chapter that the only possible approach is that of a craniofacial team. After all the team members have examined the patient, and with the invaluable help of modern imaging, a plan of treatment is drawn up by the plastic surgeon and the neurosurgeon to incorporate all the morphological and functional aspects of the correction. These operations are too complex to be performed without significant experience of the problems involved. Such experience can only be obtained if these types of operations are performed in a limited number of centers.

REFERENCES

1. Apert, E.: De l'acrocephalosyndactalie. Bull. Soc. Med. Hop. Paris, 23:1310, 1906.
2. Brueton, L. A., Van Herwerden, L., Chotai, K. A., et al.: The mapping of a gene for craniosynostosis: Evidence for linkage of the Saethre-Chotzen syndrome to distal chromosome 7p. J. Med. Genet. 29:681–685, 1992.
3. Cohen, M. M., Jr.: Craniosynostosis: Diagnosis, evaluation and management. New York, Raven Press, 1986.
4. Cohen, M. M., Jr., Jirasek, J. E., Guzman, R. T., et al.: Holoprosencephaly and facial dysmorphia: Nosology, etiology and pathogenesis. Birth Defects, 7:125, 1971.
5. Converse, J. M., Ransohoff, J., Matthew, E., et al.: Ocular hypertelorism and pseudohypertelorism. Advances in surgical treatment. Plast. Reconstr. Surg., 45:1, 1970.
6. Crouzon, O.: Dysostose craniofaciale héréditaire. Bull. Soc. Med. Hôp. Paris, 33:545, 1912.
7. David, D. J., Moore, M. H., and Cootes, R. D.: Tessier clefts revisited with a third dimension. Cleft Palate J. 26:163, 1989.
8. De Myer, W., Zeman, W., and Palmer, C. A.: The face predicts the brain: Diagnostic significance of median facial anomalies for holoprosencephaly (arrhinencephaly). Pediatrics, 34:256, 1964.
9. Gault, D., Renier, D., Marchac, D., et al.: Intracranial volume in children with craniosynostosis. J. Craniofac. Surg., 1:1–3, 1990.
10. Gault, D., Renier, D., Marchac, D., et al.: Intracranial pressure and intracranial volume in children with craniosynostosis. Plast. Reconstr. Surg., 90:377–381, 1992.
11. Gillies, H. D., and Harrison, S. M.: Operative correction by osteotomy of recessed malar maxillary compound in a case of oxycephaly. Br. J. Plast. Surg., 2:123, 1950.
12. Kawamoto, H.: Rare craniofacial clefts. In McCarthy, J., ed.: Plastic Surgery. Philadelphia, W. B. Saunders, 1990, pp. 2922–2973.
13. Le Merrer, M., Ledinot, V., Renier, D., et al.: Conseil génétique dans les craniosténoses: Bilan d'une étude prospective réalisée avec le groupe d'études sur les malformations craniofaciales. J. Genet. Hum., 36:293–306, 1988.
14. Lajeunie, E., Le Merrer, M., and Bonaïti-Pellie, C.: A genetic study of nonsyndromic coronal craniosynostosis. Am. J. Genet., 1995 (in press).
15. Marchac, D., and Renier, D.: Le front flottant, trâitement précoce des faciocraniosténoses. Ann. Chir. Plast., 24:21, 1979.
16. Marchac, D., and Renier, D.: Craniofacial Surgery for Craniosynostosis. Boston, Little, Brown, & Co., 1982, p. 125.
17. Marchac, D., and Renier, D.: Early monobloc frontofacial advancement. In Marchac, D., ed.: Craniofacial Surgery: Proceedings of the First International Congress of Cranio-maxillo-facial Surgery. Berlin, Springer-Verlag, 1987, pp. 130–136.
18. Marchac, D., and Renier, D.: Craniosynostosis and craniofacial dysostosis. In Mastery of Plastic and Reconstructive Surgery. Boston, Little, Brown, 1994, pp. 499–515.
19. Marchac, D., Cophignon, J., Achard, E., et al.: Orbital expansion for anophthalmia and mino-orbitism. Plast. Reconstr. Surg., 59:486, 1977.
20. Mühlbauer, W., Anderl, H., and Marchac, D.: Complete frontofacial advancement in infants with craniofacial dysostosis: Transactions of the Eighth International Congress of Plastic Surgery, Montreal. Montreal, McGill University, 1983, pp. 318–320.
21. Ortiz-Monasterio, F., Fuente del Campo, A., and Carillo, A.: Advancement of the orbits and the midface in one piece, combined with frontal repositioning for the correction of Crouzon's deformities. Plast. Reconstr. Surg., 6:507, 1978.
22. Patten, B. M.: Human Embryology. 3rd ed. New York, McGraw-Hill, 1968.
23. Raveh, J., and Vuillemin, T.: Advantages of an additional subcranial approach in the correction of craniofacial deformities. J. Craniomaxillofac. Surg., 16:350, 1988.
24. Renier, D.: Intracranial pressure in craniosynostosis pre- and postoperative recordings: Correlation with functional results. In Persing, J. A., Edgerton, M. T., and Jane, J. A., eds.: Scientific Foundations and Surgical Treatment of Craniosynostosis. Baltimore, Williams & Wilkins, 1989, pp. 263–269.
25. Renier, D., and Marchac, D.: Craniofacial surgery for craniostenosis. Morphological and functional results. Ann. Acad. Med. Singapore, 17:415–426, 1988.
26. Renier, D., Brunet, L., and Marchac, D.: IQ and craniostenosis: Evolution in treated and untreated cases. In Marchac, D., ed.: Craniofacial Surgery. Berlin, Springer-Verlag, 1987, pp. 114–117.
27. Renier, D., Sainte-Rose, C., Marchac, D., et al.: Intracranial pressure in craniostenosis. J. Neurosurg., 57:370–377, 1982.
28. Renier, D., Sainte-Rose, C., and Marchac, D.: Intracranial pressure in craniostenosis: 302 recordings. In Marchac, D., ed.: Craniofacial Surgery. Proceedings of the First International Congress of Cranio-maxillo-facial Surgery. Berlin, Springer-Verlag, 1987, pp. 110–113.
29. Sedano, H. O., Cohen, M. M., Jr., Jirasek, J., et al.: Frontonasal dysplasia. J. Pediatr., 76:906, 1970.
30. Tessier, P.: Osteotomies totales de la face: Syndrome de Crouzon, syndrome d'Apert, oxycephalies, scaphocephalies, turricephalies. Ann. Chir. Plast., 12:273, 1967.
31. Tessier, P.: Experience in the treatment of orbital hypertelorism. Plast. Reconstr. Surg., 53:4, 1974.
32. Tessier, P.: Anatomical classification of facial, craniofacial and laterofacial clefts. J. Maxillofac. Surg., 4:69, 1976.
33. Tessier, P. L.: Facial bipartition: A concept more than a procedure. In Marchac, D., ed.: Proceedings of the First International Congress of the International Society of Cranio-maxillo-facial Surgery. Berlin, Springer-Verlag, 1987, pp. 217–245.
34. Tessier, P., Guiot, J., Rougerie, J. P., et al.: Ostéotomies cranio-naso-orbito-faciales: Hypertelorisme. Ann. Chir. Plast., 12:103, 1967.
35. Van der Meulen, J.: Medial faciotomy. Br. J. Plast. Surg., 32:339, 1979.
36. Van der Meulen, J., and Vaandrager, J. M.: Surgery related to the correction of hypertelorism. Plast. Reconstr. Surg., 71:6, 1983.
37. Van der Meulen, J., Mazzola, R., Stricker, M., et al.: Classification of craniofacial malformations. In Stricker, M., Van der Meulen, J., and Raphael, B., eds.: Craniofacial Malformations. Edinburgh, Churchill Livingstone, 1980, pp. 149–309.
38. Wilson, J. G.: Abnormalities of intrauterine development in nonhuman primates. Acta Endocrinol. Suppl. (Kbh.), 166:261, 1972.

CHAPTER 42

Congenital and Acquired Abnormalities of the Craniovertebral Junction

The first anatomical description of the "manifestation of occipital vertebrae" was attributed to Meckel in 1815 by Gladstone and Erickson-Powell.[100] In 1830, it was Bell who first described the clinical and pathological development of "spontaneous atlantoaxial dislocations" as the result of destruction of the transverse ligament that "holds the process of the dentata in its place. In consequence of the failure of the support, the process was thrown back so as to compress the spinal marrow."[19] After this, detailed anatomical and autopsy studies were reported in reference to abnormalities of the craniovertebral junction. As their clinical implications became increasingly apparent, they were discussed more frequently.[38, 153, 164] The clinical significance became appreciated after the classic radiological studies on basilar invagination by Chamberlain in 1939.[42] The early classification of atlantoaxial abnormalities was made by Greenberg in 1968.[107] It was then that the abnormalities of the craniovertebral junction emerged from the realm of anatomical and pathological curiosity to the clinical field of practical neuroscience.

The term "craniovertebral junction" refers to the occipital bone that surrounds the foramen magnum and the atlas and the axis vertebrae.[29, 151] These bones and the ligamentous complex surrounding them form a funnel-shaped enclosure through which the medulla oblongata continues into the cervical spinal cord. Surgical treatment of conditions affecting the craniovertebral junction usually consisted of a posterior decompression by enlargement of the foramen magnum and removal of the posterior arch of the atlas vertebra.* However, the mortality and morbidity associated with such treatment was high for patients with irreducible lesions with cervicomedullary compression. A surgical physiological approach based on an understanding of the craniocervical dynamics, the site of encroachment, and

the stability of the craniovertebral junction was adopted at the University of Iowa Hospitals and Clinics in 1977.[193] Since then, 2,100 patients with neurological symptoms and signs secondary to an abnormality of the craniocervical region have been investigated. Of these, 810 have undergone surgical treatment by the author. The pathology of these abnormalities was extensive and complex. They are easily understood, and their treatment is simplified if one has a knowledge of the bony anatomy, the biomechanics, and the embryology of the region.[283]

Anatomy of the Craniovertebral Junction

Bone-Ligament Complex

The occipital bone surrounds the foramen magnum and constitutes the posterior portion of the skull base (Fig. 42–1). The sagittal diameter of the foramen magnum is approximately 35 ± 4 mm.[29, 65, 283, 285] The paired occipital condyles are located on the caudal aspect of the foramen magnum; they are oval in configuration with a caudal convexity, are covered with cartilage, and articulate with the superior facets of the atlas vertebra. The occipital condyles are partially everted and converge anteriorly. They are connected by a thin rim of bone fused to the basicranium called the condylus tertius or the third occipital condyle. A pit situated behind each occipital condyle receives the posterior portion of the superior articular facet of the atlas when the head is extended.[251]

The atlas vertebra (C1) acts as a washer between the cervical spine and the skull. It is an irregular ring that has two separate, lateral masses, which form two fifths of the circumference. The superior articular facets are dorsal to the lateral atlantal masses and are oval, elon-

---

*See references 16, 54, 58, 107, 143, 164, 193, 198, and 288.

A. H. Menezes

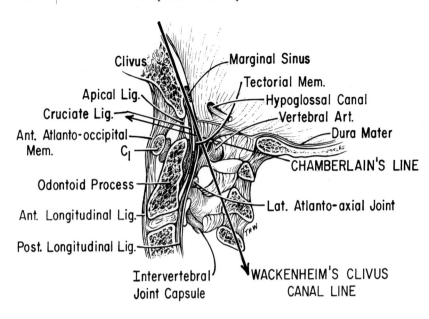

Figure 42–1

Anatomical relationships at the craniovertebral junction.

gated, and deeply concave to adapt to the contour of the occipital condyles. The inferior articular facets are concave in the sagittal direction and slightly convex in the transverse plane.

The inferior and superior zygapophyses of the atlas and the zygapophyses of the axis are unique among the spinal vertebrae because they are located ventral to the exits of the spinal nerve roots. A groove for the vertebral artery is present at the rostral base of the posterior atlantal arch. The first spinal nerve runs parallel to the vertebral artery in this groove. A concave indentation in the posterior surface of the anterior atlantal arch is a site for odontoid articulation.

The odontoid process projects cephalad from the body of the axis and its ventral surfaces and makes contact with the anterior arch of the atlas vertebra. The articulation between the atlas and the dens is lined by synovial bursae, which communicate with the bursae behind the odontoid process, forming a circumferential bursa.

The atlanto-occipital joint capsules provide poor stability because of their laxity.[98] The paired capsules are attached above the margin of the occipital condyle, and they attach caudal to the articular facets, to the lateral masses. These capsules are reinforced laterally by the occipitoatlantal ligament, which passes from the transverse process to the jugular process.

The atlantoaxial complex is unique among the intervertebral joints in that it is horizontally oriented. The lateral facet joints are relatively flat and allow for a pivoting motion at the atlantodental articulation, which is permitted by the special ligamentous support. The articular capsules of the lateral atlantal facets surround the articular surfaces and are strengthened by atlantoaxial ligaments (Fig. 42–2). These are oblique fibers that run from the tectorial membrane to reinforce the joint. The second cervical nerve exits from the cervical canal immediately adjacent and dorsal to the joint capsules.

The occipitoatlantal ligament and the atlantoaxial ligaments are present both anteriorly and posteriorly. The transverse atlantal ligament is a band 3 to 5 mm in thickness that originates from the tubercles and the inner aspect of the lateral masses of the atlas vertebra. This ligament maintains close apposition to the odontoid and keeps it in proximity to the anterior arch of the atlas, permitting axial rotation. Strong vertical fascicles blend with the transverse ligament dorsally. The alar ligaments originate in the superolateral aspects of the dens and encircle the medial aspect of each occipital condyle. These ligaments restrain and do not permit the anterior dislocation of the atlas and axis.

By itself, the geometry of the craniocervical complex is meant to provide mobility at the cost of stability. However, the complex is maintained in a clamplike vise by the craniocervical musculature, which assists in stabilization of the spine, initiates movements within the joints, and maintains the fluidity of the motion complex.

Blood Supply

The blood supply to the odontoid process is from two sources.[4, 216, 242] The vertebral arteries provide anterior and posterior ascending vessels that pass ventral and dorsal to the body of the axis and the odontoid and anastomose in an apical arcade in the region of the alar ligament. These vessels supply the small perforating branches to the body of the axis and the odontoid process. In addition, the anterior ascending branches in the apical arcade receive a contribution from the carotid arteries by way of the base of the skull and the alar ligaments (Fig. 42–3). The arrangement of these blood vessels has an embryological basis. It is axiomatic that the arterial pattern to the vertebra developed to supply the centers of ossification. The cartilaginous plate that represents the intervertebral disc between the base of the dens and the body of the axis prevents development of a vascular communication between the axis and the odontoid process. Knowledge

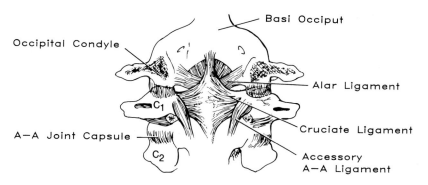

Figure 42–2

Ligaments of the occipitocervical joints viewed from within the foramen magnum.

of this anatomical and embryological basis for the vascular supply to the axis-odontoid complex is important to an understanding of the origin of os odontoideum and the formation of a sequestrum with a type II odontoid fracture.[79, 80, 122, 185]

Parke, Rothman, and Brown have demonstrated a previously undescribed system of pharyngovertebral veins with frequent lymphovenous anastomoses.[217] The periodontal venous plexus and the suboccipital epidural sinuses appear to have a direct connection with the pharyngovertebral veins. This connection may provide an additional route for septic involvement of the craniovertebral complex, which can result in osteomyelitis of the bone as well as joint effusions.

Lymphatic Drainage

The lymphatic drainage of the occipitoatlantoaxial joint complex is primarily into the retropharyngeal lymph nodes and thence into the upper deep jugular cervical chain.[2, 61, 107, 109] These nodes also receive drainage from the nasopharynx, the paranasal sinuses, and the retropharyngeal area. A retrograde infection may affect the synovial lining of the craniovertebral joint complex with a resultant inflammatory effusion, instability, and possible neurological deficit, contributing to the so-called Grisel's syndrome.[107]

Biomechanics of the Occipitoatlantal Complex

The cervical spine is the most mobile portion of the axial skeleton.[296] Relative motion of the occipitoatlantoaxial region is controlled by the geometry of the surfaces as well as the ligaments and their elastic properties.[101] The occipitoatlantoaxial complex serves as a transition zone between two completely different structures, the vertebral joints and the skull. It functions as a single unit, and the complex allows the necessary range of motion while providing support to the head.[220]

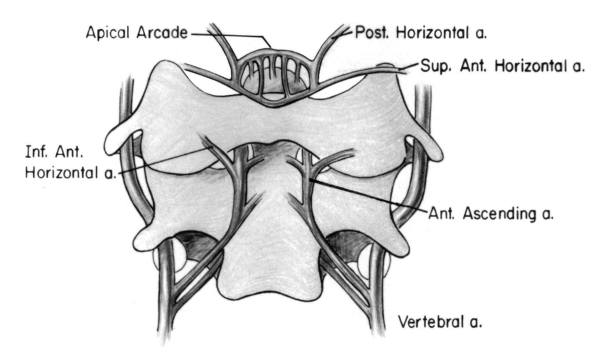

Figure 42–3

Blood supply of the odontoid process. (From Althoff, B., and Goldie, I. F.: The arterial supply of the odontoid process of the axis. Acta Orthop. Scand., 48:626, 1977, and Schiff, D., and Parke, W. J.: J. Bone Joint Surg. [Am.], 55:1450, 1975. Used by permission.)

Both occipitoatlantal and atlantoaxial articulations are involved in flexion and extension.[271] The average range of this motion at the occipitoatlantal joint is 13 to 15 degrees.[294] An additional 10 degrees of motion occurs in the atlantoaxial articulation. Flexion is limited by the tectorial membrane and by contact between the dens and the occipital basion.[130, 182, 271] Extension is restricted by the stretching of the tectorial membrane and by bony contact between the opisthion and the posterior arch of the atlas.[138, 140] In the normal adult, less than 3 mm of anterior-posterior translation occurs between the dens and the anterior ring of the atlas vertebra. This measurement may be up to 5 mm in children younger than 8 years of age. If the transverse component of the cruciate ligament has ruptured but the alar ligaments are still intact, up to 5 mm of displacement may occur at the atlantodental junction.[183, 191, 204] If both the transverse and the alar ligaments are incompetent, there is more than 5 mm of separation between the odontoid process and the anterior atlas arch.[81] Studies by Werne have demonstrated that sectioning of the alar ligament and the tectorial membrane produces instability of the occipitoatlantal joints, permitting luxation of these articulations.[294]

The anatomical configuration of the occipitoatlantal articulation precludes rotation.[101, 252] Rotation occurs only at the atlantoaxial joint. The large degree of rotation at the atlantoaxial articulation is explained by the articular surfaces, which are convex with horizontal orientation so as to allow maximal mobility. Atlantoaxial joint rotation is maximum at 37 to 42 degrees. If rotation exceeds this range, an interlocking of the lateral inferior facet of the atlas over the superior articular facet of the axis vertebra occurs.[250, 296] If the transverse ligament is deficient, the anterior arch of the atlas subluxates forward, producing a unilateral dislocation, and the facet interlocks at a rotation of less than 42 degrees. However, if the transverse ligament remains intact, there is no subluxation between the odontoid process and the anterior atlas arch up to a higher degree of rotation.[79]

Rotation of the atlantoaxial joint greater than 32 to 35 degrees produces an angulation of the contralateral vertebral artery.[250] With more rotation, there is stretching of the vertebral artery, and, at 45 degrees, the ipsilateral artery may demonstrate an angulation and subsequent occlusion. This phenomenon has implications in cervical traction, cranial manipulations, wrestling and football injuries, and sudden rotation of the head, such as may occur during general anesthesia.*

The lateral rotation of the neck can approach 90 degrees.[101] Even though half of this occurs at the atlantoaxial joint and the remainder at the lower cervical spine, after 20 to 30 degrees of rotation of the skull and upper cervical spine, the lower cervical vertebrae rotate in decreasing amounts to achieve the 90-degree rotation. This phenomenon is caused by the muscular contraction and tone produced in vivo by compressive forces across the cervical motion segment. The initial axial twist produces a threshold value that overcomes

the interlocking stiffening of the subaxial segments, allowing for the completion of the rotation to 90 degrees.

It is generally believed that there is no lateral bending of the atlantoaxial complex.[94, 271] Translatory movements in the occipitoatlantoaxial complex are small. The term "translation" refers to motion along an axis. At the occiput-atlas level, translation is normally 1 mm, and any motion greater than this is considered to be clinically significant.[292] This is especially important in cases of assimilation of the atlas associated with nonsegmentation of the C2–C3 vertebrae. In this situation, a dynamic load is thrown onto the atlantoaxial complex, with subsequent translation of the odontoid process and progression of the atlantoaxial instability.[189]

The simultaneous occurrence of translation and rotation is called "coupling."[296] This occurs at the atlantoaxial joint primarily as a result of the geometry of the facet articulations. With axial rotation of the atlas around the axis, there is an associated upward and transverse motion of the dens in relation to the atlas. Rotatory luxations of the atlas beyond 34 to 40 degrees produce excessive translation of the axis-dens process, with a relative descent of the cervicomedullary junction. Because of this, a misdiagnosis of Chiari I malformation or cerebellar tumor on magnetic resonance imaging has been made in patients with rotatory luxations of the atlas on the axis.[52, 74, 283]

In vitro studies of the craniovertebral junction indicate that application of very small loads to this complex results in significant rotation, flexion, and extension in comparison with the lower cervical spine.[101] However, in vivo observation shows that this is not the case. The principle of muscular action must therefore be responsible for holding the head firmly onto the neck and preventing these abnormal excursions.[189] If the protective muscles are relaxed or inadequately developed, as in the case of a young child, the craniovertebral junction becomes inherently less stable.[98, 223] In children, this instability may result in part from small occipital condyles and an almost horizontal plane of articulation between the cranium and the skull. The complete development of the occipital condyles with advancing age produces more vertical orientation of this joint plane. As muscular development occurs, there is less tendency for instability at the craniocervical junction.

Embryology and Development of the Craniovertebral Junction

Congenital anomalies of the base of the skull and the atlanto-occipital region involve both the osseous structures and the nervous system. The frequent occurrence of patterns with various combinations suggests an interrelationship, if not a common cause, of the origin and development of these structures.[107, 125, 189] A review of the embryology that includes the developmental sequence and timing of events in this region is necessary; a simplified version is outlined in Table 42–1.

---

*See references 15, 21, 188, 209, 246, 261, and 285.

Table 42–1
EMBRYOLOGY AND DEVELOPMENT OF THE CRANIOVERTEBRAL JUNCTION

Sclerotomes	Divisions	Subdivisions	Formations
Occipital First and second Third Fourth "proatlas"	Hypocentrum Centrum		Basiocciput Exoccipital centers (jugular tubercles) Anterior tubercle clivus Apical ligament Apex of dens
	Neural arch	Ventral rostral	Occipital condyles, third condyle U-shape of foramen magnum Alar and cruciate ligaments
		Dorsal caudal	Posterior arch of atlas (C1) Lateral atlantal masses
Spinal 1st	Hypocentrum persists Centrum Neural arch		Atlas anterior arch Dens Posterior inferior atlas arch
Spinal 2nd	Hypocentrum disappears Centrum Neural arch		Body of axis Facets, posterior arch of axis

Anomalies of the craniovertebral junction appear to be caused by faulty development of the cartilaginous neurocranium and the adjacent vertebral skeleton during the early embryonic weeks. The mesoderm caudal to the base of the plate condenses into four occipital somites.[27, 91] These are the precursors of the occipital sclerotomes (Fig. 42–4). The occipital sclerotomes fuse to form a single mass that extends around the neural tube at the region of the foramen magnum. These sclerotomes correspond to the segmental nerves that later form the hypoglossal nerve, which then passes by means of individual foramina through the bone.[29] The first two occipital sclerotomes ultimately form the basi-

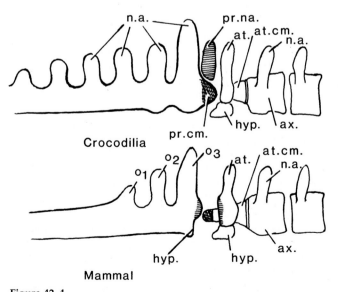

Figure 42–4
Schematic drawing of the supine median craniovertebral articulation in the crocodile and the paired articulations in mammals (at, atlas; ax, axis; cm, centrum; hyp, hypocentrum; na, neural arch; o, occipital neural arch; pr cm, proatlas centrum; pr na, proatlas neural arch).

occiput. The third occipital sclerotome is responsible for the exoccipital centers that form the jugular tubercles.

The proatlas is the key to understanding the embryology of this region and is the fourth occipital sclerotome.[38, 91, 204, 290] The hypocentrum of the fourth occipital sclerotome forms the anterior tubercle of the clivus. The centrum itself forms the apical cap of the dens and the apical ligaments. The neural arch component of the proatlas divides into rostral ventral components and caudal dorsal portions. The anterior, U-shaped margin of the foramen magnum is formed by the rostral ventral component; this structure also forms the occipital condyles and the third condyle, which may be present in the midline. The alar and cruciate ligaments are formed by condensation of the lateral portions of the proatlas. The caudal dorsal division of the neural arch of the proatlas forms the lateral atlantal masses and the superior portion of the posterior arch of the atlas.

The atlas vertebra is formed primarily by the first spinal sclerotome and differs from the remaining spinal vertebrae in that the centrum separates to fuse with the axis body, forming the midportion of the odontoid process.[166, 207] At an early stage, a hypochordal bow is found in front of each vertebral segment; it subsequently disappears except for that part which forms the anterior arch of the atlas. The neural arch of the first spinal sclerotome forms the posterior inferior portion of the atlas arch. The hypochordal bow of the proatlas itself may survive and join with the anterior arch of the atlas to form a variant, which as such may exist between the clivus or the posterior arch of the atlas and the apical segment of the odontoid process.

The hypocentrum of the second spinal sclerotome disappears in embryogenesis. The centrum forms the body of the axis vertebra, and the neural arch develops into the facets and the posterior arch of the axis.[78] As has been described, the body of the dens develops from the first sclerotome, and the terminal portion of the odontoid arises from the proatlas (Fig. 42–5). The most inferior portion of the axis is formed by the second spinal sclerotome.

The odontoid process at birth is separated from the body of the axis vertebra by a cartilaginous band that represents a vestigial disc, referred to as a neurocentral synchondrosis. This structure lies below the level of the superior facets of the axis vertebra and does not represent the anatomical base of the dens. The neurocentral synchondrosis is present in almost all children but disappears after 8 years of age.[252, 283, 285] At birth, there should be a recognizable odontoid process, even though it is not fused to the base of the axis. The tip of the odontoid process is not ossified at birth and is represented by a small ossification center, which is usually seen at 3 years of age and is called the ossiculum terminale; it fuses with the remainder of the dens by age 12. If it fails to fuse with the odontoid process, it is called an ossiculum terminale persistens and as such has little significance.

Classification of Abnormalities of the Craniocervical Junction

A wide variety of congenital, developmental, and acquired abnormalities exist at the craniocervical junction. These may occur singly or as more than one anomaly in the same individual, and their pathology is extensive. For purposes of understanding and discussion of craniocervical junction abnormalities, these entities have been subdivided into separate categories (Table 42–2). It must be appreciated that there is overlapping within these classifications.

Diagnosis of Craniovertebral Abnormalities

Symptoms and Signs

Perhaps the most interesting feature of craniovertebral abnormalities is the diversity of their presenta-

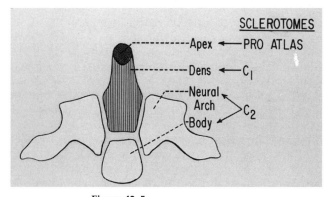

Figure 42–5
Development of the axis vertebra.

Table 42–2

CLASSIFICATION OF CRANIOVERTEBRAL JUNCTION ABNORMALITIES

Congenital Anomalies and Malformations of the Craniovertebral Junction
A. Malformations of the occipital bone
  1. Manifestations of occipital vertebrae
    a. Clivus segmentation
    b. Remnants around foramen magnum
    c. Variants at atlas
    d. Dens segmentation anomalies
  2. Basilar invagination
  3. Condylar hypoplasia
  4. Assimilation of atlas
B. Malformations of atlas
  1. Assimilation of atlas
  2. Atlantoaxial fusion
  3. Aplasia of atlas arches
C. Malformations of axis
  1. Irregular atlantoaxial segmentation
  2. Dens dysplasias
    a. Ossiculum terminale persistens
    b. Os odontoideum
    c. Hypoplasia-aplasia
  3. Segmentation failure of C2–C3

Developmental and Acquired Abnormalities of the Craniovertebral Junction
A. Abnormalities at the foramen magnum
  1. Secondary basilar invagination (e.g., Paget's disease, osteomalacia, rheumatoid cranial settling)
  2. Foraminal stenosis (e.g., achondroplasia)
B. Atlantoaxial instability
  1. Errors of metabolism (e.g., Morquio's syndrome)
  2. Down's syndrome
  3. Infection (e.g., Grisel's syndrome)
  4. Inflammatory (e.g., rheumatoid arthritis)
  5. Traumatic occipitoatlantal and atlantoaxial dislocations; os odontoideum
  6. Tumors (e.g., neurofibromatosis, syringomyelia)
  7. Miscellaneous (e.g., fetal warfarin syndrome, Conradi's syndrome)

tions.[14, 44, 164, 181, 283] Each abnormality may vary in degree of deformity, in clinical effects, and in its pattern of association with neighboring skeletal structures.[193] Compromise of the cervicomedullary junction results in a multiplicity of symptoms and signs involving dysfunction of one or more of the associated formations—the brain stem, the cervical spinal cord, the cranial nerves, the cervical nerve roots, or the vascular supply to these structures. The neurological symptoms are the result of direct compression of the neural tissue by bone and soft tissue at the craniovertebral junction or compromise of the vertebral anterior spinal and perforating arteries to the cervicomedullary junction. Each step of the pathological progression of hindbrain herniation syndromes, hydromyelia, and foramen magnum constriction due to basilar invagination presents with its own characteristic features.

The symptoms of craniovertebral dysfunction can be insidious and at times can present with false localizing signs.[63, 195, 267] In rare instances, a rapid neurological progression is followed by sudden death.[233] Frequently, there is an antecedent history of minor trauma, which then sets off a pattern of symptoms and signs that progress at a galloping pace.

General Physical Examination

An abnormal general appearance, most often involving the neck, is seen in patients with congenital abnormalities of the craniovertebral junction.[102, 104] The most common finding is atlanto-occipital fusion, which has a high incidence in patients with Klippel-Feil syndrome (Figs. 42–6). The classic triad of the Klippel-Feil syndrome consists of a low posterior hairline, a short neck, and limitation of neck motion.[10, 20, 56, 146, 167] The head may be cocked to one side or the other, as in patients with rotatory luxation of the atlas on the axis.[106, 192, 245]

The Klippel-Feil syndrome is associated with deficits in the genitourinary and cardiopulmonary systems as well as with congenital defects of the skeletal and nervous systems.* Facial asymmetry and webbing of the neck, scoliosis, and Sprengel's shoulder deformity may be present. It is not uncommon to see children with a small dysmorphic stature.[167] The skeletal dysplasias associated with abnormal bone metabolism or architecture result in structure weakness and collapse of the skeletal elements. Patients with achondroplasia, spondyloepiphyseal dysplasia, and related diseases associated with dwarfism have increased incidences of craniovertebral abnormalities.† Rheumatoid arthritis is associated with a 25 per cent prevalence of craniovertebral involvement.[12] If unexplained neurological deficits are present in association with these syndromes and diseases, the possibility of abnormalities of the craniovertebral junction should be entertained.

Myelopathy

The most common neurological deficit in the author's series of 2,100 patients with craniocervical

---

*See references 10, 125, 137, 169, 201, 211, and 251.
†See references 1, 8, 20, 32, 41, 67, 95, 103, 115, 172, 193, 195, 235, 269, and 270.

abnormalities was myelopathy, and the most common symptom was neck pain. The symptoms may be subtle and nonspecific. False localizing signs are common, and motor deficits include monoparesis, hemiparesis, paraparesis, and quadriparesis. Myelopathy mimicking the "central cord syndrome" is often seen in patients with basilar invagination.[192, 283] Central cord necrosis has been reported by several investigators.[196, 202, 286] Studies in these patients have suggested that the venous drainage of the cervical gray matter is rostral in direction, between the first thoracic vertebra and the atlas, and that separate drainage exists for the gray and the white matter of the spinal cord.[280] This may partially explain the central cord syndrome. Autopsy examinations have demonstrated a selective vulnerability of the spinal cord gray matter to compressive and anoxic changes. Additional anoxic changes may occur because of reduced blood flow from the penetrating arteries of the spinal cord that are on a plane perpendicular to the compressive flattening forces.[31, 103] Autopsy studies of patients with high cervical myelopathy secondary to occipitoatlantoaxial dislocations have shown demyelination of the posterior columns and cortical spinal tracts associated with gliosis of the gracile and cuneate nuclei.[103, 202]

Sensory abnormalities are usually manifested by deficits relating to posterior column dysfunction.[12, 55] Hypalgesia reflecting spinal thalamic dysfunction is unusual and was a finding in only 7 per cent of the author's patients. A high incidence of bladder dysfunction parallels the motor deficits.

In patients with rheumatoid arthritis, an erroneous diagnosis of entrapment neuropathy, rheumatoid peripheral neuropathy, vasculitis, or progression of the rheumatoid disease is not uncommon. Because of the severe deforming effects of the rheumatoid arthritis, hyperreflexia and the Babinski sign are of major importance in identifying those patients who have myelopathy.[194]

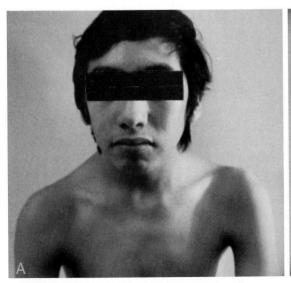 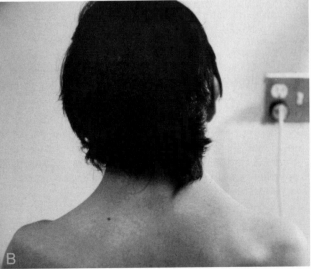

Figure 42–6

A. Klippel-Feil syndrome in a 14-year-old boy. Notice the short neck and atrophy around the shoulder girdle. *B.* Posterior view illustrating webbed neck, low hairline, and atrophy around the shoulders.

Brain Stem and Cranial Nerve Dysfunction

Brain stem and cranial nerve deficits are evidenced by abnormalities such as sleep apnea and dysphagia.[20, 41, 116] Not uncommonly, internuclear ophthalmoplegia is present, leading to a misdiagnosis of mesencephalic and upper pontine disturbance. Downbeat nystagmus is present in strictly compressive lesions of the craniocervical border with or without an associated Chiari malformation.[46, 185]

In the author's series, the most common cranial nerve dysfunction was a hearing loss, which occurred in 22 per cent of patients, with an increased prevalence in patients with Klippel-Feil syndrome. A unilateral or bilateral paralysis or dysfunction of the soft palate and the pharynx was associated with repeated bouts of aspiration pneumonia as well as poor feeding and inability to gain weight. The vascular symptoms, such as intermittent attacks of altered consciousness, confusion, transient loss of visual fields, and vertigo, occurred in 20 per cent of children with abnormalities of the craniocervical junction. This, at times, was provoked by extension of the head or rotation, as with manipulation of the head and neck. A similar occurrence was seen in adults.

Vascular Symptoms

The vascular symptoms include syncope, vertigo, intermittent periods of altered consciousness, episodic paresis, confusion, and transient loss of visual fields.[185] These symptoms have been documented in the author's series and those of several others. Symptoms related to the vertebral artery circulation may be associated with turning of the head.[85, 209] The excessive mobility of the unstable occipitoatlantoaxial joint may cause repeated trauma to the anterior spinal artery as well as to its perforating branches to the upper cervical cord and medulla.[261]

An important symptom is basilar migraine, which is not uncommon in children who have basilar invagination with atlas assimilation and compression of the medulla and the vertebrobasilar artery tree.[185]

Neck Symptoms

Suboccipital pain was reported in 82 per cent of patients in the author's series. The pain was typically described as originating in the suboccipital region with radiation to the vertex of the skull in the distribution of the greater occipital nerve. Occipital pain was present in all patients with rheumatoid arthritis; this symptom is attributable to irritation of the second cervical nerve as it exits the spinal canal immediately adjacent to the joint capsule of the atlantoaxial epiphyseal joint.[283]

Nasopharyngeal infection in the pediatric age group, especially in children younger than 10 years of age, is an important sign. The cervical musculature plays a supportive role only after this age. A majority of patients reported in the literature who had cranioverte-bral junction instability and neck infection were younger than 10 years of age.[294, 298]

Neuroradiological Investigations of Craniovertebral Junction Abnormalities

The diagnosis of a craniovertebral junction lesion should be considered if a constellation of symptoms and signs referable to the medulla oblongata, high cervical spinal cord, and cerebellum exists. The factors that influence treatment are the reducibility of the lesion, the presence of associated neural lesions, the mechanics of compression, and the presence of abnormal ossification centers and epiphyseal growth plates with anomalous development.[192, 193]

The term "reducibility" refers to the ability to achieve reduction so as to have a normal osseous alignment, thereby relieving compression on the neural structures. The direction of encroachment could be ventral, dorsal, or dorsoventral, as well as superior and lateral. An important association with neural abnormalities, such as the hindbrain herniation (Chiari) syndrome, syringohydromyelia, or vascular abnormalities, is taken into consideration in guiding the primary route of treatment.

These factors are determined by plain radiography, which must include a lateral view of the skull showing the cervical spine, the anteroposterior or open mouth view, and oblique views of the cervical spine.[192] Supplementary views, such as a Towne view and the anteroposterior projection of the foramen magnum, are done as necessary. Sophisticated pleuridirectional tomography is less often performed at this time.[65, 229] This allows the examiner to measure the craniocervical relationships and dimensions (Figs. 42–7 and 42–8). The relationships commonly visualized at the craniovertebral border on lateral and anteroposterior projections are shown in Tables 42–3 and 42–4.[144, 277, 286, 297] The slice thickness on polytomography is 1 mm; sections are usually obtained with 5-mm separations to study the anteroposterior and lateral appearance of the craniocervical region. This is done with the neck in both flexed and extended positions so as to obtain an understanding of the biomechanics. Lateral tomography images of the craniocervical region are obtained starting from one atlas articular process and going to the other articular process. This gives an idea about the stability of the region.

Although both plain tomography and computed tomography can outline the bony abnormality, cerebrospinal fluid enhancement with iohexol provides excellent anatomical details of both the neural structure abnormality and the bony distortion on computed tomography.[151, 154, 157, 229, 283] Axial views provide confirmation in another dimension.[187]

Magnetic resonance imaging is an ideal tool to use after plain radiography has been done.[185] It identifies the neural abnormalities as well as the osseous com-

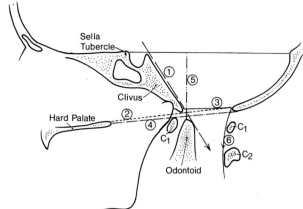

Figure 42–7

Lateral craniometry with points of reference.

① Wackenheim Clivus Canal Line   ④ McGregor Line
② Chamberlain Line   ⑤ Height Index of Klaus
③ McRae Line   ⑥ Spinous Interlaminar Line
                                                    (Posterior Canal Line)

Table 42–3
CRANIOMETRIC LINES IN LATERAL VIEW

Synonyms	Definition	Normal Measurements	Implications
Wackenheim's line (clivus canal line)	Line drawn along clivus into cervical canal	Odontoid tip is ventral and tangential to this line	Odontoid process transects the line in basilar invagination or forward position of skull
Chamberlain's line (palato-occipital line)	Joins posterior pole of hard palate to opisthion	Tip of dens 3.6 mm below this line	Odontoid process bisects the line in basilar invagination
McRae's line (foramen magnum line)	Joins anterior and posterior edges of foramen magnum (basion to opisthion)	Tip of dens does not exceed this line	If effective sagittal canal diameter is less than 20 mm, neurological symptoms occur
McGregor's line (basal line)	Hard palate to lowest point of occipital bone	Tip of dens should not exceed 5 mm above the line	Line position varies with flexion-extension—hence, not important
Height index of Klaus	Distance between tip of dens and tuberculum-cruciate line	40—41 mm	<30 mm seen in basilar invagination
Spinolamellar line (spinous interlaminar line)	Line drawn from interoccipital ridge above and down along the fused spinous processes of C2 and C3	Should intersect posterior arch of atlas	If atlas is fused, posterior arch is anterior to the line; posterior compression of spinal cord may occur

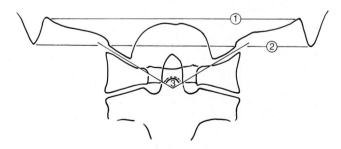

Figure 42–8

Craniometry lines and angles in anteroposterior view.

① Fishgold Diagastric Line
② Fishgold Bimastoid Line
③ Schmidt—Fischer Angle
    (angle of axes of Atlanto—occipital joints)

Table 42–4
CRANIOMETRIC LINES AND ANGLES IN ANTEROPOSTERIOR VIEW

Synonyms	Definition	Normal Measurements	Implications
Fishgold's diagastric line (biventer line)	Joins the fossae for diagastric muscles on undersurface of skull just medial to mastoid process	Dens tip should not project above this line; central axis of dens should be perpendicular to the line	Corresponds to McRae's line on lateral view; may be oblique in unilateral condylar hypoplasia; oblique odontoid suggests paramedian abnormality
Fishgold's bimastoid line	Line connecting tips of mastoid process	Runs across atlanto-occipital joints; line is 10 mm below diagastric line	Odontoid tip may be 10 mm above the line
Schmidt-Fischer angle (angle of axes of atlanto-occipital joints)	Angle of axes of atlanto-occipital joints	124–127 degrees; should be measured in plane of dens on tomography	Angle is wider in condylar hypoplasia

pression. In the examination, flexion and extension views are required to obtain visualization in the parasagittal dimension with the T1- and T2-weighted modes; these are supplemented by the axial views. The effects of cervical traction can also be documented with magnetic resonance imaging. Each of these techniques provides complementary information to define the craniovertebral abnormality.

In all the techniques of investigation, dynamic flexion-extension studies are necessary to assess the stability and the angular-osseous relationships of the neural structures, as well as to provide information regarding reducibility and the position of fixation should this be essential. The effects of cervical traction must be documented, not only with plain radiography but also with magnetic resonance imaging, to confirm the relief of neural compromise and the restored relationships of the craniovertebral complex.

Vertebral angiography and magnetic resonance angiography have been used in selected cases to identify a proven obstruction or one that occurs with dynamic changes of the craniovertebral region. An unexplained neurological sign or symptom that cannot be accounted

for by the previously mentioned studies requires angiography. In basilar invagination with atlas assimilation and in rotational luxation of the atlas on the axis vertebra, vertebral artery distortion and occlusions are not uncommon. Information about the location of these vessels and the possible kinks that occur with changes in position must be available to the treating physician before therapy is begun.

Pathology Affecting the Craniocervical Junction

DEVELOPMENTAL AND ACQUIRED ABNORMALITIES OF THE CRANIOVERTEBRAL JUNCTION

Manifestations of Occipital Vertebrae

Malformations and anomalies of the most caudal of the occipital sclerotomes (the proatlas) are collectively called "manifestations of occipital vertebrae." These

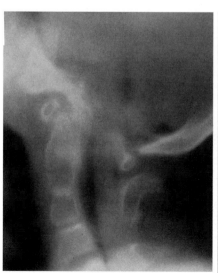
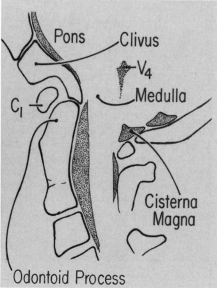

Figure 42–9

Lateral midline gas myelotomography in a 13-year-old boy with basilar migraine and paraparesis. The abnormal clivus-odontoid-atlas articulation indents the medulla oblongata, making the cervical cord taut.

may be represented as ridges or bony outgrowths to the margins of the foramen magnum.[285, 290] A significant abnormality is a pseudojoint formed by an abnormal articulation between the clivus, the anterior arch of the atlas, and the apical segment of the clivus.[192] Even though the bony abnormality is situated extracranially at the anterior margin of the foramen magnum, an abnormal angulation of the craniovertebral junction does occur with ventral compression at the cervicomedullary junction (Fig. 42–9). A normal clivus canal angle should not be less than 150 degrees in flexion.[65] This particular abnormality is often associated with a Chiari malformation and syringohydromyelia (Fig. 42–10). If the hypochordal bow assumes a large, knobby configuration, it has been called a third condyle and may in itself form an abnormal articulation, as previously described.[27, 285] This condition has been associated with os odontoideum.

Abnormal segmentation of the clivus is extremely rare and should not be mistaken for the spheno-occipi-

tal suture line. This suture line usually fuses after the 12th year. An example of this anomaly is shown in a boy with severe spastic quadriparesis (Fig. 42–11A and B). The proatlas component of the dens has failed to separate from the portion that forms the basiocciput to the clivus. The anterior arch of the atlas does rest above the axis body, and the neurocentral synchondrosis of the axis itself is well visualized in this illustration. The abnormality moved in unison with the clivus, grossly distorting the cervicomedullary junction ventrally (see Fig. 42–11C and D). This anomaly is similar to the appearance of the reptilian spine in lower vertebrates.

Abnormalities of clivus segmentation may result in bifid clivus, and failure of fusion of the occipital sclerotomes in the midline contributes to this. Failure of fusion of the first and second occipital sclerotomes produces a bipartite clivus.

It must be kept in mind that the occipital sclerotome is functionally a vertebra. Marin-Padilla and Marin-

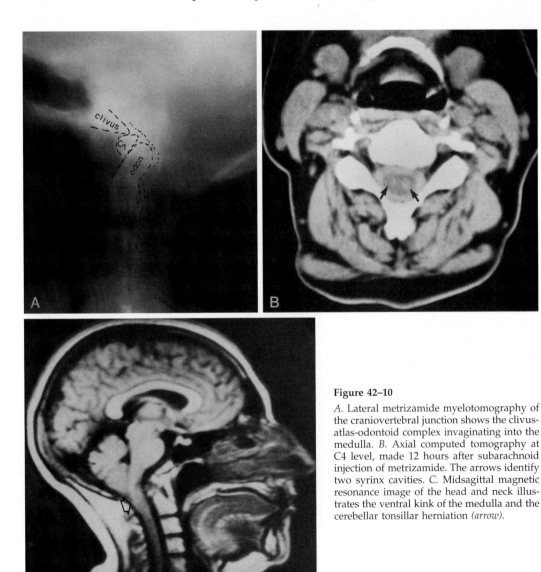

Figure 42–10

A. Lateral metrizamide myelotomography of the craniovertebral junction shows the clivus-atlas-odontoid complex invaginating into the medulla. *B.* Axial computed tomography at C4 level, made 12 hours after subarachnoid injection of metrizamide. The arrows identify two syrinx cavities. *C.* Midsagittal magnetic resonance image of the head and neck illustrates the ventral kink of the medulla and the cerebellar tonsillar herniation *(arrow).*

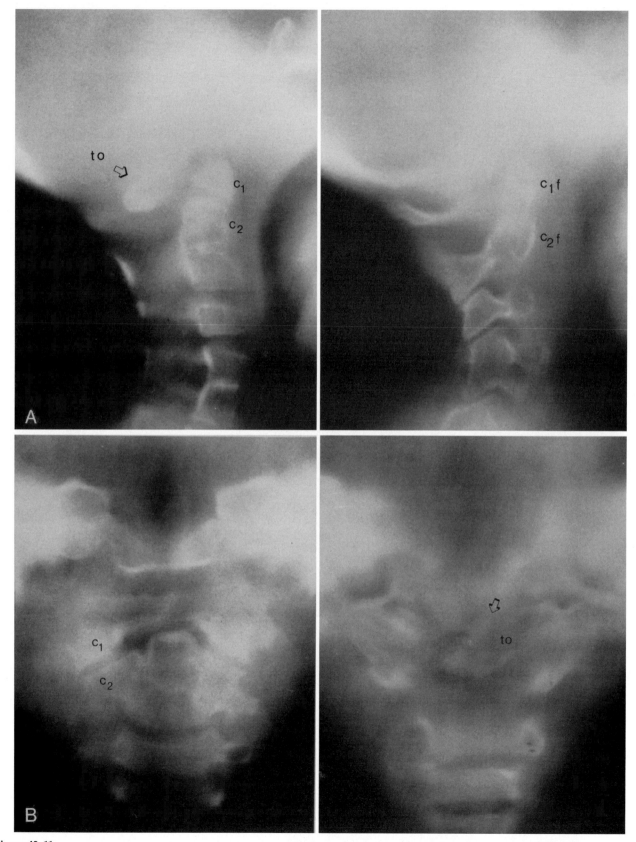

Figure 42–11

A. Lateral craniovertebral junction tomography in midsagittal *(left)* and facet planes *(right)*. The atlas anterior arch (C1) sits over the axis (C2). The terminal odontoid process (to) is fused with the clivus and protrudes into the foramen magnum. The lateral arches of the atlas and axis continue to the facet articulations (C1$_f$ and C2$_f$). *B.* Frontal tomography of the craniovertebral junction *(left)* shows the anterior arch of the atlas to be in the same plane *(right)* as the odontoid process. Tomography in a more dorsal plane shows the fusion of the terminal odontoid *(arrow)* to the clivus.

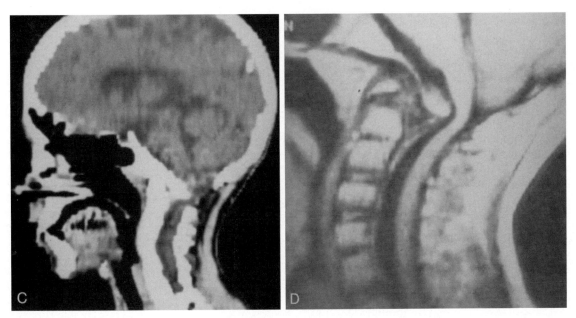

Figure 42–11 *Continued*
C. Reconstructed midsagittal computed tomography shows the severe cervicomedullary ventral bony compression. *D.* Midsagittal T1-weighted magnetic resonance image of the craniovertebral junction reveals the neural structures to be compressed and distorted by the central bony protrusion.

Padilla have demonstrated that the basichondrocranium of a fetus with a hindbrain malformation such as the Chiari malformation is shorter than normal and is elevated in relation to the axis of the vertebral column.[170] The shortness of the basichondrocranium is thought to be caused by underdevelopment of the occipital bone, especially noticeable in its basal component. The basic defects supposedly result in a short and small posterior fossa, inadequate to contain the developing nervous structures of that region. Their theory is that the developing cerebellum is then displaced downward to an anomalous position just above the foramen magnum, and the developing medulla is compressed and crowded into the small posterior fossa. The lordotic elevation of the basichondrocranium is supposedly responsible for the reduction of the pontine flexure and the increased angle of the cervical flexure of the hindbrain found in these fetuses. The elevation of the odontoid process could be explained by the depression of the underdeveloped basiocciput, resulting in a form of basilar impression often seen in clinical Chiari malformations. These same changes have been reproduced experimentally in pregnant hamsters with a single dose of vitamin A, early during the morning of the eighth day of gestation. This produces typical Chiari I and Chiari II malformations as well as various types of axial skeletal dysraphic disorders known to be associated with the human disease.[189]

Basilar Invagination

The terms "basilar invagination," "basilar impression," and "platybasia" are often used erroneously. Basilar invagination refers to the primary form of basilar impression, which consists of a distinct developmental defect of the chondrocranium, often associated

with other anomalies of the notochord in the region of the craniovertebral junction, such as occipitalization of the atlas and Klippel-Feil syndrome. Basilar invagination is also associated with anomalies of development of the epicaudal neuraxis such as the Chiari malformations, syringobulbia, and syringomyelia. The prevalence of neurodysgenesis is between 25 and 30 per cent in basilar invagination.*

The term "basilar impression" refers to the secondary, acquired form of basilar invagination that is caused by softening of the bone.[129] This condition occurs in hyperparathyroidism, rickets, osteomalacia, Paget's disease, Hurler's syndrome, and other diseases such as the Hajdu-Cheney syndrome.†

The term "platybasia" refers only to an abnormally obtuse basilar angle formed by joining the plane of the clivus with the plane of the anterior fossa of the skull.[65] This angle is of anthropological significance only. No symptoms or signs can be attributed to platybasia alone. It is not a measure of basilar invagination, although it may be associated with invagination. Confusion between basilar impression and platybasia dates to Chamberlain's paper published in 1939.[42]

Schmidt and Fischer published a detailed analysis of basilar invagination in 1960.[244] In this anomaly, all three parts of the occipital bone (basiocciput, exoccipital bone, and supraoccipital bone) are deformed. Two types of basilar invagination are recognized.[114, 243, 244, 280] In the anterior variety, there is a shortening of the basiocciput such that the clivus is short and horizontally oriented, displacing the plane of the foramen magnum rostrally in relation to the spinal column; this is

---

*See references 36, 39, 56, 58, 69, 125, 183, 192, 200, and 204.
†See references 37, 43, 115, 150, 192, 218, 222, and 280.

often associated with platybasia. In this situation, the posterior fossa structures are crowded. In the second type of basilar invagination, called paramedian invagination, there is associated hypoplasia of the exoccipital bones. Condylar hypoplasia may be such that the clivus becomes dorsally displaced into the posterior fossa, and it may be of normal length. The clivus invagination is compensated for by an excessive downward curvature of the lateral squamous-occipital bones. The distinction between these two types is not as clinically important as was initially thought, because a mixture often does occur.[180, 285] Basilar invagination is often associated with other craniovertebral abnormalities, particularly the degrees of assimilation of the atlas, defective fusion of the vertebrae, remnants of occipital vertebrae, blocked vertebrae, and other vertebral malformations.

The radiological diagnosis of basilar invagination is based on a pathological alteration in the craniometric relationships visualized on plain radiography, pleuridirectional tomography, computed tomography, and magnetic resonance imaging. Basilar invagination should be suspected if the lateral atlantoaxial articulations cannot be properly visualized on the open mouth (anteroposterior) projection of the upper cervical spine. The tip of the dens should normally not exceed the bimastoid line by more than 10 mm. The digastric or biventer line is approximately 10 mm rostral to the bimastoid line and should not be crossed by the normal dens.[83] Multiple reference lines identify basilar invagination on roentgenography projections. The tip of the odontoid process should usually be below Chamberlain's line and never more than 2.5 mm above it.[42] McRae's line represents a plane of the foramen magnum and should not be invaded by the dens under normal circumstances.[182] The index of Klaus is reduced to less than 30 mm in cases of basilar invagination.[144]

The foramen magnum normally has an average sagittal diameter of 35 mm. According to McRae and subsequent authors, including the present author, sagittal reduction of the foramen magnum to less than 19 mm produces neurological deficits.[181]

In basilar invagination, there is elevation of the floor of the posterior fossa. This may be simulated by an abnormally short clivus that results in an upward elevation of the anterior aspect of the foramen magnum (Fig. 42–12). The elevation of the floor of the posterior fossa is most prominent around the foramen magnum, so the margins curve upward, whereas the lateral portions of the posterior fossa may curve downward. Thus, the space within the posterior fossa is compromised to a varying extent.[189] Abnormalities such as the Chiari malformation and syringohydromyelia occur in 25 to 35 per cent of these patients (Fig. 42–13). An excessive amount of granulation tissue may build up around the odontoid process if chronic instability is present, as is seen with assimilation of the atlas and subsequent invagination. This, in itself, may act as a space-occupying mass in the anterior portion of the foramen magnum. In addition, fibrous bands and dural adhesions are common in the posterior cervicomedullary junction and around the cerebellar tonsils in both primary and secondary basilar invagination.[192] A severe form of basilar invagination may occur after childhood diseases of bone such as renal rickets, although later the patient may not show any other manifestations of this disease. The basilar invagination in these circumstances is difficult to differentiate from the primary adult form because maturation of bone has occurred.[283] The anterior aspect of the posterior fossa is markedly elevated, with resultant deformity of the petrous bone and the exoccipital bone, producing an upward invagination of the upper cervical spine (Fig. 42–14).

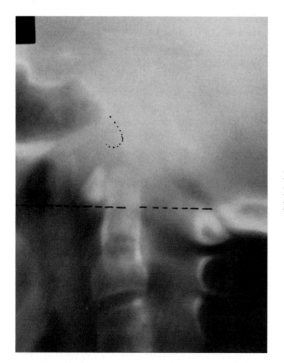

Figure 42–12

Midline lateral tomography of the craniovertebral junction shows a short clivus and platybasia. The odontoid tip is well above Chamberlain's line.

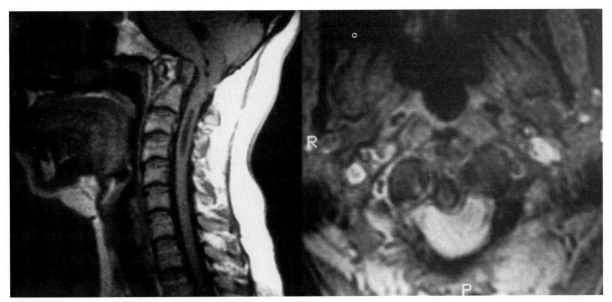

Figure 42–13

Composite of midsagittal T1-weighted magnetic resonance images of the craniovertebral and cervical spine region (*left*) and axial T2-weighted magnetic resonance images through the plane of the foramen magnum (*right*). Atlas assimilation, basilar invagination indenting the medullar oblongata, and cerebellar tonsillar herniation are present. Notice the upper cervical syringohydromyelia.

Basilar impression is the consequence of bone softening secondary to disease. Stenosis of the cervical canal and foramen magnum may occur. Treatment consists of recognition of the underlying pathology, relief of compression, and prevention of worsening of the problem by fusion and bracing.

Achondroplasia deserves mention because it is characterized by dysplasia of endochondral bone formation and is a genetic dominant disorder. Cervicomedullary dysfunction secondary to bony stenosis of the foramen magnum or to compression of the dorsal cervicomedullary junction by intradural bands has led to significant mortality within the first 2 years of life.[230, 236]

Condylar Hypoplasia

Condylar hypoplasia is often involved in malformations of the craniovertebral junction that form the paramedian type of basilar invagination. The occipital condyles are flattened, leading to an elevated position of the atlas and axis vertebrae.[65, 83, 245, 285] Transitional stages exist between condylar hypoplasia and basilar invagination. Condylar hypoplasia limits movement of the atlanto-occipital joint and at times may lead to vertebral artery compression as a result of the backward glide of the occiput. An asymmetrical flattening of the occipital condyle may produce compensatory scoliotic changes in the cervical spine. The angle of Schmidt and Fischer is wider than 125 degrees in this circumstance.[244] The medially placed occipital condyles result in a marked reduction in the transverse diameter of the foramen magnum, with a resultant lateral medullary compression that may be compounded by an already existing hindbrain malformation[238] (Fig. 42–15).

Assimilation of the Atlas and Irregular Segmentations

Atlas assimilation is defined as failure of segmentation between the fourth occipital sclerotome and the first spinal sclerotome. This anomaly occurs in 0.25 per cent of the population.[255] It may be bilateral, unilateral, segmental, or focal. In some instances, a complete atlas assimilation is seen.[38, 153, 183] In most cases, this anomaly is associated with other abnormalities such as basilar invagination and the Klippel-Feil syndrome. In the published series by McRae and Barnum in 1953, there was fusion between the second and third cervical vertebrae in 18 of 25 patients with atlas assimilation.[183] In the author's series of 242 patients with atlas assimilation, segmentation failure of the second and third cervical vertebrae was seen in 92 individuals.[189] In all these 92 patients, a Chiari malformation existed (Fig. 42–16). In addition, a paramesial invagination was present in one third of the patients with the Chiari malformation in this group. Reducible atlantoaxial or basilar invagination was present in 80 per cent of the children affected before 14 years of age. As age progressed, the lesion became irreducible. In partially reducible lesions, there was prolific granulation tissue around the dislocation, and this was soft and vascular. In irreducible lesions, the granulation tissue was tough and fibrotic. Additional findings in irreducible basilar invagination with atlas assimilation were a horizontally oriented clivus and grooves present behind the occipital condyle–lateral mass of the assimilated atlas to accommodate the superior facets of the axis vertebra.

A combination of assimilation of the atlas and segmentation failures between the second and third cervical vertebrae results in progressive laxity of the atlantodental joint with development of luxation be-

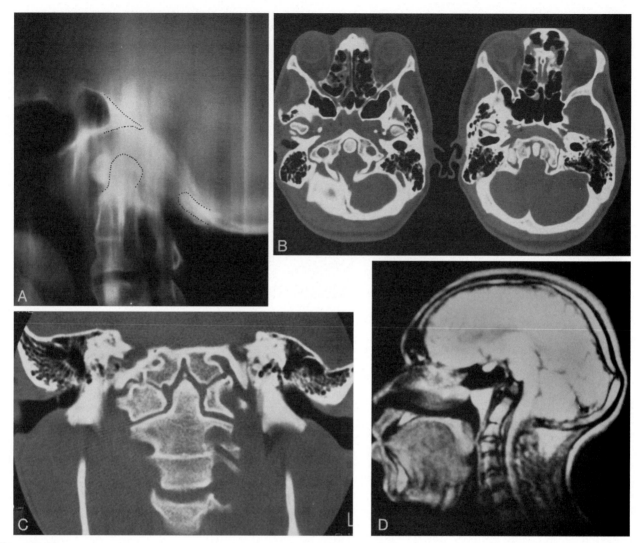

Figure 42–14

A. Lateral midline laminagraphy of the craniovertebral junction demonstrates an elevation of the short clivus and the upper cervical spine. The patient had spastic quadriparesis. *B.* Axial computed tomography of the skull base reveals elevation of the anterior aspect of the posterior fossa. The foramen magnum is small. The odontoid process is in the plane of the petrous bone. *C.* Coronal plane computed tomography through the odontoid process shows the marked elevation of the occipital condyles and upper cervical spine. *D.* Midsagittal magnetic resonance imaging of the head and cervical canal demonstrates severe basilar invagination and rostral displacement of the diencephalon and brain stem.

tween the atlas and axis in childhood. The instability causes progressive proliferation of granulation tissue.[108, 189] Remodeling of the inferior surface of the foramen magnum leads to bony indentation between the assimilated atlas and the superior facets of the axis, which are in an abnormal position; this results in an irreducible state. The odontoid invagination, combined with the abnormal clivus, leads to progressive neural compromise. Children become symptomatic at adolescence (Fig. 42–17).

Acute trauma, as with flexion-extension injuries, and chronic trauma, as with the carrying of loads on the head in developing countries, have been implicated in precipitation of symptoms of atlantoaxial instability.[288] However, the stage is originally set by the developmental abnormality.

Irregular segmentation of the atlas or the axis may be associated with assimilation or unilateral fusion be-

tween the atlas and axis vertebrae. These fusions are rare and are associated with other abnormalities of the cervical spine as well as with abnormal distortion around the foramen magnum (Fig. 42–18).

ANOMALIES OF THE ODONTOID PROCESS

Aplasia

Aplasia or hypoplasia of the dens is a special form of dysplasia. This expresses itself in different degrees.* Rudimentary dens with excessive dysplasia that does not reach the upper edge of the anterior arch of the atlas may be associated with atlantoaxial instability.[99, 205]

---

*See references 65, 87, 102, 192, 195, and 233.

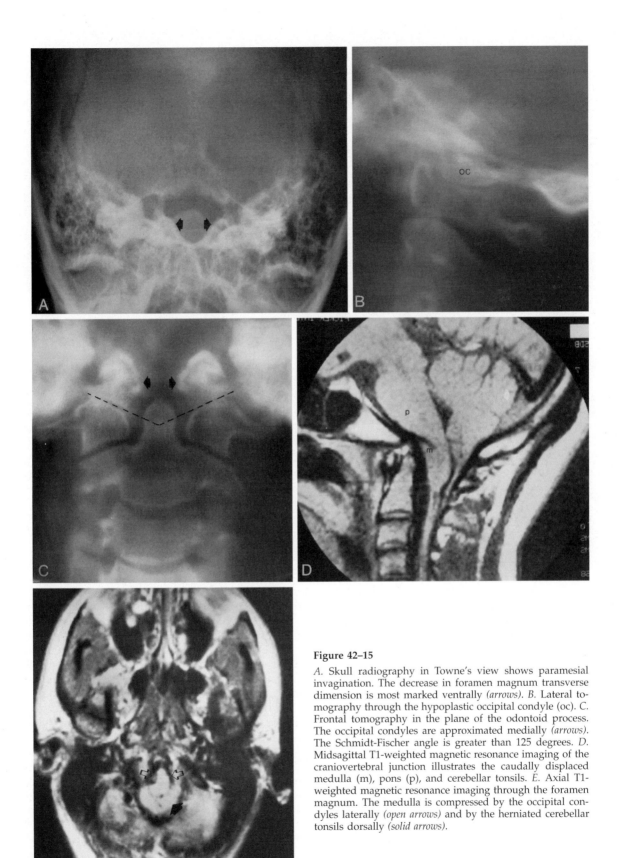

Figure 42–15

A. Skull radiography in Towne's view shows paramesial invagination. The decrease in foramen magnum transverse dimension is most marked ventrally *(arrows)*. *B.* Lateral tomography through the hypoplastic occipital condyle (oc). *C.* Frontal tomography in the plane of the odontoid process. The occipital condyles are approximated medially *(arrows)*. The Schmidt-Fischer angle is greater than 125 degrees. *D.* Midsagittal T1-weighted magnetic resonance imaging of the craniovertebral junction illustrates the caudally displaced medulla (m), pons (p), and cerebellar tonsils. *E.* Axial T1-weighted magnetic resonance imaging through the foramen magnum. The medulla is compressed by the occipital condyles laterally *(open arrows)* and by the herniated cerebellar tonsils dorsally *(solid arrows)*.

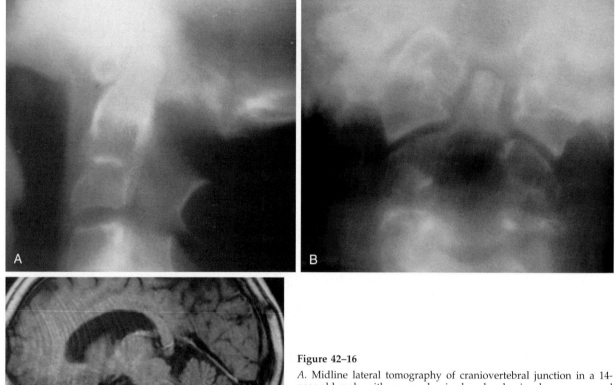

Figure 42–16

A. Midline lateral tomography of craniovertebral junction in a 14-year-old male with syncopal episodes, dysphagia, sleep apnea, and arm weakness. Notice the atlas assimilation and C2–C3 segmentation failure. *B.* Frontal tomography through the odontoid shows the lateral atlantal masses incorporated with the occipital condyles. *C.* T1-weighted midsagittal magnetic resonance imaging of the head and upper cervical spine shows atlas assimilation, abnormal clivus-odontoid articulation, near-horizontal clivus, and a small posterior fossa. The cerebellar tonsils extend below C2, and the pontine–medulla oblongata angle is 105 degrees.

Here the cruciate and alar ligaments are unable to contribute to the stabilization of the joint. Extensive hypoplasia may also be combined with congenital forms of os odontoideum that are very rare.[285] Significant vascular compromise on stretching and distortion of the vertebral artery may occur with odontoid dysplasias. A chronic atlantoaxial dislocation in this situation may result in the formation of granulation tissue at the site of the luxation, causing an hourglass constriction of the neural structures (Fig. 42–19).

Os Odontoideum

The term "os odontoideum" was coined by Giacomini in 1886.[96] This refers to an independent bone seen cranial to the axis in place of the dens. The bone is not an isolated dens but exists apart from a hypoplastic dens. Radiographically, the os odontoideum has rounded, smooth cortical borders that are separated by a variable gap from the small odontoid process.* It is

usually located in the position of the normal odontoid tip or near the base of the occiput in the area of foramen magnum, where it may fuse with the clivus. The gap between the free ossicle and the axis usually extends above the level of the superior facets of the axis. This leads to incompetence of the cruciate ligament and atlantoaxial instability.*

Two types of os odontoideum exist: dystopic and orthotopic.[285] In dystopic os odontoideum, the ossicle lies near the basion (inferior end of the clivus) and fuses with the occipital bone with time.[80] It moves in unison with the clivus (Fig. 42–20). The posterior arch of the atlas is always hypoplastic, and the anterior arch is hypertrophied. In contradistinction, the orthotopic variety has an ossicle that lies in the position of the normal dens and moves in unison with the atlas and axis vertebrae instead of with the clivus (Fig. 42–21).[186]

It may be difficult to differentiate an os odontoideum from a long-standing odontoid fracture by radiography. In traumatic nonunion, the gap between the frac-

---

*See references 9, 65, 68, 79, 108, 122, 125, 180, 181, 185, 252, 301, and 306.

*See references 16, 18, 54, 89, 113, and 260.

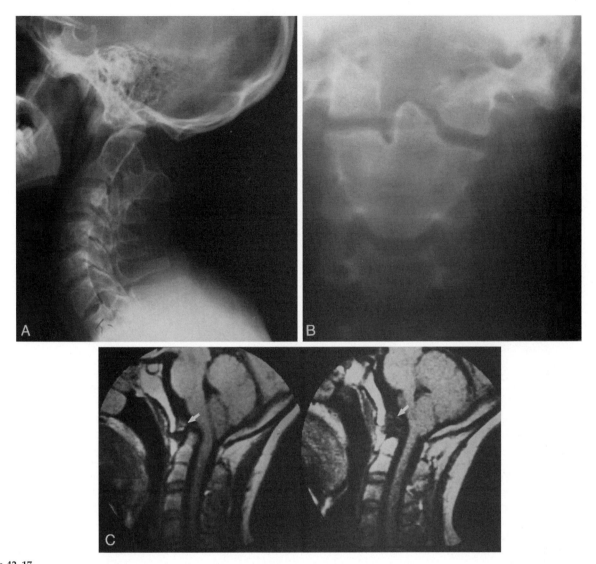

Figure 42–17

A. Lateral cervical spine roentgenography in a 16-year-old girl with excruciating neck pain and arm weakness. There is marked angulation at the atlantoaxial junction, and atlas assimilation is evident. *B.* Frontal tomography shows the lateral atlantal masses incorporated with the occiput. Segmentation failure of C2 and C3 is present. *C.* T1-weighted midsagittal and parasagittal magnetic resonance imaging of the craniocervical region with the use of a compatible halo traction device. Irreducible compression of the cervicomedullary junction is caused by the odontoid and granulation tissue *(white arrow).*

ture fragments is characteristically irregular and extends into the body of the axis, below the level of the superior facets of the axis. The bone fragments appear to match up, and no marginal cortex surrounds the lesion.

The cause of os odontoideum has been variably explained on embryological, traumatic, and vascular bases. The proponents of an embryological origin believe that failure of the dens fusion to the axis body is a causative factor.* The arguments against an embryological origin are best conceptualized by an understanding of the embryogenesis. In os odontoideum, there is invariably a gap of the dens attachment to the axis body, and a neurocentral synchondrosis is always seen. If the defect were indeed congenital, remnants

attached to the axis body would be absent, and the segmentation defect would extend into the axis body or be located caudal to the superior facets of the axis. Instead, the osseous defect is at or rostral to the level of the superior facets of the axis. A traumatic origin for os odontoideum has been well documented by several authors and was noted in more than one third of the present author's patients.* This evidence is based on radiological demonstration of a normal odontoid process in children before cervical trauma. After trauma, radiography demonstrated an os odontoideum. A history of cervical trauma was elicited by the author in one third of the patients with os odontoideum who were younger than 4 years of age. These children had been treated with either traction or immo-

---

*See references 100, 107, 188, 238, 251, 302, and 306.

*See references 78, 79, 87, 122, 128, 185, 190, 232, and 285.

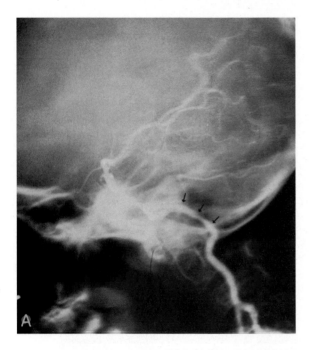

Figure 42–18

A. Lateral vertebral angiography in a 12-year-old girl with glossopharyngeal and vagus nerve dysfunction, downbeat nystagmus, quadriparesis, and Sprengel's deformity. The distal vertebral artery is irregular and dorsally displaced *(arrows).*

bilization for an odontoid fracture or atlantoaxial instability. Age is indirect evidence suggesting an acquired origin for the os odontoideum, based on the observation that the majority of patients with os odontoideum are adolescents or young adults. It is believed that after fracture or vascular compromise at the base of the odontoid process, a separation of the bone fragments may occur.[79, 122, 185] With time, the alar ligaments that are attached to the rostral odontoid process distract the separated bone fragments away from the axis toward the occiput. The intact blood supply to the os odontoideum through the apical arcade may explain the hypertrophy that is often present.

A traumatic or vascular origin is supported by the author's case of a 13-year-old girl who had a 6-month history of progressive quadriparesis. At 3 years of age, she was treated with immobilization of the cervical spine for atlantoaxial dislocation after injury (Fig. 42–22A). An intact odontoid process was seen on radiography. Roentgenography evaluation 10 years later showed that there was a dystopic os odontoideum where the ossicle had fused to the clivus (see Fig. 42–22B). Flexion and extension radiography demonstrated the instability of the craniovertebral junction (see Fig. 42–22C). The metrizamide contrast studies showed ventral compression of the cervicomedullary junction in flexion (see Fig. 42–22D).

The incidence of os odontoideum is increased in patients with Down's syndrome, spondyloepiphyseal dysplasia, or Morquio's syndrome and after upper respiratory tract infections.* The natural history of patients with os odontoideum suggests that these individuals have a potentially precarious existence. Minor trauma is commonly associated with the onset of symptoms that may vary from transitory paretic episodes to severe myelopathy. The poor results of opera-

tive intervention with an unstable craniovertebral junction secondary to os odontoideum have led authors to believe that the best course of treatment for patients without neurological deficit is watchful waiting and inactivity.[198, 265] The author disagrees with that opinion, as do others, if instability is present.[79, 122, 185]

The craniovertebral joint biomechanics in each individual situation must be thoroughly assessed before operation is undertaken in these patients.[188] A ventral decompression is necessary in those patients with irreducible os odontoideum with basilar invagination that is accompanied by chronic granulation tissue acting as a mass (Fig. 42–23). In 50 per cent of patients, the os odontoideum is not a causative factor of the ventral compression, but rather the dislocated axis body compresses the upper cervical cord. If ventral compression can be reduced in the flexed or extended position, a posterior fixation of the occiput to the upper cervical spine is essential. Placement of an odontoid screw through the axis body into the dystopic os odontoideum cannot be accepted; this procedure is fraught with danger because the cruciate ligament prevents satisfactory reduction.[112] In the orthotopic variety of os odontoideum, an atlantoaxial arthrodesis is the operation of choice.

The natural history of os odontoideum is one in which minor trauma is commonly associated with the onset of symptoms. Stabilization should be offered to all children with os odontoideum and abnormal biomechanics.

BASILAR IMPRESSION

Basilar impression is a consequence of bone softening secondary to diseases such as Paget's disease, osteomalacia, hyperparathyroidism, osteogenesis imper-

*See references 1, 2, 9, 18, 97, 152, 162, and 191.

Text continued on page 1061

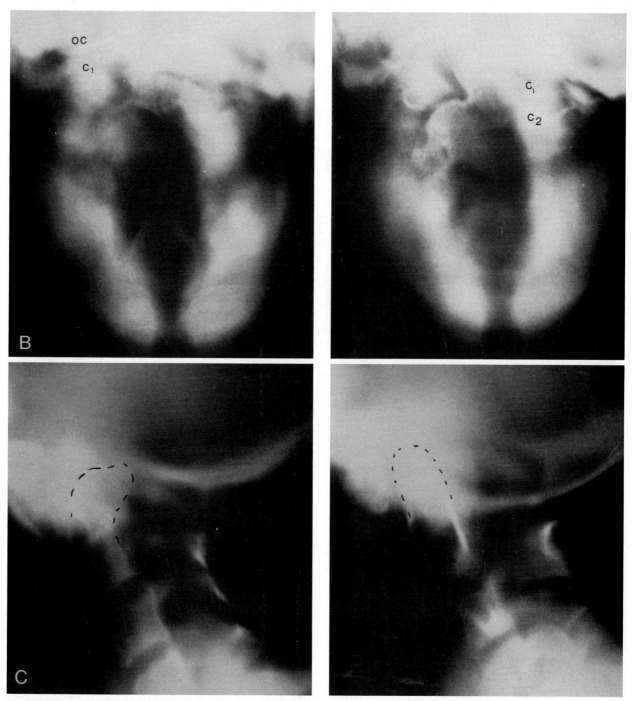

Figure 42-18 *Continued*

B. Frontal tomography images through the odontoid process show unilateral fusion of occipital bone (oc) and atlas (L) and atlantoaxial (C1–C2) fusion on the opposite side (R). *C.* Lateral midline and paramedian tomography images show the irregular, hooked, invaginated odontoid process in the foramen magnum.

Illustration continued on following page

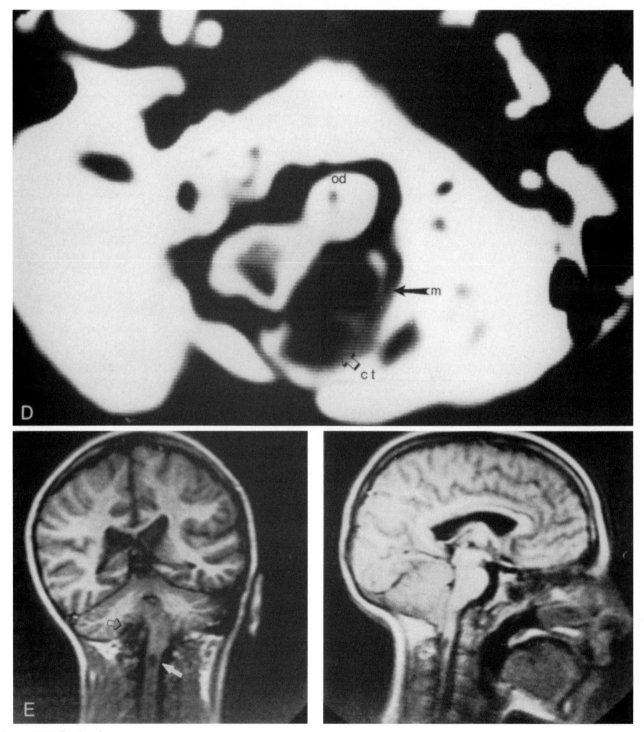

Figure 42-18 *Continued*

D. Metrizamide computed myelotomography in the axial plane of the foramen magnum. The odontoid process (od) and its base occupy the ventral half of the foramen magnum, displacing the caudal medulla (m) and cerebellar tonsils *(arrow,* ct). *E.* T1-weighted magnetic resonance images in the coronal plane (L) and midsagittal plane (R). The occipitoatlantal fusion indents the pontomedullary junction laterally *(open arrow)*. A syrinx cavity *(solid arrow)* and Chiari I malformation are seen.

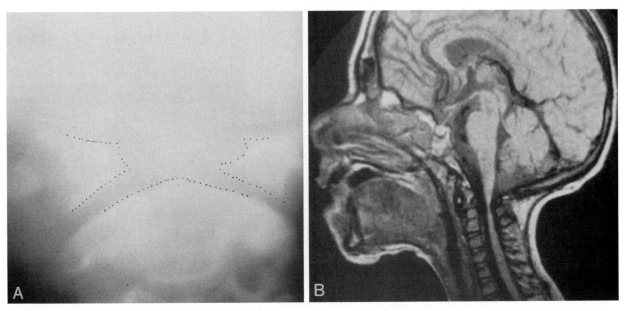

Figure 42–19

A. Frontal tomography of the upper cervical spine at the level of an absent dens. This 15-year-old girl was quadriplegic and on a ventilator. *B.* Midsagittal T1-weighted magnetic resonance imaging of the head and cervical spine demonstrates an hourglass constriction of the spinal cord at the level of the absent dens. The compression was caused by granulation tissue from chronic instability (found at operation).

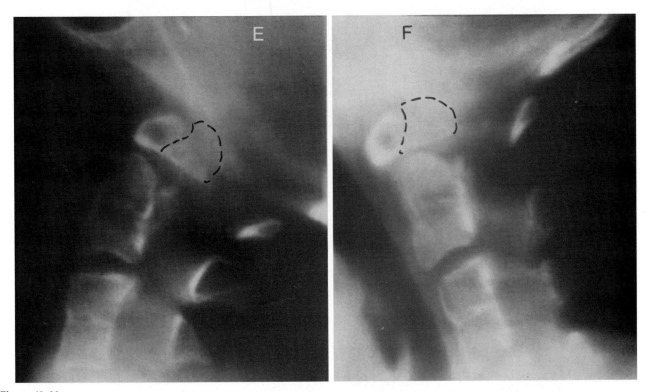

Figure 42–20

Lateral tomography of dystopic os odontoideum in extension (E) and in flexion (F) shows the varied dynamics of compromise of the spinal canal. The os moves in conjunction with the clivus and produces ventral cervicomedullary compression, which is maximal in extension, less severe in flexion.

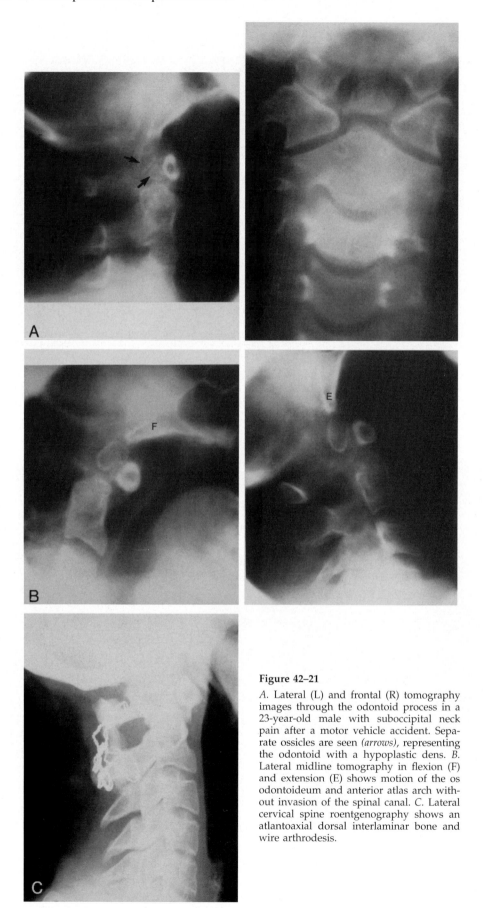

Figure 42–21

A. Lateral (L) and frontal (R) tomography images through the odontoid process in a 23-year-old male with suboccipital neck pain after a motor vehicle accident. Separate ossicles are seen *(arrows)*, representing the odontoid with a hypoplastic dens. *B.* Lateral midline tomography in flexion (F) and extension (E) shows motion of the os odontoideum and anterior atlas arch without invasion of the spinal canal. *C.* Lateral cervical spine roentgenography shows an atlantoaxial dorsal interlaminar bone and wire arthrodesis.

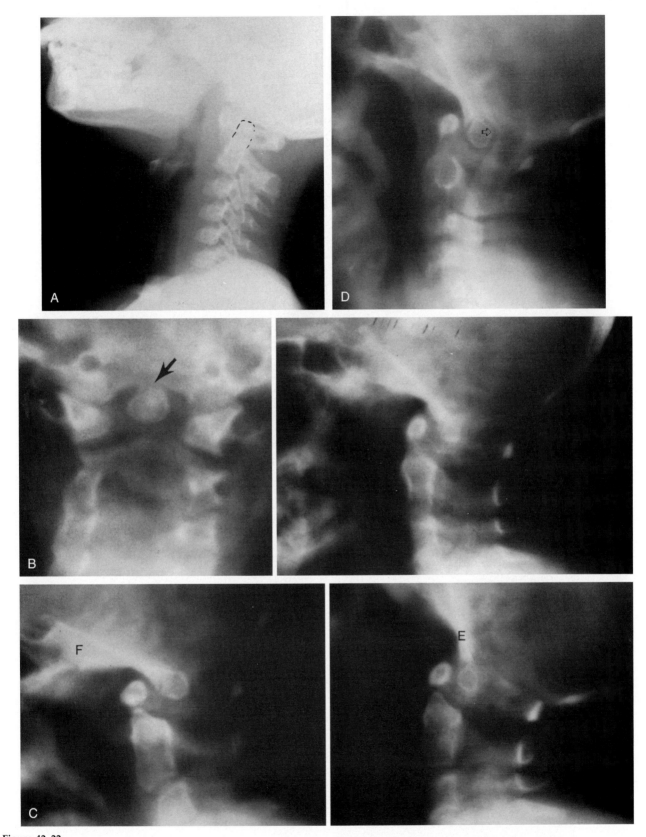

Figure 42–22

A. Lateral cervical spine radiography in a 3-year-old girl after neck trauma. The odontoid process is intact, and atlantoaxial instability is present. *B.* This child presented 10 years later with quadriparesis. Frontal (L) and lateral (R) tomography through the dystopic os odontoideum *(arrow)* show fusion of the ossicle to the basion. *C.* Flexion (F) and extension (E) tomography in the lateral projection through the dystopic os odontoideum show it to move with the clivus. The ventral alignment is best in extension. *D.* Lateral midline metrizamide myelotomography of the craniovertebral junction shows severe ventral indentation *(open arrow)* of the cervicomedullary junction by the dystopic os odontoideum in the neutral position.

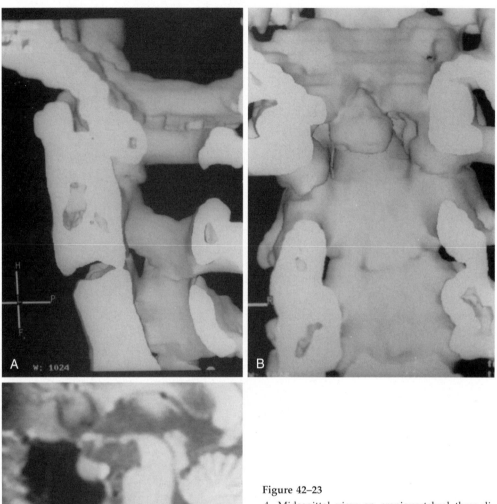

Figure 42–23

A. Midsagittal view on craniovertebral three-dimensional computed tomography in a 21-year-old woman. She had diminished gag response, episodic left arm and leg paresis, and spasticity in all limbs. The cruciate ligament was found to be in front of the os odontoideum at ventral decompression. *B.* Three-dimensional computed tomography shows the os odontoideum attached to the clivus and behind the hypoplastic dens. *C.* T1-weighted midsagittal magnetic resonance imaging shows the dystopic os odontoideum invaginating into the ventral medulla. Notice the Chiari I malformation.

fecta, renal rickets, and achondroplasia.* In an analysis of 210 patients with basilar invagination by Bares, 17 had basilar impression or secondary invagination.[14] Twenty-five cases of developmental stenosis of the cervical canal were associated with and further complicated by the basilar invagination. Fibrous bands and dural adhesions of the dorsal cervicomedullary junction were often present with basilar impression.

Paget's Disease

Paget's disease involving the craniovertebral junction results in basilar impression, as originally described by Wycis.[303] The foramen magnum tends to flatten and the anteroposterior diameter to diminish (Fig. 42–24). An axial invagination with cranial upward migration is the next progression, and it causes neural bony compression and changes in the cerebrospinal fluid dynamics.[36] It is not uncommon to see syringohydromyelia complicating distorted brain stem and cervical cord.[189]

The incidence of basilar impression with Paget's disease is high.[215] Twenty-seven of a series of 75 patients with Paget's disease reported by Poppel and co-workers had a significant degree of basilar impression.[222] The incidence was equal in males and females, and basilar impression usually became symptomatic after 40 years of age. Bull and associates discussed the radiological changes in 64 patients with Paget's disease, with emphasis on basilar impression.[36]

An important medical breakthrough has been the

*See references 37, 86, 88, 90, 120, 142, 165, 195, 235, 247, and 257.

successful treatment of Paget's disease with calcitonin and diphosphate.[49, 184] Although Paget's disease affects the middle-aged and elderly population, with a greater prevalence in the older age group, occasionally adolescents are seen with severe secondary basilar impression and pontomedullary dysfunction.

Osteogenesis Imperfecta

Osteogenesis imperfecta describes a group of inherited disorders characterized by excessive bone fragility with susceptibility to fracture.[291] This syndrome has been subdivided into osteogenesis imperfecta congenita, characterized by fractures at birth or during early infancy, and osteogenesis imperfecta tarda, in which the onset of fractures is in childhood. The fractures have been variously attributed to a decreased external volume of the bone itself, reduction in the tensile strength in each lamina, and deficiency in mineral and matrix content. Impingement of the spinal cord is usually secondary to vertebral column collapse and severe kyphosis and kyphoscoliosis. Platybasia becomes evident, with flattening of the vertex and prominence of the occiput leading to the term "tam-o'-shanter head."[120] These changes result in an abnormal configuration of the brain stem and in severe cases may result in an acute flexion angulation between midbrain and pons and also between pons and medulla (Fig. 42–25). A secondary aqueductal stenosis has been seen.[120, 224] The angulation of the superior cerebellar peduncles and the brachium conjunctivum leads to increased neurological deficit.[86, 221, 224, 263] Upper cervical cord compression as a cause of death in osteogenesis

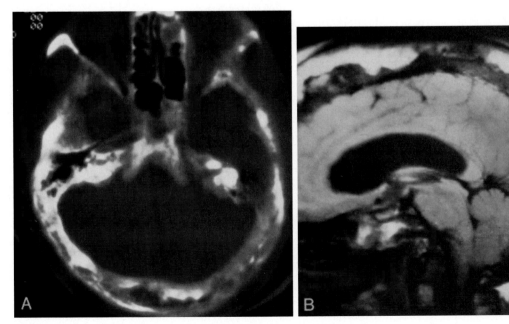

Figure 42–24

A. Axial computed tomography through the base of the skull viewed through bone windows. There is an irregular calvarial thickening with a "moth-eaten" appearance in this patient with Paget's disease. B. Midsagittal T1-weighted magnetic resonance imaging of the head reveals the significant elevation of the anterior portion of the posterior fossa bony structures with odontoid invagination. The aqueduct is markedly compressed, as is the third ventricle, with lateral ventricular enlargement. The medulla is distorted by the clivus-odontoid complex. Notice the high signal intensity in the calvaria and bone expansion.

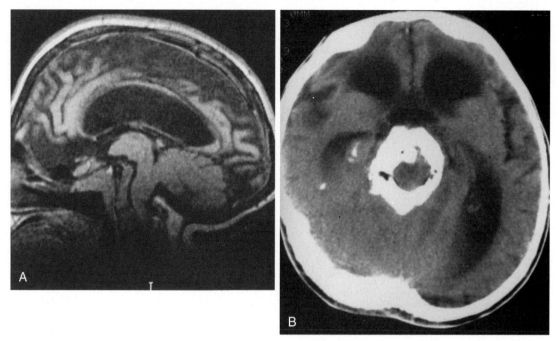

Figure 42–25

A. T1-weighted midsagittal magnetic resonance imaging of the head in a 13-year-old child with osteogenesis imperfecta. Difficulty in swallowing and progressive quadriparesis were the presenting symptoms. Notice the small, elongated posterior fossa, the upward position of the atlas and axis body, the severe basilar impression, and the acute angle of the pontine medullary flexure. Secondary aqueductal stenosis has led to hydrocephalus. *B.* Axial computed tomography scan of the head through the level of the foramen of Monro. Notice the hydrocephalus and presence of the axis vertebra in this plane, reflecting the extreme invagination.

imperfecta has been documented by several authors.[218] A variety of systemic treatments have been undertaken, including vitamin D, calcitonin, fluoride, and hormones.[95] Osteogenesis imperfecta remains the most serious form of the lethal short-limbed dwarfisms and crippling skeletal dysplasias.

Suboccipital decompression, as described by Hunt and Dekaban in 1982, grants only temporary respite, with subsequent full-blown brain stem dysfunction and death.[134] In such situations, it is imperative that a ventral decompression be accomplished first.[120] This is extremely difficult by the transoral or transpharyngeal route and requires either a transpalatal approach or a LeForte I drop-down maxillotomy. Posterior decompression and occipitocervical fixation are mandatory. The author has conducted a follow-up of patients with osteogenesis imperfecta as they developed cranial settling. The secondary invagination has been arrested with aggressive occipitocervical bracing, leading to a regression of the neurological symptoms.

Achondroplasia

Achondroplasia is the most common form of short-limbed dwarfism.[67] Defects in the rate of enchondral ossification result in a variety of skeletal malformations, usually recognizable at birth. Achondroplasia is differentiated from pseudoachondroplasia and the other osteochondral dysplasias by the inheritance pattern, clinical presentation, and distinct radiological features. Generalized spinal stenosis with spinal cord compression occurs and often requires surgical decom-

pression.[66, 236, 256, 266] Abnormalities in the formation of the basiocciput, the exoccipital bone, and the craniovertebral junction can result in foramen magnum stenosis and cervicomedullary compression.[114] These patients may present with severe respiratory compromise and myelopathy.[8, 41, 47]

The prevalence of achondroplasia has been estimated at 0.03 to 0.05 per cent of live births.[200] In familial cases, the mode of inheritance is autosomal dominance; however, the majority of cases appear to present a new mutation. Murdock and colleagues reported on 148 patients, of whom 31 had one or both parents affected and 117 had no family history of achondroplasia.[200] If both parents are affected, the patient is said to have homozygous achondroplasia, and such patients exhibit a high incidence of death in their first year. Persons with heterozygous achondroplasia have a better chance of survival and make up a majority of reported cases. Patients with achondroplasia who survive the first year have a good chance of continuing in good health.[124, 165] Mental development is usually normal, although growth is slow and ceases early, with an average height of 129 cm in males and 122 cm in females.

Diagnostic morphological features of achondroplasia are manifested at birth. Shortened limbs, large trunk and head, frontal bossing, midfacial recession with coarse facial features, and exaggerated lumbar lordosis are common manifestations. The neurological manifestations of achondroplasia are related to the abnormalities of the cranial base, compression of the neurovascular structures, and hydrocephalus. Enchondral bone formation in the cranial base leads to a shortened basicranium, shallow posterior fossa, shortened clivus, and abnormal basal spinal relationships. Foramen magnum stenosis is common and results from a combination of defective enchondral bone growth and abnormal placement and premature fusion of the basal synchondrosis.[258] Reported neurological symptoms include quadriparesis, paraparesis, feeding problems, poor head control, hypotonia, dysphagia, and delayed motor developmental milestones. Respiratory difficulties, including apneic spells and cyanosis, are common. Patients may later present with occipitocervical pain and myelopathy with incontinence, ataxia, spasticity, and hyperreflexia.

The reported radiological abnormalities of the cervicomedullary region in patients with achondroplasia include foramen magnum stenosis with paramesial invagination, a teardrop shape to the foramen magnum,

and obliteration of the subarachnoid spaces.[142, 236, 245] Ventral and dorsal cervicomedullary compression is associated with indentation of the pons by the basilar invagination and dorsal compression by the thickened exoccipital bone and the posterior arch of C1 (Fig. 42–26A through C). There is an abnormal, high position of the basilar artery and the shortened clivus.

Respiratory compromise is usually caused by brain stem compression but may be secondary to upper airway obstruction or chest wall deformities.[239, 272] Decompression of the posterior fossa and the treatment of compression of the cervicomedullary junction in achondroplasia have met with success and must address the removal of the constricting bony elements.[185, 248] The bone components that require resection may include the posterior rim of the foramen magnum, the surrounding occipital bone, and the dorsal bony elements

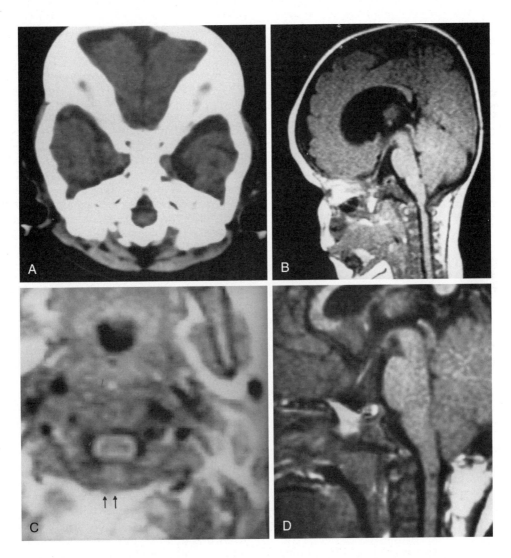

Figure 42–26

A. Axial computed tomography through the plane of the foramen magnum in a 22-month-old child with achondroplasia. Notice the pear-shaped stenotic opening. The patient had previously been shunted for hydrocephalus. She held her head flexed and was moderately quadriparetic with sleep apnea. *B.* T1-weighted midsagittal magnetic resonance imaging of the head and neck. Notice the dorsal cervicomedullary compression. *C.* T1-weighted axial magnetic resonance imaging through the atlas vertebra. Notice the lack of cerebrospinal fluid and dorsal indentation by the thickened, inwardly bent atlas arch *(arrows)*. *D.* T1-weighted midsagittal magnetic resonance imaging of the cervicomedullary region made 3 months after decompression of the dorsal foramen magnum and atlas with duraplasty. The neurological examination was normal.

of C1 and C2. The lateral margins of the decompression must extend to the medial aspect of the occipital condyles bilaterally. The dura must be opened and replaced so as not to have new bone formation, which would re-exaggerate the tight stenosis (see Fig. 42–26D).

Ventriculomegaly is seen in the majority of achondroplasia patients, and symptomatic hydrocephalus may occur in 15 to 50 per cent of these patients.[60, 236] Enlargement of the ventricular system may be caused by venous congestion secondary to stenosis of the jugular foramen, distortion of the brain stem with the obstruction of the basilar cisterns, or obstruction of the foramina of Luschka and Magendie as a result of foramen magnum stenosis. Ventricular shunting is usually reserved for demonstrated symptomatic hydrocephalus in patients with achondroplasia, because the ventriculomegaly usually arrests with time. Attention has been drawn to the inward indentation of the posterior arch of C1, which further adds to cervicomedullary compression, including the thickened fibrous epidural bands. These require resection at the time of posterior fossa decompression before duraplasty.

Renal Rickets

Softening of bone from the metabolic effects of renal rickets and, in some cases, the malabsorption syndrome usually occurs in the first 2 years of life.[185, 283] The bone changes of rickets are known to "heal" and may erroneously suggest that basilar invagination with rickets is congenital rather than developmental. Stenosis of the high cervical canal is associated with this disease.

SPECIFIC CONDITIONS

Down's Syndrome

Down published the first comprehensive review of the syndrome that subsequently bore his name in 1866.[190] The easily recognized features of Down's syndrome are the characteristic facial features, hypotonia, mental retardation, ligamentous laxity, and transverse palmar creases. Almost every organ is involved. This syndrome is the most commonly recognizable chromosomal abnormality in humans, the incidence being 1 in 700 live births.[225, 226, 268] Craniovertebral instability in Down's syndrome has received increasing interest since the 1961 report by Spitzer and colleagues of occipitoatlantal dislocation in nine of 26 patients investigated with Down's syndrome.[268] However, atlantoaxial instability in Down's syndrome has been described for the most part after the initial publication by Tishler and Martelle in 1965.[282]

Interest in the cause of ligamentous laxity, radiological assessment, and the natural history of atlantoaxial and occipitoatlantal instability in Down's syndrome led to the realization that atlantoaxial instability occurs in approximately 14 to 24 per cent of patients, although the prevalence of symptomatic atlantoaxial instability is believed to be less than 1 per cent.[82, 133, 175, 226] The

prevalence of bony anomalies such as os odontoideum, hypoplastic odontoid process, ossiculum terminale, and rotatory atlantoaxial luxation in patients with Down's syndrome has caused some concern regarding participation of these children in Special Olympics. The Committee on Sports Medicine of the American Academy of Pediatrics recommended, in 1984, that an operative stabilization of the cervical spine should be considered if the atlantodental space is greater than 4.5 mm.[5] Subsequently, several series reporting the incidence of atlantoaxial instability and the lack of attendant neurological signs and symptoms have, unfortunately, resulted in the belief that these children do not need treatment. Pessimistic reports on the outcome of arthrodesis of the cervical spine in patients with Down's syndrome have also added to this misconception.[190]

To determine the natural history of atlantoaxial instability, Burke and co-workers studied 32 individuals with Down's syndrome, only one of whom showed atlantoaxial instability initially.[37] However, at follow-up 13 years later, seven patients had developed a predental space of more than 5 mm. Two patients underwent atlantoaxial arthrodesis, and one succumbed to the disease before treatment. These researchers concluded that atlantoaxial instability is chronic and progressive, requiring serial examinations. Three of the 32 individuals in this study developed an acquired odontoid abnormality of os odontoideum. Review of the initial radiography results showed that these abnormalities were not present in 1970, providing further evidence that os odontoideum is a developmental phenomenon rather than a congenital one.

In 1985, Braakhakke and colleagues reviewed the literature on patients with symptomatic Down's syndrome presenting with myelopathy secondary to atlantoaxial instability.[28] They found that, of 20 patients described in detail, 9 had an odontoid abnormality consisting of hypoplasia or os odontoideum. Special attention should therefore be given to os odontoideum in Down's syndrome. It appears that these children suffer repeated minor trauma, which may lead to unsuspected fractures of the odontoid with secondary pull of the alar and apical ligaments.[79, 185] The superior segment receives its blood supply from the occipital artery and the apical arcade. The cruciate ligament then becomes grossly incompetent, which leads to atlantoaxial dislocation, possibly with further migration of the odontoid process into the foramen magnum and ventral cervicomedullary compression. However, os odontoideum is seen in only a few patients with Down's syndrome.

In the author's experience between 1979 and 1993, 23 symptomatic patients with Down's syndrome and cervicomedullary compromise were encountered.[190] A fixed atlantoaxial luxation was seen in 10 patients, of whom 6 developed a precipitous onset of cervicomedullary compression. Occipitoatlantal instability was present in 13, and an associated rotatory luxation was present in 10. The average predental space was 8 mm in the neutral position in 20 individuals. Two adolescents had previously undergone atlantoaxial dorsal fusion, with subsequent progressive basilar invagination caused by unrecognized occipitoatlantal instability. Os odontoideum was seen in 4 of the 23 individuals. An irreducible invagination was present in 4 patients and was treated with anterior decompression followed by dorsal occipitocervical fixation. The occipitocervical fixation was used in a total of 13 individuals (Fig. 42–27). Atlantoaxial dorsal fusion was performed in 10, and 2 patients with acute rotatory luxation of C1 and C2 were treated with immobilization alone. Halo immobilization in two individuals after dorsal occipitocervical fixation induced anterior fusion at the craniocervical complex, indicating active vertebral ligamentous pathology. The results of stabilization have been excellent. The techniques of occipitocervical fusion and atlantoaxial fixation are described elsewhere in this chapter. Bilateral intralaminar fusion is accomplished with the use of full-thickness rib graft as donor bone, individually secured to the lateral portions of the lamina of C1 and C2 by transfixation of the donor bone graft with sublaminar cables; this technique allows for spacing and prevention of flexion, extension, and lateral rotation. An upward extension of this procedure anchors the occipital squama if an occipitocervical fixation is mandated.

Special mention should be made of the immune system in Down's syndrome patients.[160, 249] Immune system dysfunction has been implicated in the increased prevalence of respiratory infections and of acute lymphocytic leukemia. Studies of the polymorphonuclear phagocytic systems of patients who have Down's syndrome have shown impaired monocyte and neutrophil chemotaxis and a decreased ability to undergo phagocytosis. The T-cell–dependent limb of the immune system has also been shown to have quantitative and qualitative deficiencies, with decrease in the number of T-lymphocytes. The functional capacity of the lymphocytes is also diminished by decreased synthesis of lymphokines and of the secretory products of these cells. These products may affect the initial inflammatory stage of bone graft incorporation. The ultimate result is that the patient's ability to mount an effective inflammatory host response is impaired, and this impairment ultimately affects the incorporation of the bone graft. This may be the reason that these individuals have a high failure rate in some series, especially during the phasic period, during which their immune systems are at a low point.[249]

From review of the literature and the author's experience, cranial settling, reducible basilar invagination, and anterioposterior or lateral cranial dislocation of the spine in Down's syndrome individuals are indications for occipitocervical fusion. Atlantoaxial fusion is performed in individuals in whom the instability is limited to the atlas and axis vertebrae. Failure to maintain proper immobilization results in resorption of the bone grafts, progressive dislocation, and nonunion.

Mucopolysaccharidosis

The mucopolysaccharidoses are primary metabolic abnormalities of complex carbohydrate metabolism.

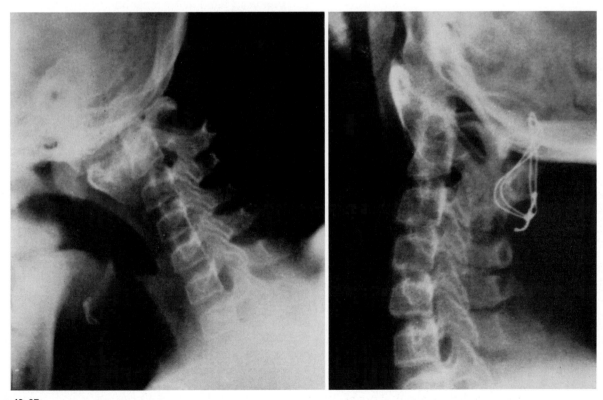

Figure 42–27

Preoperative *(left)* and postoperative *(right)* lateral cervical roentgenography in a 9-year-old girl with Down's syndrome. An occipitoatlantoaxial instability is present preoperatively but is reduced in the postoperative study. Wire and bone occipitoatlantoaxial dorsal arthrodesis is seen *(right)*.

These are inherited storage diseases manifested by mental retardation, macrocephaly, clouded cornea, skeletal dysplasia, and dwarfism. Generalized laxity is thought to contribute to the atlantoaxial luxation described in a variety of mucopolysaccharidoses. In 1969, Blaw and Langer reported on eight patients with Brailsford-Morquio disease who had undergone neurological follow-up.[24] All eight had radiological evidence of absence of the odontoid process or hypoplasia and a thoracic gibbus deformity. Four of these patients had evidence of cervical cord compression secondary to atlantoaxial dislocation, which commonly occurs in Morquio's syndrome by 7 years of age. This is secondary to cervical myelopathy as well as the effects of chest constriction on the respiratory system and resultant hypoxia. The failure of development of the dens may be a cause for spastic quadriparesis in Hurler's syndrome.[32]

Patients with type VI mucopolysaccharidosis (Maroteaux-Lamy syndrome) with high cervical myelopathy have also been described.[18, 132, 221, 289] The anesthesia complications obviously are great, because a number of these children require general anesthesia for numerous surgical procedures. A bright star on the horizon is the current success with bone marrow transplantation, which has been recognized as the treatment of choice for mucopolysaccharidosis, particularly Hurler's syndrome. Eight affected individuals have undergone therapy at the author's parent institution, with regression in the facial and organ abnormalities and improvement in the craniocervical anatomy.

BONE DYSPLASIAS

Skeletal dysplasias are divided into five categories based on the international nomenclature of constitutional diseases of bone: osteochondral dysplasias, dysostoses, idiopathic osteolyses, chromosomal aberrations, and primary metabolic abnormalities.[66, 67, 124] Osteochondral dysplasia and dysostosis account for the largest and most complex entities. Each category is further subdivided into numerous subcategories and individual diagnoses. Osteochondral dysplasias are defined as abnormalities of cartilage or bone. This category includes achondrogenesis, thanatophoric dysplasia, chondrodysplasia punctata, achondroplasia, dystrophic dysplasia, spondyloepiphyseal dysplasia, and multiple epiphyseal dysplasias.[236, 304]

The dysostoses are defined as malformations of individual bones or combinations of bones. Carpenter's syndrome, Crouzon's syndrome, and Apert's syndrome, Klippel-Feil syndrome, and Sprengel's deformity all fall in this category. Idiopathic osteolyses include spondyloepiphyseal dysplasia tarda, fibrous dysplasia, neurofibromatosis, osteogenesis imperfecta, and the multicentric forms such as Hajdu-Cheney syndrome.*

Primary metabolic and chromosomal abnormalities are numerous.[17, 254, 278] The metabolic abnormalities include problems with phosphorus and metabolism, such as rickets and pseudohypoparathyroidism. Abnormalities of calcium and phosphorus metabolism lead to bone softening and a secondary form of invagination. This may be paramesial, which is common with achondroplasia, or it may be caused by an upward inbending of the exoccipital bone, forming a shelf. Atlantoaxial instability is much more common (Fig. 42–28).

INFLAMMATORY CONDITIONS

Grisel's Syndrome

Grisel's syndrome is defined as a spontaneous subluxation of the atlantoaxial joint secondary to parapharyngeal infection.[109, 126, 274] The pathology of inflammatory subluxation seen in this syndrome has been ascribed to metastatic inflammation that causes ligamentous stretching and subluxation, muscle spasm, and regional hyperemia with decalcification of ligamentous structures.[161, 262, 295] More recently, Parke and colleagues described a parapharyngeal-paravertebral venous complex that could provide a direct hematogenous route for inflammatory exudates to access the atlantoaxial articulations.[217] These draining venous complexes allow communication of the posterior-superior nasopharynx and the lateral pharyngeal recesses with the venous plexuses around the odontoid process and in the upper cervical epidural sinuses.

In the author's experience, Grisel's syndrome has been associated with tonsillitis, mastoiditis, retropharyngeal abscess, otitis media, and infected apical tooth abscesses. A review of the literature shows that the majority of patients affected are children younger than 12 years of age. This may be explained by the greater ligamentous laxity and the vascularity of the atlas in the pediatric population.

In 1987, Wilson and co-workers reviewed 62 cases of nontraumatic subluxation of the atlantoaxial articulation that fulfilled the otolaryngological criteria for Grisel's syndrome.[298] This included 14 children who developed subluxation after surgical procedures for tonsillectomy, adenoidectomy, mastoiditis, and the resection of a pharyngeal rhabdomyosarcoma. Twelve children had symptoms of pharyngitis or cervical adenitis, seven had tonsillitis, and seven harbored cervical abscesses. There were five children with acute rheumatic fever and four with acute mastoiditis. Several patients were assigned the diagnosis of nonspecific parapharyngeal infection. The neurological deficit ranged from paresthesias to quadriplegia, suggesting compression of the cervicomedullary junction or arterial compromise.

The anatomical types of dislocation may be divided into atlantoaxial dislocations, which may be in the anterior, posterior, or transverse rotary direction, and occipitoatlantoaxial dislocations. In the latter, a vertical migration of the odontoid process may occur with cranial settling or a forward-to-backward sliding relationship between the affected vertebrae, or both.[283] Torticollis and an abnormal head position are the most

---

*See references 115, 124, 263, 266, 269, 270, and 278.

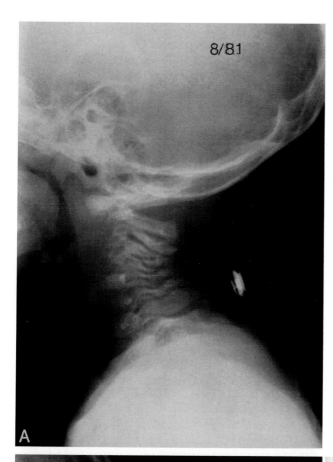

Figure 42–28

A. Lateral cervical spine radiography in a 2-year-old boy with fetal warfarin syndrome who presented with sudden paraparesis. Atlantoaxial instability is present, and there is a "ragged" appearance to the vertebral bodies, several of which are not visualized. *B.* Lateral flexion *(left, F)* and extension *(right, E)* radiography of the cervical spine shows the reducible atlantoaxial instability and development of vertebral bodies 5 years later. A dorsal C1–C2–C3 arthrodesis was performed.

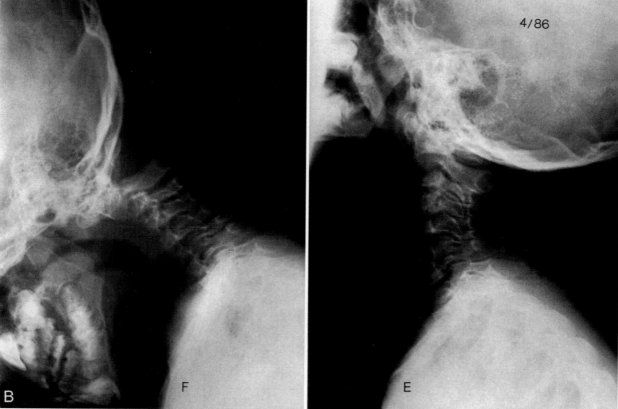

common presenting symptoms, which also include pain and tenderness in the upper cervical region that are aggravated by motion.[61, 206] The severe subluxations may produce symptoms and signs of cervical cord compression.[108]

The sedimentation rate is invariably elevated when this syndrome is associated with infection. Lateral cervical radiography demonstrates the dislocation, the presence of cervical spasm, and, at times, prevertebral soft tissue masses. It is important to define any evidence of osteomyelitis or bone erosion by the appropriate examinations. Needle biopsy of prevertebral masses is essential to confirm the presence of a pyogenic focus and to obtain specimens for bacterial culture. Appropriate antibiotics must be administered as early as possible for treatment of the primary infection. Reduction of dislocation by manipulation with skeletal traction is reserved only for the gross dislocations. Otherwise, immobilization in a Philadelphia collar or a sterno-occipital mandibular immobilizer brace is sufficient. However, in occipitocervical dislocations, halo immobilization is essential. The source of the infection must be treated. It is only rarely necessary to perform fusion.

Rheumatoid Arthritis

Rheumatoid arthritis is a chronic relapsing inflammatory arthritis, usually affecting multiple diarthrodial joints, with a varying degree of systemic involvement. Joints, articular tissues, serosae, and the eyes are commonly affected, but the spectrum of organ damage may be vast, particularly if vasculitis develops in the late stage.[308] Rheumatoid arthritis of the cervical spine was first described as a clinical entity by Garrod in 1890.[93] In his series of 500 patients, 178 had involvement of the cervical spine. According to Conlon, Isdale, and Rose, if lateral radiography were performed, 6 to 7 per cent of the general population would be found to be affected.[48] According to Sharp and Purser, rheumatoid involvement of the cervical spine occurs in 80 to 88 per cent of individuals.[253] The activity of rheumatoid arthritis in the cervical spine appears to begin early in the disease and progresses in relation to the peripheral involvement.[148] In the initial studies by Conlon and coworkers, it was believed that involvement of the cervical spine did not cause neurological deficits. This led to the common erroneous belief that treatment of rheumatoid involvement of the craniovertebral junction should be one of watchful expectancy. It was left to Matthews in 1974 to look at the same cohort of patients with rheumatoid arthritis published by Conlon, Isdale, and Rose.[177] Of the initial 74 patients, only 52 were left for evaluation after 5 years; several had expired. The prevalence of progressive atlantoaxial subluxation among the remaining patients was 25 per cent, and cranial settling was present in 18 per cent.

In studying the natural history of rheumatoid arthritis and the craniovertebral junction, Winfield and associates evaluated 100 patients with rheumatoid arthritis diagnosed within 1 year of onset.[299] On 5-year follow-up, 12 patients had experienced atlantoaxial subluxation of more than 7 mm, and a subaxial subluxation had occurred in 20. In three individuals, vertical subluxation had occurred. Pellicci and colleagues studied patients with rheumatoid arthritis during a 5-year period.[219] Mortality was 17 per cent, compared with 9 per cent for the same age group without rheumatoid disease. During the study period, subluxation was worsened in 80 per cent, and new subluxations occurred in 27 per cent. In the postmortem study of 104 patients with rheumatoid arthritis, Mikulowski and coworkers found atlantoaxial dislocation with cervicomedullary compression in 11.[196] Myelomalacia was present in two individuals, and cerebral vertebral artery vascular complications of the dislocation had occurred in three others.

It is important for the clinician to appreciate the potential severity of this disease and to plan therapy accordingly. It has now been confirmed that, once cervical myelopathy is established, mortality is common. Marks and Sharp in 1981 studied 31 patients with rheumatoid arthritis and cervical myelopathy.[171] Nineteen died within 6 months of presentation. All 19 were untreated or treated with a cervical collar. Only fusion provided a chance of survival in the remainder. It is essential for the treating physician to examine the natural history of cervical rheumatoid disease to determine the likelihood of neurological deterioration or death.[59, 63] This information underlies a decision as to whether surgical intervention is necessary and effective.[194, 241]

Pathogenesis

The peak incidence of rheumatoid arthritis is in the fourth through the sixth decades. Females outnumber males by a ratio of two to one.[307] Although the cause is unknown, it has been postulated that rheumatoid arthritis develops after an environmental exposure, such as an infection, in genetically predisposed individuals.[259] Rheumatoid arthritis is associated with the class II histocompatibility antigen HLA-DR4.[51]

Although the inciting cause of inflammation in rheumatoid arthritis is unknown, the inflammatory process itself is well described. Initially, lymphocytes proliferate in the synovium, and polymorphonuclear leukocytes predominate in the synovial fluid. The leukocytes release hydrolytic enzymes, oxygen radicals, and arachidonic acid metabolites that produce inflammation and cause tissue damage. Lymphokinens, produced by mononuclear cells, stimulate antibody production and the release of additional degradation products. Influx of fluid and the varied inflammatory mediators produce the erythema and swelling, characteristic of rheumatoid synovitis.[11, 307] Rheumatoid pannus then forms in the inflamed joint from proliferating fibroblasts and inflammatory cells, and this is actually granulation tissue.[12] This pannus produces collagenase and other proteolytic enzymes capable of destroying adjacent cartilage, tendons, and bone. Tendon ruptures, ligamentous laxity, loss of cartilage, and bone erosion follow. In general, joints that ultimately develop severe destruction become symptomatic within the first year of the disease onset.

The clinical manifestations of rheumatoid arthritis include constitutional symptoms, arthritis, and, in a few individuals, extra-articular involvement.[7, 135] Fatigue is common and may be disabling. Acute inflammatory arthritis is usually accompanied by early morning stiffness. Extra-articular manifestations are myriad and usually occur in patients with more severe arthritis and high titers of rheumatoid factor. Pericarditis is common and usually asymptomatic; myocarditis and coronary vasculitis are rare. Pulmonary manifestations of rheumatoid arthritis include pulmonary nodules, rheumatoid fibrosis, pleural effusions, and involvement of the upper airway so as to have floppy arytenoid cartilages. Ocular involvement includes keratoconjunctivitis, scleritis, and episcleritis.

The cervical spine is among the most common sites affected because of the large number of synovial joints present.[11, 22, 25, 48, 147] There is a predilection for involvement of the craniocervical junction.[293, 300] Lesions from the joints of Luschka extend into the disc spaces and into the vertebral bodies, but without osteophytosis; this is pathognomonic of the rheumatoid process, in contradistinction to osteoarthritis. Movement is therefore retained, and subluxations are common. However, in children, growth is deficient, and apophyseal joints tend to fuse, causing limitation of neck motion.

Atlantoaxial subluxation is initiated by loss of tensile strength and stretching of the transverse ligament caused by destructive inflammatory changes from the rheumatoid process as well as secondary degenerative changes in the tissues from vasculitis. Similar changes occur in the anterior and posterior synovial joints of the odontoid process and in the lateral atlantoaxial and occipitoatlantal joints. This chronic inflammatory process results in erosive changes in the adjacent bone and formation of granulation tissue in synovial joints. Bone changes in the odontoid process include loss of volume, osteoporosis, angulation of the softened bone, and occasional fractures. All these contribute to atlantoaxial dislocation. As previously mentioned, osteophyte formation does not occur in rheumatoid arthritis because of the deficient osteogenesis. Laxity of the transverse ligament results in an excessive dynamic loading of the lateral occipitoatlantal and atlantoaxial joints which have already been affected by the disease.[240] These changes result in a transverse rotatory luxation of the atlas and axis vertebrae.[117]

In addition to atlantoaxial dislocation, vertical penetration of the odontoid process into the foramen magnum or basilar impression may occur.* The invagination is secondary to loss of bone in the lateral mass of the atlas vertebra with subsequent rostral migration of the axis vertebra. The lateral atlantal mass may fracture, with lateral displacement to the bone fragment. Other destructive changes are severe. The occipital condyles may completely erode through the lateral masses of the atlas, separating and displacing them into an anterior and posterior component. The anterior

component telescopes caudally over the axis body, and the posterior component migrates upward.

In rheumatoid cranial settling, excessive proliferation of granulation tissue occurs, which, together with the invagination of the odontoid process, produces ventral cervicomedullary compression.[194] A thickened fibrous shell may envelop the odontoid process, through which bone spicules have been reported to penetrate into the tectorial membrane and subsequently become imbedded in the ventral aspect of the pons and medulla, which have been displaced dorsally. Occasionally, dural nodules and pachymeningitis may occur secondary to the rheumatoid process.

Radiological Findings

The radiological changes of rheumatoid arthritis closely reflect the latter stages of the pathological processes just described.[210] Between 1977 and 1994, 780 symptomatic patients with rheumatoid arthritis were evaluated by the author. They ranged in age from 10 to 82 years. Three categories of abnormalities were recognized from a radiological-pathological standpoint. Atlantoaxial instability was recognized in 366 patients, cranial settling in 387, and primary abnormality of rheumatoid granulation tissue in 27 individuals. The author has operated on 332 of these patients.

Atlantoaxial instability in adult patients with rheumatoid arthritis can be of great magnitude, although it may cause few symptoms. An anterior atlantoaxial instability was seen in 326 of 366 individuals, a posterior atlantoaxial instability in 3, and a primarily rotatory luxation in 37. In most patients, reduction was possible with traction and adjustments in alignment, except if tough pannus or a complex lateral or rotary component was present. Patients with long-standing reducible instability of more than 8 mm excursion developed large pannuses (Fig. 42–29).

The radiological changes associated with cranial settling consist of erosion with compression of the lateral atlantal masses, downward separation of the anterior arch of the atlas from the clivus so that the anterior atlas arch descends onto the axis body, and displacement of the posterior arch of the atlas rostrally and ventrally, which causes a decrease in the anteroposterior diameter of the spinal canal (Fig. 42–30).[194] As a result, the dens penetrates into the foramen magnum. In severe cases, the occipital condyles seem to descend onto the axis body slopes, with further erosion of the lateral masses of the atlas, completing the picture of rheumatoid "basilar invagination" (Fig. 42–31).

Based on flexion and extension lateral radiography, there was evidence of atlantoaxial instability in all individuals with cranial settling in the author's series. The odontoid process had penetrated through the foramen magnum into the posterior fossa in varying degrees, ranging from 6 mm to 33 mm. An acceptable reduction was not achieved, despite prolonged traction, if the odontoid process had penetrated more than 15 mm above the foramen magnum or if the pannus was large, the odontoid process had fractured, or the odontoid had reached an intra-arachnoid location (Fig. 42–32).

---

*See references 25, 26, 45, 50, 73, 178, and 275.

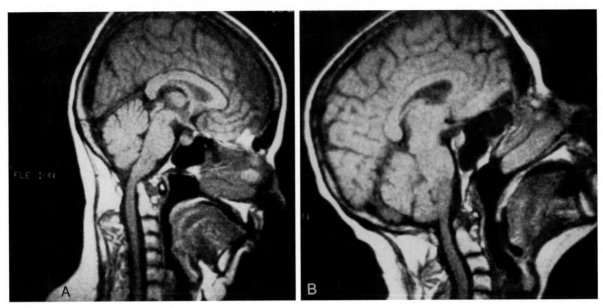

Figure 42–29

T1-weighted midsagittal magnetic resonance imaging of the head and neck in the flexed (A) and extended positions (B). This 52-year-old patient with rheumatoid arthritis had occipital headaches and neck pain. Notice the reducible atlantoaxial dislocation in the extended position.

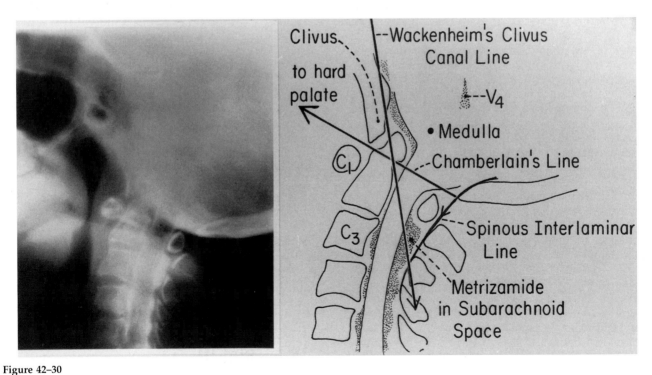

Figure 42–30

Lateral metrizamide myelotomography of the craniovertebral junction in a 48-year-old patient with rheumatoid arthritis shows cranial settling with basilar impression and a ventral position of the posterior atlantal arch. Both dorsal and ventral compression of the cervicomedullary junction are present.

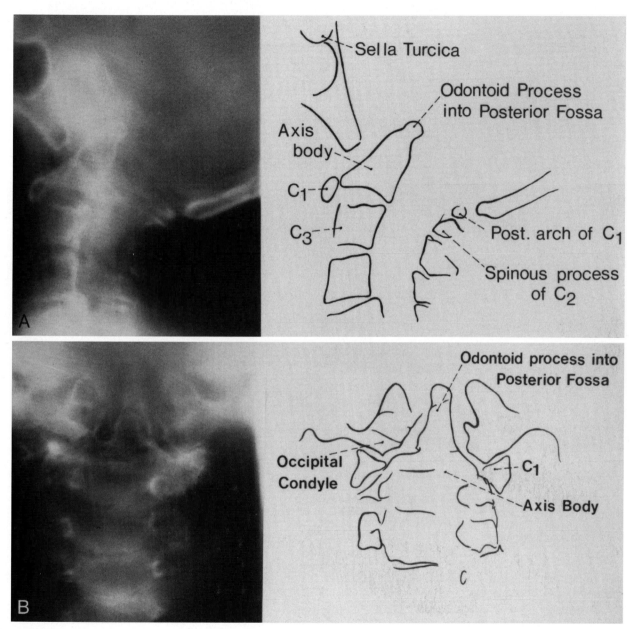

Figure 42–31

A. Midline lateral tomography of the craniovertebral junction in a 64-year-old patient with rheumatoid arthritis and quadriparesis with vagal, hypoglossal, and glossopharyngeal nerve paralysis. The odontoid process extends 22 mm into the posterior fossa. The anterior atlantal arch is located at the C2–C3 interspace. *B.* Frontal tomography through the occipital condyles. Erosion and outward displacement of the lateral atlantal masses is seen, as is a descent of the occipital condyle onto the axis, with ascent of the odontoid process.

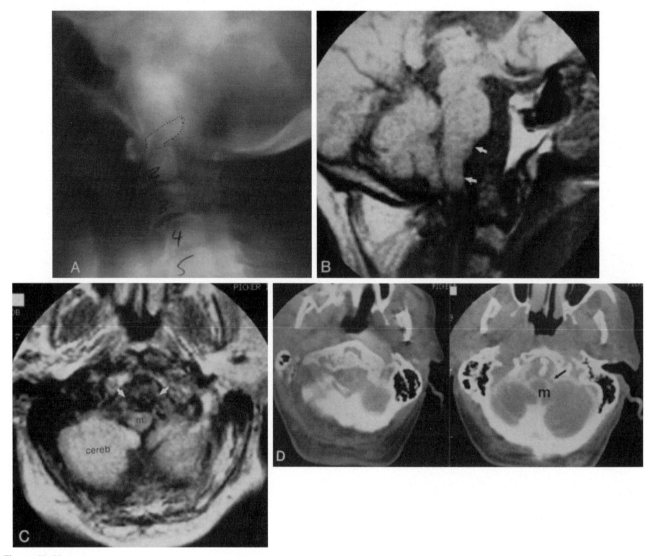

Figure 42–32

A. Lateral midline tomography at the craniovertebral junction. The invaginated odontoid process is fractured at the base. *B.* T1-weighted midsagittal magnetic resonance imaging of the posterior fossa reveals the distorted medulla oblongata displaced dorsally by a mass *(white arrows).* The osteoporotic odontoid process in the mass is not identified. *C.* Axial T1-weighted magnetic resonance imaging through the caudal medulla (m). A mass *(white arrows)* behind the clivus is compressing the medulla and flattening its ventral surface. *D.* Metrizamide axial computed tomography through the caudal medulla (m). The mass behind the medulla and the clivus contains the obliquely oriented odontoid process surrounded by granulation tissue. Notice the position of the vertebral arteries *(arrow).*

In several individuals, an irreducible cranial settling was encountered because the occipital condyles were impacted into the superior slopes of the axis vertebra. Complex cranial settling with posterior dislocation was considered to be potentially lethal at any time because of the distraction of the vertebral artery complexes (Fig. 42–33). In such cases, a fusion procedure was considered mandatory immediately. Complex cranial settling with occipitoaxial rotatory luxation was seen in a few patients (Fig. 42–34).

Rheumatoid granulation tissue arising from the synovial joint at the craniovertebral junction is an integral part of the rheumatoid process.[176] Varying amounts of tissue are seen with atlantoaxial instability and cranial settling. However, one may encounter an exuberant tissue reaction that causes severe irreducible ventral cervicomedullary compression (Fig. 42–35). This reac-

tion was seen in 27 individuals. A common denominator on frontal radiography is the atrophic, irregular odontoid process surrounded by the "moth-eaten" appearance of the medial aspect of the lateral atlantal masses. This is best appreciated on coronal computed tomography. The bony abnormality is less appreciated on magnetic resonance imaging.

Signs and Symptoms

The most frequent symptom of occipitoatlantoaxial dislocation is occipital pain with radiation toward the vertex. This was present in 90 per cent of patients with cranial settling and in 60 per cent of patients with atlantoaxial subluxation in the author's series. Myelopathy was found in 75 per cent of individuals with cranial settling and in 60 per cent of patients with

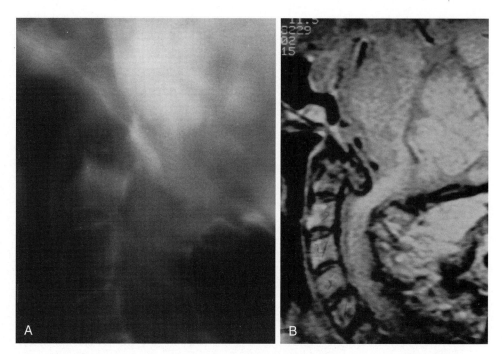

Figure 42–33

A. Midline lateral craniovertebral tomography in a 72-year-old patient with rheumatoid arthritis. A posterior occipitocervical dislocation is seen, and the odontoid process is almost replaced by granulation. *B.* Midsagittal magnetic resonance imaging of the cervicomedullary junction reveals ventral compression by the anterior atlantal arch caused by the posterior occipitocervical dislocation.

atlantoaxial luxation. Because of the deforming effects of peripheral rheumatoid arthritis in the extremities, erroneous diagnoses of entrapment neuropathy, vasculitis, rheumatoid peripheral neuropathy, and "rheumatoid progression of the disease" are common, even though cervicomedullary compression is the cause of the deterioration. Brain stem dysfunction was present in 50 per cent of the patients with cranial settling. The cranial nerves most affected were the hypoglossal, glossopharyngeal, and trigeminal nerves.

Treatment of Rheumatoid Involvement of the Craniovertebral Junction

It is essential for the treating physician to examine the natural history to prevent the likelihood of neurological deterioration or death. It is evident from the volume of literature that the primary indication for surgical intervention is neurological dysfunction and pain. An anterior atlantoaxial subluxation requires attention if the predental space is greater than 7 to 8 mm and neuroradiological studies show impingement on the cervicomedullary junction or vertical subluxation with cranial settling and involvement of the brain stem and cervical cord. Rheumatoid arthritis patients with a predental space of more than 7 to 8 mm ultimately develop neurological deficits. Cranial settling is recognized as being progressive and can be fatal. However, the abnormality can be reduced with halo traction in 80 per cent of individuals, who then need only occipitocervical stabilization. In the remaining patients, a ventral decompression is necessary before the dorsal fixation. Osteopenia and loss of the atlantal lateral masses makes screw fixation untenable. Odontoid fracture with posterior occipitocervical and atlantoaxial dislocation is rare but requires immediate decompression and fusion without traction. Internal fusion in patients with cranial settling and active pannus may cause regression of the ventral soft mass but does not cause the tough pannus and the invagination to disappear.[308]

Most patients who are to be treated for craniovertebral involvement in rheumatoid arthritis should have an attempt to realign the osseous anatomy so to produce relief of the neural compression. This is done by head positioning and cervical traction. However, the latter is contraindicated in posterior occipitoatlantal dislocations or complex rotatory luxations. All individuals undergoing cervical traction should be observed in a monitored care setting with pulse oximetry and the facility to monitor respiratory function. Traction is applied by means of a crown halo ring, as opposed to two-point pivot traction systems such as the Gardner-Wells or Vinke tongs. Traction is begun at 5 to 7 lb and gradually increased to 11 to 12 lb over a span of 3 to 4 days. Periodic radiological evaluation is essential to identify the degree of reduction and to plan changes in the vector or force of distraction applied. In most individuals, neutral to mild extension is necessary. If the reduction has not occurred by the end of 5 days, the lesion is considered to be irreducible, especially in the conditions previously described. Reducible lesions are managed with a fusion stabilization procedure; irreducible lesions require decompression according to the manner in which the encroachment has occurred, followed by fusion stabilization.

In individuals with gross instability or with complex forms of craniovertebral involvement, instrumentation of the craniovertebral junction may be necessary. Contoured loop instrumentation is used to fixate the skull to the upper cervical vertebrae.[168, 191, 228, 239] As in all fusions, it is essential that long-term stability be achieved with osseous construct, and the instrumentation is only a temporizing feature until bony integration has taken place.[227]

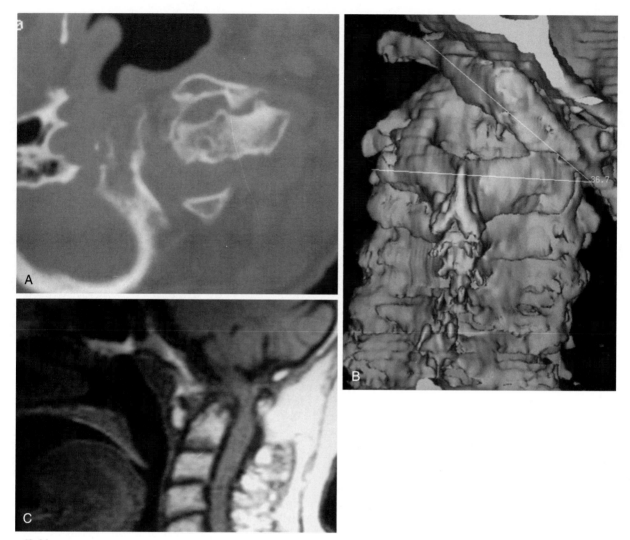

Figure 42–34

A. Axial computed tomography at the craniovertebral border in a 66-year-old female with rheumatoid disease. Notice that the right lateral border of the foramen magnum, the anterior atlantal arch and the axis body are in the same plane; this signifies rotary occipitoatlantoaxial dislocation with impaction. *B.* Three-dimensional computed tomography of the cervical spine reveals rotary atlantoaxial and lateral dislocation. *C.* T1-weighted midsagittal magnetic resonance imaging of the craniovertebral region demonstrates cranial settling with severe neural compression ventrally and dorsally.

MISCELLANEOUS INFLAMMATORY CONDITIONS AFFECTING THE CRANIOVERTEBRAL JUNCTION

The spondyloarthropathies are a group of related disorders characterized by peripheral inflammatory arthritis, inflammation of sacroiliac joints, a tendency toward diffuse spinal involvement, and sometimes extra-articular features including ocular abnormalities. The rheumatoid factor is usually absent. The pathological changes occur not only in the joints but also in the attachments of ligaments to bone. The conditions that affect the craniovertebral junction are psoriatic arthropathy, ankylosing spondylitis, enteropathic arthropathy including Crohn's disease and ulcerative colitis, and reactive disease including Reiter's syndrome.* The au-

thor has encountered calcium pyrophosphate deposition in the synovial joints around the odontoid process, which caused masses to occur, with the term "pseudogout" being employed.[72, 208, 231] Ankylosing spondylitis usually spares the atlantoaxial joints; this leads to an excessive dynamic load at this level, with subsequent dislocation and further progression, including secondary basilar invagination.[173, 174] One has to wonder about the axial load that is transmitted to the craniocervical junction in view of the spine acting as one segment.

Psoriatic arthropathy occurs in 7 per cent of patients with psoriasis.* The skin changes usually precede the onset of arthritis. Spine involvement develops in about 20 per cent of patients with psoriatic arthritis. Psoriatic arthritis affecting the craniocervical junction acts much like the ankylosing spondylitis.

---

*See references 105, 145, 149, 156, 159, and 174.

*See references 23, 70, 76, 77, 119, 284, and 305.

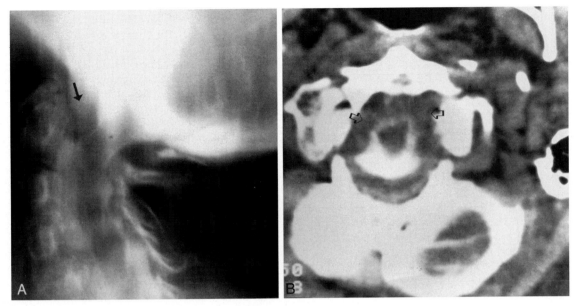

Figure 42–35

A. Metrizamide myelotomography in the lateral projection shows a soft-tissue granulation mass *(arrow)* behind the lower clivus and axis body that displaces the cervicomedullary junction dorsally. The odontoid is eroded. *B.* Metrizamide computed myelotomography at the foramen magnum. The granulation arising from the synovial joints surrounds the caudal medulla ventrally and laterally *(open arrows)*.

Inflammatory bowel disease is associated with spondyloarthropathy in 15 to 20 per cent of affected individuals.[105, 141, 179] The incidence is higher in Crohn's disease and ulcerative colitis. The triad of arthritis, urethritis, and ocular disease, referred to as Reiter's syndrome, is usually not seen simultaneously. The arthropathy is usually acute and may be associated with reactive arthritis, possibly to gonococcus, beta-hemolytic streptococcus, or *Clostridium difficile.* As a result of the synovitis, atlantoaxial luxation may occur with startling repetitiveness. The author has seen three such individuals. A detailed description of the spondyloarthropathy is given in Chapter 97.

TRAUMATIC LESIONS OF THE CRANIOVERTEBRAL JUNCTION

The literature concerning traumatic injuries to the occipitoatlantoaxial complex is limited. The conditions are not uncommon, and they appear to be associated with an extremely high mortality at the scene of the incident.[3, 35] As a result, this is presumed to be a rare occurrence.

Injury of the occipitoatlantoaxial complex can be divided into the osseous, the ligamentous, and the complex.[252, 264, 283] Osseous injuries include occipital condyle fractures, the Jefferson fracture, and odontoid fractures. Ligamentous injuries are divided into occipitoatlantal dislocation and atlantoaxial dislocation. Complex injuries are far more extensive and include the traumatic spondylolisthesis of C2 ("hangman's fracture"), the transaxial cervicomedullary junction injury, and combined osteoligamentous disruptions. A significant number of these ligamentous injuries occur in children,

whereas the fractures are more prone to occur in adults. A more detailed description is found in Chapters 85 and 86.

Treatment of Craniovertebral Abnormalities

Before the introduction of skeletal traction, treatment of occipitoatlantoaxial joint disorders was marked by failure to achieve reduction except for acute dislocations. Later, it became apparent that both acute and chronic dislocations could be reduced even years after the onset of symptoms.[164] The early operative procedures consisted of posterior decompression of the cervicomedullary junction, with or without fusion for stabilization. Posterior decompression in patients with irreducible compression of neural structures at the craniocervical area was often associated with a high operative risk and a low incidence of improvement.[16, 108, 227, 288] When a Chiari malformation was present and associated with "central cord syndrome," posterior decompression resulted in improvement in only one third of patients; the remainder either became worse or remained unchanged.[39, 238] Hemorrhage was reported to occur within the medulla and upper cervical spinal cord after posterior decompression for basilar invagination or other ventral compression.[288] No single anterior or posterior operative procedure can be used for all patients with craniospinal abnormalities. It is necessary to select the operation or combination of operative procedures for each patient based on a clear understanding of the functional anatomy and pathophysiology in this region.

The treatment of craniovertebral junction abnormalities has been divided into management of deformities that can be realigned, with relief of the compression on the neural structures, and management of deformities that are irreducible.[193] The primary aim of treatment in patients with reducible deformity is stabilization. An external immobilization is accomplished in patients with inflammatory states to allow for reconstitution of bones and ligaments. In others, a posterior fixation is essential. Operative decompression of the cervicomedullary junction is necessary in patients with irreducible lesions (Fig. 42–36). The surgical approaches are further subdivided into the ventral, lateral, and dorsal decompression categories.* If instability is present after either of these modes of decompression, a posterior fixation for stabilization is required.[187] An anterior fusion procedure alone does not allow for stability at the occipitocervical junction.[26, 75, 191] The reader is referred to Chapter 140 for a more detailed description of the surgical approaches toward decompression.

REDUCIBLE LESIONS REQUIRING IMMOBILIZATION ALONE

The patients in this category are those with acute traumatic atlantoaxial luxations, nontraumatic postinflammatory instabilities of the craniocervical region, or acute ligamentous injuries.[192] Most of these individuals require skeletal traction with a crown halo ring. Traction is applied in graded increments up to 8 to 9 lb in graded increments. The halo ring with pin fixation has the advantage of being able to be incorporated into a body brace without change of the ring. Titanium and graphite alloy halo devices are now available; they prevent distortion during the magnetic resonance imaging or computed tomography studies that may be required after the patient has been treated. The halo brace fixation is preferred for immobilization of the craniocervical junction because of its superiority in preventing motion.[121, 139] After reduction has been achieved, immobilization is maintained for 8 to 10 weeks, after which radiological evidence of stability is required. If stability has not been achieved, a posterior fixation becomes essential.

REDUCIBLE LESIONS REQUIRING POSTERIOR FUSION

The majority of the author's patients required skeletal traction; only a few realigned with head position alone. Cervical traction, even in the most difficult and complex circumstances, should not be carried out for more than 5 to 6 days. If reduction is not possible, decompression must be accomplished. In those individuals in whom a fusion must be made, both anatomical and biomechanical abnormalities must be taken into consideration. Occipitocervical and atlantoaxial fusions have been performed by ventral and dorsal routes.

Several new techniques have the attraction of immediate stabilization with "heavy metal" incorporation and require closer inspection.

A variety of techniques for fusion in the craniocervical region have been described. In general, all levels demonstrating instability need to be spanned in the fusion construct. Certain exceptions exist; for example, in patients with unstable dystopic os odontoideum and rheumatoid cranial settling, the occiput must be incorporated.

Occipitocervical fusion and atlantoaxial fusion are usually performed by the posterior routes. Anterior approaches and fusions have been less frequently described. Difficulties inherent to fusion of this crucial region have led to the development of a number of techniques and innovations, both in the approach and in the instrumentation used. As with any fusion, long-term stability is achieved on osseous union. The goal of instrumentation is to provide immediate stability until a bony fusion is obtained. Repeated stress fatigue and ultimate failure of the fusion construct occurs if bone fusion is not achieved.

Occipitocervical Fusion

Occipitocervical fusion by use of a fibular graft in the management of trauma to the craniocervical region was described by Foerster in 1927.[84] Innovations subsequently described involve the choice of grafting material, placement of stabilization wires, use of methyl methacrylate, and choice of craniocervical instruments. Incorporation of the occiput in a craniocervical fusion is required in the presence of occipitocervical instability.[237]

The most frequent cause of craniocervical instability is rheumatoid arthritis; trauma and inflammatory states are also common. Congenital and developmental anomalies causing occipitocervical instability include atlas assimilation, os odontoideum and bony dysplasias, achondroplasia, and spondyloepiphyseal dysplasia. Instability may result from erosion secondary to primary or metastatic tumor and has also been encountered in the mucopolysaccharidoses, Paget's disease, and osteogenesis imperfecta.

Most patients with occipitoatlantal instability require preoperative and intraoperative traction with a halo ring apparatus. Usually 6 to 7 lb of intraoperative traction is sufficient for combined occipitocervical and atlantoaxial instability. With isolated occipitoatlantal instability, the patients must be placed initially in a halo vest and the posterior struts removed. This allows for some degree of fixation during the operation in a very unstable situation. Fiberoptics-guided awake intubation is performed, with reassessment of neurological function after final positioning but before the induction of general anesthesia.

A midline incision is made from the inion to the spinous process of the fourth cervical vertebra. A subperiosteal dissection exposes the occiput and the laminae of the upper cervical vertebrae. The spinous process of the axis can be stabilized with a towel clip to avoid excessive motion during dissection.[123] The poste-

---

*See references 50, 57, 77, 92, 108, 123, 186, and 273.

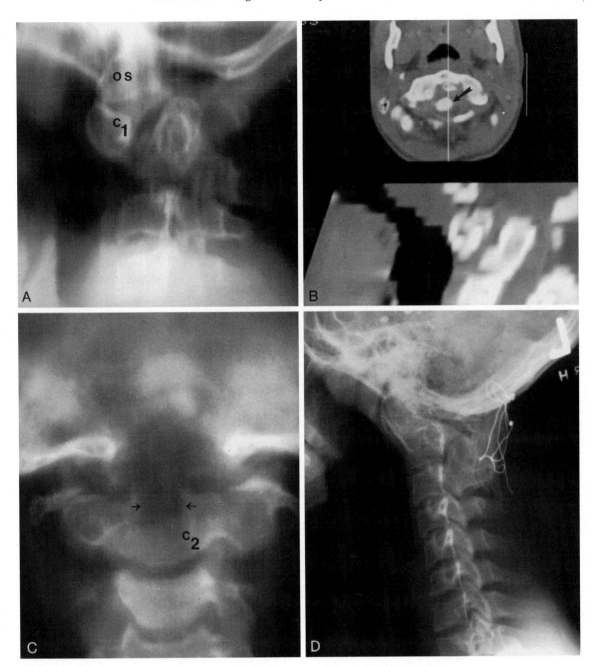

Figure 42–36

A. Lateral laminagraphy of the upper cervical spine reveals a dystopic os odontoideum (os) with axis displacement in a rostrodorsal direction. The effective canal diameter is 6 mm at the atlas level (C1). *B.* Axial computed tomography at the atlas level reveals the axis body to be occupying the middle of the spinal canal *(arrow)*. This is correlated on the reformatted sagittal images. *C.* Frontal tomography through the area of resection of the os odontoideum and axis body *(between arrows)*. *D.* Lateral cervical spine radiography 1 year after transoral resection of the os and axis body and subsequent occipitoatlantoaxial dorsal bony fusion.

rior rim of the foramen magnum is excised by use of a high-speed drill and fine rongeurs.[203] A burr hole is placed approximately 25 mm to either side of the midline and 20 mm above the rim of foramen magnum (Fig. 42–37). Soft cable or braided no. 22 wire is then passed extradurally from the trephined hole to the midline to achieve occipital anchorage for the donor graft material or instrumentation device.[276] An attractive alternative is the stainless steel or titanium cable system; these cables are strong and extremely flexible. A cable or braided wire can then be passed beneath

the laminae of the axis and atlas on either side. The exposed laminae, spinous processes, and occipital bone are carefully decorticated to facilitate fusion. Bone grafts, usually full thickness rib or iliac crest, are then applied to the occiput, atlas, and axis, with sublaminar wires at each level passed through the graft. The cables or wires are tightened in alternating fashion, securing the graft into position (Fig. 42–38*A* and *B*). This method of sublaminar wiring applies equally well in the fixation in occipitocervical arthrodesis. Bone pieces are then packed at the donor-recipient bone interface. Post-

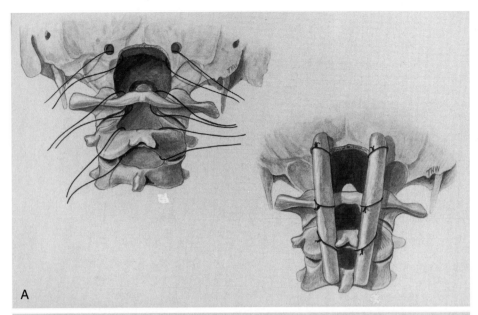

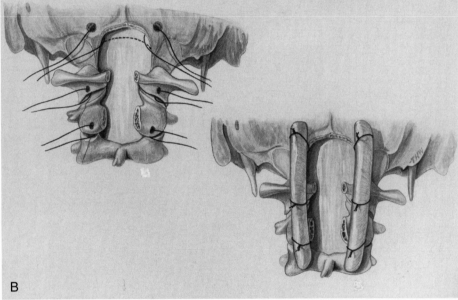

Figure 42–37

A. Illustrations of the technique of dorsal occipitocervical bone fusion. Notice the small posterior foramen magnum decompression and sublaminar wire-cable anchorage. *B.* Illustrations of the technique of dorsal occipital-lateral facet cervical fusion. This procedure is essential to accommodate decompression of the posterior fossa and laminectomies.

operative halo vest immobilization is essential for 5 to 6 months to ensure osseous integration (see Fig. 42–38*C*).

The author's series of more than 600 fusions at the craniocervical junction include a personal series of 335 patients who required occipitocervical fixations. The majority of rheumatoid patients had methylmethacrylate supplementation for internal stabilization and only a fitted occipitocervical brace for immobilization (Fig. 42–39).[187, 194] Complete fusion was achieved in 98 per cent. A fibrous union occurred in 2 per cent. An additional 106 patients had occipitocervical bony fusion and halo immobilization. Two failures occurred (a child with Down's syndrome and another with spondyloepiphyseal dysplasia). These results exceed the expectation of the 1979 review by Sherk, in which a failure rate of 20 per cent was recognized in 380 cases reviewed in the literature.[255]

Hamblen described 13 patients who required occipi-

tocervical fusion; 12 of the 13 had improvement in their neurological condition after operation.[118] All obtained a successful fusion, although three suffered graft fractures at 18 months to 4 years after operation. In the series by Lee and associates, seven patients underwent occipitocervical fusion, and two failed to obtain a stable fusion despite 6 weeks of postoperative immobilization and traction.[158] In Larsson and Toolamen's series of 34 patients with atlantoaxial subluxation and rheumatoid arthritis, six patients required occipitocervical fusion for basilar invagination.[155] Twenty-eight patients underwent atlantoaxial fixation with intraoperative traction. A soft collar was used for postoperative immobilization. The failure rate of 40 per cent ascribed to the operative technique and poor postoperative care.

Aprin and Harf discussed the indications for occipitocervical fusion in relation to atlantoaxial instability in patients with congenital and acquired atlantoaxial dislocation.[6] They suggested that the occiput be in-

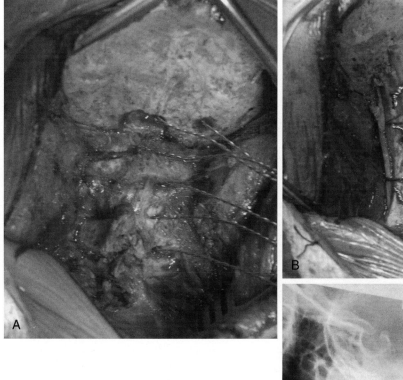

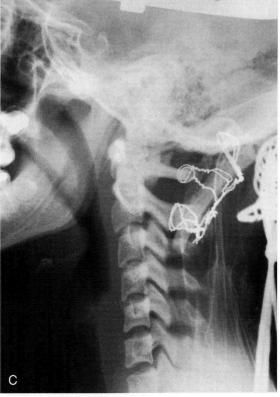

Figure 42–38

A. Operative photograph of dorsal occipitocervical fusion. The foramen magnum decompression and occipital trephination have been made on the left. Notice the braided wire for gaining occipital purchase and the sublaminar wires. *B.* Operative photograph of dorsal occipitocervical rib graft and braided wire fusion. Notice the transfixing of the donor bone with the wire. In children, the wires are not tied to each other. *C.* Lateral cervical radiography after dorsal occipitocervical fusion and in halo immobilization.

cluded in patients with rheumatoid arthritis, a basilar invagination, congenital anomalies of the atlanto-occipital interface, deficiency in the posterior arch of the atlas, irreducible atlantoaxial luxation, and significant bony destruction.

Methylmethacrylate has been used by several authors to supplement fusions of the craniocervical region.* Brattstrom and Granholm's technique, described in 1976, combines methylmethacrylate and bone fusion.[30] Sublaminar wires are passed through the occiput

and C1 and around a Steinmann pin passed transversely though the base of the C2 spinous process. Bone chips are packed while the opposite side is encased in acrylic cement. In 27 of 28 patients, improvement was seen postoperatively. Two incidents of wound infection and one of breakage occurred.

The technique described by Grob and colleagues employs screws placed into the occiput with sublaminar wires on either side that affix bone grafts to one side and acrylic cement to the other.[110, 111] The fact that the load is focused on the screws leaves much to be desired.[234]

---

*See references 30, 34, 40, 45, 71, 163, and 212.

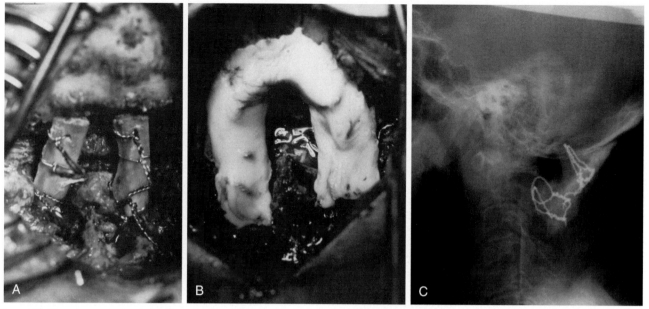

Figure 42–39

A. Operative photograph of dorsal occipitocervical fusion in a 66-year-old rheumatoid patient. The rib grafts are in place bilaterally, with elongated stubs of wire left for embedding the methylmethacrylate. *B.* Operative view of methylmethacrylate "horseshoe" reinforcement of the bone and wire fusion. *C.* Lateral cervical radiography made 3 days after dorsal occipitoatlantoaxial fusion with bone and wire and methylmethacrylate.

Occipitocervical Fusion with Contoured Loop or Rod

Segmental fixation devices have been applied to the occipitocervical region in a variety of methods. The concept of loop instrumentation fixation of the dorsal craniocervical area was initially put forth by Ransford and colleagues and subsequently modified by others.[228] In 1988, Ito and co-workers described the use of the Luque segmental instrumentation device for occipitocervical fusion in 13 patients with rheumatoid arthritis.[136] He used a Luque rod shaped like an inverted

U and contoured to the region. A bony fusion was documented in 12 patients.

Papadopoulos and colleagues described their use of a three-eighths inch contoured and threaded Steinmann pin to perform an occiput-to-C5 fusion in a 10-year-old child with traumatic occipitoatlantal dislocation.[214] Segmental sublaminar wiring was used, and a C1 laminectomy was performed. The patient was immobilized for 3 months in a halo vest. The child was neurologically normal at the end of 3 months, with the exception of a decreased range of motion in the craniocervical axis. Similar techniques have been de-

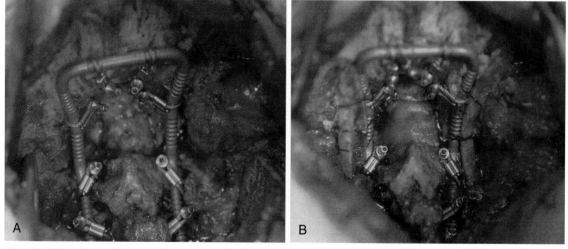

Figure 42–40

A. Operative photograph of occipitocervical fusion with the use of a custom titanium threaded-loop instrument and "cables" to anchor to the recipient occiput and upper cervical laminae. *B.* Bone grafts are added to the fusion construct lateral to the titanium loop, in apposition to the recipient occiput and dorsal laminar surfaces of the atlas and axis vertebrae.

scribed by Sakou and by MacKenzie and their colleagues.[168, 239]

The author uses a similar technique involving two trephine placements on either side of the midline occiput to support the transverse portion of a U-shaped contoured loop. Occipital purchase must anchor the transverse bar of the loop as well as the vertical component, so occipital cables are needed on either side (Fig. 42–40). Bone grafts are laid around the metallic instrumentation and secured. Osseous construct integration occurs within 3 to 4 months. The availability of titanium loop instrumentation allows for immediate fixation with the advantage of permitting magnetic resonance imaging.

Occipitocervical Plate Fusion

Several authors have described fixation devices that use T- or Y-shaped plates. Heywood and colleagues reported 14 cases of occipitocervical instability treated by occipitocervical fusion with the use of a T-shaped plate and a screw device.[127] Five of the 14 had prior failed fusion attempts. A midline incision exposed the external occipital protuberance in the upper cervical laminae. The T-shaped plate was molded to fit the occipitocervical contour. Screws were placed in the occiput with bicortical purchase and into the spinous process of C2. Sublaminar wire was passed around the axis to affix it to the plate. Cancellous strip grafts were placed from the occiput to the axis after decortication.

Grob and co-workers described posterior occipital fusion by use of a Y-shaped plate and transarticular atlantoaxial screw fixation in an attempt to avoid complications related to the passage of sublaminar wiring.[111] Their technique involved placing screws into the posterior caudal aspect of the axis and into the lateral

atlantal masses under fluoroscopy guidance. A Y-shaped plate was then fashioned and attached to the occiput with bicortical screw purchase. If bone grafting was required, the plate could be extended to include lower levels if necessary. Fourteen patients were treated in this manner, including seven with rheumatoid arthritis, four with degenerative joint disease, two with traumatic injury, and one with osteomyelitis. Six underwent fusion from the occiput to C6 and one from the occiput to T1. All achieved a solid fusion and were rated as successful. On follow-up, one patient was had loosening of the screw but did not require additional intervention. The technique fails to appreciate the underlying osseous pathology in rheumatoid cranial settling, in which there is always loss of the atlantal lateral masses leading to downward occipital condylar descent. Placement of a transarticular C1–C2 screw cannot have atlantal purchase in such a case and defeats the purpose of the procedure. Several such "plate procedures" have the same problem.[234]

Atlantoaxial Fusion

Fusion of the atlas to the axis is indicated in patients with documented atlantoaxial instability, usually defined as 5 mm or greater in children and 3 mm or greater in adults. Atlantoaxial fusion can be elected in cases of isolated atlantoaxial instability if the occipital atlantal segment is not involved or is not anticipated to become involved in the disease process (Fig. 42–41). Atlantoaxial instability can result from congenital, traumatic, inflammatory, or neoplastic processes, as can occipitoatlantal instability. Congenital atlantoaxial instability, such as odontoid aplasia and hypoplasia of the odontoid process and os odontoideum, are not infrequent. Nonunion of an odontoid process fracture

Figure 42–41

Lateral cervical radiography obtained preoperatively *(left)* and postoperatively *(right)* in a patient with rheumatoid arthritis and Felty's syndrome. The severe anterior atlantoaxial dislocation was thought to be asymptomatic, and the quadriparesis was attributed to short bowel syndrome. Notice the reduced dislocation *(right)* and dorsal interlaminar arthrodesis supplemented with methylmethacrylate.

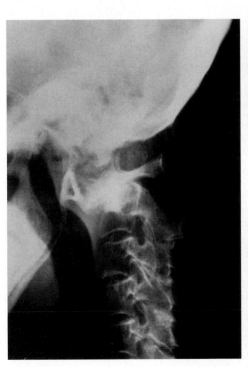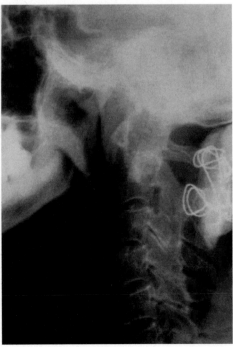

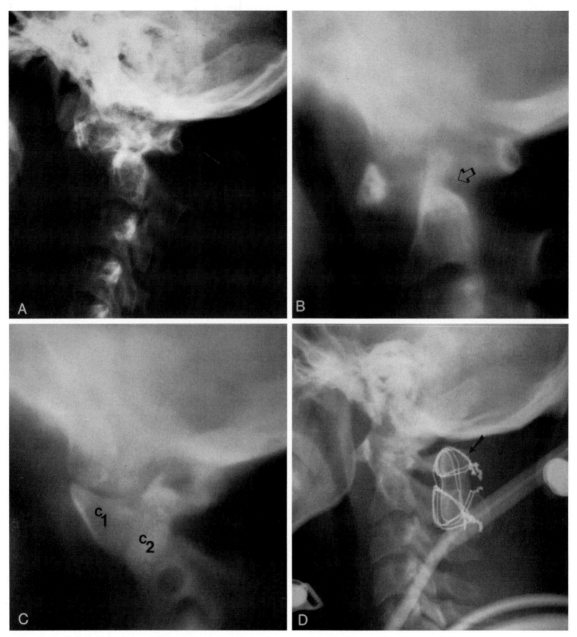

Figure 42–42

A. Atlantoaxial luxation seen on lateral cervical spine radiography in a 26-year-old quadriplegic with rheumatoid arthritis. *B.* Midline lateral craniovertebral tomography. Notice the excavation of the cruciate ligament *(open arrow)* in the atrophic odontoid base and the widened predental space. *C.* Lateral craniovertebral tomography through the lateral articulations. The lateral atlantal masses articulate with the nonarticular portion of the axis. *D.* Postoperative lateral cervical spine radiography documents the realignment of the atlantoaxial articulation by posterior wire and bone fusion *(arrow)*. The patient recovered neurological function.

with or without rupture of the transverse ligament is a frequent cause of traumatic atlantoaxial instability.

Gallie has described a technique to provide short- and long-term stabilization of the C1–C2 region by the use of sublaminar wire and cortical cancellous bone graft material between the posterior atlas and axis arches.[90] Fielding described the application of this technique in 11 patients with irreducible atlantoaxial rotatory luxation, which was successful in more than 90 per cent.[80] Waddell reported on 16 patients treated with Gallie-type C1–C2 fusion for type II odontoid fracture.[287] Fifteen of the 16 patients obtained a solid

bony fusion with no increase in the neurological deficit. One patient required reoperation for unsatisfactory alignment, and one with spinous process fracture of C2 required reoperation and augmentation with methylmethacrylate. The author concluded that C1–C2 arthrosis is justified as a primary therapy based on low morbidity and high fusion rates.

Santavirta and colleagues described the use of C1–C2 fusion in rheumatoid arthritis patients in a series of papers.[240] They reviewed 38 patients treated for craniovertebral instability secondary to rheumatoid arthritis, 24 of whom underwent a Gallie-type fusion. Twelve obtained a solid fusion, but four had a fibrous union, and eight had pseudoarthrosis. These authors believe that steroids prompted the occurrence of pseudoarthrosis. That statement could apply to all series of rheumatoid patients, and therefore effective intraoperative and postoperative management is critical.

The present author uses the technique of bilateral interlaminar rib graft over the dorsal lateral arches and fixation with braided sublaminar wire or soft cable that transfixes the graft. This technique allows for "spacing" and realignment, prevents flexion and extension over the fusion segments, and resists axial rotation.[187] All of these are desirable prerequisites (Fig. 42–42).

Several attempts to modify the techniques of Brooks and Jenkins and of Gallie have failed to show fusion rates superior to those previously described.* Papadopoulos and associates had a failure rate of 4 of 17 rheumatoid patients in whom the procedure was carried out.[213]

Atlantoaxial Fusion with Posterior Interlaminar Clamps

Posterior atlantoaxial fusion can be accomplished with the use of interlaminar clamps. Various constructs have been designed to avoid passage of sublaminar wire; for example, hooks placed under the lamina coupled with an adjustable central screw.[53, 131, 197, 199] This type of instrumentation is used primarily in the lower cervical spine. Use of such devices entails lower dorsal element compression, but at the atlantoaxial level it serves to increase the downward descent of the atlas anterior arch and to promote vertical odontoid penetration in patients with rheumatoid arthritis. The "toggle" effect of such clamps is easily visualized; attempts to overcome the effect led to the imbedding of the screws and clamps in methylmethacrylate.

Atlantoaxial Transarticular Screw Fixation

This procedure was first described by Barbour in 1971 and has the advantage of fusing the atlantoaxial interface when the posterior elements of the axis or atlas are unsuitable for other posterior procedures.[13] This technique can provide immediate, rigid internal fixation and can be coupled with bone grafting and sublaminar or spinous process wiring. It is accomplished under fluoroscopy guidance and requires a thorough understanding of the bony relationship to avoid injury to the adjacent neurovascular structures.

The technique requires a midline posterior approach, with the insertion point of the screw being on the dorsal aspect of the axis at the junction of the lamina and articular mass. A guide hole is drilled in the sagittal plane to avoid damage to the vertebral artery laterally and to avoid entering the spinal canal medially. This guide hole crosses the atlantoaxial joint and enters the articular process of the atlas in its midposition. An appropriately chosen 3.5-mm cortical screw is inserted

to affix the articular masses of the atlas and axis vertebrae.

A bone graft is then fashioned and secured with sublaminar or spinous process wires as indicated by the anatomy. Patients may be immobilized postoperatively in a cervical collar until bony fusion has occurred. Among the 161 patients described by Grob, 61 individuals had post-traumatic instability, 51 had rheumatoid arthritis, 20 had congenital anomalies, 18 had pseudoarthrosis after previous fusion attempts, 7 had degenerative osteoarthritis, 2 had atlantoaxial instability after infection, and 2 had bony tumors.[112] The follow-up period was 24 months. There were no vertebral artery injuries reported. However, one patient suffered hypoglossal nerve paralysis. A stable union and radiological evidence of fusion was documented in 153 patients. Broken screws were noted in three patients, and three others had loosening. Vertebral artery injuries have, however, been reported in a significant number of patients, mandating that computed tomography studies and confirmation of the position of the vertebral arteries be accomplished before any attempt at transarticular screw fixation of the atlantoaxial complex.

REFERENCES

1. Afshani, E., and Girdany, B. R.: Atlanta-axial dislocation in chondrodysplasia punctata. Radiology, 102:399–401, 1972.
2. Ahlback, S., and Collert, S.: Destruction of the odontoid process due to atlantoaxial pyogenic spondylitis. Acta Radiol. Diagn., 10:394–400, 1970.
3. Alker, A. J., Oh, Y. S., and Leslie, E. V.: High cervical spine and craniocervical junction injuries in fatal traffic accidents: A radiological study. Orthop. Clin. North Am., 9:1003–1010, 1978.
4. Althoff, B., and Goldie, I. F.: The arterial supply of the odontoid process of the axis. Acta Orthop. Scand., 48:622–626, 1977.
5. American Academy of Pediatrics Committee on Sports Medicine: Atlantoaxial instability in Down's syndrome. Pediatrics, 74:152, 1984.
6. Aprin, H., and Harf, R.: Stabilization of atlantoaxial instability. Orthopedics, 11:1687–1693, 1988.
7. Arnett, F. C., Edworthy, S. M., Bloch, D. A., et al.: The American Rheumatism Association 1987 revised criteria for the classification of rheumatoid arthritis. Arthritis Rheum., 31:315–324, 1988.
8. Aryanpur, J., Hurko, O., Francomano, C., et al.: Craniocervical decompression for cervicomedullary compression in pediatric patients with achondroplasia. J. Neurosurg., 73:375, 1990.
9. Bach, A., Barraquer-Bordas, L., Barraquer-Ferr, et al.: Delayed myelopathy following atlanto-axial dislocation by separate odontoid process. Brain, 78:537–553, 1955.
10. Baga, N., Chusid, E. L., and Miller, A.: Pulmonary disability in the Klippel-Feil syndrome. Clin. Orthop., 67:105–110, 1969.
11. Ball, J.: The articular pathology of rheumatoid arthritis. In Carter, M. E., ed.: Radiological Aspects of Rheumatoid Arthritis. Amsterdam, Excerpta Medica, 1964, pp. 25–39.
12. Ball, J., and Sharp, J.: Rheumatoid arthritis of the cervical spine. In Hill, A. G. S., ed.: Modern Trends in Rheumatology. 2nd ed. London, Butterworth, 1971, pp. 117–138.
13. Barbour, J. R.: Screw fixation and fractures of the odontoid process. S. Aust. Chir., 5:20–24, 1971.
14. Bares, L.: Basilar impression and the so-called associated anomalies. Eur. Neurol., 13:92–100, 1975.
15. Barton, J. W., and Margolis, M. R.: Rotational obstruction of the vertebral artery at the atlanto-axial joint. Neurol. Radiol., 9:117, 1975.
16. Barucha, E. P., and Dastur, H. M.: Craniovertebral anomalies. Brain, 87:469–480, 1964.

---

*See references 33, 61, 62, 64, 90, and 281.

17. Becker, M. H., Genieser, N. B., Finegold, M., et al.: Chondrodysplasia punctata: Is maternal Warfarin therapy a factor? Am. J. Disabled Child., 129:356–359, 1975.

18. Beighton, P., and Craig, J.: Atlanta-axial subluxation in the Morquio syndrome. J. Bone Joint Surg. [Br.], 55:478–481, 1973.

19. Bell, C.: In Longman, Rees, Orme, et al., ed.: The Nervous System of the Human Body. London, 1830, pp. 403–406.

20. Bergstrom, K., Laurent, U., and Lundberg, P. O.: Neurological symptoms in achondroplasia. Acta Neurol. Scand., 47:59–70, 1971.

21. Bernini, F. P., Elefante, R., Smaltino, F., et al.: Angiographic study on the vertebral artery in cases of deformities of the occipitocervical joint. A.J.R., 107:526–529, 1969.

22. Bland, J. H.: Rheumatoid arthritis of the cervical spine [Review]. J. Rheumatol., 1:319–342, 1974.

23. Blau, R. H., and Kaufman, R. L.: Erosive and subluxing cervical spine disease in patients with psoriatic arthritis. J. Rheumatol., 4:111–117, 1987.

24. Blaw, M. E., and Langer, L. O.: Spinal cord compression in Morquio-Brailsford's disease. J. Pediatrics, 74:593–600, 1969.

25. Bohlman, H. H.: Atlantoaxial dislocations in the arthritic patient: Report of 45 cases. Orthop. Trans., 2:197, 1978.

26. Bonney, G.: Stabilization of the upper cervical spine by the transpharyngeal route. Proc. R. Soc. Med., 63:896–897, 1970.

27. Bosma, J. F.: Symposium on development of the basicranium. In Bosma, J. F., ed.: DHEW Publication No. (NIH) 76-989. Bethesda, U. S. Dept. of Health, Education, and Welfare, National Institutes of Health, 1976, pp. 700–710.

28. Braakhekke, J. P., Gabreels, F. J., Renier, W. O., et al.: Craniovertebral pathology in Down's syndrome. Clin. Neurol. Neurosurg., 87:173–179, 1985.

29. Brasch, J. C.: Cunningham's manual of practical anatomy. London, Oxford University Press, 1958, pp. 258–295.

30. Brattstrom, H., and Granholm, L.: Atlanto-axial fusion in rheumatoid arthritis: A new method of fixation with wire and bone cement. Acta Orthop. Scand., 47:619–628, 1976.

31. Breig, A., Turnbull, I., and Hassler, O.: Effects of mechanical stresses on the spinal cord in cervical spondylosis: A study on fresh cadaver material. J. Neurosurg., 25:45-56, 1966.

32. Brill, C. B., Rose, J. S., Godmillow, L., et al.: Spastic quadriparesis due to Cl–C2 subluxation in Hurler Syndrome. J. Pediatr., 92:441–443, 1978.

33. Brooks, A. L., and Jenkins, E. B.: Atlanto-axial arthrodesis by the wedge compression method. J. Bone Joint Surg. [Am.], 60:279–284, 1978.

34. Bryan, W. J., Inglis, A. E., Sculco, T. P., et al.: Methyl methacrylate stabilization for enhancement of posterior cervical arthrodesis in rheumatoid arthritis. J. Bone Joint Surg. [Am.], 64:1045–1050, 1982.

35. Bucholz, R. W., and Burkhead, W. F.: The pathological anatomy of fatal atlanto-occipital dislocations. J. Bone Joint Surg. [Am.], 61:248–250, 1979.

36. Bull, J. W. D., Nixon, W. L. B., and Pratt, R. T. C.: The radiological criteria and familiar occurrence of primary basilar impression. Brain, 78:229–247, 1955.

37. Burke, S. W., French, H. A., Roberts, et al.: Chronic atlantoaxial instability in Down's syndrome. J. Bone Joint Surg. [Am.], 67:1356–1360, 1985.

38. Bystrow, A.: Assimilation des atlas und manifestation des pro atlas. Ztschr. Fd. Ges. Anat. (Abt. 1), 95:210–242, 1931.

39. Caetano de Barros, M., Farias, W., Ataide, L., et al.: Basilar impression and Arnold-Chiari malformation. J. Neurol. Neurosurg. Psychiatry, 31:596–605, 1968.

40. Cameron, H. U., Jacob, R., MacNab, I., et al.: Use of polymethylmethacrylate to entrance screw fixation in bone. J. Bone Joint Surg. [Am.], 57:655–656, 1975.

41. Carson, B., Winfield, J., Wang, H., et al.: Surgical management of cervicomedullary compression in achondroplastic patients. Basic Life Sci., 48:207, 1988.

42. Chamberlain, W. E.: Basilar impression (platybasia). Yale J. Biol. Med., 11:487, 1938–1939.

43. Cheney, W. D.: Acro-osteolysis. A.J.R., 94:595, 1965.

44. Christophidis, N., and Huskinsson, E. C.: Misleading symptoms and signs of cervical spine subluxation in rheumatoid arthritis. B.M.J., 285:364–365, 1982.

45. Clark, C. R., Goetz, D. D., and Menezes, A. H.: Arthrodesis of the cervical spine in rheumatoid arthritis. J. Bone Joint Surg. [Am.], 71:381–392, 1989.

46. Cogan, D. G., and Barrows, L.: Platybasia and Arnold-Chiari malformation. Arch. Ophthalmol., 52:13–29, 1954.

47. Cohen, M. E., Rosenthal, A. D., and Matson, D. D.: Neurological abnormalities in achondroplastic children. J. Pediatr., 71:367–372, 1967.

48. Conlon, P. W., Isdale, I. C., and Rose, B. S.: Rheumatoid arthritis of the cervical spine: An analysis of 333 cases. Ann. Rheum. Dis., 25:120–126, 1966.

49. Craig, J. B., and Hodkinson, M. J.: Paraplegia in Paget's disease of the vertebral column. S. Afr. Med. J., 67:103, 1985.

50. Crockard, H. A., Essigman, W. K., Stevens, J. M., et al.: Surgical treatment of cervical cord compression in rheumatoid arthritis. Ann. Rheum. Dis., 44:809–816, 1985.

51. Cush, J. J., and Lipsky, P. E.: The immunopathogenesis of rheumatoid arthritis: The role of cytokines in chronic inflammation. Clin. Aspects Autoimmun., 1:2–13, 1987.

52. Custis, D. L., and Verbrugghen, A.: Basilar impression resembling cerebellar tumor. Arch. Neurol. Psychiatry, 52:412–415, 1944.

53. Cybulski, G. R., Stone, J. L., Crowell, R. M., et al. Use of Halifax interlaminar clamps for posterior C1–C2 arthrodesis. Neurosurgery, 22:429–431, 1988.

54. Dastur, D. K., Wadia, N. H., DeSai, A. D., et al.: Medullospinal compression due to atlanto-axial dislocation and sudden haematomyelia during decompression. Brain, 88:897–924, 1965.

55. Davis, F. W., Jr., and Markley, H. E.: Rheumatoid arthritis with death from medullary compression. Ann. Intern. Med., 35:451–454, 1951.

56. Dawson, E. G., and Smith, L.: Atlanto-axial subluxation in children due to vertebral anomalies. J. Bone Joint Surg. [Am.], 61:582–587, 1979.

57. DeAndrade, J. R., and MacNab, I.: Anterior occipito-cervical fusion using an extrapharyngeal exposure. J. Bone Joint Surg. [Am.], 51:1621–1626, 1969.

58. DeBarros, M. C., DaSilva, W. F., DeAzevedo, H. C., et al.: Basilar impression and Arnold-Chiari malformation. J. Neurol. Neurosurg. Psychiatry, 31:596–605, 1968.

59. Delamarter, R. B., Dodge, L., Bohlman, H. H., et al.: Postmortem neuropathologic analysis of eleven patients with paralysis secondary to rheumatoid arthritis of the cervical spine. Orthop. Trans., 12:54, 1988.

60. Depresseuz, J. C., Carlier, A., and Stevenaert, A.: CSF scanning in achondroplastic children with cranial enlargement. Dev. Med. Child. Neurol., 17:224–228, 1975.

61. DesFosses, P.: Torticollis nasopharyngien par luxation de l'atlas. Presse Med., 25:586–590, 1932.

62. Dickman, C. A., Sonntag, V. K., Papadopoulos, S. M., et al. The interspinous method of posterior atlantoaxial arthrodesis. J. Neurosurg., 74:190–198, 1991.

63. DiLorenzo, N., Fortuna, A., and Guidetii, B.: Craniovertebral junction malformations: Clinicoradiological findings, long term results and surgical indication in 63 cases. Neurosurgery, 57:603–608, 1982.

64. Dodge, L. D., Bohlman, H. H., and Rechtine, G. R.: Paralysis secondary to rheumatoid arthritis: Pathogenesis and results of treatment. Orthop. Trans., 11:473, 1987.

65. Dolan, K. D.: Cervicobasilar relationships. Radiol. Clin. North Am., 15(2):155–166, 1977.

66. Dubousset, J.: Cervical abnormalities in osteochondroplasia. Basic Life Science, 48:207, 1988.

67. Dutton, R. V.: A practical radiologic approach to skeletal dysplasias in infancy. Radiol. Clin. North Am., 25:1211, 1987.

68. Dyck, P.: Os odontoideum in children: Neurological manifestations and surgical management. Neurosurgery, 2:93–99, 1978.

69. Dyste, G. N., and Menezes, A. H.: Presentation and management of pediatric Chiari malformations without myelodysplasia. Neurosurgery, 23:589, 1988.

70. Dzioba, R. B., and Benjamin, J.: Spontaneous atlantoaxial fusion in psoriatic arthritis. Spine, 10:102–103, 1985.

71. Eismont, F. J., and Bohlman, H. H.: Posterior methylmethracrylate fixation for cervical trauma. Spine, 6:347–362, 1980.

72. El-Khoury, G. Y., Tozzi, J. E., Clark, C. R., et al.: Massive calcium

pyrophosphate crystal deposition at the craniovertebral junction. Am. J. Radiol., 145:777–778, 1985.

73. El-Khoury, G. Y., Wener, M. H., Menezes, A. H., et al.: Cranial settling in rheumatoid arthritis. Radiology, 137:637–642, 1980.

74. Englander, O.: Nontraumatic occipito-atlanto-axial dislocation: A contribution to the radiology of the atlas. Br. J. Radiol., 15:341–345, 1942.

75. Estridge, M. N., and Smith, R. A.: Transoral fusion of odontoid fracture [Case report]. J. Neurosurg., 27:462–465, 1967.

76. Fam, A. G., and Cruickshank, B.: Subaxial cervical subluxation and cord compression in psoriatic spondylitis. Arthritis Rheum., 25:101–106, 1982.

77. Fang, H. S. Y., and Ong, A. B.: Direct anterior approach to the upper cervical spine. J. Bone Joint Surg. [Am.], 44:1588–1604, 1962.

78. Fielding, J. W.: Disappearance of the central portion of the odontoid process. J. Bone Joint Surg. [Am.], 44:1588–1604, 1962.

79. Fielding, J. W., and Griffin, P. P.: Os odontoideum. An acquired lesion. J. Bone Joint Surg. [Am.], 56:187–190, 1974.

80. Fielding, J. W., Hensinger, R. N., and Hawkins, R. J.: Os odontoideum. J. Bone Joint Surg. [Am.], 62:376–383, 1980.

81. Fielding, J. W., Cochron, G. B., Lawsing JF, III, et al.: Tears of the transverse ligament of the atlas: A clinical and biomechanical study. J. Bone Joint Surg. [Am.], 56:1683–1691, 1974.

82. Finerman, G. A., Sakai, D., and Weingarten, S.: Atlanto-axial dislocation with spinal cord compression in a mongoloid child. J. Bone Joint Surg. [Am.], 58:408–409, 1976.

83. Fischgold, H., and Metzger, J.: Etude radiotomographique de l'impression basilaire. Rev. Rheumat., 19:261–264, 1952.

84. Foerster, O.: Die Leitungsbahnen des Schmerzge-fuhls und die chirurgische Behandlung der Schmerz-zustaude. Berlin, Urban & Schwarzenberg, 1927, p. 266.

85. Ford, F. R.: Syncope, vertigo and disturbance of vision resulting from intermittent obstruction of the vertebral arteries due to defect in the odontoid process and excessive mobility of the second cervical vertebra. Bull. Johns Hopkins Hosp., 91:168–173, 1952.

86. Frank, E., Bergerm, T., and Tew, J. M., Jr.: Basilar impression and platybasia in osteogenesis imperfecta tarda. Surg. Neurol., 17:116, 1982.

87. Freiberger, R. H., Wilson, P. D., Jr., and Nicholas, J. A.: Acquired absence of the odontoid process: A case report. J. Bone Joint Surg. [Am.], 47:1231–1234, 1965.

88. Fremion, A. S., Garg, B. P., and Kalsbeck, J.: Apnea as the sole manifestation of cord compression in achondroplasia. J. Pediatr., 104:398–401, 1984.

89. Fromm, G. H., and Pitner, S. E.: Late progressive quadriparesis due to odontoid agenesis. Arch. Neurol., 9:291–296, 1963.

90. Gallie, W. F.: Fractures and dislocations of the cervical spine. Am. J. Surg., 46:495–499, 1939.

91. Ganguly, D. N., and Roy, K. K.: A study on the craniovertebral joint in the man. Anat. Anz., 114:433–452, 1964.

92. Gardner, W. J., and Goodall, R. J.: The surgical treatment of Arnold-Chiari malformation in adults. J. Neurosurg., 7:199–206, 1950.

93. Garrod, A. E.: In Griffin, C., ed.: A Treatise on Rheumatism and Rheumatoid Arthritis. London, 1890, pp. 1–342.

94. Gehweiler, J. A., Osborne, R. L., and Becker, R. F., eds.: Atlantoaxial rotary fixation. In The Radiology of Vertebral Trauma. Philadelphia, W. B. Saunders, 1980, pp. 145–147.

95. Gertner, J. M., and Root, L.: Osteogenesis imperfecta. Orthop. Clin. North Am., 21:151, 1990.

96. Giacomini, C.: Sull' esistenza dell' "os odontoideum" nell' uomo. Gior. Accad. Med. Torino, 49:24–28, 1886.

97. Giblin, P. E., and Mitchell, L. J.: The management of atlantoaxial subluxation with neurologic involvement in Down's syndrome: A report of two cases and review of the literature. Clin. Orthop., 140:66–71, 1979.

98. Gilles, R. H., Bina, M., and Sotrel, A.: Infantile atlanto-occipital instability: The potential danger of extreme extension. Am. J. Disabled Child., 133:30–37, 1979.

99. Gillman, E. L.: Congenital absence of the odontoid process of the axis: Report of a case. J. Bone Joint Surg. [Am.], 41:345–348, 1959.

100. Gladstone, J., and Erickson-Powell, W.: Manifestation of occipi-

tal vertebra and fusion of atlas with occipital bone. J. Anat. Physiol., 49:190–199, 1914–1915.

101. Goel, V. K., Clark, C. R., Gallaes, K., et al.: Movement-rotation relationships of the ligamentous occipito-atlanto-axial complex. J. Biomech., 21:678, 1988.

102. Goldberg, M. J.: Orthopaedic aspects of bone dysplasia. Orthop. Clin. North Am., 7:445–456, 1976.

103. Gooding, M. R., Wilson, C. B., and Hoff, J. T.: Experimental cervical myelopathy: Effects of ischemia and compression of the canine cervical spinal cord. J. Neurosurg., 43:9–17, 1975.

104. Gorlin, R. J., Cohen, M., and Wolfson, J.: Tricho-rhino-phalangeal syndrome. Am. J. Disabled Child., 118:595–602, 1969.

105. Gravallese, E. M., and Kantrowitz, F. G.: Arthritic manifestations of inflammatory bowel disease. Am. J. Gastroenterol., 83:703–709, 1988.

106. Greeley, P. W.: Bilateral (ninety degree) rotary dislocation of the atlas upon the axis. J. Bone Joint Surg. [Am.], 12:958–962, 1930.

107. Greenberg, A. D.: Atlanto-axial dislocations. Brain, 91:655–684, 1968.

108. Greenberg, A. D., Scoville, W. B., and Davey, L. M.: Trans-oral decompression of the atlantoaxial dislocation due to odontoid hypoplasia: Report of two cases. J. Neurosurg., 28:266–269, 1968.

109. Grisel, P.: Enucleation de l'atlas et torticollis nasopharyngien. Presse Med., 38:50–56, 1930.

110. Grob, D., Dvorak, J., Gschwend, N., et al.: Posterior occipito-cervical fusion in rheumatoid arthritis. Arch. Orthop. Trauma Surg., 110:38–44, 1990.

111. Grob, D., Dvorak, J., Panjabi, M., et al.: Posterior occipitocervical fusion: A preliminary report of a new technique. Spine, 16(Suppl. 3):917–924, 1991.

112. Grob, D., Jeannert, B., Aebi, M., et al.: Atlantoaxial fusion with transarticular screw fixation. J. Bone Joint Surg. [Br.], 73:972–976, 1991.

113. Grote, W., Romer, F., and Bettag, W.: Der ventrale Zugang zum Dens epitropheus. Langenbecks Arch. Chir., 331:266–269, 1968.

114. Gulati, D. R., and Rout, D.: Atlantoaxial dislocation with quadriparesis in achondroplasia. J. Neurosurg., 40:394–396, 1974.

115. Hajdu, N., and Kauntze, R.: Carnioskeletal dysplasia. Br. J. Radiol., 21:42, 1948.

116. Hall, C. W., and Danoff, D.: Sleep attacks: Apparent relationship to atlanto-axial dislocation. Arch. Neurol., 32:57–58, 1975.

117. Halla, J. T., Fallak, S., and Hardin, J. T.: Nonreducible rotational head tilt and lateral mass collapse: A prospective study of frequency, radiographic findings, and clinical features in patients with rheumatoid arthritis. Arthritis Rheum., 25:1316–1324, 1982.

118. Hamblen, D. L.: Occipito-cervical fusion: Indications, technique and results. J. Bone Joint Surg. [Br.], 49:33–45, 1967.

119. Hanly, J. G., Rusell, M. I., and Gladman, D. D.: Psoriatic spondyloarthropathy: A long-term prospective study. Ann. Rheum. Dis., 47:386–393, 1988.

120. Harkey, H. L., Crockard, H. A., Stevens, J. M., et al.: The operative management of basilar impression in osteogenesis imperfecta. Neurosurgery, 27:782, 1990.

121. Hartman, J. T., Palumbo, F., and Hill, B. J.: Line radiography of the braced normal cervical spine: A comparative study of five commonly used cervical orthosis. Clin. Orthop., 109:97–102, 1975.

122. Hawkins, R. J., Fielding, W., and Thompson, W. J.: Os odontoideum: Congenital or acquired [Case report]. J. Bone Joint Surg. [Am.], 58:413–414, 1976.

123. Hayakan, A. T., Kamikan, A. T., Ohnishi, T., et al.: Prevention of postoperative complications after a transoral transclival approach to basilar aneurysms. J. Neurosurg., 51:699–703, 1981.

124. Hecht, J. T., and Butler, I. J.: Neurologic morbidity associated with achondroplasia. J. Child Neurol., 5:84, 1990.

125. Hensinger, R. N.: Osseous anomalies of the craniovertebral junction. Spine, 11:323, 1986.

126. Hess, J. H., Bronstein, I. P., and Abelson, S. M.: Atlanta-axial dislocations: Unassociated with trauma and secondary to inflammatory foci in the neck. Am. J. Disabled Child., 49:1137–1147, 1935.

127. Heywood, A. W., Learmonth, I. D., and Thomas, M.: Internal fixation for occipito-cervical fusion. J. Bone Joint Surg. [Br.], 70:708–711, 1988.

128. Hikuda, S., Ota, H., Okake, N., et al.: Traumatic atlantoaxial dislocation causing os odontoideum in infants. Spine, 5:207–210, 1980.

129. Hinck, V. C., Hopkins, C. E., and Savara, B. S.: Diagnostic criteria of basila impression. Radiology, 76:572–585, 1961.

130. Hohl, M., and Baker, H. R.: The atlanto-axial joint. J. Bone Joint Surg. [Am.], 46:1739–1746, 1964.

131. Holness, R. O., Huestis, W. S., Howes, W. J., et al.: Posterior stabilization with an interlaminar clamp in cervical injuries: Technical note and long term experience with the method. Neurosurgery, 14:318–322, 1984.

132. Holzgreve, W., Grope, H., and VonFigwrak, E.: Morquio syndrome: Clinical findings in 11 patients with mucopolysaccharidosis Type IVA and two with mucopolysaccharidosis Type IVP. Hum. Genet., 57:360–365, 1981.

133. Hungerford, G. D., Akkaraju, V., Rawe, S. E., et al.: Atlanto-occipital and atlanto-axial dislocations with spinal cord compression in Down's syndrome: A case report and review of the literature. Br. J. Radiol., 54:758–761, 1981.

134. Hunt, T. E., and Dekaban, A. S.: Modified head-neck support for basilar invagination with brain stem compression. Can. Med. Assoc. J., 126:947, 1982.

135. Hurd, E. R.: Extraarticular manifestations of rheumatoid arthritis. Semin. Arthritis Rheum., 8:151–176, 1979.

136. Itoh, T., Tsuji, H., Katsh, Y., et al.: Occipito-cervical fusion reinforced by Luque segmental spinal instrumentation for rheumatoid disease. Spine, 13:1234–1238, 1988.

137. Jarvis, J. F., and Sellaus, S. L.: Klippel-Feil deformity associated with congenital conductive deafness. J. Laryngol. Otol., 88:285–289, 1974.

138. Jirout, J.: Changes in the atlas-axis relationships on lateral flexion of the head and neck. Neuroradiology, 6:215–218, 1973.

139. Johnson, R. M., Hart, D. L., Simmons, E. F., et al.: Cervical orthoses: A study comparing their effectiveness in restricting cervical motion in normal subjects. J. Bone Joint Surg. [Am.], 59:332–339, 1977.

140. Jones, M. D.: Cineradiographic studies of the normal cervical spine. Calif. Med., 93:293, 1960.

141. Jordan, J. M., Obeid, L. M., and Allen, N. B.: Isolated atlantoaxial subluxation as the presenting manifestation of inflammatory bowel disease. Am. J. Med., 80:517–520, 1988.

142. Kao, S. C., Waziri, M. H., and Smith, W. L.: MR imaging of the craniovertebral junction, cranium, and brain in children with achondroplasia. A.J.R., 153:565, 1989.

143. Klaus, E.: Rontgendiagnostik der platybasie und basilaren impression. Fortschr. Rontgenstr., 86:460–469, 1957.

144. Klaus, E., and Lehman, W.: Familliares Vorkomer bei basilarer impression. Acta Univ. Palacki. Olomuc. Fac. Med., 46:115, 1967.

145. Klemp, P., Meyers, D. L., and Keyzer, C.: Atlanto-axial subluxation in systemic lupus erythematosus [Case report]. S. Afr. Med. J., 52:331–332, 1977.

146. Klippel, M., and Feil, A.: Un cas d'absence des vertebres cervicales avec cage thoracique remontant jusqu'a base du craine. Nouv. Icon. Selpetriere, 25:223–250, 1912.

147. Konttinnen, Y., Santavirta, S., Bergroth, V., et al.: Inflammatory involvement of the cervical spine ligaments in rheumatoid arthritis. Acta Orthop. Scand., 57:587, 1986.

148. Krane, S. M., and Simon, L. S.: Rheumatoid arthritis: Clinical features and pathogenetic mechanisms. Med. Clin. North Am., 70:263–284, 1986.

149. Kransdorf, M. J., Wehrle, P. A., and Moser, R. P., Jr.: Atlanto-axial subluxation in Reiter's syndrome. Spine, 13:12–14, 1988.

150. Kurimoto, M., Ohara, S., and Takaku, A.: Basilar impression in osteogenesis imperfecta tarda [Case report]. J. Neurosurg., 74:136, 1991.

151. LaMasters, D. L., and DeGrott, J.: Normal craniovertebral junction. In Newton, T. H., and Potts, D. G., eds.: Modern Neuro-Radiology. Vol. 1, Ch. 3. San Anselmo, Clavadel Press, 1983, pp. 31–53.

152. Langer, L. O., and Carey, L. S.: The roentgenographic features of the KS-mucopolysaccharidosis of Morquio (Morquio-Brailsford's disease). A.J.R., 47:1–12, 1966.

153. Lanier, R. R., Jr.: Anomalous cervico-occipital skeleton in man. Anat. Rec., 73:189–207, 1939.

154. Larsson, E. M., Holtas, S., and Zygmunt, S.: Pre- and postoperative MR imaging of the craniocervical junction in rheumatoid arthritis. A.J.N.R., 10:89–94, 1989.

155. Larsson, S. E., and Toolamen, F.: Posterior fusion for atlanto-axial subluxation in rheumatoid arthritis. Spine, 11:525–530, 1986.

156. Latchaw, R. E., and Meyer, G. W.: Reiter's disease with atlanto-axial subluxation. Radiology, 126:303–304, 1978.

157. Lee, B. C. P., Deck, M. D. F., Kneeland, J. B., et al.: MR imaging of the craniocervical junction. Am. J. Neuroradiol., 6:209–213, 1985.

158. Lee, P. C., Chun, S. Y., and Loeng, J. C.: Experience of posterior surgery in atlanto-axial instability. Spine, 9:231–239, 1984.

159. Leventhal, M. R., Magurie, J. K., and Christian, C. A.: Atlantoaxial rotary subluxation in ankylosing spondylitis [Case report]. Spine, 15:1374–1376, 1990.

160. Levin, S.: The immune system and susceptibility to infections in Down's syndrome. In McCoy, E. E., and Epstein, C. J., eds.: Oncology and Immunology of Down's Syndrome. New York, Liss, 1987, pp. 143–162.

161. Lippmann, R. K.: Arthropathy due to adjacent inflammation. J. Bone Joint Surg. [Am.], 5:967–979, 1953.

162. Lipson, S. J.: Dysplasia of the odontoid in Morquio's syndrome causing quadriparesis. J. Bone Joint Surg. [Am.], 59:340–344, 1977.

163. Lipson, S. J.: Occipitocervical fusion using wired metal mesh and methacrylate backed bone graft. Orthop. Trans., 9:141, 1985.

164. List, C. F.: Neurologic syndromes accompanying developmental anomalies of occipital bone, atlas and axis. Arch. Neurol. Psychiatry, 45:577–616, 1941.

165. Luyendijk, W., Matricali, B., and Thomeer, R. T. W. M.: Basilar impression in an achondroplastic dwarf: Causative role in tetraparesis. Acta Neurochir., 41:243–253, 1978.

166. MacAlister, A.: Notes on the development and variations of the atlas. J. Anat. Physiol., 27:519, 1892–1893.

167. MacEwen, D.: The Klippel-Feil Syndrome. J. Bone Joint Surg. [Br.], 57:261–267, 1975.

168. MacKenzie, A. I., Uttley, D., Marsh, H. T., et al.: Craniocervical stabilization using Luque/Hartshill rectangles. Neurosurgery, 26:32–36, 1990.

169. MacKlenburg, R. S., and Krueger, P. M.: Extensive genito-urinary anomalies associated with Klippel-Feil Syndrome. Am. J. Disabled Child., 128:92–93, 1974.

170. Marin-Padilla, M., and Marin-Padilla, T.: Morphogenesis of experimentally induced Arnold-Chiari malformation. J. Neurol. Sci., 50:29–55, 1981.

171. Marks, J. S., and Sharp, J.: Rheumatoid cervical myelopathy. Q. J. Med., 199:307–319, 1981.

172. Maroteaux, P., and Lamy, M.: Hurler's disease, Morquio's disease, and related mucopolysaccharidoses. J. Pediatr., 67:312–323, 1965.

173. Martel, W.: The occipito-atlanto-axial joints in rheumatoid arthritis and ankylosis spondylitis. A.J.R., 86:223–240, 1961.

174. Martel, W., and Page, J. W.: Cervical vertebral erosions and subluxations in rheumatoid arthritis and ankylosing spondylitis. Arthritis Rheum., 3:546–556, 1960.

175. Martel, W., and Tishler, J. M.: Observations on the spine in mongoloidism. A.J.R., 97:630–638, 1966.

176. Mathews, J. A.: Atlanta-axial subluxation in rheumatoid arthritis. Ann. Rheum. Dis., 28:260–266, 1969.

177. Mathews, J. A.: Atlanta-axial subluxation in rheumatoid arthritis: A 5-year follow-up study. Ann. Rheum. Dis., 33:526–531, 1974.

178. Mayer, J. W., Messner, R. P., and Kaplan, R. J.: Brain stem compression in rheumatoid arthritis. J.A.M.A., 236:2094–2095, 1976.

179. McEwen, C., DiTata, D., and Lengg, C.: Ankylosing spondylitis and spondylitis accompanying ulcerative colitis, regional enteritis, psoriasis and Reiter's disease: A comparative study. Arthritis Rheum., 14:291–318, 1971.

180. McGregor, M.: The significance of certain measurements of the skull in the diagnosis of basilar impression. Br. J. Radiol., 21:171–181, 1948.

181. McRae, D. L.: Bony abnormalities in the region of the foramen magnum: Correlation of the anatomic and neurologic findings. Acta Radiol., 40:335–355, 1953.

182. McRae, D. L.: The significance of abnormalities of the cervical spine. A.J.R., *84*:3–25, 1960.
183. McRae, D. L., and Barnum, A. S.: Occipitalization of the atlas. A.J.R., *70*:23–46, 1953.
184. Melick, R. A., Ebeling, P., and Hjorth, R. J.: Improvement in paraplegia in vertebral Paget's disease treated with calcitonin. B.M.J., *1*:627, 1976.
185. Menezes, A. H.: Os odontoideum: Pathogenesis, dynamics and management. In Marlin, A. E., ed.: Concepts in Pediatric Neurosurgery. Vol. 8. Basel, Karger, 1988, pp. 133–145.
186. Menezes, A. H.: Anterior approaches to the craniocervical junction. In Congress of Neurological Surgeons: Clinical Neurosurgery. Vol. 37., Ch. 36. New York, Williams & Wilkins, 1991, pp. 756–769.
187. Menezes, A. H.: Surgical approaches to the craniocervical junction. In Frymoyer, J., ed.: The Adult Spine: Principles and Practice. Vol. 2., Ch. 46. New York, Raven Press, 1991, pp. 967–986.
188. Menezes, A. H.: Complications of surgery at the craniovertebral junction: Avoidance and management. Pediatr. Neurosurg., *17*:254, 1992.
189. Menezes, A. H.: Normal and abnormal development of the Craniocervical Junction. In Hoff, J. T., Crockard, A., Hayward, R., eds.: Neurosurgery: The Scientific Basis of Clinical Practice. 2nd ed. Ch. 15. London, Blackwell Scientific, 1992, pp. 63–83.
190. Menezes, A. H., and Ryken, T. C.: Craniovertebral abnormalities in Down's syndrome. Pediatr. Neurosurg., *18*:24–33, 1992.
191. Menezes, A. H., and Ryken, T. C.: Instrumentation of the craniocervical region. In Benzel, E., ed.: Spinal Instrumentation. Park Ridge, IL, American Association of Neurological Surgeons, 1994, pp. 47–62.
192. Menezes, A. H., and VanGilder, J. C.: Anomalies of the craniovertebral junction. In Youmans, J., ed.: Neurological Surgery. 3rd ed. Vol. 2, Ch. 45. Philadelphia, W. B. Saunders, 1990, pp. 1359–1420.
193. Menezes, A. H., Graf, C. J., and Hibri, N.: Abnormalities of the craniovertebral junction with cervicomedullary compression. Childs Brain, *7*:15–30, 1980.
194. Menezes, A. H., VanGilder, J. C., Clark, C. R., et al.: Odontoid upward migration in rheumatoid arthritis: An analysis of 45 patients with cranial settling. J. Neurosurg., *63*:500–509, 1985.
195. Michie, I., and Clark, M.: Neurological syndromes associated with cervical and craniocervical anomalies. Arch. Neurol., *18*:241–247, 1968.
196. Mikulowski, P., Wollheim, F. A., Rotmil, P., et al.: Sudden death in rheumatoid arthritis with atlanto-axial dislocation. Acta Med. Scand., *198*:445–451, 1975.
197. Mills, K. L., Scotland, T. R., Wardlaw, D., et al.: An implant clamp for atlanto-axial fusion. J. Neurol. Neurosurg. Psychiatry, *51*:450–451, 1988.
198. Minderhoud, J. M., Braakman, R., and Penning, L.: Os odontoideum: Clinical, radiological and therapeutic aspects. J. Neurol. Sci., *8*:521–544, 1969.
199. Mitsui, H.: A new operation for atlanto-axial arthrodesis. J. Bone Joint Surg. [Br.], *66*:422–425, 1984.
200. Murdoch, J. L., Walker, B. A., Hall, J. G., et al.: Achondroplasia: A genetic and statistical survey. Ann. Hum. Genet., *33*:227–236, 1970.
201. Nagib, M. G., Maxwell, R. E., and Chou, S. N.: Klippel-Feil syndrome in children: Clinical features and management. Childs Nerv. Syst., *1*:255–263, 1985.
202. Nakano, K. K., Schoene, W. C., Baker, R. A., et al.: The cervical myelopathy associated with rheumatoid arthritis: Analysis of 32 patients with 2 postmortem cases. Ann. Neurol., *3*:144–151, 1978.
203. Newman, P., and Sweetnam, R.: Occipito-cervical fusion: An operative technique and its indications. J. Bone Joint Surg. [Br.], *51*:423–431, 1969.
204. Nicholson, J. T., and Sherk, H. H.: Anomalies of the occipitocervical articulation. J. Bone Joint Surg. [Am.], *50*:295–304, 1968.
205. Ochiai, Y., Yamamoto, M., Takeshita, K., et al.: Myelopathy in infancy complicating congenital atlantoaxial dislocation. Am. J. Disabled Child., *130*:1270–1271, 1976.
206. Odelberg-Johnson, A.: A case of cervical spondylarthritis after tonsillectomy. Acta Orthop. Scand., *2*:302–306, 1931.
207. Oetterking, B.: On the morphological significance of certain craniovertebral variation. Anat. Rec., *25*:339–348, 1923.
208. Ogata, M., Ishikawa, K., and Ohira, T.: Cervical myelopathy in pseudogout. J. Bone Joint Surg. [Am.], *66*:1301–1303, 1984.
209. Okawara, S., and Nibbelink, D.: Vertebral artery occlusion following hyperextension and rotation of the head. Stroke, *5*:640–642, 1974.
210. O'Leary, P., Ranawat, C. S., and Pellicci, P. M.: The cervical spine in rheumatoid arthritis. Contemp. Surg., *7*:13–17, 1975.
211. Palant, D. I., and Carter, B. L.: Klippel-Feil syndrome and deafness. Am. J. Disabled Child., *123*:218–221, 1972.
212. Panjabi, M. M., Hopper, W., White, A. A., III, et al.: Posterior spine stabilization with methylmethacrylate: Biomechanical testing of a surgical specimen. Spine, *2*:241–247, 1977.
213. Papadopoulos, S. M., Dickman, C. A., and Sonntag, V. K.: Atlantoaxial stabilization in rheumatoid arthritis. J. Neurosurg., *74*:1–7, 1991.
214. Papadopoulos, S. M., Dickman, C. A., Sonntag, V. K., et al.: Traumatic atlanto-occipital dislocation with survival. Neurosurgery, *28*:574–579, 1991.
215. Paradis, R. W., and Sax, D. S.: Familial basilar impression. Neurology, *22*:554–560, 1972.
216. Parke, W. W.: The vascular relations of the upper cervical vertebrae. Orthop. Clin. North Am., *9*:879–889, 1978.
217. Parke, W. W., Rothman, R. H., and Brown, M. D.: The pharyngovertebral veins: An anatomical rationale for Grisel's syndrome. J. Bone Joint Surg. [Am.], *66*:568, 1984.
218. Pauli, R. M., and Gilbert, E. F.: Upper cervical cord compression as a cause of death in osteogenesis imperfecta type II. J. Pediatr., *108*:579, 1986.
219. Pellicci, P. M., Ranawat, C. S., Tsairis, P., et al. A prospective study of the progression of rheumatoid arthritis of the cervical spine. J. Bone Joint Surg. [Am.], *63*:342–346, 1981.
220. Penning, L.: Normal movements of the cervical spine. A.J.R., *130*:317–326, 1978.
221. Pizzutillo, P. D., Osterkamp, J. A., Scott, C. I., et al.: Atlantoaxial instability in mucopolysaccharidosis type VII. J. Pediatr. Orthop., *9*:76, 1989.
222. Poppel, M. H., Jacobson, H. G., Duff, B. K., et al.: Basilar impression and platybasia in Paget's disease. Radiology, *61*:639–644, 1953.
223. Potter, E. L., and Craig, J. M.: Pathology of the Fetus and the Infant. 3rd. ed. Chicago, Year Book Medical, 1975, pp. 550–557.
224. Pozo, J. L., Crockard, H. A., and Ransford, A. O.: Basilar impression in osteogenesis imperfecta: A report of three cases in one family. J. Bone Joint Surg. [Br.], *66*:233, 1984.
225. Pueschel, S. M., and Scola, F.: Atlantoaxial instability in individuals with Down's syndrome: Epidemiologic, radiographic and clinical studies. Pediatrics, *80*:555, 1987.
226. Pueschel, S. M., Herndon, J. H., Gelch, M. M., et al.: Symptomatic atlanto-axial subluxation in persons with Down's syndrome. J. Pediatr. Orthop., *4*:682–688, 1984.
227. Ranawat, C. S., O'Leary, P., Pellici, P., et al.: Cervical spine fusion in rheumatoid arthritis. J. Bone Joint Surg. [Am.], *61*:1003–1010, 1979.
228. Ransford, A. 0., Crockard, H. A., Pozo, J. L., et al.: Craniocervical instability treated by contoured loop fixation. J. Bone Joint Surg. [Am.], *68*:173–177, 1986.
229. Redlund-Johnell, I., and Pettersson, H.: Radiographic measurements of the craniovertebral region. Acta Radiol. Diagn., *25*:23–28, 1984.
230. Reid, C. S., Pyeritz, R. E., Kopits, S. E., et al.: Cervicomedullary compression in young patients with achondroplasia: Value of comprehensive neurologic and respiratory evaluation. J. Pediatr., *110*:522, 1987.
231. Resnick, D., and Pineda, C.: Vertebral involvement in calcium pyrophosphate dehydrate crystal deposition disease. Radiology, *153*:55–60, 1984.
232. Ricciardi, J. E., Kaufer, H., and Louis, D. S.: Acquired os odontoideum following acute ligament injury [Case report]. J. Bone Joint Surg. [Am.], *58*:410–412, 1976.
233. Rowland, L. P., Shapiro, J. H., and Jacobson, H. G.: Neurological syndromes associated with congenital absence of the odontoid process. Arch. Neurol. Psychiatry, *80*:286–291, 1958.
234. Roy-Camille, R., and Mazel, C.: Stabilization of the cervical

spine with posterior plates and screws. *In* Camins, M. B., and O'Leary, P. F., eds.: Disorders of the Cervical Spine. Baltimore, Williams & Wilkins, 1992, pp. 577–591.

235. Rush, P. J., Berbrayer, D., and Reilly, B. J.: Basilar impression and osteogenesis imperfecta in a 3 year old girl: CT and MRI. Pediatr. Radiol., *19*:142, 1989.

236. Ryken, T. C., and Menezes, A. H.: Cervicomedullary compression in achondroplasia. J. Neurosurg., *81*:43–48, 1994.

237. Sadeghpour, E., Noer, H. R., and Mahinpour, E. S.: Skull-C2 fusion in rheumatoid patients with atlanto-axial subluxation. Orthopaedics, *4*:1369–1374, 1981.

238. Saez, R. J., Onofrio, B. M., and Yanaghihara, T.: Experience with Arnold-Chiari malformation, 1960 to 1970. J. Neurosurg., *45*:416–422, 1976.

239. Sakou, T., Kawaida, H., Morizono, Y., et al.: Occipitoatlantoaxial fusion utilizing a rectangular rod. Clin. Orthop., *239*:136–144, 1989.

240. Santavirta, S., Sandelin, J., and Slatis, P.: Posterior atlanto-axial subluxation in rheumatoid arthritis. Acta Orthop. Scand., *56*:298–301, 1985.

241. Saway, P. A., Blackburn, W. D., Halla, J. T., et al.: Clinical characteristics affecting survival in patients with rheumatoid arthritis undergoing cervical spine surgery: A controlled study. J. Rheumatol., *16*:890–896, 1989.

242. Schiff, D. C. M., and Parke, W. W.: The arterial blood supply of the odontoid process (dens). Anat. Rec., *172*:399–400, 1972.

243. Schmidt, H., and Fischer, E.: Über zwei ver schiedene Formen der primaren basilaren impression. Fortschr. Rontgenstr., *88*:60–66, 1958.

244. Schmidt, H., and Fischer, E.: Über partielle einseitige synostosen zwischen Atlas und Axis. Fortschr. Rontgenstr., *92*:380–384, 1960.

245. Schmidt, H., Sartor, K., and Heckl, R. W.: Bone malformation of the craniocervical region. *In* Vinken, P. J., and Bruyn, A. W., eds.: Handbook of Clinical Neurology. Vol. 32. Amsterdam, Elsevier North-Holland, 1978, pp. 1–83.

246. Schneider, R. C., and Schemm, G. W.: Vertebral artery insufficiency in acute and chronic spinal trauma, with special reference to the syndrome of acute central cervical spinal cord injury. J. Neurosurg., *18*:348–360, 1961.

247. Schuller, A.: Diagnosis of "Basilar Impression." Radiology, *34*:214–216, 1940.

248. Scott, R. M.: Foramen magnum decompression in infants with homozygous achondroplasia [Letter]. J. Neurosurg., *72*:519, 1990; also Comment in J. Neurosurg., *70*:126, 1989.

249. Segal, L. E., Drummond, D. S., Zanotti, R. M., et al.: Complications of posterior arthrodesis of the cervical spine in patients who have Down's syndrome. J. Bone Joint Surg. [Am.], *73*:1547–1554, 1991.

250. Selecki, B. R.: The effects of rotation of the atlas on the axis: Experimental work. Med. J. Aust., *1*:1012, 1969.

251. Shapiro, R., and Robinson, F.: Anomalies of the craniovertebral border. A.J.R., *127*:281–287, 1976.

252. Shapiro, R., Youngberg, A. S., and Rothman, S. L. G.: The differential diagnosis of traumatic lesions of the occipito-atlanto-axial segment. Radiol. Clin. North Am., *11*:505–526, 1973.

253. Sharp, J., and Purser, D. W.: Spontaneous atlanto-axial dislocation in ankylosing spondylitis and rheumatoid arthritis. Ann. Rheum. Dis., *20*:47–77, 1961.

254. Shaul, W. L., Emery, H., and Hall, J.: Chondrodysplasia punctata and maternal Warfarin use during pregnancy. Am. J. Disabled Child., *129*:360–362, 1975.

255. Sherk, H. H.: Atlantoaxial instability and acquired basilar invagination in rheumatoid arthritis. Orthop. Clin. North Am., *9*:1053–1063, 1978.

256. Shikata, J., Yamamuro, T., Idia, H., et al.: Surgical treatment of achondroplastic dwarfs with paraplegia. Surg. Neurol., *29*:125, 1988.

257. Shoenfeld, Y., Fried A. and Ehrenfeld, N. E.: Osteogenesis imperfecta: Review of the literature with presentation of 29 cases. Am. J. Disabled Child., *129*:679, 1975.

258. Sillence, D. O., Senn, A. S., and Danks, D. M.: Genetic heterogeneity in osteogenesis imperfecta. J. Med. Genet., *16*:101, 1979.

259. Silman, A. J.: Rheumatoid arthritis and infection: A population approach. Ann. Rheum. Dis., *48*:707–710, 1989.

260. Silvernail, W. I., Brown, R. B., and Pool, C. C.: Medullospinal decompression and fusion for atlanto-axial dislocation due to hypoplastic separate odontoid. Pa. Med., *75*:58–60, 1972.

261. Singer, W. D., Haller, J. S., and Wolpert, S. M.: Occlusive vertebrobasilar artery disease associated with cervical spine anomaly. Am. J. Disabled Child., *129*:492–495, 1975.

262. Skok, P., Kapp, J., and Troland, C. E.: Spontaneous dislocation of the atlas: Case reports. J. Neurosurg., *21*:219–222, 1964.

263. Smith, R.: Osteogenesis imperfecta: Clin. Rheum. Dis., *12*:655, 1986.

264. Spence, K. F., Decker, S., Scott, K. W., et al.: Bursting atlantal fracture associated with rupture of the transverse ligament. J. Bone Joint Surg. [Am.], *52*:543–549, 1970.

265. Spierings, E. H., and Braakman, R.: The management of os odontoideum: Analysis of 37 cases. J. Bone Joint Surg. [Br.], *64*:422–428, 1982.

266. Spillane, J. D.: Three cases of achondroplasia with neurological complications. J. Neurol. Neurosurg. Psychiatry, *15*:246–252, 1952.

267. Spillane, J. D., Pallis, C., and Jones, A. M.: Developmental abnormalities in the region of the foramen magnum. Brain, *80*:11–48, 1957.

268. Spitzer, R., Rabinowitch, J. Y., and Wybar, K. C.: A study of the abnormalities of the skull, teeth and lenses in mongolism. Can. Med. Assoc. J., *84*:567–572, 1961.

269. Spranger, J. W., and Langer, L. O.: Spondyloepiphyseal dysplasia congenita. Radiology, *94*:313–322, 1970.

270. Spranger, J., Langer, L. O., and Wiedemann, H. R.: Spondyloepiphyseal dysplasia congenita. *In* Bone Dysplasia. Stuttgart, Gustav Fischer Verlag, 1974, pp. 95–103.

271. Steel, H. H.: Anatomical and mechanical considerations of the atlanto-axial articulations. J. Bone Joint Surg. [Am.], *50*:1481–1488, 1968.

272. Stokes, D. C., Phillips, J. A., Leonard, C. O., et al.: Respiratory complications of achondroplasia. J. Pediatr., *102*:534–538, 1983.

273. Sukoff, M. H., Kadin, M. M., and Moran, T.: Transoral decompression for myelopathy caused by rheumatoid arthritis of the cervical spine [Case report]. J. Neurosurg., *37*:493–497, 1972.

274. Sullivan, A. W.: Subluxation of the atlanto-axial joint: Sequel to inflammatory processes of the neck. J. Pediatr., *35*:451–469, 1949.

275. Swinson, D. R., Hamilton, E. B. D., Mathews, J. A., et al.: Vertical subluxation of the axis in rheumatoid arthritis. Ann. Rheum. Dis., *31*:359–363, 1972.

276. Taitsman, J. P., and Saha, S.: Tensile strength of wire-reinforced bone cement and twisted stainless steel wire. J. Bone Joint Surg. [Am.], *59*:419–425, 1977.

277. Tanzer, A.: Die basilare impression. Radiol. Clin., *25*:135–142, 1956.

278. Tasker, W. G., Mastfi, A. R., and Gold, A. P.: Chondroystrophia calcificans congenita (dysplasia epiphysalis punctata): Recognition of the clinical pitures. Am. J. Disabled Child., *119*:122–127, 1970.

279. Taylor, A. R., and Byrnes, D. P.: Foramen magnum and high cervical cord compression. Brain, *97*:473–480, 1974.

280. Taylor, A. R., and Chakravorty, B. C.: Clinical syndromes associated with basilar impression. Arch. Neurol., *10*:475–484, 1964.

281. Thompson, R. C., and Meyer, T. J.: Posterior surgical stabilization for atlantoaxial subluxation in rheumatoid arthritis. Spine, *10*:598–601, 1985.

282. Tishler, J., and Martel, W.: Dislocation of the atlas in mongolism. Radiology, *84*:904–906, 1965.

283. VanGilder, J. C., Menezes, A. H., and Dolan, K.: Craniovertebral Junction Abnormalities. Mt. Kisco, NY, Futura, 1987, pp. 1–255.

284. Vasey, F. B.: Psoriatic arthritis. *In* Schumacher, H. R., ed.: Primer in the Rheumatic Diseases. 9th ed. Atlanta, Arthritis Foundation, 1988.

285. VonTorklus, D., and Gehle, W., eds: The upper cervical spine: Regional anatomy, pathology and traumatology. *In* A Systemic Radiological Atlas and Textbook. New York, Grune & Stratton, 1972, pp. 1–99.

286. Wackenheim, A.: Radiologic diagnosis of congenital forms, intermittent forms and progressive forms of stenosis of the spinal canal of the level of the atlas. Acta Radiol. Diagn., *9*:481–486, 1969.

287. Waddell, J. P., and Reardon, A. P.: Atlantoaxial arthrodesis to treat odontoid fractures. Can. J. Surg., *26*:355–257.

288. Wadia, N. H.: Myelopathy complicating congenital atlanto-axial dislocation: A study of 28 cases. Brain, *90*:449–474, 1967.

289. Wald, S. L., and Schmidek, H. H.: Compressive myelopathy associated with type VI mucopolysaccharidosis (Maroteaux-Lamy syndrome). Neurosurg., *14*:83, 1984.

290. Warkany, J.: Congenital Malformations. Chicago, Year Book Medical Publishers, 1971, pp. 768–781.

291. Weil, V. H.: Osteogenesis imperfecta: Historical background. Clin. Orthop., *159*:6, 1981.

292. Weisel, S. W., and Rothman, R. H.: Occipitoatlantal hypermobility. Spine, *4*:187, 1979.

293. Weissman, B. N. W., Alliabadi, P., Weinfeld, M. S., et al.: Prognostic features of atlanto-axial subluxation in rheumatoid arthritis patients. Radiology, *144*:745–751, 1982.

294. Werne, S.: Studies in spontaneous atlas dislocation: The craniovertebral joints. Acta Orthop. Scand. Suppl., *23*:11–83, 1957.

295. Wetzel, F. T., and LaRocca, H.: Grisel's syndrome: A review. Clin. Orthop., *240*:141–152, 1989.

296. White, A. A., III, and Panjabi, M. M.: The clinical biomechanics of the occipito-atlantoaxial complex. Orthop. Clin. North Am., *9*:867–878, 1978.

297. Wholey, M. H., Bruwer, A. J., and Baker, H. L.: The lateral roentgenogram of the neck with comments on the atlanto-odontoid-basion relationship. Radiology, *71*:350–356, 1958.

298. Wilson, B. C., Jarvis, B. L., and Handon, R. C.: Nontraumatic subluxation of the atlantoaxial joint: Grisel's syndrome. Ann. Otol. Rhinol. Laryngol., *96*:705, 1987.

299. Winfield, J., Cooke, D., Brook, A. S., et al.: A prospective study of the radiological changes in early rheumatoid disease. Ann. Rheum. Dis., *40*:109–114, 1981.

300. Winfield, J., Cooke, D., Brook, A. S., et al.: A prospective study of the radiological changes in the cervical spine in early rheumatoid arthritis. Ann. Rheum. Dis., *42*:613–618, 1983.

301. Wittek, A.: Ein Fall Von Distensionsluxation in atlanto-epistropheal gelenke. Munch. Med. Wschr., *55*:1836–1837, 1908.

302. Wollin, D. G.: The os odontoideum: Separate odontoid process. J. Bone Joint Surg. [Am.], *45*:1459–1471, 1963.

303. Wycis, H. T.: Basilar impression platybasia: A case secondary to advanced Paget's disease with severe neurological manifestations. Successful surgical result. J. Neurosurg., *1*:299, 1944.

304. Wynne-Davies, R., Hall, C. M., Young, I. D.: Pseudoachondroplasia: Clinical diagnosis at different ages and comparison of autosomal dominant and recessive types. A review of 32 patients (26 kindreds). J. Med. Genet., *23*:425, 1986.

305. Yadon, R., Dumas, J. M., and Karsh, J.: Lateral subluxation of the cervical spine in psoriatic arthritis. Arthritis Rheum., *26*:109–111, 1983.

306. Zingesser, L. H.: Radiological aspects of anomalies of the upper cervical spine and craniocervical junction. Clin. Neurosurg., *20*:220–231, 1972.

307. Zvaifler, N. J.: Rheumatoid arthritis: Epidemiology, etiology, rheumatoid factor, pathology, pathogenesis. *In* Schumacher, H. R., ed.: Primer on the Rheumatic Diseases. 9th ed. Atlanta, Arthritis Foundation, 1988.

308. Zygmunt, S., Saveland, H., Brattstrom, H., et al.: Reduction of rheumatoid periodontoid pannus following posterior occipitocervical fusion visualized by magnetic resonance imaging. Br. J. Neurosurg., *2*:315–320, 1988.

Syringomyelia, Chiari Malformation, and Hydromyelia

Definitions

SYRINGOMYELIA AND HYDROMYELIA

Strictly defined, "syringomyelia" is a tubular cavitation (i.e., cyst) of the spinal cord extending over many segments.[14] As such, the term does not specify the location of this cavity with respect to the central canal and does not describe the histology of the wall of the cyst nor the character of the fluid within the cyst; it also does not concern itself with the cause or pathogenesis of the cyst. For this reason, syringomyelia is an all-inclusive term, embracing cysts of diverse nature, including cerebrospinal fluid containing post-traumatic cysts, cysts associated with abnormalities at the craniovertebral junction, and cysts associated with intramedullary tumors. "Hydromyelia," a term introduced by Simon, is more specific and was used to describe intramedullary cavities thought to represent a distended central canal, lined by ependyma, and containing fluid identical with cerebrospinal fluid.[72] The distinction was drawn between hydromyelia, as here described, and syringomyelia, reported as a condition in which the cyst was located within the actual substance of the cord, that is, a cyst that was not simply an expansion of the central canal, and therefore lined by glial tissue rather than ependyma.

Current usage employs the term syringomyelia for all cysts of the spinal cord, with the exception of most cysts associated with intramedullary tumors whose xanthochromic, proteinaceous fluid can be regarded as a product of the tumors, analogous to certain cystic glial tumors of the cerebrum. This more general definition of syringomyelia is supported by the observations that cysts that might have originated from the central canal may expand in an irregular pattern throughout the spinal cord, although mostly sparing the posterior columns; as they expand they may leave only scattered islands of their former ependymal lining, much of the remainder of the surface being glial. The hydrodynamics of the lesions all seem identical as judged by modern flow-gated imaging techniques.[33] Communication with the fourth ventricle, once thought common in hydromyelia (although d'Angers called it syringomyelia), is recognized as being infrequent.[59, 77] For this reason, syringomyelia is the term generally used in the medical literature today to describe intramedullary cysts with cerebrospinal fluid–like content, thus excluding tumor cysts and parasitic cysts. Syringomyelia is used in this sense throughout the remainder of this chapter.

Syringobulbia represents an upward extension of the cystic cavity into the brain stem.[86]

HINDBRAIN HERNIATION (CHIARI MALFORMATION)

The strict definition of hindbrain herniation is that provided by Chiari in his 1891 publication, which was based on a study of autopsy material.[17] It represents downward displacement of portions of the cerebellum, the fourth ventricle, and pons, ranging in degree from type I (elongation of the cerebellar tonsils into conical extensions that accompany the medulla into the cervical canal) to type II (downward displacement of the vermis, fourth ventricle, and lower brain stem into the spinal canal) and type III (displacement of nearly the entire cerebellum as well as the fourth ventricle into the cervical canal). All of these degrees of cerebellar displacement, or ectopia, were believed to be the result of hydrocephalus. Slight dilatation of the central canal was noted in 3 of 14 type I cases, while intramedullary cysts were described in association with the type II and type III abnormalities. Chiari's original type I case was in a 17-year-old young woman; the other types were described in infants.[17] Chiari's later publication ex-

U. Batzdorf

panded on his early descriptions and included additional patients.[18]

The early contribution of Cleland as well as the later contribution by Arnold are recognized, but the preferred designation of Chiari malformation is now generally used.[3, 22] Current usage of the term "Chiari malformation" recognizes that downward displacement of the cerebellar tonsils and hindbrain may exist with or without an associated intramedullary cyst, although at present one can only speculate on the explanation for these two variants. Furthermore, it is now established that the Chiari malformation is only one of numerous abnormalities that may exist at the craniovertebral junction and which may be associated with an intramedullary cavity. Lastly, it is by no means clear that cerebellar tonsil displacement is always in the nature of a "mal-formation," and numerous instances of cerebellar ectopia following lumbar cerebrospinal fluid shunting are now documented.[20, 21, 34, 63] Current usage of the "type" designations also tends to be less rigid; thus, type I cases often show some downward displacement of the fourth ventricle by magnetic resonance imaging and on surgical exploration and there is a gradient of progressively more severe tonsillar ectopia.[55] Type I abnormalities are seen in children as young as 10 years old. The type II malformation is characterized by downward displacement of the cerebellar vermis, fourth ventricle, and brain stem below the foramen magnum; although the tonsils may be below the foramen magnum, they are described as rudimentary in some cases.[18] The displaced vermis and fourth ventricle characterize this abnormality. The most severe form of cerebellar ectopia, designated as Chiari type III, is identified in infants. Most of the cerebellum and brain stem are displaced below the foramen magnum. It appears to be incompatible with normal life if left untreated, and even with appropriate treatment these infants have a poorer prognosis than patients with type I and II malformations.

SHUNT-RELATED HINDBRAIN HERNIATION

Descent of the cerebellar tonsils after shunting of lumbar subarachnoid fluid out of the spinal canal may result in tonsillar descent, as first described by Fischer and associates.[34] With magnetic resonance imaging, more recent reports have shown that tonsillar descent is quite common in children who have undergone lumbar cerebrospinal fluid shunting[20]; syringomyelic cavities may also develop in this situation.[34] The tonsillar descent is reversible, so that when the lumbar shunt is eliminated, the tonsils appear to have the ability to return to their former, strictly intracranial, position.[63]

Anatomy and Physiology

The evolution of concepts of the pathophysiology of syringomyelia and hindbrain herniation can best be considered from three different perspectives: (1) mechanisms for hindbrain herniation and tonsillar descent, (2) mechanisms by which fluid may enter the spinal cord, and (3) the behavior of fluid within the spinal cord cystic cavities.

PROPOSED MECHANISMS FOR HINDBRAIN HERNIATION AND TONSILLAR DISPLACEMENT

Chiari believed that hydrocephalus, which he diagnosed at autopsy in all 14 of his type I cases and in all 7 of his type II cases, was the primary event and pushed the brain out of the skull.[18] He suggested that perhaps hydrocephalus developed earlier in fetal life in the type II cases, thereby accounting for the two different types. Penfield and Coburn, and later Lichtenstein, believed that tethering of the spinal cord by a myelomeningocele pulled the brain stem and tonsils through the foramen magnum with axial growth.[50, 64] A variant of this concept was proposed by Roth, who envisioned that the myelomeningocele prevents normal downward migration of the neuraxis, resulting in an upward push of the cervical-medullary junction with resulting kinking of the brain stem and "overflow" of the cerebellar tonsils through the foramen magnum.[67] The experimental work of Goldstein and Kepes puts such theories in doubt.[39]

Patten, as well as Daniel and Strich, favored the concept that hindbrain herniation represented a failure of the normal brain stem flexures to form in embryonic life[24, 61]; the not infrequent occurrence of associated abnormalities of bone structure, such as basilar invagination, atlanto-occipital assimilation, and the midline posterior fossa keel, and the abnormalities of the dura, such as the vascular lakes between the dural leaves, have been cited in support of this theory.

Müller and O'Rahilly postulated a disproportional development in size of the posterior fossa contents and the enclosing skull.[57] The finding of a small or shallow posterior fossa in patients with Chiari malformation has been cited in support of this concept. Gardner believed there was failure of development of the normal outlet foramina of the fourth ventricle and that the arterial pulse wave was transmitted to the cerebrospinal fluid, impacting the tonsils into the foramen magnum.[36, 38] Van Hoytema and van den Berg postulated that the posterior medullary velum remains intact in Chiari II malformations, resulting in downward prolongation of the vermis with growth.[74]

A pressure gradient between the intracranial and spinal compartments resulting in downward herniation of the medulla, which then becomes draped over the cervical dentate ligaments, was cited by Emery and Mackenzie.[32] The tonsils were believed to be pulled down secondarily. Williams believes that birth trauma may be an etiological factor, with local tonsillar edema and arachnoid scarring, perhaps aided by excessive head molding, setting the stage for tonsillar impaction.[81]

Carmel believes that the pathogenesis of the type I

and type II malformation have little in common and cites morphogenetic evidence in support of this argument.[16] McLone and Knepper believe that lack of distention of the embryonic and fetal ventricular system in the presence of a myelomeningocele is the underlying mechanism for the development of the Chiari II malformation.[52]

MECHANISMS FOR ENTRY OF FLUID INTO THE SPINAL CORD

Different explanations have been offered for the presence or entry of fluid into the spinal cord in patients with hindbrain herniation associated with syringomyelia as well as for those patients with primarily spinal forms of cyst formation.

Chiari believed that fluid was present in the cord because of persistence of an embryological state: embryological hydromyelia associated with hydrocephalus.[17, 18] Gardner believed that the arterially generated pulse wave deflected cerebrospinal fluid into the central canal of the cord through an opening near the obex because the normal outlet foramina of the fourth ventricle were not open.[36, 38] Isotope studies showing cerebrospinal fluid flow into the central canal have been cited in support of this concept.[43]

Ball and Dayan, noting evidence that only about 10 per cent of patients show a communication between the fourth ventricle and the syringeal cavity, proposed that subarachnoid fluid dissects into the cord along the Virchow-Robin spaces when tonsillar impaction prevents upward escape of the fluid[5]; secondary entry of this fluid into the central canal was envisioned. Aboulker suggested a somewhat similar concept, with fluid believed to enter the cord along the dorsal roots.[1] The now well-recognized phenomenon of transparenchymal migration of water-soluble contrast lends support to these concepts.[4] Oldfield and colleagues, on the other hand, postulate that, in the presence of tonsillar impaction, systolic pressure waves on the surface of the cord may force cerebrospinal fluid into the cord along perivascular and interstitial spaces.[59]

Cardiac-gated cine-mode magnetic resonance imaging confirms the existence of cerebrospinal fluid flow velocity profile abnormalities at the foramen magnum in patients with Chiari I malformation.[2] This development of magnetic resonance imaging technology is based on the sensitivity of T2-weighted images to fluid motion, with loss of signal when motion exceeds a certain threshold. Using cine-magnetic-resonance data acquisition, fluid motion can be recorded as a function of the cardiac cycle.[33]

Williams proposed that subarachnoid fluid is forced upward past the tonsils with coughing or Valsalva maneuvers by distention of epidural veins but that the tonsils act as a ball valve and prevent fluid from returning along the same pathway, creating a pressure differential[81]; instead, the cerebrospinal fluid is sucked into the central canal as a result of this craniospinal pressure dissociation.

Milhorat and co-workers have suggested that fluid

produced by the ependyma accumulates when viral ependymitis scars over the outlet of the central canal at its most rostral end.[56] Cerebrospinal fluid production by the ependyma of the central canal had been proposed by Cornil and Mosinger.[23]

In the case of post-traumatic spinal cord cavitation, it has been suggested that tissue necrosis and hematomyelia occurring after a cord injury are the precursors of an intramedullary cyst, which presumably develops as the blood elements are resorbed.[11, 89] The appearance of post-traumatic spinal cord cavitation after very minor spinal trauma raises questions about this theory, or at least its general applicability.[9, 47] It is likely that subarachnoid scarring develops after trauma and can act in a manner analogous to hindbrain herniation to impede rapid pressure equilibration within the subarachnoid space proximal and distal to the scar (spinal-spinal pressure dissociation). This circumstance may then also favor entry of fluid into the spinal cord by one of the mechanisms cited earlier. Work in the author's laboratory and the study of Cho and associates support the concept that subarachnoid scarring plays a major role in the development of post-traumatic spinal cord cavitation.[19, 76] The sometimes sizable subarachnoid cysts or pouches resulting from scar adhesions may be considered as acting in a manner analogous to the cerebellar tonsils in reducing normal cerebrospinal fluid flow (Fig. 43–1A).

MECHANISMS FOR EXPANSION OF FLUID CAVITIES WITHIN THE CORD

It is generally accepted that, at least in some situations, a fluid cavity within the cord, once established, will expand. Certain slitlike cavities imaged in the vicinity of osteophytic bars of the cervical spine may represent exceptions, perhaps because there is little or no associated arachnoid scarring. Undoubtedly, in the majority of patients with spine injury, cyst formation does not occur, perhaps for similar reasons. Various theories have been proposed for the mechanisms by which an intramedullary cyst once formed may expand. Gardner proposed progressive dissection from above through the opening at the rostral end of the central canal.[36, 37] Ball and Dayan postulated that fluid dissecting into the cord parenchyma would ultimately coalesce and rupture into the central canal.[5] Aboulker's theory was similar.[1]

Williams and associates proposed a type of to-and-fro fluid dissection within the cord in response to pressure differentials initiated by epidural venous distention occurring after normal physiological events such as coughing and straining.[89] Enzmann's observation on flow patterns of cerebrospinal fluid as visualized by cardiac-gated cine-mode magnetic resonance imaging support the concept that very different cerebrospinal fluid flow forces apply to subarachnoid cerebrospinal fluid and fluid within the cystic cavity.[33] The study by Oldfield and co-workers provides evidence that a systolic pressure wave of the subarachnoid cerebrospi-

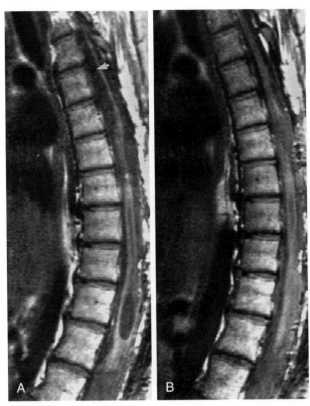

Figure 43–1

A. Thoracic spine magnetic resonance image of a 28-year-old woman who had undergone multiple resections of a spinal cord ependymoma. Note the large distended subarachnoid pouch anterior to the spinal cord (*arrow*) and the more distal syrinx cavity. The patient presented with increasing lower extremity dysfunction. Sagittal T1-weighted magnetic resonance image. B. Postoperative image showing collapse of the syrinx cavity after drainage of the subarachnoid pouch into the pleural cavity. There was no recurrence of tumor. The syrinx itself was not directly approached. Sagittal T2-weighted magnetic resonance image obtained 2 months after surgical procedure.

nal fluid, applied against the surface of the spinal cord, will force syrinx fluid downward within the cyst.[59]

Types of Syringomyelia

Although it is not known exactly why fluid enters into the spinal cord in patients who develop syringomyelia, there appears to be a feature common to all patients who develop syringomyelia: significant, but not necessarily hydrodynamically total, obstruction of the subarachnoid space, which may be quite focal and which prevents the normally near-instantaneous pressure equilibration under such physiological circumstances as coughing or straining. Two general anatomical sites are recognized at which such abnormalities may be associated with syringomyelia: the craniocervical junction and the spinal level. Abnormalities at the craniocervical junction include the following:

1. Bone abnormalities: basilar invagination, platybasia, bone tumors

2. Arachnoid scarring: post-traumatic, postinfectious, postinflammatory

3. Subarachnoid space compression due to hindbrain and cerebellar tonsil or vermis impaction

4. Fourth ventricle cysts (Dandy-Walker)

5. Tumors, extrinsic and intrinsic, at the craniovertebral junction

Abnormalities at the spinal level include the following:

1. Post-traumatic arachnoid scarring, including postsurgical scarring

2. Postinflammatory arachnoid scarring

3. Subarachnoid space compression due to tumor

4. Subarachnoid space compression or scarring in relation to spondylitic disease

Natural History

IN INFANTS: CHIARI II MALFORMATION

All infants with myelomeningocele have magnetic resonance imaging evidence of Chiari II malformation.[68] In the experience of Vandertop and colleagues, 21 per cent of 405 patients with myelomeningocele developed symptoms related to a Chiari II malformation.[75] More than 90 per cent of these children develop hydrocephalus.[15] Park, as well as DiRocco, noted that signs of Chiari malformation develop in some patients with myelomeningocele even though their hydrocephalus is well controlled.[25, 60] Hindbrain dysfunction was found to be responsible for 73 per cent of deaths of children with myelomeningocele.[68]

A review of a group of 17 infants with Chiari II malformation aged 1 month or younger showed that 71 per cent presented with swallowing difficulty, 59 per cent with stridor, 29 per cent with apneic spells, 12 per cent with aspiration, 18 per cent with weak cry, and 53 per cent with arm weakness.[75] These symptoms may be due to both cranial nerve palsies and direct brain stem compression or distortion. The respiratory and swallowing difficulties may lead to a fatal outcome. Occasionally a patient will survive infancy, and limb weakness and spasticity then appear to dominate the clinical picture.[15, 16]

Menezes and associates reported treating six infants with Chiari III malformation but did not detail their mode of presentation or outcome.[55]

IN ADULTS

Hindbrain Herniation (Chiari Malformation) Cerebellar Ectopia Without Syringomyelia

The diagnosis of Chiari I malformation, also variously referred to as hindbrain herniation and cerebellar ectopia, is being made with increased frequency since the availability of magnetic resonance imaging. Many of the patients now diagnosed and treated would, in

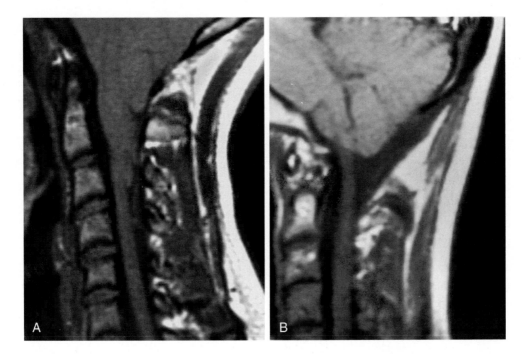

Figure 43–2

A. Chiari II malformation in a 20-year-old man who had undergone repair of a myelomeningocele and ventricular shunting at birth with recognition of the Chiari malformation at birth. He presented with symptoms of headache sometimes accompanied by lethargy and vomiting and of tingling with occasional spasm of the hands. All symptoms improved after decompressive laminectomy at C1 to C3 with placement of a dural graft. *B.* A 38-year-old woman presented with long-standing symptoms of suboccipital headache. Chiari I malformation without syringomyelia was found. Note the enlarged cisterna magna that resulted from dural decompression, leaving the arachnoid intact. Her headache resolved after surgery. Sagittal T1-weighted magnetic resonance image obtained 9 months after surgery.

previous years, have been treated rather less effectively with medication for "tension headache" or headache of unknown origin (Fig. 43–2).

It remains very difficult to determine whether tonsillar descent and impaction in a given patient would progress if untreated and whether such a patient would develop syringomyelia over the course of time. Patients seen in the author's clinic seem to fall into two groups. One group presents with suboccipital headache as the primary complaint; these patients have mostly small but significant degrees of tonsillar descent. The second, less common group includes patients with headache and lower cranial nerve symptoms; extensive tonsil molding and descent is seen in this group of patients. If left untreated, the patients in this second group would appear to be at risk of sudden death due to medullary compression. The forces of intracranial fluid dynamics favor progressive tonsillar impaction, once the process has started. Cough headache may be a particularly noteworthy and characteristic symptom in this group of patients.[82]

Hindbrain Herniation (Chiari Malformation) with Syringomyelia

The natural history of this group of patients is probably related mostly to the potential for enlargement of the syringomyelic cavity. Coughing and other physiological Valsalva-like maneuvers have the potential not only of acting on the tonsils but also of producing sudden rostrocaudal extension of a distended syringomyelic cavity, with resulting increase in neurological deficit. The clinical history of many patients reveals evidence of such progressive neurological impairment, which is often insidious but sometimes clearly associated with coughing episodes.[35] Very few patients with a distended syringeal cavity are left untreated today, and it is therefore impossible to state whether a patient with numbness in one upper extremity found to have a small cervical cavity extending over two spinal segments would ultimately evolve into a severely disabled, wheelchair-bound patient with claw hands and a holocord syrinx. Very few patients are now seen for the first clinic visit with such advanced disability (Fig. 43–3A). The clearest evidence for the potential progression of an intraspinal cyst comes from the documentation of patients with post-traumatic syringomyelia, many of whom were already under neurological surveillance when progression became evident. The hydrodynamics of an intramedullary cystic cavity studied by Williams, Enzmann, and Oldfield and associates allow us to understand readily how progressive extension of a syringomyelic cavity could take place.[33, 59, 81, 82]

PRIMARILY SPINAL FORMS

Barnett and Jousse called attention to the potential for sudden progression of so-called post-traumatic syringomyelia, although earlier instances of such had

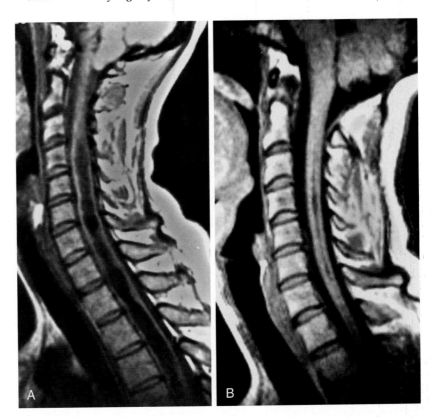

Figure 43–3

A. Distended syrinx cavity in a 44-year-old woman, extending from C3–C4 to T6. Note the characteristic Chiari I malformation with pointed tonsil tips that extend to the inferior margin of the C1 arch. *B.* Postoperative image showing collapse of the syrinx cavity and partial ablation of the cerebellar tonsils; in this patient titanium clips were applied to compress very gliottic tonsil tips. There is a generous cisterna magna. Midsagittal T1-weighted magnetic resonance image obtained 30 months after surgical procedure.

been recorded and were summarized by them.[9] The same authors also noted the frequently prolonged time interval (often measured in years) between spine injury and the development of neurological manifestations of a progressive process. Barnett and Jousse also described three patients with less severe spinal injuries who later developed syringomyelia.[11] The author has had experience with patients who have had seemingly trivial spine injuries without any initial neurological deficit who developed typical syringomyelia after an interval of years.[47] The intramedullary cysts that develop in patients after tuberculous meningitis probably also evolve over a period of months or years and also have the potential for gradual enlargement. Unrelenting or progressive spinal pain may be a manifestation of dural stretching due to a distended intramedullary cyst. Progression of neurological deficit after severe spinal injury classically occurs in a cephalad direction. Focal adherence of the arachnoid at the point of injury can sometimes be demonstrated by myelography or magnetic resonance imaging in the post-traumatic patient, while multiple sites of arachnoid scarring may be seen in post-tuberculous syringomyelia.

Syringomyelia may occur after surgical removal of spinal cord tumors (see Fig. 43–1*A*). The most flagrant example of this was encountered in a patient whose surgery for excision of a cervical meningioma was complicated by a wound infection and meningitis. Scar tissue formation compromising the subarachnoid space at the level of surgery can be envisioned to produce conditions analogous to those seen after spine trauma or infection. Undoubtedly, individuals differ greatly in the tendency to develop arachnoid scar tissue, even

under essentially similar provocative circumstances. Spinal cord tumors may, however, also be associated with true syringomyelia. An extensive spinal cord cyst, not contiguous to the tumor nodule, was encountered in a patient with a thoracic hemangioblastoma and gradually resolved after the tumor had been excised. Focal compression of the subarachnoid space by a tumor can be conceived of as setting up conditions similar to those described in other situations of primarily spinal syringomyelia, although one would hope that scarring has not taken place, so that the underlying mechanism is reversible once the tumor has been removed.

"ARRESTED HYDROMYELIA" AND SLITLIKE CAVITIES

As our experience with magnetic resonance imaging increases, it appears that there are some patients who have intramedullary cystic cavities that appear nondistended. A number of these slitlike cavities have been seen in juxtaposition to spondylotic bars in the cervical region. Clinically, these patients have so far been found to be stable, and conceivably they can be monitored over a period of time with additional magnetic resonance imaging. It is not understood why the cavities remain undistended and thus not subject to the forces that produce dissection in a rostrocaudal direction, as in the case of a distended cavity. We do not as yet know whether there might be a fluid equilibrium state in these patients, not present in patients with a distended syrinx cavity, allowing the cyst-filling dynamics to be "arrested." It is also quite possible that these patients have less complete obstruction of the subarachnoid space, whether by compression or scarring, than those whose intramedullary cysts progressively expand. In situations in which a cyst fails to expand, or contract postoperatively, there could theoretically also be a factor of reduced spinal cord compliance.

Diagnosis and Clinical Presentation

HINDBRAIN HERNIATION (CHIARI I MALFORMATION) INCLUDING SYRINGOMYELIA

Most reports of symptoms and signs seen in patients with Chiari malformation or hindbrain herniation do not distinguish between symptoms seen in patients without and with syringomyelia.[30, 35, 62, 69] In part, this is because in patient series compiled before the routine use of magnetic resonance imaging syringomyelia often was not or could not be diagnosed with certainty before surgical exploration. Syringobulbia was even more difficult to diagnose on clinical grounds alone. In the author's experience with a small number of patients who had only tonsillar descent without syringomyelia, headache was clearly the dominant symptom. The headache was suboccipital and exacerbated by exertion, coughing, and straining, as had been pointed out by other authors previously.[35] It was quite often severe and debilitating to the point of interfering greatly with a patient's life and work. Lower cranial nerve symptoms were present in only one of these patients without syringomyelia, a person with severe molding of the tonsils down to C2.

Headache of the same character is also a very significant symptom in patients who have hindbrain herniation as well as syringomyelia. Table 43–1 summarizes the presenting symptoms in four larger series that, however, do not distinguish between symptoms in the syringomyelic group from those with simple tonsillar descent.

The shoulder girdle sensory deficit often takes on the classic "suspended sensory deficit" pattern first described by Gowers.[40]

Some authors prefer to group these symptoms into broader syndrome categories:

	Saez et al.[69] (%)	Paul et al.[62] (%)
Foramen magnum compression	38.3	22.0
Paroxysmal intracranial hypertension	21.7	37.0
Central cord disturbance	20.0	65.0
Cerebellar dysfunction	10.0	11.0
Spasticity	6.7	
Bulbar palsy	3.3	

Certainly differences in the proportion of patients with hindbrain herniation alone and those with an associated syringomyelia would explain some of the differences noted in the incidence of various clinical symptoms.

CLINICAL PRESENTATION OF HINDBRAIN HERNIATION IN INFANCY (CHIARI II MALFORMATION)

Many of the infants with Chiari II malformation are born with a myelomeningocele; all infants with myelomeningocele were found to have a Chiari II malformation by magnetic resonance imaging criteria.[68] Hydrocephalus is almost always present in these infants.[15] The clinical picture has already been noted in the section on natural history. Newborns often present with severe respiratory stridor, apnea, facial nerve palsies, lack of gag reflex, and quadriparesis.[68] DiRocco points out that symptoms appear to stabilize or even improve after the first year of life[25]; a small number of infants, however, die of respiratory problems early in life. Nystagmus is described as relatively frequent; opisthotonus is also seen in a significant number of these infants.

In older children the presentation is less acute and is manifested by nystagmus, weakness or spasticity of the upper limbs, and limb or truncal ataxia as well as neck pain and swallowing difficulties.[68] Cranial lacunae, or Lückenschädel, are seen in a large number of children with Chiari II malformations.[16, 52] Scoliosis often develops as the child grows.[43, 44, 80] The typical pattern of shoulder girdle sensory deficit may also be seen in children.[44] An overall mortality of 34 per cent was noted in one series of children with Chiari II malformation.[62]

IMAGING

Syringomyelia is best demonstrated by magnetic resonance imaging, which will also disclose most of the associated soft tissue abnormalities at the craniocervical junction, such as hindbrain herniation and a retained rhombic roof. Plain radiographs of the skull and upper cervical spine are very helpful in revealing bone abnormalities of the skull and craniocervical junction, including platybasia, a midline keel, and assimilation of the atlas. Occasionally, plain radiographs reveal an anomalous course of the vertebral artery by the presence of vascular ostia in the lamina of C1. Only patients who cannot undergo magnetic resonance imaging should be studied by myelography and delayed (4- to 12-hour) computed tomography. Accumulation of contrast medium within the cyst is seen in many, but evidently not all, intramedullary cysts.[4, 33]

Water-soluble contrast myelography also plays a role in the diagnosis of post-traumatic spinal cord cavitation. Observation of the flow of contrast medium under fluoroscopy may demonstrate a focal area of subarachnoid scarring, which has direct implications for the treatment of this type of syringomyelia.

Cardiac-gated cine-mode magnetic resonance T2-weighted imaging permits a study of cerebrospinal fluid flow patterns.[33, 59] It is becoming more important in distinguishing hydrodynamically active syrinx cavities from cavities with little pulsatile flow, which may also be expected to show less benefit from surgical

Table 43-1

MOST COMMON PRESENTING SYMPTOMS IN PATIENTS WITH CHIARI MALFORMATION WITH AND WITHOUT SYRINGOMYELIA*

Author	No. of Patients	Age Range in Years	Headache (%)	Neck Pain (%)	Limb Pain Arm/Leg (%)	Limb Weakness (%)	Limb Numbness (%)	Unsteadiness or Vertigo Ataxia (%)	Leg Stiffness (%)	Blurred Vision or Diplopia (%)	Dysphagia (%)	Tinnitus (%)	Vomiting (%)	Dysarthria (%)	Oscillopsia (%)
Foster & Hudgson[35]	100	6–63	14	24	16/—		28	3	42	4					6
Saez et al.[69]	60	10–69	42	23 17†	23/5	32	47	42	7	23	27	8		3	
Paul et al.[62]	71	15–66	34	13	8/3	56	52	40		13	8‡	7	5	4	
Dyste et al.[30]	50	1–57	24	18	12/4	60	34	32		6	6	2	2	4	

*Percentages are rounded to nearest integer.
†Suboccipital pain listed separately.
‡Listed as dysphasia.

therapy.[33] This diagnostic technique also may prove helpful in evaluating patients with simple tonsillar descent and distinguishing those with abnormal cerebrospinal fluid flow dynamics, who might benefit from surgery. Patients with normal cerebrospinal fluid dynamics would be unlikely to change with surgery.[2]

Pathology

Different types of pathological processes at the craniovertebral junction can produce the conditions that favor development of a syrinx cavity. These include the following:

1. Abnormalities of the bone structure around the foramen magnum, skull base, and upper cervical spine; abnormalities of the dura in the region of the foramen magnum such as dural bands and venous lakes[62]
2. Arachnoid scarring at the fourth ventricle outlet–tonsillar area
3. Hindbrain herniation
4. Fourth ventricle cysts (Dandy-Walker) and retained rhombic roof
5. Neoplasms at the craniovertebral junction, including extrinsic and intrinsic tumors

Whereas Chiari described and classified the degrees of hindbrain herniation, pathologists, surgeons, and modern imaging specialists have subsequently been able to add to the spectrum of more subtle associated derangements of anatomy seen with the so-called Chiari malformation.[71] Communication of the cyst with the fourth ventricle, assumed by Gardner to be present in all instances, is in fact seen in at most 10 per cent of patients who have a Chiari malformation with syringomyelia.[77] Oldfield and associates were not able to demonstrate such a communication in any of their patients.[59] In some individuals the cerebellar tonsils may be invested with densely scarred arachnoid, while in many other adult patients the tonsils, "jammed" into the foramen magnum, can be gently mobilized from the medullary-spinal junction and separated from each other. The tips of the tonsils can often be gliotic; in one patient the author encountered a small piece of cerebellar tissue that had been amputated by chronic compression. Beaking of the midbrain tectum is often recognized on magnetic resonance images. The fourth ventricle is displaced caudad to varying degrees, and with this downward elongation of the brain stem the cranial nerves may also be placed on stretch. Similarly, the upper cervical spinal roots angulate upward to reach their exit foramina. There may be a Z-shaped deformity at the medullary-cervical junction, occasionally seen on magnetic resonance images.[32] Large, distended cysts may show "haustrations" or more-or-less complete septations, which may represent stages in the rostrocaudal expansion of the cystic cavity. The septations may appear complete on a particular sagittal image, although in fact extending only part way across a cavity. Incomplete drainage of a complex cyst, however, suggests that some cavities are truly septate.

In Chiari type II anomalies a retained posterior medullary velum may be seen; major downward displacement of the cerebellar vermis, fourth ventricle, and brain stem is encountered in this anomaly; the foramen magnum is generally enlarged and medullary kinking is seen.[16, 68]

The histopathology of the cyst varies from a more-or-less complete ependymal lining to scattered few islands of ependyma in the wall of the cystic cavity.[76]

The pathology of primary spinal syringomyelia seems invariably to involve at least partial obliteration of the subarachnoid space. This may take the form of very focal arachnoid scarring at the site of a spine injury; scarring may extend over many spinal levels in patients who had tuberculous meningitis. Gliotic changes of an injured cord with foci of discoloration may be recognized in the post-traumatic case. Extensive changes reflecting cord injury may be seen on histology. The cysts associated with primary spinal forms of syringomyelia are often septate or multichambered, and occasionally two parallel cavities running in a rostrocaudal direction are seen. Rarely, spontaneous drainage of syringeal cavities has been reported, but to the author's knowledge an opening of a syrinx cavity into the subarachnoid space has never been demonstrated in a neuropathological specimen.[70] Communication with the fourth ventricle has been reported in a post-traumatic syrinx cavity.[58]

Treatment Modalities

DECOMPRESSION

A basic assumption underlying the treatment of syringomyelia is that most, if not all, forms of syringomyelia are related to at least partial obstruction of the subarachnoid space by an intradural or extradural mechanism. The exceptions to this assumption possibly include the unusual congenital syringomyelia seen with some severe forms of hindbrain herniation. Cystic spinal cord tumors are not included in this discussion because the primary treatment of these lesions consists of tumor excision. Syringomyelia treatment is therefore directed at decompression with restoration of unimpeded cerebrospinal fluid flow through the subarachnoid space. With the exception of infants with Chiari II malformation, in most patients with hindbrain herniation and other abnormalities at the craniovertebral junction, the surgical approach consists of enlarging the foramen magnum ("suboccipital craniectomy") and accomplishing a dural or intradural decompression by one of the techniques described later.[12, 13] In patients with platybasia and other odontoid abnormalities, the compression appears to be anterior, and Menezes and colleagues have treated such patients successfully by odontoid resection.[55] The mechanism by which restoration of unimpeded cerebrospinal fluid flow in the subarachnoid space acts to eliminate an intramedullary cyst is not understood. It is, however, evident from the work of many investigators in the field that the technique is very effective[2, 59]; it has the added advantage that it allows one to disregard totally the septations in a complex cyst and avoids the need for an incision into the spinal cord.

Although decompressive surgery for infants with Chiari II malformation has strong advocates, there is still disagreement on the efficacy of surgery, and some authors question whether cervical decompression in newborns alters the course of the disease.[53, 55, 60, 75]

Ventricular cerebrospinal fluid shunting is indicated in those patients with Chiari I malformation who have associated hydrocephalus and is part of the treatment of most infants with Chiari II malformation with myelomeningocele.[60]

Post-traumatic syrinx cavities with focal scarring of the arachnoid may also be treated by decompression, with laminectomy over the area of scarring, intradural lysis of adhesions, and dural expansion for fluid to pass the former area of subarachnoid constriction.[42, 84]

FLUID DIVERSION

Diversion of fluid trapped within the spinal cord has been carried out for many years, beginning with shunting this fluid into the subarachnoid space.[73] Because the subarachnoid space may be scarred over an extended area and because of possibly less favorable pressure relationships when fluid is shunting from cyst to subarachnoid compartments, techniques of shunting from the cyst into the peritoneal or pleural cavities were introduced.[31, 88] In most situations, shunting should not be considered the preferred primary approach to syringeal cavities. The reasons for this include the risk of shunt obstruction as glial tissue grows into the shunt openings, shunt dislocation and shunt infection, incomplete drainage of a complex septate cyst, and the possibility that an extracavitary shunt tube may act to tether the cord or generate shear stresses on the cord as the patient moves about. In addition, myelotomy may add further neurological deficit.[66] In certain situations, however, shunting cerebrospinal fluid is the only or best available option. These situations include patients in whom decompressive procedures have failed and some patients with postinflammatory syringeal cavities. At times, the subarachnoid scar that develops after trauma or repeat surgery can be so dense that it favors development of a subarachnoid fluid collection proximal to the scar in conjunction with a more distally situated syrinx cavity. A possible causal relationship between such a subarachnoid cyst, which may itself act as a compressive entity, and a more distal syrinx cavity has already been alluded to. The role of endoscopic assistance in placement of shunts is being investigated at several centers.[45]

Techniques
POSTERIOR DECOMPRESSION

There are several variations of the general technique of posterior decompression for hindbrain herniation (Chiari malformation) and other abnormalities at the craniovertebral junction associated with syringomyelia.*

Bone

All procedures in adults include a bony decompression, which is preferably considered an enlargement of the foramen magnum, rather than a posterior fossa craniectomy. The decompression is 2.5 to 3.0 cm in diameter and the same measurement upward from the rim of the foramen magnum. A high-speed nitrogen-driven drill is helpful to thin out the bone in the size of the planned decompression; the bone is then removed in piecemeal fashion, taking care to protect the underlying dura from injury, since frayed dura is difficult to close at the end of the procedure. The posterior arch of C1 is removed to a width of approximately 2.5 cm, that is, no wider than the craniectomy; a partial or complete laminectomy of C2 is performed if this is necessary to unroof the cerebellar tonsils.

Dura

The dura is opened in Y-shaped manner, with the vertical limb over the upper cervical cord and an oblique extension in the direction of each cerebellar hemisphere. The dura is carefully separated from the underlying arachnoid, which is left intact, if possible, at this stage of the procedure. The dural edges are tacked to adjacent soft tissues with temporary sutures to maintain the exposure. Occasionally, tight horizontal dural bands are encountered, which may compress the tonsils, and these must be sectioned. Dural vascular lakes may be seen, which require extensive dural coagulation.

Arachnoid
Arachnoid Intact

In the modification first described by Logue and Edwards and subsequently also used by Lapras, the arachnoid is left intact.[48, 51] The author has used this procedure only in patients with hindbrain herniation of small degree, and in the absence of syringomyelia. When the arachnoid is left intact, the dural edges should be stitched back at several points with permanent suture material. The exposed arachnoid and dural edge are covered with fibrin glue reconstituted from autologous cryoprecipitate and commercial thrombin with calcium. This added measure helps reduce cerebrospinal fluid seepage through the arachnoid. A lumbar drain has been left in place for 3 days in some of these patients as added protection against accumulation of cerebrospinal fluid in the suboccipital-cervical soft tissues. This procedure may be used in selected cases; it should not be used when there is a suggestion of a membrane over the fourth ventricle outlets or of any other intradural pathological process by magnetic

_____

*See references 12, 13, 15, 30, 46, 51, 59, 60, 62, 75, and 85.

resonance imaging. Oldfield and associates have further modified this procedure and have placed a dural graft over the intact arachnoid after establishing, by ultrasound, that pulsatile compression of the spinal cord and syrinx disappeared when the posterior fossa dura was opened.[59] Based on the author's observations, this modification appears helpful.

Arachnoid Opening

A midline arachnoid opening is made under magnification. As the arachnoid is elevated, attached strands of arachnoid come into view and are divided. The arachnoid is held to the dural edge with temporary metal clips; Williams prefers to excise the arachnoid insofar as possible.[85]

Occasionally, the arachnoid is densely adherent to the cerebellar tonsils, which are held down against the medulla and upper cervical cord by an investment of scar tissue. If the tonsils cannot be elevated readily, further arachnoid dissection should not be undertaken because of the risk of serious injury to the lower brain stem. Splitting of the vermis under ultrasound guidance to reach the fourth ventricle is the recommended procedure in this situation, with a catheter (ventricular end of a shunt device) left in the fourth ventricle, while the distal end is appropriately shortened and left in the cervical subarachnoid space. The tube must be anchored to the dura or the arachnoid with fine suture material.

Intradural Assessment and Definitive Treatment

The objective of the posterior fossa approach to hindbrain herniation is to provide easy flow of cerebrospinal fluid from the fourth ventricle into the cervical subarachnoid space. As noted earlier, a variety of abnormalities may be encountered that can produce partial hindrance to cerebrospinal fluid flow. The most commonly encountered is impaction of the tonsils, which have been jammed into the foramen magnum. There are a number of maneuvers that can be carried out to facilitate cerebrospinal fluid flow from the fourth ventricle. The tonsils can be shrunk by touching the dorsal and medial surface of each tonsil with bipolar coagulation (Fig. 43–4A).[13, 41] Care must be taken to avoid injury to major vessels, such as the posterior inferior cerebellar artery; a subpial resection of the tonsils should be done if the tonsils are so gliotic that they do not shrink in response to bipolar coagulation; occasionally even after subpial resection, the remaining tissue will not collapse. In this situation a nonferromagnetic clip may be applied across the emptied tonsil envelope. Sometimes there is an opportunity to place a fine suture (5-0) from the arachnoid at the medial edge of the tonsil to the dural edge, thereby holding the tonsils apart and permitting cerebrospinal fluid egress from the fourth ventricle. A similar maneuver can be used in some situations in which a firm membrane covers the outlet foramina of the fourth ventricle (see Fig. 43–4B). The surgeon should be able to visualize the inferior apex of the fourth ventricle, with perhaps some choroid plexus, at the completion of this procedure.

Many surgeons no longer attempt to plug the presumed or actual opening at the obex.[12, 15, 59, 85] The maneuver is associated with higher morbidity (see the section on complications) and probably does not address the mechanism of cyst-filling operant in most patients.

Closure

It is preferred to close the dura by interposing an autologous fascia lata graft. The dural patch is sutured in with a running, locked 4-0 suture, placed in such a manner as to incorporate the edge of the retracted arachnoid (see Fig. 43–4C). All temporary metal clips holding the arachnoid are now removed. After harvesting the premeasured fascia lata, the fatty layer is carefully dissected off the "inside" surface and the dural graft is sewn in watertight fashion, with the suture line challenged by a Valsalva maneuver. The patch, however, should not be taut but allowed to billow or luff, so that when filled with cerebrospinal fluid it will be well away from the neural structures. Fibrin glue layered over the fascia lata patch and dural closure may help reinforce the dural seal. To prevent the muscle closure from pressing against the dural graft, only the fascia is sutured, and deep approximating sutures in the muscle itself are avoided.

Williams leaves the dura and arachnoid open and stitches the dura to adjacent soft tissues.[85] He closes only the fascia in watertight fashion. This technique has been employed in four patients, including two whose posterior fossa pathology included extensive vascular lakes between the leaves of the dura, so that coagulation for hemostasis left too little intact dura to place a suture line. When the dura has been left open, patients may experience more nausea, occasionally with vomiting, and headache in the early postoperative period. The long-term results of therapy, however, appear to be the same as for patients treated with a dural graft.

Posterior Decompressive Surgery in Newborns

There are certain important differences in the surgical management of Chiari II malformation in infants as compared with older children and adults. Several authors recommend that a decompressive procedure be done as soon as the diagnosis is made.[29, 75] As in older children and adults, the decompression procedure should be performed with the infant in the prone position. The experience at the Toronto Hospital for Sick Children with newborns points out that it is not necessary to enlarge the foramen magnum because it was already enlarged and because the compression of the brain stem occurred at the upper cervical level.[75] A tight fibrous band under the arch of C1 was found in 59 per cent of their patients; a cervical laminectomy with midline dural opening was carried out until the

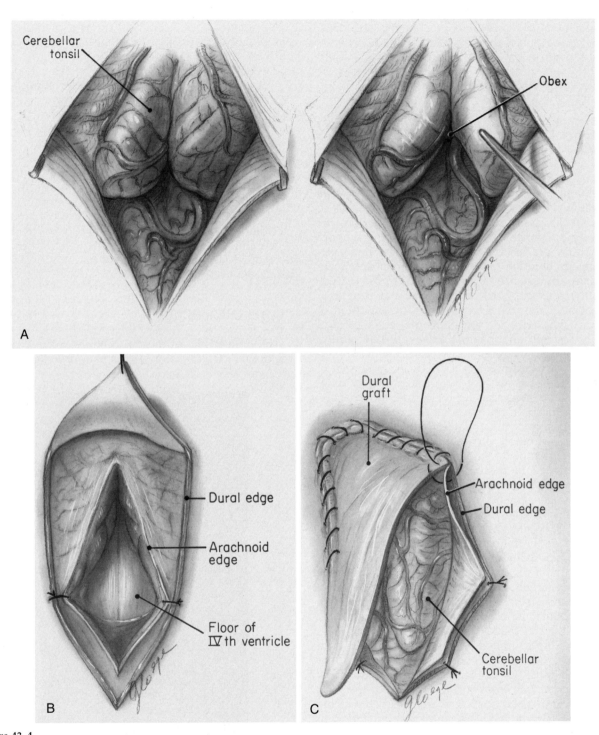

Figure 43–4

A. Coagulation of the tips of the cerebellar tonsils (dorsal and medial aspects) with bipolar current. *B.* Placement of permanent retraction sutures when the arachnoid is adherent to the tonsils or when there is a firm retained rhombic roof; this maneuver exposes the fourth ventricle. *C.* Closure of the posterior fossa dura incorporating the retracted arachnoid into the dural closure. (*A* From Batzdorf, U.: Syringomyelia related to abnormalities at the level of the craniovertebral junction. *In* Batzdorf, U., ed.: Syringomyelia: Current Concepts in Diagnosis and Treatment. Baltimore, Williams & Wilkins, 1991. © 1991, the Williams & Wilkins Co., *B* and *C* from Batzdorf, U.: Chiari I malformation with syringomyelia: Evaluation of surgical therapy by magnetic resonance imaging. J. Neurosurg., *68*:726–730, 1988. Reprinted by permission.)

cerebellar tongue was completely unroofed and normal cord was seen; this required varying levels of laminectomy, extending as far as C6 in 2 of 17 patients. Dissection of the arachnoid should be limited to that necessary to ensure ready drainage of cerebrospinal fluid from the fourth ventricle.[16] The dura was closed with fascia or a lyophilized dural graft.

Posterior Decompressive Approach for Primary Spinal Syringomyelia

One may assume a concept of spinal-spinal pressure dissociation, analogous to the craniospinal pressure dissociation enunciated by Williams with respect to syringomyelia associated with abnormalities at the craniocervical junction.[81] Thus, an area of arachnoid scarring may prevent the normal nearly instantaneous pressure equilibration throughout the spinal subarachnoid space in response to physiological forces that increase the pressure, such as exertion and coughing. Extrapolating from the experience with restoration of an open subarachnoid space at the craniocervical junction, several investigators have applied similar concepts to focal spinal lesions associated with syringomyelia.[42, 84] Demonstration of a relatively focal area of subarachnoid space scarring by myelography or magnetic resonance imaging is a prerequisite to undertaking this approach. In the presence of a complete subarachnoid block to contrast material, myelography may have to be performed above and below the block to define the extent of the subarachnoid scar. The situation encountered in postinflammatory syringomyelia, in which extensive subarachnoid scarring may be present over long segments of the spine (e.g., in posttuberculous syringomyelia), does not lend itself to this approach. The surgical technique consists of performing a laminectomy over the area of arachnoid scarring, undertaking an intradural lysis of arachnoid adhesions under magnification, and creating, in effect, a meningocele that acts as a fluid bypass at the level of arachnoid scarring. Williams has described his technique in detail[83]; he essentially leaves the dura open and closes the soft tissues over the defect.

In the author's limited experience with this technique, autologous fascia lata dural graft is sutured into the dural defect. The areolar tissue layer is carefully dissected away from the "inside" surface of the graft before the graft is sutured in place. Very convincing evidence of clinical improvement and elimination of the intraspinal cyst on postoperative magnetic resonance images has been seen. The technique would appear to offer advantages over shunting such cysts as a primary surgical approach.

Decompressive Surgery for Syringobulbia

Decompressive surgery for syringobulbia follows the same considerations detailed for syringomyelia.[86]

ANTERIOR DECOMPRESSION

As noted earlier, in a small number of patients the pathological process at the craniovertebral junction underlying the development of syringomyelia is anterior and related to the dens. This can be seen in patients with platybasia, basilar invagination, or abnormalities of the dens, which produce anterior compression of the subarachnoid space, not necessarily accompanied by hindbrain herniation (Fig. 43–5). Resection of the odontoid by the transoral approach has been performed in these patients, with collapse of the syringeal cavity demonstrated by magnetic resonance imaging in 5 of 7 children treated by Menezes.[54] In instances in which there is craniocervical instability, odontoid resection must be followed by a C1–C2 stabilization procedure. Occipital-cervical fixation was, in fact, performed on all seven children who had undergone a ventral transoral decompression. The technique of odontoid resection is discussed in Chapter 42.

FLUID DIVERSION

The indications for these procedures were discussed previously. Historically, aspiration, drainage, myelo-

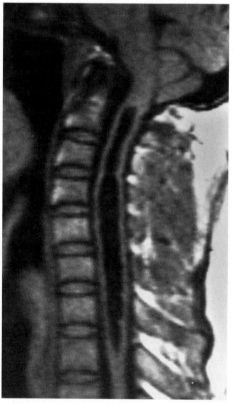

Figure 43–5

A 35-year-old man presented with upper extremity sensory deficit and gait ataxia. There is significant ventral indentation of the brain stem by the high-riding odontoid, with shallow angulation of brain stem relative to cervical cord, as seen in basilar invagination. Sagittal T1-weighted magnetic resonance image before transoral decompression, which was followed by C1–C2 fusion. (Courtesy of J. Patrick Johnson, M.D., Los Angeles, California.)

tomy, and a variety of devices and tubes, as well as different extraspinal drainage sites have been used for diversion of fluid from a syringeal cavity.[47] Aspiration and myelotomy have failed as long-term therapeutic measures. Transection of a nonfunctional spinal cord through the cyst (cordectomy) has few indications even in a patient with a total and fixed motor and sensory deficit.[28] The opening into the cyst at the level of cord transection may not remain open. These older forms of therapy have fallen into disuse in the modern era. Improved biocompatible materials for cyst shunts, microsurgical technique, and magnetic resonance imaging to validate the outcome of surgical therapy have limited the currently used diversion methods to three procedures.

Subarachnoid Shunt

The major advantage of shunting the syringeal cavity to the subarachnoid space is that the procedure is limited to a single incision and does not require awkward positioning of the patient on the operating table. The procedure requires special care in positioning the distal end of the catheter into the subarachnoid, rather than the subdural, space.[73] When subarachnoid shunts have been performed for post-traumatic and postinflammatory syringomyelia, it is sometimes difficult to find an unscarred area of the subarachnoid space for placement of the distal end of the catheter. This may account for the disappointing results of this system of drainage in some earlier uses of the technique.[31] Some authors have reported better results with subarachnoid shunts, but even the best available studies predate the routine use of magnetic resonance imaging to validate the effectiveness of this form of drainage.

Extraspinal Shunts

Syringoperitoneal and syringopleural shunts have the advantage that even extensive subarachnoid scarring does not affect the drainage system.* In both situations the system will be under slightly negative pressure, aiding drainage. Syringopleural shunting does not require awkward positioning or repositioning of the patient on the operating table and is carried out with the patient prone, the position that surgeons are most familiar with and in which potentially abnormal anatomical relationships are most likely to be recognized.[88] All the disadvantages of shunting, enumerated previously, apply equally to the two systems. One of the major problems noted, incomplete drainage of a complex (i.e., septated) cyst, can be very troublesome and may necessitate multiple shunt drainage tubes in one patient.

For a syringoperitoneal shunt the patient is placed in the prone position as for a syringopleural shunt, with the shunt tube buried subcutaneously before the patient is repositioned in the lateral position and redraped; alternatively, the patient may be placed in the lateral position and secured to the table, supported on a bean bag covered with sheepskin. This permits some turning to facilitate exposure of the spine and abdomen.

The approach to the syringeal cavity is through a standard one- to one-and-one-half-level laminectomy performed over the most caudal point of the cyst.[47] Meticulous hemostasis is essential before the dura is opened; several temporary dural retention sutures are placed once the dura has been opened in the midline. The myelotomy may be carried out through the root entry zone area of an analgesic limb or through a midline incision into the cord. Intraoperative ultrasound is often invaluable in locating the cyst.[26] The advantages of using ultrasound are such as to justify starting even a syringoperitoneal shunt with the patient in prone position. With the patient well secured to the table, it is possible to tilt the table away from the surgeon by several degrees. This position is more comfortable and makes it easier to fill the wound with saline for ultrasound evaluation. The size of the myelotomy opening should admit whichever catheter is used without forcing the surgeon to manipulate or distort the cord while introducing the catheter. In this respect some catheters are easier to introduce than others. K- or T-shaped catheters, as well as straight catheters, are available for drainage of intramedullary cysts.[6]

A K- or T-shaped catheter should be introduced by folding one side limb against the "stem" of the shunt tubing, rather than forcing the catheter in some other way. The author's preference is for straight catheters because they are significantly easier to introduce. The tube is anchored to the dura with several of the dural closing sutures (Fig. 43–6). Standard shunt technique is then used to pass the tubing subcutaneously and to connect the syrinx catheter to a previously placed valveless (no resistance) peritoneal catheter. When a syringopleural shunt is to be placed, a similar valveless catheter, premeasured in length, is secured to the syrinx catheter and is introduced through an intercostal incision, over the upper edge of the lower rib, while the lung is temporarily deflated. The lung is reinflated immediately before wound closure. Flow restricting valves of the type used for hydrocephalic shunts are not used, since the volume of fluid produced is very small and a valve would add too much resistance to the system.

Results

Treatment outcome is generally expressed in clinical improvement. In syringomyelia, modern imaging techniques permit determination of decreasing the size of the syrinx cavity after treatment and possibly even recognition of cerebrospinal fluid flow normalization.[2, 12] Results of treatment can therefore be considered from both the clinical and the imaging points of view.

HINDBRAIN HERNIATION (CHIARI MALFORMATION)

Adults

Unfortunately reports of larger series in the literature do not always clearly distinguish separate groups of

---

*See references 6, 7, 31, 47, 65, and 88.

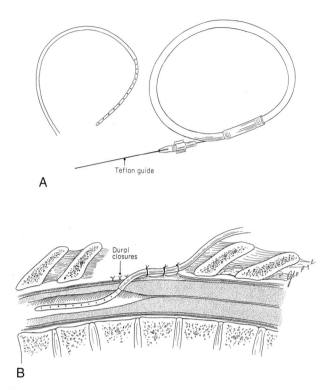

A

B

Figure 43–6

A and B. Shunt catheter with multiple perforations along its thin intracyst portion (1.5 mm diameter); tip rigidity during insertion is maintained with a Teflon guide. (Custom Device, PS Medical, Goleta, California.)

patients, such as those with hindbrain herniation only versus those who also have syringomyelia. Some of the larger series have combined different treatment modalities, and it is sometimes difficult to get a clear idea of important technical details of treatment in subgroups of patients.

Chiari I Malformation Without Syringomyelia

A group of 12 adult patients with Chiari I malformation who had only hindbrain herniation without syringomyelia were treated by the author. Eleven patients had a Chiari I abnormality; one, who had undergone a myelomeningocele repair and ventricular shunt in infancy, presented with symptoms of a Chiari II malformation at age 20. All except the patient with the Chiari II malformation underwent enlargement of the foramen magnum (suboccipital craniectomy) and C1 laminectomy. The breakdown by procedure type and the results are described in Table 43–2. Eight patients, including the patient with the Chiari II malformation, underwent intradural exploration as described previously with placement of a dural graft. All but one patient had postoperative magnetic resonance imaging, and all showed satisfactory decompression (see Fig. 43–2B). An additional three pediatric patients underwent a suboccipital decompression procedure for simple hindbrain herniation.

Complications. There was one death in this group

of patients, a 68-year-old man who had a cardiopulmonary arrest on the second postoperative day after an initially benign course. Autopsy demonstrated a significant epidural hematoma. This operation had been performed in the sitting position, which may have obscured a potential bleeding site. None of the posterior fossa procedures for Chiari malformation have been performed in the sitting position since 1986. As noted, four patients underwent bony decompression with opening of the dura, leaving the arachnoid intact. Postoperatively, closed lumbar drainage was used for 3 days in this group of patients. One of these patients developed tonsillar impaction 2 weeks after surgery and required re-exploration with tonsillar resection and dural grafting. It is believed that this complication may be related to greater than recognized cerebrospinal fluid drainage in this patient, whose obesity led to multiple attempts at lumbar puncture when the drain was placed.

One patient had extensive vascular lakes between the dural leaves and underwent a suboccipital procedure as described by Williams, leaving the dura and arachnoid open.[85] This patient required a second operation to reduce the size of a very large "cisterna magna" causing chronic local suboccipital pain.

Chiari I Malformation with Syringomyelia

The results of treatment in selected larger groups of adult patients with hindbrain herniation and syringomyelia are summarized in Table 43–3 (see Figs. 43–3A and B). The results of the author's group of patients, reflecting specific neurological manifestations, are provided in Table 43–4.

Change in the magnetic resonance images of the 30 patients for whom a postoperative scan was available showed significant improvement in 19, partial improvement in 8, and minimal or no improvement in 3. Six of the 36 patients underwent a posterior fossa procedure as a secondary procedure (one had undergone a prior posterior fossa procedure, the others had shunting or marsupialization of the syrinx cavity). Of the patients who underwent a secondary posterior fossa procedure, only two of six had an overall satisfactory outcome, including significant improvement in the magnetic resonance images (in one of these the syrinx-

Table 43–2

ADULT CHIARI I MALFORMATION WITHOUT SYRINGOMYELIA: RESULTS OF SUBOCCIPITAL DECOMPRESSION

Surgical Technique	No.	Complications	Improved	No Change	Worse	Dead
Dural graft	8*	1	7			1
Arachnoid intact	4*	1	3	1		
Dura-arachnoid left open	1	1		1		

*One patient underwent a dural graft procedure subsequent to a decompression with intact arachnoid 2 weeks before (see complications).

Table 43–3

OUTCOME OF SURGICAL PROCEDURES FOR CHIARI MALFORMATION WITH SYRINGOMYELIA: SELECTED LITERATURE

Author (Reference)	Year	Features of Surgery[a]	Number of Patients	Improved	No Change	Clinical Outcome Worse	Died	Lost	Required Secondary Procedure
Hankinson[b]	1970	FMD, obex plug	39[c] } 6[d]	37	6	2	0		2[d]
Logue and Edwards[51]	1981	FMD, DO, arachnoid intact	25	9	13	3	0		3
		FMD, DO, arachnoid dissected, obex plug	26	9	11	6	0		
		FMD, syringostomy	7	1	3	2	1		
Cahan and Bentson[e]	1982	FMD	1		1				
		FMD, obex plug	13 }	3	9	11	0	2	2
		FMD, obex plug, fourth vent, drain	12						
Peerless and Durward[f]	1983	FMD	10	3	5	2	0		10
		FMD, obex plug	16	10	4	2	0		
		FMD, obex plug, fourth vent, drain	8	8	0	0	0		
Levy et al.[49]	1983	FMD	25	11	8	6	6[i]		11[g]
		FMD, obex plug	60	29	16	15			
Dyste et al.[30]	1989	FMD, DG[a]	6	4		2	0		1
		FMD, obex plug, fourth vent, drain, DG	32	28	3	1	0		
Total patients			286	152	79	52	7	2	29
(Percent)			(100)	(53)	(26)	(18)	(2)	(1)	
Obex plug			206	124	49	37	0		
(Percent)			(102)[h]	(60)	(24)	(18)			
FMD			67	27	27	13	0		
(Percent)			(99)[h]	(40)	(40)	(19)			

[a]FMD = foramen magnum decompression; DO = dura left open; vent = ventricle; DG = dural graft specified.
[b]Hankinson, J.: Syringomyelia and the surgeon. *In* Williams, D., ed.: Modern Trends in Neurology. Vol. 5. London, Butterworths, 1970, pp. 127–148.
[c]Chiari patients only.
[d]Arachnoiditis cases.
[e]Cahan, L. D., and Bentson, J. R.: Considerations in the diagnosis and treatment of syringomyelia and the Chiari malformation. J. Neurosurg., *57*:24–31, 1982.
[f]Peerless, S. J., and Durward, Q. J.: Management of syringomyelia: A pathophysiological approach. Clin. Neurosurg., *30*:531–576, 1983.
[g]Shunted; not specified how many underwent fourth ventricle shunt as part of primary procedure.
[h]Percents do not equal 100% because of rounding.
[i]Deaths in total group of FMD and FMD with obex plug; deaths not included in the 85 patients whose clinical outcomes were evaluated.
Modified from Batzdorf, U.: *In* Batzdorf, U., ed.: Syringomyelia: Current Concepts in Diagnosis and Treatment. Baltimore, Williams & Wilkins, 1991, p. 176. Copyright © 1991, the Williams & Wilkins Co., Baltimore. Reprinted by permission.

subarachnoid shunt had fallen out, the other had undergone a lumboperitoneal shunt); the remainder of the patients continued to be quite symptomatic and as a group also showed less significant improvement in their magnetic resonance images.

Menezes and co-workers found that 7 of 55 patients with Chiari malformation required transoral resection of the dens for ventral decompression of the cervical-medullary junction.[55] These patients subsequently underwent posterior fossa decompression and occipito-cervical fusion. All patients had resolution of their brain stem signs and cervical myelopathy.

The procedure of terminal ventriculostomy has generally fallen into disuse.[87]

In the experience of Dyste and associates, symptomatic improvement after effective treatment was greatest with respect to pain (81.5 per cent) and motor weakness (70 per cent) and less with respect to cranial nerve dysfunction (18 per cent) and sensory deficits (6 per cent).[30] Other studies have confirmed that pain re-

Table 43–4

CHIARI MALFORMATION WITH SYRINGOMYELIA: RESULTS OF POSTERIOR FOSSA DECOMPRESSION IN 36 CONSECUTIVE PATIENTS*

Symptom	No. of Patients With Symptoms Present Preoperatively	Clinical Outcome Improved	No Change	Worse	Unknown
Headache and/or spinal pain	20	18	2		
Dysesthetic pain	19	11	7	1	
Extremity weakness	22	13	8		1
Sensory deficit	33	10	21		2
Spasticity	11	7	4		

*All but one patient, who had extensive dural venous lakes, underwent placement of a dural graft; in this patient the dura was left open.

sponds best[13]; considerable improvement in spasticity has also been noted (7 of 11 patients). Sensory deficit shows the least improvement.

Complications. Complications of posterior fossa decompression procedures were analyzed in detail by Williams and by Menezes and include deaths and neurological deficit as well as respiratory and cardiac irregularities.[37, 49, 54, 62, 79] When the dura is left open, patients may develop postoperative fever, vomiting, and headache, which gradually subsides.

Ptosis or sag of the cerebellum poses difficult management problems because the newly incarcerated cerebellum recreates conditions permitting pressure dissociation and allows refilling of the syrinx cavity.[27, 55] The condition is believed to result from an excessively large posterior fossa craniectomy.

Pseudomeningocele has been a complication in 3 of 36 patients who underwent placement of a dural graft. The author now uses only autologous fascia lata for the dural closure and reinforces the dural seal with fibrin glue prepared from autologous cryoprecipitate whenever the latter is available. Two of 36 patients in whom posterior fossa decompression with intradural exploration were performed as the primary procedure subsequently required syrinx shunting because of persistent symptoms. One of these patients, in retrospect, probably had a primarily spinal form of syringomyelia with mild tonsillar descent.

Every patient undergoing posterior fossa decompression is advised that a shunting procedure may be necessary should the decompression fail.

Infants and Children

Results in infants and children with hindbrain herniation have been described in several recent reports.

All patients with Chiari II malformations who have undergone closure of a myelomeningocele and who have hydrocephalus undergo ventricular shunting.[60, 75] Hydrocephalus develops in more than 90 per cent of these children.[15] As pointed out by Park and co-workers, symptoms of Chiari malformation may be precipitated by increased intracranial pressure due to shunt malfunction and respond to shunt revision.[60] Unfortunately, some children develop symptoms of lower cranial nerve and brain stem dysfunction in spite of good control of their hydrocephalus.

Carmel believed that only a small number of children with type II anomalies require direct posterior fossa surgery, the majority responding to shunting.[15] McLone and Naidich stated that it remained open to question whether posterior fossa and cervical decompression in neonates with type II anomalies alter the course of the disease.[53]

Dyste and Menezes described results in 16 patients younger than age 20, of whom 11 had a Chiari I malformation, 3 had a Chiari II malformation, and 2 had a Chiari III malformation.[29] Ventriculoperitoneal shunting for hydrocephalus had been performed in 2 of these patients; 3 patients underwent a ventral brain stem decompression. Fifteen of the patients underwent foramen magnum decompression; 14 became asymp-

tomatic or experienced improvement, while the condition remained stable in the 2 others. Some children had almost immediate neurological improvement after decompression. These authors state that children who became asymptomatic with surgical treatment were those who were treated early in the course of their disease, leading to the recommendation that children with symptomatic Chiari malformation undergo surgery early in the hope of maximizing the outcome. Postoperative magnetic resonance images showed collapse of the syringeal cavity.

The results of surgical therapy in a group of symptomatic newborns with Chiari II malformation reported from the Toronto Hospital for Sick Children were equally encouraging.[75] Seventeen infants underwent upper cervical laminectomy to unroof the descended hindbrain completely. Of the 15 patients who survived, all showed complete recovery. The two deaths were the result of respiratory arrest 8 months after decompression and shunt infection with peritonitis almost 7 years after surgery. These authors also emphasize the importance of early recognition and prompt treatment for more complete and rapid recovery.

The results of Lapras and co-workers are generally similar, although they reported a higher operative mortality (25 per cent) in newborns, with much better outcome in children older than 2 years of age who underwent surgery.[48]

Lapras and co-workers treated 13 patients with opening of the dura, leaving the arachnoid intact, while 5 others with associated aqueductal stenosis underwent exploration of the fourth ventricle with cannulation of the aqueduct, leaving a tube from the third ventricle to the cervical subarachnoid space. Two patients died of sudden decompensation of their hydrocephalus. In 2 patients with associated syringomyelia, a second procedure, a syrinx to subarachnoid shunt, was performed at the same time as the posterior fossa decompression.

Primary Spinal Forms of Syringomyelia

It is difficult to arrive at a clear picture of the results of treatment of primary spinal syringomyelia. The most common form of this condition is post-traumatic syringomyelia, detailed by Barnett and Jousse.[9–11] Since most of these patients have significant spinal cord dysfunction due to their injury, the assessment of treatment outcome is more difficult. Other significant variables relate to the spinal level of the original injury, spine angulation, and the large variety of surgical procedures carried out. These include cordectomy, intraspinal and extracavitary shunting procedures, as well as decompressive procedures, as described in preceding sections. Overall improvement or neurological stabilization has been reported in as high as 80 per cent of patients.[6]

Barnett and Jousse reported on three "partial" paraplegic patients who all showed some improvement with catheter drainage[10]; four complete paraplegics showed improvement with spinal cord transection or catheter insertion. Tator and colleagues reported excellent clinical results in four post-traumatic patients treated by subarachnoid shunting of the syrinx cavity.[73]

In the author's experience, six patients who underwent cyst to peritoneal shunting all showed improvement, although two of these patients have subsequently developed evidence of shunt failure; one underwent reoperation (Fig. 43–7).[47] Barbaro and colleagues reported on six post-traumatic patients, three of whom were believed to have a good result after syringoperitoneal shunting.[7]

Williams advocated shunting into the pleural cavity.[88] His series included nine patients with post-traumatic syringomyelia, four of whom had an initial good response; one subsequently deteriorated acutely, a fair result was noted in another four patients, and one had a poor result. The author's own experience confirms a generally good response (see Figs. 43–1A and B).

Selected patients who underwent decompressive procedures as described previously also have shown a satisfactory early response.

In all groups of patients, periodic monitoring with magnetic resonance imaging after surgery is extremely useful; it should be done whenever there is evidence of neurological deterioration.

The results of treatment of patients with syringomyelia secondary to adhesive arachnoiditis of infectious or inflammatory origin have been disappointing.[7, 8, 73] This discouraging outcome undoubtedly relates to the long rostrocaudal extent of adhesions and potential interference with spinal fluid dynamics, the often complex, septate structure of the cysts, and the sometimes severe myelomalacia.

There is as yet no consensus regarding the management of the slitlike syrinx cavities seen in the cervical region in a very small number of patients with cervical spondylosis. It is a good general policy to monitor these patients with an occasional magnetic resonance image. In all the author's patients, including one who underwent a posterior decompressive procedure, the size of the syrinx cavity has remained unchanged.

Unfortunately, a few patients whose syrinx cavity has collapsed by magnetic resonance criteria, continue to show disabling symptoms, particularly dysesthetic pain.

Complications. Complications of therapy have consisted of shunt malfunction, neurological deterioration related to shunt placement, as well as delayed deterioration possibly related to tethering of the cord by the shunt tubing, infection, and mechanical distortion by a T drain.[7, 78, 88] One of the author's patients developed a spinal cord abscess following a shunt infection but was successfully treated with excision of the shunt tip and antimicrobial therapy.

REFERENCES

1. Aboulker, J.: La syringomyélie et les liquides intra-rachidiens. Neurochirurgie, 25(Suppl. 1):9–144, 1979.
2. Armonda, R. A., Citrin, C. M., Foley, K. T., et al.: Quantitative cine-mode MRI of Chiari I malformations: An analysis of CSF dynamics. Neurosurgery, 35:214–224, 1994.
3. Arnold, J.: Myelocyste, Transposition von Gewebskeimen und Sympodie. Beitr. Path. Anat., 16:1–28, 1894.
4. Aubin, M. L., Vignaud, J., Jardin, C., et al.: Computed tomograph in 75 clinical cases of syringomyelia. Am. J. Neurorad., 2:119–204, 1981.
5. Ball, M. J., and Dayan, A. D.: Pathogenesis of syringomyelia. Lancet, 2:799–801, 1972.
6. Barbaro, N. M.: Surgery for primarily spinal syringomyelia. In Batzdorf, U., ed.: Syringomyelia: Current Concepts in Diagnosis and Treatment. Baltimore, Williams & Wilkins, 1991.
7. Barbaro, N. M., Wilson, C. B., Gutin, P. H., et al.: Surgical treatment of syringomyelia: Favorable results with syringoperitoneal shunting. J. Neurosurg., 61:531–38, 1984.
8. Barnett, H. J. M.: Syringomyelia associated with spinal arachnoiditis. In Barnett, H. J. M., Foster, J. B., and Hudgson, P., eds.: Syringomyelia. London, W. B. Saunders, 1973.
9. Barnett, H. J. M., and Jousse, A. T.: Syringomyelia as a late sequel to traumatic paraplegia and quadriplegia: Clinical features. In Barnett, H. J. M., Foster, J. B., and Hudgson, P., eds.: Syringomyelia. London, W. B. Saunders, 1973.
10. Barnett, H. J. M., and Jousse, A. T.: Nature, prognosis and management of post-traumatic syringomyelia. In Barnett, H. J. M., Foster, J. B., and Hudgson, P., eds.: Syringomyelia. London, W. B. Saunders, 1973.
11. Barnett, H. J. M., and Jousse, A. T.: Posttraumatic syringomyelia (cystic myelopathy). In Vinken, P. J., and Bruyn, G. W., eds.: Handbook of Clinical Neurology. Amsterdam, North Holland Publishing, 1976.
12. Batzdorf, U.: Chiari I malformation with syringomyelia: Evaluation of surgical therapy by magnetic resonance imaging. J. Neurosurg., 68:726–730, 1988.
13. Batzdorf, U.: Syringomyelia related to abnormalities at the level of the craniovertebral junction. In Batzdorf, U., ed.: Syringomyelia: Current Concepts in Diagnosis and Treatment. Baltimore, Williams & Wilkins, 1991.
14. Blackwood, W., and Corsellis, J., eds.: Greenfield's Neuropathology. 3rd ed. London, E. Arnold, 1976.
15. Carmel, P. W.: Management of the Chiari malformation in childhood. Clin. Neurosurg., 30:385–406, 1983.
16. Carmel, P. W.: The Chiari malformations and syringomyelia. In

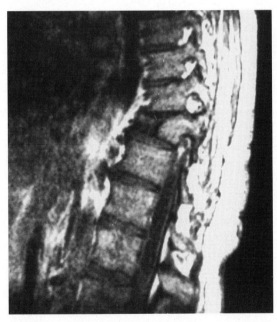

Figure 43–7

Post-traumatic syringomyelia in a 42-year-old man 5 years after a motor vehicle accident in which he sustained almost total motor and sensory loss with a wedge-type compression fracture at T10 with permanent kyphotic deformity of the thoracic spine. Patient presented with low back pain and loss of the slight residual motor and sensory function. He showed little, if any, response to shunting of the syrinx cavity into the peritoneal cavity. Sagittal T1-weighted magnetic resonance image before shunting procedure.

Hoffman, H. J., and Epstein, F., eds.: Disorders of the Developing Nervous System: Diagnosis and Treatment. Boston, Blackwell Scientific, 1986.

17. Chiari, H.: Ueber Veränderungen des Kleinhirns infolge von Hydrocephalie des Grosshirns. Dtsch. Med. Wochenschr., 42:1172–1175, 1891.
18. Chiari, H.: Ueber Veränderungen des Kleinhirns, des Pons und der Medulla oblongata in Folge von genitaler Hydrocephalie des Grosshirns. Denkschr. Akad. Wiss. Wien, 63:71–116, 1896.
19. Cho, K. H., Iwasaki, Y., Imamura, H., et al.: Experimental model of posttraumatic syringomyelia: The role of adhesive arachnoiditis in syrinx formation. J. Neurosurg., 80:133–139, 1994.
20. Chumas, P. D., Armstrong, D. C., Drake, J. M., et al.: Tonsillar herniation: The rule rather than the exception after lumboperitoneal shunting in the pediatric population. J. Neurosurg., 78:568–573, 1993.
21. Chumas, P. D., Kulkarni, A. V., Drake, J. M., et al.: Lumboperitoneal shunting: A retrospective study in the pediatric population. Neurosurgery, 32:376–383, 1993.
22. Cleland, J.: Contribution to the study of spina bifida, encephalocele, and anencephalus. J. Anat. Physiol., 17:257–291, 1883.
23. Cornil, L., and Mosinger, M.: Sur les processus proliferatifs de l'ependyme médullaire (rapports avec les tumeurs intramédullaires et la syringomyélia). Rev. Neurol., 1:749–754, 1933.
24. Daniel, P. M., and Strich, S. J.: Some observations on the congenital deformity of the central nervous system known as the Arnold-Chiari malformation. J. Neuropathol. Exp. Neurol., 17:255–266, 1958.
25. DiRocco, C., and Rende, M.: Chiari malformations. In Raimondi, A. J., Choux, M., and DiRocco, C., eds.: The Pediatric Spine II: Developmental Anomalies. New York, Springer-Verlag, 1989.
26. Dohrmann, G. J., and Rubin, J. M.: Intraoperative ultrasound imaging of the spinal cord: Syringomyelia, cysts and tumors: A preliminary report. Surg. Neurol., 18:395–399, 1982.
27. Duddy, M. J., and Williams, B.: Hindbrain migration after decompression for hindbrain hernia: A quantitative assessment using MRI. Br. J. Neurosurg., 5:141–152, 1991.
28. Durward, Q. J., Rice, G. P., Ball, M. J., et al.: Selective spinal cordectomy: Clinicopathological correlation. J. Neurosurg., 56:359–367, 1982.
29. Dyste, G. N., and Menezes, A. H.: Presentation and management of pediatric Chiari malformations without myelodysplasia. Neurosurgery, 23:589–597, 1988.
30. Dyste, G. N., Menezes, A. H., and VanGilder, J. C.: Symptomatic Chiari malformations: An analysis of presentation, management, and long-term outcome. J. Neurosurg., 71:159–168, 1989.
31. Edgar, R. E.: Surgical management of spinal cord cysts. Paraplegia, 14:21–27, 1976.
32. Emery, J. L., and MacKenzie, N.: Medullo-cervical dislocation deformity (Chiari II deformity) related to neurospinal dysraphism (meningomyelocele). Brain, 96:155–162, 1973.
33. Enzmann, D. R.: Imaging of syringomyelia. In Batzdorf, U., ed.: Syringomyelia: Current Concepts in Diagnosis and Treatment. Baltimore, Williams & Wilkins, 1991.
34. Fischer, E. G., Welch, K., and Shillito, J., Jr.: Syringomyelia following lumboureteral shunting for communicating hydrocephalus. J. Neurosurg., 47:96–100, 1977.
35. Foster, J. B., and Hudgson, P.: The clinical features of communicating syringomyelia. In Barnett, H. M. J., Foster, J. B., and Hudgson, P., eds.: Syringomyelia. London, W. B. Saunders, 1973.
36. Gardner, W. J.: Hydrodynamic mechanism of syringomyelia: Its relationship to myelocele. J. Neurol. Neurosurg. Psychiatry, 28:247–256, 1965.
37. Gardner, W. J., and Angel, J.: The mechanism of syringomyelia and its surgical correction. Clin. Neurosurg., 6:131–140, 1959.
38. Gardner, W. J., Abdullah, A. F., and McCormack, L. J.: The varying expressions of embryonal atresia of the 4th ventricle in adults: Arnold-Chiari malformation, Dandy-Walker syndrome, "arachnoid" cyst of the cerebellum, and syringomyelia. J. Neurosurg., 14:591–605, 1957.
39. Goldstein, F., and Kepes, J. J.: The role of traction in the development of the Arnold-Chiari malformation: An experimental study. J. Neuropathol. Exp. Neurol., 25:654–666, 1966.
40. Gowers, W. R.: A Manual of Diseases of the Nervous System. Vol. 1. London, Churchill, 1886, pp. 433–443.

41. Halamandaris, G. G., and Batzdorf, U.: Adult Chiari malformation. Contemp. Neurosurg., 11(26), 1989.
42. Halamandaris, G. G., and Batzdorf, U.: The role of subarachnoid decompression in the treatment of syringomyelia with arachnoiditis [Poster presentation]. Atlanta, GA, Congress of Neurological Surgeons, 1989.
43. Hall, P. V., Lindseth, R. E., Campbell, R. L., et al.: Myelodysplasia and developmental scoliosis: A manifestation of syringomyelia. Spine, 1:48–56, 1976.
44. Hoffman, H. J.: Syringomyelia in childhood. In Batzdorf, U., ed.: Syringomyelia: Current Concepts in Diagnosis and Treatment. Baltimore, Williams & Wilkins, 1991.
45. Huewel, N., Perneczky, A., Urban, V., et al.: Neuroendoscopic technique for the operative treatment of septated syringomyelia. Acta. Neurochir., 54(Suppl.):59–62, 1992.
46. Isu, T., Sasaki, H., Takamura, H., et al.: Foramen magnum decompression with removal of the outer layer of the dura as treatment for syringomyelia occurring with Chiari I malformation. Neurosurgery, 33:845–850, 1993.
47. LaHaye, P. A., and Batzdorf, U.: Posttraumatic syringomyelia. West. J. Med., 148(6):657–663, 1988.
48. Lapras, C., Guilburd, J. N., and Patet, J. D.: La malformation de Chiari type II. Neurochirurgie, 34(Suppl. 1):53–58, 1988.
49. Levy, W. J., Mason, L., and Hahn, J. F.: Chiari malformation presenting in adults: A surgical experience in 127 cases. Neurosurgery, 12:377–90, 1983.
50. Lichtenstein, B. W.: Distant neuroanatomic complications of spina bifida (spinal dysraphism). Arch. Neurol. Psychiatry, 47:195–214, 1942.
51. Logue, V., and Edwards, M. R.: Syringomyelia and its surgical treatment: An analysis of 75 patients. J. Neurol. Neurosurg. Psychiatry, 44:273–284, 1981.
52. McLone, D. G., and Knepper, P. A.: The cause of Chiari II malformation: A unified theory. Pediatr. Neurosci., 15:1–12, 1989.
53. McLone, D. G., and Naidich, T. P.: Myelomeningocele. In Hoffman, H. J., and Epstein, F., eds.: Disorders of the Developing Nervous System: Diagnosis and Treatment. Boston, Blackwell Scientific, 1986.
54. Menezes, A. H.: Chiari I malformations and hydromyelia. Pediatr. Neurosurg., 92:146–154, 1991.
55. Menezes, A. H., Smoker, W. R. K., and Dyste, G. N.: Syringomyelia, Chiari malformations, and hydromyelia. In Youmans, J., ed.: Neurological Surgery. 3rd ed. Philadelphia, W. B. Saunders, 1990.
56. Milhorat, T. H., Miller, J. I., Johnson, W. D., et al.: Anatomical basis of syringomyelia occurring with hindbrain lesions. Neurosurgery, 32:748–754, 1993.
57. Müller, F., and O'Rahilly, R.: The human chondrocranium at the end of the embryonic period, proper, with particular reference to the nervous system. Am. J. Anat., 159:33–58, 1980.
58. Oakley, J. C., Ojemann, G. A., and Alvord, E. C.: Posttraumatic syringomyelia. J. Neurosurg., 55:276–81, 1981.
59. Oldfield, E. H., Muraszko, K., Shawker, T. H., et al.: Pathophysiology of syringomyelia associated with Chiari I malformation of the cerebellar tonsils: Implications for diagnosis and treatment. J. Neurosurg., 80:3–15, 1994.
60. Park, T. S., Hoffman, H. S., Hendrick, E. B., et al.: Experience with surgical decompression of the Arnold-Chiari malformation in young infants with myelomeningocele. Neurosurgery, 13:147–152, 1983.
61. Patten, B. M.: Embryological stages in the establishing of myeloschisis with spina bifida. Am. J. Anat., 93:365–395, 1953.
62. Paul, K. S., Lye, R. H., Strang, F. A., et al.: Arnold-Chiari malformation. J. Neurosurg., 58:183–187, 1983.
63. Payner, T., Prenger, E., Berger, T. S., et al.: Acquired Chiari malformations: Incidence, diagnosis and management. Neurosurgery, 34:429–434, 1994.
64. Penfield, W., and Coburn, D. F.: Arnold-Chiari malformation and its operative treatment. Arch. Neurol. Psychiatry, 40:328–336, 1938.
65. Phillips, T. W., and Kindt, G. W.: Syringoperitoneal shunt for syringomyelia: A preliminary report. Surg. Neurol., 16:462–466, 1981.
66. Rhoton, A. L., Jr.: Microsurgery of Arnold-Chiari malformation in adults with and without hydromyelia. J. Neurosurg., 45:473–483, 1976.

67. Roth, M.: Cranio-cervical growth collision: Another explanation of the Arnold-Chiari malformation and of basilar impression. Neuroradiology, *28*:187–194, 1986.
68. Ruge, J. R., Masciopinto, J., Storrs, B. B., et al.: Anatomical progression of the Chiari II malformation. Child's Nerv. System, *8*:86–91, 1992.
69. Saez, R. J., Onofrio, B. M., and Yanagihara, T.: Experience with Arnold-Chiari malformation 1960 to 1970. J. Neurosurg., *45*:416–422, 1976.
70. Santoro, A., Delfini, R., Innocenzi, G., et al.: Spontaneous drainage of syringomyelia: Report of two cases. J. Neurosurg., *79*:132–134, 1993.
71. Sherman, J. L., Barkovich, A. J., and Citrin, C. M.: The MR appearance of syringomyelia: New observations. A.J.R., *148*:381–391, 1987.
72. Simon, T.: Über Syringomyelie und Geschwulstbildung im Rückenmark. Arch. Psychiatrie Nervenkrankh, *5*:120–163, 1875.
73. Tator, C. H., Meguro, K., and Rowed, D. W.: Favorable results with syringosubarachnoid shunts for treatment of syringomyelia. J. Neurosurg., *56(4)*:517–523, 1982.
74. van Hoytema, G. J., and van den Berg, R.: Embryological studies of the posterior fossa in connection with Arnold-Chiari malformation. Dev. Med. Child Neurol., *11*(Suppl.):61–76, 1966.
75. Vandertop, W. P., Asai, A., Hoffman, H. J., et al.: Surgical decompression for symptomatic Chiari II malformation in neonates with myelomeningocele. J. Neurosurg., *77*:541–544, 1992.
76. Vinters, H. V.: Neuropathology of syringomyelia. *In* Batzdorf, U., ed.: Syringomyelia: Current Concepts in Diagnosis and Treatment. Baltimore, Williams & Wilkins, 1991.
77. West, R. J., and Williams, B.: Radiographic studies of the ventricles in syringomyelia. Neuroradiology, *20*:5–16, 1980.
78. Wester, K., Pedersen, P. H., and Kräkenes, J.: Spinal cord damage caused by rotation of a T-drain in a patient with syringoperitoneal shunt. Surg. Neurol., *31*:224–227, 1989.
79. Williams, B.: A critical appraisal of posterior fossa surgery for communicating syringomyelia. Brain, *101*:223–250, 1978.
80. Williams, B.: Orthopaedic features in the presentation of syringomyelia. J. Bone Joint Surg. [Br.], *61*:314–323, 1979.
81. Williams, B.: On the pathogenesis of syringomyelia: A review. J. R. Soc. Med., *73*:798–806, 1980.
82. Williams, B.: Simultaneous cerebral and spinal fluid pressure recordings: II. Cerebrospinal dissociation with lesions at the foramen magnum. Acta. Neurochir. (Wien), *59*:123–142, 1981.
83. Williams, B.: Syringomyelia. Neurosurg. Clin. North Am., *1*:653–685, 1990.
84. Williams, B.: Post-traumatic syringomyelia (cystic myelopathy). *In* Frankel, H. L., ed.: Handbook of Clinical Neurology. Vol. 17. Spinal Cord Trauma. Amsterdam, Elsevier Science Publishing, 1992.
85. Williams, B.: Surgery for hindbrain related syringomyelia. *In* Symon, L., et al., eds.: Advances and Technical Standards in Neurosurgery. Vol. 20. New York, Springer-Verlag, 1993.
86. Williams, B.: Surgical treatment of syringobulbia. Neurosurg. Clin. North Am., *4*:553–571, 1993.
87. Williams, B., and Fahy, G.: A critical appraisal of "terminal ventriculostomy" for the treatment of syringomyelia. J. Neurosurg., *58*:188–197, 1983.
88. Williams, B., and Page, N.: Surgical treatment of syringomyelia with syringopleural shunting. Br. J. Neurosurg., *1*:63–80, 1987.
89. Williams, B., Terry, A. F., Jones, F., et al.: Syringomyelia as a sequel to traumatic paraplegia. Paraplegia, *19*:67–80, 1981.

PART VII

Vascular Disease

CHAPTER 44

Pathophysiology and Clinical Evaluation of Ischemic Cerebrovascular Disease

Cerebrovascular disease encompasses all pathological processes that result from a disturbance of blood vessels within or supplying the brain. It is a source of mortality and profound morbidity that remains pervasive in the modern world. In developed nations, diseases of the cerebrovasculature rank behind only heart disease and cancer as a cause of death. The majority of cerebrovascular diseases are ischemic in nature, and the remainder comprise syndromes of vessel rupture. Stroke is a generic term that may include all of these maladies. However, in this chapter, "stroke" refers only to ischemic brain injury or infarction.

Epidemiology

Annually, 250,000 to 500,000 Americans suffer a stroke.[4, 210] For many, the outcome is fatal; however, some 2 million stroke survivors remain chronically disabled.[15] The cost to individuals and society in terms of acute care resources, rehabilitation, chronic care, and lost productivity is enormous.

Thirty-day case-fatality rates for cerebral infarction are 10 to 15 per cent.[20, 21, 174] In the initial hours to days after infarction, direct neurological injury may cause death. Thereafter, immobility and related medical complications such as pneumonia, sepsis, and pulmonary embolism lead to deterioration or demise. Death from cardiovascular disease predominates in long-term survivors.[64]

It is noteworthy that mortality rates for stroke have declined steadily since the turn of the century.[205, 209] Historically, this trend has reflected a decreasing incidence of stroke. More recently, incidence rates of stroke have plateaued or even increased by some reports.[33, 122] Changes in measured stroke incidence may reflect improved diagnostic imaging capabilities, which allow for detection of ischemic events of marginal clinical impact. The recent decline in stroke mortality parallels an apparently diminishing stroke severity.[209] Mortality rate declines may also be caused in part by recognition and modification of risk factors and improved medical care.[137]

Risk Factors

Efforts to minimize the occurrence and effects of brain ischemia necessitate a knowledge of risk factors for this condition (Table 44–1). Numerous factors that influence the risk of stroke have been identified. Among these are hypertension, cardiac disease, diabetes mellitus, and cigarette smoking. Hypertension is the prominent risk factor for all forms of stroke. A decreasing incidence and falling mortality of stroke have been attributed largely to better treatment of hypertension.[44, 107, 131, 196] Cardiac disease, particularly congestive heart failure, left ventricular hypertrophy, and arrhythmia, has been strongly correlated with the risk of stroke.[115] Diabetes mellitus has been established as an independent risk factor for atherosclerotic brain infarction, as has the adverse central nervous system effect of cigarette smoking.[3, 211] Smokers have a two- to threefold greater risk of stroke than nonsmokers.[3] The role of other factors, such as elevated serum cholesterol and lipid levels, alcohol consumption, physical inactivity, obesity, and oral contraceptive use, is less well defined. Although variations in stroke incidence related to geographical location, climate, and socioeconomic status have been observed, the significance of such trends is not known. Still other factors, such as advanced age, male sex, black race, and familial predisposition, increase the risk for cerebral infarction.[65, 66, 145, 148, 169]

R. A. Ratcheson • S. P. Kiefer • W. R. Selman

Table 44–1
RISK FACTORS FOR CEREBRAL ISCHEMIA

Established	
Treatable	*Not Treatable or Value of Treatment Not Established*
Hypertension	Age and gender
Cardiac disease	Race
Cigarette smoking	Familial attributes
Elevated hematocrit	Diabetes mellitus
Sickle cell disease	
Possible	
Treatable	*Not Treatable or Value of Treatment Not Established*
Elevated cholesterol, lipids	Geographic location
Alcohol consumption	Climate
Oral contraceptives	Socioeconomic factors
Sedentary lifestyle	Elevated fibrinogen
Obesity	

Modified from Dyken, M. L., Wolf, P. A., Barnett, H. J. M., et al.: Risk factors in stroke: A statement for physicians by the subcommittee on risk factors and stroke of the stroke council. Stroke 15:1105, 1984.

Pathophysiology of Cerebral Ischemia

The brain requires a continuous supply of nutrients and oxygen to maintain its complex array of functions. Although the human brain comprises only 2 per cent of the total body weight, it utilizes 20 per cent of the cardiac output to supply its voracious needs. These demands and requirements place nervous system tissues in a particularly vulnerable circumstance. Limitations or alterations in blood flow can create profound disturbances in brain function and structural integrity. The physiological and clinical outcomes of an ischemic event are functions of both the degree and duration of blood flow reduction.

Some reductions in blood flow may be well tolerated because compensatory mechanisms limit the effects of diminished blood supply on the neural parenchyma. Ischemia may foster or intensify metabolic derangements. Hypoxia, hypercarbia, and acidosis promote local vasodilatation, increasing cerebral blood volume. The overwhelming of this vasodilatory capacity leads to enhanced extraction of oxygen from the capillary blood supply.[159] As the duration or extent of ischemia increases, compensatory responses are unable to maintain cellular homeostasis. Without nourishment, cells are unable to generate the energy stores required for processes such as protein synthesis, membrane maintenance, and ion balance. Inhibition of protein synthesis compromises cell manufacturing and enzyme-mediated cell processes, leading to diminished cytoskeletal integrity. Ischemia-induced changes in membrane permeability allow for net ion influx, resultant cellular edema, and further energy consumption as efforts ensue to reconstitute ion gradients.[180] Adenosine triphosphate–dependent ion pumps may fail, further ravaging electrochemical gradients. In the absence of bloodborne oxygen, anaerobic glycolysis ensues, generating acid byproducts. Unhindered progression of these cellular pathological events may ultimately result in tissue death.

Progressive ischemia first alters neuronal functioning and later threatens cell viability. Blood flow thresholds in reference to dysfunction have been defined (Fig. 44–1). Below a level of approximately 20 mL per 100 g per minute, electrophysiological and functional deficits begin to emerge.[179] Animal studies have revealed that at 15 to 18 mL per 100 g per minute of blood flow (approximately 25 per cent of control levels), synaptic transmission is lost.[32, 94] Levels below 10 mL per 100 g per minute (18 per cent of control levels) may render neurons incapable of maintaining membrane integrity, resulting in cell death.[18, 31] Astrup and co-workers have defined tissues perfused at a level between these extremes as the *ischemic penumbra*.[18] These are regions that are electrophysiologically quiescent but nonetheless potentially viable. Continued or worsening ischemia may subject such neuronal tissues to irreversible injury and subsequent infarction. However, reperfusion or pharmacological therapy may offer a return to states of normal function. Time thresholds for viability in penumbral tissues are not well defined. Siesjö has postulated that different time thresholds exist for reperfusion and for pharmacological therapeutics.[180]

Factors Influencing Ischemia

The consequences of a lesion in a cerebral blood vessel are variable. One afflicted individual may be profoundly affected, whereas another may demonstrate few or no sequelae. A number of factors, both anatomical and functional, influence the occurrence and implications of cerebral ischemia.

ANATOMICAL VARIABILITY

Considerable variation exists in the territorial supply of cerebral vessels and the nature of subserved tissues.

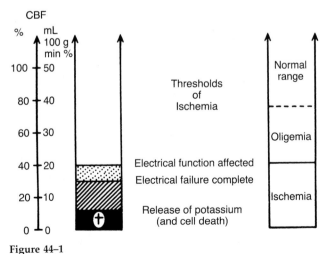

Figure 44–1

Neuronal dysfunction in reference to cerebral blood flow thresholds. (From Astrup, J., Symon, L., Branston, N. M., et al.: Cortical evoked potential and extracellular K⁺ and H⁺ at critical levels of brain ischemia. Stroke, 8:56, 1977. Reprinted by permission.)

However, many studies and textbooks have minimized these variabilities. Large differences in arterial territories from person to person are appreciated, and it is also likely that the boundaries between vascular supplies vary within the same individual, being dynamic rather than static.[23, 194] Cerebral blood vessels should not be viewed in isolation but as part of a larger vascular network. Anastomoses serve to connect adjacent vessels comprising this system. Alterations in hemodynamic conditions may enhance or limit baseline arterial territories through these anastomotic channels. Hemodynamic changes may derive from differences in systemic blood pressure or from acquired vessel pathology as may occur in atherosclerosis or hypertension. A cerebral blood vessel may nourish different regions of the brain in different persons, or even in the same person at different times, creating a range of functional disturbances in the setting of occlusive or flow-limiting lesions.

COLLATERAL CIRCULATION

Numerous anatomical considerations are important in determining whether ischemia occurs and, if so, to what extent tissue is damaged. Highly significant is collateral circulation. The presence of adequate supplementary blood flow through alternate channels can abort ischemia or limit its manifestations. Conversely, in diminished flow states, the absence of sufficient collateral flow dooms neuronal populations to dysfunction and subsequent infarction. Anastomotic networks with the capacity to provide additional flow exist in numerous forms. The extent to which such systems are developed varies from individual to individual and from region to region within a given brain. With vessel occlusion or stenosis, pressure gradients develop across existing anastomoses, permitting supplementary flow into compromised vascular regions.[138] In acute disturbances, these channels, if present, provide a defined blood flow dependent on the caliber of the vessels. The more gradual occurrence of flow obstruction allows for greater structural remodeling of collateral vessels, with resultant increases in diameter and blood-bearing capacity.[47]

In the normal adult circulation, three anatomical patterns of collateral flow are present. Anastomoses exist at extracranial sites, at the level of the circle of Willis, and within the leptomeninges. On occasion, remnants of embryonic vasculature may persist in the adult state, providing additional sources of collateral flow.

The most prominent extracranial anastomotic channels are those between external carotid artery and internal carotid artery branches. Less commonly, extracranial supply may supplement posterior circulation vessels. With proximal internal carotid artery occlusion, retrograde blood flow in the ophthalmic artery may nourish large regions of internal carotid artery territory. Prominent anastomoses are present between pterygopalatine branches of the maxillary artery and ethmoidal branches of the ophthalmic artery[143] (Fig. 44–2). Additionally, anterior portions of the superficial temporal

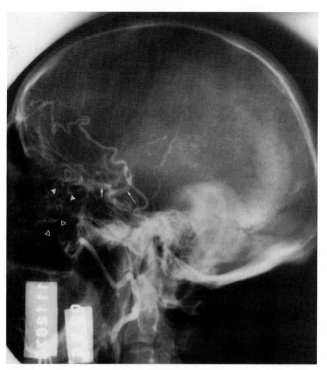

Figure 44–2

Ophthalmic-internal carotid artery collaterals. With internal carotid artery occlusion, ethmoidal ophthalmic artery branches (*solid arrowheads*) supply the intracranial circulation through the external carotid artery system (*open arrowheads*). *Short arrow*, ophthalmic artery; *long arrow*, reconstituted internal carotid artery.

artery may service assorted orbital branches. More rarely, collateral flow may be rendered by middle meningeal vessels, which supply lacrimal branches of the ophthalmic artery. Similarly, angular divisions of the facial artery may provide flow to descending nasal arteries, tributaries of the ophthalmic artery.

The circle of Willis is the most significant large-vessel collateral system in the human brain. Its configuration allows for instantaneous collateral flow if a constituent vessel or feeder becomes obstructed. Anomalies of the circle, however, are commonplace. Riggs and Rupp noted hypoplasia of one or more stem vessels within the circle of Willis in 79 per cent of studied cadaveric specimens.[168] Anterior and posterior communicating vessels are often rudimentary and of limited functional significance.[117, 168] These variations instill a delicate hemodynamic balance within the network, imparting some degree of limitation with respect to flow compensation in ischemic states.

Leptomeningeal anastomoses account for the most widespread source of collateral flow. Whereas the circle of Willis functions in the deep recesses of the brain, leptomeningeal vessels become significant in the periphery of arterial supplies. End-to-end pial anastomoses, 200 to 600 microns in diameter, are present over the surfaces of the cerebrum and cerebellum.[143] Under normal circumstances, these anastomoses are inactive. Proximal vessel occlusion, however, creates a gradient across these channels, favoring flow to the hindered circulation (Fig. 44–3). Given the small size and high

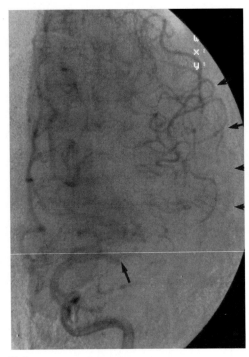

Figure 44–3

Leptomeningeal collateral vessels *(short arrows)* in the setting of middle cerebral artery occlusion *(long arrow)*.

resistance of these anastomoses, the volume of collateral flow is somewhat restricted. Although nourishment for small, focal areas may be provided through these routes, it is unlikely that these avenues can supply sufficient resources to avert destruction from large-vessel occlusive processes.[195]

Vestigial embryonic vasculature, although uncommon, is an alternative source of collateral blood flow. These arteries represent persistent large-vessel anterior-to-posterior anastomoses. The trigeminal artery is the most commonly encountered primitive vessel. It arises from the cavernous internal carotid artery and extends posteriorly to the upper basilar artery. This anomaly is observed in 0.1 to 0.2 per cent of individuals.[187] Hypoglossal, otic, and proatlantal intersegmental arteries are similar remnants that are seen less frequently.

SELECTIVE VULNERABILITY

Another consideration exists that may have an impact on the course of cerebral ischemia. Inherent differences in cells or tissues render some populations more resistant to ischemic damage and, conversely, some more susceptible. "Selective vulnerability" describes this graded response to ischemia or other harmful circumstance. Marked ischemic insults may harm multiple tissue elements; less severe disturbances may affect only the most vulnerable cells. "Selective neuronal necrosis" and "selective necrosis of the parenchyma" were terms previously used to define such injury in the brain.[178, 181]

In general, endothelial cells are believed to be less

susceptible to ischemia than glial cells, which are in turn less vulnerable than neuronal cells. Gradation of vulnerability exists even within neural tissues. One such example is found in the cerebellum. Purkinje cells are noteworthy for their special sensitivity to ischemic and hypoxic insult, whereas nearby Golgi cells are resilient by comparison.[178] Even neurons of the same type display varying degrees of vulnerability.[92, 170] Heiss and Rosner suggested that the concept of selective vulnerability can be applied not only to pathological changes but to physiological function of neurons or nervous tissue as well.[93] Studies in awake animals have confirmed that the more complex cerebral functions are impaired by lesser degrees of ischemia and that neurological deficits are progressive in the setting of progressive ischemia.[112] Whether native to the cell or a product of environment, or a combination of both, the source of this "vulnerability" remains unknown.

Clinical Evaluation of Ischemic Syndromes

HISTORY

Disturbance in consciousness or the presence of focal neurological deficits suggests nervous system compromise. Many processes may affect the brain and its related structures. However, it is the abrupt onset of signs and symptoms that characteristically signals the presence of a cerebrovascular disorder. Most commonly, these events arise within seconds or minutes; and less frequently, over the course of hours or days. Ascertainment of the temporal profile of the presenting illness is of particular importance. The length of time that a patient has been having symptoms, the frequency and duration of episodes, and the pattern of onset should be determined. The static or progressive nature of neurological dysfunction should also be elucidated. Such details help the physician to formulate a diagnosis and a conception of the disease course. Similarly, the existence of inciting or precipitating events may prove important. The location and quality of headache may have diagnostic or localizing value. Inquiry should be made regarding the presence or absence of seizure activity, infection, and pain. All aspects of neurological functioning and pertinent systemic issues should be addressed.

A thorough investigation of past medical history is considered indispensable. Identification of risk factors provides insight into the potential mechanisms and manifestations of disease. This information and other historical details serve to focus physical examination and subsequent diagnostic evaluation.

PHYSICAL EXAMINATION

A thorough general physical examination is necessary in any patient suspected of falling victim to an ischemic cerebral insult. This examination may reveal contributing systemic processes. Similarly, neurological examination often determines the location of the neural lesion and its cause. Vascular and neurovascular evaluations should be performed. Vital sign readings, auscultation, pulse survey, and thorough ophthalmoscopy should be included.

Vital sign parameters should include orthostatic indices (if not contraindicated), and blood pressure readings should be obtained from both arms. Differences in blood pressures may be indicative of occlusive disease affecting the great vessels of the chest and neck. Elevated blood pressures may be either a cause or an effect of a central nervous system lesion. Abnormal respiratory patterns are suggestive of brain stem or global central nervous system involvement and should evoke close attention to the need for supportive measures.

Auscultation begins at the heart and proceeds cephalad. Abnormalities in heart rate and rhythm or the presence of additional heart sounds, rubs, or murmurs, is suggestive of cardiac processes that may have consequences for the nervous system. Auscultation over the carotid and subclavian arteries, globes, temples, cranial vault, mastoids, and posterior cervical regions may reveal bruits. Bruits occur when blood flow becomes turbulent and causes a vessel wall to vibrate and generate sound; these may represent physiological turbulent blood flow, atherosclerotic stenotic disease, or another pathological flow state. Carotid artery bruits, often atherosclerotic in nature, become audible when the residual vessel lumen diameter approaches 2.5 to 3 mm and later disappear as the lumen is thinned to 0.5 to 0.8 mm.[125] The tightest stenoses are characterized by soft, high-pitched bruits that extend into diastole.[109] Bruits of atherosclerotic origin do not necessarily bode adversely for the vessels in which they rest or the tissues these vessels nourish. Yet, such bruits are markers for advanced atherosclerotic disease, which is known to increase the risk of stroke and cardiovascular disease.[42, 99, 212, 216]

The presence, symmetry, and quality of peripheral and central pulses should be determined. However, palpation of the internal carotid arteries in patients with suspected stenotic disease is of limited utility and presents a small, but existent, risk. Stimulation of the carotid sinus may result in syncope, cardiac arrhythmia, or arrest. The potential also exists for the dislodging of plaque material, with propagation into the cerebral circulation. The branches of the external carotid artery, however, may safely be inspected and can provide valuable information. Simultaneous bilateral palpation of the peripheral branches of the external carotid artery should seek differences in vessel caliber and pulsation. An asymmetric, bounding pulse is suspicious for internal carotid artery occlusion with development of collateral flow through the eye by means of the external carotid artery system. A diminished pulse suggests external carotid artery or common carotid artery occlusion or, in some instances, vessel inflammation.

Funduscopic examination allows for a direct view of blood vessels in a portion of the nervous system—the retina. Although these vessels may not absolutely reflect conditions in other regions of the brain, they do provide some insight into the processes affecting the cerebrovasculature. Findings in retinal blood vessels may visibly demonstrate the effects of hypertension, atherosclerosis, or embolus. Alterations in retinal vessel morphology such as arteriovenous "nicking" and "silver" and "copper" wire changes may be observed in the setting of hypertension and atherosclerosis. Numerous types of emboli may be observed. Cholesterol emboli, or Hollenhorst plaques, are most commonly encountered and are often associated with ulcerated internal carotid artery atheromata.[101] Calcific emboli originating from cardiac valves may produce segmental blockage of retinal vessels, with resultant infarction.[105, 172] Marked stasis or arterial occlusion may also result from platelet and fibrin debris, thought to arise from large-vessel mural thrombi. Findings resulting from global retinal ischemia may include fundal pallor, vessel dilatation or degeneration, exudative deposit, hemorrhage, or microaneurysm formation.

Temporal Course of Ischemia

TRANSIENT ISCHEMIC ATTACK AND REVERSIBLE ISCHEMIC NEUROLOGICAL DEFICIT

Clinical abnormalities occurring as a result of ischemia may be short-lived or permanent. "Transient ischemic attack" and "reversible ischemic neurological deficit" describe time-limited episodes of neurological impairment. The term transient ischemic attack more specifically refers to nonconvulsive, focal neurological dysfunction due to inadequate blood supply to a region of the brain, retina, or cochlea. By definition, a transient ischemic attack lasts 24 hours or less.[141] Reversible ischemic neurological deficit refers to a qualitatively similar event, but one lasting for longer than 24 hours but not more than 3 weeks.[141] Findings present for more than 3 weeks are considered permanent ischemic sequelae and indicative of stroke.

The reversibility of nervous system dysfunction after transient ischemia has been documented.[103, 104] However, radiographic and cerebral blood flow studies demonstrate a significant incidence of physical lesions in the clinical setting of transient ischemic attack.[29, 36, 198] Transient ischemic attack may therefore include a spectrum of cerebral insults. Those lasting for minutes probably represent transient ischemic processes in the traditional sense—that is, those that are functionally reversible without permanent physical sequelae. Transient ischemic attacks with a duration of many hours and reversible ischemic neurological deficits may represent another subset, one in which clinical deficits may resolve but some degree of structural integrity is lost.

The incidence of transient ischemic attacks increases markedly with advancing age.[207] Cerebral infarction frequently, but not invariably, follows transient ischemic events. The period immediately after a transient ischemic attack is thought to convey the greatest risk for subsequent stroke.[60, 134, 207] Although details of duration and frequency of transient ischemia are in general of restricted value in predicting the occurrence of infarction, "crescendo" transient ischemic attacks—those clustered in a brief interval of time—are viewed as highly threatening. Whisnant noted that 21 per cent of cerebral infarctions occurring after a transient ischemic attack ensued within the first month after symptom onset and that approximately 50 per cent occurred within the first year.[206] The North American Symptomatic Carotid Endarterectomy Trial demonstrated that those with transient ischemic attack or minor stroke and a carotid stenotic lesion of greater than 70 per cent had a 28 per cent incidence of stroke at 2 years after receiving optimal nonoperative care.[146] Stroke need not be preceded by transient ischemic episodes. Transient ischemic attacks are reported as antecedent to stroke in 9 to 26 per cent of cases.[58, 144, 207]

A transient ischemic attack is a sudden, discrete event in which neurological deficits are fulminant immediately or within minutes of onset. It typically lasts for 2 to 15 minutes and is most often a distinctive clinical entity; vague symptom complexes or alterations in consciousness are not typical. Waxing, waning, or marching of signs and symptoms is also not usually observed. Such findings may typify other disease entities, from which transient ischemic events must be differentiated. Migraine and its variants may resemble transient ischemia in presentation, as may seizure activity. Less commonly, a space-occupying lesion or metabolic disturbance may enter the differential diagnosis of transient neurological dysfunction.

Transient ischemic attacks are usually categorized as those that affect the carotid system and those that affect the vertebrobasilar circulation (Table 44–2). In patients with carotid system ischemia, history may be indicative of retinal or hemispheric involvement. Simultaneous involvement of these regions is not common. Retinal findings are those of transient monocular blindness, also referred to as amaurosis fugax. These episodes are characterized by sudden, painless, unilateral loss of vision lasting 5 to 10 minutes and disappearing quickly. Visual loss often occurs in sweeping fashion, as if a curtain or window shade were falling smoothly over the visual field, and may recede in a similar manner. Blindness may be complete, or a "grayness" or "haziness" may be present in a filmlike manner, serving to cloud vision in the eye. On occasion, a wedge of the monocular visual field may be absent, or positive visual phenomena such as sparkles or jagged bright lights may be observed.[88]

Transient hemispheric ischemia is usually manifest as hemimotor and hemisensory signs and symptoms opposite the affected cortex. The entire contralateral half of the body may be affected, although commonly the arm and face show greater involvement. Frank paralysis may be described, although motor deficits are often paretic in nature and are described as clumsiness or heaviness. Sensory complaints parallel motor difficulties and consist of paresthesia or numbness in the face or upper extremity. If the dominant hemisphere is involved, speech and language disturbance may range from minor to global. Selective abnormalities of reading, writing, or calculation have been described. Dysarthria may reflect dominant cortical impairment or simply facial weakness. Deep branches of the middle cerebral artery supply temporoparietal visual tracts whose involvement may result in quadrantal or hemianopic visual field deficits. Less commonly, confusion is observed in a carotid system transient ischemic attack.

The clinical picture of transient ischemic events in the posterior circulation is varied because of the magnitude and proximity of ascending and descending neural structures that are supplied by the vertebrobasilar system. Although solitary symptoms may be referable to carotid or vertebrobasilar circulations, it is the diversity and multiplicity of symptoms that localize ischemic processes to the posterior circulation. Vertigo and visual loss are the most common vertebrobasilar transient ischemic symptoms. Vertigo in isolation, however, should not be attributed to brain stem ischemia. Vertigo may result from peripheral vestibular dysfunction and has been described in the setting of hemispheric disturbance.[134] Similarly, visual loss may occur from anterior circulation disease or primary disorders of the optic apparatus. Manifestations of vertebrobasilar ischemia may also include headache, diplopia, ataxia, facial paresis, tinnitus, dysphagia, dysarthria, and drop attack. Circumoral sensory changes are considered specific for brain stem involvement. Sensory and motor symptoms may be bilateral or unilateral or may alternate.

Transient global amnesia is perhaps another occurrence attributable to posterior circulation ischemia. This condition, which usually occurs in the elderly, is characterized by the sudden onset of amnesia (anterograde more so than retrograde) lasting for several hours followed by a return of memory to baseline,

Table 44–2
COMMON SYMPTOMS OF TRANSIENT ISCHEMIA

Carotid Circulation	Vertebral Circulation
Transient monocular blindness, ipsilateral	Homonymous hemianopsia, unilateral or bilateral
Hemimotor loss, contralateral	Vertigo (not in isolation)
Hemisensory loss, contralateral	Diplopia
Quadrantal/hemianopic visual field defect, contralateral	Facial weakness
Dysphasia	Circumoral sensory loss and paresthesia
Dysarthria	Ataxia
Confusion (not in isolation)	Dysphagia
Combination of the above	Dysarthria
	Extremity motor/sensory loss, unilateral, bilateral, or alternating
	Drop attack
	Tinnitus
	Memory disturbance
	Combination of the above

Adapted from Adams, H. P., Jr., and Biller, J.: Ischemic cerebrovascular disease. *In* Bradley, W. G., Daroff, R. B., Fenichel, G. M., et al., eds. Neurology in Clinical Practice. Boston, Butterworth-Heinemann, 1991, pp. 907–939.

although long-term memory dysfunction is sometimes noted. The exact cause remains poorly defined; however, it is suspected that transient global amnesia is the result of ischemia in the mesial bitemporal regions, which are supplied by the distal posterior cerebral arteries. Given the propinquity of these many anatomically and functionally discrete neural tissues, it is not surprising that vertebrobasilar transient ischemic attacks may vary considerably from episode to episode, in contrast to carotid system attacks, which tend to be stereotypical and consistent from event to event.

INFARCTION

It is the presence of neuronal death, whether discovered pathologically or radiographically, and the lasting quality of neurological deficit that differentiate infarctions from transient ischemic events. The onset of stroke is most often sudden and may be followed by progression or remission of symptoms, a fluctuating course, or static findings. Evolution of stroke is frequently more protracted in the vertebrobasilar circulation than in the carotid system.[110, 111] Although a lack of progression for 24 to 72 hours is suggestive of completed stroke, it is only in retrospect that the extent and course of infarction can be fully determined.

Some strokes may not be clinically apparent and are considered "silent" (Fig. 44–4). Reviews of series of stroke and transient ischemic attack reveal that 11 to 13 per cent of patients have radiographically defined ischemic lesions unrelated to the presenting event.[43, 97] These lesions are believed to represent prior asymp-

tomatic infarction. Autopsy studies demonstrate similar findings.[55] It is presumed that "silent" infarction may have the same implications for future stroke as does symptomatic prior stroke.[97]

Stroke Mechanisms and Causes

THROMBOTIC, EMBOLIC, AND HYPOPERFUSION STATES

Numerous disease entities may produce cerebral ischemia through several mechanisms. Thrombus, embolus, and low-flow states may limit blood flow, producing local or more widespread ischemia. Although the clinical presentation of each of these conditions is considered distinct, overlapping clinical features are observed.

Arterial thrombosis is characterized by abrupt onset and gradual progression of symptoms, usually over minutes or hours. A fluctuating or stuttering course may be observed. Relation to physical activity is not usual, and infarction occurring during sleep or in the early morning hours is suggestive of thrombosis. Recovery is gradual and often incomplete. Propagation of thrombus, either anterograde or retrograde, may occur. With extension of clot, further limitation in blood flow may occur as important sources of collateral flow become obstructed. In some instances, this propagation of thrombus may be responsible for the saltatory pattern of thrombotic infarction.

Embolus is the most common mechanism of cerebral

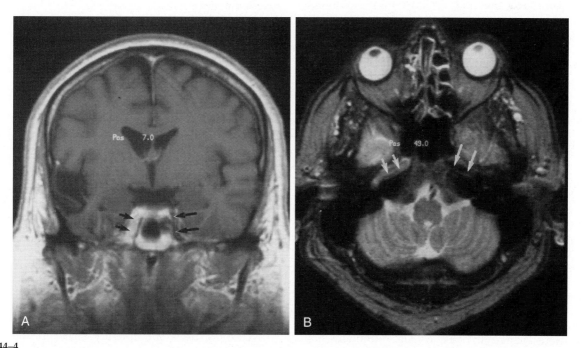

Figure 44–4

Silent infarction. A 60-year-old man with transient right arm paresthesias and no clinical history of stroke. *A.* Coronal magnetic resonance image revealing right temporal infarction. Increased signal *(short arrows)* characterizes occlusion of the right internal carotid artery. *Long arrows,* left internal carotid artery. *B.* Axial magnetic resonance image of the same patient. *Short arrows,* occluded right internal carotid artery; *long arrows,* left internal carotid artery.

infarction. Symptoms are usually of maximal severity immediately after a sudden onset. Embolic events may occur at any time, although physical activity or Valsalva maneuver may foster emboli. With lysis of emboli, rapid and dramatic improvement may be observed. Embolic vessel occlusion may damage subserved tissues as well as the endothelial cells comprising the artery or its involved branches. Breakdown of the embolus and subsequent reperfusion of injured blood vessels may allow extravasation of blood into infarcted parenchyma. Degeneration of thrombus occurs more slowly and to a lesser extent than breakdown of embolus. These observations may explain the greater incidence of hemorrhage after embolic infarction than after thrombotic infarction.

Emboli most frequently arise from the heart, from the aorta, or within the great vessels of the neck. Platelet-fibrin particles, infected or noninfected valvular vegetations, calcium deposits, cholesterol, thrombus, fat, air, neoplastic tissue, and various foreign bodies are potential emboli. Emboli may disperse throughout the entire cerebrovasculature. Seeding of specific regions or arterial distributions is proportional to the blood flow to these territories. Middle cerebral artery tissues are most commonly affected by embolic phenomena, reflecting the blood-bearing capacity of the middle cerebral artery, which is the largest source of cerebral blood supply. Emboli tend to lodge at vessel branch points. Stagnant flow beyond the embolic occlusion may nurture thrombus formation, which compounds the initial effects of the embolus.

In an absolute sense, all infarctions occur subsequent to states of hypoperfusion. Thrombosis and embolic disease result in diminished blood flow, with destruction of distal neuronal populations. Focal infarction from states of low cardiac output or systemic hypotension occurs much less commonly. In this latter situation, border zone tissues residing at the periphery of major arterial territories are most susceptible. Small declines in systemic pressure may markedly reduce flow in the high-resistance vessels serving these peripheral tissues, precipitating infarction.

CAUSES OF STROKE

Many disease entities can facilitate or promote cerebral ischemia. Some are primarily nervous system processes, and others are systemic conditions that affect neuronal tissues. Disorders such as atherosclerosis, cardiac disease, hematological abnormalities, and nonatherosclerotic vasculopathy cause the majority of stroke syndromes. Less common maladies account for the remainder of brain infarctions (Table 44–3).

Atherosclerosis is the most common cause of cerebral ischemia and infarction. Hypertension, diabetes mellitus, hyperlipidemia, and tobacco use serve to accelerate atheromatous changes in blood vessels. Although small cerebral vessels may be affected, atherosclerosis most prominently affects large intracranial and extracranial arteries. Atheromatous deposits accumulate at vessel branch points. The most common sites of involvement

Table 44–3
SOURCES OF CEREBRAL ISCHEMIA

Atherosclerosis	*Complications of Arteriography*
Thrombus	*Vasculitis*
Stenosis	Infectious
Embolus, artery-to-artery	Pyogenic
Cardiogenic	Fungal
Myocardial infarction	Parasitic
Cardiac aneurysm	Viral
Arrhythmia	Inflammatory
Cardiomyopathy	Lupus erythematosus
Septal/foraminal defects	Polyarteritis nodosa
Valvular cardiac disease	Rheumatoid arthritis
Congenital	Giant cell arteritis
Rheumatic	Takayasu's disease
Prosthetic	Granulomatous angiitis
Bacterial endocarditis	Miscellaneous
Marantic endocarditis	*Elevated Intracranial Pressure*
Cardiac diagnostic procedures	Trauma
or surgery	Mass lesion
Atrial myxoma	*Large Vessel Disorders*
Hematological Disorders	Aortic, vertebral artery, carotid
Polycythemia	artery dissection
Thrombocytosis	Traumatic
Sickle cell disease	Atraumatic
Thrombotic thrombocytopenic	Direct vessel compromise
purpura	Steal syndromes
Disseminated intravascular	*Miscellaneous Vasculopathy*
coagulation	Moyamoya
Coagulation factor abnor-	Fibromuscular dysplasia
malities	Lipohyalinosis
Other	Radiation-induced
Shock	Drug-related
Volume loss	Inherited disorders
Sepsis	Other
Cardiogenic	
Vasospasm	
Migraine	
Subarachnoid hemorrhage	

Adapted from Kiefer, S. P., Selman, W. R., and Ratcheson, R. A.: Clinical syndromes in cerebral ischemia. *In* Tindall, G. T., Barrow, D. L., Cooper, P. R., eds.: The Practice of Neurosurgery. Baltimore, Williams & Wilkins, 1995.

include the origin and cavernous portions of the internal carotid artery, the vertebral artery at its origin and junction with the basilar artery, and the bifurcation of the middle cerebral artery (Fig. 44–5). Atherosclerotic lesions create flow-limiting stenoses; however, vessel occlusion from "pure" atherosclerotic narrowing is uncommon.[82] Thrombosis can complicate atherosclerotic stenosis, producing arterial occlusion or embolization of particulate matter.

Most emboli to the brain arise within the heart. It is estimated that 75 per cent of cardiac emboli travel to the brain.[5] Mural thrombus formation may result from dilated cardiomyopathy, ventricular aneurysm, or myocardial infarction. Cerebral ischemic events follow myocardial infarction in 2 to 5 per cent of cases.[186] The risk of embolization correlates with the degree of myocardial injury. Native or prosthetic cardiac valves may serve as sources for vegetation and thrombus that may, in turn, give rise to cerebral infarction. Cardiac arrhythmias, most prominently atrial fibrillation, promote turbulent flow, encouraging embolic events. Although most systemic venous emboli are filtered in the lungs, cardiac septal defects may permit paradoxical emboli to reach the brain. Invasive cardiac procedures

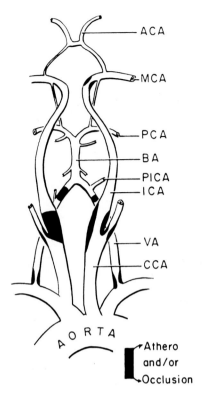

Figure 44–5

Common sites of atherosclerotic disease. ACA, anterior cerebral artery; MCA, middle cerebral artery; PCA, posterior cerebral artery; BA, basilar artery; PICA, posterior inferior cerebellar artery; ICA, internal carotid artery; VA, vertebral artery; CCA, common carotid artery. (From Fisher, C. M., Karnes, W. E., and Kubik, C. S.: Lateral medullary infarction: The pattern of vascular occlusion. J. Neuropathol. Exp. Neurol., 20:334, 1961. Reprinted by permission.)

and atrial myxoma may also give rise to cerebral emboli.

Alteration in the composition and constituents of blood may affect blood flow and delivery of nutrients. Such changes may favor ischemia and subsequent stroke. Oxygen transport is maximal when hematocrit is in the range of 30 to 32 per cent.[100, 213] Increases in the red cell component of blood may enhance blood viscosity, limiting cerebral blood flow. Similarly, thrombocytosis or derangement of blood elements, as occurs in sickle cell disease, may promote sludging, which further compromises blood flow. Abnormalities in coagulation and lytic factors as well as deficiencies in clotting inhibitors such as antithrombin III, protein C, and protein S may encourage thrombosis. Elevated fibrinogen levels have been associated with an increased risk of stroke, as have hypercoagulable states that may accompany malignancy.[114, 203, 208]

Inflammatory and infectious processes may affect the cerebral blood vessels, causing infarction. A variety of organisms, including bacteria, fungi, parasites, and viruses, can directly injure parenchyma and the vessels that supply these tissues. Infectious agents may embolize to the cerebral arteries or incite local thrombosis. Stroke may result as a consequence of systemic processes such as lupus erythematosus, polyarteritis nodosa, and rheumatoid arthritis. The mechanisms of stroke in these multisystem vasculitides may include coagulopathy, cerebral angiitis, or cardiogenic embolism. Granulomatous angiitis is a necrotizing angiopathy largely restricted to the central nervous system. Giant cell arteritis involving the temporal artery in elderly patients may extend intracranially and compromise vision. Takayasu's disease is manifest as pathological changes in the great vessels of the thorax and neck that feed the brain.

Numerous other conditions may cause stroke. Direct vessel compromise can occur from mass or trauma. Cerebral arterial spasm may result from subarachnoid hemorrhage or migraine. Vessel dissection or steal phenomena may alter blood flow to the brain (Fig. 44–6). Lipohyalinosis represents vascular change induced by hypertension that may result in infarction in small-vessel territories. Increased intracranial pressure, miscellaneous vasculopathies, and inherited disorders are among the other entities that may play a role in the development of cerebral ischemia and stroke.

Vessel Syndromes

Evaluation of nervous system ischemic events must consider not only mechanism and cause but also the site within the cerebrovasculature at which the insult occurs. Occlusion of specific vessels can produce a range of effects. Although classic syndromes are described, occlusive states may produce these syndromes in whole or in part, or they may have minimal impact. Variations in collateral blood supply and functional localization as well as differences in the duration and severity of ischemic episodes impart a wide array of injuries and associated neurological findings.

ANTERIOR CIRCULATION

Ophthalmic Artery

The ophthalmic artery, the first major branch of the internal carotid artery, arises from its anterior or anteromedial aspect. In 83 to 89 per cent of cases, the ophthalmic artery originates from the internal carotid artery as the latter emanates from the cavernous sinus.[91, 162] In the remainder, the ophthalmic artery takes off more proximally from the internal carotid artery or from another parent vessel, such as the middle meningeal artery. It closely follows the course of its ipsilateral optic nerve, entering the optic foramen to supply the globe, orbit, and surrounding periorbital tissues. As previously noted, the anastomotic network between the external and internal carotid artery systems is extensive in this region. Collateral flow through these routes may serve not only structures of the eye but also large intracranial territories. Emboli reaching the retinal vessels may result in transient monocular visual loss, which can be attitudinal or lateralized in nature.[34] Proximal occlusion of the ophthalmic artery does not cause blindness unless a thrombus extends into the

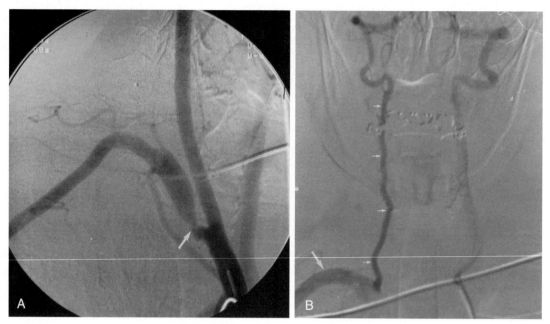

Figure 44–6

Radiographic subclavian steal. *A.* Innominate artery arteriogram demonstrates proximal right subclavian artery stenosis *(arrow). B.* Left vertebral injection of the same patient reveals retrograde filling of the right vertebral system *(short arrows)* and subsequent filling of the right subclavian artery *(long arrow).*

central retinal artery or unless propagating thrombus includes a significant number of posterior ciliary branches.[200] Historically, ophthalmic artery obliteration or trapping procedures for the treatment of carotid cavernous fistulas have not resulted in visual loss.[7, 51, 90] Other causes of monocular visual loss include vasculitis, migraine, hematological disorder, systemic hypotension, and primary ocular disease.

Posterior Communicating Artery

The posterior communicating artery originates from the dorsal, supraclinoid portion of the internal carotid artery. The vessel projects caudally and medially in close association with the oculomotor nerve and ultimately joins the posterior cerebral artery. Although the posterior communicating arteries are important segments of the circle of Willis, bridging anterior and posterior circulations, they are commonly rudimentary. Four to twelve branch vessels, termed "anterior thalamoperforating arteries," arise from the posterior communicating artery to supply the inferior optic chiasm, optic tract, tuber cinereum, mamillary bodies, anterior and ventral thalamus, subthalamus, posterior hypothalamus, and posterior limb of the internal capsule.* The largest and most constant of these vessels, referred to as the premamillary or thalamotuberal artery, supplies the anterior and lateral portions of the thalamus and hypothalamus[78, 156, 184] (Fig. 44–7). In some instances, multiple small arteries or perforators from other parent arteries nourish these regions. Clinical significance is inferred from infarction in the territory of the premamillary artery as delineated by computed

tomography studies. Associated findings include neuropsychological dysfunction characterized by perseveration, apathy, lack of spontaneity, and disorientation.[28] Mild to moderate sensory and motor disturbance may also be observed. Left-sided lesions may produce language impairment, and right-sided lesions may result in syndromes of hemineglect or spatial disorientation.[27, 28] Clinical deficit from compromise of other posterior communicating artery perforators is not well defined. The degree to which the subserved tissues are affected is largely dependent on the extent of complementary blood supply. Despite the caliber of the posterior communicating artery, the number of its perforators is relatively constant. In some instances, the diameter of the thalamoperforating vessels has been noted to exceed that of the parent posterior communicating artery.[89, 154] Therefore, the functional significance of a posterior communicating artery cannot be determined by its size alone. Surgical procedures, particularly those addressing aneurysms at the basilar apex or the posterior communicating artery's origin, must strive to avoid isolation of posterior communicating artery perforators. If possible, interruption of the posterior communicating artery should be preceded by evidence that the vessel will remain in continuity with the circle of Willis despite such a maneuver.

Anterior Choroidal Artery

The anterior choroidal artery most frequently arises from the internal carotid artery just distal to the origin of the posterior communicating artery. On occasion, two or more vessels may subserve territories supplied by the more typical single-branch anterior choroidal artery. From the internal carotid artery, the anterior

---

*See references 1, 24, 54, 116, 176, 184, 189, 204, and 215.

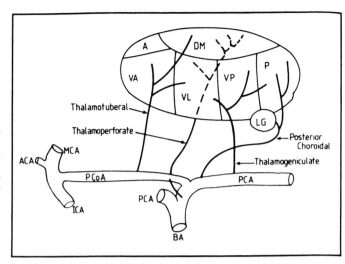

Figure 44–7

Thalamotuberal artery and associated vessels supplying the thalamic region. ICA, internal carotid artery; ACA, anterior cerebral artery; MCA, middle cerebral artery; PCoA, posterior communicating artery; PCA, posterior cerebral artery; BA, basilar artery. Thalamic nuclei: A, anterior; VA, ventral anterior; DM, dorsal medial; VL, ventral lateral; VP, ventral posterior; P, pulvinar; LG, lateral geniculate. (From Chambers, B. R., Brooder, R. J., and Donnan, G. A.: Proximal posterior cerebral artery occlusion simulating middle cerebral artery occlusion. Neurology, 41:388, 1991. Reprinted by permission.)

choroidal artery courses posteromedially below the optic tract and medial to the uncus of the temporal lobe. At the anterior margin of the lateral geniculate body, the vessel begins a posterolateral route, coursing around the cerebral peduncle to enter the choroidal fissure, subsequently terminating in the choroid plexus of the lateral ventricle. The anterior choroidal artery maintains reciprocal relationships with numerous other vessels, including the posterior cerebral artery, the posterior communicating artery, and the lateral posterior choroidal artery. Prominence of one or more of these blood supplies may diminish the realm of anterior choroidal artery supply, whereas a dominant anterior choroidal system may nourish a greater array and volume of associated tissues. Structures supplied by the anterior choroidal artery are numerous and may include portions of the temporal lobe, basal ganglia, diencephalon, and midbrain as well as components of the visual system. In detail, supplied regions include the uncus, the pyriform cortex, the posteromedial amygdala, the medial segments of the globus pallidus, the tail of the caudate, the genu and posterior aspects of the internal capsule, the lateral portions of the thalamus and subthalamus, the middle one third of the cerebral peduncle, the substantia nigra, regions of the red nucleus, the optic tract and radiations, part of the lateral geniculate body, and the choroid plexus within the anterior and inferior temporal horn of the lateral ventricle[1, 2, 24, 120, 166] (Fig. 44–8). In 1891, Kolisko outlined the areas affected by infarction in the distribution of the anterior choroidal artery, and in 1925, Foix and co-workers elucidated the clinical syndrome of anterior choroidal artery infarction.[79, 120] As classically reported, the syndrome includes contralateral hemiplegia, hemianesthesia, and hemianopsia. The motor and sensory alterations are attributed to involvement of the internal capsule and cerebral peduncle. Visual compromise reflects infarction involving the visual pathway at the level of the optic tract, optic radiation, or lateral geniculate body. This classic presentation, however, is a relatively rare occurrence, and partial syndromes are more commonly observed.[57] Other findings may include spatial or constructional apraxia in patients with

right-sided lesions. Left-sided infarction may create mild degrees of language dysfunction. Pseudobulbar mutism has been described in patients with bilateral anterior choroidal artery distribution infarction.[96] Infarction in the regions supplied by the anterior choroidal artery is said to result most often from small-vessel disease, changes wrought by atherosclerosis, and chronic hypertension.[35, 95] Such changes are likely to be diffuse, serving to limit collateral blood flow from the reciprocal vessels. Under more normal circumstances, proximal occlusion of the anterior choroidal artery may be well tolerated. Historically, such occlusion has been used to treat the tremor and rigidity of parkinsonism.[45, 46, 163] Clinical and pathological review of these cases has revealed a wide range of effects from these procedures, varying from little or no injury to infarction in the subserved tissues. Such findings illustrate the variability in anterior choroidal artery distribution as well as the importance of associated collateral and complementary blood supplies.

Anterior Cerebral Artery

At the level of the anterior perforated substance, the internal carotid artery terminates, bifurcating into the middle cerebral artery and the smaller, medially positioned, anterior cerebral artery. From its origin, the anterior cerebral artery courses anteromedially over the optic nerve and chiasm to reach the interhemispheric fissure. This initial horizontal portion is termed the A_1 segment; it extends from the carotid terminus to the level of the anterior communicating artery. The anterior cerebral artery distal to the communicating vessel (the A_2 segment) projects anterosuperiorly in front of the lamina terminalis and genu of the corpus callosum. Further anterior cerebral artery segments extend superiorly and posteriorly, supplying the frontal pole, approximately three quarters of the medial surface of the hemisphere, and parasagittal frontal and parietal regions (Fig. 44–9; see Fig. 44–8). The posterior extent of the anterior cerebral artery territories is dependent on the extent of supply of the posterior cerebral artery and its splenial branches.[217]

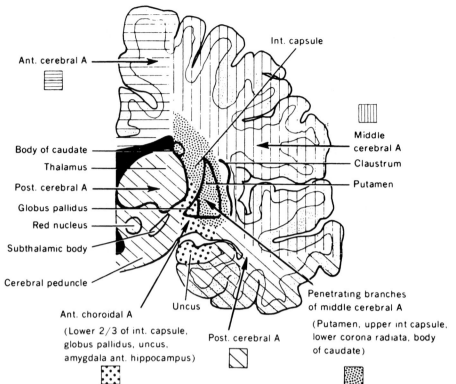

Figure 44–8

The cerebral hemisphere, coronal section, outlining the subserved territories of the major cerebral arteries. (From Adams, R. D., and Victor, M.: Principles of Neurology. 5th ed. New York, McGraw-Hill, 1993, p. 679. Reprinted by permission.)

The initial segment of the anterior cerebral artery gives rise to perforating vessels termed "medial lenticulostriate arteries" (Fig. 44–10). Commonly, 5 to 11 such vessels are described.[61, 86, 156] These vessels supply the medial portion of the anterior commissure and globus pallidus, the optic chiasm, the paraolfactory area, the anterior limb of the internal capsule, the medial inferior aspect of the putamen and head of the caudate, and the anterior hypothalamus.[61, 149, 156] Dunker and Harris have described extension of such perforators as far posteriorly as the genu of the internal capsule and the anterior thalamus.[61] Similar small vessels

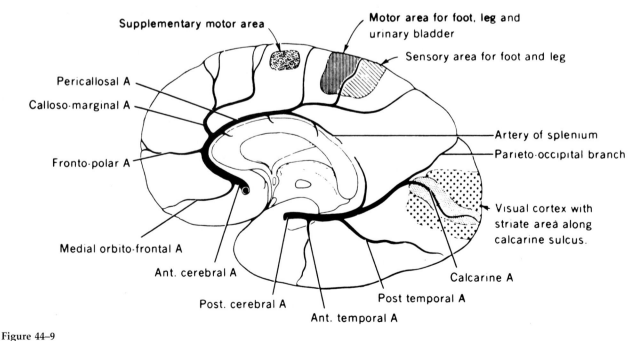

Figure 44–9

A medial view of the cerebral hemisphere, midsagittal section, detailing the course of the anterior and posterior cerebral arteries and functional localization of subserved tissues. (From Adams, R. D., and Victor, M.: Principles of Neurology. 5th ed. New York, McGraw-Hill, 1993, p. 680. Reprinted by permission.)

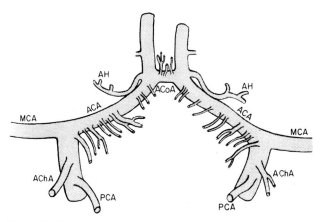

Figure 44–10

The proximal anterior intracranial circulation. The medial lenticulostriate arteries are demonstrated. MCA, middle cerebral artery; ACA, anterior cerebral artery; AChA, anterior choroidal artery; PCA, posterior communicating artery; AH, recurrent artery of Heubner. (From Dunker, R. O., and Harris, A. B.: Surgical anatomy of the proximal anterior cerebral artery. J. Neurosurg., *44*:365, 1976. Reprinted by permission.)

arise from the proximal postcommunicating anterior cerebral artery. These branches supply the anterior hypothalamus, the septum pellucidum, the pillars of the fornix, a portion of the anterior commissure, and the anterior-inferior regions of the striatum.[184] The largest of these arteries was described in 1872 by Heubner[98] (Fig. 44–11). The recurrent artery of Heubner originates at or just beyond the level of the anterior communicating artery in 86 to 92 per cent of cases.[86, 156] The vessel doubles back on the anterior cerebral artery, later accompanying the middle cerebral artery for a variable distance before entering the substance of the brain. The

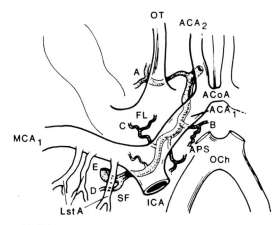

Figure 44–11

A schematic representation of the course of the recurrent artery of Heubner (*shaded vessel*): A, olfactory branch; B, anterior perforated substance branches; C, frontal branches; D, sylvian fissure branches; E, terminal branches. ICA, internal carotid artery; MCA$_1$, proximal middle cerebral artery; ACA$_1$, proximal anterior cerebral artery; ACA$_2$, distal anterior cerebral artery; ACoA, anterior communicating artery; OCh, optic chiasm; OT, olfactory tract; FL, frontal lobe; SF, sylvian fissure; Lst A, lenticulostriate arteries; APS, anterior perforated substance. (From Gomes, F., Dujovny, M., Umansky, F., et al.: Microsurgical anatomy of the recurrent artery of Heubner. J. Neurosurg., *60*:135, 1984. Reprinted by permission.)

branches of Heubner's artery have been described as supplying the anterior regions of the striatum, a small segment of outer globus pallidus, and the anterior limb of the internal capsule.[48, 61, 149, 202]

Flow-obstructing lesions in the proximal anterior cerebral artery are usually well tolerated, given the potential for collateral flow from the neighboring contralateral artery through the anterior communicating artery. Limitation in communicating artery blood supply in this circumstance can result in massive cortical and subcortical infarction and in damage to basal tissues supplied by perforating vessels. Anatomical states in which both distal anterior cerebral arteries are supplied by a single proximal segment may be associated with significant bilateral infarction in the setting of occlusion involving the initial portions of the dominant anterior cerebral artery. If compromise of the basal perforators or the recurrent artery of Heubner is observed, transient contralateral hemiparesis is the most common finding.[37] A propensity for weakness to occur in a faciobrachiocrural or faciobrachial pattern in these instances has been described.[26, 202] Involvement of the internal capsular and basal ganglionic regions in these cases has been postulated to account for these findings, which are in contrast to the primarily lower extremity deficits seen in patients with cortical lesions from more distal anterior cerebral artery lesions. Dysarthria and behavioral disturbance are also common abnormalities found in those with ischemic lesions affecting the deep anterior cerebral perforators. Transcortical motor aphasia may occur with infarction affecting the dominant hemisphere. Contralateral neglect may reflect involvement of deep nondominant structures.

Infarction caused by vessel occlusion distal to the anterior communicating artery results in sensory and motor disturbance in the contralateral body, more prominently in the lower than the upper extremity. Eye and head deviation to the side of the lesion may be observed. Language dysfunction may accompany dominant hemisphere lesions. Apraxia and spatial disorientation syndromes may attend nondominant hemisphere lesions. Contralateral hypertonia and peripheral reflex changes may be present. Primitive reflexes or frontal release signs are commonly noted. Urinary incontinence and cognitive alterations such as abulia, akinetic mutism, and profound personality changes are more common in the setting of bifrontal disease.

Anterior Communicating Artery

The anterior communicating artery is a short-vessel component of the circle of Willis that unites the paired anterior cerebral arteries at a point ventral to the lamina terminalis. Anomalies are commonplace and include vessel duplications, triplications, fenestrations, loops, and bridges.[215] The nature of the communicating artery is dependent on the character of the initial anterior cerebral artery segments (A$_1$). Not infrequently, a hypoplastic A$_1$ segment is observed and is accompanied by a generous anterior communicating artery. This configuration proves beneficial to both distal anterior cerebral artery circulations. Aneurysms in this region are commonplace. Surgical treatment of these lesions must respect the deep perforating vessels emanating from the anterior communicating artery. Failure to do so may result in altered personality, memory deficit, hemiplegia, aphasia, visual field defect, or even death.[165] Usually, 2 to 5 perforators originating from the dorsal surface of the anterior communicating artery are described.[49, 132, 165, 197] Most branches are small, ranging in size from 50 to 250 microns.[49] These branches supply the septum pellucidum, the corpus callosum, the columns of the fornix, the lamina terminalis, the paraolfactory areas, the anterior hypothalamus, the infundibulum, the cingulum, the superior surface of the optic chiasm, and portions of the ventral frontal lobes[49, 61, 156] (Fig. 44–12). In approximately 10 per cent of specimens, at least one large branch, 500 to 1,000 microns, arises from the anterior communicating artery.[61, 132] This vessel is referred to as the arteria termatica of Wilder or the median artery of the corpus callosum. It courses superiorly over the corpus callosum to supply parasagittal aspects of both hemispheres.[184]

Compromise of the perforators of the anterior communicating artery is implicated in the genesis of some memory disturbances. Studies reviewing patients with anterior communicating artery aneurysm rupture and subsequent treatment report a high incidence of memory dysfunction.* The anatomical basis for this disturbance remains ill-defined. Damage to the basal forebrain regions, including the septal nuclei, nucleus accumbens, substantia innominata, and related pathways, has been considered as a potential source of memory impairment.[50] Additional regions implicated include the cingulum, anterior hypothalamus, fornices, striatum, and ventral frontal cortical regions, or a combination of these structures.[8, 108, 197] It remains to be

---

*See references 8, 50, 81, 106, 108, and 129.

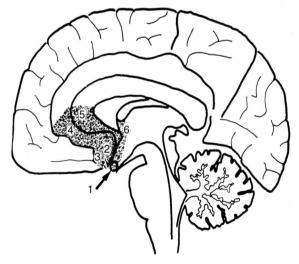

Figure 44–12

Region of supply of the anterior communicating artery perforators: 1, basal forebrain; 2, anterior cingulate; 3, anterior hypothalamus. (From Crowell, R. M., and Morawetz, R. B.: The anterior communicating artery has significant branches. Stroke, 8:273, 1977. Reprinted by permission.)

determined whether ischemia in the territory of the anterior communicating artery has a direct role in memory impairment. Physical injury from subarachnoid hemorrhage, surgical manipulation, or vasospasm may damage tissues unrelated to the deep perforators of the anterior communicating artery, tissues that may be responsible for observed memory deficits. Gade's patients who underwent trapping of anterior communicating artery aneurysms, with isolation of the anterior communicating artery and its branches from the circulation, developed a much higher incidence of postoperative amnestic syndromes than those who underwent ligation of the aneurysmal neck or related procedures.[81] These observations suggest that regions supplied by the anterior communicating artery may have a role in memory function.

Middle Cerebral Artery

The middle cerebral artery is the larger of the vessels arising from the internal carotid artery terminus, and it nourishes a larger volume of tissue than any other cerebral vessel. Its origination from the parent internal carotid artery at a less acute angle than the anterior cerebral artery, along with the massive blood flow carried by the vessel, creates a favored conduit through which emboli may be channeled. The regions supplied by proximal branches of the middle cerebral artery include deep ganglionic and capsular areas (see Fig. 44–8). More distal branches subserve the entire lateral hemisphere, with the exception of the frontal pole, occipital pole, and small parasagittal strips anteriorly and posteriorly, which are fed by the anterior and posterior cerebral systems (Fig. 44–13). From its inception, the middle cerebral artery courses horizontally and laterally, beneath the anterior perforated substance, to access the sylvian fissure. This initial or M_1 segment gives rise to lateral lenticulostriate arteries and to small branch arteries supplying the mesial anterior temporal lobe. Some 2 to 20 lenticulostriate vessels arise from the inferior surface of the middle cerebral artery (M_1), either from one or two primary trunks or as numerous twigs from the parent vessel.[133, 167, 193, 215] A reciprocal relationship or balance has been noted between the striate vessels of the anterior cerebral artery and those of the middle cerebral artery.[193, 204, 215] Prominence in one group may be manifest in the size or number of perforators from the other vessel. The middle cerebral artery lenticulostriate branches supply the substantia innominata, the lateral portion of the anterior commissure, the putamen, the lateral globus pallidus, the body and head of the caudate nucleus with exception of the anteroinferior aspect, parts of the posterior limb of the internal capsule, and the corona radiata.[56, 84, 153, 171, 184]

Near the limen insulae, the middle cerebral artery gives rise to two or more branch vessels (M_2), which continue to course laterally into the depths of the sylvian fissure. As the cortical vessels emerge from the fissure, one branch extends inferiorly, supplying the temporal and temporoparietal regions. A second artery

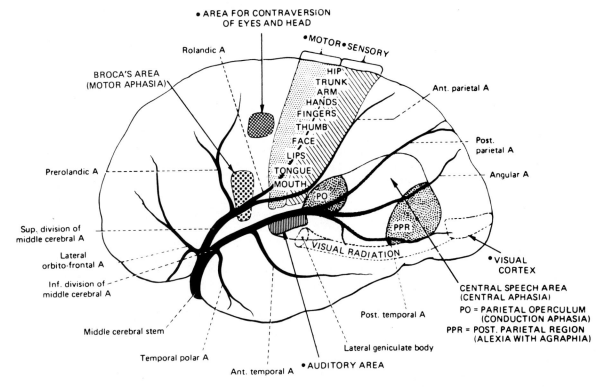

Figure 44–13

The lateral aspect of the cerebral hemisphere, demonstrating middle cerebral artery course and functional localization of subserved tissues. (From Adams, R. D., and Victor, M.: Principles of Neurology. 5th ed. New York, McGraw-Hill, 1993, p. 677. Reprinted by permission.)

ascends to provide blood flow to the expanse of the lateral frontal and parietal lobes.

Mainstem middle cerebral artery occlusion is most often embolic in nature.[70, 127] Such lesions render ischemic injury to deep perforators and cortical branches alike. The resultant clinical profile is one of contralateral hemiplegia involving the face, arm, and leg; hemisensory loss; and homonymous hemianopsia. Dominant hemisphere insult may be characterized by severe and global aphasia. Nondominant hemisphere damage produces disturbance of body image with spatial apraxia and neglect. In the acute phase, head and eye deviation to the side of the infarction may also be present, accompanied by paralysis of conjugate contralateral gaze. Massive infarction and associated edema may generate alteration in the level of consciousness from brain stem compression. Progression may lead to uncal herniation and death. Those who survive proximal middle cerebral artery occlusion often make little recovery and are relegated to an existence of disability.

Infarction in the distribution of the lateral lenticulostriate arteries is not uncommonly the result of embolus. However, small-vessel disease is considered to be a prominent cause of infarction in the territories of these perforators. Injury in this setting may affect the internal capsule and basal ganglia, with resultant mixed sensorimotor disturbance or hemiparesis involving the face, arm, and leg. Isolated sensory disturbance is infrequently observed. Higher cognitive functions are also largely preserved. Language dysfunction, if present, is transient in nature. Visual field limitation may be

indicative of injury to optic radiations in the dorsal posterior limb of the internal capsule.

Frequently, emboli traverse the middle cerebral artery main stem and subsequently compromise more distal cortical arterial segments. In these circumstances, partial syndromes predominate. Superior branch syndromes may be difficult to differentiate from mainstem occlusions. Infarction of more cephalad frontal and parietal tissues may result in severe contralateral motor and sensory loss. Changes in consciousness are less likely to be observed. Language dysfunction may initially be mixed, but it ultimately predominates as an expressive disorder. Emboli locating more distally in superior division branches serve to further restrict the clinical syndrome.

The inferior division of the middle cerebral artery is less commonly affected by such occurrences. Compromise of this portion of the middle cerebral artery may produce receptive language disorder of the Wernicke type in dominant hemisphere lesions. Characteristically, weakness is absent. Nondominant injury may result in hemineglect and spatial agnosia. Disruption of the optic radiations often results in hemianopic or quadrantal visual field deficit.

Internal Carotid Artery

The spectrum of cerebral injury in states of internal carotid artery occlusive disease is varied. Occlusion of the internal carotid artery may occur without overt clinical manifestation. In other instances, occlusion is accompanied by massive hemispheric infarction and herniation. Flow-limiting lesions of the internal carotid artery most commonly occur at its origin at the level of the common carotid artery. The carotid siphon is the next most frequent site of significant atherosclerotic occlusive disease.[74, 128] The presence of an intact circle of Willis and extracranial to intracranial avenues for collateral blood flow may abort damage to neuronal populations threatened by internal carotid artery occlusion (Fig. 44–14). If collateral flow proves inadequate, infarction that mimics mainstem middle cerebral artery occlusion is most often observed. Contralateral hemiplegia, hemisensory disturbance, and homonymous hemianopsia are characteristic. Emboli generated more proximally have a propensity for entering the middle cerebral artery circulation. Similarly, the propagation or embolization of thrombus from internal artery occlusions most profoundly disturbs middle cerebral artery territories. Blood supply to the anterior cerebral artery system is often preserved, given collateral flow through the anterior communicating artery. In states of carotid occlusion, poor anterior communicating artery supply may result in infarction of anterior cerebral and middle cerebral artery regions. In the presence of anomaly, stroke may extend beyond the usual confines. Internal carotid artery ischemia accompanied by a hypoplastic contralateral anterior cerebral artery segment (A_1) may result in bifrontal infarction. Internal carotid artery occlusion accompanied by a persistent fetal circulation

may also result in injury to occipital tissues usually nourished by the posterior circulation. Patients suffering infarction of large portions of a hemisphere are most often stuporous or semicomatose and have a grim prognosis.

POSTERIOR CIRCULATION

Anterior Spinal Artery

As the distal vertebral artery enters the cranium, it gives rise to an anterior spinal ramus, which courses inferiorly and medially to join its counterpart from the opposite side. This union fashions the anterior spinal artery, which then descends along the anterior median fissure of the medulla oblongata and spinal cord. In some cases, one or both rami may be absent or have an anomalous course.[85] In other instances, the rami may descend for a variable distance before uniting. The anterior spinal artery and its feeders supply the pyramids, the medial lemnisci, and, occasionally, the fibers of the hypoglossal nerves and ventrolateral portions of the inferior olivary nuclei.[52, 62] Spiller was the first to postulate a syndrome arising from occlusion of the anterior spinal artery.[182] Occlusion of one ramus may be compensated for by blood flow from the contralateral fellow; however, it can also result in contralateral hemiplegia and ipsilateral tongue weakness from involvement of corticospinal and hypoglossal fibers. These findings may be associated with contralateral loss of proprioception and vibratory sense, heralding injury to the medial lemniscus (medial medullary syndrome; Fig. 44–15). Bilateral motor and sensory deficits may occur from occlusion of the anterior spinal artery or a dominant ramus. Compromise of the anterior spinal circulation is most often seen as a result of compressive lesions at the cervicomedullary junction rather than degenerative vascular disease.[164]

Posterior Inferior Cerebellar Artery

The posterior inferior cerebellar artery is the largest branch vessel arising from the vertebral artery. Most commonly, it arises from the intracranial vertebral artery before the formation of the basilar artery. Origin below the foramen magnum or from other parent arteries has been observed. In 7 per cent of cases, the vertebral artery terminates in the posterior inferior cerebellar artery.[14] The size and territorial extent of the posterior inferior cerebellar artery are dependent on the adjacent anterior inferior cerebellar artery, to which it bears an inverse relation.

From the vertebral artery, the posterior inferior cerebellar artery travels laterally around the medulla. At the lateral margin of the medulla, it courses inferiorly to form a caudal loop in the vicinity of the cerebellar tonsil. The artery then ascends on the tonsil, initiating a cranial loop. Branches to the choroid plexus of the fourth ventricle and tonsil are given off before the vessel descends to supply the inferior vermis and cerebellar hemisphere. Posterior inferior cerebellar artery blood usually supplies the posterior medulla and cere-

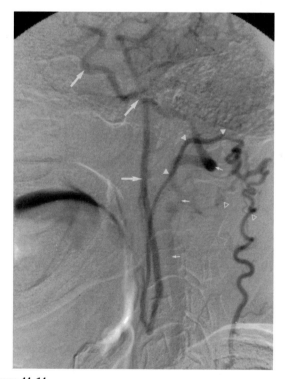

Figure 44–14

Left common carotid artery occlusion with extracranial to intracranial collateral flow. This left subclavian arteriogram reveals retrograde filling of the occipital artery (*closed arrows*) through thyrocervical and vertebral artery branches (*open arrows*). Occipital supply nourishes the internal carotid artery system (*long arrows*). Short arrows indicate vertebral artery.

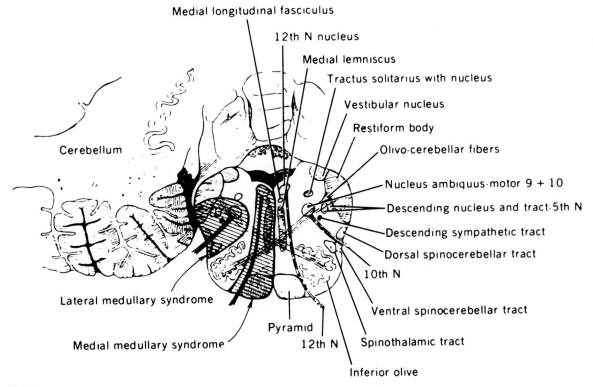

Figure 44–15

Axial section of the superior medulla oblongata. *Shaded regions* indicate topography and encompassed structures in the medial and lateral medullary syndromes. (From Adams, R. D., and Victor, M.: Principles of Neurology. 5th ed. New York, McGraw-Hill, 1993, p. 690. Reprinted by permission.)

bellum. Supply to the lateral aspects of the medulla is considered inconstant.[14, 67]

Occlusion of the proximal posterior inferior cerebellar artery or the respective vertebral artery may produce a well-recognized syndrome first elucidated by Wallenberg[199] (Fig. 44–15). This lateral medullary syndrome has many components. Injury to descending sympathetic fibers in this region is manifest as an ipsilateral Horner syndrome. Involvement of the spinothalamic tract and afferent trigeminal system produces alteration in pain and temperature sensation in the ipsilateral face and contralateral body. Nausea, vomiting, nystagmus, and vertigo typify the presence of lesions of the vestibular nuclei. Ipsilateral ataxia or hypotonia may reflect damage to the inferior cerebellar peduncle and its constituents. Hoarseness and dysphagia localize to the nucleus ambiguous or to the ninth and tenth cranial nerve fibers. Hiccups are often present, but a pathological basis for this finding remains ill-defined. Facial weakness, hearing loss, or ocular disturbance are less commonly seen and may suggest extension of the ischemic process into pontine zones.[68, 77, 173] Impairment of more distal posterior inferior cerebellar artery branch vessels results in fragmentation of the complete lateral medullary syndrome. The main posterior inferior cerebellar artery trunk ultimately gives rise to two branches, one medial and one lateral. Infarction in the lateral branch territory is likely to encompass peripheral cerebellar hemispheric regions and remains poorly defined clinically. The medial ves-

sel supplies a triangular territory with a dorsal base and a ventral apex toward the fourth ventricle[14] (Fig. 44–16). Clinical patterns in this circumstance are not constant and may include isolated vertigo, complete lateral medullary syndrome, or silent infarction.[12]

Vertebral Artery

The vertebral artery takes origin from the subclavian artery, coursing upward to traverse the transverse fo-

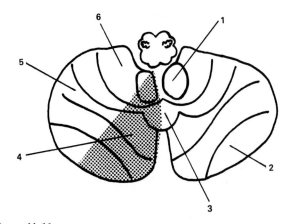

Figure 44–16

Diagrammatic representation of the territory of the medial branch of the posterior inferior cerebellar artery. (From Amarenco, P., Roullet, E., Hommel, M., et al.: Infarction in the territory of the medial branch of the posterior inferior cerebellar artery. J. Neurol. Neurosurg. Psychiatry, 53:732, 1990. Reprinted by permission.)

ramina of the sixth through first cervical vertebrae. Its path then follows horizontally along the posterior arch of the first cervical vertebra before ascending intracranially through the foramen magnum. Each vertebral artery projects anteromedially to the pontomedullary sulcus, at which both arteries unite to form the basilar artery. In its extracranial course, the vertebral artery maintains extensive anastomoses with vessels of the dorsal cervical musculature and the thyrocervical trunk. This network serves as a potential source of collateral blood flow in states of posterior circulation occlusive disease.

The vertebral arteries supply the upper aspects of the cervical spinal cord, the medulla, and a large portion of the cerebellum. Lesions affecting the vertebral artery may have a wide range of effects. Atherosclerosis most commonly affects the vertebral artery at its origin. Vertebral artery occlusion at this level is often well tolerated because of collateral flow. Intracranial vertebrobasilar occlusive disease does not afford soft tissue collateral flow, may involve vertebral branch vessels, and is more likely to cause stroke.[147] Nevertheless, as demonstrated by the use of vertebral artery ligation for unclippable posterior circulation aneurysms, vertebral artery occlusion often causes few or no sequelae.[59, 152, 183, 214] The occurrence of infarction is dependent on the extent of collateral blood supply. Vertebral artery infarction may duplicate in part or in whole the syndromes occurring from ischemia in the vertebral artery branches. Vertebral artery compromise at the level of paramedian medullary perforators results in a medial medullary syndrome that is also seen in anterior spinal artery occlusion. This condition is typified by contralateral body and ipsilateral tongue weakness as well as by contralateral diminution in proprioception and vibratory sensation. Similarly, involvement of the lateral medullary structures and cerebellum may occur. The lateral medullary or Wallenberg syndrome is described in the previous section.

Anterior Inferior Cerebellar Artery

The first major branch of the basilar artery is the anterior inferior cerebellar artery. From its inception, it courses laterally, posteriorly, and inferiorly, reaching the cerebellopontine angle, where it is closely associated with the seventh and eighth cranial nerve complex. Thereafter, it continues on to supply the flocculus and the cerebellar hemisphere.[11, 124] The extent of its supply is variable and is largely dependent on the distribution of the posterior inferior cerebellar artery. The clinical syndrome of anterior inferior cerebellar artery infarction is, as a result, protean. Generally, the anterior inferior cerebellar artery supplies the lateral and tegmental aspects of the lower pons, the superior dorsolateral medulla, and the anterior-inferior cerebellum. Within this realm reside the superior olivary nucleus, the facial nucleus, the lateral lemniscus, the eighth nerve, the vestibular nuclei, the cochlear nucleus, the trapezoid body, the spinal trigeminal tract and nucleus, the spinothalamic tract, the middle and inferior cerebellar peduncles, and, in some cases, the

lateral portion of the abducens nucleus and the central tegmental tracts.[6, 10, 14, 19, 63] Given the potential for involvement of these structures, ischemia in the distribution of the anterior inferior cerebellar artery may resemble the lateral medullary syndrome in many respects. Nausea, vomiting, vertigo, nystagmus, loss of pain and temperature sensation in the ipsilateral areas of the face and contralateral side of the body, and ipsilateral ataxia may be present. Although it has been described, Horner's syndrome does not occur commonly.[11] Peripheral facial paralysis, deafness, tinnitus, and lateral gaze palsy differentiate this syndrome from that of the posterior inferior cerebellar artery. Occlusion at the origin of the anterior inferior cerebellar artery may result in injury to the corticospinal tract, with resultant contralateral hemiparesis. The anterior inferior cerebellar artery is consistently the source of the internal auditory artery.[119, 135] With a variable collateral supply, the latter vessel nourishes the vestibulocochlear nerve complex within the internal auditory canal, whereas the inner ear is exclusively supplied by the internal auditory artery.[136] Patients suffering ischemic events in the distribution of the anterior inferior cerebellar artery or its internal auditory branch vessels are prone to deafness on the affected side.

Superior Cerebellar Artery

The paired superior cerebellar arteries are considered the most constant of the cerebellar vessels. They arise infratentorially from the rostral basilar artery. The superior cerebellar artery courses around the brain stem in the groove between the pons and the midbrain. Within the ambient cistern at the lateral margin of the brain stem, the artery follows a gentle loop, subsequently bifurcating into a medial and a lateral branch. The lateral branch encircles the cerebellum, supplying its superolateral surface and deep nuclei. The medial segment tracks around the pontomesencephalic junction to supply dorsal brain stem regions. Territory supplied by the superior cerebellar artery includes the cerebellar hemisphere, the dentate nucleus, the inferior colliculus, the superior cerebellar peduncle, the upper aspects of the middle cerebellar peduncle, the locus ceruleus, parts of the medial lemniscus, the spinothalamic tract, the lateral lemniscus, the reticulospinal tract, the mesencephalic nucleus, the tract of the trigeminal nerve, and fibers of the trochlear nerve.[13, 14, 63, 85, 184] Occlusion of the superior cerebellar artery results in contralateral dissociated hemisensory loss affecting the face, arm, trunk, and leg. Horner's syndrome and palatal myoclonus may be observed. Hearing loss, ipsilateral or contralateral, presumably resulting from damage to the cochlear nucleus or lateral lemniscal pathway, has been described.[80, 142] Other findings include gaze disorders, vertigo, nausea, vomiting, nystagmus, ipsilateral ataxia, and coarse tremor affecting the ipsilateral upper extremity.[53, 80] However, some studies have found this "classic" syndrome to occur infrequently.[13, 130, 185] In addition, it is uncommon for infarctions in the superior cerebellar artery distribution to occur in isolation.[13, 126] Most often, these lesions result from emboli that have followed the course of the basilar artery. In such cases, other blood supplies at the basilar terminus are frequently affected as well. With infarction occurring in multiple vessel territories, it is often difficult to distinguish a pure superior cerebellar artery syndrome.

Basilar Artery

The basilar artery is formed by the union of the vertebral arteries at the pontomedullary junction. The vertebral arteries are often of different caliber. In 2 to 3 per cent of individuals, a vertebral artery may be hypoplastic, lacking functional significance, or, rarely, altogether absent.[85] In still other cases, the vertebral artery may fail to join its opposite fellow, ending as the posterior inferior cerebellar artery. From its origin, the basilar artery proceeds cephalad along the ventrum of the brain stem, bifurcating into the posterior cerebral arteries at the level of the caudal midbrain. The basilar artery nourishes the pons, caudal midbrain, and large regions of the cerebellum (Fig. 44–17). Throughout its course, it gives rise to numerous pairs of paramedian penetrating vessels that supply ventral brain stem tissues. Short circumferential arteries feed anterolateral aspects of the brain stem at these same levels. Two pairs of long circumferential arteries (superior and anterior inferior cerebellar arteries) provide blood supply to dorsal mesencephalic and pontine structures in addition to a large volume of cerebellum. From the most

rostral aspects of the basilar artery, perforators variably emerge to supply subthalamic and high midbrain regions. A more extensive blood supply to these tissues is derived from the initial segments of the posterior cerebral arteries.

Atherosclerotic changes are often most pronounced in the proximal basilar artery and at the vertebrobasilar junction. Basilar ischemia may ensue at atherosclerotic sites from superimposed thrombus in the basilar artery itself or within one or both vertebral arteries. More commonly, basilar branch arteries are affected by thrombosis, sparing the trunk. The clinical findings in branch disease, however, may be difficult to differentiate from those resulting from disease affecting the basilar artery itself. Thrombus, plaque, or cardiogenic embolus may seed the posterior circulation. Injury from such insults is usually borne in the distal basilar system. Most of these emboli originate from the heart or vertebral arteries. Particles traversing the vertebral arteries meet with a capacious proximal basilar artery and continue on into the more narrow confines of the distal artery or its branch vessels (Fig. 44–18).

The basilar artery subserves brain stem nuclei and tracts, cerebellar tissues and connections, and all ascending and descending long tracts. Basilar artery ischemia may compromise some or all such structures, creating profound neurological dysfunction. In states of basilar artery occlusion, neurological signs are most often bilateral. Deficits may arise suddenly or in a more protracted fashion. Findings associated with basilar ar-

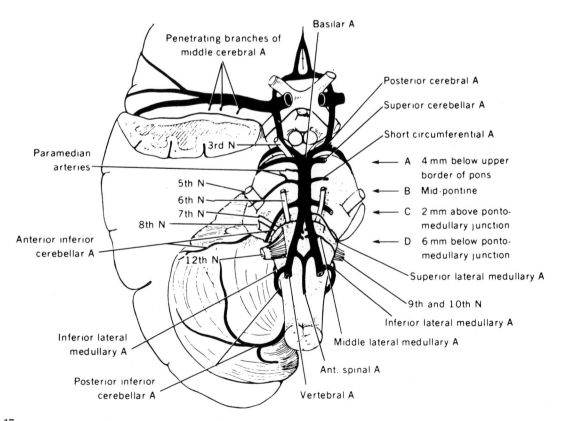

Figure 44–17

The ventral brain stem, depicting the basilar artery course. (From Adams, R. D., and Victor, M.: Principles of Neurology. 5th ed. New York, McGraw-Hill, 1993, p. 674. Reprinted by permission.)

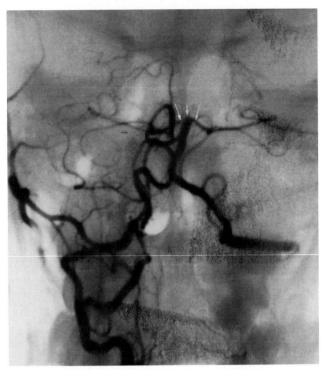

Figure 44–18

Basilar artery occlusion *(short arrow)* at the level of the anterior inferior cerebellar arteries *(long arrows).*

tery occlusion frequently evolve in a stepwise manner, developing over hours to days.[111] Patients so affected are often comatose or have markedly diminished levels of consciousness because of involvement of the midbrain reticular activating system. Lesions encompassing more caudal midbrain regions may spare reticular activating centers and vertical eye movements but interrupt lower cranial nerve and extremity motor function, producing a "locked-in" state. Emboli may be recurrent and thrombi may propagate, further impairing the basilar artery circulation and subserved tissues. Progressive infarction in the basilar artery territories is often accompanied by death. Partial basilar syndromes are more common given the frequency of lesions limited to basilar artery branch vessels. Identification of infarction locus and compromised blood supply can often be determined by the pattern of long tract and brain stem nuclei involvement. Numerous ischemic brain stem syndromes have been described.

Posterior Cerebral Artery

Of the intracranial arteries supplying the brain, the posterior cerebral artery is perhaps the most complex. In its course, the vessel serves both infratentorial and supratentorial tissues. The posterior cerebral arteries are formed at the basilar artery bifurcation, ventral to the midbrain. However, in 15 to 22 per cent of individuals, the vessel has a fetal origin, arising from the internal carotid artery.[9, 150, 176] In the normal adult configuration, initial segments of the posterior cerebral artery encircle the brain stem, nourishing mesence-

phalic and diencephalic parenchyma. More distal elements continue into the hemisphere to supply occipital and temporal regions.

The first portion of the posterior cerebral artery, extending from vessel origin to ostium of the posterior communicating artery, is referred to as the peduncular or precommunicating segment (P_1).[121] Synonymous terms are mesencephalic artery and basilar communicating artery.[117, 155] This segment gives rise to posterior thalamoperforating vessels and circumflex arteries (Fig. 44–19). An average of 3 to 4 perforators arise from each P_1 segment.[39, 176, 217] On occasion, the unilateral absence of such branches is observed, with the contralateral P_1 perforators providing supply bilaterally. The posterior thalamoperforating arteries nourish the medial margin of the cerebral peduncles, the substantia nigra, the medial tegmentum, the anterior thalamus, portions of the posterior thalamus, the hypothalamus, the subthalamus, the red nucleus, the third and fourth cranial nerve nuclei, the oculomotor nerve, the medial longitudinal fasciculus, the superior cerebellar peduncle, the pretectum, the rostromedial floor of the fourth ventricle, the anterior portion of the periaqueductal gray matter, and the posterior rim of the internal capsule.[40, 217] Short and long circumflex branches arise from the posterior cerebral artery in this P_1 segment to follow the circumference of the brain stem. The short-vessel group reaches the lateral aspect of the cerebral peduncle and, in some instances, the geniculate bodies.[217] The long circumflex arteries also travel medial to the main body of the posterior cerebral artery, persevering to reach the colliculi. These branches are sometimes termed the quadrigeminal arteries.[121, 184] The thalamogeniculate arteries originate from the posterior cerebral artery distal to its junction with the posterior communicating artery (P_2). This cluster of vessels courses superiorly to supply the geniculate bodies, the pulvinar, the brachium of the superior colliculus, other portions of the posterolateral thalamus, and the posterior limb of the internal capsule.[139, 177] The next major branches are the posterior choroidal arteries. The lateral posterior choroidal artery courses laterally and superiorly to feed portions of the temporal lobe, hippocampus, thalamus, and choroid plexus of the lateral ventricle.[161] The medial posterior choroidal artery encounters an extensive array of structures supplying regions of the diencephalon, mesencephalon, and choroid plexus of the lateral ventricle.[63, 118, 177, 217] As the final segment of the posterior cerebral artery courses around the brain stem, the vessel projects toward the calcarine fissure. Cortical branches supply the primary visual centers, the medial temporal lobe, and the splenium of the corpus callosum.

A variety of clinical effects can result from posterior cerebral artery ischemia. The degree and pattern of impairment is dependent on the location of blood flow compromise, the nature of collateral supply, and the extent of involvement of any of the numerous perforating vessels. Significant atherosclerotic disease in the posterior cerebral artery is uncommon.[157] Ischemia is most often perpetrated by emboli arising from the proximal circulation. Caplan first referred to the "top of

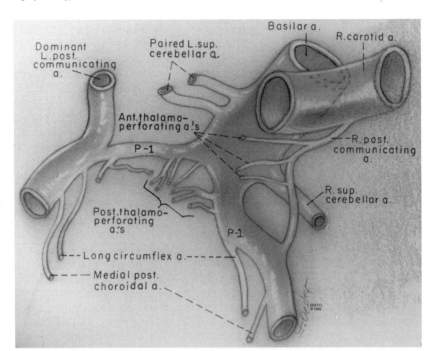

Figure 44–19

Basilar artery bifurcation. Branch vessels of the proximal posterior cerebral arteries (P₁) are shown. (From Sundt, T. M., Jr.: Surgical Techniques for Saccular and Giant Intracranial Aneurysms. Baltimore, Williams & Wilkins, 1990, p. 233. By permission of Mayo Foundation.)

the basilar" syndrome to identify signs and symptoms attributable to ischemia in the upper brain stem and hemispheric territories of the posterior cerebral artery.[38] Findings include visual and oculomotor abnormalities and alterations in consciousness and mentation. Embolic occlusion of peduncular branches of the posterior cerebral artery may explain many of the findings in this syndrome. Disturbances in ocular motility suggest injury to midbrain or tectal centers. Occlusion of long circumflex arteries may precipitate limitation in vertical gaze caused by infarction of the posterior commissure or the nuclei of Darkschewitsch or Cajal.[188] Weber's syndrome is characterized by contralateral hemimotor loss and ipsilateral third nerve palsy, which are indicative of ventral midbrain dysfunction involving the cerebral peduncle and fibers of the oculomotor nerve. Diminished consciousness or coma may result from tegmental damage with reticular activating system injury. Movement disorders, including tremor, ballism, and choreoathetosis, may be witnessed. Behavioral abnormalities with apathy and mood alteration, hypersomnia, sensory defects, and akinetic mutism characterize paramedian thalamic infarction.[40, 87] Amnestic syndromes are also commonplace.

Occlusion of thalamogeniculate branches supplying the posterocentral thalamus may produce infarction with dissociated sensory loss in the contralateral body, which may be accompanied by a transient hemiparesis. As sensation returns, it may give way to lancinating pain or paresthesia in the affected regions. This, the Dejerine-Roussy thalamic pain syndrome, may prove exceedingly refractory to treatment.

Occipital infarction resulting from posterior cerebral artery occlusion occurs infrequently. Peerless and Drake reported persistent visual field defect from occipital infarction in only 1 of 27 patients who underwent inadvertent or deliberate posterior cerebral artery occlusion.[151] Such occlusion must occur distal to the origins of the posterior choroidal vessels to prevent possible devastating infarction in these territories. If present, infarction of cortical tissues of the occipital lobe or geniculocalcarine tract characteristically results in homonymous hemianopsia. Defects in the ipsilateral nasal and contralateral temporal visual fields are largely congruent. Macular vision may be spared, given that strong collateral blood flow serves the occipital poles. Bilateral occipital infarction results in cortical blindness, with pupillary reflexes remaining intact. Behavioral disturbance, including active hallucination, confabulation, and denial of visual loss, may accompany such lesions. Prosopagnosia (the inability to recognize faces) also occurs in the setting of occipital infarction, more commonly with bilateral insults.[201] Lesions involving the splenium of the corpus callosum and adjacent occipital cortex of the dominant hemisphere allow dissociation of vision and language function. Alexia without agraphia and variable degrees of anomia, particularly for colors, can occur. Rarely, posterior cerebral artery infarction can masquerade as a middle cerebral artery stroke.[41, 102] Occipitally based visual loss may be accompanied by contralateral sensory and motor loss from infarction in the thalamus and the cerebral peduncle, parading as a more anterior lesion. As previously described, bilateral inferomesial temporal lobe ischemia is postulated to be an etiologic factor in transient global amnesia. Infarction in these territories due to posterior cerebral or basilar artery ischemia may result in profound and lasting memory disturbance.

BORDER ZONE INFARCTION

Border zone regions, less accurately termed watershed areas, reside at the periphery of adjacent vascular territories. Most prominent border zones are located between the fields of the middle cerebral artery and the anterior cerebral artery and between those of the middle cerebral artery and the posterior cerebral artery. In addition, boundary zones are also found between the major cerebellar vascular supplies, the superior cerebellar artery and the posterior inferior cerebellar artery, and at sites within the basal ganglia.[218] Border zones may also be observed between major branches of the same parent vessel, for example, subcortical areas between the deep and superficial vessels of the middle cerebral artery.[16] These zones are significant in that up to 10 per cent of brain infarctions occur in these regions.[113] By virtue of their peripheral locus, border zone tissues are characterized by sparse small-vessel collateral flow through leptomeningeal channels. These outlying territories are at foremost risk for ischemic processes. Large-vessel stenoses, thrombotic occlusions, and profound systemic hypotension, together or in isolation, are considered common etiologic factors in border zone infarction. Occlusive disease in the more distal brain circulation may also play a role.[16] Damage often occurs in the form of an elongated, sickle-shaped strip of injury extending from frontal to occipital regions.[5] In states of hypotension, these findings tend to occur bilaterally. Focal flow-limiting lesions may generate unilateral and more restricted patterns of injury. Cholesterol emboli and particles from cardiac, large-vessel, or neoplastic sources have been shown to account for a portion of these lesions.[158, 191] Hematogenous disorders are also implicated as a contributing factor for border zone infarction, particularly in the absence of hypotension, embolus, or stenosis.[190]

Lacunar Disease

A lacune is a small infarction in the deep aspects of the cerebrum or brain stem. Characteristically, such cavitary lesions range from 3 to 20 mm in diameter.[69] They are thought to represent the ischemic sequelae of occlusion of single perforating end-arteries within the brain parenchyma.

Lacunes represent 12 to 25 per cent of cerebral infarctions.[22, 30, 175] They occur in the basal ganglia and, to a lesser extent, in the thalamus, pons, internal capsule, and convoluntional white matter.[69, 192] Lacunar infarction may be silent or may present with stereotypical findings characteristic of stroke location. Headache, if present, is mild. Consciousness and higher cortical functions are not affected. Mortality is low, but morbidity may be significant. Many patients, however, ultimately recover fully. A number of common lacunar syndromes have been described.[69, 72, 73, 75, 76]

Pure motor hemiparesis may result from compromise of lateral lenticulostriate vessels supplying the posterior limb of the internal capsule. Alternatively, lacunar infarction in the basis pontis or, more rarely, in the cerebral peduncle may produce similar effects. Deficits include weakness of the face, arm, and leg on the side contralateral to the lacunar stroke. Sensation and higher functions such as language and vision are preserved.

Pure sensory stroke is associated with lacunar infarction in the ventral posterior nuclei of the thalamus or parietal white matter regions. Motor and other cortical functions are not affected. Contralateral hemisensory loss may be partial or complete.

Ataxic hemiparesis is a third commonly described lacunar syndrome. Infarction is usually localized to the pons. Contralateral motor loss is observed. The limbs and face may be affected to varying degrees. Ipsilateral limb ataxia and nystagmus suggest involvement of cerebellar connections.

Dysarthria–clumsy hand syndrome occurs with lacunar stroke in the basis pontis or genu of the internal capsule. Upper extremity weakness and clumsiness is noted. Dysarthria, dysphagia, and facial weakness may occur and reflect corticobulbar involvement.

Small-vessel disease, attributed to chronic vasculopathic changes wrought by atherosclerosis and long-standing hypertension, is considered by some authorities to be the pathogenetic mechanism of infarction.[71] However, hypertension is not coexistent in all patients who suffer lacunar infarction. Clinical profiles similar to those associated with lacunar infarction may result from hemorrhage, infection, inflammatory process, or neoplasm.[17] Many patients with symptomatic lacunar infarction do not present with the classical lacunar syndromes.[192] In addition, radiological and pathological changes consistent with lacunar stroke may occur in the setting of large-vessel occlusion or from embolus derived from cardiac or large-vessel sources.[25, 83, 160] These findings challenge the concept of lacunar infarction as delineated by Fisher. Those lesions defined as lacunes may well represent a heterogeneous array of conditions, yet the term lacune, as traditionally used, implies a specific pathophysiology, radiology, and pathology with associated implications for treatment and prognosis. Confusion and ambiguity related to the term lacune can be avoided by classifying infarcts as small, medium, or large, ischemic or hemorrhagic, with location determined by clinical presentation and radiological appearance.[123] Complacency and sole reliance on antihypertensive treatment for small, deep infarctions is unfounded. These occurrences, like other forms of stroke, require individualized and aggressive management.[140]

REFERENCES

1. Abbie, A. A.: The clinical significance of the anterior choroidal artery. Brain, 56:233, 1933.
2. Abbie, A. A.: The blood supply of the lateral geniculate body, with a note of the morphology of the choroidal arteries. J. Anat., 67:491, 1932–1933.
3. Abbott, R. D., Yin, Y., Reed, D. M., et al.: Risk of stroke in male cigarette smokers. N. Engl. J. Med., 315:717, 1986.
4. Adams, H. P., Jr., and Biller, J.: Ischemic cerebrovascular disease. In Bradley, W. G., Daroff, R. B., Fenichel, G. M., et al., eds.: Neurology in Clinical Practice. Boston, Butterworth-Heinemann, 1991, pp. 907–939.
5. Adams, R. D., and Victor, M.: Principles of Neurology. 5th ed. New York, McGraw-Hill, 1993, pp. 669–748.

6. Adams, R. D.: Occlusion of the anterior inferior cerebellar artery. Arch. Neurol. Psychiatry, *49*:765, 1943.
7. Adson, A. W.: Surgical treatment of vascular diseases altering the function of the eyes. Trans. Am. Acad. Ophthal. Otolaryngol., *46*:95, 1941.
8. Alexander, M. P., and Freedman, M.: Amnesia after anterior communicating artery aneurysm rupture. Neurology, *34*:752, 1984.
9. Alpers, B. J., Beery, R. G., and Paddison, R. M.: Anatomical studies of the circle of Willis in normal brain. Arch. Neurol. Psychiatry, *81*:409, 1959.
10. Amarenco, P.: The spectrum of cerebellar infarctions. Neurology, *41*:973, 1991.
11. Amarenco, P., and Hauw, J. J.: Cerebellar infarction in the territory of the anterior and inferior cerebellar artery. Brain, *113*:139, 1990.
12. Amarenco, P., Roullet, E., Hommel, M., et al.: Infarction in the territory of the medial branch of the posterior inferior cerebellar artery. J. Neurol. Neurosurg. Psychiatry, *53*:731, 1990.
13. Amarenco, P., and Hauw, J. J.: Cerebellar infarction in the territory of the superior cerebellar artery: A clinicopathologic study of 33 cases. Neurology, *40*:1383, 1990.
14. Amarenco, P., and Hauw, J. J.: Anatomie des artères cérébelleuses. Rev. Neurol. (Paris), *145*:267, 1989.
15. American Heart Association: 1989 Stroke Facts, Dallas, 1988.
16. Angeloni, U., Bozzao, L., Fantozzi, L., et al.: Internal borderzone infarction following acute middle cerebral artery occlusion. Neurology, *40*:1196, 1990.
17. Anzalone, N., and Landi, G.: Nonischaemic causes of lacunar syndromes: Prevalence and clinical findings. J. Neurol. Neurosurg. Psychiatry, *52*:1188, 1989.
18. Astrup, J., Symon, L., Branston, N. M., et al.: Cortical evoked potential and extracellular K$^+$ and H$^+$ at critical levels of brain ischemia. Stroke, *8*:51, 1977.
19. Atkinson, W. J.: The anterior inferior cerebellar artery. J. Neurol. Neurosurg. Psychiatry, *12*:137, 1949.
20. Bamford, J., Sandercock, P., Dennis, M., et al.: Classification and natural history of clinically identifiable subtypes of cerebral infarction. Lancet, *337*:1521, 1991.
21. Bamford, J., Sandercock, P., and Dennis, M.: A prospective study of acute cerebrovascular disease in the community: The Oxfordshire Community Stroke Project, 1981–86. J. Neurol. Neurosurg. Psychiatry, *53*:16, 1990.
22. Bamford, J., Sandercock, P., Jones, L., et al.: The natural history of lacunar infarction: The Oxfordshire Community Stroke Project. Stroke *18*:545, 1987.
23. Beevor, C. E.: On the distribution of the different arteries supplying the human brain. Philos. Trans. R. Soc. Lond., *200*:1, 1909.
24. Beevor, C. E.: The cerebral arterial supply. Brain, *30*:403, 1907.
25. Bogousslavsky, J., Regli, F., and Maeder, P.: Intracranial large-artery disease and "lacunar" infarction. Cerebrovasc. Dis., *1*:154, 1991.
26. Bogousslavsky, J., and Regli, F.: Anterior cerebral artery territory infarction in the Lausanne stroke registry. Arch. Neurol., *47*:144, 1990.
27. Bogousslavsky, J., Regli, F., and Uske, A.: Thalamic infarcts: Clinical syndromes, etiology, and prognosis. Neurology, *38*:837, 1988.
28. Bogousslavsky, J., Regli, F., and Assal, G.: The syndrome of unilateral tuberothalamic artery territory infarction. Stroke, *17*:434, 1986.
29. Bogousslavsky, J., and Regli, F.: Cerebral infarct in apparent transient ischemic attack. Neurology, *35*:1501, 1985.
30. Boiten, J., and Lodder, J.: Lacunar infarcts: Pathogenesis and validity of the clinical syndromes. Stroke, *22*:1374, 1991.
31. Branston, N. M., Hope, T., and Symon, L.: Barbiturates in focal ischemia of primate cortex: Effects on blood flow distribution, evoked potential and extracellular potassium. Stroke, *10*:647, 1979.
32. Branston, N. M., Symon, L., Crockard, H. A., et al.: Relationship between the cortical evoked potential and local cortical blood flow following acute middle cerebral artery occlusion in the baboon. Exp. Neurol., *45*:195, 1974.
33. Broderick, J. P., Phillips, S. J., Whisnant, J. P., et al.: Incidence rates of stroke in the eighties: The end of the decline in stroke? Stroke, *20*:577, 1989.
34. Bruno, A., Corbett, J. J., Biller, J., et al.: Transient monocular visual loss patterns and associated vascular abnormalities. Stroke, *21*:34, 1990.
35. Bruno, A., Graff-Radford, N. R., Biller, J., et al.: Anterior choroidal artery territory infarction: A small vessel disease. Stroke, *20*:616, 1989.
36. Calandre, L., Gomara, S., Bermejo, F., et al.: Clinical-CT correlations in TIA, RIND, and strokes with minimum residuum. Stroke, *15*:663, 1984.
37. Caplan, L. R., Schmahmann, J. D., Kase, C. S., et al.: Caudate infarcts. Arch. Neurol., *47*:133, 1990.
38. Caplan, L. R.: "Top of the basilar" syndrome. Neurology, *30*:72, 1980.
39. Caruso, G., Vincentelli, F., Giudicelli, G., et al.: Perforating branches of the basilar bifurcation. J. Neurosurg., *73*:259, 1990.
40. Castaigne, P., Lhermitte, F., Buge, A., et al.: Paramedian thalamic and midbrain infarcts: Clinical and neuropathological study. Ann. Neurol., *10*:127, 1981.
41. Chambers, B. R., Brooder, R. J., and Donnan, G. A.: Proximal posterior cerebral artery occlusion simulating middle cerebral artery occlusion. Neurology, *41*:385, 1991.
42. Chambers, B. R., and Norris, J. W.: Outcome in patients with asymptomatic neck bruits. N. Engl. J. Med., *315*:860, 1986.
43. Chodosh, E. H., Foulkes, M. A., Kase, C. S., et al.: Silent stroke in the NINCDS stroke data bank. Neurology, *38*:1674, 1988.
44. Collins, R., Peto, R., MacMahon, S., et al.: Blood pressure, stroke, and coronary heart disease. Lancet, *335*:827, 1990.
45. Cooper, I. S.: Anterior choroidal artery ligation for involuntary movements. Science, *118*:193, 1953.
46. Cooper, I. S.: Ligation of the anterior choroidal artery for involuntary movements—parkinsonism. Psychiatr. Q., *27*:317, 1953.
47. Coyle, P., and Heistad, D. D.: Development of collaterals in the cerebral circulation. Blood Vessels, *28*:183, 1991.
48. Critchley, M.: The anterior cerebral artery and its syndromes. Brain, *53*:120, 1930.
49. Crowell, R. M., and Morawetz, R. B.: The anterior communicating artery has significant branches. Stroke, *8*:272, 1977.
50. Damasio, A. R., Graff-Radford, N. R., Eslinger, P. J., et al.: Amnesia following basal forebrain lesions. Arch. Neurol., *42*:263, 1985.
51. Dandy, W. E.: Treatment of carotid-cavernous arteriovenous aneurysms. Ann. Surg., *102*:916, 1935.
52. Davison, C.: Syndrome of the anterior spinal artery of the medulla oblongata. Arch. Neurol. Psychiatry, *37*:91, 1937.
53. Davison, C., Goodhart, S. P., and Savitsky, N.: The syndrome of the superior cerebellar artery and its branches. Arch. Neurol. Psychiatry, *33*:1143, 1935.
54. Dawson, B. H.: The blood vessels of the human optic chiasma and their relation to those of the hypophysis and hypothalamus. Brain, *81*:207, 1958.
55. De Reuck, J., Sieben, G., DeCoster, W., et al.: Stroke pattern and topography of cerebral infarcts: A clinicopathological study. Eur. Neurol., *20*:411, 1981.
56. De Reuck, J.: La limite du territoire profond de l'artère sylvienne chez l'homme. Acta Anat. (Basel), *74*:30, 1969.
57. Decroix, J. P., Graveleau, P. H., Masson, M., et al.: Infarction in the territory of the anterior choroidal artery. Brain, *109*:1071, 1986.
58. Dennis, M. S., Bamford, J. M., Sandercock, P. A. G., et al.: Incidence of transient ischemic attacks in Oxfordshire, England. Stroke, *20*:333, 1989.
59. Drake, C. G.: Ligation of the vertebral (unilateral or bilateral) or basilar artery in the treatment of large intracranial aneurysms. J. Neurosurg., *43*:255, 1975.
60. Duncan, G. W., Pessin, M. S., Mohr, J. P., et al.: Transient cerebral ischemic attacks. Adv. Intern. Med., *21*:1, 1976.
61. Dunker, R. O., and Harris, B.: Surgical anatomy of the proximal anterior cerebral artery. J. Neurosurg., *44*:359, 1976.
62. Duret, H.: Artères nourric ières du bulbe rachidien. Arch. Physiol. Norm. Pathol., *5*:97, 1873.
63. Duvernoy, H. M.: Human Brainstem Vessels. Berlin, Springer-Verlag, 1978.
64. Dyken, M. L.: Stroke risk factors. *In* Norris, J. W., and Hachinski, V. C., eds.: Prevention of Stroke. New York, Springer-Verlag, 1991, pp. 83–101.

65. Dyken, M. L., Wolf, P. A., Barnett, H. J. M., et al.: Risk factors in stroke: A statement for physicians by the subcommittee on risk factors and stroke of the stroke council. Stroke, 15:1105, 1984.

66. Eckstrom, P. T., Brand, F. R., Edlavitch, S. A., et al.: Epidemiology of stroke in a rural area. Public Health Rep., 84:878, 1969.

67. Escourolle, R., Hauw, J. J., DerAgopian, P., et al.: Les infarctus bulbaires. J. Neurol. Sci., 28:103, 1976.

68. Fisher, C. M., and Tapia, J.: Lateral medullary infarction extending to the lower pons. J. Neurol. Neurosurg. Psychiatry, 50:620, 1987.

69. Fisher, C. M.: Lacunar strokes and infarcts: A review. Neurology, 32:871, 1982.

70. Fisher, C. M.: The anatomy and pathology of the cerebral vasculature. In Meyer, J. S., ed.: Modern Concepts of Cerebrovascular Disease. New York, Spectrum, 1975, pp. 1–41.

71. Fisher, C. M.: The arterial lesions underlying lacunes. Acta Neuropathol. (Berl.), 12:1, 1969.

72. Fisher, C. M.: A lacunar stroke: The dysarthria—clumsy hand syndrome. Neurology, 17:614, 1967.

73. Fisher, C. M., and Cole, M.: Homolateral ataxia and crural paresis: A vascular syndrome. J. Neurol. Neurosurg. Psychiatry, 28:48, 1965.

74. Fisher, C. M., Gore, I., Okabe, N., et al.: Atherosclerosis of the carotid and vertebral arteries: Extracranial and intracranial. J. Neuropathol. Exp. Neurol., 24:455, 1965.

75. Fisher, C. M.: Pure sensory stroke involving face, arm and leg. Neurology, 15:76, 1965.

76. Fisher, C. M., and Curry, H. B.: Pure motor hemiplegia of vascular origin. Arch. Neurol., 13:30, 1965.

77. Fisher, C. M., Karnes, W. E., and Kubik, C. S.: Lateral medullary infarction: The pattern of vascular occlusion. J. Neuropathol. Exp. Neurol., 20:323, 1961.

78. Foix, C., and Hillemand, P.: Les syndromes de la région thalamique. Presse Méd., 1:113, 1925.

79. Foix, C. H., Chavany, J. A., Hillemand, P., et al.: Obliteration de l'artère choroidienne anterieure: Ramollissement cerebral hémiplégie, hémianesthesie et hémianopsie. Soc. d'Ophtal., 27:221e, 1925.

80. Freeman, W., and Jaffe, D.: Occlusion of the superior cerebellar artery. Arch. Neurol. Psychiatry, 46:115, 1941.

81. Gade, A.: Amnesia after operations on aneurysms of the anterior communicating artery. Surg. Neurol., 18:46, 1982.

82. Gautier, J. C., and Mohr, J. P.: Intracranial internal carotid artery disease. In Barnett, H. J. M., Mohr, J. P., Stein, B. M., et al., eds.: Stroke. Pathophysiology, Diagnosis, and Management. New York, Churchill Livingstone, 1986, pp. 337–349.

83. Ghika, J., Bogousslavsky, J., and Regli, F.: Infarcts in the territory of the deep perforators from the carotid system. Neurology, 39:507, 1989.

84. Ghika, J. A., Bogousslavsky, J., and Regli, F.: Deep perforators from the carotid system. Arch. Neurol., 47:1097, 1990.

85. Gillilan, L. A.: The correlation of the blood supply of the human brain stem with clinical brain stem lesions. J. Neuropathol. Exp. Neurol., 23:78, 1964.

86. Gomes, F. B., Dujovny, M., Umansky, F., et al.: Microanatomy of the anterior cerebral artery. Surg. Neurol., 26:129, 1986.

87. Gomez, C. R., Hogan, P. A., Cruz-Rodriguez, R. F., et al.: Altered sensorium, confusion, and vertical gaze paresis: The top of the basilar syndrome. South. Med. J., 81:842, 1988.

88. Goodwin, J. A., Gorelick, P. B., and Helgason, C. M.: Symptoms of amaurosis fugax in atherosclerotic carotid artery disease. Neurology, 37:829, 1987.

89. Grand, W., and Hopkins, L. N.: The microsurgical anatomy of the basilar artery bifurcation. Neurosurgery, 1:128, 1977.

90. Hamby, W. B.: Carotid-cavernous fistula. J. Neurosurg., 21:859, 1964.

91. Hayreh, S. S., and Dass, R.: The ophthalmic artery: I. Origin and intra-cranial and intra-canalicular course. Br. J. Ophthalmol., 46:65, 1962.

92. Heiss, W. D.: Flow thresholds of functional and morphological damage of brain tissue. Stroke, 14:329, 1983.

93. Heiss, W. D., and Rosner, G.: Functional recovery of cortical neurons as related to degree and duration of ischemia. Ann. Neurol., 14:294, 1983.

94. Heiss, W. D., Hayakawa, T., and Waltz, A. G.: Cortical neuronal function during ischemia: Effects of occlusion of one middle cerebral artery on single-unit activity in cats. Arch. Neurol., 33:813, 1976.

95. Helgason, C., Caplan, L. R., Goodwin, J., et al.: Anterior choroidal artery-territory infarction. Arch. Neurol., 43:681, 1986.

96. Helgason, C. M.: A new view of anterior choroidal artery territory infarction. J. Neurol., 235:387, 1988.

97. Herderscheê, D., Hijdra, A., Algra, A., et al.: Silent stroke in patients with transient ischemic attack or minor ischemic stroke. Stroke, 23:1220, 1992.

98. Heubner, J. B. O.: Zur Topographie der Ernährungsgebiete der einzelnen Hirnarterien. Zentralbl. Med. Wiss., 10:817, 1872.

99. Heyman, A., Wilkinson, W. E., Heyden, S., et al.: Risk of stroke in asymptomatic persons with cervical arterial bruits. N. Engl. J. Med., 302:838, 1980.

100. Hint, H.: The pharmacology of dextran and the physiological background for the clinical use of rheomacrodux and macrodux. Acta Anaesthesiol. Belg., 19:119, 1968.

101. Hollenhorst, R. W.: Significance of bright plaques in the retinal arterioles. J.A.M.A., 178:123, 1961.

102. Hommel, M., Besson, G., Pollak, P., et al.: Hemiplegia in posterior cerebral artery occlusion. Neurology, 40:1496, 1990.

103. Hossmann, K. A., and Kleihues, P.: Reversibility of ischemic brain damage. Arch. Neurol., 29:375, 1973.

104. Hossmann, K. A., and Sato, K.: Recovery of neuronal function after prolonged cerebral ischaemia. Science, 168:375, 1970.

105. Hoyt, W. F.: Ocular symptoms and signs. In Wylie, E. J., and Ehrenfeld, W. K., eds.: Extracranial Occlusive Cerebrovascular Disease: Diagnosis and Management. Philadelphia, W. B. Saunders, 1970.

106. Hütter, B. O., and Gilsbach, J. M.: Cognitive deficits after rupture and early repair of anterior communicating artery aneurysms. Acta Neurochir. (Wein), 116:6, 1992.

107. Hypertension Detection and Follow-up Program Cooperative Group: Five-year findings of the hypertension detection and follow-up program: III. Reduction in stroke incidence among persons with high blood pressure. J.A.M.A., 247:633, 1982.

108. Irle, E., Wowra, B., Kunert, H. J., et al.: Memory disturbances following anterior communicating artery rupture. Ann. Neurol., 31:473, 1992.

109. Janeway, R.: The art of listening. Curr. Concepts Cerebrovasc. Dis., 4:17, 1971.

110. Jones, H. R., and Millikan, C. H.: Temporal profile (clinical course) of acute carotid system cerebral infarction. Stroke, 7:64, 1976.

111. Jones, H. R., Jr., Millikan, C. H., and Sandok, B. A.: Temporal profile (clinical course) of acute vertebrobasilar system cerebral infarction. Stroke, 11:173, 1980.

112. Jones, T. H., Morawetz, R. B., Crowell, R. M., et al.: Thresholds of focal cerebral ischemia in awake monkeys. J. Neurosurg., 54:773, 1981.

113. Jorgensen, L., and Torvik, A.: Ischaemic cerebrovascular diseases in an autopsy series: Part 2. Prevalence, location, pathogenesis and clinical course of cerebral infarcts. J. Neurol. Sci., 9:285, 1969.

114. Kannel, W. B., Wolf, P. A., Castelli, W. P., et al.: Fibrinogen and risk of cardiovascular disease: The Framingham Study. J.A.M.A., 258:1183, 1987.

115. Kannel, W. B., Wolf, P. A., and Verter, J.: Manifestations of coronary disease predisposing to stroke: The Framingham Study. J.A.M.A., 250:2942, 1983.

116. Kaplan, H. A., and Ford, D. H.: The Brain Vascular System. New York, Elsevier, 1966.

117. Kaplan, H. A.: Collateral circulation of the brain. Neurology, 11:9, 1961.

118. Khan, N. M.: The blood supply of the midbrain in man and monkey [Doctoral thesis]. London, University of London, 1969.

119. Kim, H. N., Kim, Y. H., Park, I. Y., et al.: Variability of the surgical anatomy of the neurovascular complex of the cerebellopontine angle. Ann. Otol. Rhinol. Laryngol., 99:288, 1990.

120. Kolisko, A.: Über die Beziehung der Arteria choroidea anterior zum hinteren Schenkel der inneren Kapsel des Gehirns. Vienna, A. Hoelder, 1891.

121. Krayenbühl, H. A., and Yasargil, M. G.: Cerebral Angiography. 2nd ed. Philadelphia, J. B. Lippincott, 1968.

122. Kuller, L. H.: Incidence rates of stroke in the eighties: The end of the decline in stroke? Stroke, 20:841, 1989.

123. Landau, W. M.: Au clair de lacune: Holy, wholly, holey logic. Neurology, 39:725, 1989.

124. Lazorthes, G.: Vascularisation et circulation cérébrales. Paris, Masson, 1961.

125. Lees, R. S., and Kistler, J. P.: Carotid phonoangiography. In Bernstein, E. F., ed.: Non-invasive Diagnostic Techniques in Vascular Disease. St. Louis, C. V. Mosby, 1978, pp. 187–194.

126. Levine, S. R., and Welch, K. M. A.: Superior cerebellar artery infarction and vertebral artery dissection. Stroke, 19:1431, 1988.

127. Lhermitte, F., Gautier, J. C., and Derouesné, C.: Nature of occlusions of the middle cerebral artery. Neurology, 20:82, 1970.

128. Lhermitte, F., Gautier, J. C., and Derouesné, C.: Anatomie et physiopathologie des stenoses carotidiennes. Rev. Neurol. (Paris), 115:641, 1966.

129. Lindqvist, G., and Norlén, G.: Korsakoff's syndrome after operation on ruptured aneurysm of the anterior communicating artery. Acta Psychiatr. Scand., 42:24, 1966.

130. Macdonell, R. A. L., Kalnins, R. M., and Donnan, G. A.: Cerebellar infarction: Natural history, prognosis, and pathology. Stroke, 18:849, 1987.

131. Management Committee: The Australian therapeutic trial in mild hypertension. Lancet, 1:1261, 1980.

132. Marinkovic, S., Milisavljevic, M., and Marinkovic, Z.: Branches of the anterior communicating artery: Microsurgical anatomy. Acta Neurochir. (Wein), 106:78, 1990.

133. Marinkovic, S. V., Kovacevic, M. S., and Marinkovic, J. M.: Perforating branches of the middle cerebral artery. J. Neurosurg., 63:266, 1985.

134. Marshall, J.: The natural history of transient ischemic cerebrovascular attacks. Q. J. Med., 33:309, 1964.

135. Martin, R. G., Grant, J. L., Peace, D., et al.: Microsurgical relationships of the anterior inferior cerebellar artery and the facial-vestibulocochlear nerve complex. Neurosurgery, 6:483, 1980.

136. Mazzoni, A.: Internal auditory artery supply to the petrous bone. Ann. Otol. Rhinol. Laryngol., 81:13, 1972.

137. McGovern, P. G., Burke, G. L., Sprafka, J. M., et al.: Trends in mortality, morbidity, and risk factor levels for stroke from 1960 through 1990: The Minnesota heart survey. J.A.M.A., 268:753, 1992.

138. Meyer, J. S., and Denny-Brown, D.: The cerebral collateral circulation: 1. Factors influencing collateral blood flow. Neurology, 7:447, 1957.

139. Milisavljevic, M. M., Marinkovic, S. V., Gibo, H., et al.: The thalamogeniculate perforators of the posterior cerebral artery: The microsurgical anatomy. Neurosurgery, 28:523, 1991.

140. Millikan, C., and Futrell, N.: The fallacy of the lacune hypothesis. Stroke, 21:1251, 1990.

141. Millikan, C., Bauer, R., Goldschmidt, J., et al.: A classification and outline of cerebrovascular diseases: II. Stroke, 6:514, 1975.

142. Mills, C. K.: Hemianesthesia to pain and temperature and loss of emotional expression on the right side, with ataxia of the upper limb on the left: The symptoms probably due to a lesion of thalamus or superior peduncles. J. Nerv. Ment. Dis., 35:331, 1908.

143. Mishkin, M. M., and Schreiber, M. N.: Collateral circulation. In Newton, T. H., and Potts, D. G., eds.: Radiology of the Skull and Brain: Angiography. St. Louis, C. V. Mosby, 1974, pp. 2344–2374.

144. Mohr, J. P., Caplan, J. W., Melski, R. J., et al.: The Harvard Cooperative Stroke Registry: A prospective registry. Neurology, 28:754, 1978.

145. Nichaman, M. Z., Boyle, E., Jr., Lesesne, T. P., et al.: Cardiovascular disease mortality by race: Based on a statistical study in Charleston, South Carolina. Geriatrics, 17:724, 1962.

146. North American Symptomatic Carotid Endarterectomy Trial Collaborators: Beneficial effect of carotid endarterectomy in symptomatic patients with high-grade carotid stenosis. N. Engl. J. Med., 325:445, 1991.

147. Ojemann, R. G., Heros, R. C., and Crowell, R. M.: Surgical Management of Cerebrovascular Disease. 2nd ed. Baltimore, Williams & Wilkins, 1988, pp. 103–119.

148. Ostfield, A. M., Shekelle, R. B., Klawans, H., et al.: Epidemiology of stroke in an elderly welfare population. Am. J. Public Health, 64:450, 1974.

149. Ostrowski, A. Z., Webster, J. E., and Gurdjian, E. S.: The proximal anterior cerebral artery: An anatomic study. Arch. Neurol., 3:661, 1960.

150. Pedroza, A., Dujovny, M., Artero, J. C., et al.: Microanatomy of the posterior communicating artery. Neurosurgery, 20:228, 1987.

151. Peerless, S. J., and Drake, C. G.: Surgical techniques of posterior cerebral aneurysms. In Schmidek, H. H., and Sweet, W. H., eds.: Operative Neurosurgical Techniques. 2nd ed. Philadelphia, W. B. Saunders, 1988, pp. 973–989.

152. Pelz, D. M., Viñuela, F., Fox, A. J., et al.: Vertebrobasilar occlusion therapy of giant aneurysms. J. Neurosurg., 60:560, 1984.

153. Percheron, G.: Les artères du thalamus humain: Les artères choroidiennes. Rev. Neurol. (Paris), 133:547, 1977.

154. Percheron, G.: Les artères du thalamus humain. II: Les artères du thalamus. Rev. Neurol. (Paris), 132:297, 1976.

155. Percheron, G.: Étude anatomique du thalamus de l'homme adulte et de sa vascularisation artérielle. Paris, Thése de Médecine, 1966.

156. Perlmutter, D., and Rhoton, A. L., Jr.: Microsurgical anatomy of the anterior cerebral-anterior communicating-recurrent artery complex. J. Neurosurg., 45:259, 1976.

157. Pessin, M. S., Kwan, E. S., DeWitt, L. D., et al.: Posterior cerebral artery stenosis. Ann. Neurol., 21:85, 1987.

158. Pollanen, M. S., and Deck, J. H. N.: The mechanism of embolic watershed infarction: Experimental studies. Can. J. Neurol. Sci., 17:395, 1990.

159. Powers, W. J.: Cerebral hemodynamics in ischemic cerebrovascular disease. Ann. Neurol., 29:231, 1991.

160. Pullicino, P. M., Nelson, R. F., Kendall, B. E., et al.: Small deep infarcts diagnosed on computed tomography. Neurology, 30:1090, 1980.

161. Pullicino, P. M.: The course and territories of cerebral small arteries. In Pullicino, P. M., Caplan, L. R., Hommel, M., eds.: Advances in Neurology. New York, Raven Press, 1993, pp. 11–39.

162. Punt, J.: Some observations on aneurysms of the proximal internal carotid artery. J. Neurosurg., 51:151, 1979.

163. Rand, R. W., Brown, W. J., and Stern, W. E.: Surgical occlusion of anterior choroidal arteries in parkinsonism. Neurology, 6:390, 1956.

164. Reinmuth, O. M., and Karanjia, P. N.: Neurological evaluation in cerebrovascular disease. In Fein, J. M., and Flamm, E. S., eds.: Cerebrovascular Surgery. New York, Springer-Verlag, 1985, pp. 129–179.

165. Rhoton, A. L., Jr., and Perlmutter, D.: Microsurgical anatomy of anterior communicating artery aneurysms. Neurol. Res., 2:217, 1980.

166. Rhoton, A. L., Jr., Fujii, K., and Fradd, B.: Microsurgical anatomy of the anterior choroidal artery. Surg. Neurol., 12:171, 1979.

167. Rhoton, A. L., Jr., Saeki, N., Perlmutter, D., et al.: Microsurgical anatomy of common aneurysm sites. Clin. Neurosurg., 26:248, 1979.

168. Riggs, H. E., and Rupp, C.: Variation in form of circle of Willis. Arch. Neurol., 8:24, 1963.

169. Robins, M., and Baum, H. M.: The national survey of stroke. Stroke, 12(Suppl 1):1–45, 1981.

170. Rosner, G., Graf, R., Kataoka, K., et al.: Selective functional vulnerability of cortical neurons following transient MCA-occlusion in the cat. Stroke, 17:76, 1986.

171. Rosner, S. S., Rhoton, A. L., Jr., Ono, M., et al.: Microsurgical anatomy of the anterior perforating arteries. J. Neurosurg., 61:468, 1984.

172. Russell, R. W. R., and Cantab, M. D.: The source of retinal emboli. Lancet, 2:789, 1968.

173. Sacco, R. L., Freddo, L., Bello, J. A., et al.: Wallenberg's lateral medullary syndrome: Clinical-magnetic resonance imaging correlations. Arch. Neurol., 50:609, 1993.

174. Sacco, R. L., Wolf, P. A., Kannel, W. B., et al.: Survival and recurrence following stroke. Stroke, 13:290, 1982.

175. Sacco, S. E., Whisnant, J. P., Broderick, J. P., et al.: Epidemiological characteristics of lacunar infarcts in a population. Stroke, 22:1236, 1991.

176. Saeki, N., Rhoton, A. L., Jr.: Microsurgical anatomy of the upper basilar artery and the posterior circle of Willis. J. Neurosurg., 46:563, 1977.

177. Schlesinger, B.: The Upper Brain Stem in the Human: Its Nuclear Configuration and Vascular Supply. Berlin, Springer-Verlag, 1976.

178. Scholz, W.: Selective neuronal necrosis and its topistic patterns in hypoxemia and oligemia. J. Neuropathol. Exp. Neurol., 12:249, 1953.

179. Sharbrough, F. W., Messick, J. M., and Sundt, T. M., Jr.: Correlation of continuous electroencephalograms with cerebral blood flow measurements during carotid endarterectomy. Stroke, 4:674, 1973.

180. Siesjö, B. K.: Pathophysiology and treatment of focal cerebral ischemia: Part I. Pathophysiology. J. Neurosurg., 77:169, 1992.

181. Spielmeyer, W.: Histopathologie des Nervensystems. Berlin, Springer-Verlag, 1922.

182. Spiller, W. G.: The symptom complex of a lesion of the uppermost portion of the anterior spinal and adjoining portion of the vertebral arteries. J. Nerv. Ment. Dis., 35:775, 1908.

183. Steinberg, G. K., Drake, C. G., and Peerless, S. J.: Deliberate basilar or vertebral artery occlusion in the treatment of intracranial aneurysms. J. Neurosurg., 79:161, 1993.

184. Stephens, R. B., and Stilwell, D. L.: Arteries and Veins of the Human Brain. Springfield, Charles C Thomas, 1969.

185. Sypert, G. W., and Alvord, E. C.: Cerebellar infarction: A clinicopathologic study. Arch. Neurol., 32:357, 1975.

186. Thompson, P. L., and Robinson, J. S.: Stroke after acute myocardial infarction: Relation to infarct size. B.M.J., 2:457, 1978.

187. Tomsick, T. A., Lukin, R. R., and Chambers, A. A.: Persistent trigeminal artery: Unusual associated abnormalities. Neuroradiology, 17:253, 1979.

188. Toole, J. F., and Cole, M.: Ischemic cerebrovascular disease. In Baker, A. B., and Baker, L. H., eds.: Clinical Neurology. Hagerstown, MD, Harper & Row, 1976, pp. 15–16.

189. Toole, J. F., and Patel, A. N.: Cerebrovascular Disorders. 2nd ed. New York, McGraw-Hill, 1974, pp. 12–34.

190. Torvik, A.: The pathogenesis of watershed infarcts in the brain. Stroke, 15:221, 1984.

191. Torvik, A., and Skullerud, K.: Watershed infarcts in the brain caused by microemboli. Clin. Neuropathol., 1:99, 1982.

192. Tuszynski, M. H., Petito, C. K., and Levy, D. E.: Risk factors and clinical manifestations of pathologically verified lacunar infarctions. Stroke, 20:990, 1989.

193. Umansky, F., Gomes, F. B., Dujovny, M., et al.: The perforating branches of the middle cerebral artery. J. Neurosurg., 62:261, 1985.

194. Van der Zwan, A., Hillen, B., Tulleken, C. A. F., et al.: Variability of the territories of the major cerebral arteries. J. Neurosurg., 77:927, 1992.

195. Vander Eecken, H. M., and Adams, R. D.: Anatomy and functional significance of the meningeal anastomoses of the human brain. J. Neuropathol. Exp. Neurol., 12:132, 1953.

196. Veterans Administration Cooperative Study Group on Antihypertensive Agents: Effects of treatment on morbidity in hypertension. II. Results in patients with diastolic blood pressure averaging 90 through 114 mm Hg. J.A.M.A., 213:1143, 1970.

197. Vincentelli, F., Lehman, G., Caruso, G., et al.: Extracerebral course of the perforating branches of the anterior communicating artery: Microsurgical anatomical study. Surg. Neurol., 35:98, 1991.

198. Vorstrup, S., Hemmingsen, R., Henriksen, L., et al.: Regional cerebral blood flow in patients with transient ischemic attacks studied by xenon-133 inhalation and emission tomography. Stroke, 14:903, 1983.

199. Wallenberg, A.: Acute bulbäraffection (embolie der art cerebellar post inf sinistr?). Arch. F. Psychiatr., 27:504, 1895.

200. Walsh, F. B., and Hoyt, W. F.: Vascular lesions and circulatory disorders of the nervous system: Ocular signs. In Clinical Neuro-Ophthalmology. 3rd ed. Baltimore, Williams & Wilkins, 1969, pp. 1629–1925.

201. Walsh, K. W.: Two posterior neuropsychological syndromes revisited. Tohoku J. Exp. Med., 161:121, 1990.

202. Webster, J. E., Gurdjian, E. S., Lindner, D. W., et al.: Proximal occlusion of the anterior cerebral artery. Arch. Neurol., 2:29, 1960.

203. Welin, L., Svärdsudd, K., Wilhelmsen, L., et al.: Analysis of risk factors for stroke in a cohort of men born in 1913. N. Engl. J. Med., 317:521, 1987.

204. Westberg, G.: Arteries of the basal ganglia. Acta Radiol., 5:581, 1966.

205. Whelton, P. K.: Declining mortality from hypertension and stroke. South Med. J., 75:33, 1982.

206. Whisnant, J. P.: Epidemiology of stroke: Emphasis on transient cerebral ischemic attacks and hypertension. Stroke, 5:68, 1974.

207. Whisnant, J. P., Matsumoto, N., and Elveback, L. R.: Transient cerebral ischemic attacks in a community. Rochester, Minnesota, 1955 through 1969. Mayo Clin. Proc., 48:194, 1973.

208. Wilhelmsen, L., Svärdsudd, K., Korsan-Bengtsen, K., et al.: Fibrinogen as a risk factor for stroke and myocardial infarction. N. Engl. J. Med., 311:501, 1984.

209. Wolf, P. A., D'Agostino, R. B., O'Neal, M. A., et al.: Secular trends in stroke incidence and mortality: The Framingham Study. Stroke, 23:1551, 1992.

210. Wolf, P. A.: An overview of the epidemiology of stroke. Stroke, 21(Suppl 2):4, 1990.

211. Wolf, P. A., D'Agostino, R. B., Kannel, W. B., et al.: Cigarette smoking as a risk factor for stroke: The Framingham Study. J.A.M.A., 259:1025, 1988.

212. Wolf, P. A., Kannel, W. B., Sorlie, P., et al.: Asymptomatic carotid bruit and risk of stroke: The Framingham Study. J.A.M.A., 245:1442, 1981.

213. Wood, J. H., and Kee, D. B., Jr.: Hemorheology of the cerebral circulation in stroke. Stroke, 16:765, 1985.

214. Yamada, K., Hayakawa, T., Ushio, Y., et al.: Therapeutic occlusion of the vertebral artery for unclippable vertebral aneurysm: Relationship between site of occlusion and clinical outcome. Neurosurgery, 15:834, 1984.

215. Yasargil, M. G., Smith, R. D., Young, P. H., et al.: Microneurosurgery. New York, Thieme-Stratton, 1984, pp. 54–168.

216. Yatsu, F. M., and Hart, R. G.: Asymptomatic carotid bruit and stenosis: A reappraisal. Stroke, 14:301, 1983.

217. Zeal, A. A., and Rhoton, A. L., Jr.: Microsurgical anatomy of the posterior cerebral artery. J. Neurosurg., 48:534, 1978.

218. Zülch, K. J.: Die Pathogenese von Massenblutung und Erweichung unter besonderer Berücksichtigung klinischer Gesichtspunkte. Acta Neurochir., 7(Suppl):51, 1961.

CHAPTER 45

Medical Management of Acute Cerebral Ischemia

Stroke continues to be a major public health problem. Indeed, it is the most common life-threatening neurological disease. Primary care physicians often believe that stroke is an untreatable disease and have a nihilistic approach toward stroke victims. As a result, patients with strokes are left untreated in the emergency department for hours while those with other "curable diseases" are treated. Consequently, the ischemic brain process is left unchallenged and rapidly involves possibly salvageable brain tissue. However, now there is reason for optimism. A new era for stroke management is emerging in which stroke can be treated acutely and aggressively, similar to ischemic heart disease. The reasons for this optimism are multiple. Identification and treatment of stroke risk factors has resulted in a decline in mortality from stroke.[155] The understanding of the pathophysiology of ischemic brain mechanisms has progressed dramatically during the past decade. Consequently, pharmaceutical companies have developed a large number of promising agents that may be used in the treatment of stroke. Animal studies have clearly demonstrated that the brain ischemic cascade can be retarded with new therapies, and the process of taking these therapies from "bench to bedside" has begun. The large number of new clinical stroke trials attests to the fact that it is now believed that stroke is a treatable disease and the major disability that has occurred in the past secondary to stroke may now be prevented by aggressive anti-stroke therapy. In this chapter background information about the epidemiology of stroke, treatable risk factors, and the basic pathophysiology of ischemic stroke is provided. Preliminary results of current major clinical stroke trials are also detailed if available.

Epidemiological Aspects of Stroke

Stroke continues to be the third leading cause of death in North America. The incidence of stroke averages 180 per 100,000 population per year worldwide, with a prevalence of 500 to 600 per 100,000 population per year. American Heart Association figures estimate that there are almost 500,000 new strokes yearly in the United States and almost 3 million stroke survivors.[97, 114] Stroke is more often disabling than fatal; thus it is a major reason for patients requiring institutionalization. Consequently, the annual health care costs attributed to stroke are more than 3 billion dollars per year.[1] The incidence of stroke has decreased over the past decades, mainly owing to the identification and treatment of stroke risk factors; however, recently the incidence of stroke has leveled off while the mortality secondary to stroke continues to decrease slowly. Recurrence rates for stroke range from 4 to 14 per cent per year, and 5-year survival after stroke averages 56 per cent in men and 64 per cent in women.[115]

Classification of Stroke

The syndrome of stroke can be defined as an abrupt onset of a focal neurological deficit, the origin of which can be traced to either the occlusion of a cerebral vessel or the spontaneous rupture of an intracranial vessel with hemorrhage into the brain parenchyma or the subarachnoid space. Retrospective analysis of large groups of stroke patients has demonstrated that infarction accounts for about 75 per cent of all stroke syndromes.[4] Intracerebral hemorrhage is responsible for approximately 11 per cent, and subarachnoid hemorrhages account for about 5 per cent of all strokes. Hence, ischemic stroke constitutes the most common disabling and lethal neurological disease of adult life.

A focal neurological symptom lasting less than 24 hours is defined as a transient ischemic attack, whereas if the deficit lasts longer, cerebral infarction is diagnosed. Cardioembolism accounts for 15 to 30 per cent, atherosclerotic infarction accounts for 14 to 40 per cent,

B. Tranmer • *C. E. Gross* • *G. W. Kindt* • *M. Bednar*

and lacunar infarction accounts for 15 to 30 per cent of cerebral infarction. Infarction of undetermined causes may include as many as 30 per cent of cases.[40]

Primary Stroke Prevention

A major reduction in stroke morbidity and mortality has occurred over the past few decades mainly because of the identification and treatment of stroke risk factors.

Hypertension. Hypertension, after age, is the most powerful risk factor.[157] The risk of stroke rises proportionately with increasing blood pressure. Men with systolic blood pressures between 160 and 180 mm Hg have about four times the risk of stroke compared with men with blood pressures less than 160 mm Hg.[118] In addition, a 5- to 6-mm Hg reduction in diastolic blood pressure correlates with a 42 per cent reduction in stroke rate over a 2- to 3-year period.[25]

Smoking. Cigarette smoking increases the risk for stroke by about 50 per cent.[120] Smoking is associated with an acceleration of carotid artery atherosclerosis that is independent of age, hypertension, and diabetes.[34] Also, smoking is associated with cardiac disease, which in turn increases the risk for stroke.

Diabetes. The incidence of stroke is increased by 2.5 to 3.5 times in diabetic patients.[74, 84] In the Framingham study the stroke risk as a result of diabetes was found in both men and women, did not decrease with age, and was independent of hypertension.[114] Kiers and colleagues found a correlation among admission glucose concentration, diabetes, and poor stroke outcome in a prospective study of patients with acute stroke.[74] Laboratory data clearly demonstrate that hyperglycemia aggravates ischemic damage in focal ischemia, but glucose management in acute stroke is still controversial and clinical studies are required.[20, 29, 31]

Lipids. The relationship between serum cholesterol, serum lipids, and stroke has been debated in the past. However, elevated serum levels of cholesterol have been demonstrated to be a risk factor for transient ischemic attack and ischemic stroke.[109] Also, progression of carotid atherosclerosis is directly related to cholesterol and low-density lipoproteins and inversely related to high-density lipoproteins.[114]

Cardiac Disease. An increasing risk of ischemic stroke is clearly associated with cardiac disease. Atrial fibrillation, valvular heart disease, myocardial infarction, and congestive heart failure are all recognized as potential causes of cardioembolism. Atrial fibrillation is associated with a fivefold increase in stroke.[156, 157] Myocardial infarction is associated with a fivefold increase in stroke rate, and coronary artery disease plus congestive heart failure is associated with a fourfold increase in stroke rate.[118, 157]

Secondary Stroke Prevention (After Transient Ischemic Attack or Ischemic Stroke)

Aspirin is the most widely used antiplatelet agent in patients with transient ischemic attacks or ischemic stroke. Four of the largest clinical trials (United Kingdom Transient Ischemic Attack Aspirin Trial and European, French, and Canadian Aspirin trials) all found aspirin to be of benefit, with results ranging from 20 to 50 per cent.[19, 37, 51, 149] The Swedish Aspirin Low-Dose Trial demonstrated a significant reduction (18 per cent) in minor strokes or transient ischemic attacks in patients taking 75 mg of aspirin versus placebo.[137] In the United Kingdom Transient Ischemic Attack Aspirin Trial, patients with transient ischemic attacks or minor stroke were randomly selected to receive 600 mg of aspirin twice daily, 300 mg of aspirin once a day, or a placebo.[149] A 15 per cent reduction in major stroke, myocardial infarction, and vascular death was noted in the aspirin-treated patients. However, gastrointestinal side effects also occurred in this group. The optimal dose for aspirin remains controversial. The Dutch Transient Ischemic Attack Trial showed no significant difference in vascular events (including stroke) in patients taking 30 mg of aspirin per day and those taking 283 mg per day.[36]

Ticlopidine is a newer antiplatelet agent that has been shown to be beneficial in the prevention of stroke after transient ischemic attack and ischemic stroke. It appears to be more effective than aspirin, with a 20 to 30 per cent reduction over aspirin in stroke or stroke death.[44, 61] Patients receiving the greatest benefit of ticlopidine are women; those failing aspirin therapy; patients with vertebrobasilar insufficiency, hypertension, or diabetes; and patients without major carotid stenosis.[50] At the present time, ticlopidine is reserved for those patients who continue to have ischemic symptoms while on aspirin therapy.

Pathophysiology of Ischemic Stroke

A brief review of the pathophysiology of ischemic stroke is presented so that the following described strategies of managing acute cerebral ischemia can be better understood.

CEREBRAL AUTOREGULATION AND BLOOD FLOW REGULATION

The brain requires approximately 15 per cent of the resting cardiac output (approximately 750 mL per minute), and 20 per cent of the inspired oxygen at rest, despite accounting for only 2 per cent of total body weight. The brain has no appreciable stores of glycogen and is therefore totally dependent on the oxidative phosphorylation of glucose for adenosine triphosphate production.[123, 124] Resting cerebral blood flow in the human brain is 50 to 55 mL per 100 g of brain tissue per minute with gray matter blood flow higher than the white matter blood flow.

The brain possesses the ability to autoregulate that, as Johnson describes, is the "intrinsic tendency of an organ to maintain constant blood flow despite changes in arterial perfusion pressure."[69] The brain is able to maintain a constant cerebral blood flow despite changes in arterial perfusion pressure in order to maintain an adequate cerebral perfusion. Under normal circumstances, the cerebrovascular resistance varies to maintain a constant cerebral blood flow over a wide range of changes in blood pressure and cardiac output.[145] However, there are specific factors that may alter cerebral blood flow in normal brain. The blood flow of the brain is coupled to neuronal activity and metabolism.[122] A local increase in cerebral blood flow does occur during direct electrical excitation, seizures, and even mental activity.[106, 107, 117] Cerebral activity decreases during barbiturate anesthesia and depressed states of cerebral activity.[72]

Alterations in partial pressure of arterial carbon dioxide have profound effects on cerebral blood flow.[73] Hypercapnia is associated with arterial smooth muscle relaxation, which decreases cerebrovascular resistance, resulting in an increase in cerebral blood flow. Lassen reported that this cerebrovascular response was mediated by the influence of carbon dioxide on the periarteriolar pH.[81] Oxygen, or more accurately the lack of oxygen, also has profound effects on cerebral blood flow.[88] Levels of partial pressure of oxygen below 50 to 60 mm Hg profoundly increase cerebral blood flow. At less than 50 mm Hg there is a decrease in cortical pH, which is associated with an increase in blood flow, and therefore it is believed that pH is probably also involved in the process of hypoxic vasodilatation.

Lassen has proposed that neuronal metabolism is coupled to cerebral blood flow by lactic acid production because as lactic acid accumulates, extracellular pH decreases and vascular dilatation follows.[81] However, experimental data demonstrate that cerebral blood flow regulation may be more complex than this and a number of neuropeptides may also be involved in the vasodilatation process. Neuropeptides such as substance P and vasoactive intestinal peptide have been shown to affect cerebral blood flow, and adenosine has been shown to be a powerful dilator of cerebral vessels.[88]

DYSREGULATION AND ISCHEMIC STROKE

During cerebral ischemia, autoregulation is impaired.[104, 132] Cerebral blood flow passively follows changes in systemic arterial blood pressure. Cerebrovascular reactivity to carbon dioxide is also impaired.[152] If flow is restored, an intense hyperemia occurs that some suggest is the result of vasomotor paralysis associated with severe focal lactic acidosis. Experimental and clinical data also suggest that changes in cardiac output affect cerebral blood flow in ischemic brain. In normal brain, changes in cardiac output do not affect cerebral blood flow; but in ischemic brain, increases in cardiac output produce significant increases in cerebral blood flow.[83, 145] Occlusion of a single major cerebral artery produces a localized area of reduced perfusion that is surrounded by brain, with normal conducting vessels attempting to supply this ischemic area through

anastomotic channels. The microcirculatory changes in this area of ischemia have been well documented by Sundt and Waltz.[134, 153] The first changes that occur on the cortex after vessel occlusion are darkening of the venous blood, a decrease in the velocity of the blood flow, and sludging. At this time there is slight dilatation of the arteries and arterioles. Severe ischemia is indicated by the ensuing cortical pallor. Vessels that are associated with the ischemic cortical pallor constrict in response to some unknown vasospastic substance. Edema also develops in this area of ischemia. With the restoration of blood flow to the ischemic area, the chain of events is reversed. Reactive hyperemia is often observed, with marked vasodilatation of the vessels and the appearance of red venous blood.

Metabolic changes have also been studied during cerebral ischemia. After vessel occlusion, the adenosine triphosphate level progressively decreases and the tissue concentration of phosphocreatine is readily reduced to zero. Lactic acid levels increase quickly, leading to a fall in extracellular pH. Increases in free fatty acid content also occur during cerebral ischemia (Fig. 45–1).[86] If perfusion is restored within a certain time period, all values will return to control level.[122] During focal cerebral ischemia, obstruction of a major cerebral artery in focal ischemia does not necessarily lead to irreversible damage to the dependent region of the brain. Location and size of the obstructed artery are

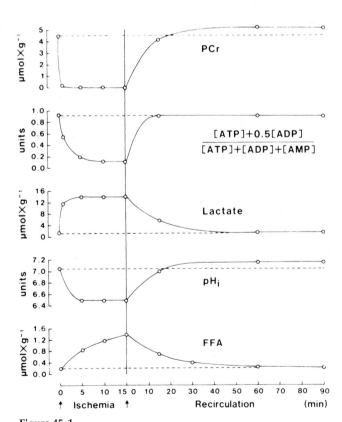

Figure 45–1

Changes in cerebral cortical concentrations of phosphocreatine (PCr), lactate, free fatty acids (FFA), adenylate energy charge, and intracellular pH (pH$_i$) during and after transient complete ischemia. (From Siesjo, B. K.: Cerebral circulation and metabolism. J. Neurosurg., 60:883–908, 1984. Reprinted by permission.)

important factors to determine the degree of ischemic change, but also of extreme importance is the availability of collateralization to the ischemic area. In the cerebral hemispheres, extensive collateralization may occur among the anterior, middle, and posterior cerebral arteries and also through the leptomeningeal arteries. Occlusive lesions of the middle cerebral artery tend to cause greater infarction of the basal ganglia than the cerebral cortex.[150] The reason for this is that the pial arteries have much greater potential for providing collateral blood flow to the cortex than to the deeper brain structures.

THRESHOLDS OF CEREBRAL ISCHEMIA

The understanding of the pathophysiology of acute cerebral ischemia has been aided by the recognition of two major concepts: thresholds of cerebral ischemia and ischemic penumbra.[6, 63, 70, 85, 92] Specific thresholds of cerebral blood flow exist for various neuronal functions (Fig. 45–2). That is, if blood flow falls below the threshold for electrical function, cortical function ceases; however, the neurons remain viable until blood flow falls even farther to the threshold for membrane pump failure, or if blood flow is increased the electrical function of that neuron may recover. The degree of permanent damage within an ischemic area of brain is a function of both the degree and the duration of the ischemic blood flow. The ischemic penumbra has been defined as the area of ischemic brain that is perfused at cerebral blood flow values below threshold for electrical function but greater than the threshold for membrane pump failure, and therefore these neurons (idling neurons) remain viable but nonfunctioning.[6] The implication is that if blood flow is restored to these neurons cortical function will be restored, and it is this principle on which current stroke therapy is based.

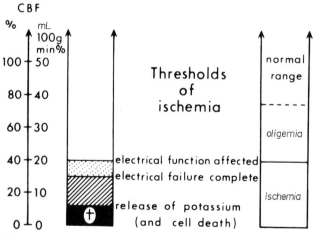

Figure 45–2

Levels of ischemic thresholds for neuronal electrical activity and for membrane pump failure (release of K⁺). CBF, cerebral blood flow. (From Astrup, J., Symon, L., Branston, N. M., et al.: Cortical evoked potential and extracellular K⁺ and H⁺ at critical levels of brain ischemia. Stroke, 8:51–57, 1977. Reprinted by permission.)

Thresholds for Neurological Function

In the awake monkey stroke model, Jones and associates demonstrated that no deficits developed at local cerebral blood flow values above 23 mL per 100 g per minute.[70] When flow decreased below this level, immediate limb weakness occurred; and as flow decreased further, limb function deteriorated further.

Thresholds of Neuronal Electrical Activity

Both clinical and experimental data have shown that the critical flow for cortical electrical activity ranges between 15 and 20 mL per 100 g per minute.[10, 133] During carotid artery occlusion, local cerebral artery blood flow studies and electroencephalography show that amplitude of the latter decreases when flows fall below 20 mL per 100 g per minute and becomes isoelectric at values of 15 to 16 mL per 100 g per minute. In the primate model for cerebral artery occlusion, Branston and associates found that somatosensory evoked potentials were sustained with cerebral blood flow down to levels of 20 mL per 100 g per minute but that evoked responses declined sharply with flows of 14 to 16 mL per 100 g per minute.[10] Therefore, the flow threshold for failure of neuronal electrical function is believed to be 15 to 18 mL per 100 g per minute.[64]

Thresholds for Membrane Pump Failure

When local cerebral blood flow is further reduced to a level of about 10 mL per 100 g per minute, an increase in extracellular potassium concentration can be measured.[9] This level of cerebral blood flow has been considered to be the point at which potassium is released from adenosine triphosphate–depleted cells and has been labeled as the threshold for membrane failure. The increases in extracellular potassium concentration are accompanied by cellular uptake of calcium and glial uptake of sodium, chloride, and water.[122]

Threshold for Cerebral Infarction

Experimental data suggest that infarct size correlates with the reduction of regional blood flow and that an infarct will develop only if flow is reduced below 12 mL per 100 g per minute for 2 hours or longer.[92] Flows of 17 to 18 mL per 100 g per minute during permanent middle cerebral artery occlusion have led to large infarctions; however, in primates, restoration of flow within 1 to 2 hours after middle cerebral artery occlusion can result in full recovery of neurological function and prevent tissue damage.[27, 28, 70] The development of infarction, therefore, is a function of the intensity and duration of the ischemia. From experimental data, a graph of infarction thresholds has been developed by Jones and associates.[70]

Ischemic Penumbra

The ischemic penumbra is defined as ischemic tissue that is at risk for infarction but is potentially salvageable (Fig. 45–3).[6, 55, 123] It is believed that in the ischemic penumbra cerebral blood flow is between 10 and 20 mL per 100 g per minute. Voltage-sensitive calcium channels are activated during the penumbra phase, and the binding of dihydropyridines to these channels has been quantitated in vivo. Experiments show that the response of the dihydropyridines to reperfusion can distinguish penumbra regions that have maintained the potential to be salvaged from those that have lost it.[56, 66] The duration of ischemia that allows tissue to maintain reversibility depends on the degree to which cerebral blood flow is suppressed (Fig. 45–4). During middle cerebral artery occlusion the penumbra is only gradually recruited into an irreversible stage, and therefore time is available to salvage these cells. It is probably only the penumbra that is treatable during acute ischemic stroke and at which the stroke therapies are aimed.

Reperfusion of cerebral tissue usually follows focal cerebral ischemia, be it following an ischemic stroke in which an embolus dissolves in the middle cerebral artery or during planned cerebral ischemia in the operating room when a proximal cerebral vessel that has been clamped is unclamped and perfusion is allowed to occur. A number of experimental studies have examined the reperfusion phenomenon, and it has been demonstrated in the primate that ischemia of less than 1 hour followed by reperfusion is generally well tolerated. It is known, however, that the process of reperfusion may be a double-edged sword.[32, 85, 123] Although blood flow to the brain can restore the delivery of vital substrates to the brain, it has been observed that reperfusion of the middle cerebral artery after 6 hours may be associated with massive swelling and secondary damage referred to as reperfusion injury. Such damage may be due to the resupply of water and osmotic equivalents or of oxygen that may trigger pro-

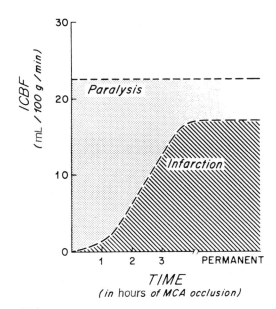

Figure 45–4

Ischemic and infarction thresholds. Jones and co-workers demonstrated that the transition from ischemia to infarction is a function of both the degree and the duration of ischemia. When cerebral blood flow falls below about 23 mL per 100 g per minute, reversible paralysis occurs. When cerebral blood flow falls below 10 mL per 100 g per minute for 2 hours or 18 mL per 100 g per minute permanently, irreversible infarction occurs. (From Jones, T. H., Morawetz, R. B., Crowell, R. M., et al.: Thresholds of focal cerebral ischemia in awake monkeys. J. Neurosurg., 54:773–782, 1981. Reprinted by permission.)

duction of injurious free radicals.[121] Thus, brain tissue during an ischemic stroke may be damaged by the lack of oxygen or glucose (ischemic injury) or reperfusion injury. Potential anti-ischemic agents may be effective in stroke by protecting against either the ischemic or the reperfusion injury.

MECHANISMS OF ISCHEMIC NEURONAL DAMAGE: THE ISCHEMIC CASCADE

Once cerebral blood flow decreases to a critical level and the energy stores of the cell are depleted, membrane failure occurs. A derangement of the pump-leak relationship for ions follows and triggers an ischemic cascade that results in an ischemic injury (Fig. 45–5). Accumulating evidence suggests that excitatory amino acids play a crucial role in the initiation of various pathophysiological events that ultimately lead to neuronal death during cerebral ischemia.[22, 113, 121, 146] The neurotoxic effects of excitatory amino acids are thought to be mediated by overstimulation of glutamate receptors, causing a massive influx of calcium ions into the cell.[89] Under physiological conditions, energy is necessary to maintain the ionic gradient between cytosolic calcium concentration (10^{-7}) and extracellular calcium concentration (10^{-3}). Calcium is allowed to enter cells only through specific channels (gates), and adenosine triphosphate is needed to transport calcium out of the cytosol into the extracellular space. Under ischemic conditions, however, the neuronal membrane depolar-

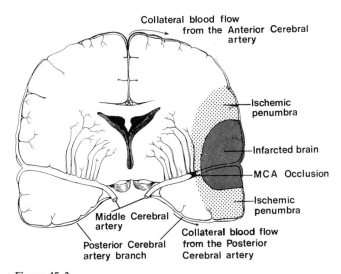

Figure 45–3

Ischemic penumbra in middle cerebral artery (MCA) distribution. After occlusion of the middle cerebral artery, an area of infarction is surrounded by a region of brain containing neurons that are viable but not functioning. This area is kept viable by blood flow through collateral pial vessels.

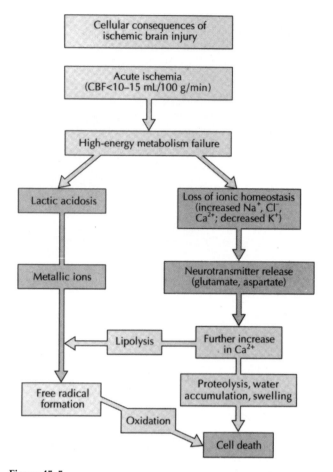

Figure 45–5

Cellular consequences of ischemic brain injury. (Redrawn from Fisher, M.: Medical therapy for ischemic stroke. *In* Fisher, M., and Bogousslavsky, J., eds.: Current Review of Cerebrovascular Disease. Philadelphia, Current Medicine, 1993, pp. 158–170.)

izes and a massive influx of calcium enters into the neurons through a number of processes, including voltage-sensitive calcium channels and receptor-operated calcium channels (Fig. 45–6).[130] Calcium is also released during ischemia from intracellular stores such as the endoplasmic reticulum. This massive increase in cytosolic calcium leads to a cascade of events that inhibits mitochondrial function, and thus energy production ceases and, as well, lipases, proteases, and nucleases are activated, ultimately leading to the cell's death.

There are at best three types of voltage-sensitive calcium channels (L—long lasting, T—transient, N—neuronal).[79] Of these, only the L channel has been shown to be modulated by calcium agonists and antagonists. It can potentially reduce ischemic brain injury by directly blocking the influx of calcium into the cell or by indirectly decreasing the release of neural transmitters such as glutamate.[124] A number of L-channel antagonists have been identified, such as dihydropyridines (nimodipine), phenylalkylamines (Verapamil), and benzothiazepines (diltiazem).[79] It has also been hypothesized that calcium channel blockers may protect against ischemic injury by reducing the vascular vasoconstriction that occurs early in the ischemic

injuries. Calcium entry into the ischemic neuron may also occur through receptor-operated calcium channels such as glutamate receptors that are linked to ion channels. Glutamate is an excitatory amino acid that has been linked to ischemic neuronal death (Fig. 45–7).[146] At least three subtypes of glutamate receptors have been identified: (1) *N*-methyl-D-aspartate receptor; (2) kainate, an α-amino-3-hydroxyl-5-methyl-4-isoxazole propenate receptor; (3) metabotropic receptor.[125] During the ischemic process there is an excess release of excitatory amino acids, including glutamate, and it is believed that this glutamate activates the receptors, thus allowing a massive influx of calcium into the cell. The *N*-methyl-D-aspartate glutamate receptor gates a channel permeable to both monovalent cations and calcium. The α-amino-3-hydroxy-5-methyl-4-isoxazole propenate receptor is linked to a channel providing a nonselective conductance mechanism for monovalent cations sodium and potassium. By allowing sodium to enter through the opening of the channel, depolarization of membrane occurs, and this sets the stage for further influx of calcium through voltage-sensitive calcium channels.

Nitric oxide is emerging as one of the major neurotransmitters in the central and peripheral nervous systems.[129] It has been implicated as a mediator of neuronal destruction in cerebral ischemia. Evidence has shown that nitric oxide mediates the same neurotoxic effects as glutamate.[30] Nitric oxide synthase is activated by calcium binding to calmodulin associated with the enzyme. *N*-methyl-D-aspartate receptor activation triggers a massive influx of calcium into neurons, and nitric oxide is formed and diffuses to adjacent cells to kill them.[42] This hypothesis is supported by the ability of nitric oxide synthase inhibitors to block the neurotoxic actions of glutamate and the receptor in brain cultures.

The massive increase in cytosolic calcium during the ischemic process activates degradative enzymes, including lipases, proteases, and endonucleases, which catabolize cellular membranes and neurofilaments.[121, 123] A loss of membrane phospholipids increases the permeability of mitochondrial membranes that interferes with residual oxidative phosphorylation. There is also an accumulation of free fatty acids from membrane phospholipid degradation that are thought to be oxidized through cyclooxygenase or lipoxygenase pathways during reperfusion. The net result of these pathways is the production and release of prostaglandins, leukotrienes, and free radicals. Thromboxane A_2 is a potent vasoconstrictor, leukotrienes alter membrane permeability and lead to vasoconstriction, and free radicals destroy cellular membranes.

Potential Strategies for the Treatment of Acute Cerebral Ischemia

As detailed earlier, the pathophysiology of cerebral ischemia is very complex, and it is unlikely that a

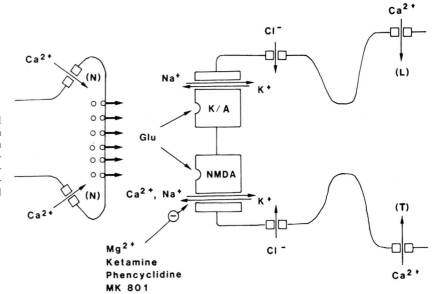

Figure 45–6

Schematic diagram illustrating presynaptic and postsynaptic ion channels with emphasis on voltage-sensitive and agonist-operated calcium channels. NMDA, N-methyl-D-aspartate receptor. (From Siesjo, B. K.: Review article: Pathophysiology and treatment of focal cerebral ischemia. J. Neurosurg., 77:169–184, 1994. Reprinted by permission.)

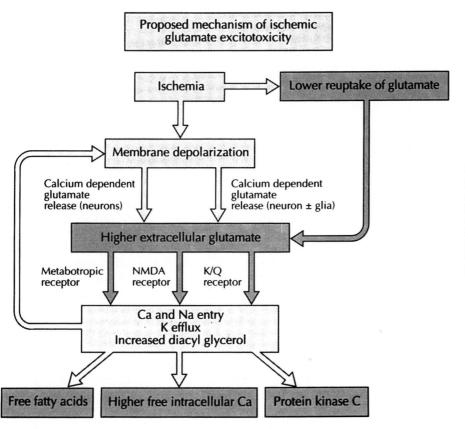

Figure 45–7

Proposed mechanisms of glutamate excitotoxicity in ischemia. (Redrawn from Sharma, M., and Hakim, A. M.: The neuroscience of cerebral ischemia. *In* Fisher, M., and Bogousslavsky, J., eds.: Current Review of Cerebrovascular Disease. Philadelphia, Current Medicine, 1993, pp. 15–22. Reprinted by permission.)

single "magic bullet" will be discovered that will cure a patient of ischemic stroke. In all likelihood, a combination of therapies will be necessary to salvage the ischemic brain. A combination of the following therapeutic modalities should be considered (Table 45–1).

1. Acute resuscitation
2. Reperfusion of the ischemic brain
3. Decreasing cerebral metabolic demands
4. Inhibition of the degradative ischemic cascade

ACUTE RESUSCITATION OF THE STROKE PATIENT

Acute cerebral ischemia is a neurological emergency and must be recognized as such. The management of the stroke patient deserves the same urgency and vigilance as that of the patient who has acutely experienced a traumatic brain injury. Appropriate brain resuscitation can prevent secondary injury to the brain and may even prevent progression of the initial ischemic insult. Secondary insults such as hypoxia, hypotension, hypovolemia, decreased cardiac output, hyperthermia, and hyperglycemia have been shown to be detrimental to injured brain and can potentially be prevented by routine resuscitative procedures. Maintenance of an adequate airway and of proper ventilation is mandatory. Supplementary oxygen, proper head positioning, and frequent suctioning may be all that is necessary to ensure proper blood oxygenation in the "typical stroke patient." However, in the unconscious patient, intubation and mechanical ventilation may be required.

Cerebral ischemia is extremely sensitive to fluctuations in blood pressure and cardiac output. In ischemic brain tissue, autoregulation fails and cerebral blood flow varies directly with blood pressure. A decrease in blood pressure aggravates cerebral ischemia, and elevations in blood pressure increase the cerebral blood flow to the poorly perfused tissues.[59] This has been demonstrated both clinically and in the laboratory setting.[8, 77] Fein and Boulos demonstrated significant

Table 45–1
MANAGEMENT OF ACUTE CEREBRAL ISCHEMIA

1. Acute resuscitation of the stroke patient
   a. Maintenance of airway and adequate ventilation
   b. Maintenance of adequate blood volume and blood pressure
   c. Correction of hyperglycemia, hyperthermia, and low cardiac output
2. Reperfusion of ischemic brain
   a. Thrombolytic therapy
   b. Hypervolemic hemodilution
   c. Anticoagulation
3. Decreasing cerebral metabolic demands
   a. Hypothermia
   b. Barbiturates
4. Inhibition of the degradative ischemic cascade
   a. Calcium antagonists
   b. Excitatory amino acid antagonists
   c. Free radical scavengers

increases in cerebral blood flow in a monkey vasospasm model following induced hypertension.[39] Hope and associates were able to show significant increase in cerebral blood flow and improvement in somatosensory evoked potentials after metaraminol bitartrate (Aramine) infusion in ischemic brain tissue following middle cerebral artery occlusion.[67] Hayashi and colleagues clearly demonstrated the benefit of elevated blood pressure following middle cerebral artery occlusion in an awake primate stroke model.[62] After induced hypertension, neurological status improved, local cerebral blood flow increased, and infarction size decreased. Although hypertensive therapy can improve cerebral blood flow in ischemic brain, the risks of this therapy should be realized. Elevation of blood pressure is hazardous in a patient with an unclipped cerebral aneurysm. Also the risk of hemorrhage into ischemic brain is a well-known complication of this treatment and may be particularly hazardous in patients with large areas of ischemic damage. Several authors have noted an increase in brain edema leading to rapid deterioration when blood pressure was elevated late in the course of cerebral ischemia.[9, 64] In addition, induced hypertension may be hazardous to elderly patients with cardiac problems.

As the brain autoregulates cerebral blood flow to changes in systemic blood pressure, it also regulates cerebral blood flow with respect to cardiac output. In ischemic brain, this regulatory process is lost and cerebral blood flow changes directly with changes in cardiac output.[83, 100, 145] Cardiac output varies directly with volume status and can also be abnormally low in elderly stroke patients with congestive heart failure or cardiac arrhythmias. Thus, in stroke patients, maintaining adequate intravascular volume is important and correcting cardiac abnormalities may prevent further ischemic damage. A central venous line or even a Swan-Ganz catheter may be necessary in patients when fluid status or even cardiac status is a concern.

The temperature of the stroke victim is also critical in the acute phase of ischemia.* Hypothermia of even 2 to 3° C has been shown in the laboratory to be very protective while elevation of temperature above 37° C aggravates ischemic brain injury. Stroke patients may become dehydrated or develop lung congestion during the early phases of their "expectant" stroke therapy; thus, the hypovolemia and elevated temperature may only worsen the already present brain injury.

Glucose control may also become a routine in the management of these patients (Fig. 45–8).[24, 31, 95, 154] In animal studies, an elevated blood glucose level has been shown to worsen experimental cerebral ischemia. Clinically, patients with ischemic symptoms who also had elevated blood glucose levels on admission to a hospital had worse clinical neurological outcomes than those patients without elevated blood glucose values.[20, 29] It is thus recommended that a stroke patient not receive high-glucose–containing solutions and that the blood glucose level be maintained as close to nor-

---

*See references 12, 16–18, 23, 26, 47, 110, and 162.

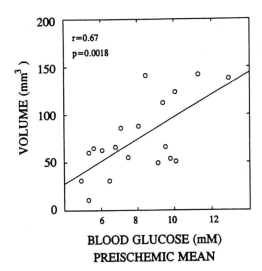

Figure 45–8

In a rat model of focal cerebral ischemia, the cerebral infarction volume correlated with the preischemia blood glucose levels. Linear regression R = .67, P = .0018. (From Hamilton, M. G., Tranmer, B. I., and Auer, R. N.: Insulin-induced hypoglycemia reduces cerebral infarction due to transient focal ischemia. J. Neurosurg., 82:262–268, 1995. Reprinted by permission.)

mal as possible. Insulin may even play a role if blood sugar levels remain high despite glucose restriction.[82]

REPERFUSION OF THE ISCHEMIC BRAIN

Thrombolytic Therapy

Increasing laboratory and clinical experience with thrombolytic agents such as urokinase, streptokinase, and recombinant tissue plasminogen activator has demonstrated significant and sustained neurological improvement when the thrombolytic treatment has been initiated in the first few hours.[11, 33, 52, 93, 151] The thrombolytic agents appear to be effective in producing recanalization of the thrombosed cerebral vessel, but the risk of reperfusion hemorrhage remains significant. It remains uncertain which agent is the most effective and safest, when this agent should be given, and what is the best route of administration.

The earlier thrombolytic studies were not performed with clot-specific thrombolytic agents such as streptokinase and urokinase. Improvement in the thrombolytic process has been achieved with serine proteases (included in the endogenous thrombolytic system). Recombinant tissue plasminogen activator is now produced in vitro.[94] It is a relatively clot-specific agent initially used in the treatment of myocardial infarction and infarction due to intracoronary thrombosis. Much of the initial work with thrombolysis was done in the coronary patient. Streptokinase and recombinant tissue plasminogen activator appear to be equally effective in the treatment of acute myocardial infarction. Stroke, especially hemorrhagic stroke, and other bleeding side effects are a major concern for myocardial infarction patients given fibrinolytic therapy.[127] Some reports suggest that the clot-specific recombinant tissue plasmino-

gen activator is associated with a higher intracerebral hemorrhage rate than streptokinase.

The initial work with streptokinase and urokinase in human ischemic stroke was disappointing, and it was thought that the relatively fibrin-specific recombinant tissue plasminogen activator would be more effective and be associated with fewer hemorrhagic side effects. Initial animal studies were performed by Zivin and co-workers, and it was shown that if the activator was given up to 45 minutes after the onset of stroke there was an improved neurological outcome without increasing hemorrhagic risk.[163] Overgaard and co-workers, in an embolic stroke model, provided evidence that recombinant tissue plasminogen activator induced clot lysis, reduced infarction size, improved neurological outcome, and reduced mortality.[102]

A multicenter, phase I trial evaluated the safety and efficacy of intravenous administration of recombinant tissue plasminogen activator in the treatment of acute ischemic stroke.[11, 57] Of the 74 patients treated within 90 minutes, major neurological improvement at 2 hours occurred in 30 per cent, and at 24 hours it occurred in 46 per cent. Neurological deterioration occurred in 11 per cent (2 patients with intracerebral hemorrhage). Asymptomatic bleeding occurred in 4 per cent and was not dose related. Symptomatic bleeding correlated with total dose given. Of the 20 patients treated at 91 to 180 minutes, 2 had fatal intracerebral hemorrhages and 3 had major neurological improvement at 24 hours. In three other studies based on angiographic criteria for the diagnosis of arterial occlusion, it was given intravenously within 6 hours of the onset of stroke.[33, 101, 151] Recanalization was demonstrated angiographically in 25 to 50 per cent, asymptomatic hemorrhagic conversion occurred in 30 to 40 per cent, hemorrhage causing deterioration or death occurred in 10 per cent, and good clinical outcome was noted at 24 hours in 40 per cent. There has also been a renewed interest in urokinase and streptokinase.[52, 93] Beneficial results have been reported when these agents have been given intraarterially.

The use of thrombolytic agents has been encouraging in the treatment of both myocardial infarction and ischemic stroke, but clinical randomized trials are continuing in an attempt to clear the controversy surrounding this treatment.

Hypervolemic Hemodilution Therapy

Hypertensive hypervolemic hemodilution is an effective treatment for cerebral ischemia secondary to cerebral vasospasm.[45, 71, 76, 77] Both elevation of blood pressure and colloidal volume expansion augment cerebral blood flow to ischemic brain, and the clinical outcome of patients with cerebral vasospasm has improved since this therapy has become popular. In the 1970's, with the use of artificially induced hypertension in the treatment of patients with ischemic deficits associated with vasospasm, Kindt and associates became aware that most of the patients were hypovolemic. It was also noticed that once therapy used to increase intravascular volume was instituted, both the amount and the duration of vasopressor therapy could be reduced. Subsequently, these researchers demonstrated that intravascular volume expansion, independent of induced hypertension, was effective in treating the ischemia secondary to vasospasm.[75, 108] Thus, colloidal volume expansion with or without hypertensive therapy has become a popular and successful method of treating ischemic neurological deficits associated with cerebral vasospasm (Fig. 45–9).

Intravascular volume expansion has also become recognized as a therapy for acute ischemic stroke. Clinical trials by Gilroy and co-workers, Gottstein and colleagues, Strand and associates, and Tranmer and colleagues have demonstrated favorable results using volume expansion in patients with acute cerebral ischemia.[46, 49, 131, 143] However, randomized multicenter trials have failed to demonstrate a benefit in patients treated with hemodilution.[131, 146] In both the Scandinavian Stroke Study Group and the Italian Acute Stroke Study Group there was no significant improvement in morbidity or decrease in mortality in the treatment group. However, one single-center randomized trial has demonstrated benefits with hemodilution. Goslinga and associates (the Amsterdam Stroke Study) performed a prospective single-center randomized clinical trial in which custom-tailored hemodilution with albumin and crystalloids was given to patients with acute ischemic stroke.[48] They demonstrated a significant ($P < .005$) reduction in mortality at 3 months and an increase in independence at home in the treatment group.

The efficacy of colloidal volume expansion has

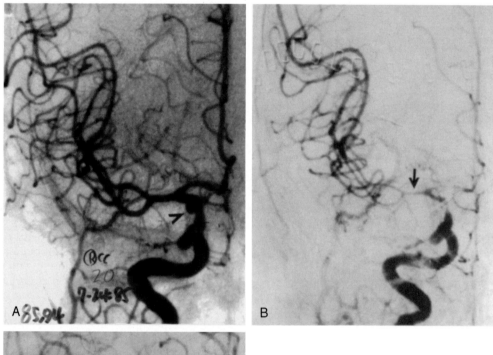

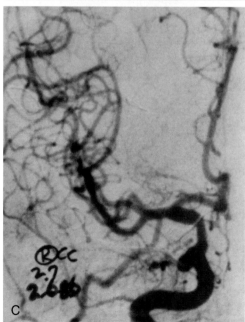

Figure 45–9

Case report, cerebral vasospasm treated with hypertension and volume expansion. *A.* A 34-year-old woman presented with a grade II (Hunt's classification) subarachnoid hemorrhage from a posterior communicating artery aneurysm. *B.* The aneurysm was clipped on day 3, but on the fifth postoperative day she suddenly became hemiplegic. The angiogram demonstrates severe vasospasm of the supraclinoid internal carotid artery and the proximal middle cerebral artery. *C.* After intensive volume expansion and hypertensive therapy her deficits resolved. The angiogram shows normal intracranial vessels.

been demonstrated experimentally using many stroke models.[144, 159] In a primate model of middle cerebral artery occlusion, colloidal volume expansion with hetastarch has been shown to increase cerebral blood flow to the ischemic brain as well as improve the electroencephalographic power data in the ischemic brain.[144] In a rat model of middle cerebral artery occlusion, the animals that were volume expanded with hetastarch showed increases in cerebral blood flow in ischemic brain and also reduction in the size of the brain infarction.[100]

The mechanism by which colloidal volume expansion increases local cerebral blood flow and decreases infarction volume remains controversial. Wood and Feischer coined the term "hypervolemic hemodilution" and have demonstrated that local cerebral blood flow correlates inversely with both hematocrit and blood viscosity and is directly related to total blood volume.[158] Dextran has also been shown to have antisludging effects by charge-coating the red cells and platelets, thus inhibiting their aggregation.[159] As well, colloidal volume expansion also augments cardiac output according to the Frank-Starling curve. Studies have shown that increases in cardiac output during volume expansion are closely followed by increases in local cerebral blood flow in ischemic brain.[100, 145] In both the primate stroke model and the rat stroke model, Tranmer and associates have demonstrated that in normal brain, changes in cardiac output did not alter cerebral blood flow; however, in ischemic brain, cerebral blood flow changed passively as cardiac output increased and decreased (Fig. 45–10).[100, 145] It is hypothe-

sized that this hyperdynamic cardiovascular response to colloidal volume expansion increases cardiac output and pulse pressure, which thus increases the pulsatile nature of cerebral blood flow, resulting in more effective blood flow in the ischemic brain. Benefits of pulsatile perfusion have been demonstrated during both cardiopulmonary bypass and ischemic stroke.[142]

Regardless of the mechanism by which it is achieved, an increase in intravascular volume has been shown to benefit patients with cerebral ischemia secondary to either cerebral occlusive disease or cerebral vasospasm. The risk of this therapy has been found to be minimal. Hemorrhagic complications have not been a problem. Cerebral edema of the ischemic brain has also generally not been a problem clinically or experimentally. Colloidal volume expansion does play a role in the treatment of acute ischemic stroke; however, the agents to be used, doses to be given, and timing of the therapy remain controversial. Central venous pressure monitoring or even the use of Swan-Ganz catheters is suggested to accurately monitor fluid status and critically titrate cardiac function.

Anticoagulation

Many clinicians continue to use anticoagulation (heparin) as a treatment for acute cerebral ischemic stroke. Evidence of the usefulness of this therapy is, however, not compelling. Only two clinical trials in the computed tomography era have evaluated the usefulness of heparin anticoagulation in the treatment of acute stroke.[21, 35] Unlike thrombolytic therapy, anticoag-

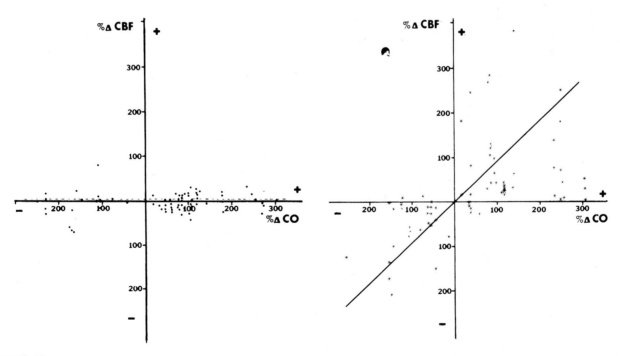

Figure 45–10

Graphs depict autoregulatory responses to cardiac output (CO) variations in nonischemic brain regions (left, $r = .00$) and ischemic brain regions (right, $r = .89$). % change CBF, % change in cerebral blood flow; % change CO, % change in cardiac output. (From Tranmer, B. I., Keller, T., and Kindt, G. W.: Loss of cerebral regulation during cardiac output variations in focal cerebral ischemia. J. Neurosurg., 77:253–259, 1992. Reprinted by permission.)

ulation with heparin is not intended to dissolve thrombus but to impair the thrombogenesis created by the clotting cascade. One clinical study randomized 45 patients with cardioembolic stroke to immediate anticoagulation with intravenous heparin versus delayed anticoagulation with warfarin after 14 days.[21] Of the 24 patients randomized to early anticoagulation there were no recurrences and no hemorrhages during the 2-week study. Of the 21 patients randomized to receive delayed anticoagulation, 2 had early recurrent embolism, 2 had hemorrhagic conversion, and 2 died. This study was terminated early because of the strong trend toward the benefit of early anticoagulation with heparin. In the second study the effect of intravenous heparin within 48 hours of onset of ischemic stroke was studied.[35] The effect of the heparin was compared with that of a placebo. There was no significant difference in stroke progression or death after 7 days, and there was also no difference in functional level seen after 1 year. However, significantly more deaths occurred in the group on heparin at 1 year. Thus, heparin was believed not to be useful for the treatment of acute ischemic stroke.

The complication rate of anticoagulation in acute ischemic stroke is significant. The incidence of major brain hemorrhage in the anticoagulated stroke patient varies widely but is generally reported to be 5 to 15 per cent. Based on the previously discussed study, early anticoagulation with heparin is believed to be the appropriate treatment for patients who have suffered a cardioembolic stroke. This therapy should be instituted only after computed tomography has ruled out an intracerebral hemorrhage or a large cerebral infarction.

DECREASING CEREBRAL METABOLIC DEMANDS

Cerebral ischemia is the result of an imbalance between supply and demand of blood flow and its nutrients. If reperfusion of the cerebral tissue cannot occur soon enough, then cerebral protection by decreasing the cerebral metabolic demands may help preserve brain tissue until reperfusion can occur. Hypothermia and barbiturates have been recognized in the past as agents that do decrease cerebral metabolic demands and have been studied as cerebral protectors.

Hypothermia

The technique of hypothermia was probably the first method of cerebral protection. Over the past 30 years neurosurgeons, cardiovascular surgeons, and anesthesiologists have used hypothermia to protect the brain during periods in which the cerebral circulation had to be greatly reduced or eliminated to permit proper surgical access.[78, 86, 112] It has been thought that hypothermia decreases the cerebral metabolic rate. Hagerdal and associates demonstrated that cerebral oxygen metabolism decreased in a linear fashion during temperature reduction from 37 to 22° C.[54] At 22° C the local cerebral blood flow and metabolic rates were reduced

to about 25 per cent of normal. Ganshirt and associates demonstrated that survival time after total cerebral ischemia was a function of the depth of hypothermia and concluded that optimal brain protection was produced at temperatures between 27° and 30° C.[41] However, the clinical usefulness of profound hypothermia has been limited by the adverse side effects associated with the severity and duration of hypothermia. Cardiac arrhythmias and cardiac arrests have been encountered during neurosurgical operations especially if the temperature was allowed to drop near the threshold for cardiac arrhythmias (27° C). Pulmonary complications such as pneumonia and neurogenic pulmonary edema have also been attributed to hypothermia.

There has been a revival of interest in hypothermia in the treatment of cerebral ischemia since animal experiments have shown that a reduction of brain temperature of only 2° C effectively protects neurons against cerebral ischemia.[16, 17, 47] Ridenour and associates demonstrated that mild hypothermia reduced infarction size during focal ischemia, and Zhang and colleagues demonstrated that hypothermia implemented 1 hour after ischemia dramatically reduced ischemic neuronal injury.[110, 162] Hypothermia has also been shown to protect against ischemia during transient global ischemia.[17] The mechanism by which hypothermia is protective may not be as simple as saying it decreases the cerebral metabolic rate. Busto and associates produced hypothermia in a rat stroke model and found that the release of glutamate and dopamine was dramatically reduced during hypothermic ischemia.[18] The mechanism of reduced release may be the inhibition of protein kinase C translocation to the plasma membrane by hypothermia. Studies have also demonstrated the deleterious effect of mild (2° C) hyperthermia, which accelerates and worsens cell damage during experimental ischemia.

Clinical studies using mild hypothermia during acute stroke and also during traumatic brain injury are underway. For the time being, maintenance of euthermia and certainly reduction of hyperthermia in the patient with ischemic stroke should be done to reduce progression of the ischemic insult. Hypothermia is effective during planned cerebral ischemia, that is, during temporary clipping of cerebral vessels or extracranial vessels during carotid endarterectomy.

Barbiturates

Barbiturates have been reported to provide effective cerebral protection if given before or soon after the onset of cerebral ischemia in animal studies.[65, 91, 128] Cerebral protection using barbiturates has also been shown to be of clinical benefit.[90, 98] Although it does appear that barbiturates have some protective efficacy during temporary focal ischemia, it also seems likely that their efficacy in the older literature has been overstated. Hypothermia may have accounted for some of the brain protection that was attributed to barbiturates in these older studies.[65, 128]

INHIBITION OF THE DEGRADATIVE ISCHEMIC CASCADE

Calcium Antagonism

As previously discussed, studies in experimental cerebral ischemia have demonstrated that calcium influx into cells and liberation of intracellular stores of calcium activate proteases and phospholipases that produce cytotoxic free radicals and leukotrienes, resulting in cell death. The critical rise in intracellular free calcium concentration during ischemia occurs through voltage-dependent calcium channels, receptor-operated calcium channels, and release from endoplasmic reticulum.[79, 89]

Calcium antagonists may beneficially modulate ischemic brain damage either by increasing blood flow through the vasodilatation of cerebral vessels or by protecting the neurons by blocking calcium entry into the cell during ischemia or by antagonizing the intracellular action of calcium. Of the three types of voltage-dependent calcium channels only the L type has been modulated by a calcium channel blocker. Nimodipine, a dihydropyridine compound, has been the calcium channel blocker that has received the most attention.[3, 53, 60, 138, 161] Nimodipine has been demonstrated to protect against the ischemic effect of vasospasm and is commonly used in patients with subarachnoid hemorrhage.[138] Despite encouraging results using nimodipine in animal stroke models, results of clinical stroke trials have been mixed.[2, 43] Initial studies by Gelmers showed that nimodipine, 30 mg four times a day, given within 24 hours of the stroke significantly reduced morbidity.[43] However, three more studies have not shown any positive effects of nimodipine.[7, 87, 147] In the most recent study, the American Nimodipine Study Group (a randomized double-blind trial), it was suggested that nimodipine may be effective in patients with moderate deficits who are treated within 12 hours of the ischemic event.[3] Nicardipine, another voltage-dependent calcium channel blocker, has been studied in a safety trial, but side effects such as hypotension and tachycardia were noted.[160] Preliminary results with intracellular antagonist BAPTA, an intracellular calcium chelator, have been encouraging in a rat stroke model, and AT877, a protein kinase inhibitor, has been demonstrated to be a cerebral protector in a rat stroke model and also an effective antispasm drug when used in patients with vasospasm.[99, 119, 148] Like other calcium antagonists, AT877 may protect the ischemic neuron by a reduction in cerebrovascular resistance.

Excitatory Amino Acid Antagonists

The blockade of the voltage-sensitive calcium channel alone during cerebral ischemia may not be sufficient to dramatically affect the rapid rise in intracellular calcium. Activation of receptor-operated calcium channels by excitatory amino acids, especially glutamate, appears to be an important inducer of intracellular calcium, and it is hypothesized that blockade of these channels may protect the ischemic neuron.[79, 89, 130] The receptor-operated calcium channels include N-methyl-D-aspartate, α-amino-3-hydroxyl-5-methyl-4-isoxazole propenate, and metabotropic subtypes.[125] The N-methyl-D-aspartate channels can be blocked by both noncompetitive (MK801) and competitive antagonists. The agent MK801 and dextromethorphan significantly decrease neuronal damage in experimental ischemia.[103, 105, 126, 136] Although these antagonists have been shown to be experimentally beneficial during moderate ischemia, reproducible protection has not been reported in models of severe ischemia.[13] The protective effect of MK801 may be due to its hypothermic effect on the animals as opposed to a direct cytoprotective effect.[12, 26] The α-amino-3-hydroxyl-5-methyl-4-isoxazole propenate antagonist 2,3-dihydroxyl-6-nitro-7-sulfamoyl-benzoquinoxaline has been shown to be a powerful cerebral protector during severe forebrain ischemia and during transient focal ischemia.[14, 15] Clinical trial is necessary to study these agents for both safety and efficacy in humans.

Free Radical Scavengers

Free radical generation during ischemia and reperfusion is believed to be the final common pathway for neuronal damage during ischemic stroke. Free radical scavengers such as tirilazad and superoxide dismutase have been shown to be protective in animal models.[58] A phase III trial studying the efficacy of tirilazad in patients with subarachnoid hemorrhage has been completed and demonstrated a 44 per cent decrease in morbidity secondary to vasospasm.[38] A clinical stroke trial is also underway to evaluate the efficacy of tirilazad in ischemic stroke. Mannitol is a hydroxyl free radical scavenger and is routinely given by neurosurgeons intraoperatively during "planned" vessel occlusion during aneurysm surgery.

Current Strategies for Planned Cerebral Ischemia (Cerebral Protection)

Not infrequently neurosurgeons encounter a situation of vascular occlusion in which the potential for cerebral ischemia is anticipated a priori. Included among these situations are temporary occlusions of the carotid artery during carotid endarterectomy and also temporary occlusion of the cerebral vessels during the technique of temporary clipping during aneurysm surgery. These situations give the neurosurgeon a unique opportunity to draw on the significant body of laboratory and clinical data on cerebral protection and to use planned techniques for cerebral protection. Many of the agents or techniques that have been disappointing in their post hoc efficacy for the treatment of acute ischemic stroke are, in fact, potentially good cerebral protectants when pre-emptively applied in anticipation of ischemia. Suzuki is one of the pioneers of cerebral protection for planned cerebral ischemia having introduced his "Sendai cocktail," which contained mannitol, vitamin E, and phenytoin.[135] The authors' practical experiences and strategies for cerebral protection for planned cerebral ischemia are detailed in this section. Commonly used techniques by the authors include hypothermia, colloidal volume expansion, induced hypertension, barbiturate coma, and perfluorocarbons (Fluosol).

HYPOTHERMIA

Recent laboratory research has shown that hypothermia (34 to 35° C) is a powerful cerebral protector.[16, 23, 47] In most examples of planned cerebral ischemia, modest hypothermia can be effective; it is not necessary to cool the patient to the level of 30° C when cardiac arrhythmias may occur. The authors also believe that the indication for full hypothermic cardiac arrest and cardiac bypass support is limited. Inducing mild hypothermia when the patient is under general anesthesia is usually simply a matter of keeping the room cool as well as using a cooling blanket on the patient.

COLLOIDAL VOLUME EXPANSION

Colloidal volume expansion is an important first step common to cerebral protection.[75, 143] The intravascular system needs to be fully primed if one is to take full advantage of cardiovascular manipulation to overcome ischemic conditions. Titrating the intravascular volume to the maximum without threatening the pumping action of the heart requires attention to the Starling curve, which requires placement of a central venous line or a Swan-Ganz catheter. Colloid agents such as albumin or hetastarch are more useful than crystalloids as volume expanders. Blood and blood products have also been used as volume expanders, although they are not as effective as colloid agents such as hetastarch. Colloid agents such as albumin or plasminate have a relatively short intravascular half-life. Low-molecular-weight dextran has a reasonable half-life and improves rheology, but allergic reactions with the contaminating high- and middle-molecular-weight dextrans have been encountered. Dextran has also been associated with a hemostatic defect attributed to an acquired form of von Willebrand's disease. Additionally, it has at times created an osmotic block in the renal tubules resulting in oliguria and anuria and, because of the size of the molecule, dialysis is ineffective in treating the problem. Hetastarch has been the authors' usual choice for colloidal volume expansion. Hetastarch, or hydroxyethyl starch, is a synthetic polymer with a 30-hour intravascular half-life. The authors' experience suggests that hetastarch stays within the intravascular space better than albumin; thus, leakage of the colloid agent through a damaged blood-brain barrier is rare.[141] Coagulopathies, however, have been encountered that are due to a direct effect of hetastarch on factor VIII and to the dilutional impact on the other clotting factors. The recommended limit for hetastarch in any 24-hour period is 1,200 mL. If more than 1,200 mL in a 24-hour period is necessary for volume expansion, then it is supplemented with albumin. Not infrequently patients with cardiac problems are in need of hyperdynamic therapy, and cardiac complications can occur. For prolonged therapy, such as in the vasospasm patient, the authors have frequently found it necessary to digitalize patients to maintain them in an optimal hyperdynamic state. Another drug that has been particularly useful and supplements colloidal volume expansion is dobutamine,[83] which, in addition to colloid volume expansion, can further augment cardiac output.

INDUCED HYPERTENSION

Induced hypertension is used by the authors during carotid endarterectomy and occasionally during temporary clipping for aneurysm surgery. There are a number of excellent drugs that can be used to induce hypertension; and if the patient's blood volume has expanded adequately, less of the drug is necessary to obtain the desired effect. Short-term therapy is best accomplished with phenylephrine (Neo-Synephrine). This agent is easily titrated, and its effect is rapidly terminated (less than 10 minutes) on discontinuation of the drip. Most vascular beds are constricted by this drug except for the coronary and cerebral vasculature, and cardiac irritation is minimal. For longer therapy, dopamine is the drug of choice because of its minimal effect on the renal vasculature. During carotid endarterectomy the authors try to maintain mean arterial blood pressure at 20 to 30 mm Hg above the patient's normal mean blood pressure.

BARBITURATE COMA

During carotid endarterectomy barbiturate coma is used occasionally. If lateralization of the electroencephalogram occurs during cross-clamping of the carotid artery, and this does not respond to induced hypertension, then barbiturate coma is induced as 15- to 60-second burst suppression on the electroencephalogram. The usual induction dose of thiopental is 1,000 to 1,200 mg given in 250- to 500-mg boluses. As burst suppression shortens, further boluses of thiopental are given, and the total dose of thiopental required to maintain burst suppression through the period of carotid cross-clamping is usually 2,500 to 3,500 mg. The initial experience with barbiturates as a cerebral protector did not include volume expansion. Without volume expansion, approximately 15 per cent of the patients required barbiturates. With colloidal volume expansion, only 2 per cent of the patients have required barbiturate cerebral protection during carotid surgery.

PERFLUOROCARBONS

Although available for clinical practice, perfluorocarbons as blood substitutes have not proven particu-

Table 45–2
CURRENT STROKE TRIALS

Name of Trial	Protocol
Thrombolytic Therapy	
Multicenter Acute Stroke Trial	A randomized, controlled, double-blind study of streptokinase (1.5 MU), aspirin (300 mg/d × 10 d), or their combination or neither on mortality and severe disability. Therapy will be initiated within 6 hours of acute ischemic stroke with final assessment at 6 months.
Australian Stroke Trial	Patients are randomized in a double-blind fashion to receive streptokinase vs. placebo within 4 hours of the acute ischemic event.
European Cooperative Acute Stroke Study	Randomized, double-blind study with tissue plasminogen activator treatment (1.1 mg/kg over 1 hr) begun within 6 hours of the ictus. Patients are evaluated 90 days following treatment. Preliminary data suggest that this treatment is safe.
National Institute of Neurological Disease and Stroke Recombinant Tissue Plasminogen Activator Stroke Trial	Randomized, double-blind study in which patients receive 0.9 mg/kg tissue plasminogen activator vs. placebo within 3 hours of the ischemic event. Patients are examined for neurological improvement at 14 hours and for neurological improvement/functional outcome at 7 to 10 days and at 3 months.
Thrombolytic Therapy in Acute Ischemic Stroke	Randomized, double-blind, placebo-controlled study with tissue plasminogen activator treatment (0.9 mg/kg) begun within 5 hours of the ictus. Patients will be examined for neurological improvement 30 days after therapy.
Overview Analysis of Completed, Randomized Trials of Thrombolysis in Acute Ischemic Stroke (streptokinase, urokinase, tissue plasminogen activator, plasmin)	Analysis demonstrates a significant reduction of 56% in the odds of death or deterioration after thrombolytic treatment.
Free Radical Scavengers/Inhibitors of Lipid Peroxidation	
Efficacy of Tirilazad Mesylate (U74006F) in Acute Stroke	A randomized trial of tirilazad mesylate with treatment initiated within 12 hours of the ischemic event.
Antiplatelet/Antithrombin Therapy	
Britton Study	Aspirin (325 mg/d) vs. placebo.
National Stroke Study of China	Patient randomized to receive either aspirin (325 mg/d × 100 d) vs. placebo.
International Stroke Trial	A multicenter, randomized study, using a 3 × 5 factorial design examining low-dose aspirin (300 mg/d) vs. two doses of subcutaneous heparin (5,000 vs 12,500 units). Time to treatment will be within 48 hours of the event and will continue for 14 days.
Ticlid Angiology	Patients randomized received ticlid (250 mg bid × 21 d) vs. placebo. The study demonstrated a significant improvement in neurological outcome in the acute period.
Fraxiparine (Low-Molecular-Weight Heparin) in Stroke Study	This trial will examine low-molecular-weight heparin vs. placebo.
ORG10172 in Acute Stroke Treatment	Multicenter, randomized placebo-controlled trial of the low-molecular-weight heparinoid ORG10172 in acute progressing stroke. Patients will be randomized within 24 hours of the ischemic event and continue treatment for 7 days.
Excitatory Amino Acid Antagonists	
Dextromethorphan	A small cohort of patients previously experiencing a hemispheric stroke were given oral dextromethorphan for 3 weeks. No evidence of toxicity was noted.
CGS 19755 Acute Stroke Trial	A double-blind, multicenter, placebo-controlled pilot study, evaluating safety and tolerability of two intravenous bolus doses of CGS 19755 in acute stroke.
Ganglioside Therapy	
Italian Acute Stroke Study	This study randomized patients, within 12 hours of the ischemic event to receive ganglioside-1, hemodilution, both, or neither. Treatment continued for 15 days, with final evaluation at 120 days. There was no difference in mortality. Although early neurological improvement was noted, this was not significant at the 120-day time point.
Monoganglioside Stroke Trial	This is a randomized, placebo-controlled multicenter study. Treatment will begin within 5 hours of the ictus. Neurological status and mortality rates will be assessed 4 months after initiation of treatment.
Ancrod	
Stroke Treatment with Ancrod Trial	A multicenter, phase III, placebo-controlled study. Patients are treated within 3 hours of acute ischemic stroke and given ancrod over a 5-day period. Neurological assessment is performed 3 months after the initiation of treatment.
Hemorrheological	
Randomized Study of Hemodilution Therapy in Acute Ischemic Stroke	Patients undergoing venesection and 10% dextran for volume replacement were noted to have significant improvement at the 1-year follow-up, though there was no diffference in mortality rate.
Calcium Entry Blockers	
Trials of the United Kingdom for Stroke Treatment	Patients randomized to receive either nimodipine or placebo. Although improvement was noted at 21 days in the active treatment group, no significant difference was noted at follow-up week 24.
American Nimodipine Study Group	In this randomized, double-blind, multicenter clinical trial, patients were randomized to receive either placebo or nimodipine (60, 120, or 240 mg/d × 21 d). Nimodipine had no overall effect when treatment was begun within 48 hours.
Serotonin Receptor Antagonists	
Praxilene in Stroke Treatment in Northern Europe	Comparison of Praxilene (specific serotonin S_2-receptor antagonist) vs. placebo.

larly useful in the treatment of stroke.[140] Their expense precludes their general use in trauma resuscitation; however, with the current problems of bloodborne viral infections a resurgence may occur. Although the authors' experience with this preparation is limited, they have used Fluosol in two patients whose hyperdynamic therapy required anemia-threatening volume expansion but whose religion precluded the use of blood. Results were dramatic on both occasions, with almost immediate resolution of evolving neurological deficit. Fluosol, in combination with a colloid volume expander, with its improved rheology through hemodilution in addition to the improved oxygen-carrying capacity, may prove beneficial in the treatment of cerebral ischemia in the future.

CAROTID ENDARTERECTOMY

The authors' approach to cerebral ischemic protection during carotid cross-clamping is based on the use of colloidal volume expansion and preoperative cardiological evaluation. Approximately 500 mL of hetastarch or albumin is given before surgery and at least 250 to 500 mL is given intraoperatively. Electroencephalography is used by some of the authors. The authors favor isoflurane anesthesia for ease in monitoring an active electroencephalogram and because of its potential cerebral protecting effect.[96] After heparinization, the external carotid artery is clamped and the clamp left for the duration of the operation. For the initial electroencephalography, only the common carotid artery is clamped in addition to the external carotid artery. This allows removal of the clamp if necessary with minimal threat of plaque fracturing and possible embolization into the internal carotid artery. Just before cross-clamping of the common carotid artery, the systolic blood pressure is raised to 130 mm Hg with phenylephrine. If lateralization of the electroencephalogram is noted on cross-clamping, the clamps are removed and the systolic blood pressure is raised to 180 to 200 mm Hg and the clamps reapplied. If lateralization persists at this point or if evidence of cardiac strain is demonstrated on the electrocardiogram, barbiturate burst suppression is induced on the electroencephalogram with thiopental. The authors also perform carotid endartectomy with the patient under mild hypothermia.

TEMPORARY CLIPPING DURING ANEURYSM SURGERY

Colloidal volume expansion is initiated with a unit of albumin or hetastarch during anesthetic induction with critical control of blood pressure being observed. Every effort is made to avoid extreme blood pressure swings, and the target blood pressure is usually the preoperative pressure. Isoflurane anesthesia is preferred.[96] The authors use mannitol, 1 g per kg, which is given at the same time as the burr holes are initiated and spinal drainage is implemented to ensure brain relaxation. The cerebrospinal fluid drainage is not be-

gun until the dura is opened. Limiting the drainage to 20 mL at a time serves to keep the surgeon and the anesthesiologist critically appraised of the total cerebrospinal fluid drainage throughout the case. Mild hypothermia is used during most of the aneurysm cases. Hypotension is avoided whenever possible. The authors prefer temporary clipping to induced hypotension. With temporary clipping, induced hypertension to systolic pressure of 140 to 150 mm Hg is imposed for the duration of temporary clipping. If prolonged temporary clipping is anticipated, especially on the dominant middle cerebral artery, the patient is given a 500-mg bolus of thiopental before clipping and each 30 minutes thereafter until the clips are removed. Laboratory experimental work suggests that repeated interrupted temporary clipping is safer than a continuous, long, single episode of temporary clipping.[139] Before temporary clipping, mannitol, 0.5 g per kg, is given because of its ability to increase cerebral blood flow in ischemic brain.

Current Research

Information on the current research being done in clinical stroke trials is presented in Table 45–2.

REFERENCES

1. Adelman, S. M.: The national survey of stroke: Economic impact. Stroke, 12(Suppl.): 1–69, 1981.
2. Allen, G. S., Ahns, H. S., Prezrosi, T. J., et al.: Cerebral artery spasm: A controlled trial of nimodipine in patients with subarachnoid hemorrhage. N. Engl. J. Med., 308:619–624, 1983.
3. American Nimodipine Study Group: Clinical trial of Nimodipine Study Group: Clinical trial of Nimodipine and acute ischemic stroke. Stroke, 23:3–9, 1992.
4. Anderson, G. L., Whisnant, J. P.: A comparison of trends in mortality from stroke in the United States and Rochester, Minnesota. Stroke, 13:804–809, 1982.
5. Argentino, C., Sacchette, I. M. L., Toni, D., et al.: GM1 ganglioside therapy in acute ischemic stroke. Stroke, 20:1143–1149, 1988.
6. Astrup, J., Siesjo, B. K., and Symon, L.: Thresholds in cerebral ischemia: The ischemic penumbra. Stroke, 12:723–725, 1981.
7. Bogousslavsky, J., Regli, F., Zumstein, V., et al.: Double-blind study of nimodipine in non-severe stroke. Eur. Neurol., 30:23–26, 1990.
8. Boisvert, D. P., Overton, T. R., Weir, B. K., et al.: Cerebral arterial response to induced hypertension following subarachnoid hemorrhage in the monkey. J. Neurosurg., 49:75–83, 1978.
9. Branston, N. M., Hope, D. T., and Symon, L.: Barbiturates in focal ischemia of primate cortex: Effects of blood flow distribution, evoked potential and extracellular potassium. Stroke, 10:647–653, 1979.
10. Branston, N. M., Symon, L., Crockard, H. A., et al.: Relationship between the cortical evoked potential and local cortical blood flow following acute middle cerebral artery occlusion in the baboon. Exp. Neurol., 45:195–208, 1974.
11. Brott, T. G., Haley, E. C., Levy, D. E., et al.: Urgent therapy for stroke: I. Pilot study of tissue plasminogen activator administered within 90 minutes. Stroke, 23:632–639, 1992.
12. Buchan, A., and Pulsinelli, W. A.: Hypothermia but not the N-methyl-D-aspartate antagonist, MK-801, attenuates neuronal damage in gerbils subjected to transient global ischemia. J. Neurol. Sci., 10:311–316, 1990.
13. Buchan, A., Li, H., and Pulsinelli, W.: The N-methyl-D-aspartate

antagonist, MK 801, fails to protect against neuronal damage caused by transient, severe forebrain ischemia in adult rats. J. Neurol. Sci., 11:1049–1056, 1991.

14. Buchan, A. M., Li, H., Cho, S. H., et al.: Blockade of AMPA receptor prevents CA, hippocampal injury following severe but transient forebrain ichemia in adult rats. Neurosci. Lett., 132:255–258, 1991.

15. Buchan, A. M., Zue, D., Huan, Z. G., et al.: Delayed AMPA receptor blockade reduces cerebral infarction induced by focal ischemia. Neurol. Res., 2:473–476, 1991.

16. Busto, R., Dietrich, W. D., Globus, M. Y. T., et al.: Small differences in intraischemic brain temperature critically determine the extent of ischemic neuronal injury. J. Cereb. Blood Flow Metab., 7:729–738, 1987.

17. Busto, R., Dietrich, W. D., Globus, M. Y. T., et al.: Post ischemic moderate hypothermia inhibits CA 1 hippocampal ischemic neuronal injury. Neurosci. Lett., 101:299–304, 1989.

18. Busto, R., Globus, M. Y. T., Dietrich, W. D., et al.: Effect of mild hypothermia on ischemia induced release of neurotransmitters and free fatty acid in rat brain. Stroke, 20:904–910, 1989.

19. Canadian Cooperative Study Group: A randomized trial of aspirin and sulfinpyrazone in threatened stroke. N. Eng. J. Med., 299:53–59, 1978.

20. Candelise, L., Landi, G., Orazio, E., et al.: Prognostic significance of hyperglycemia in acute stroke. Arch. Neurol., 42:661–663, 1985.

21. Cerebral Embolism Study Group: Immediate anti-coagulation of embolic stroke: A randomized trial. Stroke, 14:668–676, 1983.

22. Choi, D. W.: Cerebral hypoxia: Some new approaches and unanswered questions. J. Neurosci., 10:2493–2501, 1990.

23. Chopp, M., Knight, R., Tidwell, C. D., et al.: The metabolic effects of mild hypothermia on global cerebral ischemia and recirculation in the cat: Comparison to normothermia and hyperthermia. J. Cereb Blood Flow Metab., 9:141–148, 1989.

24. Chopp, M., Welch, K. M., Tidwell, C. D., et al.: Global cerebral ischemia and intracellular pH during hyperglycemia and hypoglycemia in cats. Stroke, 19:1383–1387, 1988.

25. Collins, R., Peto, R., MacMahon, S., et al.: Blood pressure, stroke and coronary heart disease: II. Short-term reductions in blood pressure: Overview of randomized drug trials in their epidemiological contex. Lancet, 335:827–838, 1990.

26. Corbett, D., Evans, S., Thomas, C., et al.: MK-801 reduces cerebral ischemic injury by inducing hypothermia. Brain Res., 524:300–304, 1990.

27. Crowell, R. M., Marcoux, F. W., and DeGirolami, U.: Variability and reversibility of focal cerebral ischemia in unanesthetized monkeys. Neurology, 31:1295–1302, 1981.

28. Crowell, R. M., Olsson, Y., Klatzo, I., et al.: Temporary occlusion of the middle cerebral artery in the monkey: Clinical and pathological observations. Stroke, 1:439–448, 1970.

29. Davalos, A., Cendra, E., Teruel, J., et al.: Deteriorating ischemic stroke: Risk factors and prognosis. Neurology, 40:1865–1869, 1990.

30. Dawson, V. L., Dawson, T. M., London, E. D., et al.: Nitric oxide mediates glutamate neurotoxicity in primary cortical culture. Proc. Natl. Acad. Sci. USA, 88:6368–6371, 1991.

31. de Courten-Myers, G., Myers, R. E., and Schoolfield, L.: Hyperglycemia enlarges infarct size in cerebrovascular occlusion in cats. Stroke, 19:623–630, 1988.

32. DeGirolami, U., Crowell, R. M., and Marcoux, F. W.: Selective necrosis and total necrosis in focal cerebral ischemia: Neuropathologic observations on experimental middle cerebral artery occlusion in the macaque monkey. J. Neuropathol. Exp. Neurol., 43:57–71, 1984.

33. Del Zoppo, G. H. L., Poeck, K., Pessin, M. S., et al.: Recombinant tissue plasminogen activator in acute thrombotic and embolic stroke. Ann. Neurol., 32:78–86, 1992.

34. Dempsey, R. J., and Moore, R. W.: Amount of smoking independently predicts carotid artery atherosclerosis severity. Stroke, 23:693–696, 1992.

35. Duke, R. J., Bloch, F. R., Turpie, A. G. G., et al.: Intravenous heparin for the the prevention of stroke progression in acute partial stable stroke: A randomized controlled trial. Ann. Intern. Med., 105:825–828, 1986.

36. Dutch Transient Ischemic Attack Trial Study Group: A compari-

son of two doses of aspirin (30 mg versus 283 mg a day) in patients after a transient ischemic attack or minor ischemic stroke. N. Engl. J. Med., 325:1261–1266, 1991.

37. ESPS Group: The European Stroke Prevention Study. Stroke, 21:1122–1130, 1990.

38. European/Australian Study Group: Tirilazad in subarachnoid hemorrhage [Abstract]. Presented before the Xth International Congress of the World Federation of Neurological Surgeons, 1993.

39. Fein, J. M., and Boulos, R.: Local cerebral blood flow in experimental middle cerebral artery vasospasm. J. Neurosurg., 39:337–347, 1973.

40. Foulkes, M. A., Wolf, P. A., Price, T. R., et al.: The stroke bank design: Methods and baseline characteristics. Stroke, 19:547, 1988.

41. Ganshirt, H., Hirsch, H., Krenkel, W., et al.: Uber de Einfluss der Temperatursenkung auf die Erholungsfahigkeit des Warmblutergehirns. Arch Exp. Path. Pharmakol., 222:431–449, 1954.

42. Garthwaite, J.: Glutamate, nitric oxide and cell-cell signalling in the nervous system. Trends Neuro. Sci., 14:60, 1991.

43. Gelmers, H. J., Gorter, K., de Weerdt, C. J., et al.: A controlled trial of nimodipine in acute stroke. N. Engl. J. Med., 318:203–207, 1988.

44. Gent, M., Glakely, J. A., Easton, J. D., et al.: The Canadian American Ticlopidine Study (CATS) in thromboembolic stroke. Lancet, 1:1215–1220, 1989.

45. Gianotta, S. L., McGillicuddy, J. E., and Kindt, G. W.: Diagnosis and treatment of postoperative cerebral vasospasm. Surg. Neurol., 8:286–290, 1977.

46. Gilroy, J., Barnhart, J. I., and Meyer, J. S.: Treatment of acute stroke with dextran 40. J.A.M.A., 210:293–298, 1969.

47. Ginsberg, M. D., Sternau, L. L., Globus, M. Y. T., et al.: Therapeutic modulation of brain temperature: Relevance to ischemic brain injury. Cerebrovasc. Brain Metab. Rev., 4:189–225, 1992.

48. Goslinga, H., Eijzenbach, V., Heuvelmans, J. H. A., et al.: Custom-tailored hemodilution with albumin and crystalloids in acute ischemic stroke. Stroke, 23:181–188, 1992.

49. Gottstein, V., Selmeyer, I., and Heuss, A.: Treatment of acute cerebral ischemia with low molecular dextran: Results of a retrospective study. Dtsch. Med. Wochenschr., 101:223–227, 1976.

50. Grotta, J. C., Norris, J. W., and Kamm, B.: Prevention of stroke with ticlopidine: Who benefits most? Neurology, 42:111–115, 1992.

51. Guiraud-Chaumeil, B., Rascol, A. D., Boneu, B., et al.: Prevention des recidivés des accidents vasculaires cérébraux ischemiques parles anti-agrégants plaquettaires. Rev. Neurol., 5:367–385, 1982.

52. Hacke, W., Zeumer, H., Ferbert, A., et al.: Intra-arterial thrombolytic therapy improves outcome in patients with acute vertebrobasilar occlusive disease. Stroke, 19:1216–1222, 1988.

53. Hadley, M. N., Zabramski, J. M., Spetzler, R. F., et al.: The efficacy of intravenous nimodipine in the treatment of focal cerebral ischemia in a primate model. Neurosurgery, 25:63–70, 1989.

54. Hagerdal, M., Harp, J., Nilsson, L., et al.: The effect of induced hypothermia upon oxygen consumption in the rat brain. J. Neurochem., 24:311–316, 1975.

55. Hakim, A. M.: The cerebral ischemic penumbra. Can. J. Neurol. Sci., 14:557–559, 1987.

56. Hakim, A. M., and Hogan, M. J.: In vivo binding of nimodipine in the brain: I. The effect of focal cerebral ischemia. J. Cereb. Blood Flow Metab., 11:762–779, 1991.

57. Haley, E. C., Levy, D. E., Brott, T. G., et al.: Urgent therapy for stroke: II. Pilot study of tissue plaminogen activator administered 91–180 minutes from onset. Stroke, 23:641–645, 1992.

58. Hall, E. D., and Yonkers, P. A.: Attenuation of post-ischemic cerebral hypoperfusion by the 21-aminosteroid U74006F. Stroke, 19:340–344, 1988.

59. Harper, A. M.: Autoregulation of cerebral blood flow: Influence of the arterial blood pressure on the blood flow through the cerebral cortex. J. Neurol. Neurosurg. Psychiatry, 29:398–403, 1966.

60. Harper, A. M., Craigen, L., and Kazda, S.: Effect of the calcium antagonist nimodipine on cerebral blood flow and metabolism in the primate. J. Cereb. Blood Flow Metab., 1:349–356, 1981.

61. Hass, W. K., Easton, H. D., Adams, H. P., et al.: The Ticlopidine Aspirin Stroke Study Group: A randomized trial comparing ticlopidine hydrochloride with aspirin for the prevention of stroke in high-risk patients. N. Engl. J. Med., *321*:501–507, 1989.

62. Hayashi, S., Nehls, D. G., Kieck, C. F., et al.: Beneficial effects of induced hypertension on experimental stroke in awake monkeys. J. Neurosurg., *60*:151–157, 1984.

63. Heiss, W. D.: Flow thresholds of function and morphological damage of brain tissue. Stroke, *14*:329–331, 1983.

64. Heiss, W. D., Hayakawa, T., and Waltz, A. F.: Patterns of changes of blood flow and relationships to infarction in experimental cerebral ischemia. Stroke, *7*:454–459, 1976.

65. Hoff, J. T., Smith, A. L., Hankinson, H. L., et al.: Barbiturate protection from cerebral infarction in primates. Stroke, *6*:28–33, 1975.

66. Hogan, M. J., Gjedde, A., and Hakim, A. M.: In vivo binding of nimodipine in the brain: II. Binding kinetics in focal cerebral ischemia. J. Cereb. Blood Flow Metab., *11*:771–778, 1991.

67. Hope, D. T., Branston, N. M., and Symom, L.: Restoration of neurological function with induced hypertension in acute experimental cerebral ischemia. Acta Neurol. Scand., *56* (Suppl. 64):506–507, 1977.

68. Italian Acute Stroke Study Group: The Italian hemodilution trial on acute stroke. Stroke, *19*:145, 1988.

69. Johnson, P. C.: Review of previous studies and current theories of autoregulation. Circ. Res., *15*(Suppl. 1):2–9, 1964.

70. Jones, T. H., Morawetz, R. B., Crowell, R. M., et al.: Thresholds of focal cerebral ischemia in awake monkeys. J. Neurosurg., *54*:773–782, 1981.

71. Kassel, N. F., Saski, T., Colohan, A. R. T., et al.: Cerebral vasospasm following aneurysmal subarachnoid hemorrhage. Stroke, *16*:562–572, 1985.

72. Kety, S. S.: The physiology of the human cerebral circulation. Anesthesiology, *10*:610–614, 1949.

73. Kety, S. S., and Schmidt, C. F.: The effects of altered arterial tensions of carbon dioxide and oxygen on cerebral blood flow and cerebral oxygen consumption of normal young men. J. Clin. Invest., *27*:484–492, 1948.

74. Kiers, L., Davis, S. M., Larkins, R., et al.: Stroke topography and outcome in relation to hyperglycemia and diabetes. J. Neurol. Neurosurg. Psychiatry, *55*:263–270, 1992.

75. Kindt, G. W., McGillicuddy, J. E., Giannotta, S. L., et al.: The reversal of neurologic deficit in patients with acute cerebral ischemia by profound increases in intravascular volume. In Gotoh, F., Nagai, H., Tazake, Y., eds.: Cerebral Blood Flow and Metabolism. Copenhagen, Munksgaard, 1979, pp. 468–469.

76. Kindt, G. W., McGillicuddy, J. E., Pritz, M. B., et al.: Hypertension and hypervolemia as therapy for patients with vasospasm. In Wilkins, R. H., ed.: Cerebral Arterial Spasm. Baltimore, Williams & Wilkins, 1980, pp. 659–664.

77. Kosnick, E. J., and Hunt, W. E.: Postoperative hypertension in the management of patients with intracranial arterial aneurysms. J. Neurosurg., *45*:148–154, 1976.

78. Kramer, R. S., Sanders, A. P., Leshage, A. M., et al.: The effect of profound hypothermia on preservation of cerebral ATP content during cerebral arrest. J. Thorac. Cardiovasc. Surg., *56*:699–709, 1968.

79. Krieglstein, J., Karkoutly, C., Seifel Nasr, M., et al.: Ischemic brain damage and the role of calcium. In Traber, J., Gispen, W. H., eds.: Nimodipine and Central Nervous System Function: New Vistas. Stutgart, Schattauer, 1989, pp. 101–108.

80. Kuwashima, J., Makamura, K., and Fujitani, B.: Relationship between cerebral energy failure and free fatty acid accumulation following prolonged brain ischemia. Jpn. J. Pharmacol., *28*:277–287, 1978.

81. Lassen, N. A.: Brain extracellular pH: The main factor controlling cerebral blood flow. Scand. J. Clin. Lab. Invest., *22*:247–251, 1968.

82. LeMay, Dr., Gehua, L., Zelenock, G. B., et al.: Insulin administration protects neurologic function in cerebral ischemia in rats. Stroke, *19*:1411–1419, 1988.

83. Levy, M. L., Rabb, C. H., Zelman, V., et al.: Cardiac performance enhancement from dobutamine in patients refractory to hypervolemic therapy for cerebral vasospasm. J. Neurosurg., *79*:494–499, 1993.

84. Mamot, M. G., Poulter, N. R.: Primary prevention of stroke. Lancet, *339*:344–347, 1992.

85. Marcoux, F. W., Morawetez, R. B., Crowell, R. M., et al.: Differential regional vulnerability of transient focal cerebral ischemia. Stroke, *13*:339–346, 1982.

86. Marshall, S. B., Owens, J. C., and Swan, H.: Temporary circulatory occlusion to the brain of the hypothermic dog. Arch. Surg., *72*:98–106, 1956.

87. Martinz-Vila, E., Guillen, F., Villanueva, J. A., et al.: Placebo controlled trial of nimodipine in the treatment of acute ischemic cerebral infarction. Stroke, *21*:1023–1028, 1990.

88. McDowall, D. G.: Inter-relationships between blood oxygen tensions and cerebral blood flow. In Payne, J. P., Hill, O. W., eds.: Oxygen Measurements in Blood and Tissues. London, Churchill Livingstone, 1966, p. 205.

89. Meyer, F. B.: Calcium, neuronal hyperexcitability and ischemic injury. Brain Res. Rev., *14*:227–243, 1989.

90. Michenfelder, J. D.: A valid demonstration of barbiturate-induced brain protection in man—at last. Anesthesiology, *64*:140–142, 1986.

91. Michenfelder, J. D., Milde, J. H., Sundt, T. M., Jr.: Cerebral protection by a barbiturate anesthesia: Use of middle cerebral artery occlusion in Java monkeys. Arch. Neurol., *33*:345–350, 1976.

92. Morawetz, R. B., Crowell, R. H., DeGirolami, U., et al.: Regional cerebral blood flow thresholds during cerebral ischemia. Fed. Proc., *38*:2493–2494, 1979.

93. Mori, E., Tabuchi, M., Yoshida, T., et al.: Intracarotid urokinase with thromboembolic occlusion of the middle cerebral artery. Stroke, *19*:802–812, 1988.

94. Nader, J., and Bogousslavsky, J.: Treatment of acute cerebral infarction. Curr. Opin. Neurol. Neurosurg., *6*:51–54, 1993.

95. Nedergaard, M., Jakobsen, J., and Diemer, N. H.: Autoradiographic determination of cerebral glucose content, blood flow, and glucose utilization in focal ischemia of the rat brain: Influence of the plasma glucose concentration. J. Cereb. Blood Flow Metab., *8*:100–108, 1988.

96. Newberg, L. A., and Michenfelder, J. D.: Cerebral protection by isoflurane during hypoxemia or ischemia. Anesthesiology, *59*:29–35, 1983.

97. 1992 Heart and Stroke Facts. Dallas, American Heart Association, 1991.

98. Nussmeier, N. A., Arlund, C., and Slogoff, S.: Neuropsychiatric complications after cardiopulmonary bypass: Cerebral protection by barbiturate. Anesthesiology, *64*:165–170, 1986.

99. Ohtaki, M., and Tranmer, B.: Pre-treatment of transient focal cerebral ischemia with the calcium antagonist AT877. J. Cereb. Blood Flow Metab., *13*(Suppl. 1):S652, 1993.

100. Ohtaki, M., and Tranmer, B.: Role of hypervolemic hemodilution in focal cerebral ischemia of rats. Surg. Neurol., *40*:196–206, 1993.

101. Okada, U., Sadoshima, S., and Nakane, H.: Early computerized tomographic findings for thrombolytic therapy in patients with acute brain embolism. Stroke, *23*:20–23, 1992.

102. Overgaard, K., Sereghy, T., Boysen, G., et al.: Reduction of infarct volume and mortality by thrombolysis in a rat embolic stroke model. Stroke, *23*: 1167–1174, 1992.

103. Ozyurt, E., Graham, D. I., Woodruff, G. N., et al.: Protective effect of glutamate antagonist MK 801 after induction of ischemia. J. Cereb. Blood Flow Metab., *8*:138–143, 1988.

104. Paulson, O. B.: Cerebral apoplexy (stroke): Pathogenesis, pathophysiology and therapy as illustrated by regional blood flow measurements in the brain. Stroke, *2*:327–360, 1971.

105. Park, C. K., Nehls, D. G., Graham, D. I., et al.: Focal cerebral ischemia in the cat: Treatment with glutamate antagonist MK-801 after induction of ischemia. J. Cereb. Blood Flow Metab. *8*:757–762, 1988.

106. Penfield, W., VonSantha, K., and Cipriani, A.: Cerebral blood flow during induced epileptiform seizures in animals and man. J. Neurophysiol., *2*:257–267, 1939.

107. Plum F., Posner, J. B., and Troy, B.: Cerebral metabolic and circulatory responses to induced convulsions in animals. Arch. Neurol., *18*:1–13, 1968.

108. Pritz, M. B., Giannotta, S. L., Kindt, G. W., et al.: Treatment of patients with neurological deficits associated with cerebral

vasospasm by intravascular volume expansion. Neurosurgery, 3:364–368, 1978.

109. Qizilbash, N., Jones, L., Warlow, C., et al.: Fibrinogen and lipid concentrations as risk factors for transient ischemic attacks and minor ischemic stroke (published erratum appears in B.M.J. 303:968). B.M.J., 303:605–609, 1991.

110. Ridenour, T. R., Warner, D. S., Todd, M. M., et al.: Mild hypothermia reduces infarct size resulting from temporary but not permanent focal ischemia in rats. Stroke, 23:733–738, 1992.

111. Rocca, W. A., Dorsey, F. C., Grigolett, O. F., et al.: Design and baseline results of the monosialoganglioside early stroke trial. Stroke, 23:519–526, 1992.

112. Rosomoff, H. L.: Hypothermia and cerebrovascular lesions: II. Experimental interruption followed by induction of hypothermia. Arch. Neurol. Psychiatry, 78:454–464, 1957.

113. Rothman, S. M., and Olney, J. W.: Glutamate and the pathophysiology of hypoxic ischemic brain damage. Ann. Neurol., 19:105–111, 1986.

114. Sacco, R. L.: Current epidemiology of stroke. In Fisher, M., and Bogousslavsky, J., eds.: Current Review of Cerebrovascular Disease. Philadelphia, Current Medicine, 1993.

115. Sacco, R. L., Wolf, P. A., Kannel, W. B., et al.: Survival and recurrence: The Framingham Study. Stroke, 13:290–295, 1982.

116. Scandinavian Stroke Study Group: Multicenter trial of hemodilution in acute ischemic stroke: I: Results in the total patient population. Stroke, 18:691–699, 1987.

117. Schmidt, C. F., and Hendrix, J. P.: The action of chemical substances on cerebral blood vessels. Res. Publ. Assoc. Res. Nerv. Ment. Dis., 18:229–276, 1937.

118. Shaper, A. G., Phillips, A. N., Pocock, S. J., et al.: Risk factors for stroke in middle aged British men. B. M. J., 301:1111–1115, 1991.

119. Shibuya, M., Suzuki, Y., and Sugita, K.: Effect of AT877 on cerebral vasospasm after aneurysmal subarachnoid hemorrhage. J. Neurosurg., 76:571–577, 1992.

120. Shinto, R., and Beevers, G.: Meta-analysis of relation between cigarette smoking and stroke. B.M.J., 298:789–794, 1989.

121. Siesjo, B. K.: Cell damage in the brain: A speculative synthesis. J. Cereb. Blood Flow Metab., 1:155–185, 1981.

122. Siesjo, B. K.: Cerebral circulation and metabolism. J. Neurosurg., 60:883–908, 1984.

123. Siesjo, B. K.: Pathophysiology and treatment of focal cerebral ischemia: I. Pathophysiology [Review article]. J. Neurosurg., 77:169–184, 1992.

124. Siesjo, B. K.: Pathophysiology and treatment of focal cerebral ischemia: II. Mechanisms of damage and treatment [Review article]. J. Neurosurg., 77:337–354, 1992.

125. Seisjo, B. K., and Begstsson, F.: Calcium fluxes, calcium antagonist and calcium related pathophysiology in brain ischemia, hypoglycemia, and spreading depression: A unifying hypothesis. J. Cereb. Blood Flow Metab., 9:127–140, 1989.

126. Simon, R. P., Swan, J. H., Friffith, T., et al.: Blockade of N-methyl-D-aspartate receptors may protect against ischemic damage in the brain. Science, 226:850–852, 1984.

127. Sloan, M. A., and Gore, J. M.: Ischemic stroke and intracranial hemorrhage following thrombolytic therapy for acute myocardial infarction: A risk-benefit analysis. Am. J. Cardiol., 69:21A–38A, 1992.

128. Smith, A. L., Hoff, J. T., Nielson, S. L., et al.: Barbiturate protection in acute focal cerebral ischemia. Stroke, 5:1–7, 1974.

129. Snyder, S. H.: Janus basis of nitric oxide. Nature, 363:577, 1993.

130. Snyder, S. H., and Reynolds, I. J.: Calcium-antagonist drugs: Receptor interactions that clarify therapeutic effects. N. Engl. J. Med., 313:995–1002, 1985.

131. Strand, T., Asplund, K., Erickson, S., et al.: A randomized controlled trial of hemodilution therapy in acute ischemic stroke. Stroke, 15:980–989, 1984.

132. Strandgaard, S., and Paulson, O. B.: Cerebral autoregulation. Stroke, 15:413–416, 1984.

133. Sundt, T. M., Jr.: The ischemic tolerance of neural tissue and the need for monitoring and selective shunting during carotid endarterectomy. Stroke, 14:93–98, 1983.

134. Sundt, T. M., and Waltz, A. G.: Cerebral ischemia and reactive hyperemia: Studies of cortical blood flow and microcirculation before, during and after temporary occlusion of middle cerebral artery of squirrel monkeys. Circ. Res., 28:426–433, 1971.

135. Suzuki, J., Kwak, R., and Okudairo, Y.: The safe time limit of temporary clamping of cerebral arteries in the direct surgical treatment of intracranial aneurysm under moderate hypothermia. Tohoku J. Exp. Med., 127:1–7, 1979.

136. Swan, J. H., and Meldrum, B. S.: Protection by NMDA antagonists against selective cell loss following transient ischemia. J. Cereb. Blood Flow Metab., 10:343–351, 1990.

137. Swedish Aspirin Low-Dose Trial Collaborative Group: Swedish Aspirin Low-Dose Trial (SALT) of 75 mg aspirin as secondary prophylaxis after cerebrovascular ischemic events. Lancet, 338:1345–1349, 1991.

138. Teasdale, G., Sokard, J., Shaw, D., et al.: Treatment of subarachnoid hemorrhage with calcium-antagonist: A large randomized controlled trial. Presented before the International Symposium on Cerebral Ischemia and Calcium. Chiemsee, West Germany, June 12–15, 1988, p. 9.

139. Tranmer, B. I., and Ohtaki, M.: Continuous vs. repetitive ischemia in the rat model of cerebral ischemia. J. Cereb. Blood Flow Metab., Supplement S638, 1993.

140. Tranmer, B. I., Iacobacci, R., and Feiler, S.: The effect of Fluosol-DA and Hetastarch on local CF, cortical O_2 availability and computerized EEG data during cerebral ischemia. Neurol. Res., 12:17–22, 1990.

141. Tranmer, B. I., Iacobacci, R., and Kindt, G. W.: Effect of crystalloid and colloid infusions on ICP and computerized EEG data in dogs with vasogenic edema. Neurosurgery, 25:173–179, 1989.

142. Tranmer, B. I., Gross, C. E., Kindt, G. W., et al.: Pulsatile vs nonpulsatile blood flow in the treatment of acute cerebral ischemia. Neurosurgery, 19:724–731, 1986.

143. Tranmer, B. I., Keller, T. S., Gross, C. E., et al.: Acute middle cerebral artery occlusion: Experience with volume expansion therapy. Neurosurgery, 18:397–401, 1986.

144. Tranmer, B. I., Keller, T. S., Kindt, G. W., et al.: Blood volume expansion with hetastarch in acute ischemic stroke: Effects on local cerebral blood flow and computer mapped EEG. Neurol. Res., 8:177–182, 1986.

145. Tranmer, B. I., Keller, T. S., Kindt, G. W., et al.: Loss of cerebral regulation during cardiac output variations in focal cerebral ischemia. J. Neurosurg., 77:213–259, 1992.

146. Troy, D. W., Koh, J. Y., and Peters, S.: Pharmacology of glutamate neurotoxicity in cortical cell culture: Attenuation by NMDA antagonist. J. Neurol. Sci., 8:185–196, 1988.

147. Trust Study Group: Randomized double-blind placebo controlled trial of nimodipine in acute stroke. Lancet, 336:1205–1209, 1990.

148. Tymianski, M., Wallace, M. C., Uno, M., et al.: Successful treatment of experimental focal ischemic stroke by intracellular calcium chelation. J. Cereb. Blood Flow Metab., 1(Suppl. 1):S638, 1993.

149. UK-TIA Study Group: United Kingdom transient ischemic attack (UK-TIA) aspirin trial: Interim results. B. M. J., 296:316–320, 1988.

150. Vander Eecken, H. R., and Adams, R. D.: The anatomy and functional significance of the meningeal arterial anastomosis of the human brain. J. Neuropathol. Exp. Neurol., 12:132–157, 1953.

151. von Kummer, R., and Hacke, W.: Safety and efficacy of intravenous tissue plasminogen activator and heparin in acute middle cerebral artery stroke. Stroke, 23:646–652, 1992.

152. Waltz, A. G.: Effect of blood pressure on blood flow in ischemic and non-ischemic cerebral cortex: The phenomena of autoregulation and luxury perfusion. Neurology, 18: 613–621, 1968.

153. Waltz, A. G., and Sundt, T. M., Jr.: The microvasculature and microcirculation of the cerebral cortex after arterial occlusion. Brain, 90:681–696, 1967.

154. Welch, F. A., Ginsberg, M. D., Rieder, W., et al.: Deleterious effect of glucose pretreatment on recovery from diffuse cerebral ischemia in the cat. II. Regional metabolite levels. Stroke, 11:355–363, 1980.

155. Whisnant, J. P.: The decline of stroke. Stroke, 15:160–168, 1984.

156. Wolf, P. A., Abbott, R. D., and Kannel, W. B.: Atrial fibrillation as an independent risk factor for stroke: The Framingham Study. Stroke, 22:983–988, 1991.

157. Wolf, P. A., Belanger, A. J., and D'Agostino, R. B.: Management of risk factors. Neurol. Clin., 10: 177–191, 1992.

158. Wood, J. H., and Feischer, A. S.: Observations during hypervo-

lemic hemodilution of patients with acute focal cerebral ischemia. J.A.M.A., *248*:2999–3004, 1982.

159. Wood, J. H., Simeone, F. A., Fink, B. A., et al.: Correlative aspects of hypervolemic hemodilution law: Molecular weight dextran infusions after experimental cerebral arterial occlusion. Neurology, *34*:24–34, 1984.

160. Yatsu, F.: Nicardipine in acute stroke. *In* Hartman, A., Kuchinsky, W., eds. Cerebral Ischemia and Calcium. Berlin, Stringer-Verlag, 1989.

161. Yuematsu, D., Greenberg, J. H., Hickey, W. F., et al.: Nimodipine attenuates both increase in cytosolic free calcium and histologic damage following focal cerebral ischemia and reperfusion in cats. Stroke, *20*:1531–1535, 1989.

162. Zhang, R. L., Chopp, M., Chen, H., et al.: Post-ischemic (one hour) hypothermia significantly reduces ischemic cell damage in rats subjected to two hours of middle cerebral artery occlusion. Stroke, *24*:1235–1240, 1993.

163. Zivin, J., Lyden, P. D., DeGirolami, U., et al.: Tissue plasminogen activator reduction of neurological damage after experimental embolic stroke. Arch. Neurol., *17*:196–201, 1988.

Extracranial Occlusive Disease of the Carotid Artery

Stroke is a major health care problem; it is the third leading cause of death and the primary cause of disability in the United States.[86] In 1989, more than 350,000 individuals in this country suffered an ischemic stroke, and more than 150,000 died.[4] At present, there are more than 3 million American stroke survivors.[28] From an economic standpoint, annual costs of stroke in the United States are estimated at more than $30 billion, including both direct health care costs and lost productivity.[4]

Several reports have documented a progressive decline in stroke mortality from 1960 to 1980, attributed to improvements in diagnosis, acute care, and control of various risk factors, especially hypertension.[45, 46, 80] However, the overall incidence of stroke, especially ischemic stroke, has remained constant in recent years.[80] Current estimates of stroke incidence range from 12 per 100,000 (for women 30 to 49 years of age) to 809 per 100,000 (for men 70 to 74 years of age).[80] Although most population data do not differentiate ischemic from hemorrhagic stroke, or lacunar from hemispheric infarction, they nevertheless point out the continuing importance of stroke as a major health care concern in this country. Because no effective therapy currently exists for completed stroke, treatment of this disorder is predicated on identification of individuals at risk and institution of preventative measures.

Carotid Occlusive Disease and Stroke

The association between atheromatous disease of the cervical carotid artery and increased stroke risk has been recognized since the early 1900's, but it was not fully appreciated until Fisher described the syndrome in 1951.[41] Initial estimates of stroke risk associated with carotid stenosis were based in large part on population studies, retrospective analyses, or nonsurgical trials

that failed to distinguish stroke type or distribution.[22, 121, 123] A multidisciplinary panel summarized this data in 1988 and estimated stroke rates to be 6 to 7 per cent per year for symptomatic carotid stenosis and 2 to 3 per cent per year for asymptomatic stenosis.[21] Data from three subsequent published surgical trials for high-grade symptomatic stenosis demonstrated ipsilateral stroke rates considerably higher than those estimates, ranging from 10 per cent per year to 15 to 17 per cent per year.[38, 78, 89] For asymptomatic carotid stenosis, Norris and colleagues estimated that cerebral ischemic events occur at a rate of 10.5 per cent per year in patients with more than 75 per cent stenosis.[88] In the Veterans Administration Asymptomatic Stenosis Trial, nonsurgical patients with more than 50 per cent stenosis had ipsilateral cerebral ischemic events at a rate of approximately 5 per cent per year and strokes at 2 per cent per year.[55] These findings emphasize the high degree of association between carotid stenosis and stroke and the need for evaluation of patients with these lesions.

Rationale for Surgical Treatment of Cerebrovascular Disease

Since the reports of successful carotid endarterectomy in 1954, this operation has been commonly applied as a prophylactic measure for prevention of cerebral ischemia.[35] The rationale for carotid endarterectomy was based on the concept that removal of the stenotic, atheromatous lesion would eliminate a potential source of emboli and improve cerebral blood flow. Similar reasoning was applied for extracranial-to-intracranial bypass procedures as a prophylactic measure in the setting of cervical carotid occlusion or intracranial stenosis. Reports of retrospective surgical series for endarterectomy and the bypass procedure sug-

---

M. R. Mayberg

gested an acceptable level of morbidity compared with an indeterminate natural history of untreated lesions.[13, 105, 106, 108, 121]

As indications for carotid endarterectomy and the extracranial-to-intracranial bypass were expanded to include a variety of lesions and clinical presentations, both operations became increasingly used, until almost 100,000 endarterectomies and 4,000 bypass procedures were performed in the United States in 1984.[34] However, reports of considerably higher surgical morbidity for endarterectomy and a less malignant natural history of carotid stenosis led several authors to question the efficacy of carotid endarterectomy.* Simultaneously, concerns were raised regarding the effectiveness of extracranial-to-intracranial bypass in preventing strokes. Since that time, data from several prospective trials have objectively defined specific indications for surgery in the setting of cervical carotid occlusive disease and better described the natural history of this disorder.[36, 38, 78, 89]

Pathological Features of Cervical Atheromatous Disease

THE ATHEROSLCEROTIC LESION

Atherosclerosis is a diffuse disorder affecting the walls of medium and large muscular and elastic arter-

---

*See references 10, 15, 19, 20, 34, 101, and 118.

ies that is characterized by a spectrum of pathological lesions.[6] The fatty streak is the initial manifestation of atherosclerosis; it is composed of focal accumulations of intimal smooth muscle cells in association with plasma-derived lipids (primarily cholesterol). Fatty streaks are apparent in humans by 10 years of age and may progress or regress according to unknown factors.[42] Fibrous plaques, representing the next stage in the development of atheromatous lesions, are characterized by lipid and cell debris surrounded by smooth muscle cells, lipid-laden macrophages (foam cells), collagen, proteoglycans, and fibrous tissue. Fibrous plaques typically create varying degrees of concentric or eccentric arterial stenosis.

The final stage of atheroma development is the complicated lesion (Fig. 46–1), which is a fibrous plaque with various degenerative components, including ulceration, intramural hemorrhage, calcification, and thrombosis.[42] Risk factors associated with the development of atherosclerosis include age, male gender, serum lipids, hypertension, family history, diabetes, and tobacco exposure. However, factors leading to the establishment and progression of dynamic atheromatous lesions are multifactorial, involving complex interactions between elements of the arterial wall, circulating blood, inflammation, hereditary factors, and environmental exposure.[71]

ATHEROSCLEROTIC DISEASE IN THE CRANIOCERVICAL CIRCULATION

Although occlusive diseases of the craniocervical vasculature may be caused by a variety of disorders,

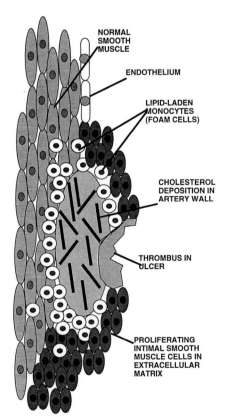

NORMAL SMOOTH MUSCLE

ENDOTHELIUM

LIPID-LADEN MONOCYTES (FOAM CELLS)

CHOLESTEROL DEPOSITION IN ARTERY WALL

THROMBUS IN ULCER

PROLIFERATING INTIMAL SMOOTH MUSCLE CELLS IN EXTRACELLULAR MATRIX

Figure 46–1

Schematic representation of the histological appearance of a typical carotid artery atheroma. Notice the cholesterol accumulation in the arterial wall and within accumulating macrophages (foam cells) in the lesion. Proliferation of smooth muscle cells and deposition of extracellular matrix contribute to the intimal accumulation. A complex ulcer contains fibrin-platelet thrombus.

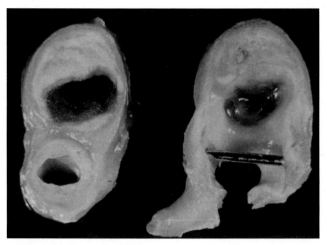

Figure 46–2

Postmortem specimen of carotid artery bifurcation. Notice the distribution of atheromatous narrowing of the common, internal, and external carotid arteries and thrombus in the residual lumen of the internal carotid artery.

the great majority of strokes in this setting are related to atheromatous narrowing of these arteries[42, 71] (Fig. 46–2). Atherosclerosis has a relatively consistent pattern of occurrence in the craniocervical circulation; lesions are almost invariably present at multiple sites.[42] These include the origins of the carotid and vertebral arteries, the carotid bifurcations, the cavernous internal carotid artery, the basilar artery, and the middle cerebral arteries. Significant atheromatous disease in these sites is highly associated with the presence of similar lesions in the coronary circulation.[105] At the carotid bifurcation, stenotic lesions typically involve the distal common carotid artery and the proximal segment of the internal carotid artery, extending along the posterior wall. The propensity for the development of atheromas at these sites suggests the role of local flow characteristics in the development of lesions.[125]

HEMODYNAMIC FACTORS IN THE CEREBRAL CIRCULATION

Controversy exists regarding the importance of hemodynamically significant stenosis in carotid artery disease. Flow remains relatively constant in a larger artery, with progressive stenosis until internal diameter is reduced to approximately 70 per cent of normal (more than 90 per cent reduction in lumen cross-sectional area).[84] After that point, progressive reduction in diameter causes marked diminution in flow. Several studies have demonstrated an association between high-grade carotid stenosis and stroke risk.[38, 78, 89]

The concept of hemodynamically significant stenosis in the carotid artery has fostered the rationale of endarterectomy and extracranial-to-intracranial bypass as means to augment ipsilateral cerebral blood flow. However, several lines of evidence discount this theory. The anterior cerebral circulation has ample collateral supply from a variety of sources, including the circle of Willis, the external carotid artery, and the superficial pial vessels. Most carotid artery occlusions are asymptomatic, and significant changes in ipsilateral cerebral blood flow with intraoperative clamping of the common carotid artery (i.e., both internal and external carotid arteries) occur in fewer than 15 per cent of cases.[109, 122] By symptomatic presentation or pathological criteria, the majority of cerebral ischemic events correspond to embolic phenomena.[41] Intra-arterial thrombosis and embolism are complex processes regulated by interactions among circulating blood elements, the luminal surface, and local blood flow characteristics including rate and turbulence; high-grade stenosis at the site of a complex atheromatous lesion probably promotes thrombus formation by all of these mechanisms[124] (Figs. 46–3 and 46–4). In this regard, carotid endarterectomy may act to prevent stroke by eliminating sites of potential thrombosis rather than by augmentation of cerebral blood flow.

Other Causes of Cervical Carotid Stenosis

FIBROMUSCULAR DYSPLASIA

Fibromuscular dysplasia is a noninflammatory vasculopathy characterized by arterial stenosis at specific

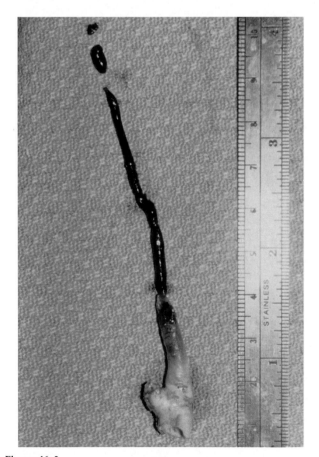

Figure 46–3

Surgical specimen after endarterectomy. A long intraluminal thrombus extends distally from the end of the internal carotid artery plaque.

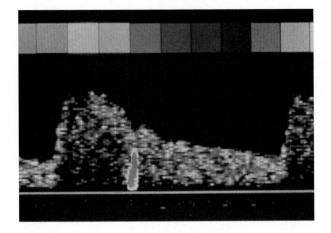

Figure 46–4

Transcranial Doppler recording of an intraluminal embolus in a patient with carotid artery dissection. The embolus is represented by the sharply demarcated positive signal occurring at the end of systole in this case.

sites in the systemic vasculature.[95] The most commonly affected sites are the renal and cervical carotid arteries, and it represents the second most common cause of extracranial carotid stenosis.[76] Although the specific incidence is not known, it most commonly afflicts young white females (20 to 50 years of age). The hallmark pathological lesion involves fibroplasia of the media or, less commonly, of the intima, with interspersed luminal constrictions and aneurysmal outpouchings that produce a typical "string of beads" appearance on angiography. Fibromuscular dysplasia involves the carotid artery in 17 to 25 per cent of cases, usually at the level of C2–C3, with sparing of the proximal internal carotid artery at the bifurcation.[27] In most cases, the lesions are bilateral, and the vertebral arteries are frequently involved. There is a high association between fibromuscular dysplasia and intracranial aneurysms, with coincidence estimated at 20 to 40 per cent.[95]

Carotid fibromuscular dysplasia rarely produces complete occlusion; controversy remains as to whether cerebral ischemic symptoms are hemodynamic or caused by embolism. In this regard, antiplatelet therapy may prove effective in preventing symptoms. Surgical treatment is limited by the nature of the pathological lesion and its extent in the distal cervical internal carotid artery. If it is symptomatic, percutaneous transluminal angioplasty may be successfully employed in the treatment.[52]

CAROTID ARTERIAL DISSECTIONS

Dissections of the cervical carotid artery have been categorized as traumatic or spontaneous. Traumatic dissections typically involve the distal extracranial internal carotid artery and are thought to originate from impingement of the artery against the C2 transverse process during rotation with extension of the neck.[83] Spontaneous dissections can be associated with atherosclerosis or fibromuscular dysplasia; the frequent relation to minor trauma suggests that their distinction from traumatic dissections may be arbitrary. Typically, both lesions present with headaches or facial pain, oculosympathetic palsy (Horner's syndrome), and, of-

ten, ipsilateral cerebral ischemia.[48] The angiography appearance of internal carotid artery dissection is characteristic, with a tapered stenosis or occlusion beginning distal to the carotid bifurcation and ending at the skull base, occasionally associated with aneurysm formation (Fig. 46–5).

The presumed mechanism of cerebral ischemia in carotid dissection is secondary to distal embolization. Surgical repair of carotid dissections is difficult because of the nature of the lesion (which often necessitates resection and interposition grafting with vein or synthetic prosthesis) and the distal extent of the lesion to the skull base.[83] For these reasons, anticoagulation therapy with heparin and subsequently, with warfarin (Coumadin) is often employed, although these measures have not been tested by clinical trial.[44] In the setting of trauma, anticoagulation may be contraindicated; surgical therapies in this case include direct repair with or without grafting, embolectomy, and, occasionally, extracranial-to-intracranial bypass.

RADIATION AND CAROTID STENOSIS

The long-term effects of radiation on larger blood vessels have not been systematically determined.[85] Several authors have demonstrated injury to elastic membranes, intimal thickening, plaque formation, and fibrosis of muscular arteries after focal irradiation at doses greater than 2,500 rad.[47, 72] At lower doses (500 to 600 rad), radiation potentiated cholesterol deposition and atherosclerotic plaque formation in uninjured cholesterolemic animals; this response was probably precipitated by an initial radiation-induced endothelial injury.[43, 63, 64, 114] Other authors have postulated injury to the vaso vasorum as the primary pathological event caused by radiation.[99]

In humans, the primary vascular manifestations of gamma irradiation typically involve the smaller blood vessels. At 3 months after high-dose irradiation, these vessels demonstrate endothelial vacuoles, intimal thickening, and damage to elastic fibers.[1, 39] This is followed by the appearance of subintimal foam cells similar to those observed in early atherosclerosis.[62] Radiation-induced injury to large arteries, on the other

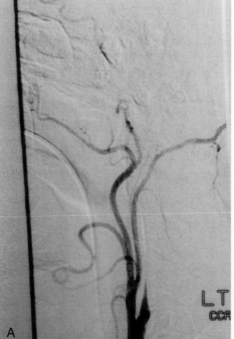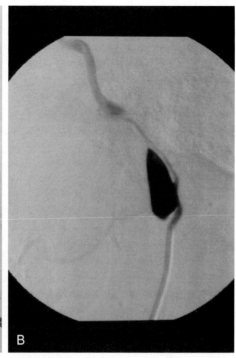

Figure 46–5

Common carotid angiograms showing typical appearances of carotid dissection. *A.* A gradual, tapered occlusion of the internal carotid artery. *B.* Pseudoaneurysm of the internal carotid artery associated with carotid dissection.

hand, is relatively uncommon.[39] Analysis in these cases is complicated by the coexistence of pre-existing atheromatous disease and local changes caused by surgery or adjacent neoplasm. Murros and Toole summarized the existing literature regarding radiation injury to large arteries and concluded that, although radiation occasionally accelerates atherosclerotic lesions, doses in excess of 5,000 rad are required to produce significant changes.[85]

Nonsurgical Therapy for Stroke Prevention

Nonsurgical prophylactic measures for stroke are reviewed in greater detail in Chapter 44. In brief, for those patients who are not suitable for carotid endarterectomy, adjunctive medical therapy may be used. Control of risk factors for stroke, including smoking cessation, antihypertensive medications, and serum lipid reduction, remains essential therapy for both surgical and nonsurgical patients. Although both warfarin and aspirin are effective in reducing stroke associated with atrial fibrillation, anticoagulants have not been shown to be beneficial in stroke prevention for carotid stenosis.[2, 17] Although aspirin has been reported to reduce stroke risk in symptomatic patients, most of these studies included myocardial or other vascular events or death as end points.[18, 22, 23] If these studies are analyzed for stroke only, the effect of aspirin was marginal, and there was no difference in efficacy between daily aspirin doses of 30 mg and 300 mg.[33] Ticlopidine, a new antiplatelet agent, was shown to slightly reduce stroke incidence when compared with aspirin in a recent prospective trial.[51] In summary, antiplatelet agents play an

adjunctive role in preventing vascular events in patients with cerebral ischemia; they should not, however, be used as an alternative to carotid endarterectomy in potential surgical candidates.

Surgery for Cerebral Ischemia: Data from Clinical Trials

THE EXTRACRANIAL-TO-INTRACRANIAL CAROTID ARTERY BYPASS TRIAL

The Extracranial-to-Intracranial Bypass Trial represented the first major study of cerebrovascular surgery in the era of modern clinical trials.[36] The conclusion that surgery provided no benefit in protection against subsequent stroke in this group of patients was controversial and has had a profound impact on clinical practice in North America.[66, 69] In addition, the trial initiated an era of intense scrutiny of cerebrovascular surgery, including the development of several clinical trials for carotid endarterectomy (see next section).

At 71 centers in the United States, Canada, Japan, and Europe, 1,377 patients with anterior circulation strokes, retinal infarction, or transient ischemic attack within 3 months of presentation were randomized to surgical (n = 663) or nonsurgical (n = 714) treatment. Qualifying lesions included middle cerebral artery stenosis or occlusion and cervical internal carotid artery occlusion or stenosis above the C2 vertebral body. Patients were followed for 5 years, and primary end points were designated as fatal or nonfatal stroke (including all vascular distributions).

At an average follow-up of 55.8 months, extracranial-to-intracranial carotid artery bypass provided no significant protection against stroke in any distribution, against ipsilateral stroke, or against stroke and death. Technical results of surgery were excellent, with 96 per cent of anastomoses patent on postoperative angiogram. Perioperative major stroke and death occurred in 4.5 per cent; however, one third (10 of 30) of these strokes occurred before surgery and were included in an intent-to-treat analysis. In the equivalent time period, 1.3 per cent of nonsurgical patients had major strokes. By 60 months, there was no significant difference in stroke rate between surgical and nonsurgical groups (20 and 18 per cent, respectively). Subgroup analysis showed no benefit for surgery based on the site or severity of lesions on arteriography, the presence of carotid artery occlusion, the temporal pattern of presenting symptoms, or the size and location of the participating center. Outcome appeared to be worse after surgery in patients with middle cerebral artery stenosis and in those with persistent ischemic symptoms after carotid occlusion. Analysis that excluded surgical patients with preoperative stroke did not affect outcome. There was no benefit in terms of functional status for patients receiving extracranial-to-intracranial bypass. The researchers concluded that bypass surgery was ineffective in preventing cerebral ischemia in patients with atherosclerotic disease in the carotid and middle cerebral arteries.[36]

The Extracranial-to-Intracranial Bypass Trial was widely criticized on several grounds.[11, 13, 29, 66] The ratio of persistently symptomatic versus asymptomatic patients studied was relatively low, and fewer than one symptomatic patient per center per year were entered into the trial. A telephone survey of 57 participating centers revealed that, during the period of the trial, with 1,255 patients entered into the study, more than twice as many patients (2,572) received surgery outside of the trial.[107] These data contradicted those in the published report, which described only 115 patients refusing entry and 52 patients with surgery outside of the trial.[36] The ultimate fate of eligible nonrandomized patients and the possibility that randomized patients represented a distinct subgroup (perhaps at lower risk) raise significant questions about the validity of the conclusions for this study.

TRIALS FOR CAROTID ENDARTERECTOMY

Carotid endarterectomy has been applied for a variety of clinical presentations and anatomical lesions; specifics of cerebral ischemic syndromes are reviewed in detail in Chapter 44. Briefly, clinical indications for endarterectomy may be classified generally as asymptomatic cartoid stenosis or symptomatic carotid stenosis. In most settings, asymptomatic carotid stenosis is determined by the demonstration of arterial narrowing through noninvasive testing or angiography. Symptomatic carotid stenosis usually refers to ischemia (transient ischemic attack, amaurosis fugax, or completed stroke) in the distribution of the ipsilateral stenotic internal carotid artery.[92] Ischemia of the posterior circulation and nonfocal neurological symptoms have less commonly been considered as indications for carotid endarterectomy. Angiography considerations in carotid endarterectomy include degree of carotid stenosis, presence of ulceration at the stenotic site, presence of additional lesions in the craniocervical circulation (e.g., tandem lesions or contralateral carotid stenosis), and extent of collateral flow or intra-arterial emboli assessed by noninvasive means.[68] As discussed in the section on preoperative assessment, patients with carotid artery disease have a propensity for concomitant coronary, peripheral vascular, and pulmonary disease, and surgical indications must be carefully weighed against potential risk.[105] The combinations of clinical presentation, anatomical lesions, and operative risk create a wide variety of situations, which limits generalizations regarding indications for carotid endarterectomy.

Until recently there was little objective data concerning the natural history of untreated carotid stenosis, the risk of endarterectomy in widespread practice, and the protective effect of surgery in preventing stroke. By 1995, six prospective, randomized, multicenter carotid endarterectomy trials reported their results.* The cumulative data from these studies should provide a basis for objective determination of the indications for carotid endarterectomy.

EARLY TRIALS FOR CAROTID ENDARTERECTOMY

Results of three randomized trials for carotid endarterectomy were published before 1991. The Joint Study of Extracranial Arterial Occlusion involved 24 centers in the United States.[40] From 1962 to 1968, 316 patients with transient ischemic attack and carotid stenosis were randomized to surgical or nonsurgical therapy. At a mean follow-up of 42 months, stroke had occurred in 19 (11 per cent) of 167 surgical patients, compared with 18 (12 per cent) of 145 nonsurgical patients. In the endarterectomy group, the majority of strokes (13 of 19) occurred in the perioperative period, with a relatively low subsequent stroke rate (approximately 1.5 per cent per year). This study was flawed by a number of methodological errors, including limited sample size, lack of follow-up for eligible nonrandomized patients, variability in stroke diagnosis, and inconsistency of adjunctive therapies. Shaw and colleagues published a limited trial involving 41 symptomatic patients in Great Britain.[100] This trial was terminated because of an excessive perioperative stroke rate (25 per cent) among participating surgeons.

Perhaps the only meaningful data from early prospective randomized trials for carotid endarterectomy concerned the relatively low (1 to 2% per year) risk of subsequent stroke in those patients surviving surgery. Owing to methodological flaws, other data regarding comparisons between surgical and nonsurgical therapy in these studies must be discounted.

---

*See references 9, 25, 38, 55, 57, 78, and 89.

TRIALS FOR ASYMPTOMATIC CAROTID STENOSIS

The CASANOVA Study (Table 46–1) randomized patients with asymptomatic carotid stenosis (greater than 50 but less than 90 per cent stenosis) to either immediate carotid endarterectomy (n = 206) or no immediate surgery (n = 204); the latter group included some patients who underwent delayed surgery after developing ischemic symptoms, progressive severe stenosis, bilateral stenosis, or contralateral stenosis.[25] At 3-year follow-up, using death or new stroke as end points, there was no difference in outcome between the immediate surgery group and the other group of patients (10.7 versus 11.3 per cent, respectively). However, almost half of the patients in the "no immediate surgery" group eventually did have an endarterectomy for one of the reasons stated. The unusual study design for this trial considerably lessens its statistical validity.

The Veterans Administration Asymptomatic Stenosis Trial randomized patients with asymptomatic carotid stenosis (greater than 50 per cent) to operative (n = 211) or nonoperative (n = 233) therapy.[55, 117] At a mean follow-up of 4 years, the combined incidence of ipsilateral neurological ischemic events (transient ischemic attack and stroke) was reduced in the surgical group compared with the medical group (8 and 20.6 per cent, respectively; P < 0.001). However, the sample size was not sufficient to provide statistical power to show a difference in stroke alone. The ipsilateral stroke rate in the surgical group was 4.7 per cent (including perioperative strokes), compared with 9.4 per cent in the medical group (P = 0.056). However, if perioperative mortality (1.9 per cent) is added to the surgical stroke rate, the difference between the two groups was not statistically significant.

The Asymptomatic Carotid Atherosclerosis Study is the largest of the three asymptomatic stenosis trials and substantiated the hypothesis that carotid endarterectomy may prevent stroke in certain patients with asymptomatic carotid stenosis.[9] Among 1662 individuals randomized with high-grade carotid stenosis (>60% diameter reduction by ultrasound and/or angiography), there was a projected overall 53 per cent relative risk reduction in ipsilateral stroke over 5 years (mean follow-up was 2.7 years) in patients receiving carotid endarterectomy (5.1%) compared to unoperated patients (11.0%). The stroke risk reduction was more prominent in men and was apparently independent of degree of stenosis or contralateral carotid artery disease. A substantial portion of the surgical risk was attributable to angiography (1.2% stroke rate), and the initial risk for surgery plus angiography was offset by a constant risk of stroke at approximately 2.2 per cent per year in the nonsurgical group. The surgical benefit was apparent by 10 months and was statistically significant at 3 years.

The Mayo Asymptomatic Carotid Endarterectomy Trial was stopped shortly after initiation because of increased frequency of a secondary end point (myocardial infarction) in the surgical group.[119]

TRIALS FOR SYMPTOMATIC CAROTID STENOSIS

The European Carotid Surgery Trial (Table 46–2) enrolled patients with mild (less than 30 per cent), moderate (30 to 69 per cent), or severe (70 to 99 per cent) carotid stenosis, who were then randomized to surgical or nonsurgical treatment.[38] Interim analysis of 2,200 patients (mean follow-up, 2.7 years) led to premature termination of the trial for the mild and severe stenosis groups. Among 374 randomized patients with mild stenosis, there was no significant difference in ipsilateral stroke between the surgical and nonsurgical groups. More treatment failures occurred in the surgery group, and this was attributed to the 2.3 per cent risk of death or disabling stroke during the first 30 days

Table 46–1

PROSPECTIVE RANDOMIZED TRIALS OF CAROTID ENDARTERECTOMY FOR ASYMPTOMATIC STENOSIS

Trial	Stenosis Criteria	Aspirin	Computed Tomography	Follow-Up	Estimated Sample Size	Primary End Points
CASANOVA Trial	50–90% by noninvasive measurement	1,000 mg/day + Dipyridamole 225 mg/day	Yes	3 yr	400 (410)	TIA, stroke, or death
Veterans Administration Asymptomatic Stenosis Trial	>50% by angiography	1,300 mg/day	No	5 yr	500 (444)	TIA or stroke in distribution of randomized artery; death <30 d after randomization
Asymptomatic Carotid Atherosclerosis Study	>60% by angiography in surgery group only	325 mg/day	Yes	5 yr	1800 (1662)	TIA or stroke in distribution of randomized artery; death <30 d after randomization
Mayo Asymptomatic Carotid Endarterectomy Trial	>50% by noninvasive measurement	80 mg/day (nonsurgical group only)	Option	2 yr	900	TIA, reversible ischemic neurological deficit, stroke, or death

TIA, transient ischemic attack.

Table 46–2

PROSPECTIVE TRIALS OF CAROTID ENDARTERECTOMY FOR SYMPTOMATIC STENOSIS

Trial	Stenosis Criteria	Aspirin	Computed Tomography	Follow-Up	Projected Sample Size	Primary End Points
European Carotid Surgery Trial	0–99% by angiography	Discretion	Yes	5 yr	2,200 (<30%* 374†) (>70%* 395†)	Ipsilateral stroke
North American Symptomatic Carotid Endarterectomy Trial	30–99% by angiography	Discretion	Yes	5 yr	3,000 (>70%* 659†)	Ipsilateral stroke; stroke-related death; death <30 d after randomized
Veterans Administration Symptomatic Stenosis Trial	50–99% by angiography	325 mg/day	Yes	3 yr	500 (192)	Ipsilateral stroke or crescendo TIA; death <30 d after randomization

TIA, transient ischemic attack.
*Percentage of stenosis.
†Number of patients entered into study.

after surgery. Among those with severe stenosis, however, surgery was shown to be beneficial in preventing stroke. There was a 7.5 per cent risk of ipsilateral stroke or death within 30 days of surgery, but at 3 years of follow-up, the surgery group had an additional 2.8 per cent risk of stroke (total, 10.3 per cent), compared with 16.8 per cent in the nonsurgery group ($P < .0001$). More importantly, the risk of death or ipsilateral disabling stroke was reduced from 11 per cent in the nonsurgery group to 6 per cent in the surgery group. Patient entry for patients with moderate stenosis continues in this trial.

The North American Symptomatic Carotid Endarterectomy Trial prematurely stopped randomizing patients with carotid stenosis greater than 70 per cent as a result of the overwhelming stroke risk reduction observed in the surgical group.[89] A total of 659 patients in this category of stenosis were randomized to surgical (n = 331) or nonsurgical (n = 328) therapy. At a mean follow-up of 24 months, ipsilateral stroke was noted in 26 per cent of nonsurgical patients, compared with 9 per cent of patients with endarterectomy, for an overall risk reduction of 17 per cent (relative risk reduction, 71 per cent). The benefit for surgical patients was highly significant ($P < .001$) for a variety of outcomes, including stroke in any territory, major stroke, and major stroke or death from any cause. A perioperative morbidity-mortality rate of 5.8 per cent was rapidly surpassed in the nonsurgical group, so that surgical benefit was apparent by 3 months. In addition, the protective effect of surgery was durable over time, with few strokes noted in the endarterectomy group beyond the perioperative period. Functional disability (assessed by a standardized disability scale) was significantly less in the surgery group over time ($P < 0.001$). Multivariate analysis demonstrated that surgical benefit was independent of a variety of concurrent demographic variables such as age, sex, and risk factors for stroke. There was a direct correlation between surgical benefit and the degree of stenosis on angiography. Post hoc analysis showed the following clinical features were related to increased stroke risk in the nonsurgical

group: evidence of ulceration on angiography, contralateral carotid occlusion, and hemispheric (as opposed to retinal) ischemia as a presenting symptom. This trial group continues to randomize symptomatic patients with carotid stenosis (30 to 69 per cent); the benefit of carotid endarterectomy in this group of patients remains indeterminate.

Enrollment in the *Veterans Administration Symptomatic Stenosis Trial* was stopped based on preliminary data consistent with the findings of the North American Symptomatic Carotid Endarterectomy Trial.[78] Subsequent analysis demonstrated a statistically significant reduction in ipsilateral stroke or crescendo transient ischemic attack for patients with carotid stenosis greater than 50 per cent, two thirds of whom demonstrated internal carotid artery stenosis greater than 70 per cent on angiography. A total of 193 men aged 35 to 82 years (mean, 64.2 years) were randomized to surgical (n = 91) or nonsurgical (n = 98) treatment. Duplex ultrasound examination was performed in 152 patients who subsequently underwent cerebral angiography; there was poor accuracy in the lower ranges of stenoses, especially underestimation of degrees of stenosis between 30 and 49 per cent. Complications of surgery other than end points were relatively infrequent and included respiratory insufficiency requiring extended intensive care monitoring (5 per cent), minor to moderate wound hematoma (5 per cent), cranial nerve deficit (5 per cent), myocardial infarction (2 per cent), and pulmonary embolism (1 per cent).

At a mean follow-up of 11.9 months, there was a significant reduction in stroke or crescendo transient ischemic attack in patients receiving carotid endarterectomy compared with nonsurgical patients (7.7 versus 19.4 per cent, respectively), for a risk reduction of 11.7 per cent (relative risk reduction, 60 per cent; $P = .028$). Among subgroups, the benefit of surgery was most prominent among patients with transient ischemic attack, compared with patients with transient monocular blindness or stroke, although these differences were not statistically significant. There was a positive correlation between the degree of carotid stenosis and the subsequent risk of stroke. For patients with carotid stenosis greater than 70 per cent, surgery provided a risk reduction for stroke or crescendo transient ischemic attack of 14.8 per cent ($P = .01$). The benefit for surgery was apparent as early as 2 months after randomization and persisted over the entire period of follow-up. The efficacy of carotid endarterectomy was durable, with only one ipsilateral stroke beyond the 30-day perioperative period. Discounting one preoperative stroke, a perioperative morbidity of 2.2 per cent and mortality of 3.3 per cent (total, 5.5 per cent) was achieved in multiple centers among relatively high-risk patients.

INDICATIONS FOR CAROTID ENDARTERECTOMY—CONCLUSIONS

Several notable features are common to the symptomatic stenosis trials. First, carotid endarterectomy provided a profound protection against subsequent ipsilateral stroke or crescendo transient ischemic attack in patients with high-grade symptomatic stenosis. The stroke risk reduction was realized early after surgery, persisted over extended periods, and was independent of other risk factors. Second, stroke rates in the nonsurgical group considerably exceeded those reported from previous prospective and retrospective studies. Symptomatic patients receiving aspirin in previous prospective multicenter trials had annual stroke rates ranging from 3 to 7 per cent, compared with rates between 15 and 20 per cent in unoperated patients from the North American Symptomatic Carotid Endarterectomy Trial and the Veterans Administration Symptomatic Stenosis Trial.[14, 18, 23] Third, the inaccuracy of carotid duplex ultrasound noted in the latter trial suggests that symptomatic patients with intermediate degrees of stenosis by duplex ultrasound should have definitive assessment by angiography before determination of therapy. Finally, efficacy for carotid endarterectomy in these trials depended on an acceptable level of perioperative morbidity and mortality.

For asymptomatic stenosis, the data are less conclusive. Based on the results of prospective trials, carotid endarterectomy in patients with asymptomatic stenosis should be determined on the basis of multiple factors, including degree of stenosis, whether there has been progression of stenosis, degree of stenosis in the contralateral carotid artery, assessment of cerebral circulatory reserve and collateral flow, presence of silent infarcts on computed tomography, and ulceration at the site of stenosis.[9, 87, 88, 96] Most importantly, the operation should be performed for asymptomatic stenosis only in low-risk patients; that is, when the surgical morbidity does not exceed 3 to 4 per cent.[21] This determination of risk is highly dependent on preoperative assessment of the patient.

Preoperative Assessment for Carotid Endarterectomy

HISTORY OF PRESENTING SYMPTOMS

The considerable risk of stroke in patients with high-grade carotid stenosis mandates accurate diagnosis of potential causes, although the cause of cerebral ischemia may be indeterminate in up to 40 per cent of cases.[67] Careful history should be taken in all patients and should include risk factors, family history, and the nature and timing of the presumed event.[56] In many cases, ischemia from small vessel disease can be differentiated from large vessel pathology on the basis of clinical presentation, although the two entities frequently coexist.[112] Tobacco abuse in particular has been highly associated with stroke risk in carotid stenosis.[56, 78] Cardiac assessment is an essential component of the work-up for cerebrovascular ischemia, owing to the prevalence of coexistent coronary artery disease.[105]

Clinical and pathological features of cerebral ischemia are described in Chapter 44. Symptoms of anterior circulation ischemia are typically classified as transient ischemic attacks, amaurosis fugax (transient monocular blindness), or completed stroke.[92] The distribution of those presenting syndromes was relatively consistent among the three symptomatic endarterectomy trials: transient ischemic attack, 35 to 40 per cent; transient monocular blindness, 35 to 40 per cent; completed stroke, 20 to 25 per cent.[38, 78, 89] All three trials showed a high incidence of stroke in close temporal proximity to the presenting symptoms in nonsurgical patients. This observation corresponds to that in the retrospective analysis by Whisnant and co-workers, in which the risk of stroke for untreated transient ischemic attack was increased by a factor of 120, compared with the age-adjusted population, in the first 30 days after symptoms appeared.[121] This finding implies that patients with suspected cerebral ischemia should be evaluated with some urgency for potential surgical intervention.

ASSESSMENT OF PERIOPERATIVE RISK

The efficacy of carotid endarterectomy is dependent on selection of patients with appropriate indications and minimization of perioperative risk. Owing to the concurrence of other significant medical disorders with carotid stenosis, all patients evaluated for carotid endarterectomy require a thorough preoperative medical evaluation.[105] Particular attention should be paid to cardiac status; cardiological consultation for all patients is recommended. The initial cardiac work-up should include electrocardiography and echocardiography; these studies can also delineate potential cardiogenic sources of emboli.[2] Medical therapy for existing medical disorders should be maximized before surgery. Sundt and colleagues have addressed preoperative risk by a careful retrospective analysis. Based on medical, neurological, and angiographic risk factors, patients can be categorized according to perioperative risk (Table 46–3) to determine those best suited for surgical intervention.

NONINVASIVE EVALUATION

Ultrasound evaluation of carotid artery morphology and flow has been widely accepted as a noninvasive

Table 46–3

PERIOPERATIVE RISK FACTORS FOR PATIENTS WHO ARE CANDIDATES FOR CAROTID ENDARTERECTOMY

Risk Grade	Neurological Status	Medical Risk	Angiographic Risk	Morbidity/ Mortality (%)
I	Stable	No	No	<1
II	Stable	No	Yes	1.8
III	Stable	Yes	Yes or no	4.0
IV	Unstable	Yes or no	Yes or no	8.5

Neurological Instability: Progressive deficit, infarct <7 days previously, transient ischemic attack within 24 hours, crescendo transient ischemic attack.

Medical Risk Factors: Angina, recent myocardial infarction, congestive heart failure, severe hypertension, advanced chronic obstructive pulmonary disease, age >70 years, severe obesity.

Angiographic Risk Factors: Occlusion of opposite internal carotid artery, stenosis of ipsilateral internal carotid artery at siphon, extension of plaque proximally or distally from bifurcation, high cervical bifurcation, intraluminal thrombus.

Adapted from Sundt, T. M., Jr., Sandok, B. A., and Whisnant, J. P.: Carotid endarterectomy: Complications and preoperative assessment of risk. Mayo Clin. Proc., 50:301–306, 1975.

measure and has largely supplanted prior techniques such as oculoplethysmography.[91] Conventional B-mode ultrasound provides highly accurate determination of vessel wall thickness and, to a lesser extent, plaque morphology.[111] The combination of B-mode ultrasound and Doppler analysis (duplex ultrasound) provides an assessment of flow that aids in determination of the degree of stenosis. The accuracy of duplex analysis may be affected by several factors, including plaque asymmetry, low velocities, calcium in the arterial wall, patient motion, and extension of the lesion distally in the cervical internal carotid artery.[103] Duplex ultrasound may be more sensitive than angiography in determining the presence of ulceration.[98] In determining the accuracy of duplex ultrasound, the inherent variability among readers and among sonographers, particularly the latter, must be considered.[110] Although several laboratories have demonstrated a high degree of accuracy for duplex ultrasound, two multicenter trials have shown surprisingly low sensitivity and specificity for this modality, especially in the intermediate ranges of stenosis.[78, 89] These data suggest that patients with symptoms of cerebral ischemia should not necessarily be excluded from consideration for carotid endarterectomy solely on the basis of duplex examination.

Transcranial Doppler ultrasound is a new modality that enables the noninvasive determination of blood velocity (and, indirectly, of flow) in major intracranial arteries by means of range-gated ultrasound.[87] In addition to velocity, considerable information can be gained regarding collateral flow patterns, pulse-wave analysis ("pulsatility index"), and intracranial stenosis.[87] Evocative tests such as carbon dioxide inhalation or acetazolamide (Diamox) challenge can be used to determine autoregulation and hemodynamic reserve.[61] In addition, detection of small, frequently asymptomatic emboli by transcranial Doppler ultrasound can greatly aid in determination of the locus of the embolic source and the response to therapy (e.g., anticoagulation).[68] It can

also be used to monitor middle cerebral artery velocity and embolic events during carotid endarterectomy and to determine postoperative changes in cerebral hemodynamics.[49, 79]

Other noninvasive means to measure cerebral blood flow have aided in the diagnosis of cerebral ischemia. Although positron emission tomography provides a quantitative measurement of cerebral blood flow and of cerebral metabolism, its usefulness is limited by the scarcity of scanners, the cost, and the practical considerations of using radionuclides.[77] The xenon–computed tomography technique provides an anatomical correlate of cerebral blood flow with quantitative measurement but has not been widely applied.[124] Single photon emission computed tomography is a widely available technique for nonquantitative assessment of regional cerebral blood flow that may be useful in determining hemodynamic changes after endarterectomy.[94]

RADIOLOGICAL ASSESSMENT

All patients evaluated for carotid endarterectomy should have preoperative computed tomography or magnetic resonance imaging of the head. These studies effectively rule out other lesions (e.g., tumor, hematoma) as a cause of symptoms, delineate the presence of hemorrhagic infarction or cerebral edema, and demonstrate the existence of previous cerebral infarctions.

CONVENTIONAL CEREBRAL ANGIOGRAPHY

Angiography is an essential component of the preoperative evaluation for endarterectomy. Although current angiography techniques have less than 1 per cent major morbidity, the procedure is nevertheless invasive and must be performed in the hospital setting.[116] In addition to defining cervical carotid stenosis, ulceration, and intraluminal thrombus, angiography demonstrates other potentially significant lesions of the craniocervical circulation and provides information about collateral flow patterns (Fig. 46–6). In this regard, it is important that the entire cerebral vasculature be studied by angiography.

Per cent stenosis of the internal carotid artery lesion is usually calculated as the ratio of the narrowest diameter of the stenotic artery in one plane to the diameter of the "normal" artery (Fig. 46–7). "Normal" has been interpreted as the imaginary outline of the carotid bulb, although most recent studies have used the internal carotid artery distal to the stenotic lesion as the denominator.[78, 89] Variations in the interpretation of stenosis by angiography have been estimated at 15 per cent between readers, and at 10 per cent for interpretations by the same reader at different times, for stenosis greater than 50 per cent.[26] In addition, ulcerations and focal stenotic "webs" are often poorly visualized by angiography, leading to underestimation of arterial disease.[37] In spite of the lower sensitivity of angiography

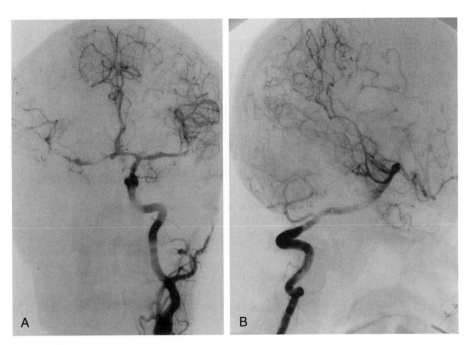

Figure 46–6

Cerebral angiograms showing extensive collateral flow to the right hemisphere after right carotid artery occlusion. *A.* The anteroposterior left carotid injection shows collateral filling of the right middle cerebral artery from the left through the anterior communicating artery. *B.* The lateral vertebral injection shows forward filling of left middle cerebral branches through the posterior communicating artery.

in these respects, it remains the "gold standard" for evaluation of stenosis in the craniocervical circulation for suspected cerebral ischemia.

MAGNETIC RESONANCE ANGIOGRAPHY

Magnetic resonance angiography is a powerful, noninvasive imaging technique well suited for the rapid laminar flow of the carotid artery.[5] It is based on standard magnetic resonance principles but uses special imaging coils and protocols for data analysis (e.g., time-of-flight analysis). Two-dimensional magnetic resonance angiography images are reconstructions of a series of thin transverse slices. These are very sensitive for low-flow states but are limited by lower resolution overall and decreased contrast when flow is parallel to the slice. Three-dimensional magnetic resonance angiography images provide excellent resolution and high sensitivity to flow in any direction; however, there is

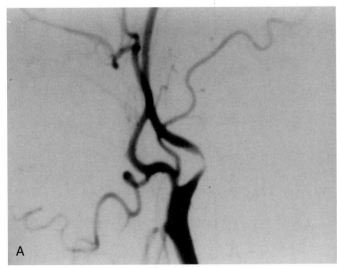

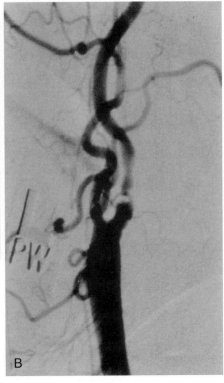

Figure 46–7

Lateral angiograms of cervical carotid artery showing varied appearance of critical stenosis of the internal carotid artery. *A.* Smoothly tapered segmental narrowing. *B.* Sharply demarcated stenosis.

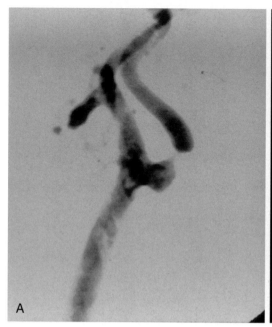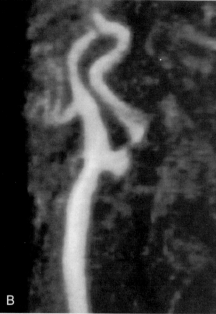

Figure 46–8

Comparison of conventional angiography (A) and magnetic resonance angiography (B) for high-grade carotid stenosis.

poor contrast in low-flow states. Because the use of either image type alone results in problems with interpretation, it is recommended that both images be obtained for a full evaluation.[5] Although it is still being refined, the resolution of magnetic resonance angiography is comparable to that of standard angiography for carotid artery imaging (Fig. 46–8), with a sensitivity of 90 per cent compared with angiography. The accuracy and safety of magnetic resonance angiography suggest that it may soon become the imaging modality of choice for assessment of carotid artery stenosis.[7]

Timing of Surgical Intervention for Cerebral Ischemia

Several prospective studies have showed a high incidence of stroke in close temporal proximity to the presenting symptoms.[78, 89] This observation corresponds to those reported in a retrospective analysis by Whisnant and colleagues, in which the risk of stroke for patients with untreated transient ischemic attack was markedly increased compared with age-adjusted population in the first 30 days after symptoms appeared.[120] This finding implies that patients with suspected cerebral ischemia should be evaluated with some urgency for potential surgical intervention. Those patients with fluctuating neurological deficits or crescendo transient ischemic attacks are at particular risk and should receive surgical evaluation on an emergency basis.[122]

Some controversy exists regarding the timing of surgery for patients with recent completed stroke and fixed neurological deficit.[73] Although these patients have increased surgical risk (see Table 46–3), they are also at increased risk for an additional stroke, and no data support the current practice of delaying surgery

for several weeks.[78, 89, 105] At present, the author recommends proceeding directly with surgery in appropriate patients after stroke unless there exists significant neurological disability (i.e., inability to function independently) or computed tomography evidence of edema or hemorrhage. Rapid emergent endarterectomy in the setting of acute carotid occlusion and major deficit may occasionally yield beneficial outcomes.[81]

Surgical Technique

Considerable variation exists among surgeons with regard to specific techniques used in carotid endarterectomy. Prospective trials to date have not standardized surgical technique among participating surgeons; analysis of complication rates associated with technical factors in these studies is retrospective and of less validity.[57] In addition, the low rate of perioperative complications in those studies reporting detailed surgical results further limits any meaningful comparisons.[78, 116] In general, the experience of the surgeon with a specific protocol supersedes other technical considerations in the determination of perioperative morbidity. The technique described in this section should serve as a general guideline for the operative and perioperative care of patients having endarterectomy.

ANESTHETIC CONSIDERATIONS AND POSITIONING

Most surgeons perform carotid endarterectomy with the patient under general anesthesia, although excellent results have been presented in individual series with regional anesthesia.[32] Regardless of technique, the principal goals of anesthetic management are to maintain adequate cerebral and myocardial perfusion. In addition to routine monitors, intra-arterial pressure monitoring facilitates the meticulous control of blood pressure. Central venous pressure catheters or Swan-Ganz catheters are often used in patients with increased cardiac risk.

Induction of general anesthesia is usually accomplished with either an ultrashort-acting barbiturate or etomidate; intravenous narcotics and lidocaine are often added to blunt the stimulation of intubation. Although most volatile anesthetics provide some protection from cerebral ischemia by depressing the cerebral metabolic rate, isoflurane has been shown to be modestly superior in decreasing the frequency of cerebral ischemia during carotid endarterectomy.[82] Mechanical ventilation is adjusted to maintain normocapnia as determined by arterial blood gas analysis. The blood pressure should be maintained at or slightly above the patient's awake pressure. However, a high cerebral perfusion pressure may increase cardiac work and lead to myocardial ischemia in some patients. Vasoactive drugs should be available to treat either hypertension or hypotension. If a barbiturate or etomidate is used to achieve cerebral metabolic protection at the time of carotid cross-clamping, it should be given well in advance to ensure adequate brain tissue levels. The use of glucose-containing fluids is discouraged.

The patient is placed in the supine position with the head turned away from the side of the operation (Fig. 46–9). A small roll is placed beneath the shoulders to put the neck in slight extension and facilitate full exposure of the carotid bifurcation. The operative field should extend from the mastoid process superiorly to the sternal notch inferiorly; care should be taken during surgical preparation to avoid dislodging emboli by vigorous scrubbing. Instillation of local anesthetic into the superficial cervical plexus may reduce general anesthetic requirements. If a vein patch is to be used (see

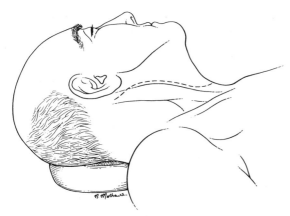

Figure 46–9

The patient is placed in the supine position with a small roll beneath the shoulder and the head turned away from the side of the operation. The incision runs along the anterior border of the sternocleidomastoid muscle and curves posteriorly 1 cm below the angle of the mandible to avoid injury to the facial nerve. (From Barrow, D. L.: Carotid endarterectomy: Technical aspects and perioperative management. *In* Awad, I. A., ed.: Cerebrovascular Occlusive Disease and Brain Ischemia. Park Ridge, IL, American Association of Neurological Surgeons, 1991, p. 169. Reprinted by permission.)

Patch Angioplasty), the ipsilateral leg is prepared for saphenous vein graft.

OPERATIVE PROCEDURE

The procedure is performed with the use of loupe magnification with a headlight, although the operating microscope is an excellent alternative.[102] The magnification and illumination provided by these adjuncts ensures identification of critical structures in the operative field, meticulous removal of loose fragments from the luminal surface, and precise suturing of the arteriotomy. An incision is made along the anterior border of the sternocleidomastoid muscle, curving posteriorly toward the mastoid process about 1 cm below the angle of the mandible (see Fig. 46–9); this enables distal exposure of the internal carotid artery without injury to the mandibular ramus of the facial nerve. Attempts should be made to identify and protect the greater auricular nerve at the superior margin of the incision. Meticulous hemostasis is maintained throughout the procedure with bipolar cautery. The platysma is incised, and the dissection is carried along the medial border of the sternocleidomastoid muscle. Usually, an avascular plane is extant, and little cautery is required.

At this point in the dissection, the ansa cervicalis of the cervical plexus is often encountered. Although it is safe to section this nerve, the author prefers to mobilize it medially; this enables medial retraction of the hypoglossal nerve at its junction with the ansa during dissection of the distal internal carotid artery. Care should be taken to keep the medial blade of self-retaining retractors in the superficial layers of the wound, because deeper placement can cause injury to the recurrent laryngeal or superior laryngeal nerve.

Beneath the sternocleidomastoid muscle, the internal jugular vein is encountered. The common facial branch of this vein, which courses medially, is doubly ligated and divided, and the vein is gently retracted laterally. At this point, the carotid artery can be gently palpated, and the carotid sheath is visible. Care must be taken during dissection of the carotid sheath because, on rare occasions, the vagus nerve is located anterior to the artery. Before manipulation of the carotid artery in the region of the bifurcation, lidocaine (2 per cent Xylocaine) without epinephrine is instilled into the carotid sinus and along the course of the nerve of Hering to minimize bradycardia and hypotension resulting from stimulation of these structures. The carotid sheath is opened inferiorly along the anterior surface of the artery to the level of the omohyoid muscle. Before further dissection is undertaken, proximal control of the common carotid artery is obtained by careful dissection of the posterior wall from the underlying vagus nerve and passage of a vessel loop. Superiorly, the superior thyroid artery, external carotid artery, and internal carotid artery are dissected in the region of the bifurcation (Fig. 46–10).

Dissection is then carried distally along the internal carotid artery. Extreme care must be taken to identify the hypoglossal nerve early in the dissection, because

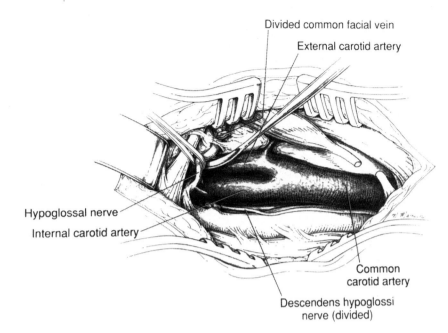

Divided common facial vein

External carotid artery

Hypoglossal nerve

Internal carotid artery

Common carotid artery

Descendens hypoglossi nerve (divided)

Figure 46–10

After division of the common facial vein, the carotid sheath is opened to expose common, internal, and external carotid arteries. The hypoglossal nerve at the superior margin of the dissection can be gently retracted medially. (From Barrow, D. L.: Carotid endarterectomy: Technical aspects and perioperative management. *In* Awad, I. A., ed.: Cerebrovascular Occlusive Disease and Brain Ischemia. Park Ridge, IL, American Association of Neurological Surgeons, 1991, p. 171. Reprinted by permission.)

it crosses the distal internal carotid artery. On occasion, it can be mobilized and gently retracted medially for better distal exposure. The carotid plaque can often be gently palpated to determine its distal end; usually, it extends further along the posterior wall of the artery. Dissection must be carried to at least 1 cm distal to the end of the plaque to allow for posterior wall extension and placement of a shunt, if necessary. Circumferential dissection around the internal carotid artery for placement of an umbilical tape is done only at the site of the tape position. A Rumel tourniquet is fashioned by placing the umbilical tapes on the internal carotid and common carotid arteries through a segment of rubber tubing. Dissection is then completed around the external carotid artery and superior thyroid artery, which are isolated with vessel loops.

At this point, the anesthesiologist is instructed to give 100 U per kg of heparin as a bolus. The blood pressure is maintained at or slightly above awake baseline, and the electroencephalography results are examined. During a 5-minute interval after the heparin is administered and before the artery is clamped, it is also helpful to review with the scrub nurse the instruments to be used and the order of use. The shunt tubing is filled with heparinized saline and clamped to ensure that there are no intraluminal bubbles, and it is compared with the internal carotid artery to ensure proper sizing.

The internal carotid artery is clamped first; the author prefers to use an aneurysm clip because it has a lower profile and is less traumatic to the vessel. The common carotid artery is then clamped with an angled or straight Fogarty Hydragrip clamp, and the external carotid artery and superior thyroid artery are clamped with aneurysm clips. An arteriotomy is started about 1 cm proximal to the bifurcation in the midline of the

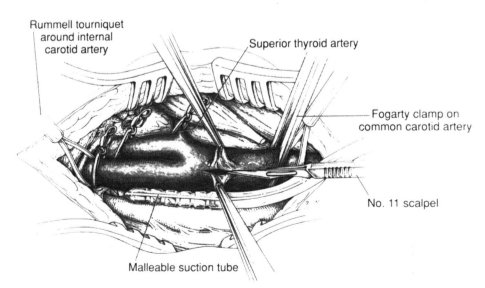

Rummell tourniquet around internal carotid artery

Superior thyroid artery

Fogarty clamp on common carotid artery

No. 11 scalpel

Malleable suction tube

Figure 46–11

Clamps have been applied to the common, internal, and external carotid arteries and the superior thyroid artery. Notice the tourniquets on the common carotid artery and internal carotid artery for potential shunt placement. The arteriotomy incision is initiated in the midline of the common carotid artery just below the bifurcation. (From Barrow, D. L.: Carotid endarterectomy: Technical aspects and perioperative management. *In* Awad, I. A., ed.: Cerebrovascular Occlusive Disease and Brain Ischemia. Park Ridge, IL, American Association of Neurological Surgeons, 1991, p. 172. Reprinted by permission.)

Figure 46–12

The arteriotomy is extended distally in the midline of the internal carotid artery with Potts scissors. The incision is continued until normal intima is encountered on the anterior wall of the artery. Plaque usually extends slightly more distally on the posterior wall of the artery. (From Barrow, D. L.: Carotid endarterectomy: Technical aspects and perioperative management. *In* Awad, I. A., ed.: Cerebrovascular Occlusive Disease and Brain Ischemia. Park Ridge, IL, American Association of Neurological Surgeons, 1991, p. 172. Reprinted by permission.)

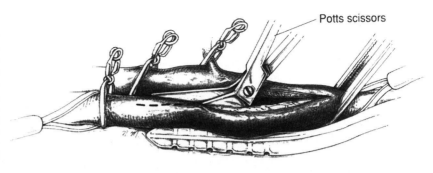

common carotid artery (Fig. 46–11). The incision is carried through the arterial wall until plaque is encountered, and a smooth plane is developed between plaque and artery wall. Some surgeons prefer to include the full thickness of the plaque in the arteriotomy incision; however, the author believes the dissection is made more accurate by removing the plaque without incising it.

At this point, the electroencephalogram is again examined to determine whether shunt placement is necessary (see Intraoperative Monitoring and Shunt Use). If no changes have occurred, dissection is carried distally along the plaque with a no. 4 Penfield dissector, and the arteriotomy is completed with a Potts scissors (Fig. 46–12). The arteriotomy should extend along the anterior midline of the internal carotid artery until normal intima beyond the plaque is reached. Circumferential dissection of the plaque is then accomplished at the proximal end, a curved clamp is placed between plaque and artery wall, and the plaque is sharply incised with a scalpel. Care must be taken to ensure that the remaining plaque in the common carotid artery has a smooth edge (Fig. 46–13). The plaque is then dissected free from the arterial wall with the Penfield dissector to the bifurcation and into the external carotid artery. It is often helpful to have the assistant temporarily release the external carotid artery clamp as dissection proceeds up that artery and the plaque is gently torn free from its distal attachment.

A critical part of the dissection involves the distal attachment of the plaque to normal intima of the internal carotid artery. By gentle dissection and proximal traction on the plaque, it will usually tear away from its distal attachment and leave a firm, adherent, normal intima. If the intima at this site is not adherent, it should be further resected or, less commonly, tacked to the arterial wall with a 6–0 Prolene suture.

After the plaque has been removed, the luminal surface is carefully inspected while the assistant continuously irrigates the site with heparinized saline. Small bits of debris that become apparent during this maneuver should be meticulously removed under magnified vision to create a lumen that is as smooth as possible. The arteriotomy is then closed with a running 6–0 Prolene suture from the distal to the proximal end (Fig. 46–14). Extreme care must be taken to approximate the edges with small, equal bites so that no regions of stenosis are created. Just before final suturing at the proximal end of the arteriotomy, the internal carotid artery clamp is briefly released. The resulting backflow of blood ensures that the artery is patent and flushes any residual debris from the lumen. The superior thyroid artery clamp is removed as the final suture is placed in order to have continuous backflow of blood and to prevent entraining of air into the lumen. The clamps are then removed in the following order: external carotid artery, common carotid artery, internal carotid artery. This sequence ensures that any potential embolic material is flushed into the external artery circulation. The arteriotomy is covered with oxidized cellulose, and gentle pressure is applied to the wound with a sponge for about 1 minute. Meticulous hemostasis is maintained during closure; occasionally, a small drain is placed in the superficial wound.

Figure 46–13

The plaque has been excised in the common carotid artery and distally into the internal and external carotid arteries. The distal end of the common carotid plaque is trimmed to provide a smooth margin. (From Barrow, D. L.: Carotid endarterectomy: Technical aspects and perioperative management. *In* Awad, I. A., ed.: Cerebrovascular Occlusive Disease and Brain Ischemia. Park Ridge, IL, American Association of Neurological Surgeons, 1991, p. 174. Reprinted by permission.)

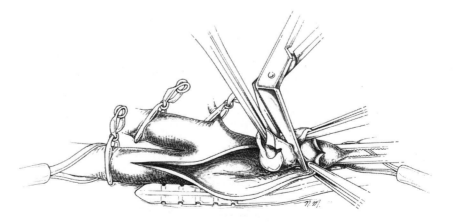

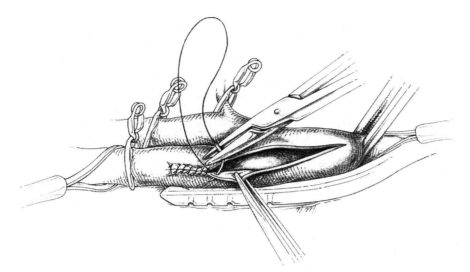

Figure 46–14

The arteriotomy is closed with a running 6–0 Prolene suture. Care must be taken to ensure a precise approximation of the edges without compromise of the lumen at any point. (From Barrow, D. L.: Carotid endarterectomy: Technical aspects and perioperative management. *In* Awad, I. A., ed.: Cerebrovascular Occlusive Disease and Brain Ischemia. Park Ridge, IL, American Association of Neurological Surgeons, 1991, p. 175. Reprinted by permission.)

INTRAOPERATIVE MONITORING AND SHUNT USE

Intraoperative monitoring provides an assessment of cerebral blood flow during endarterectomy and may facilitate the decision of whether to employ a shunt during carotid cross-clamping. Direct measurement of cerebral blood flow with diffusion techniques such as xenon-133 are somewhat cumbersome and require special operating room facilities. Electroencephalography is widely available and correlates well with diminished hemispheric cerebral blood flow but may not reflect regional ischemia or embolic events.[104] Somatosensory evoked potential monitoring may be more sensitive in this regard.[3] Transcranial Doppler ultrasound can demonstrate both embolic events and diminished velocity in the middle cerebral artery during cross-clamping, but it has a lower sensitivity than electroencephalography.[49] Although determination of internal carotid artery stump pressure is widely employed, it correlates poorly with cerebral blood flow and is not recommended as a sole measure of intraoperative monitoring.[109] Intraoperative monitoring demonstrates significant reductions in cerebral blood flow during carotid cross-clamping in 10 to 24 per cent of cases, depending on the monitoring modality used.[109] Presumably, these patients are at risk for hemodynamic ischemic infarction at this time, although short-acting barbiturates may attenuate cerebral metabolic demands during cross-clamping.[102]

The use of a shunt during carotid endarterectomy is controversial, with various authors advocating no shunting, uniform shunting, and selective shunting based on monitoring.[59, 102, 104] The potential disadvantages of shunts are dislodgment of embolic material during placement, need for additional distal exposure, and limited visualization at the critical distal margin of the plaque. For these reasons, the author restricts use of a shunt to those situations in which cerebral ischemia is demonstrated by electroencephalography or other monitoring techniques. Electroencephalography changes that occur at the time of carotid artery cross-clamping (manifested by decrease in higher frequencies or decrease in amplitude, or both) sometimes spontaneously resolve with elevation of the blood pressure. If changes persist longer than 60 to 90 seconds, the arteriotomy is extended through the plaque along its entire length with Potts scissors to expose the normal intima of the distal internal carotid artery. The distal end of the saline-filled and clamped shunt tubing is carefully inserted into the internal carotid artery, which is briefly opened to permit shunt passage, then secured in place with a tourniquet. Backflow is ascertained by brief removal of the shunt clamp, and the proximal shunt is then inserted into the common carotid artery in a similar fashion. The shunt clamp is then removed, and flow through the shunt is documented with Doppler ultrasound. The midportion of the shunt is then retracted to the side to enable plaque removal as described. At the final stage of arteriotomy suturing, the shunt is removed by reversing the steps listed for insertion.

PATCH ANGIOPLASTY

The routine use of vein or synthetic patch angioplasty in carotid endarterectomy has been advocated, but patch grafts of various types were used in only 14 per cent of cases in a multicenter trial.[8, 12, 78, 106] Angioplasty provides theoretical advantage compared with direct closure by maintaining a larger lumen and improving flow patterns at the distal end of the arteriotomy, thus limiting acute occlusion or restenosis at this site.[8, 12] On the other hand, patch angioplasties require additional cross-clamping time and are susceptible to aneurysmal dilatation and rupture, especially patches from smaller veins.[8] The author advocates routine use of vein angioplasty only for recurrent or radiation-induced carotid stenosis.

Postoperative Care

The attention to detail that is necessary during the endarterectomy procedure must be maintained throughout the postoperative period, because many complications occur during this time. All patients should be observed in an intensive care unit for 24 to 48 hours after the procedure with sequential neurological examinations by nursing staff. Blood pressure should be rigidly controlled in the approximate preoperative range with continuous monitoring by arterial catheter; hemodynamic parameters are similarly monitored by Swan-Ganz catheter in selected patients. Intravenous fluids, pressors, inotropes, and antihypertensive agents are routinely administered to optimize these indices. Postoperative electrocardiography and chest radiography should be performed for all patients. Urine output and serum electrolytes are monitored during the period of intensive care. The cervical wound is repeatedly examined for enlargement or superficial bleeding. Aspirin therapy is initiated immediately after surgery, and stable patients are usually discharged to home within 3 to 5 days.

Complications of Endarterectomy

CEREBRAL INFARCTION

Cerebral infarction as a consequence of intraoperative or postoperative ischemia is an often devastating complication of carotid endarterectomy (Table 46–4). In a retrospective review, Sundt and associates estimated the incidence of perioperative ischemia after endarterectomy at 2.5 per cent for reversible deficits, 1.3 per cent for minor stroke, and 2.9 per cent for major stroke (4.2 per cent for all strokes).[105] These figures are comparable to perioperative (30-day) stroke rates in the Veterans Administration Asymptomatic Stenosis Trial (2.4 per cent) and the Veterans Administration and North American endarterectomy trials for asymptomatic stenosis (2.2 and 5.5 per cent, respectively).[78, 89, 116]

Strict adherence to the surgical technical details described here is essential for minimization of perioperative cerebral infarction. Intraoperative ischemia as a result of hemodynamic consequences can be minimized by monitoring and shunting or by strategies

Table 46–4
COMPLICATIONS OF CAROTID ENDARTERECTOMY

Cerebral Infarction
   Intraoperative
   Postoperative
Intracerebral Hemorrhage
Myocardial Infarction
Wound
   Hematoma
   Infection
Cranial Nerve Injury
   Hypoglossal
   Vagus
   Facial
   Greater auricular
   Glossopharyngeal
Recurrent Carotid Stenosis

for cerebral metabolic protection. Distal embolic events during the procedure are reduced by careful handling of vessels during dissection, heparin anticoagulation, application and removal of clamps in specific order, meticulous attention to the luminal surface, and back-bleeding from the internal carotid artery before closure. Technical aspects of the procedure also determine embolic or thrombic events in the postoperative period; factors such as stenosis at the arteriotomy site, residual intraluminal debris, or an intimal flap all predispose to subsequent events. Not reversing heparin anticoagulation may allow formation of a nonthrombogenic luminal surface over several hours.[31] In addition, maintenance of adequate blood pressure in the postoperative period may reduce thrombosis caused by low flow in the artery.

INTRACEREBRAL HEMORRHAGE

The occurrence of postoperative intracerebral hemorrhage after carotid endarterectomy has been related to inadequate control of hypertension.[24, 115] However, early reports of this complication (before the advent of computed tomography) probably included patients with unrecognized preoperative hemorrhagic infarcts. The incidence of intracerebral hemorrhage is increased in patients with critical carotid stenosis; this is probably related to chronic impairment of cerebral autoregulation.[16]

CRANIAL NERVE INJURIES

Injuries to cervical cranial nerves are a common consequence of carotid endarterectomy. The reported incidence of cranial neuropathy after endarterectomy varies depending on how vigorously these deficits are sought, but they have been estimated to complicate 12 to 20 per cent of cases.[30, 53, 70] The majority of cranial nerve injuries after endarterectomy are transient and of minor clinical consequence; nevertheless, they are often disturbing to the patient and can be minimized by attention to surgical detail. In general, the use of bipolar coagulation is imperative after dissection has proceeded below the level of the sternocleidomastoid muscle. Precise coagulation of vascular structures adjacent to nerves can provide better visualization and mobilization and reduces direct injury from spread of monopolar current. Second, the use of magnified vision is essential for this operation. Magnifying loupes or an operating microscope should be used throughout the dissection as well as during the arteriotomy and closure. Third, traction on nerves should be minimized or avoided if possible. If a nerve must be displaced, it should be mobilized along a length that is sufficient to allow it to be moved with very little traction. Similarly, a stay suture carefully placed adjacent to the artery in the carotid sheath can often serve to rotate the artery and bring it into better view without excessive nerve traction.

Injury to the *hypoglossal nerve* is usually manifest as

unilateral tongue weakness with dysarthria and chewing difficulty.[30] The frequency and significance of hypoglossal nerve injury mandates the identification of this structure early in the dissection of the carotid complex. The hypoglossal nerve can often be located by following the descendens hypoglossi to its origin from the hypoglossal nerve. Although the descendens hypoglossi can be sectioned without apparent deficit, the author has found it most helpful to dissect this structure so that it can be retracted medially. In this manner, the hypoglossal nerve can also be displaced gently in a medial direction, exposing the internal carotid artery well above the bifurcation. The origin of the descendens hypoglossi should be verified before it is sectioned, because, on rare occasions, an aberrant vagus nerve can be located anterior to the carotid artery. In those cases in which the descendens hypoglossi cannot be retracted medially, it can usually be sharply dissected from the hypoglossal nerve as a distinct bundle of fibers and retracted laterally for better internal carotid artery exposure.

Injuries to the *vagus nerve* or its branches occur in up to 6 per cent of cases and are usually manifest as dysphagia or hoarseness caused by unilateral vocal cord dysfunction or dysphagia.[53] Vagus nerve injuries caused by either superior or recurrent laryngeal nerve traction can be minimized by early identification of the vagus in the carotid sheath and careful placement of medial retractor blades. The anomalous course of the vagus nerve, which may rarely be located anterior to the carotid artery, is a potential cause of injury to this nerve and its important branches to the larynx. Injury to the nerve in its usual posterior location may occur during dissection posterior to the carotid bifurcation or during application of clamps to either the common carotid or the internal carotid artery. There is an increased risk of vagus nerve injury during operation for recurrent stenosis; this observation also holds true for carotid endarterectomy performed after local irradiation or other surgical procedures in the neck. In this setting, the author restricts circumferential dissection of the carotid artery to the point at which clamps will be applied, taking extreme care to identify the nerve at these sites. Again, the importance of careful retractor placement must be stressed with regard to the superior laryngeal and recurrent laryngeal nerves. Although the lateral blade of the lower self-retaining retractor may be placed quite deeply adjacent to the carotid artery, the medial blade should always be placed superficially above the platysma to avoid inadvertent traction on these nerves. Because of the disabling consequences of bilateral vocal cord palsies, laryngoscopy to assess vocal cord function should be performed before the second procedure of bilateral endarterectomies is begun. This measure should routinely be undertaken in such a circumstance, regardless of the apparent absence of any other clinical evidence for pre-existing vocal cord dysfunction.

Injury to the *mandibular branch of the facial nerve* produces a transient or occasionally a permanent paresis that can be cosmetically disfiguring. It is important to curve the skin incision posteriorly toward the mastoid process at the superior margin of the incision, so that it lies 1 to 2 cm below the angle of the mandible. Another potential cause of injury to this nerve occurs if a hand-held retractor is placed beneath the mandible; this should be avoided. Adequate exposure of the internal carotid artery can usually be obtained through other measures, such as splitting the belly of the digastric muscle or further extending the dissection at the superior margin of the incision.

Transection of the *greater auricular nerve* or the *superficial cervical plexus* produces anesthesia and, occasionally, disturbing paresthesias. Injury to the greater auricular nerve often produces an analgesia of the ear and periauricular region. This nerve can be sectioned and usually regenerates; occasionally, the author has anastomosed the nerve after sectioning, with excellent results. If possible, it is preferable to dissect this nerve both medially and laterally from the incision and mobilize it away from the upper carotid artery, thereby avoiding sectioning.

Rarely, the *glossopharyngeal nerve* is encountered at extreme distal internal carotid dissections to the base of the skull. Injury to this nerve produces significant dysphagia.

MYOCARDIAL INFARCTION

As previously discussed, there is a high association between carotid stenosis and coronary vascular disease. Sundt and colleagues reported a myocardial infarction rate of less than 1 per cent, primarily in the high-risk (grade III and IV) patients.[105] Other series have reported considerably higher rates of postoperative myocardial infarction, ranging as high as 6 per cent.[19] In the prospective carotid endarterectomy trials describing this data, the incidence of myocardial infarction was reported at 2.5 per cent (Veterans Administration Asymptomatic Stenosis Trial) and 1 per cent (Veterans Administration Symptomatic Stenosis Trial).[78, 116]

WOUND HEMATOMA

Because of the use of anticoagulants and antiplatelet agents in the perioperative period, wound hematomas of varying degree are relatively frequent after carotid endarterectomy.[58] Most are self-limited and can be closely watched. If the hematoma presents as an expanding mass in the neck, emergent return to the operating room for evacuation and establishment of airway may be necessary.

WOUND INFECTION

Presumably because of the rich vascular supply to the neck, wound infection in carotid endarterectomy is uncommon, with the reported incidence less than 1 per cent.[75] Those factors that predispose to infection are systemic risk factors, such as diabetes, and the use of a prosthetic patch for angioplasty. In this setting, the infection may present as a false aneurysm.

RECURRENT CAROTID STENOSIS

The histopathology of recurrent carotid stenosis is distinct from that of the primary atheromatous lesion. In recurrent stenosis, the luminal narrowing is secondary to proliferation of intimal smooth muscle cells. These lesions usually produce a smooth narrowing, which may explain the relative lack of symptoms in recurrent disease. Whereas the incidence of restenosis by noninvasive or angiography testing has been reported at 10 to 50 per cent for primary closure, symptomatic recurrences are in the range of 1 to 2 per cent.[93] Several authors have suggested that use of a vein patch angioplasty may reduce the incidence of recurrent stenosis.[12, 108] In most cases, recurrent stenosis occurs within 6 to 12 months and can be followed with sequential noninvasive testing in asymptomatic patients. In patients with inadequate collateral supply and in symptomatic patients, vein patch angioplasty is mandatory at the time of reoperation for restenosis.

Future Directions in the Treatment of Extracranial Carotid Occlusive Disease

PERCUTANEOUS TRANSLUMINAL CAROTID ANGIOPLASTY

Primarily used for distal lower extremity and coronary stenoses, percutaneous transluminal angioplasty has also been advocated for use on the extracranial and intracranial vasculature.[54, 60, 90, 113] However, the potential efficacy of percutaneous transluminal angioplasty and the natural history of intracranial atheromatous lesions dilated by percutaneous transluminal angioplasty can be inferred only from experience in other vascular territories.[97] Carotid angioplasty may potentially be complicated by recurrent stenosis or distal embolism. In coronary vessels, percutaneous transluminal angioplasty has been associated with acute occlusion rates of 2 to 4 per cent and delayed restenosis of up to 30 per cent, usually within the first 6 months.[74] With advances in catheter technology, the risks of distal embolism during percutaneous transluminal angioplasty have been reduced; nevertheless, rigorous clinical trials are needed to confirm the safety and efficacy of percutaneous transluminal angioplasty for preventing stroke.

ADVANCES IN NONINVASIVE IMAGING

Advanced noninvasive imaging modalities are likely to play an increasing role in the assessment of patients with cerebrovascular disease.[77] Magnetic resonance angiography, determination of cerebral blood flow by single photon emission computed tomography, and transcranial Doppler ultrasound detection of embolic sources and hemodynamic reserve should further delineate the pathogenesis of cerebral ischemia and augment the clinical decision-making process in preoperative, intraoperative, and postoperative situations.[65, 68, 94] Adjunctive medical therapy to control risk factors for stroke and to prevent restenosis at the endarterectomy site may further improve long-term outcome in patients after endarterectomy.[50]

REFERENCES

1. Ackerman, L. V.: The pathology of radiation effect on normal and neoplastic tissue. A.J.R., *114*:447–459, 1972.
2. Albers, G. W., Sherman, D. G., Gress, D. R., et al.: Stroke prevention in nonvalvular atrial fibrillation: A review of prospective randomized trials. Ann. Neurol., *30*:511–518, 1991.
3. Amantini, A., Bartelli, M., Descisciolo, G., et al.: Monitoring of somatosensory evoked potentials during carotid endarterectomy. J. Neurol., *239*:241–247, 1992.
4. American Heart Association: 1989 Stroke Facts. Dallas, 1989.
5. Anderson, C., Saloner, D., Lee, R. E., et al.: Assessment of carotid artery stenosis by MR angiography: Comparison with x-ray angiography and color-coded Doppler ultrasound. A.J.N.R., *13*:989–1003, 1992.
6. Anonymous: Arteriosclerosis: Report by National Heart and Lung Institute Task Force on Arteriosclerosis. Vol. 2. US Dept. of Health, Education, and Welfare publication NIH 72–219. Washington DC, Government Printing Office, 1971.
7. Anson, J., Heiserman, J. E., Drayer, B. P., et al.: Surgical decisions on the basis of magnetic resonance angiography of the carotid arteries. Neurosurgery, *3*:335–343, 1993.
8. Archie, J. R., Jr., and Green, J. J., Jr.: Saphenous vein rupture pressure, rupture stress, and carotid endarterectomy vein patch reconstruction. Surgery, *107*:389–396, 1990.
9. The Asymptomatic Carotid Atherosclerosis Study Group: Endarterectomy for asymptomatic carotid stenosis. J.A.M.A. *273*:1421–1428, 1995.
10. The Asymptomatic Cervical Bruit Study Group: Natural history and effectiveness of aspirin in asymptomatic patients with cervical bruits. Arch. Neurol., *48*:683–686, 1991.
11. Ausman, J. I., and Diaz, F. G.: Critique of the extracranial-intracranial bypass study. Surg. Neurol., *26*:218–221, 1986.
12. Awad, I. A., and Little, J. R.: Patch angioplasty in carotid endarterectomy: Advantages, concerns and controversies. Stroke, *20*:417–422, 1989.
13. Awad, I. A., and Spetzler, R. F.: Extracranial-intracranial bypass surgery: A critical analysis in light of the international cooperative study. Neurosurgery, *19*:655–664, 1986.
14. Barnett, H. J. M.: A randomized trial of aspirin and sulfinpyrazone in threatened stroke. N. Engl. J. Med., *299*:53–59, 1978.
15. Barnett, H. J. M., Plum, F., and Walton, J. N.: Carotid endarterectomy: An expression of concern. Stroke, *15*:941–943, 1984.
16. Bernstein, M., Fleming, J. F. R., and Deck, J. H. N.: Cerebral hyperperfusion after carotid endarterctomy: A cause of cerebral hemorrhage. Neurosurgery, *15*:50–56, 1984.
17. The Boston Area Anticoagulation Trial for Atrial Fibrillation Investigators: The effect of low-dose warfarin on the risk of stroke in patients with nonrheumatic atrial fibrillation. N. Engl. J. Med., *323*:1505–1511, 1990.
18. Bousser, M. G., Eschwege, E., Hagvenau, M., et al.: "AICLA" controlled trial of aspirin and dipyridamole in the secondary prevention of atherothrombotic cerebral ischemia. Stroke, *14*:5–14, 1983.
19. Brott, T., and Thalinger, K.: The practice of carotid endarterectomy in a large metropolitan area. Stroke, *15*:950–955, 1984.
20. Busuttil, R. W., Baker, J. D., Davidson, R. K., et al.: Carotid artery stenosis-hemodynamic significance and clinical course. J.A.M.A., *245*:1438, 1981

21. Callow, A. D., Caplan, L. R., Correll, J. W., et al.: Carotid endarterectomy: What is its current status? Am. J. Med., *85*:835–838, 1988.

22. Canadian Cooperative Stroke Study Group: A randomized trial of aspirin and sulfinpyrazone in threatened stroke. N. Engl. J. Med., *299*:53–59, 1978.

23. Candelise, L., Landi, G., et al.: A randomized trial of aspirin and sulfinpyrazone in patients with TIA. Stroke, *13*:175–179, 1982.

24. Caplan, L. R., Skillman, J., Ojemann, R., et al.: Intercerebral hemorrhage following carotid endarterectomy: A hypertensive complication. Stroke, *9*:457, 1978.

25. CASANOVA Study Group: Carotid surgery versus medical therapy in asymptomatic carotid stenosis. Stroke, *22*:1229–1235, 1991.

26. Clagett, P. G., Youkey, J. R., Brigham, R. A., et al.: Asymptomatic cervical bruit and abnormal ocular pneumoplethysmography: A prospective study comparing two approaches to management. Surgery, *96*:823–830, 1984.

27. Corrin, L. S., Sandok, B. A., and Houser, W.: Cerebral ischemic events in patients with fibromuscular dysplasia. Arch. Neurol., *38*:616–618, 1981.

28. Dawson, D. A., and Adams, P. F.: Current estimates from the National Center for Health Statistics. Vital Health Stat., *10*:164, 1987.

29. Day, A. L., Rhoton, A. L., Jr., and Little, J. R.: The extracranial-intracranial bypass study. Surg. Neurol., *22*:222–226, 1986.

30. Dehn, T. C. B., and Taylor, G. W.: Cranial and cervical nerve damage associated with carotid endarterectomy. Br. J. Surg., *70*:365–368, 1983.

31. Dirrenberger, R. A., and Sundt, T. M., Jr.: Carotid endarterectomy: Temporal profile of the healing process and effects of anticoagulation therapy. J. Neurosurg., *48*:201–219, 1978.

32. Donato, A. T., and Hill, S. L.: Carotid arterial surgery using local anesthesia: A private practice retrospective study. Am. Surg., *58*:446–450, 1992.

33. The Dutch TIA Trial Study Group: A comparison of two doses of aspirin (30 mg vs. 283 mg a day) in patients after a transient ischemic attack or minor ischemic stroke. N. Engl. J. Med., *325*:1261–1266, 1991.

34. Dyken, M. L., and Pokras, R.: The performance of endarterectomy for disease of the extracranial arteries of the head. Stroke, *15*:948–950, 1984.

35. Eastcott, H. G., Pickering, G. W., and Rob, C. G.: Reconstruction of internal carotid artery in a patient with intermittent attacks of hemiplegia. Lancet, *2*:994–998, 1954.

36. ECIC Bypass Study Group: Failure of extracranial-intracranial arterial bypass to reduce the risk of ischemic stroke: Results of an international randomized trial. N. Engl. J. Med., *313*:1191–1200, 1985.

37. Estol, C., Claassen, D., Hirsch, W., et al.: Correlative angiographic and pathologic findings in the diagnosis of ulcerated plaques in the carotid artery. Arch. Neurol., *48*:692–694, 1991.

38. European Carotid Surgery Trialists' Collaborative Group: European Carotid Surgery Trial: Interim results for symptomatic patients with severe (70–99%) or with mild (0–29%) carotid stenosis. Lancet, *337*:1235–1243, 1991.

39. Farjardo, L. F.: Morphologic patterns of radiation injury. *In* Vaeth, J. M., and Meyer, J. L., eds.: Radiation Tolerance of Normal Tissues. Front. Radiat. Ther. Oncol., *23*:75–84, 1989.

40. Fields, W. S., Maslenikov, V., Meyer, J. S., et al.: Joint Study of Extracranial Arterial Occlusion: V. Progress report of prognosis following surgery or nonsurgical treatment for transient cerebral ischemic attacks and cervical carotid artery lesions. J.A.M.A., *211*:1993–2003, 1970.

41. Fisher, C. M.: Transient monocular blindness associated wtih hemiplegia. Arch. Ophthalmol., *47*:167–203, 1952.

42. Fisher, C. M., Gore, I., Okabe, N., et al.: Atherosclerosis of the Carotid and Vertebral Arteries: Extracranial and Intracranial. J. Neuropathol. Exp. Neurol., *24*:455–476, 1965.

43. Fonkalsrud, E. W., Sanchez, M., Zerubavel, R., et al.: Serial changes in arterial structure following radiation therapy. Surg. Gynecol. Obstet., *145*:395–400, 1977.

44. Friedman, W. A., Day, A. L., Quisling, R. G., et al.: Cervical carotid dissecting aneurysms. Neurosurgery, *7*:207–214, 1980.

45. Garraway, W. M., Whisnant, J. P., and Drury, J.: The continuing decline in the incidence of stroke. Mayo Clin. Proc., *58*:520–526, 1983.

46. Gillum, R. F., Gomez-Martin, O., Kottke, T. E., et al.: Acute stroke in a metropolitan area, 1970 and 1980: The Minnesota Heart Survey. J. Chronic Dis., *38*:8911–8918, 1985.

47. Gold, H.: Production of arteriosclerosis in the rat: Effects of x-ray and high-fat diet. Arch. Pathol. Lab. Med., *71*:268–273, 1961.

48. Greiner, A. L.: Spontaneous dissecting aneurysms of the cervical internal carotid artery. Stroke, *7*:6, 1976.

49. Halsey, J. H., McDowell, H. A., and Gelman, S.: Transcranial Doppler and rCBF compared in carotid endarterectomy. Stroke, *17*:1206–1208, 1986.

50. Harker, L. A., Bernstein, E. F., Dilley, R. B., et al.: Failure of aspirin plus dipyridamole to prevent restenosis after carotid endarterectomy. Ann. Intern. Med., *116*:731–736, 1992.

51. Hass, W. K., Easton, J. D., Adams, H. P., Jr., et al.: A randomized trial comparing ticlopidine hydrochloride with aspirin for the prevention of stroke in high-risk patients. N. Engl. J. Med., *321*:501–507, 1989.

52. Hasso, A. N., Bird, R. C., Zinke, D. E., et al.: Fibromuscular dysplasia of the internal carotid artery: Percutaneous transluminal angioplasty. A.J.R., *136*:955–960, 1981.

53. Hertzer, N. R., Feldman, B. J., Beven, E. G., et al.: A prospective study of the incidence of injury to the cranial nerves during carotid endarterectomy. Surg. Gynecol. Obstet., *151*:781–784, 1980.

54. Higashida, R. T., Hieshima, G. B., Tsai, F. Y., et al.: Transluminal angioplasty of the vertebral and basilar artery. A.J.N.R., *8*:745–749, 1987.

55. Hobson, R., Weiss, D., Fields, W., et al. Efficacy of carotid endarterectomy for asymptomatic carotid stenosis. N. Engl. J. Med., *328*:221–227, 1993.

56. Homer, D., Ingall, T. J., Baker, H. L., et al.: Serum lipids and lipoproteins are less powerful predictors of extracranial carotid artery atherosclerosis than are cigarette smoking and hypertension. Mayo Clin. Proc., *66*:259–267, 1991.

57. Howard, V. J., Toole, J. F., Grizzle, J., et al.: Comparison of multicenter study designs for investigation of the efficacy of carotid endarterectomy. Stroke, *23*:583–593, 1992.

58. Imparato, A. M., Riles, T. S., Ramariz, A. A., et al.: Early complications of carotid surgery. Int. Surg., *69*:223–229, 1984.

59. Javid, H., Ormand, C. S., Williams, S. D., et al.: Seventeen year experience with routine shunting in carotid artery surgery. World J. Surg., *3*:167–178, 1979.

60. Kachel, R., Basche, S., Heerklotz, I., et al.: Percutaneous transluminal angioplasty (PTA) of supra-aortic arteries especially the internal carotid artery. Neuoradiology, *33*:191–194, 1991.

61. Kamik, R., Valentin, A., Ammerer, H. P., et al.: Evaluation of vasomotor reactivity by transcranial Doppler and acetazolamide test before and after extracranial intracranial bypass in patients with internal carotid artery occlusion. Stroke, *23*:812–817, 1992.

62. Kirkpatrick, J. B.: Pathogenesis of foam cell lesions in irradiated arteries. Am. J. Pathol., *50*:291–309, 1967.

63. Konings, A. W. T., Smit Sibinga, C. T., and Lamberts, H. B.: Initial events in radiation-induced atheromatosis. Strahlenther. Onkol., *156*:134–138, 1980.

64. Lamberts, H. D., and de Boer, W. G. R. M.: Contributions to the study of immediate and early x-ray reactions with regard to chemoprotection: VII. X-ray-induced atheromatous lesions in the arterial wall of cholesterolemic rabbits. Int. J. Radiat. Biol., *9*:165–174, 1965.

65. Lane, J. I., Flanders, A. E., Doan, H. T., et al.: Assessment of carotid artery patency on routine spin-echo MR imaging of the brain. A.J.N.R., *12*:819–826, 1991.

66. Langfitt, T., Goldring, S., and Zervas, N.: The extracranial-intracranial bypass study: A report of the committee appointed by the American Association of Neurologic Surgeons to examine the study. N. Engl. J. Med., *316*:817–820, 1987.

67. Lanzino, G., Andreoli, A., Di Pasquale, G., et al.: Etiopathogenesis and prognosis of cerebral ischemia in young adults: A survey of 155 treated patients. Acta Neurol. Scand., *84*:321–325, 1991.

68. Lash, S., Newell, D., Mayberg, M. M., et al.: Artery to artery cerebral emboli detection with transcranial Doppler: Analysis of eight cases. J. Stroke Cerebrovasc. Dis., *3*:15–22, 1993.

69. Leape, L. L., Park, R. E., Solomon, D. H., et al.: Relation between

surgeon's practice volumes and geographic variation in the rate of carotid endarterectomy. N. Engl. J. Med., 321:653–657, 1989.

70. Liapsis, D. C., Satiani, B., Florance, C. L., et al.: Motor speech malfunction following carotid endarterectomy. Surgery, 89:56–59, 1981.

71. Lie, J. T.: Pathology of occlusive disease of the extracranial arteries. In Sundt, T. M., Jr., ed.: Occlusive Cerebrovascular Disease. Philadelphia, W. B. Saunders, 1987, pp. 19–37.

72. Lindsay, S., Kohn, H. I., Dakin, R. L., et al.: Aortic arteriosclerosis in the dog after localized aortic x-irradiation. Circ. Res., 10:51–60, 1962.

73. Little, J. R., Moufarrij, N. A., and Furlan, A. J.: Early carotid endarterectomy after cerebral infarction. Neurosurgery, 24:334–338, 1989.

74. Liu, M. W., Roubin, G. S., and King, S. B.: Restenosis after coronary angioplasty: Potential biologic determinants and the role of intimal hyperplasia. Circulation, 79:1374–1387, 1989.

75. Lusby, R. J., and Wylie, E. J.: Complications of carotid endarterectomy. Surg. Clin. North Am., 63:1293–1302, 1983.

76. Luscher, T. F., Lie, J. T., Stanson, A. W., et al.: Arterial fibromuscular dysplasia. Mayo Clin. Proc., 62:931–952, 1987.

77. Mayberg, M. R., and Newell, D. W.: Advances in non-invasive imaging. In Selman, W., ed.: Clinical Neurosurgery. Baltimore, Williams & Wilkins, 1990, pp. 166–179.

78. Mayberg, M. R., Wilson, S. E., Yatsu, F., et al.: V. A. Cooperative Studies Program No. 309: The role of carotid endarterectomy in preventing cerebral ischemia from symptomatic carotid stenosis. J.A.M.A., 266:3289–3294, 1991.

79. McDowell, H. A., Jr., Gross, G. M., and Halsey, J. H.: Carotid endarterectomy monitored with transcranial Doppler. Ann. Surg., 215:514–518, 1992.

80. McGovern, P. G., Burke, G. L., Sprafka, J. M., et al.: Trends in mortality, morbidity, and risk factor levels for stroke from 1960 through 1990. J.A.M.A., 268:753–759, 1992.

81. Meyer, F. B., Sundt, T. M., Jr., Piepgras, D. G., et al.: Acute Carotid Occlusion. In Sundt, T. M., Jr., ed.: Occlusive Cerebrovascular Disease. Philadelphia, W. B. Saunders, 1987, pp. 269–279.

82. Michenfelder, J. D., Stundt, T. M., Fode, N., et al.: Isoflurane when compared to enflurane and halothane decreases the frequency of cerebral ischemia during carotid endarterectomy. Anesthesiology, 67:336, 1987.

83. Mokri, B., Piepgras, D. G., and Houser, O. W.: Traumatic dissections of the extracranial internal carotid artery. J. Neurosurg., 68:189–197, 1988.

84. Moore, W. S., and Malone, J. M.: Effect on flow rate and vessel calibre on critical arterial stenosis. J. Surg. Res., 26:1, 1979.

85. Murros, K. E., and Toole, J. F.: The effect of radiation of carotid arteries. Arch. Neurol., 46:449–455, 1989.

86. National Center for Health Statistics: Advance report of final mortality statistics, 1986. Monthly Vital Stat. Rep., 40:1–55, 1992.

87. Newell, D. W., and Aaslid, R.: Transcranial Doppler. New York, Raven Press, 1992.

88. Norris, J. W., Zhu, C. Z., Bornstein, N. M., et al.: Vascular risks of asymptomatic carotid stenosis. Stroke, 22:1485–1490, 1991.

89. North American Symptomatic Carotid Endarterectomy Trial Collaborators: Beneficial effect of carotid endarterectomy in symptomatic patients with high-grade stenosis. N. Engl. J. Med., 325:445–453, 1991.

90. O'Leary, D. H., and Clouse, M. E.: Percutaneous transluminal angioplasty of the cavernous carotid artery for recurrent ischemia. A.J.N.R., 5:644–5, 1984.

91. O'Leary, D. H., Potter, J. E., and Clouse, M. E.: Non-invasive tests as an indicator of carotid stenosis. Acta Radiol., 369:11–13, 1986.

92. Pessin, M. S., Duncan, G. W., Mohr, J. P., et al.: Clinical and angiographic features of carotid transient ischemic attacks. N. Engl. J. Med., 296:358–362, 1977.

93. Piepgras, D. G., Sundt, T. M., Jr., Marsh, W. R., et al.: Recurrent carotid stenosis: Results and complications of 57 operations. Ann. Surg., 203:205–213, 1986.

94. Ramsay, S. C., Yeates, M., Lord, R. S., et al.: Use of technetium-HMPAO to demonstrate changes in cerebral blood flow reserve following carotid endarterectomy. J. Nucl. Med., 32:1382–1386, 1991.

95. Reisner, A., and Barrow, D. L.: Neurosurgical aspects of fibromuscular dysplasia. In Barrow, D. L., ed.: Perspect. Neurol. Surg., 2:27–54, 1991.

96. Roederer, G. O., et al.: The natural history of carotid disease in asymptomatic patients with cervical bruits. Stroke, 15:605–613, 1984.

97. Rostomily, R. C., Mayberg, M. R., Eskridge, J., et al.: Resolution of petrous internal carotid artery stenosis after transluminal angioplasty. J. Neurosurg., 76:520–523, 1992.

98. Rubin, J. R., Bondi, J. A., and Rhodes, R. S.: Duplex scanning versus conventional arteriography for the evaluation of carotid artery plaque morphology. Surgery, 102:749–755, 1987.

99. Rubin, P., and Casarett, G. W.: Clinical Radiation Pathology. Philadelphia, W. B. Saunders, 1968, pp. 43–51.

100. Shaw, D. A., Venables, G. S., Cartilidge, N. E. F., et al.: Carotid endarterectomy in patients with transient cerebral ischemia. J. Neurol. Sci., 64:45–53, 1984.

101. Slavish, L. G., Nicholas, G. G., and Gee, W.: Review of a community hospital experience with carotid endarterectomy. Stroke, 15:956–959, 1984.

102. Spetzler, R. F., Martin, N., Hadley, M. N., et al.: Microsurgical endarterectomy under barbiturate protection: A prospective study. J. Neurosurg., 65:63–73, 1986.

103. Strandness, D.: Noninvasive tests for carotid disease: Conventional Doppler ultrasound. In Barnett, H., ed.: Stroke: Pathophysiology, Diagnosis, and Management. New York, Churchill Livingstone, 1986.

104. Sundt, T. M.: The ischemic tolerance of neural tissue and the need for monitoring and selective shunting during carotid endarterectomy. Stroke, 14:93–98, 1983.

105. Sundt, T. M., Sandok, B. A., and Whisnant, J. P.: Carotid endarterectomy: Complications and preoperative assessment of risk. Mayo Clin. Proc., 50:301–306, 1975.

106. Sundt, T. M., Whisnant, J. P., Houser, O. W., et al.: Prospective study of the effectiveness and durability of carotid endarterectomy. Mayo Clin. Proc., 65:625–635, 1990.

107. Sundt, T. M., Jr.: Was the international randomized trial of extracranial-intracranial arterial bypass representative of the population at risk? N. Engl. J. Med., 316:814–816, 1987.

108. Sundt, T. M., Jr., Houser, O. W., Whisnant, J. P., et al.: Correlation of postoperative and two-year follow-up angiography with neurological function in 99 carotid endarterectomies in 86 consecutive patients. Ann. Surg., 203:90–100, 1986.

109. Sundt, T. M., Jr., Sharbrough, F. W., Piepgras, D. G., et al.: Correlation of cerebral blood flow and electroencephalographic changes during carotid endarterectomy, with results of surgery and hemodynamics of cerebral ischemia. Mayo Clin. Proc., 56:533–543, 1981.

110. Sutton-Tyrrell, K., Wolfson, S. K., Jr., Thompson, T., et al.: Measurement variability in duplex scan assessment of carotid atherosclerosis. Stroke, 23:215–220, 1992.

111. Tanganelli, P., Bianciardi, G., Centi, L., et al.: B-mode imaging and histomorphometric evaluation of carotid atherosclerosis. Angiology, 41:908–914, 1990.

112. Tegeler, C. H., Shi, F., and Morgan, T.: Carotid stenosis in lacunar stroke. Stroke, 22:1124–1128, 1991.

113. Theron, J., Raymond, J., Casaco, A., et al.: Percutaneous angioplasty of atherosclerotic and postsurgical stenosis of carotid arteries. A.J.N.R., 8:495–500, 1987.

114. Tiamson, E., Anzola, E., Fritz, K., et al.: The effect of low dosage irradiation on rabbit atherosclerosis. Circulation, 37(Suppl):VI-25, 1968.

115. Towne, J. B., and Bernhard, V. M.: The relationship of postoperative hypertension to complications following carotid endarterectomy. Surgery, 88:575–580, 1980.

116. Towne, J. B., Weiss, D. G., and Hobson, R. W.: First phase report of cooperative Veterans Administration Asymptomatic Carotid Stenosis Study: Operative morbidity and mortality. J. Vasc. Surg., 11:252–259, 1990.

117. A Veterans Administration Cooperative Study: Role of carotid endarterectomy in asymptomatic carotid stenosis. Stroke, 17:534–539, 1986.

118. Warlow, C.: Carotid endarterectomy: Does it work? Stroke, 15:1068–1076, 1984.

119. Wiebers, D. O.: Effectiveness of carotid endarterectomy for

asymptomatic carotid stenosis: Design of a clinical trial. Mayo Clin. Proc., *64*:897–904, 1989.

120. Whisnant, J. P., Matsomoto, N., and Elveback, L. R.: Transient cerebral ischemic attacks in a community. Mayo Clin. Proc., *48*:194–198, 1973.

121. Whisnant, J. P., Sandok, B. A., and Sundt, T. M.: Carotid endarterectomy for unilateral carotid system transient cerebral ischemia. Mayo Clin. Proc., *58*:171–175, 1983.

122. Wilson, S. E., Mayberg, M. R., and Yatsu, F. R.: Defining the indications for carotid endarterectomy. Surgery, *104*:932–933, 1988.

123. Wolf, P. A., Kannel, W. B., and McGee, D. L.: Epidemiology of Strokes in North America. In Barnett, H. J. M., Mohr, J. P., Stein, B. M., et al., eds.: Stroke: Pathophysiology, Diagnosis and Management. New York, Churchill Livingstone, 1986, pp. 3–30.

124. Yonas, H., Steed, D. L., Latchaw, R. E., et al.: Relief of nonhemispheric symptoms in low flow states by anterior circulation revascularization: A physiologic approach. J. Vasc. Surg., *5*:289–297, 1987.

125. Zarin, C. K., Giddens, D. P., Bharadvaj, B. K., et al.: Carotid bifurcation atherosclerosis: Quantitative correlation of plaque localization with flow velocity profiles and wall shear stress. Circ. Res., *53*:502, 1983.

CHAPTER 47

Extracranial Occlusive Disease of the Vertebral Artery

The syndrome of vertebrobasilar ischemia has been a source of confusion and misunderstanding since Kubick and Adams made the first pathological observation of thrombosis of the basilar artery.[23] Millikan and Seikert were the first to describe the syndrome that is now accepted as representing ischemic disease of the brain stem.[24] Multiple diagnostic techniques have been used in the evaluation of patients with vertebrobasilar insufficiency, including angiography, Doppler ultrasound, transcranial Doppler ultrasound, computed tomography, magnetic resonance imaging, and magnetic resonance angiography. Cerebral angiography remains the gold standard in the anatomical determination of occlusive lesions of the posterior circulation.

Numerous medical approaches have been used in the management of patients with vertebrobasilar disease and have had variable degrees of success. In 1955, Millikan and co-workers proposed the use of anticoagulation to treat patients suspected clinically of having basilar artery thrombosis.[24, 25] Their approach decreased the incidence of brain stem infarction in symptomatic patients by 50 per cent, but since most patients did not undergo angiographic examination, it was not possible to determine what condition was treated. Surgical approaches to the vertebrobasilar circulation have included intracranial and extracranial procedures. Surgeons have been uniformly encouraged by the symptomatic improvement observed in their patients; however, no agreement exists among neurologists and neurosurgeons about the potential benefit obtained by any surgical procedure used to treat patients with ischemia of the posterior circulation.

Until better medical treatment protocols are devised and until surgeons develop objective standards to evaluate surgical results, it will be difficult to resolve the current questions regarding the management of patients with vertebrobasilar ischemic disease.

Anatomical Features

The vertebrobasilar system is formed by the confluence of the vertebral arteries, which arise from the subclavian artery on the left and from the brachiocephalic artery on the right (Fig. 47–1). The vertebral arteries have four distinct anatomical portions. The first or proximal portion extends from the origin of the vertebral artery to the foramen transversarium of C6. The second or intraosseous portion consists of the section of the vertebral artery that traverses the foramina transversaria of C6 through C1. The third or atlantal portion extends from the exit of the vertebral artery at the C1 foramen to its entry into the dura through the atlanto-occipital membrane. The fourth or intradural portion is the subarachnoid section of the vertebral artery from its point of entry through the dura to its convergence with the opposite vertebral artery to become the basilar artery.[4]

The vertebrobasilar junction is located at the level of the midpons. The basilar artery then extends from the midpons to the upper midbrain; here, it bifurcates, giving rise to the two posterior cerebral arteries. The main arteries arising from the vertebrobasilar system are the posterior inferior cerebellar artery (from the vertebral arteries), the anterior inferior cerebellar artery (from the midportion of the basilar artery), and the superior cerebellar arteries (from the distal basilar artery before its termination). Although these three pairs of vessels are the main arteries originating from the vertebrobasilar system, numerous short and intermediate circumferential arteries, as well as perforators, originate directly from the basilar and vertebral arteries.[10, 23] The entire brain stem, the cerebellum, the occipital lobes, and part of the temporal lobes are supplied by the vertebrobasilar circulation.

The carotid circulation connects with the vertebro-

F. G. Diaz · R. R. Johnson

basilar circulation at the level of the posterior cerebral arteries, normally via the posterior communicating arteries. The posterior cerebral arteries develop embryologically from the internal carotid arteries at the level of the posterior communicating arteries. These primitive posterior cerebral arteries join with the basilar artery at the level of its terminal bifurcation, eventually becoming the P_1 or proximal portion of the posterior cerebral arteries. After embryonic development is complete, the carotid origin of the posterior cerebral artery regresses and becomes the posterior communicating artery. In most cases, the P_1 portion of the posterior cerebral artery then enlarges to form the proximal portion of the artery; however, in 25 per cent of patients, this segment remains incompletely developed or atrophies. Communication with the anterior circulation through the posterior communicating artery is functional in only 65 per cent of individuals.[10, 20] Four normal embryological arterial connections may persist after birth in some individuals (Fig. 47–2). These arteries are the trigeminal artery, which connects the intracavernous portion of the carotid artery to the tip of the basilar artery; the otic artery, which joins the intrape-

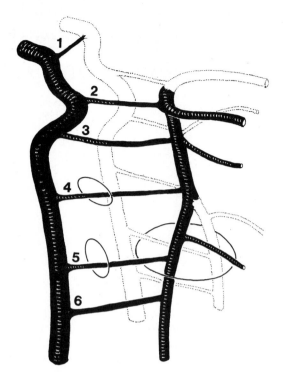

Figure 47–2

Normal embryological connections of the vertebrobasilar system and the internal carotid artery system. Anterior communicating artery (1). The posterior communicating artery connects the supraclinoid internal carotid artery to the P_1 segment of the posterior cerebral artery (2). The trigeminal artery connects the cavernous internal carotid artery to the top of the basilar artery (3). The otic artery connects the petrous internal carotid artery to the proximal basilar artery via the vidian canal (4). The hypoglossal artery connects the distal extracranial internal carotid artery to the intracranial vertebral artery via the hypoglossal canal (5). The proatlantal artery connects the distal extracranial carotid artery to the third portion of the vertebral artery (6).

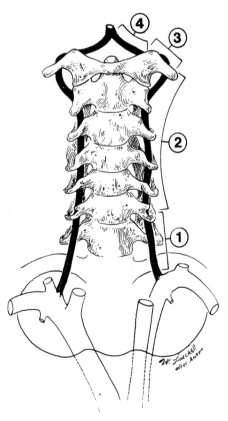

Figure 47–1

Anatomical diagram of the vertebrobasilar system. The vertebral arteries arise from the brachiocephalic trunk on the right and from the aortic arch on the left. The vertebral arteries have four distinct portions: the first portion from their origin to the entry into the foramen transversarium of C6 (1); the second portion from the C6 foramen to the C1 foramen (2); the third portion from the exit of the C1 foramen to their entry through the atlanto-occipital membrane (3); and the fourth portion from the entry through the dura to the vertebrobasilar junction (4).

trous carotid artery to the midportion of the basilar artery; the hypoglossal artery, which connects the extracranial internal carotid artery to the intracranial vertebral artery; and the proatlantal artery, which links the extracranial internal carotid artery to the extracranial vertebral artery at the C2 level.[35] The trigeminal artery is purely subarachnoid and is easy to identify intracranially. The otic artery is partly intrapetrous, coursing through the vidian canal to become subarachnoid and join the midportion of the basilar artery. The hypoglossal artery is initially extracranial in origin and gains access to the intracranial cavity through the hypoglossal canal. The proatlantal artery is entirely extracranial.

The extracranial vertebral artery is surrounded by an extensive venous plexus that extends from the third portion of the artery and follows the artery into and throughout the second portion as it travels through the foramina transversaria. It drains into the vertebral vein at the level of the sixth or seventh transverse process, which subsequently drains into the subclavian vein.

Pathological Features

The vertebrobasilar circulation may be affected by a variety of processes, of which arteriosclerosis plays the most important role.[29, 30, 35] Schwartz and Mitchell described arteriosclerotic lesions at the origin of the vertebral artery as the most common abnormality found in a large group of unselected autopsies.[30] Second in frequency were arteriosclerotic deposits in the second portion of the vertebral artery, as the artery passes through the foramina transversaria. It is uncertain why the intraosseous portion of the vertebral artery in the foramina transversaria is a site of deposition of arteriosclerotic material. It is intuitively possible that the segmental damping effect of the pulsatile expansion of the artery may contribute to the deposition of lipids in the wall. Third in frequency with respect to arteriosclerotic plaque formation is the vertebrobasilar junction, probably because of the flow turbulence that develops as the two vertebral arteries come together to form the basilar artery. Arteriosclerotic lesions at other levels are less frequent and include the point of entry of the vertebral artery through the dura, and the middle and distal portions of the basilar artery.[5, 20, 23, 24, 30] The frequency of atherosclerosis in the vertebral artery is variable and in general is lesser than that in the carotid artery territory.[35]

Other pathological conditions of the vertebrobasilar system include spontaneous dissection of the vertebral arteries with the formation of pseudoaneurysms and complete occlusion (Fig. 47–3). Spontaneous dissection is frequently observed in association with fibromuscular hyperplasia of the vertebral arteries or the carotid arteries.[24, 29] Fibromuscular changes have been observed at all levels of the first three portions of the vertebral

artery but have not been reported in the fourth portion. Spontaneous dissections observed in association with fibromuscular disease have occurred mostly in the distal second and third portions of the vertebral artery.[24, 29]

Direct trauma to the vertebral artery caused by penetrating wounds or severe cervical spine fracture-dislocations can result in occlusion, dissecting pseudoaneurysms, or arteriovenous fistula of the vertebral artery.[27] Traumatic occlusion or dissection of the vertebral arteries, which may extend into the basilar artery, has been reported after chiropractic manipulation of the neck.[27] The effect of trauma to the vertebral arteries induced by chiropractic manipulation is not necessarily age-dependent or related to pre-existing pathology. The mechanism proposed for the injury relates to the areas of fixation of the artery at the level of the foramina transversaria and to the sudden traction that is introduced. Since the artery is tethered at two fixed points within its intraosseous course, the sudden stretch of the artery between these two points causes the vessel to tear and allows traumatic dissection and occlusion of the artery to occur.

External encroachment on the vertebral artery from osteophytic spurs arising from the cervical vertebrae may compress the second portion of the vertebral artery and produce symptoms of vertebrobasilar insufficiency generally associated with dynamic changes in the position of the cervical spine.[19, 31] These changes are most frequently seen in individuals with severe spondylitic and osteoarthritic spurs and are frequently missed when arteriography is performed on a patient

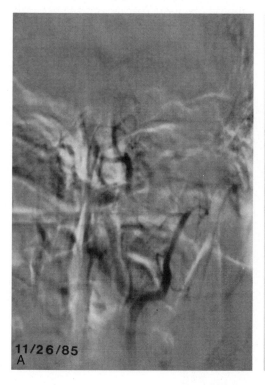 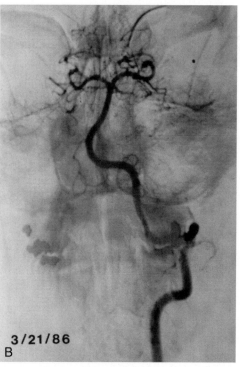

Figure 47–3

Spontaneous dissection of the vertebral artery. *A.* Selective left vertebral angiography demonstrates high-grade stenosis of the distal vertebral artery at the atlanto-occipital membrane, with slight distal filling of the vertebrobasilar junction. *B.* Selective left vertebral arteriography performed 4 months after the initial study and following treatment with full anticoagulation demonstrates spontaneous recanalization of the vertebral artery.

who is in the resting state. It is necessary to perform dynamic angiography with the head turned in the direction known to induce the symptoms.

Compression of the vertebral artery at C6 by ligamentous bands from the anterior scalene muscle also can cause vertebrobasilar insufficiency.[31] In patients with osteophytic spurs that compress the second portion of the vertebral artery and in those with ligamentous bands that compress the artery as it enters the C6 foramen, it frequently is possible to precipitate the symptoms with rotation of the neck. In these patients, dynamic angiography done while the neck is rotated in the direction that produces the symptoms usually reveals the exact level of the occlusion.

The subclavian steal syndrome is a clinical entity associated with symptoms of vertebrobasilar insufficiency, and it is generally provoked by active use of the left arm.[9, 18] The increased demand for blood triggered by the activity, coupled with the occlusion of the subclavian artery before the origin of the left vertebral artery, results in the shunting of blood into the left subclavian artery through many muscular collaterals and in the reversal of flow in the left vertebral artery. The left vertebral artery carries flow from the intracranial circulation to the left arm (Fig. 47–4). The flow reversal in these circumstances is generally well tolerated, as long as the patient is not using the left arm repeatedly or to the point of causing an increase in arterial demand. When the demand for blood flow in the left arm increases, more arterial flow is diverted from the cerebral circulation; this causes partial ischemia of the brain stem.

Most emboli in the vertebrobasilar territory originate from sources other than the vertebral artery itself, including the cardiac valves or areas of previous myocardial infarction; atrial thrombi; atrial myxomas; arterio-sclerotic plaques of the aorta, subclavian, or innominate arteries; and pathological emboli of systemic origin.[29]

Clinical Features

The syndrome of vertebrobasilar insufficiency is characterized by intermittent episodes of neurological dysfunction that usually include multiple symptoms. The symptoms usually are repetitive, but they can be progressive or can occur as a single, sudden, severe event with resultant complete and permanent neurological dysfunction. The syndrome of vertebrobasilar insufficiency can be observed in patients who have at least two of the following symptoms: (1) motor or sensory symptoms, or both, occurring bilaterally during the same attack; (2) ataxia of gait; (3) diplopia; (4) dysarthria; (5) dysmetria; and (6) bilateral homonymous hemianopsia.[36] Additional symptoms compatible with this syndrome are vertigo, tinnitus, multiple cranial nerve involvement (usually contralateral to the major sensory deficit), and motor involvement of the extremities. Dizziness by itself, syncope, drop attacks, and transient global amnesia do not form part of the syndrome of vertebrobasilar insufficiency. If any of these symptoms occurs alone, other causes besides vertebrobasilar insufficiency should be considered.[29, 36] No study has correlated any specific combination of symptoms and the angiographic findings observed in patients with vertebrobasilar insufficiency.

The differential diagnosis of vertebrobasilar disease should exclude cardiac problems such as dysrhythmias, myocardial insufficiency, and the presence of emboli. Emboli of cardiac origin may arise from a prior myocardial infarction, from valvular disease, or from

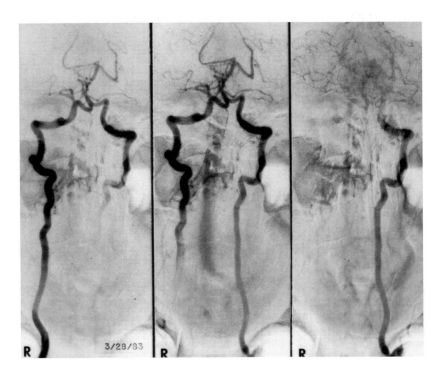

Figure 47–4

Vertebral artery steal. Selective sequential right vertebral angiography reveals filling of the right vertebral artery, with initial crossover through the vertebrobasilar junction and eventual filling of the entire left vertebral artery. Steal resulted from complete occlusion of the subclavian artery before the origin of the vertebral artery.

subacute bacterial endocarditis. Any potential hematological problem associated with the development of hypercoagulability, including thrombocytosis, sickle cell disease, or macroglobulinemias, should be ruled out. Women who smoke, who are taking contraceptives, and who present with events of basilar migraine may develop symptoms that mimic vertebrobasilar ischemia. Bleeding disorders characterized by intraparenchymal hemorrhages could result in the development of sudden neurological dysfunction in the vertebrobasilar distribution. The abrupt onset of symptoms and the severity of the clinical picture would be comparable only with thrombosis of the basilar artery with complete loss of function of the brain stem.

Other processes that may resemble the vertebrobasilar insufficiency syndrome include demyelinating disease (which usually occurs in younger individuals) and intracranial neoplasms, such as tumors of the cerebellopontine angle region or intra-axial tumors of the cerebellum. In some cases, Ménière's syndrome could mimic vertebrobasilar insufficiency and, therefore, must be excluded.

Since the differential diagnosis can be difficult, complete ancillary tests are necessary to rule out other problems. Routine laboratory examinations required include a complete differential blood count as well as a blood smear and complete coagulation profile, a metabolic battery, 12-lead electrocardiography, and Holter monitoring for 24 or 36 hours. Computed tomography excludes most intracranial sources of nonvascular structural pathology.[29] With the recent introduction of positron emission tomography, the metabolic function of the brain stem or cerebellum can be determined; however, this modality's application to the study of vertebrobasilar ischemic disease has been limited. Magnetic resonance imaging has improved diagnostic capabilities and scanning resolution in patients evaluated for vertebrobasilar insufficiency (Fig. 47–5). Not only do the resolution capabilities of the technique permit the study of the anatomical characteristics of the brain stem and the cerebellum, as with computed tomography, but they also permit the metabolic study of these structures with magnetic resonance spectroscopy.

Selective cerebral angiography is the most definitive diagnostic tool for establishing the nature of the vascular involvement in the patient with vertebrobasilar insufficiency (Fig. 47–6).[10, 13, 20] Currently, angiography has an acceptable overall mortality of 0.6 per cent, with a rate of major complications of less than 1 per cent.[5] The introduction of intra-arterial digital cerebral angiography and nonionic contrast agents has reduced further the incidence of postangiography problems. Digital angiography obtains excellent diagnostic images with relatively low doses of contrast medium and reduces the contrast load required in patients with serious renal or cardiac problems who may be at risk if large volumes of contrast material are used. An interesting diagnostic tool for vascular imaging that is now undergoing development is magnetic resonance angiography. This procedure does not require the administration of contrast material and is noninvasive. As the diagnostic accuracy and precision of magnetic resonance angiography increase, it will become the ideal diagnostic tool for evaluating the cerebral circulation. Current limitations with magnetic resonance angiography include the relative inability to perform a selective study of one arterial territory at a time; difficulty in separating the arterial, capillary, and venous phases; and the relative conglomeration of vessels seen on the monitoring screen. Future developments should permit the selective visualization of individual vessels as well

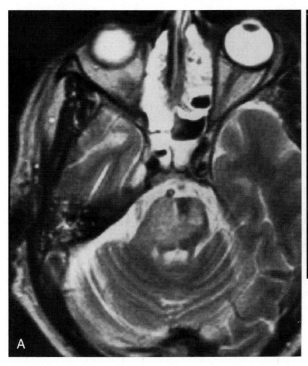

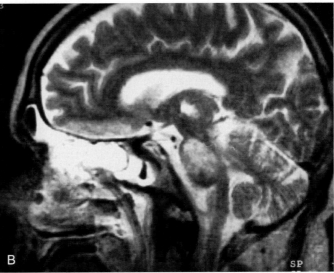

Figure 47–5

Magnetic resonance imaging in patient with basilar artery thrombosis. *A.* This axial scan demonstrates extensive high-intensity signal in the entire ventral portion of the pons, with more significant changes on the right side. *B.* The sagittal scan demonstrates the extent of the ischemic changes to include the entire pons in a rostrocaudal direction.

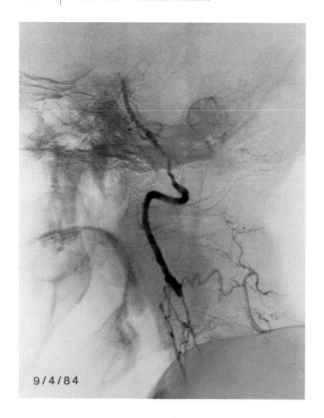

9/4/84

Figure 47–6

Selective cerebral angiography. Selective arteriography of the cerebral vessels allows the precise localization of lesions affecting the vertebral artery. In this patient with complete proximal occlusion of both vertebral arteries, right carotid artery injection with delayed subtraction technique demonstrates persistent patency of the right vertebral artery through muscular collaterals.

as three-dimensional imaging of the vascular territories in relation to selected cerebral structures.

Medical Management

The medical management of patients with vertebrobasilar insufficiency has progressed little since the mid-1950's. In the 1950's, Millikan and co-workers introduced systemic anticoagulation to treat patients with vertebrobasilar ischemic symptoms.[25] They observed a decline in the mortality rate from 43 per cent in an untreated group of patients to 24 per cent in a group of patients treated with heparin. Angiography was not performed on any of their patients, other major causes of symptoms were not ruled out, and patients were not randomly assigned to treatment groups. All patients were assumed to have impending basilar occlusion before the treatment started, but no definitive clinical study was performed to document their conclusions. Whisnant and associates reported a decreased incidence of brain stem stroke from 35 per cent to 15 per cent within 4 years in patients with symptoms of vertebrobasilar ischemia who received oral anticoagulants.[36] A treatment group and a control group were chosen, but most patients had not undergone angiographic examination and were not assigned randomly to the two treatment groups.

Other forms of treatment, such as the administration of antiplatelet agents, are used to treat patients with vertebrobasilar disease; however, the effectiveness of this treatment in averting strokes cannot be reliably predicted in an individual patient. In patients with

angiographically confirmed impending basilar artery occlusion caused by a local thrombus or from a systemic embolus, systemic or locally infused streptokinase and urokinase have been used. The hemorrhagic complications resulting from the systemic administration of these drugs and their limited efficacy have discouraged their use. The local application of streptokinase has met with some success and has led to the administration of tissue plasminogen activator in a similar manner. The cost of tissue plasminogen activator has been a major limiting factor in its use. Comparative studies that have evaluated the differences between it and streptokinase in cardiac patients have not shown either to have a significant benefit over the other for intravascular clot lysis.

Strict blood pressure control should be discouraged in patients who have angiographically demonstrated, hemodynamically significant lesions of the vertebrobasilar tree. In patients with severe lesions, a significant drop in blood pressure could acutely alter the perfusion to the ischemic brain and create a watershed area of ischemia.[16, 29] Hypertension in these patients could reflect ischemia of the brain stem.

Surgical Management

The surgical management of patients with vertebrobasilar insufficiency has been controversial since Crawford and colleagues reported the surgical approach to lesions of the extracranial vertebral artery in 1958.[13] Initial surgical procedures, including endarterectomy of the vertebral artery origin through the vertebral artery wall or through the subclavian artery, were poorly received.[16, 17, 21] These procedures were associated with many complications, including occlusion of the vertebral artery, postoperative hematomas, phrenic nerve paresis, lymphoceles, and chyle fistulae. It was not until the early 1970's that Edwards and Wright reported a successful series of proximal extracranial vertebral artery reconstructions for the treatment of patients with vertebrobasilar insufficiency.[17]

Several procedures for treating extracranial lesions of the vertebral artery are currently in use. The most common is the transposition of the vertebral artery from its origin to a new location, generally the ipsilateral common carotid artery.[9, 16, 17] The vertebral artery is exposed through a supraclavicular incision made 2 cm above the clavicle and just across the midline. The surgeon approaches the prevertebral fascia by dissecting the space medial to the sternocleidomastoid muscle, thus exposing the common carotid artery, the jugular vein, and the vagus nerve. The sympathetic ganglia and their branches are found immediately beneath the prevertebral fascia, directly over the anterior scalene muscle. The ascending pharyngeal artery and the posterior cervical arteries are frequently in the operative field adjacent to the cervical sympathetic plexus. The vertebral artery can be found as it travels from its origin to the foramen transversarium of C6, lateral to the longus colli muscle, medial to the anterior scalene muscle, and deep to the vertebral vein and sympathetic chain (Fig. 47–7).

Care must be taken to identify the thoracic duct as it enters the angle formed by the confluence of the jugular vein and the subclavian vein. The lymphatic duct generally is formed by three or four small branches that enter the venous angle from a deep to a more superficial location. When the vertebral artery

origin is dissected, the lymphatics are generally clearly visible with loupe magnification. The lymphatics are larger on the left side than on the right but should and can be identified on either side. The lymphatic ducts should be identified, and transfixion ligated to prevent the ultimate development of a chyle fistula or a chyle cyst. Lymphatics do not coagulate well and must be ligated if satisfactory control of them is to be achieved. Once the lymphatics are ligated, they can be transected to expose the origin of the vertebral artery.

When exposing the vertebral artery on the right side, it is important to devote special attention to the retraction exerted on the trachea and the esophagus. The recurrent laryngeal nerve is located in the tracheoesophageal groove and is very close to the area of exposure after it loops around the subclavian artery to return to the larynx. On the left side, the recurrent laryngeal nerve is more lax because it loops around the aortic arch, and thus the trachea can be retracted with greater freedom. Extreme retraction of the recurrent laryngeal nerve results in paresis of the ipsilateral vocal cord, which in most cases is temporary but in a small percentage may be permanent.

Length of vertebral artery sufficient for an anastomosis may be gained by means of dissection of the entire vertebral artery from its origin to the foramen transversarium. The vertebral artery is located directly below the vertebral vein, and many times it is completely covered by the vein. To expose the artery, it is necessary to coagulate and transsect the vein. Coagulation of the vein may be difficult because it forms a plexus that surrounds the artery as it exits the foramen transversarium. Coagulation of the vein can be difficult, since the vein is sometimes densely adherent to the artery. Careful separation of the vein is required before it can be coagulated. The vertebral artery is transsected after

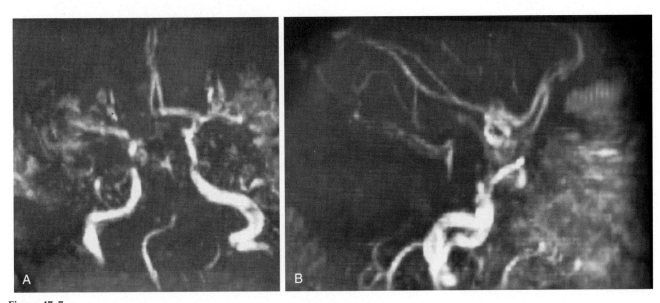

Figure 47–7

Cerebral magnetic resonance arteriography. *A.* This anteroposterior view of the intracranial circulation on magnetic resonance angiography demonstrates with clarity the absence of the proximal portion and minimal filling of the top of the basilar artery. Note also the absence of the right A_1 segment of the anterior cerebral artery. *B.* Lateral magnetic resonance angiography demonstrates complete occlusion of the proximal basilar artery, with distal recanalization of the basilar artery and posterior cerebral arteries via patent posterior communicating arteries.

it has been ligated at its origin and temporarily clipped at the foramen transversarium. A fish-mouth stoma is prepared on the free end of the vertebral artery, and the common carotid artery is then clamped proximally and distally. A fenestration is made on the lateral wall of the carotid artery, and an end-to-side anastomosis between the vertebral and the common carotid arteries is completed under magnification (Fig. 47–8).

Transposition of the subclavian artery to the common carotid artery has been performed for patients with subclavian steal syndrome secondary to subclavian artery occlusion.[17] This procedure is preferable to the vertebral artery–to–carotid artery transposition in patients who have intermittent claudication of the upper extremity. Other angioplastic procedures of the vertebral artery origin include vertebral endarterectomy, patch grafting of the vertebral artery origin with removal of the atherosclerotic plaque, and angioplastic reconstruction, which widens and shortens the vertebral artery in patients with poststenotic ectasia of the first portion of the vertebral artery.[21]

Saphenous vein grafts and prosthetic grafts have been placed from the subclavian artery to the vertebral artery or from the common carotid artery to the vertebral artery distal to the area of stenosis.[8, 15] The vertebral artery is exposed in the same manner as that described for the vertebral artery–to–carotid artery transposition. Then, a saphenous vein graft is obtained from the lower portion of the leg. The greater saphenous vein may be found immediately posterior to the medial malleolus and superficial to the medial malleolar ligament. The graft is obtained in a conventional manner, and care should be taken to cauterize or ligate side branches without damaging the vein wall. It is also important not to strip the vein clean of all periadventitial tissue, since this could damage the vasa vasorum and result in endothelial necrosis. When the dissection is completed, the vein should be gently distended with warm heparinized blood or saline with the use of a pressure-regulated balloon providing no more than 200 to 300 mm of water pressure. The vein is then stored in cold heparinized blood or saline until it is needed. The distal portion of the vein must be identified so that the anastomosis is performed with proper orientation of the valves.

In patients in whom the graft will be placed from the carotid artery to the vertebral artery, the carotid artery has been exposed during the initial dissection. In patients in whom the anastomosis of the graft is to come from the subclavian artery, it is necessary to disinsert the two heads of the sternocleidomastoid muscle to expose the length of the subclavian artery. The vertebral artery is then temporarily occluded at the foramen transversarium and ligated at the origin. The proximal end is transsected, a fish-mouth stoma is made, and an end-to-end anastomosis is completed with the vein graft. Next, the proximal anastomosis is performed either on the carotid artery or on the subclavian artery in a manner similar to that described for the vertebral artery–to–carotid artery transposition. Special

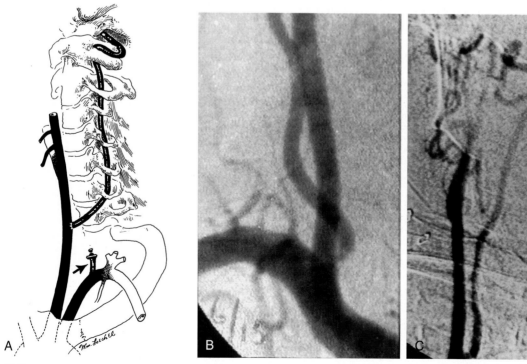

Figure 47–8

Vertebral artery-to-carotid artery transposition. *A.* The surgeon identifies origin of the vertebral artery by locating the angle formed by the anterior scalene muscle and the longus colli muscle and by following the artery in a proximal direction to its origin. The origin of the vertebral artery is ligated, and the end of the artery is anastomosed to the side of the common carotid artery. *B.* Preoperative selective digital subtraction angiography demonstrates stenosis of the origin of the right vertebral artery. *C.* Intraoperative digital subtraction angiography of the right carotid artery demonstrates recanalization of the vertebral artery through a patent vertebral artery–to–carotid artery transposition.

care must be taken to back-bleed the anastomosis before the last suture is closed so that air and possible thrombi can exit the artery.

Balloon angioplasties have been successfully performed at the origin of the vertebral artery and in the subclavian artery proximal to the origin of the vertebral artery. However, the rate of recurrence of occlusion is nearly 35 per cent within the first 6 months after angioplasty.

Decompressive procedures have been used to treat lesions in the second portion of the vertebral artery. Fibrous bands originating from the anterior scalene muscle can easily be released at the level of entry of the vertebral artery into the C6 foramen.[12, 16, 21] Decompressive osteotomies of the foramina transversaria can be performed at a single level or at multiple levels throughout the course of the vertebral artery from C6 to C1 foramina via an anterior or lateral route.[19, 31] When the foramina are removed for decompression, it is necessary to remove the periosteum that surrounds the vertebral artery; if the periosteum is not removed, then the areas of constriction could persist. In some patients, it is not possible to remove all areas of stenosis in the second portion of the vertebral artery. In such patients, it is possible to perform a high vertebral artery–to–carotid artery transposition to the external or the internal carotid arteries.

Vascular reconstruction with the use of a long saphenous vein graft or a prosthetic graft traveling from the subclavian artery or the common carotid artery to the vertebral artery distal to the point of stenosis has been reported for patients with arteriosclerotic areas of stenosis in the second portion of the vertebral artery.[11, 12] Anastomosis of a branch or the trunk of the external carotid artery to the second portion of the vertebral artery has also been reported.[12, 26] To accomplish these procedures, the anterior surfaces of one or two of the foramina above the level of stenosis are exposed through an anterior incision made along the sternocleidomastoid muscle. The common carotid artery and the bifurcation are dissected in the usual manner and retracted laterally to expose the deep cervical fascia. The transverse processes are identified, and the longus colli muscle is dissected from the anterior surface of the transverse process. The anterior and lateral walls of the transverse processes are removed, and the periosteum adjacent to the vertebral artery canal is resected. The venous plexus surrounding the vertebral artery is carefully separated, cauterized, and transsected to expose the vertebral artery. It is usually necessary to remove two or three foramina to expose a sufficient length of the vertebral artery.

When the vertebral artery is free, several management options are available. Whenever possible, the surgeon may dissect out the plaque by inverting the vertebral artery and gradually separating the plaque until it feathers out; alternatively, he or she may remove the plaque by creating a longitudinal arteriotomy, dissecting the plaque out in a conventional manner, and closing the artery. Either maneuver would leave sufficient vertebral artery length for a transposition to the carotid bifurcation (Fig. 47–9). If the surgeon believes

that it is not possible to resect the plaque and mobilize a length of vertebral artery sufficient to perform a transposition, then it is necessary to perform either saphenous vein grafting from the carotid artery or an end-to-side anastomosis to the second portion of the vertebral artery from one of the major branches of the external carotid artery—either the occipital artery or the ascending pharyngeal artery.

For arteriosclerotic lesions in the first or second foraminal level of the vertebral artery, it is sometimes possible to perform an anastomosis of the occipital artery or saphenous vein grafting to the third portion of the vertebral artery. The vertebral artery is exposed through an anterolateral incision that extends from the anterior border of the sternocleidomastoid muscle below the angle of the jaw to the highest point of the mastoid bone along the path of the external occipital artery. To expose the occipital artery, the mastoid attachment of the sternocleidomastoid muscle is transsected and the posterior portion of the digastric muscle is disinserted. The superior and inferior oblique muscles are transsected at the level of the lateral mass of C1 as the vertebral artery exits from the foramen. The vertebral artery is freed of the surrounding vertebral venous plexus and dissected from the foramen transversarium of C1 to its entrance into the skull at the atlanto-occipital membrane. If the segment of vertebral artery dissected is not long enough for the anastomosis, the atlanto-occipital membrane and dura mater may be opened to expose the fourth portion of the vertebral artery. Temporary clips are applied at the most proximal and distal ends of the vertebral artery, a longitudinal arteriotomy is performed, and an end-to-side anastomosis is completed with the occipital artery or a saphenous vein graft (Fig. 47–10).

Vertebral endarterectomies have been performed in patients with highly stenotic areas in the third and fourth portions of the vertebral artery usually associated with contralateral or high-grade stenosis or with vertebral artery occlusion.[1, 5] The vertebral artery is approached through a suboccipital craniotomy performed with the patient lying in a three-quarter prone position. A midline or paramedian approach is used and extended laterally until the vertebral artery is exposed and dissected from its exit at the first transverse process to its entry into the atlanto-occipital membrane. The vertebral artery is surrounded by a venous plexus that must be carefully dissected, cauterized, and transsected. When dissection is complete, the dura is opened from the midline in the direction of the vertebral artery entry. The perimedullary portion of the vertebral artery is dissected to expose the origin of the posterior inferior cerebellar artery. If a vertebral endarterectomy is required, the artery can be clipped proximally at C1 and distally before the posterior inferior cerebellar artery. A longitudinal arteriotomy is made, and the plaque is dissected under microscopic magnification. After the plaque is removed, the arteriotomy is closed with running 6–0 or 7–0 polypropylene sutures (Fig. 47–11). During the occlusion period, patients receive an intravenous bolus of 250 mg of

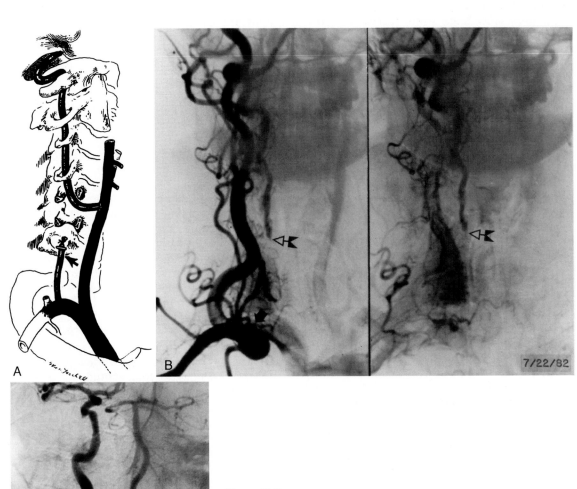

Figure 47–9

Endarterectomy of the second portion of the vertebral artery, and vertebral artery–to–carotid artery transposition. *A.* The surgeon exposes the second portion of the vertebral artery by removing the artery from the bony canal. The artery is ligated at its proximal end, and an endarterectomy is performed by means of reversing the artery on itself. The plaque is removed from within, and an end-to-side anastomosis is performed from the vertebral artery to the common carotid or the internal carotid artery. *B.* Selective arteriography of the right innominate artery demonstrates complete occlusion of the proximal vertebral artery, with recanalization of the second portion of the artery through muscular collaterals. *C.* Selective postoperative arteriography of the right carotid artery demonstrates recanalization of the entire vertebral artery after a successful endarterectomy and vertebral artery–to–carotid artery transposition.

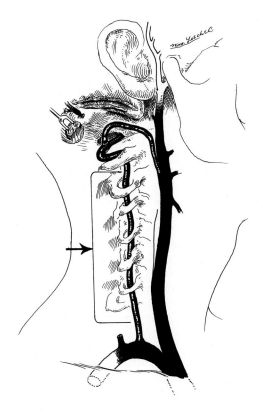

Figure 47–10

Anastomosis of the occipital artery to the distal vertebral artery. The occipital artery is dissected on the dorsal surface of the temporo-occipital area and followed proximally, with transsection of the insertion of the sternocleidomastoid muscle. The third portion of the vertebral artery can be found after the oblique muscles covering the atlanto-occipital membrane have been separated. An anastomosis is completed on the third portion of the vertebral artery.

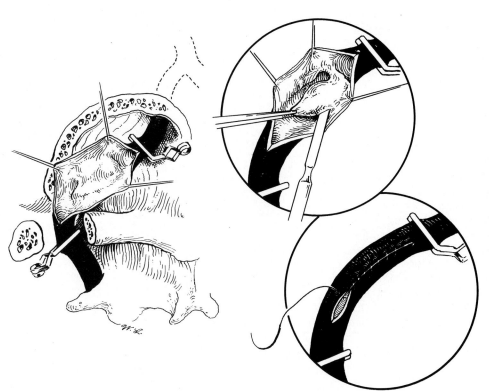

Figure 47–11

Distal vertebral artery endarterectomy. The third and fourth portions of the vertebral artery are dissected, and the vertebral artery is isolated between temporary clips. An endarterectomy is completed, and the arteriotomy is closed with a running suture.

thiopental, 100 mg of lidocaine (Xylocaine), and 5,000 U of heparin.

Sundt attempted balloon dilatation of the distal vertebral artery under direct observation but observed significant problems following the angioplasty, including vertebral artery dissections, thrombosis, and perforation.[32] Sundt abandoned the use of intracranial vertebral angioplasty following this dismal experience. The results for endarterectomy were initially promising, but further experience revealed the occurrence of many complications, including brain stem infarctions such as those found by Sundt during balloon angioplasties. Neither endarterectomy nor angioplasty of the distal vertebral artery is now recommended.

Various forms of extracranial-intracranial anastomoses have been described for the management of patients with bilateral distal lesions of the vertebral artery, including anastomosis of the occipital artery to the posterior inferior cerebellar artery or to the second portion of the anterior inferior cerebellar artery, and anastomosis of the superficial temporal artery to the superior cerebellar artery or to the posterior cerebral artery.* The saphenous vein graft may be used to join the extracranial carotid artery to the posterior cerebral artery or to the superior cerebellar artery.[33, 34]

The surgical results for patients who had an extracranial reconstructive procedure of the vertebral artery have been encouraging, with a neurological morbidity of 2 per cent and a mortality of 1 per cent.[14] The intracranial reconstructive procedures, including angioplasties of the fourth portion of the vertebral artery and all types of extracranial-to-intracranial anastomoses, have been associated with a greater incidence of complications.[6] The greatest number of complications were observed in patients who had unstable neurological syndromes with signs of progressing ischemia or stroke in evolution.

Conclusions

Current information indicates that the stroke risk for untreated patients symptomatic for vertebrobasilar ischemia is 35 per cent within 4 years after the onset of symptoms.[36] The risk of stroke decreased by 50 per cent in symptomatic patients treated with anticoagulants, although no angiographic evidence exists that these patients had significant arterial lesions compatible with their symptomatology.[36] The surgical morbidity for patients with angiographically proven, significant vertebrobasilar lesions is 5 per cent, and the surgical mortality 3 per cent.[4, 15] Since no controlled study has compared the best medical treatment with the best surgical treatment, the approach to each patient must be individualized. Intuitively, it is reasonable to treat patients medically. If medical therapy fails in otherwise untreatable patients, surgery may then be justified.

*See references 2, 3, 4, 7, 22, 28, 33, and 34.

REFERENCES

1. Allen, G. S., Cohen, R. J., and Preziosi, T. J.: Microsurgical endarterectomy of the intracranial vertebral artery for vertebrobasilar transient ischemic attacks. Neurosurgery, 8:56, 1981.
2. Ausman, J. I., Nicoloff, D. M., and Chou, S. N.: Posterior fossa revascularization: Anastomosis of vertebral artery to PICA with interposition radial artery graft. Surg. Neurol., 9:281, 1978.
3. Ausman, J. I., Diaz, F. G., de los Reyes, R. A., et al.: Anastomosis of occipital artery to anterior inferior cerebellar artery for vertebrobasilar junction stenosis. Surg. Neurol., 16:69, 1981.
4. Ausman, J. I., Diaz, F. G., de los Reyes, R. A., et al.: Microsurgical techniques on cerebral revascularization. Henry Ford Hosp. Med. J., 31:3, 1983.
5. Ausman, J. I., Diaz, F. G., Pearce, J. E., et al.: Endarterectomy of the vertebral artery from C2 to posterior inferior cerebellar artery intracranially. Surg. Neurol., 18:400, 1982.
6. Ausman, J. I., Diaz, F. G., Vacca, D. F., et al.: Superficial temporal artery and occipital artery bypass pedicles to superior, anterior inferior and posterior inferior cerebellar arteries for vertebrobasilar insufficiency. J. Neurosurg., 72:554, 1990.
7. Ausman, J. I., Lee, M. C., Klassen, A. L., et al.: Stroke: What's new? Cerebral revascularization. Minn. Med., 59:223, 1976.
8. Berguer, R., and Bauer, R. B.: Vertebral artery reconstruction: A successful technique in selecting patients. Ann. Surg., 193:441, 1981.
9. Bohmfalk, G. L., Storey, J. L., Brown, W. E., et al.: Subclavian steal syndrome: Parts 1, 2. J. Neurosurg., 51:628, 1979.
10. Caplan, L. R., and Rosenbaum, A. E.: Role of cerebral angiography and vertebrobasilar occlusive disease. J. Neurol. Neurosurg. Psychiatry, 38:601, 1975.
11. Clark, K., and Perry, M. O.: Carotid vertebral anastomosis: An alternate for repair of the subclavian steal syndrome. Ann. Surg., 163:414, 1966.
12. Corkill, G., French, B. N., Michas, C., et al.: External carotid–vertebral artery anastomosis for a vertebrobasilar insufficiency. Surg. Neurol., 7:109, 1977.
13. Crawford, E. S., DeBakey, M. E., and Fields, W. S.: Roentgenographic diagnosis and surgical treatment of basilar artery insufficiency. J.A.M.A., 166:509, 1958.
14. Diaz, F. G., and Ausman, J. I.: Surgical therapy in vascular brain stem diseases. In Hofferberth, B., Brune, G. G., Sitzer, G., et al., eds.: Vascular Brain Stem Diseases. Basel, Karger, 1990, pp. 270–281.
15. Diaz, F. G., Ausman, J. I., de los Reyes, R. A., et al.: Surgical correction of lesions affecting the vertebral artery. Surg. Forum, 33:495, 1982.
16. Diaz, F. G., Ausman, J. I., Shrontz, C., et al.: Combined reconstruction of the vertebral and carotid artery in one single procedure. Neurosurgery, 12:629, 1983.
17. Edwards, W. H., and Wright, R.: A new surgical technique for relief for subclavian stenosis. Hosp. Pract., 7:78, 1972.
18. Fisher, D. M.: A new vascular syndrome: The subclavian steal. N. Engl. J. Med., 265:912, 1961.
19. Hardin, C.: Vertebral artery insufficiency produced by cervical osteoarthritic spurs. Arch. Surg. (Chicago), 90:629, 1965.
20. Hass, W. K., Fields, W. B., North, R. R., et al.: Joint study of extracranial arterial occlusion: II. Arteriography, techniques, sites and complications. J.A.M.A., 203:96, 1968.
21. Imparato, A. M.: Surgery for extracranial cerebrovascular insufficiency. In Ransohoff, J., ed.: Modern Techniques in Surgery: Neurosurgery. Installment II. Mount Kisco, Futura, 1980, pp. 1–38.
22. Kodadad, G.: Occipital artery–posterior inferior cerebellar artery anastomosis. Surg. Neurol., 5:225, 1976.
23. Kubick, C. S., and Adams, R. D.: Occlusion of the basilar artery: A clinical and pathological study. Brain, 69:73, 1946.
24. Millikan, C. H., and Seikert, R. G.: Studies in cerebrovascular disease: I. The syndrome of intermittent insufficiency of the basilar arterial system. Mayo Clin. Proc., 3:61, 1965.
25. Millikan, C. H., Siekert, R. G., and Shick, R. M.: Studies in cerebrovascular disease: III. The use of anticoagulant drugs in the treatment of insufficiency or thrombosis within the basilar arterial system. Mayo Clin. Proc., 30:116, 1955.
26. Pritz, M. B., Chandler, W. F., and Kindt, G. W.: Vertebral artery

disease: Radiologic evaluation, medical management, and microsurgical treatment. Neurosurgery, *9*:524, 1981.

27. Rosenwasser, R., Delgado, T., and Buchheit, W.: Cerebrovascular complications of closed neck and head trauma: Injuries to the carotid artery. Surg. Rounds, *12*:56, 1983.

28. Roski, R. A., Spetzler, R. F., and Hopkins, L. N.: Occipital artery to posterior inferior cerebellar artery bypass for vertebrobasilar ischemia. Neurosurgery, *10*:44, 1982.

29. Sahs, A. L., and Hartmann, E. C.: Fundamentals of Stroke Care. Washington, D.C., U.S. Department of Health, Education and Welfare Publication (HRA) 76-14016, 1976.

30. Schwartz, C. J., and Mitchell, J. R. A.: Atheroma of the carotid and vertebral artery systems. B.M.J., *2*:1057, 1961.

31. Sheehan, S., Bauer, R., and Meyer, J. S.: Vertebral artery compression in cervical spondylosis. Neurology (Minneap.), *70*:968, 1960.

32. Sundt, T. M.: Transluminal angioplasties for basilar artery stenosis. Mayo Clin. Proc., *55*:673, 1981.

33. Sundt, T. M., Jr., Whisnant, J. P., Piepgras, D. G., et al.: Intracranial bypass grafts for vertebrobasilar ischemia. Mayo Clin. Proc., *53*:12, 1978.

34. Sundt, T. M., Jr., Whisnant, J. P., Piepgras, D. G., et al.: Interposition saphenous vein grafts for advanced occlusive disease and large aneurysms in the posterior circulation. J. Neurosurg., *56*:205, 1982.

35. Taveras, J. M., and Wood, E. H.: Diagnostic Neuroradiology. Vol. 2. Baltimore, Williams & Wilkins, 1976, pp. 543–986.

36. Whisnant, J. P., Cartlidge, N. E. F., and Elvebach, L. R.: Carotid and vertebrobasilar transient ischemic attacks: Effects of anticoagulants, hypertension, and cardiac disorders on survival and stroke occurrence [A population study]. Ann. Neurol., 3:107, 1978.

Operative Management of Intracranial Arterial Occlusive Disease

The surgical management of intracranial arterial occlusive disease has markedly changed over the past decade primarily because of a clearer understanding of the natural history of this condition, improved medical management, and the evolution of endovascular therapeutic techniques. We currently consider only a very select group of patients with intracranial arterial occlusive disease and resultant cerebral ischemia for operative treatment, and selection criteria and treatment modalities remain evolutionary.

Focal Ischemia and the Therapeutic Window

The pathophysiology and medical management of cerebral ischemia have been discussed previously (see Chapters 44 and 45). These subjects are briefly summarized here only as a basis for surgical considerations that may be applicable to acute and subacute or chronic ischemia discussed in subsequent sections.

THERAPEUTIC WINDOW

Although the phenomenon may vary with the underlying pathological process and arterial territory, there is now considerable clinical and experimental evidence supporting the concept that focal cerebral ischemia exists as a dense ischemic focus (umbra) surrounded by a less dense ischemic zone (penumbra). Neurons within the umbra of profound focal ischemia become threatened after only a few minutes and will not survive unless reperfusion is established early after the ictus. However, neuropil within the penumbra may have a considerably longer viability. This window of

opportunity for penumbral viability has been termed the "therapeutic window," and current therapy is directed toward limiting the damage and salvaging the cells in this border-zone ischemic area within this time frame. The magnitude of the therapeutic window is variable and is determined by the severity of the ischemic insult, which, to a large degree, is dependent on the duration of ischemia and the extent of collateral flow.[4, 14, 43, 44]

FOCAL ISCHEMIA

At the cellular level, the secondary factors most implicated in the evolution of focal ischemic injury include increases in intracellular cytosolic calcium, acidosis, and the production of free radicals.[43, 44] Salvage of ischemic tissue during the therapeutic window has two areas of focus: maximizing perfusion and minimizing the secondary effects of ischemia.

Maximizing perfusion includes improving natural collateral flow using such measures as hemodilution, enhancement of cerebral perfusion pressure, and avoidance of cerebral vasoconstriction as may occur with profound hyperventilation. Anticoagulant therapy may be beneficial in preventing recurrence or progression of the thromboembolic process, but its beneficial effect remains unproven and therapy in the acute setting carries some risk for secondary hemorrhagic and, rarely, thrombotic complications.[5] Also, perfusion may be maximized by instigating reperfusion techniques such as intravenous or intra-arterial thrombolytic therapies and surgical re-establishment of flow.

Measures of theoretical benefit under investigation to protect viable neurons against the secondary effects of ischemia include hypothermia, inhibitors of excitatory amino acids, calcium channel blockers, ganglio-

D. G. Piepgras • J. L. D. Atkinson

sides, lazaroides, free radical scavengers, and inhibitors of lipid peroxidation.[14, 44]

Acute Symptomatic Ischemia

Acute cerebral ischemia due to intracranial arterial occlusion encompasses a variety of causes. Innovative medical therapies may eventually prove beneficial for a wide spectrum of acute focal ischemia. There are few situations in which surgery is indicated, although in certain cases of major intracranial arterial occlusion, emergent surgical therapy, either endovascular or transcranial, becomes a consideration.

Most intracranial nonlacunar ischemic arterial occlusions are due to complications of atheromatous disease in the extracranial cerebral vessels or elsewhere with secondary intracranial embolic occlusion.[10, 16] Angiographic studies have demonstrated arterial occlusions in up to 76 per cent of middle cerebral artery distribution ischemia, of which 25 to 35 per cent will reperfuse naturally within 48 hours and 95 per cent by 2 to 3 weeks.[6, 7, 41] Rapid dissolution of middle cerebral artery thrombus or migration of embolus with resolution of major neurological deficits has been documented.[35] Likewise, recanalization of middle cerebral artery occlusions within 8 hours in conjunction with collateral flow has been demonstrated to have a favorable impact on infarct size and neurologic outcome.[41, 46] Although lysis of acute intracranial arterial embolic occlusions often occurs spontaneously, the time course is often outside the critical therapeutic window, and the natural history of acute middle cerebral artery occlusion is characteristically one of a major, though variable, neurological deficit.[11, 15, 49, 50] Hemorrhagic transformation may complicate embolic arterial occlusion and may be related to factors other than recanalization, such as age and the size of the infarct.[37] The use of anticoagulant, notably heparin, in acute stroke is controversial and probably increases the risk for hemorrhagic infarction. In rare cases, heparin may actually precipitate arterial occlusion secondary to heparin-induced thrombosis.[5]

Practical guidelines for the management of patients with acute ischemic stroke have been reviewed and well summarized; the reader is referred to this publication for a discussion of the generally accepted medical as well as surgical treatments and their rationale.[1]

Surgical interventions have attempted to target early reperfusion of focally ischemic tissue during the therapeutic window when potentially viable cells may be salvaged. In the experimental setting, the benefit of early reperfusion has been consistently demonstrated, whereas in the clinical experience, the effects have been less dramatic and less consistent, undoubtedly related in part to variability of mechanisms and degree of ischemic insult.[45–47]

In the following sections, we propose criteria for selection of patients and surgical techniques that may be utilized in the treatment of acute and subacute or chronic focal cerebral ischemia and life-threatening infarction.

SURGICAL INTERVENTION FOR REVASCULARIZATION

Extracranial-to-intracranial bypass has been advocated in the treatment of acute cerebral ischemia but realistically is probably justified in only exceptional circumstances.[8, 47, 48] In select cases, surgery for acute cerebral ischemia may involve techniques of embolectomy, endarterectomy, or primary vessel repair. Pharmacological thrombolysis constitutes an attractive alternative to open embolectomy, with these agents being administered either intravenously or through selective angiographic catheterization of the occluded vessel. Optimism exists for pharmacological thrombolytic therapy in acute ischemia since this form of therapy has proven beneficial in acute coronary artery thrombosis.[3, 13, 20, 34, 39]

Selective endovascular techniques for delivery of thrombolytic agents have shown promise, particularly in anecdotal cases, most of which have involved thromboembolic stroke in hospitalized patients and those undergoing endovascular procedures. Whether such therapy could consistently be carried out within a therapeutic window for a broader spectrum of strokes and whether it might prove more efficacious than systemically administered thrombolytic therapy remains uncertain.[22, 23, 53, 54] Neuroprotective agents may augment the benefit from thrombolytic therapy.[30, 42] Thrombolytic therapy is not without significant risks, and large-scale clinical trials will be necessary to define the indications and patient selections to determine its role in acute cerebral ischemia.[13, 31, 39] In our limited experience, although thrombolytic therapy may be effective in achieving reperfusion (Fig. 48–1), in certain acute thrombotic conditions this is not always possible, especially in the situation of a well-organized embolus as may originate from a chronic cardiac thrombus.

In cases of embolic middle cerebral occlusion, which are defined in the acute setting with angiography, it is our policy to attempt selective arterial catheterization and pharmacological thrombolytic therapy unless there exist clear contraindications. If thrombolytic therapy does not prove beneficial after a limited attempt, particularly in cases in which an organized cardiac thrombus is suspected, consideration is given to surgical embolectomy.

The role of surgical treatments in acute major cerebral ischemia has always been controversial, and while intracranial middle cerebral artery embolectomy has been performed with moderate and sometimes dramatic success in small case series, it must be admitted that these patients are highly selected.[17, 20, 34] Only rarely has embolectomy been carried out in other intracranial vessels.[33] Our experience comprises a series of somewhat greater than 20 cases of middle cerebral embolectomy performed over the past 25 years.[34] Based on this experience and the experimental evidence in the focal ischemia/reperfusion model, we believe that if revascularization and reperfusion can be done within a 6- to 8-hour therapeutic window, the outcome is superior to that of the natural history. In very select cases with even longer periods of ischemia, embolectomy and

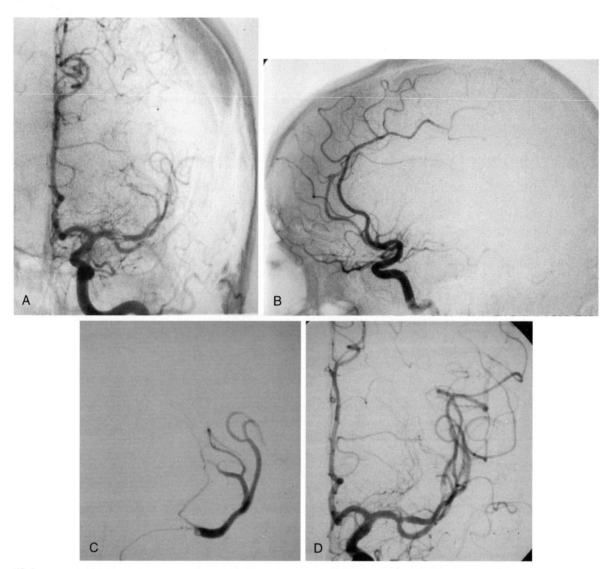

Figure 48–1

Left carotid angiogram demonstrating acute thrombus in the proximal middle cerebral artery segment with markedly slow filling of the distal segments. *A.* Anteroposterior view. *B.* Lateral view. This study was done within 6 hours of the onset of the stroke. *C.* Intra-arterial selective infusion of urokinase. *D.* Anteroposterior view after urokinase infusion.

restoration of flow may achieve good results. When done using microsurgical technique, our experience is that a solitary middle cerebral embolus can be successfully extracted, the adjacent propagated clot removed, and flow restored with patency preserved in the majority of cases. Nevertheless, this surgery should be considered far from routine and seems indicated only in those patients in whom a middle cerebral trunk occlusion is identified angiographically within a few hours of onset. Special consideration must be given to the makeup of the embolus and whether it proves responsive to medical thrombolytic therapy.[9, 12, 36, 38, 39]

Operative Technique

Operative preparations for middle cerebral embolectomy are performed under normocarbic general anesthesia often supplemented with barbiturate infusion for cerebral protection and induced hypertension to maximize cerebral collateral flow until flow can be restored through the occluded segment. The procedure is performed through a pterional craniotomy, exposing the middle cerebral artery and, if necessary, the carotid bifurcation in the opened sylvian fissure. The location of the occlusion is predicted by preoperative angiography, but it can usually also be readily identified at the middle cerebral bifurcation as a pale focus within the arterial wall. A proximal dark discoloration is typically present, owing to the stagnant column of blood proximal to the site of occlusion.

Temporary vascular clips are placed proximal and distal to the site of obstruction. We prefer to make a longitudinal arteriotomy just distal to the embolus preferably in a large M_2 branch. The embolus can then be gently milked out of the bifurcation and extracted. In some cases, however, it is necessary to extend the arteriotomy into the M_1 segment for complete removal of the embolus. Antegrade and retrograde flow is then sequentially restored by release of the temporary clips to wash out remaining propagated thrombus. (Failure to achieve good flow has been the exception in our experience and usually indicates more extensive embolization with a failure to either restore patency or improve the patient's neurological condition.) The arteriotomy is then closed simply with 9–0 or 10–0 monofilament sutures (Fig. 48–2). Normotension is maintained postoperatively.

Our results with 20 patients undergoing emergency intracranial embolectomy are summarized in Table 48–1. Before surgery, each of these patients manifest a severe neurological deficit, including hemiplegia and a reduced level of consciousness. Aphasia was present in those patients with dominant hemisphere involvement. Postoperatively, two patients (10 per cent) had an excellent outcome and five (25 per cent) made a good recovery (Fig. 48–3). Seven patients (35 per cent) achieved a fair outcome while four (20 per cent) were considered to have a poor result and two (10 per cent) died. One of the deaths and two of the poor outcomes were associated with an inability to restore flow in the middle cerebral complex. As mentioned earlier, it was found that an organized fibrin-platelet embolus was more conducive to complete removal whereas those of an atherosclerotic origin tended to be more fragmented and dispersed into the distal middle cerebral branches. This experience leads us to conclude that surgery should be reserved for those cases in which a more solid organized embolus can be anticipated, these generally being of cardiac origin. Friable atherosclerotic emboli that originate from procedures such as vascular surgery or angiography in the great vessels and carotid arteries were less amenable to complete extraction and

restoration of flow; and, therefore, these patients are less likely to be considered candidates for surgical embolectomy by our present criteria.

SURGICAL DECOMPRESSION FOR COMPLETED INFARCTION

Extensive brain infarction may be accompanied in its acute and subacute stages by swelling due to cytotoxic and vasogenic edema and occasionally associated hemorrhagic infarction. In these cases, progressive mass effect may prove life threatening, owing to increased intracranial pressure and herniation. Resection of the infarcted tissue to control increasing pressure and optimize cerebral perfusion can provide protection of uninvolved brain, patient salvage, and, depending on the extent and location of the infarction, possibly a functional recovery.

CEREBELLAR INFARCTION

Resection of cerebellar infarction has been advocated in patients in whom life-threatening deterioration is occurring from focal cerebellar swelling, herniation, and brain stem compression or secondary fourth ventricular obstruction and hydrocephalus. Particularly in those patients without primary ischemic brain stem involvement, resection of the swollen infarcted portion of the cerebellum often results in rewarding salvage.[24, 25, 32] These infarctions have been previously described simply as posterior inferior cerebellar artery distributions with or without vertebral artery involvement, but

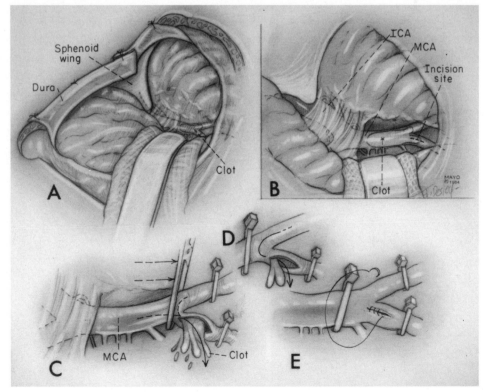

Figure 48–2

Operative sequence for middle cerebral embolectomy. The middle cerebral artery (MCA) complex is exposed through a pterional craniotomy (A). In this example the clot has involved the main trunk and extends proximally to the lenticulostriate arteries. The arteriotomy is preferably made in one of the branches of the middle cerebral artery (B). Temporary clips are placed on the branches distal to the embolus, and the clot is milked out with the aid of antegrade flow (C). With sequential removal of the clips, retrograde flow is used to remove the distal aspect of the embolus (D). The arteriotomy is closed with a running or interrupted 9–0 or 10–0 suture (E). ICA, internal carotid artery. (From Meyer, F. B., Piepgras, D. G., Sundt, T. M., Jr., et al.: Emergency embolectomy for acute occlusion of the middle cerebral artery. J. Neurosurg., 62:641, 1985. © 1984 Mayo. By permission of Mayo Foundation.)

Table 48–1
CLINICAL DATA IN 20 PATIENTS UNDERGOING EMERGENCY EMBOLECTOMY

Patient No.	Age (yr), Sex	Occlusion Site	Source of Embolus	Occlusion Time (hr)	Preoperative Collateral Flow	Backflow at Surgery	Postoperative Patency*	Operative Results†	Carotid Occlusion
1	69, F	Left branch	Heart	18	Fair	Yes	Patent	Good	No
2	57, F	Left trunk	Heart	14	Good	Yes	Patent	Good	No
3	57, M	Left trunk	Heart	8	?	Yes	Patent	Fair	No
4	68, M	Left branch	Aorta	5	Poor	None	No	Poor	No
5	65, F	Left trunk	Cardiac operation	14	Poor	Poor	—‡	Death	Yes
6	55, M	Right trunk	?	7	Fair	Yes	Patent	Fair	No
7	62, M	Left trunk	?	8	Good	Yes	Patent	Excellent	No
8	70, M	Right branch	Carotid artery	5.5	Fair	Yes	Patent	Fair	No
9	58, M	Left trunk	Aorta	6	None	None	No	Death	No
10	53, F	Left trunk	Heart	6.5	Fair	Yes	Patent	Fair	No
11	52, F	Left trunk	Heart	4.5	Poor	Yes	Patent	Fair	No
12	67, F	Left branch	Carotid artery	6.5	Good	Yes	Patent	Good	Yes
13	76, F	Left trunk	Heart	12	Good	Yes	Patent	Good	No
14	56, M	Left trunk	Carotid artery	7	Poor	Yes	Patent	Poor	Yes
15	59, F	Left trunk	Carotid artery	4.5	Fair	Yes	Patent	Poor	Yes
16	18, F	Left trunk	Aneurysm	3.5	Good	Yes	Patent	Good	No
17	31, F	Left trunk	Carotid artery	5	Good	Yes	Patent	Excellent	No
18	59, M	Left trunk	Carotid artery	3	?	Yes	Patent	Fair	Yes
19	57, M	Left trunk	Aorta	4–8	Good	Yes	Patent	Fair	Yes
20	16, M	Right trunk	Carotid artery	48	None	None	No	Poor	Yes

*Results obtained from angiography.
†Patients 3 and 15 had postoperative hemorrhagic infarctions and patient 19 had transient rhinorrhea.
‡Postoperative angiography was not performed.

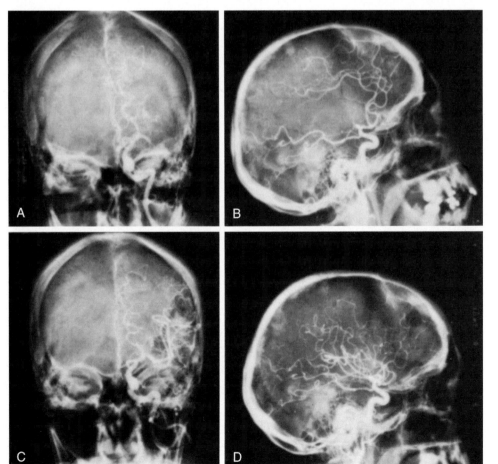

Figure 48–3

Left carotid angiograms demonstrating occlusion of the middle cerebral artery trunk. *A.* Anteroposterior view. *B.* Lateral view. The study was done within 2 hours of the onset of the stroke, which was caused by embolus of cardiac origin. *C and D.* Study done 8 days after middle cerebral embolectomy shows that all major branches of the middle cerebral artery are filling. The absence of mass effect due to cerebral edema is apparent.

more precise clinicoanatomical descriptions have now been published.[2, 21, 28] In a series of 28 postmortem specimens, cerebellar swelling was associated with multiple infarcts overlapping the posterior inferior cerebellar artery distribution with anterior inferior cerebellar artery or superior cerebellar artery territories. In a report of 13 cases of multiarterial infarctions, 8 had cerebellar swelling with tonsillar herniation.[2] Kase and co-workers studied 66 cases of cerebellar infarctions in posterior inferior cerebellar artery or superior cerebellar artery distributions to compare clinical presentation, course, and prognosis. Posterior inferior cerebellar artery infarctions tended to present as a triad of vertigo, headache, and gait imbalance at ischemic onset, and computed tomography revealed mass effect in 30 per cent, hydrocephalus in 19 per cent, and brain stem compression resulting in death in 11 per cent of the 36 patients. Patients with superior cerebellar artery infarction typically presented with acute gait disturbance, and headache and vertigo were much less common. The clinical course in these patients was typically more benign, with mass effect or hydrocephalus occurring in only 7 per cent of the 30 patients.[28]

Patients who present with major cerebellar infarction should be observed carefully for signs of brain stem compression and developing hydrocephalus on computed tomography or magnetic resonance imaging. For those progressing to obtundation due to mass effect of the infarcted hemisphere, suboccipital craniectomy and resection of the necrotic cerebellar tissue seems strongly indicated in patients who are in an otherwise good state of health.

HEMISPHERIC INFARCTION

Unlike cerebellar infarction, emergency decompression for cerebral hemispheric infarction is not widely advocated. However, if there is a reasonable possibility that the neurological deficit will be within acceptable limits, surgery may be considered in an attempt to salvage those patients who are progressing toward death due to mass effect of the infarcted tissue. In general, candidates for surgery are those of a younger age and in good general health before the ictus. Surgical therapy in this selected group of patients should be reserved for those who have failed optimal medical therapy aimed at controlling cerebral swelling. These measures include intubation, mild to moderate hyperventilation, mannitol diuresis, and, in some cases, intracranial pressure monitoring for maintenance of adequate cerebral perfusion pressure. When performed, the resection is usually limited to resection of the core areas of infarction and nonessential frontal and temporal regions, particularly the mesial temporal structures. A large craniotomy with durotomy and skin closure allowing subgaleal decompression has been advocated by some.[18, 26, 27] In very selected cases, such surgery has achieved patient salvage with preservation of a reasonable quality of life as assessed by both family and patients.[18]

Subacute and Chronic Ischemia

The role of extracranial-intracranial bypass procedures in treatment of subacute or chronic cerebral ischemia remains controversial, in part owing to limitations in defining the condition and its natural history. The International Randomized Trial for Extracranial/Intracranial Bypass for Cerebral Ischemia found no benefit from the procedure when carried out for presumed hemodynamic ischemia secondary to inaccessible internal carotid or middle cerebral artery stenosis or internal carotid artery occlusion.[48] However, valid criticisms of the study have been raised, particularly as related to patient selection criteria and cases operated outside the study.[6, 47] Studies suggest that there is a subgroup of patients with carotid occlusion or very high grade intracranial stenosis who experience recurring or progressive cerebral ischemia due to collateral failure and who carry a higher than average risk for subsequent cerebral infarction. Admittedly, this subgroup of patients is small, but their identification by clinical characteristics and supportive physiological testing seems to be possible. Patients with abnormally low cerebral reserve capacity can be identified by positron emission tomography and cerebral blood flow studies with vasodilatory challenge.[52] In such cases with progressive cerebral ischemia, which has proven refractory to optimal medical management, extracranial-intracranial bypass, particularly with superficial temporal artery–middle cerebral artery anastomosis, seems to be justified. Also, in cases of progressive cerebral ischemia due to moyamoya disease, a variety of collateral blood flow augmentation procedures seems beneficial.[29, 51] We continue to believe that extracranial-intracranial bypass utilizing superficial temporal artery–middle cerebral artery anastomosis (or rarely interposed saphenous vein grafts) is indicated in those select cases with recurrent or progressive hemodynamic cerebral ischemia due to carotid occlusion or severe intracranial stenosis. The latter instances pose a very difficult problem, owing to the inherent risk of post–bypass-induced thrombosis of the stenotic segment. In all of these instances, patient selection and a decision for surgery should be made only after more conventional medical treatment has proved ineffective and only by an experienced cerebrovascular team.

Direct intracranial arterial endarterectomy has been used in highly selected cases in which symptoms result from a focal severe stenotic atherosclerotic plaque in the middle cerebral or vertebral trunk.[3, 19] Although case reports have demonstrated that the procedure can be effective in relieving the stenosis and symptoms, this surgery should be considered very cautiously and only after other therapeutic alternatives have been exhausted. The potential for serious complications is high, especially owing to thrombosis of the operated segment, which may result from an inability to achieve a clean endarterectomy and from the relatively small diameter of the operated vessel. In those rare situations in which direct approach to such a lesion is carried out, repair with a venous patch angioplasty may be a valuable adjunct.

Early experience with endovascular transluminal angioplasty has shown good results in selected cases in which treatment of proximal vertebral as well as extracranial carotid artery stenosis was done. However, transluminal balloon angioplasty for symptomatic distal extracranial and intracranial stenoses of the carotid, vertebral, and basilar arteries has proven hazardous, with complications including arterial thrombosis, dissection, and disruption as well as distal embolization. Newer techniques involving improved microcatheter systems are being used on a very limited and investigational basis. The safety and efficacy of these techniques remains to be demonstrated, and their employment is indicated only in highly selected cases after other therapeutic measures have failed and by consensus of an experienced cerebrovascular team, including a neurologist, neurosurgeon, and endovascular neuroradiologist.

REFERENCES

1. Adams, H. P., Jr., Brott, T. G., Crowell, R. M., et al.: Guidelines for the management of patients with acute ischemic stroke. Stroke, 25:1901–1914, 1994.
2. Amarenco, P., Hauw, J. J., Henin, D., et al.: Cerebellar infarction in the territory of the posterior inferior cerebellar artery: A clinico-pathologic study of 28 cases. Rev. Neurol. (Paris), 145:277–286, 1989.
3. Anson, J. A., and Spetzler, R. F.: Endarterectomy of the intradural vertebral artery via the far lateral approach. Neurosurgery, 33:804–811, 1993.
4. Atkinson, J. L. D., Anderson, R. E., and Sundt, T. M., Jr.: The effect of carbon dioxide on the diameter of brain capillaries. Brain Res., 517:333–340, 1990.
5. Atkinson, J. L. D., Sundt, T. M., Jr., Kazmier, F. J., et al.: Heparin-induced thrombocytopenia and thrombosis in ischemic stroke. Mayo Clin. Proc., 63:353–361, 1988.
6. Ausman, J. I., and Diaz, F. G.: Critique of the extracranial-intracranial bypass study. Surg. Neurol., 26:218–221, 1986.
7. Baird, A. E., Donnan, G. A., Austin, M. C., et al.: Reperfusion after thrombolytic therapy in ischemic stroke measured by single-photon emission computed tomography. Stroke, 25:79–85, 1994.
8. Batjer, H., Mickey, B., and Samson, D.: Potential roles for early revascularization in patients with acute cerebral ischemia. Neurosurgery, 18:283–291, 1986.
9. Benomar, A., Yahyaoui, M., Birouk, N., et al.: Middle cerebral artery occlusion due to hydatid cysts of myocardial and intraventricular cavity cardiac origin: Two cases. Stroke, 25:886–888, 1994.
10. Bogousslavsky, J., Gates, P. C., Fox, A. J., et al.: Bilateral occlusion of vertebral artery: Clinical patterns and long-term prognosis. Neurology, 36:1309–1315, 1986.
11. Bozzao, L., Fantozzi, L. M., Bastianello, S., et al.: Ischaemic supratentorial stroke: Angiographic findings in patients examined in the very early phase. J. Neurol., 236:340–342, 1989.
12. Branch, C. L., Jr., Laster, D. W., and Kelly, D. L., Jr.: Left atrial myxoma with cerebral emboli. Neurosurgery, 16:675–680, 1985.
13. Brott, T. G., Haley, E. C., Levy, D. E., et al.: Urgent therapy for stroke: I. Pilot study of tissue plasminogen activator administered within 90 minutes. Stroke, 23:632–640, 1992.
14. Camarata, P. J., Heros, R. C., and Latchaw, R. E.: "Brain attack": The rationale for treating stroke as a medical emergency. Neurosurgery, 34:144–158, 1994.
15. Caplan, L., Babikian, V., Helgason, C., et al.: Occlusive disease of the middle cerebral artery. Neurology, 35:975–982, 1985.
16. Chambers, B. R., Norris, J. W., Shurvell, B. L., et al.: Prognosis of acute stroke. Neurology, 37:221–225, 1987.
17. Chou, S. N.: Embolectomy of middle cerebral artery: Report of a case. J. Neurosurg., 20:161–163, 1963.
18. Delashaw, J. B., Broaddus, W. C., Kassell, N. F., et al.: Treatment of right hemispheric cerebral infarction by hemicraniectomy. Stroke, 21:874–881, 1990.
19. de los Reyes, R. A., Bederson, J. B., and Germano, I. M.: Direct endarterectomy of the middle cerebral artery for treatment of symptomatic stenosis: Case report. Neurosurgery, 32:464–468, 1993.
20. Dolenc, V.: Middle cerebral artery embolectomy. Acta Neurochir., 44:131–135, 1978.
21. Duncan, G. W., Parker, S. W., and Fisher, C. M.: Acute cerebellar infarction in the PICA territory. Arch. Neurol., 32:364–368, 1975.
22. Haley, E. C., Jr., Levy, D. E., Brott, T. G., et al.: Urgent therapy for stroke: Pilot study of tissue plasminogen activator administered 91–180 minutes from onset. Stroke, 23:641–645, 1992.
23. Hamilton, M. G., Lee, J. S., Cummings, P. J., et al.: A comparison of intra-arterial and intravenous tissue-type plasminogen activator on autologous arterial emboli in the cerebral circulation of rabbits. Stroke, 25:651–656, 1994.
24. Heros, R. C.: Cerebellar hemorrhage and infarction. Contemp. Neurosurg., 2:1–6, 1980.
25. Heros, R. C.: Surgical treatment of cerebellar infarction: Editorial. Stroke, 23:937–938, 1992.
26. Ivamoto, H. S., Numoto, M., and Donaghy, R. M. P.: Surgical decompression for cerebral and cerebellar infarcts. Stroke, 5:365–370, 1974.
27. Kalia, K. K., and Yonas, H.: An aggressive approach to massive middle cerebral artery infarction. Arch. Neurol., 50:1293–1297, 1993.
28. Kase, C. S., Norrving, B., Levine, S. R., et al.: Cerebellar infarction: Clinical and anatomic observations in 66 cases. Stroke, 24:76–83, 1993.
29. Kinugasa, K., Mandai, S., Kamata, I., et al.: Surgical treatment of moyamoya disease: Operative technique for encephalo-duro-arterio-myo-synangiosis, its follow-up, clinical results, and angiograms. Neurosurgery, 32:527–531, 1993.
30. Komiyama, M., Nishio, A., and Nishijima, Y.: Endovascular treatment of acute thrombotic occlusion of the cervical internal carotid artery associated with embolic occlusion of the middle cerebral artery: Case report. Neurosurgery, 34:359–364, 1994.
31. Koudstaal, P. J., Stibbe, J., and Vermeulen, M.: Fatal ischaemic brain oedema after early thrombolysis with tissue plasminogen activator in acute stroke. B.M.J., 297:1571–1574, 1988.
32. Lehrich, J. R., Winkler, G. F., and Ojemann, R. G.: Cerebellar infarction with brain stem compression: Diagnosis and surgical treatment. Arch. Neurol., 22:490–498, 1970.
33. Lougheed, W. M., Gunton, R. W., and Barnett, H. J. M.: Embolectomy of internal carotid, middle, and anterior cerebral arteries: Report of a case. J. Neurosurg., 22:607–609, 1965.
34. Meyer, F. B., Piepgras, D. G., Sundt, T. M., Jr., et al.: Emergency embolectomy for acute occlusion of the middle cerebral artery. J. Neurosurg., 62:639–647, 1985.
35. Minematsu, K., Yamaguchi, T., and Omae, T.: "Spectacular shrinking deficit": Rapid recovery from a major hemispheric syndrome by migration of an embolus. Neurology, 42:157–162, 1992.
36. Morgan, M. K., and Biggs, M. T.: Direct embolectomy of the basilar artery bifurcation: Case report. J. Neurosurg., 77:463–465, 1992.
37. Okada, Y., Yamaguchi, T., Minematsu, K., et al.: Hemorrhagic transformation in cerebral embolism. Stroke, 20:598–603, 1989.
38. O'Neill, B. P., Dinapoli, R. P., and Okazaki, H.: Cerebral infarction as a result of tumor emboli. Cancer, 60:90–95, 1987.
39. Overgaard, K., Sperling, B., Boysen, G., et al.: Thrombolytic therapy in acute ischemic stroke: A Danish pilot study. Stroke, 24:1439–1446, 1993.
40. Piazza, G., and Gaist, G.: Occlusion of middle cerebral artery by foreign body embolus: Report of a case. J. Neurosurg., 17:172–176, 1960.
41. Ringelstein, E. B., Biniek, R., Weiller, C., et al.: Type and extent of hemispheric brain infarctions and clinical outcome in early and delayed middle cerebral artery recanalization. Neurology, 42:289–298, 1992.
42. Sereghy, T., Overgaard, K., and Boysen, G.: Neuroprotection by excitatory amino acid antagonist augments the benefit of thrombolysis in embolic stroke in rats. Stroke, 24:1702–1708, 1993.

43. Siesjö, B. K.: Pathophysiology and treatment of focal cerebral ischemia: I. Pathophysiology. J. Neurosurg., 77:169–184, 1992.

44. Siesjö, B. K.: Pathophysiology and treatment of focal cerebral ischemia: II. Mechanisms of damage and treatment. J. Neurosurg., 77:337–354, 1992.

45. Sundt, T. M., Jr.: Surgical Techniques for Saccular and Giant Intracranial Aneurysms. Baltimore, Williams & Wilkins, 1990.

46. Sundt, T. M., Jr., Grant, W. C., and Garcia, J. H.: Restoration of middle cerebral artery flow in experimental infarction. J. Neurosurg., 31:311–322, 1969.

47. Sundt, T. M., Jr., Piepgras, D. G., Marsh, W. R., et al.: Saphenous vein bypass grafts for giant aneurysms and intracranial occlusive disease. J. Neurosurg., 65:439–450, 1986.

48. The EC/IC Bypass Study Group: Failure of extracranial-intracranial arterial bypass to reduce the risk of ischemic stroke: Results of an international randomized trial. N. Engl. J. Med., 313:1191–1200, 1985.

49. Tomsick, T. A., Brott, T. G., Olinger, C. P., et al.: Hyperdense middle cerebral artery: Incidence and quantitative significance. Neuroradiology, 31:312–315, 1989.

50. Tranmer, B. I., Gross, C. E., Keller, T. S., et al.: Acute middle cerebral artery occlusion: Experience with volume expansion therapy. Neurosurgery, 18:397–401, 1986.

51. Ueki, K., Meyer, F. B., and Mellinger, J. F.: Moyamoya disease: The disorder and surgical treatment. Mayo Clin. Proc., 69:749–757, 1994.

52. Yonas, H., Smith, H. A., Durham, S. R., et al.: Increased stroke risk predicted by compromised cerebral blood flow reactivity. J. Neurosurg., 79:483–489, 1993.

53. Zeumer, H., Freitag, H.-J., Grzyska, U., et al.: Local intra-arterial fibrinolysis in acute vertebrobasilar occlusion: Technical developments and recent results. Neuroradiology, 31:336–340, 1989.

54. Zeumer, H., Freitag, H.-J., Zanella, F., et al.: Local intra-arterial fibrinolytic therapy in patients with stroke: Urokinase versus recombinant tissue plasminogen activator. Neuroradiology, 35:159–162, 1993.

CHAPTER 49

Moyamoya Disease

Moyamoya disease is a cerebrovascular disease that features narrowing or stenosis starting at the distal internal carotid and proximal portions of the anterior and middle cerebral arteries. It has become known, and reports have been published about it, in every part of the world.

According to Goto and associates, 1,063 patients were reported outside Japan from 1972 through 1989.[14] True distribution of moyamoya disease, however, is not certain, because some reports did not clearly differentiate moyamoya disease from moyamoya syndrome (Table 49–1).

In the definition, moyamoya phenomenon or moyamoya effect should be differentiated from moyamoya disease.[91, 93] The syndrome or effect is due to an oligemic state caused by a clear disease entity and should be called moyamoya syndrome.

History

The first report of moyamoya disease consistent with current criteria for diagnosis was reported by Takeuchi in 1961.[90] The disease showed peculiar angiographical features, as shown in Figure 49–1. The Japanese word *moyamoya* means "wavering puff of smoke" and was used to describe the abnormal vasculature at the base of the brain.

In 1960, Kudo noticed the collateral circulation in this disease and advocated the idea of occlusion of the circle of Willis.[32] In 1965, Nishimoto and Takeuchi collected 96 cases of the disease throughout Japan and reported the symptomatological outline of the disease.[64]

In 1966, Kudo published the proceedings of the 25th Congress of the Japanese Neurosurgical Society in the name of "spontaneous occlusion of the circle of Willis."[33] In these proceedings, Suzuki discussed an angiographical staging of the disease. He also named the disease as moyamoya disease because the arterial feature appeared like a puff of smoke.

In 1969, Suzuki and Takaku published a report on this disease in English by the name of moyamoya disease and the name became used in western countries and in Japan.[84] Goto organized a research committee of the disease in 1977 that was sponsored by the Ministry of Health and Welfare of Japan. This committee publishes an annual report in the name of spontaneous occlusion of the circle of Willis. Accordingly, in Japan, two names are in use.

In the early 1980's and 1990's various surgical procedures to improve the ischemic condition due to the disease were introduced and they have been revealed to be effective (Table 49–2).[105]

Epidemiology

Moyamoya disease was once believed to be specific to the Japanese.[34] After the report by Subirana in 1962, many other reports have been noted from all over the world.[14, 79] This disease, however, is most found among Japanese, and reports outside Japan are mostly from China (519 cases in the author's collection) and Korea (289 cases in the author's collection). The number of diseased patients in Japan is now estimated to be 3,300 and the annual occurrence is believed to be around 200 cases. They are distributed evenly throughout Japan, and the male-to-female ratio is 1 to 1.6. There are two peaks in incidence (Fig. 49–2).[35] The first is at about 4 years of age when the lesions usually cause ischemia. The second peak of incidence is at about 34 years of age when most of the lesions cause hemorrhage.

Y. Matsushima

Table 49–1

CRITERIA FOR THE DIAGNOSIS OF MOYAMOYA DISEASE AND MOYAMOYA SYNDROME

Moyamoya disease is a cerebrovascular disease in which the following angiographical and etiological requirements are fulfilled:
A. Angiographical requirements:
   1. Stenosis or occlusion is observed at the terminal portion of internal carotid artery and at the proximal portion of the anterior cerebral artery, the middle cerebral artery, or both.
   2. Abnormal vascular moyamoya networks are observed in the vicinity of the previously mentioned areas in the arterial phase.
   3. These findings are observed bilaterally.
B. Etiological requirements:
   Etiology is unknown, and basic disease (e.g., arteriosclerosis, meningitis, neoplasm, Down syndrome, von Recklinghausen's disease, trauma, irradiation) is ruled out.

For the patients without angiograms, angiographical findings can be replaced by the following pathological findings:
   1. Intimal thickening and resulting stenosis or occlusion are observed around the intracranial terminal portion of the internal carotid artery, usually bilaterally. They are sometimes associated with lipoid degeneration.
   2. In the main arteries (anterior cerebral, middle cerebral, and posterior communicating arteries) constructing the circle of Willis, various degree of stenoses and occlusions are observed in association with intimal fibrous thickening, winding of the internal elastic lamina, and thinning of the tunica media.
   3. Many tiny, vascular channels (perforators and anastomotic branches) are observed around the circle of Willis.
   4. Small vessels of conglomerated networks are observed in the pia mater.

Diagnosis:
   1. Definite moyamoya disease: fulfills all of the findings described in A and B.
   2. Probable moyamoya disease: fails to fulfill the criteria in A-3, but fulfills the other criteria mentioned in the definite case.
   3. Moyamoya syndrome: fulfills all or some of the findings described in A but not B.

Modified from Yonekawa, Y., Handa, H., and Okuno, T.: Moyamoya disease: Diagnosis, treatment, and recent achievements. Stroke, 1:805–829, 1986. Reprinted by permission. Copyright 1986, American Heart Association.

Yearly occurrence has been calculated as 0.07 per cent in Japan.[24] If this number is used in calculating family occurrence, the recurrence rate in siblings is calculated at about 42 times higher than that of the general population. The recurrence rate in the offspring of the proband was 34 times that of the general population. The most likely mode of inheritance of moyamoya disease is thus considered to be multifactorial.[10]

According to the case-control study of the author's 66 patients with moyamoya disease and 132 controls, there was no significant difference in the prevalence of tonsillitis, conjunctivitis, otitis media, or bronchitis. The ratio of fever of unknown cause was 2.793, and χ^2 was 7.213. The author could not find an overt relationship between head and neck infections and the disease, though some researchers put much weight on infectious disease around the face and neck.[83, 98, 100]

Etiology

Aoyagi and co-workers have established strains of smooth muscle cells derived from extracranial arteries of patients with moyamoya disease obtained at surgery.[3] The cells proliferated less in a medium supplemented with 15 per cent serum and responded poorly to the addition of platelet-derived growth factor 5 per cent serum. This factor alone did not stimulate the cells in a quiescent state to initiate DNA synthesis in moyamoya disease, though it significantly stimulated the controls. Simultaneous addition of the erythrocyte growth factor, insulin-like growth factor I, and platelet-derived growth factor stimulated the initiation of DNA synthesis in the smooth muscle cells but not as much as the platelet-derived growth factor alone in the controls. Aoyagi and co-workers suggested from these findings that a delayed repair of the injured vascular wall, and thus a slower but somewhat longer-term rate of intimal proliferation, might be present in arteries of patients with moyamoya disease.

Aoyagi and co-workers further investigated the binding and processing of iodine-125–labeled platelet-derived growth factor and the down-regulation of the factor's receptor in the smooth muscle cells of patients with moyamoya disease.[2] They showed that when these cells were exposed to lower concentrations of nonlabeled platelet-derived growth factor the percentage of remaining binding sites on the cells was significantly less than that from controls. This excess down-regulation of receptor in the smooth muscle cells may be interpreted as insufficient recycling or a decreased intracellular pool of the factor's receptor. These results provide evidence that functional alterations in vascular cells are involved in the mechanism of development of initial thickening in moyamoya disease.

Pathology

The intima of the diseased artery is thickened with fibrous tissue, and there is lamellar formation by elastic fiber proliferation (Fig. 49–3B). The cavity of the vessels is eccentrically displaced by intimal thickening. The degree of stenosis is not necessarily symmetrical. The internal elastic lamina is folded and tortuous. No inflammatory changes are observed in the vascular wall. The findings show no great difference in children or adults.

The primary lesion described earlier is seen in intracranial internal carotid arteries, the proximal portion of the main cerebral arteries, the communicating arteries, and, occasionally, the more distal cerebral arteries, external carotid system, and other parts of the body (see Fig. 49–3A). Involvement of the posterior half of the circle of Willis is not common in the early stage.

The secondary lesions are in collateral vessels, seen as the abnormal netlike vessels at the base of the brain (basal moyamoya vessels) and leptomeningeal arteries of the cerebral surface. The dilated and tortuous perforating vessels branch off the circle of Willis, anterior choroidal arteries, internal carotid arteries, and posterior cerebral arteries. These arteries form complex channels that usually connect to the distal portion of the anterior and middle cerebral arteries. These small

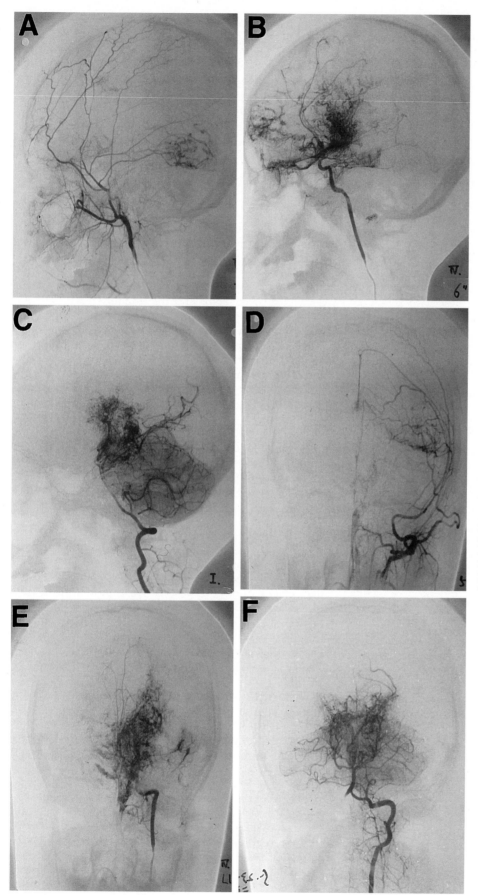

Figure 49–1

Typical angiograms of a patient with moyamoya disease. *A and D.* External carotid arteriograms, lateral and Towne's views, respectively. Marked transdural anastomoses (vault moyamoya) are observed at the temporooccipital area. *B and E.* Internal carotid arteriograms, lateral and Towne's views, respectively. Marked anterior basal moyamoya vessels are observed at the anterior basal area and ethmoidal transdural anastomoses (ethmoidal moyamoya) are observed at the frontal region. *C and F.* Vertebral arteriograms, lateral and Towne's views, respectively. Posterior basal moyamoya vessels are observed at the posterior basal area. At a little more later phase, marked leptomeningeal blood supply through the posterior cerebral artery to the anterior circulation is usually demonstrated.

Table 49–2
SURGICAL TREATMENT OF MOYAMOYA DISEASE

Procedure	Source
Direct Anastomoses	
Superficial temporal artery–middle cerebral artery anastomosis	Krayenbuehl, H.A.: Surg. Neurol., 4:353–360, 1975
Middle meningeal artery–middle cerebral artery anastomosis	Nishikawa, M., et al.: Proceedings of the 9th annual meeting of Japanese Society of Stroke Surgeons 1980, pp. 151–154
Indirect Anastomoses	
Procedures Using Dura Mater	
Durapexia	Tsubokawa, T., et al.: Neurol. Med. Chir., 6:48–49, 1964
Encephalodurosynangiosis	Wakuta, Y., et al.: Abstracts of the 9th annual meeting of the Japanese Society of Pediatric Neurosurgery, 1984, p. 56
Cranial burr holing	Endo, M., et al.: J. Neurosurg., 71:180–185, 1989
Reversed durapexia	Fujimoto, T., et al.: Abstracts of the 21st annual meeting of the Japanese Society of Pediatric Neurosurgery, 1993, p. 99.
Procedure Using Temporal Muscle	
Encephalomyosynangiosis	Karasawa, J., et al.: Neurol. Med. Chir., 17:29–37, 1977
Procedures Using Scalp Arteries	
Encephaloduroarteriosynangiosis	Matsushima, Y., et al.: Child's Nerv. Syst. (Kobe), 5:249–255, 1980
Encephaloarteriosynangiosis	Lesoin, F., et al.: Surg. Neurol., 20:318–322, 1983
Encephaloarteriosynangiosis (not that of Lesoin's)	Nakagawa, Y., et al.: Neurol. Med. Chir., 23:464–470, 1983
Encephaloarteriosynangiosis (devised especially for frontal portion)	Ichikawa, A., et al.: Neurol. Med. Chir., 29:106–112, 1989
Cerebroarteriosynangiosis	Balagura, S., et al.: Surg. Neurol., 23:270–274, 1985
Modified encephaloduroarteriosynangiosis	Rooney, C. M., et al.: J. Child. Neurol., 6:24–31, 1991
Procedure Using Omentum	
Omental transplantation	Karasawa, J., et al.: Surg. Neurol., 14:444–449, 1980
Procedure Using Galea	
Encephalogaleosynangiosis (reported as encephaloarteriosynangiosis)	Ishii, R., et al.: Stroke, 15:873–877, 1984
Procedures Using a Combination of the Above (encephalomyosynangiosis + encephaloduroarteriosynangiosis)	Nakagawa, Y., et al.: Neurol. Med. Chir., 23:464–470, 1983
Synangiodural plasty	Wanibuchi, H., et al.: Abstracts of the 44th annual meeting of the Japanese Neurosurgical Society, 1985, p. 356
Encephaloduroarteriomyosynangiosis	Kinugasa, K.: Abstracts of the 14th annual meeting of the Japanese Society of Stroke Surgeons, 1985, p. 76
Combined revascularization (extensive indirect revascularization)	Sato, H.: Abstracts of the 19th International Society of Pediatric Neurosurgery meeting. Child's Nerv. Syst. 7:281, 1991
Galeoencephaloduroarteriomyosynangiosis	Nishimoto, A.: In educational lecture at 19th annual meeting of Japanese Society of Pediatric Neurosurgery, 1991
Ribbon encephaloduroarteriomyosynangiosis	Tokunaga, K., et al.: Abstracts of the 21st annual meeting of Japanese Society of Pediatric Neurosurgery, 1993, p. 21
Nonanastomotic bypass using temporal muscle, galea, and dura mater	Hara, Y., et al.: Abstracts of the 21st annual meeting of Japanese Society of Pediatric Neurosurgery, 1993, p. 19
Others	
Cervical perivascular sympathectomy and superior cervical ganglionectomy	Suzuki, J., et al.: Child's Brain, 1:193–206, 1985

vessels seem identical with lenticulostriate arteries and thalamoperforate arteries, except for their dilatation and tortuosity. Yamashita and colleagues noticed that there were various degrees of luminal stenoses with intimal thickening and reduplication of elastic lamina, partial dilatation with discontinuity of the elastic lamina, microaneurysm formation, dilatative change of the vessels with medial fibrosis, and rupture of the vascular wall, with or without fibrin deposits.[102]

Kono and co-workers examined the brain surface of 16 patients with moyamoya disease and 14 controls.[30] Neither the vascular density nor the arteriovenous ratio differed significantly between them. All the patients with the disease showed dilatative changes of both arteries and veins, attenuation or disruption of the internal elastic lamina, and fibrous intimal thickening. These changes were more prominent in those patients who had had the disease longer. The result suggests that the prominent leptomeningeal vessels of moya-moya disease are not newly formed but are merely dilated pre-existing vessels.

Atrophic lesions were often seen in the brain. Under the vascular-rich area there was marked softening, and microscopic necrosis of the second and third layers was conspicuous.[66]

Ikeda and associates performed histopathological examination and morphometric analysis of the extracranial vessels in 13 patients with moyamoya disease.[65] They showed advanced intimal fibrous thickening similar to that of intracranial vessels and characteristic intimal fibrous nodular thickening. Organization of mural thrombi was found in the proximal portion of pulmonary arteries in 3 of the 13 patients. Morphometric analysis revealed significant intimal thickening of the pulmonary arteries ($P < .05$), renal arteries ($P < .05$), and pancreatic arteries ($P < .05$) in patients with moyamoya disease as compared with age- and sex-matched controls.

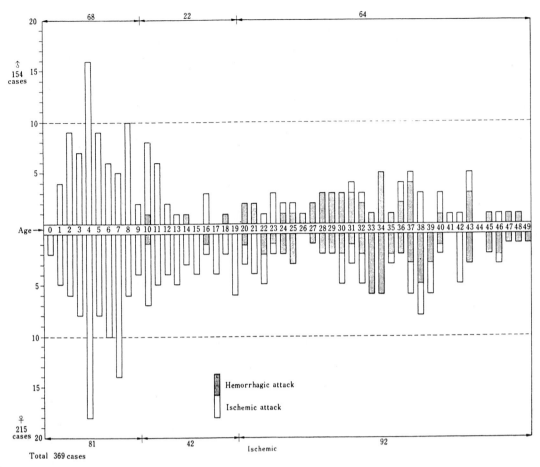

Figure 49–2

The age at onset of moyamoya disease reported by Kudo in 1976. There are two peaks of onset: one at age 4 years and the other at 34. Onset in children is ischemic, and that in adults is mostly hemorrhagic. (From Kudo, T., and Fukuda, S.: Spontaneous occlusion of the circle of Willis. Shinkei-shinpo, *20*:750–757, 1976. Reprinted by permission.)

Moyamoya disease is characterized by a slowly progressive intimal thickening of unknown etiology. This lesion usually starts at the distal end or bifurcation of the bilateral carotid arteries and spreads distally or centrifugally to the adjacent main arteries of the anterior base of the brain. The intimal thickening causes stenosis or occlusion of the proximal arteries of the anterior circulation and thus results in decrease in blood flow through the normal pathway.

There are many factors that decide the disease course and prognosis of an individual case. Among them, the most important is the nature of the primary endothelial thickening of the proximal major arteries of the anterior circulation. The next important factor is how the collateral vessels develop and compensate for the deficits in cerebral blood flow produced by the primary lesion. The third important factor is the age of the patient. According to Ogawa and associates, the hemispheric blood flow of children younger than the age of 5 years is between 2 and 2.5-fold and for the 10- to 15-year-old child it is 1.3 fold of the adult.[65] This age-associated blood requirement of the brain affects the course of the disease. Patients who had onset of the disease at age younger than 2 often have catastrophic onset, sometimes with convulsive seizures associated with in-

farction. Elapse of time, on the other hand, decreases the cerebral blood flow demand in children and may cause so-called spontaneous recovery in some cases.

Collateral pathways observed in moyamoya disease usually are prominent possibly because they develop in response to slowly progressive chronic ischemia (see Fig. 49–1). Close observation of the angiograms of patients with moyamoya disease shows collateral pathways that develop in chronic cerebrovascular insufficiency.

COLLATERAL SYSTEMS TO THE BRAIN

Collateral pathways thus observed are categorized as follows[49]:

A System (Anastomosis Intracerebralis). There are two sets of perforating arteries to the brain, one from the base of the brain and the other from the surface of the brain. They anastomose with each other at the external angle of the lateral ventricle. This anastomosis is well shown as moyamoya phenomenon in various ischemic conditions of the brain and as basal moyamoya vessels in moyamoya disease.

B System (Basal Communications). The B system

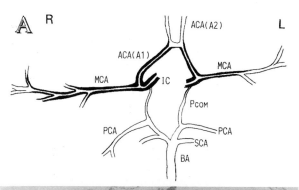

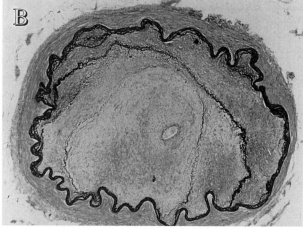

Figure 49–3

Basal main arterial tree of a patient with moyamoya disease *(A)* and a cross section of the left distal internal carotid artery of the patient *(B)*. The lumen is markedly narrowed by thick intima of sparse fibrous tissue in which thin layers of convoluted elastic fibers are arranged parallel to the elastic lamina. The internal elastic lamina is markedly tortuous, but no discontinuance is noted. Media and adventitia are well preserved. No cellular infiltration nor scar tissue is observed. The thick intima shows a ring-like pattern, suggesting intermittent deterioration of the primary lesion. ACA, anterior cerebral artery; BA, basilar artery; IC, internal carotid artery; MCA, middle cerebral artery; PCA, posterior cerebral artery; PCOM, posterior communicating artery; SCA, superior cerebellar artery.

includes the circle of Willis. The primary lesion in moyamoya disease starts and spreads mainly in the anterior half of the circle of Willis and its adjoining arteries and, later, may spread to the posterior half.[29, 73]

C System (Cortical Leptomeningeal Anastomosis). These anastomoses are end-to-end and are 200 to 600 microns in size. They are between the principal cerebral arteries on the surface of the brain (Fig. 49–4; see color section in this volume). There are marked differences in the anastomosis and thus the symptoms in patients with moyamoya disease, emboli, or cerebral vasospasm.

D System (Dural Networks). The dural arteries anastomose with each other as if the brain were covered with a mesh hat composed of the dural arteries. Therefore, if there was no subarachnoid layer of cerebrospinal fluid and if the dura was in direct physical contact with the brain, this system could be used as a collateral blood source immediately after ischemia occurred in the brain.

E System (Extracranial Networks). The blood flow

in the vascular networks of the scalp and pericranial muscle is also abundant. This blood source is usually used in both direct and indirect extracranial to intracranial bypass procedures.

F System (Functional Collateral). The increase in cerebral blood flow in hypercarbia, with acetazolamide, and after cervical sympathectomy or superior cervical ganglionectomy is due to functional and not to anatomical changes. The author calls these functional collateral vessels.

G System (Ground Communications). These collateral vessels are below the cranium. Carotid and vertebral arteries have many collateral anastomoses in the neck.

The brain is surrounded by horizontal collateral layers. These layers are connected to each other with minimal vertical collateral communications between layers forming a large total network. Arterioles in these tissues grow slowly to become visualized on angiograms. So-called vault moyamoya vessels are formed when the transdural anastomosis is perfused by the middle cerebral and the superficial temporal arteries.[29] Ethmoidal moyamoya vessels are formed when transdural anastomosis of netlike vessels in the orbit to frontal lobe are perfused from the ophthalmic artery, the anterior and posterior ethmoidal arteries, and the

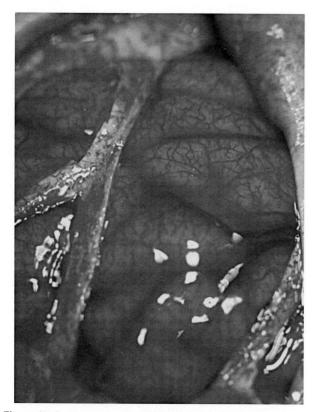

Figure 49–4

Marked leptomeningeal anastomosis of the surface of the brain observed in a moyamoya patient (see color section in this volume). This picture was taken during encephalomyosynangiosis. (From Matsushima, Y., and Inaba, Y.: The specificity of the collaterals to the brain through the study and surgical treatment of moyamoya disease. Stroke, *17*:117–122, 1986. Reproduced by permission. Copyright 1986, American Heart Association.)

external carotid arteries. Thus, transdural anastomoses are formed between the D and C systems.

SPECIFIC ANATOMY OF THE BRAIN COVERINGS

As protective coverings, the brain has a hard closed box of the skull between the D and E systems and a fluid layer of the subarachnoid space between the D and C systems. Both guard the soft and fibrin sparse brain just like the wall (the cranium) and the moat (the subarachnoid fluid space) of a castle. Vertical communications in these two tissues or spaces are so sparse and additional formation of communications is so difficult that the brain is isolated from the D and E systems that have abundant blood flow.

At an early phase of moyamoya disease, vessels at the base of the brain and leptomeningeal vessels from the posterior circulation become prominent (Fig. 49–5).[81, 82] After an interval, collateral vessels from the external carotid system come into use. They replace the intra-axial collateral vessels in the course of time. Finally, the brain becomes fed mainly by the collateral vessels from the external carotid system and the patients become stable symptomatically. This progress of

the disease is explained as follows using the nomenclature of the collateral vessels stated earlier.[49]

The primary lesion slowly and progressively occludes the anterior B system, starting at the periphery of the bilateral internal carotid artery (stage I of Suzuki). In proportion to the blood flow decrease due to this stenosis, the collateral vessels develop in the order of ease of their development. With initial B system insufficiency, both the A and C systems become used almost simultaneously and compensate for the B system insufficiency. Any failure in this compensation is expressed as an ischemic episode common to the patient with moyamoya disease. The A system becomes prominent and becomes the netlike vessels at the base of the brain (the basal moyamoya) (stage II of Suzuki). The vessels show a peculiar picture never present in normal cerebral angiograms and attracted attention of early researchers of the disease. The C system, on the other hand, did not prompt so much attention because nothing but the cortical arteries are visible on usual cerebral angiograms. As the oligemia continues, the A system becomes quite apparent (stage III of Suzuki). When the ischemic state persists further, the transdural anastomoses called the vault moyamoya and the ethmoidal moyamoya begin to be apparent in angiograms. When the transdural anastomoses between the C sys-

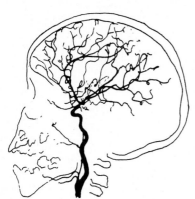

Stage I. Narrowing of carotid fork. Only the carotid fork stenosis is observed.

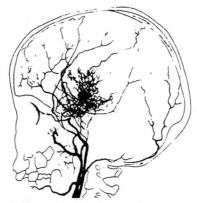

Stage III. Intensification of moyamoya. Remarkable moyamoya vessels at the base of the brain. The defection of the middle and anterior cerebral arteries is observed.

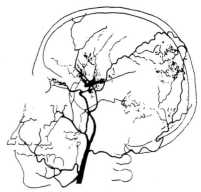

Stage V. Reduction of moyamoya. All the main cerebral arteries missing.

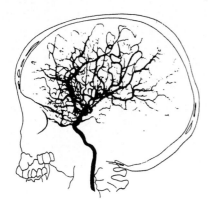

Stage II. Initiation of basal moyamoya. All the main cerebral arteries are dilated.

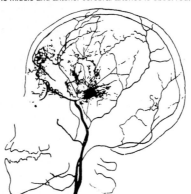

Stage IV. Minimization of Moyamoya. The defection of the posterior cerebral artery is observed.

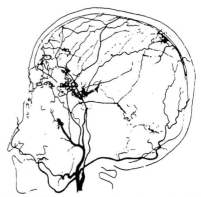

Stage VI. Disappearance of moyamoya. Cerebral blood flow supplied only from external carotid artery.

Figure 49–5

Progress of findings of angiography in patients with pediatric moyamoya disease. (From Suzuki, J., and Kodama, N.: Moyamoya disease: A review. Stroke *14*:106–107, 1983. Reprinted by permission. Copyright 1983, American Heart Association.)

tem and the D and E systems increase with time, blood flow through the external carotid system increases. So, the A system (basal moyamoya) loses their role as collateral vessels to the brain and gradually become invisible on cerebral angiography (stage IV of Suzuki).

When the blood flow required by the brain mass is adequately supplied by the collateral vessels of the external carotid system, ischemic attacks disappear and natural healing is said to have occurred (stages V and VI of Suzuki).

In many cases, progression of B system insufficiency is so rapid that irreversible ischemic change occurs in the brain before the D and E systems surmount the two obstacles of the cerebrospinal fluid layer of the subarachnoid space and the hard, closed box of the skull and form sufficient transdural anastomoses.

There are two ways to surmount these two obstacles. One is to wait for the development of collateral vessels and the decrease in the blood flow demand with age and by partially losing the brain mass by infarction; and the other is to perform surgery and surmount the obstacles by a surgical procedure. It is impossible to predict the disease course of any individual case. Waiting for the natural healing exposes the brain to an ischemic state that can lead to irreversible damage.

Clinical Features

In moyamoya disease, ischemic episodes are repeated.[36] The ischemic attacks are often of a transient nature so that the patient may be completely free of symptoms at the time of presentation or admission. The history from the family is very important and should be recorded in detail.

The age at onset and frequency, severity, and nature of the ischemic attacks, the portion of the body involved, precipitating factors, and occasion or time of the day are all to be recorded. The details of the last episode and its progress should also be recorded. It is important to know if the present neurological signs are just the residue of the last attack or the accumulated deficits from the previous attacks.

Symptoms such as sensory attacks, headache, and visual disturbance are sometimes not noticed by the family.

Moyamoya disease becomes symptomatic whenever the secondary development of collateral vessels fails in compensating the cerebral blood flow deficit produced by the slowly progressive stenotic lesion in the circle of Willis.

Based on observation of the clinical courses of 81 patients,[53] the patterns of progression can be grouped into six types (Table 49–3). Symptoms were episodic in types I and II, while some symptoms were persistent in types III and IV. Most of the symptoms were persistent in types V and VI. There was only one patient with type V disease. This patient presented with infarction in the distribution of the right middle cerebral artery at the age of 19 years. Intracerebral hematoma

Table 49–3

A NEW CLASSIFICATION OF CHILDHOOD MOYAMOYA DISEASE

Type I (TIA type)
Episodes of TIA or RIND are seen less than twice a month. No low-density area on computed tomography nor fixed neurological deficits are seen.

Type II (Frequent TIA type)
Episodes of TIA or RIND are seen more than twice a month. No low-density areas on computed tomography nor fixed neurological deficits are seen.

Type III (TIA-infarction type)
With repeated attacks like type I or II over time, visible low-density areas on computed tomography or irreversible neurological deficits on examinations occur.

Type IV (Infarction-TIA type)
The disease started as an infarction attack near its onset. Episodes of TIA or RIND and occasionally infarction are seen afterward.

Type V (Infarction type)
The disease started as an infarction attack. No ensuing attacks, or only infarction attacks, are repeated afterward.

Type VI (Ruptured collateral vascular bed type, others)
The disease is caused by hemorrhage from a vascular bed of the overgrown collateral path. Those that cannot be classified into any of the types are also included in this group.

TIA, transient ischemic attack; RIND, reversible ischemic neurological deficit.

Adapted from Matsushima, Y., Aoyagi, M., Masaoka, H., et al.: Mental outcome following encephaloduroarterioangiosis in children with moyamoya disease with the onset earlier than 5 years of age. Child's Nerv. Syst., 6:440–443, 1990. Reprinted by permission.

developed in all three patients with type VI disease, and symptoms corresponding to the site and extent of the hematoma were observed in each patient. Types V and VI correspond to so-called adult moyamoya disease and are usually observed in patients older than 20 years of age (see Fig. 49–2).

Subjects who developed symptoms when younger than 20 years of age (pediatric moyamoya patients by the author's definition) totaled 77, and they fitted the clinical patterns of types I through IV. The data on type I through type IV disease are summarized in Table 49–4.

Episodic symptoms and the initial symptom usually occurred with such activities associated with hyperventilation or with a rise in body temperature as reported by Kurokawa and co-workers.[36]

Motor disturbances occurred as the initial symptom in most patients (80.5 per cent), varying from weakness to paralysis of the extremities. These motor disturbances usually occurred as a transient ischemic attack or reversible ischemic neurological deficit and rarely as an infarction and appeared either on the same side or the opposite side or on the same or the different extremity in ensuing episodes.

Convulsions were seen in 8.6 per cent as symptoms at the onset of the disease. In six of the seven patients who had a convulsion as the initial ischemic symptom, the onset of the disease was earlier than 2 years and 4 months. The disease presented as acute infantile hemiplegia in two of these cases. There were variations from

Table 49–4

CHARACTERISTICS OF CHILDHOOD MOYAMOYA DISEASE (TYPES I THROUGH IV AND TOTAL CASES)

	Type I	Type II	Type III	Type IV	Total
No. of Cases (%)	21 (25.9%)	15 (18.5%)	17 (21.0%)	24 (29.6%)	81
Symptoms at Onset (%)	Motor disturbance (76%)	Motor disturbance (93.3%)	Motor disturbance (76.5%)	Motor disturbance (75%)	Motor disturbance (79%)
	Headache (14.3%)	Headache (6.7%)	Convulsion (17.6%)	Convulsion (16.7%)	Convulsion (8.6%)
	Involuntary movement (4.8%)				Headache (7.4%)
					Involuntary movement (2.5%)
Age at Visit (Average)	5.8–19 (10.6)	1.6–21 (9.0)	1.6–18 (10.3)	1.7–36 (9.5)	1.6–36 (10.4)
Symptoms at Visit (%)	Motor disturbance (66.7%)	Motor disturbance (66.7%)	Motor disturbance (88.2%)	Motor disturbance (100%)	Motor disturbance (81.5%)
	Headache (33.3%)	Headache (26.7%)	Mental disturbance (29.4%)	Sensory disturbance (41.7%)	Headache (27.2%)
	Involuntary movement (14.3%)	Mental retardation (13.3%)	Speech disturbance (17.6%)	Speech disturbance (33.3%)	Mental retardation (19.8%)
			Sensory disturbance (17.6%)	Mental retardation (29.2%)	Speech disturbance (17.3%)
				Headache (20.8%)	Sensory disturbance (16.0%)
				Convulsion (20.8%)	Convulsion (6.2%)
					Involuntary movement (6.2%)
Preoperative IQ/DQ (Average)	74–138 (111.4)	53–103 (88.9)	40–117 (69.8)	20–125 (63.6)	20–138 (83.6)

IQ, intelligence quotient; DQ, development quotient.

Adapted from Matsushima, Y., Aoyagi, M., Niimi, Y., et al.: Symptoms and their pattern of progression in childhood moyamoya disease. Brain Dev., 12:784–789, 1990. Reprinted by permission.

focal seizures to generalized convulsions with loss of consciousness.

It was difficult to obtain detailed descriptions of the headache that was reported in 7.3 per cent of cases. However, it was suggested that headache in this disease is closely related to intracranial oligemia, since it disappeared promptly after the revascularizing operation.

Involuntary movements seen in the author's patient were mostly choreic movements, usually of an extremity and rarely of the face; muscle tonus was usually decreased and the movements were not seen when the patient was asleep.

The incidence of intellectual impairment increased from type I to type IV, with quotients averaging 111.4, 88.9, 68.9, and 63.9, respectively. The development quotient or intelligence quotient is the most reliable and important parameter in the evaluation and follow-up of the patient. In observing patients it is difficult to detect subtle changes in neurological or mental function. Thus, periodical evaluation of the intelligence or development quotient should be done.

Hemorrhage at onset occurred in only one case of the author's 113 pediatric moyamoya cases (see Fig. 49–6). The cause of hemorrhage in later life, after pediatric moyamoya disease has symptomatically subsided, is considered to be due to aging and hypertensive loading leading to the formation of microaneurysms and rupture of these abnormal networks of basal moyamoya vessels.

Clinical Examinations

No remarkable findings are observed in the laboratory data.

COMPUTED TOMOGRAPHY

In patients with types I and II disease, computed tomography is usually normal (Fig. 49–6). In patients with types III and IV disease, often multiple hypodense infarction areas are observed at the so-called watershed zone.[48] The hypodense areas sometimes show mottled hypodensity or a honeycomb pattern. Various degrees of cerebral atrophy with widening of the subarachnoid space and the ventricles are observed. Enhanced computed tomography shows defective distal internal carotid arteries, proximal anterior cerebral and middle cerebral arteries, and, in later stages, the entire circle of Willis in some cases. Moyamoya vessels can be recognized, and in most of the cases a fraying pattern of the middle cerebral artery is visible (see Fig. 49–6D and E). In the acute phase of the ischemic episode, gyral enhancement is observed at the hypodense areas for 1 to 4 weeks after the onset of the episode (see Fig. 49–6E). The author usually avoids doing surgery while this enhancement is present on computed tomography.

Cerebral hemorrhage is usually observed near and lateral to the lateral ventricle where the perforators from the surface and the base of the brain anastomose with each other. The hemorrhage may stay as an intracerebral hematoma or easily rupture into the lateral ventricle in adult patients with moyamoya disease.

MAGNETIC RESONANCE IMAGING

New and old ischemic lesions, atrophy, and bleeding observed by computed tomography can show more clearly on magnetic resonance imaging (Fig. 49–7). Stenotic vascular lumina as well as moyamoya vessels can be seen by signal void phenomenon.

Yamada and associates studied 12 of the author's patients with three-dimensional time-of-flight magnetic resonance angiography and compared the findings

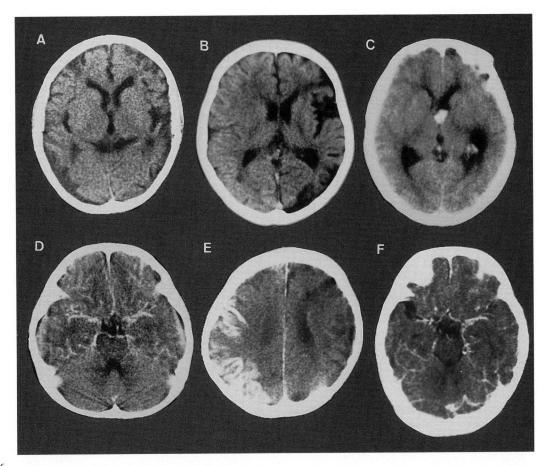

Figure 49–6
Typical findings of computed tomography in patients with moyamoya disease: Plain scans *(A through C)* and contrast medium–enhanced scans *(D through F)*. A. Infarction occurs at so-called watershed zones first and extends to the adjacent cortices. B. Widening of the ventricle and the subarachnoid space is often observed with mottled pattern or honeycomb pattern of white matter. C. Ventricular or intracerebral hemorrhage is a common occurrence in adult moyamoya disease and has been noted by the author in a 13-year-old patient. D. Defective demonstration of circle of Willis and irregular fraying pattern of the middle cerebral artery and communications from the posterior cerebral arteries are observed. E. Gyral enhancement seen 1 to 4 weeks after acute infarct. This must resolve before a surgical procedure is done. F. Prominent communications from the posterior cerebral arteries.

with results obtained with conventional angiography (see Fig. 49–7).[99] Of the total 24 supraclinoid internal carotid arteries studied, 21 arteries (88 per cent) were accurately evaluated with magnetic resonance angiography, and in three arteries the extent of occlusion was overestimated. While conventional arteriography showed basal moyamoya vessels in all 24 hemispheres, magnetic resonance angiography showed moyamoya vessels in 20 of these. Of a total of 28 large leptomeningeal and transdural collateral vessels, 18 were identified with this type of angiography. In one case, postsurgical collateral vessels were evaluated and their patency was successfully demonstrated.

ELECTROENCEPHALOGRAPHY

Kodama and co-workers studied electroencephalography in 25 children with moyamoya disease.[28] Characteristic findings of slow waves in the posterior hemisphere, centrotemporal slow waves, "re-buildup" phenomenon, and sleep spindle depression were observed. Slow waves of the posterior hemisphere were

mainly observed on electroencephalograms examined within a short time period (mean, 10 months), Centrotemporal slow waves were seen after a little longer period (mean, 28 months), and a diffuse low-voltage pattern occurred after a longer period (mean, 56 months) after the onset of the disease.

In many patients, 20 to 60 seconds after the termination of hyperventilation there was the return of high voltage slow waves. Kodama and co-workers named this the re-buildup phenomenon and observed it in 15 (75 per cent) of their 20 pediatric cases. Buildup occurs because of hypocapnic hypoxia, while the re-buildup phenomenon is considered due not only to ischemic hypoxia but also to hypoxic hypoxia due to depression of respiration after hyperventilation.[22] For moyamoya disease in childhood, the re-buildup phenomenon is pathognomonic to the disease, but close observation and care must be taken in performing the examination.

CEREBRAL BLOOD FLOW

According to Suzuki's simplified method of xenon-enhanced computed tomography for measurement of

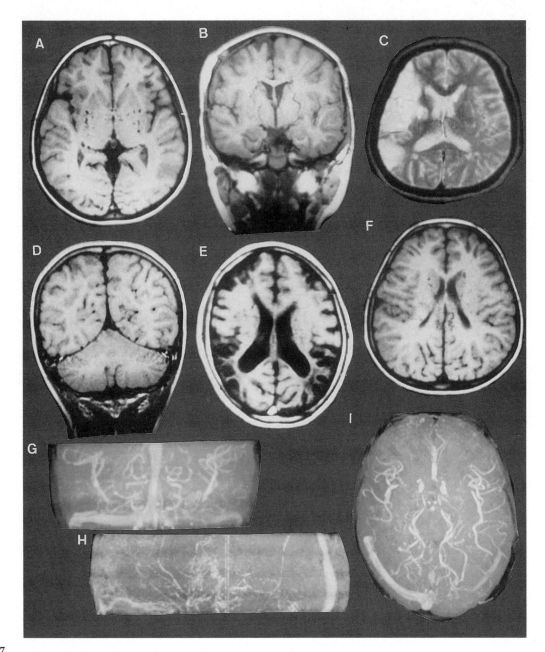

Figure 49–7

Typical magnetic resonance imaging findings of moyamoya disease. *A.* Multiple hypointensity dots of moyamoya vessels at basal ganglia are observed. *B.* Multiple moyamoya vessels are observed at basal ganglia. *C.* Watershed or adjacent ischemic lesion is demonstrated. *D.* Leptomeningeal communications from the posterior cerebral arteries are markedly dilated. *E.* Cortical hypointensity and widened subarachnoid hypointensity are marked at watershed zones. Ventricular dilatation and multiple dots at basal ganglia are also observed. *F.* Leptomeningeal communications from the posterior cerebral arteries and anterior and posterior moyamoya vessels are observed. *G through I.* Time-of-flight magnetic resonance angiograms. *G.* Stenosis of the major arteries is overestimated. Bilateral M$_1$ segments are not observed in this patient with early-stage disease in which conventional angiography demonstrates M$_1$ segment. *H.* Moyamoya vessels. *I.* Axial view of the patient shows defective anterior circle of Willis and bilateral M$_1$ segments.

cerebral blood flow, the flow in pediatric patients with moyamoya disease is characterized by a moderate to severe hypoperfusion in the frontal and temporal cortices, a subcortical ischemia, and a high flow in the central structures of the brain that involves the area of basal moyamoya (Fig. 49–8, see color section in this volume).[85, 87]

Nariai and colleagues studied vasoactivity in 16 patients with moyamoya disease.[63] The patients were subjected to xenon-enhanced computed tomography for an acetazolamide challenge test. Regional cerebral blood flow in the resting state and after injection of 20 mg per kg of acetazolamide was measured. Regional changes of resting cerebral blood flow with acetazolamide challenge were expressed as delta acetazolamide (regional cerebral blood flow after acetazolamide challenge minus the regional cerebral blood flow in the resting state). Five patients were also subjected to position emission tomography. Patients with type I disease showed low delta acetazolamide in regions where resting cerebral blood flow is low (see Fig. 49–8). The regions also well correlated to the regions where high oxygen extraction fraction and high regional cerebral blood volume were proved by positron emission tomography. Young patients with moyamoya disease have chronic low perfusion in the forebrain (see Fig. 49–8).

ANGIOGRAPHY

The findings of angiography described in Table 49–1 are indispensable for the diagnosis (see Fig. 49–1). Satoh and associates analyzed the author's 34 pediatric patients based on the primary pathological narrowing of the anterior circulation.[73] Stenosis and occlusion of the internal carotid artery bifurcation were classified in five groups: slight to moderate stenosis of internal carotid artery bifurcation (lumen greater than or equal to 10 per cent) in 10 sides; severe stenosis of the internal carotid artery bifurcation (lumen less than 10 per cent) in 12 sides; occlusion of anterior cerebral artery or middle cerebral artery in 11 sides; occlusion of the internal carotid artery or anterior and middle cerebral arteries with partial patency of the trunk of the anterior and middle cerebral artery in 20 sides; and occlusion of the internal carotid or anterior and middle cerebral arteries with no patency of the main trunk of the anterior and middle cerebral arteries in 15 sides. The blood flow to the moyamoya vessels at the base of the brain is mainly supplied from the internal carotid artery in the early stage of the disease. In a later stage, however, the blood supply is mainly from the posterior cerebral artery. No remarkable change was found in the volume of basal moyamoya vessels from early to later stages of the disease. The leptomeningeal collateral vessels, however, had a tendency to decrease during the later stage with the development of posterior cerebral artery stenosis. Interestingly, 18 occlusive lesions of the posterior cerebral artery were found in the proximal portion of the artery in eight sides (12 per cent), and in the distal portion in nine sides (13 per cent). Two aneu-

rysms in the moyamoya vessels were found in one patient among all the 34 who were studied. Collateral vessels from the external carotid artery were rare in the early stage and appeared frequently in later stages (45 to 67 per cent). The most common collateral vessels from the external carotid artery were from the anterior branch of the middle meningeal artery. Collateral vessels from the maxillary artery were seen. Collateral vessels from the superficial temporal artery and occipital artery were rare, with their frequency being less than 15 per cent.

Diagnosis

It is easy to diagnose moyamoya disease when one encounters a pediatric patient who develops ischemic attacks during hyperventilation or overexercising and whose affected side shifts from side to side. The definitive diagnosis is made by angiography.

The differential diagnosis includes acute infantile hemiplegia, epileptic seizure, alternating hemiplegia in childhood, and migraine. Moyamoya disease sometimes takes the form of acute infantile hemiplegia, especially in an infant. In both situations, angiography should be done to confirm the diagnosis.[16] There are many children with moyamoya disease who have only headache as a symptom.

The diseases from which the moyamoya syndrome should be differentiated also include meningitis; tuberculous meningitis; Down syndrome; von Recklinghausen's disease; head injury; irradiation; stenosis of the internal carotid artery due to tumor; fibromuscular dysplasia; sickle cell anemia; Fanconi's anemia; spontaneous occlusion of the internal carotid artery, anterior cerebral artery, or middle cerebral artery; policystic kidney; eosinophilic granuloma; type I glycogenosis; transient central nervous system deficits; and limb shaking.* In the adult, atherosclerosis should be excluded first.[17]

Conditions Possibly Related to Moyamoya Disease

In managing moyamoya disease one often encounters hypertensive children who have renal artery stenosis.[9, 15, 21, 103] The author has an impression that the child with moyamoya disease may have suffered frostbite. Such a case has been reported in Australia.[74]

There are two types of aneurysms associated with moyamoya disease.[95] One is saccular and occurs on the circle of Willis at the same sites as seen in the general population. However, their distribution is different. The most frequent site is the basilar tip, possibly because of a hemodynamic stress in the posterior circulation, and the second most frequent site is the internal

---

*See references 1, 4–7, 11, 26, 40–42, 46, 61, 69, 71, 72, 75, 77, 80, 94, and 97.

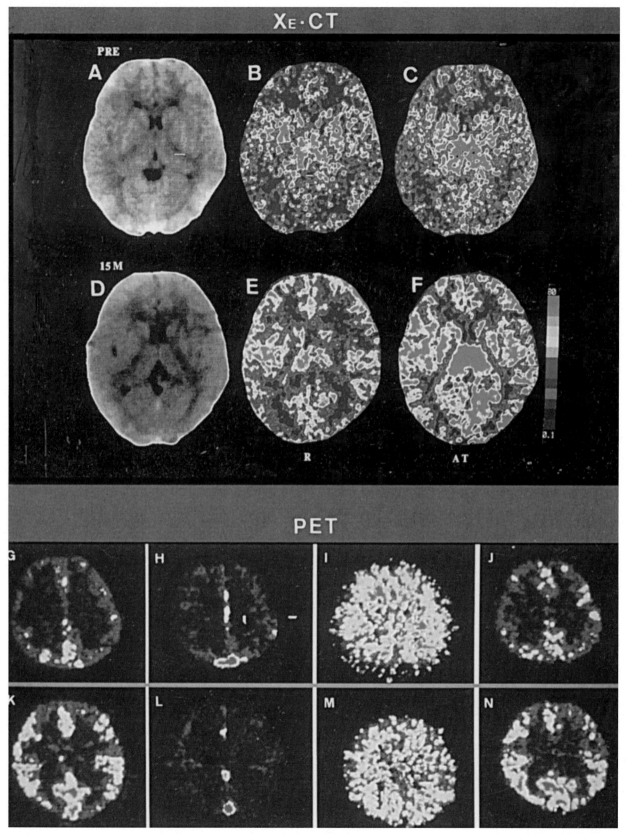

Figure 49–8

Preoperative and 15 months postoperative xenon-enhanced computed tomography and positron emission tomography of 16-year-old girl with symptomatic onset of type II disease at 11 years old (see color section in this volume). Xenon-enhanced cerebral blood flow studies: before *(A through C)* and 15 months after encephaloduroarteriosynangiosis *(D through F). (A and D,* plain scans; *B and E,* xenon-enhanced scans at rest; *C and F,* xenon-enhanced scans with acetazolamide challenge test.)* PET studies: before *(G through J)* and 15 months after encephaloduroarteriosynangiosis *(K through N). (G and K,* cerebral blood flow studies; *H and L,* cerebral blood volume studies; *I and M,* oxygen extraction factor; *J and N,* CMRO$_2$, cerebral metabolic rate for oxygen.)

carotid artery. Middle cerebral artery aneurysms are rare, and anterior communicating aneurysms have not been reported.

The second type of aneurysm associated with moyamoya disease is a small aneurysm on the basal moyamoya vessels or on other collateral vessels. These aneurysms often disappear spontaneously or after surgical revascularization. They are supposed to be the cause of intracerebral or intraventricular hemorrhage observed usually in adult patients.

Vascular malformations are sometimes associated with moyamoya disease. They are arteriovenous malformations and persistent primitive arteries.[25, 38, 39, 43]

Several other pathological processes, primary pulmonary hypertension, periodic torticolis, and growth failure have also been reported to have occurred in association with this disease.[23, 44, 104]

Anesthesia

As has been stated, the specific cerebral blood flow pattern in patients with moyamoya disease makes it necessary to take special care at the time of anesthesia. In this disease, cerebral blood flow is decreased but the reactivity of the cerebral vessels to carbon dioxide is retained. Hyperventilation decreases the cerebral blood flow and often results in neurological deterioration.

Possible factors resulting in ischemic complication during general anesthesia in moyamoya disease are hypocarbia caused by hyperventilation, hypotension and dehydration, hyperthermia, and intracerebral steal phenomenon caused by hypercarbia.

To avoid hyperventilation created mainly by crying, it is important to reassure the patient, to use heavy premedication, to use titrated doses of barbiturates in induction of anesthesia, to allow for rapid control with mask ventilation, to perform smooth intubation, and to monitor by capnography supplemented by arterial blood gas analyses to allow for real time monitoring and modulation of arterial PCO_2.[45] The author tries to keep the PCO_2 at 45 mm Hg. The PCO_2 in the author's 82 cases was kept between maximal value, 46.3 ± 6.9 mm Hg, and minimal value, 39.6 ± 5.1 mm Hg, and no intraoperative ischemic attacks were observed.

To avoid hypotension and dehydration, it is necessary to maintain appropriate hydration and to monitor arterial pressure together with routine electrocardiography, pulse oximetry, and the precordial/esophageal stethoscope. The author tries to keep the mean arterial pressure above 75 mm Hg, and the blood pressure in the series was kept between the maximal value, 138 ± 18 mm Hg, and a minimal value, 87 ± 24 mm Hg, without trouble.

Change in body temperature is one of the precipitating factors of neurological deficits in moyamoya disease.[36] Vigorous treatment of hyperthermia is necessary to decrease the cerebral consumption of oxygen. Temperature monitoring is indispensable.

One of the author's patients developed malignant hyperthermia during an operation. It was treated by discontinuing the operation, but two fatal cases have occurred in other institutions. Urinary monitoring is also necessary.

Hypocarbia induces diffuse reduction of regional cerebral blood flow without changing the regional flow pattern. On the other hand, hypercarbia induces a remarkable change of the regional flow pattern in which flow in the temporo-occipital region is increased but decreased or scarcely increased in the frontal region. The temporo-occipital lobes fed mainly by the posterior cerebral artery seem to retain carbon dioxide reactivity. In contrast, the cortical and pial arteries in the frontal region seem to be in a state of full dilatation or high vascular resistance owing to proximal vascular insufficiency. Thus, hypercarbia in excess of PCO_2 of 50 mm Hg for a long time may cause intracranial steal phenomenon and resultant ischemia.[67]

Treatment

MEDICAL TREATMENT

Vasodilators, anticoagulant drugs, antifibrinolytic drugs, hemostatic agents, anticonvulsants, corticosteroids, and suppressors of intracranial pressure have been used against symptoms of ischemic states, intracranial hemorrhage, convulsive seizures, involuntary movements, or intracranial hypertension, respectively.[8, 31, 70, 101]

SURGICAL TREATMENT

The ideal management of moyamoya disease is to treat the diseased vessel (see Table 49–2). The lesion, however, is due to a progressive pathological process of unknown etiology so that no adequate treatment is available. The next best treatment is to introduce blood from the external carotid artery system as is seen in so-called natural healing. This is to surmount the obstacles surgically before nonreversible changes occur to the brain. Anastomosis of the superficial temporal artery and middle cerebral artery and encephalomyosynangiosis were operative procedures that had been tried for moyamoya disease before the appearance of encephaloduroarteriosynangiosis. The author's operative procedure of encephaloduroarteriosynangiosis was developed to overcome problems peculiar to these two procedures.

The procedures that are most often used now are encephaloduroarteriosynangiosis and its modified or combined procedures, superficial temporal artery–middle cerebral artery bypass, encephalomyosynangiosis, and omental transplantation.

Encephaloduroarteriosynangiosis

Operative Procedure.[47, 56, 57] Any one of the three main arteries of the scalp, the anterior and posterior branches of the superficial temporal artery and the occipital artery, is available as a donor artery. The author usually uses the posterior branch of the superficial temporal artery on both sides (Fig. 49–9). Depending on the location of the ischemia and its severity, the anterior branch of the superficial temporal artery or the occipital artery is used.

The donor vessel is exposed as extensively as possible. The author's average exposure length was 9.67 ± 1.94 cm on the right (n = 42) and 9.54 ± 2.33 cm on the left (n = 40). Small branches running from the main artery are cut after ligation or coagulation. The galea is cut with a needle electrocoagulator parallel to and 5 to 7 mm apart from the artery so that a strip of galea is attached to the donor artery for its entire exposed length. A nonconductive spatula is used (Fig. 49–10). If large branches of the donor artery run parallel to or at an acute angle to the main artery, these branches are also included with the galeal strip.

The scalp artery with the strip of galea is freed from the pericranium or the fascia below and is put aside (see Fig. 49–9B). Then the fascia, the muscle, and the pericranium are cut linearly using an electrocoagulator just on the line where the donor artery was located. The pericranium and the muscle (never the donor vessel) are retracted by dermal hooks, thus exposing the skull. Two burr holes are made below the proximal and the distal ends of the freed donor artery. The two burr holes are connected by two cuts in the skull and an oval bone flap is removed (see Fig. 49–9C). The dura mater is exposed and carefully examined for large vessels. A linear incision is made, or a narrow strip of dura mater is removed. Large dural vessels or transdural anastomoses are spared (see Fig. 49–9D). The dural openings are closed by suturing the dural edge and galeal edge of the donor strip on each side. The artery and the strip of galea are merely laid on the arachnoid membrane; and no incision or injury is made to the arachnoid membrane (see Fig. 49–9E). Several dural tenting sutures are placed to avoid bleeding from abundant horizontal collateral vessels severed along the edge of the cranial window. The bone flap is shaped so as not to hinder the blood flow of the donor artery and replaced and fastened in place by sutures through drill holes. Then the wound is closed in layers (see Fig. 49–9F).

Indication for Encephaloduroarteriosynangiosis. This procedure is effective and indicated when an area of the brain has chronic low perfusion. Low cerebral blood flow itself has little to do with good revascularization, but poor reaction to the acetazolamide challenge test is significantly correlated with good revascularization. The same result was obtained by positron emission tomography. Good revascularization was obtained in such a case in which cerebral blood flow is low, oxygen extraction fraction is high, and cerebral blood volume is high.[63]

Many modified procedures have been presented. The author believes the original procedure is adequate for most cases. He performs it on any patient who has a poorly perfused area; and if the area is wide, dual procedures are performed using the anterior and posterior branches of the superficial temporal artery and

adding encephaloarteriosynangiosis or encephalogaleosynangiosis as needed.

If moyamoya disease is diagnosed, surgical treatment, which has a low rate of complications, should be performed without delay. Apparently normal patients with minimal episodic symptoms and patients with headache, seizure, or involuntary movements as their main symptoms are selected for operation.

Encephaloduroarteriosynangiosis was originally developed for the treatment of moyamoya disease in children. This operation, however, is also indicated for adult patients and for other ischemic conditions that accompany moyamoya phenomenon (moyamoya syndrome).*

Operative Results

Change in Symptoms. With the improvement of cerebral blood flow, ischemic attacks disappear swiftly.[51] Since encephaloduroarteriosynangiosis is an "indirect anastomosis," the appearance of its effects is likely to be considered delayed. Takasato and colleagues, however, reported that 12 of 25 surgical cases showed amelioration of deficits or attacks within 3 weeks.[89] Improvements began after 4 to 20 days (mean, 10.1 days). The author speculates that at the earliest stage of indirect anastomosis, spontaneous communication between the extracranial and intracranial arteries is formed by angiogenesis of wound healing in the granulation tissue of the operative wound. Such neovascular networks connect insatiably to the existing arteries in both the donor galea and the cortical surface (the author calls this the initial anastomosis). The pressure gradient between the two arterial systems ensures the constant and early flow from the external carotid to the internal carotid systems. The pathways become so adjusted that the blood flow through the anastomoses becomes increased. This hypothesis agrees with the observation that the size of the dural arteries around the operative wound started to increase beginning 2 to 3 months after encephaloduroarteriosynangiosis and with the fact that the increased regional cerebral blood flow underneath the operative site and good total hemispheric vascular reserve were obtained within 2 weeks after this procedure.[50, 86]

The symptoms of moyamoya disease have two components: the episodic ischemic attacks and the resultant neurological deficits. The author, therefore, studied the interval needed for the disappearance of the episodic ischemic attacks and the change of intelligence quotient and development quotient as results of accumulated deficits.

The cessation of episodic ischemic attacks (transient ischemic attacks, reversible ischemic neurological deficit, or infarction) indicates when an adequate blood supply to the brain has been established. The cessation of attacks is defined as such when an attack-free period lasts at least 6 months.

Ischemic attacks disappeared at a mean of 239 days after encephaloduroarteriosynangiosis. Forty-one of 56

---

*See references 13, 26, 59, 60, 78, and 96.

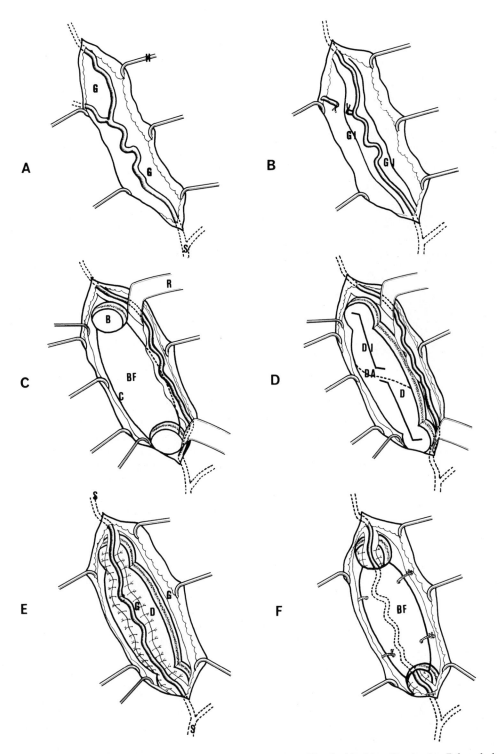

Figure 49–9

Procedures of encephaloduroarteriosynangiosis. H, hook; G, galea; S, donor artery; GI, galeal incision; R, retractor; B, burr hole; C, craniectomy; BF, bone flap; DI, dural incision; DA, dural artery; D, dura mater. *A.* A skin incision is made along a chosen scalp donor artery as long as possible, taking care not to damage the artery or to detach the artery from the galea underneath. Hemostasis of the incised edges can be obtained just by pulling the wound edges by hooks. *B.* The galea is cut with a needle electrocoagulator parallel to, but 5 to 7 mm apart from, the donor artery on both sides so that a strip of galea is attached to the donor artery over its entire length. The donor with the strip of galea (the arterial bridge) is detached from the tissue below. *C.* The arterial bridge is pulled aside by retractors. The fascia with muscle and the periosteum are cut along the line where the arterial bridge was attached and are displaced to expose the skull. Hooks are replaced so as to retract the muscle and the periosteum. Two burr holes are made beneath the proximal and the distal end of the arterial bridge. Burr holes are connected by two cuts in the skull to make an oval bone flap. *D.* A linear incision is made to the exposed dura mater, sparing large dural arteries. It is recommended that both ends of the dural incisions be cut in an L shape to widen the dural opening. Some surgeons recommended making an arachnoidal incision here, but the author does not believe in doing this, nor is too meticulous a hemostasis of the dural edge and surface recommended. *E.* The arterial bridge is put back on the exposed brain surface, and the galeal edges of the arterial bridge and the dural edges are sutured to provide a watertight closure of the dural opening. Silk rather than hyporeactive artificial suture is recommended. *F.* After placement of several dural tenting sutures along the edge of the bone window, the bone flap is shaped so as not to hinder the blood flow of the donor artery and is replaced and fastened in place by sutures through drill holes. (Reprinted by permission of the publisher from Matsushima, Y., Fukai, N., Tanaka, K., et al.: A new surgical treatment of moyamoya disease in children: A preliminary report. Surg. Neurol., 15:313–320, 1981. Copyright 1981, Elsevier Science Inc.)

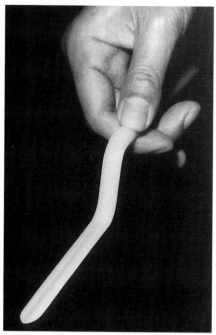

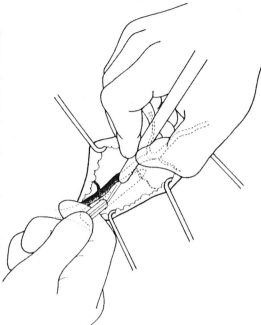

Figure 49–10

Encephaloduroarteriosynangiosis. Nonconducting spatula with a line of ditch makes it possible to cut the galea without damaging the adjoining tissue. Clear coagulated cut edge lines thus made give a good orientation at suturing the arterial bridge to the dural edges.

patients (73.2 per cent) with preoperative ischemic attacks became attack-free within a year. Thirteen patients (23.2 per cent) became attack-free within 2 years.

Fukuyama and colleagues reported that by medical treatment about half of Moyamoya patients with transient ischemic attacks became attack-free 4 to 5 years after the onset.[12] In the other half of this group, however, episodic ischemic attacks are still observed after a mean interval of 6 years and 11 months. Therefore, ischemic attacks in moyamoya disease continue for a long time in the natural course even in patients with less serious type I disease.

The disappearance of ischemic attacks in the author's operated group with more serious patients was far faster, even if the interval of mean onset to operation of 3.7 ± 3.3 years was considered. Thus, the procedure shortens the oligemic period for the developing brain in children with moyamoya disease.

The author measured the intelligence or development quotient examined by the specialists as a total functional parameter. He studied changes in development quotient for children younger than 5 years of age based on the development questionnaires of Tsumori and co-workers and the change in intelligence quotient based on the Wechsler Intelligence Scale for Children (or the Wechsler Intelligence Scale for Children—Revised) for children older than 5 years of age.

The mean development or intelligence quotient before the operation was 83.6 ± 30.0. After the operation (range, 6 months to 5 years and 5 months; mean, 2 years and 3 months) the mean quotients were 85.0 ± 31.8. Thus, there was no significant difference.

Kurokawa and colleagues reported that the intelligence of patients with moyamoya disease declined after the onset of the disease.[37] If an intelligence or development quotient of 86 or above is considered normal, then within 4 years of onset, 92 per cent of

patients were normal, between 5 and 9 years after onset 40 per cent were normal, and between 10 and 15 years only 33 per cent were normal (n = 27). Corresponding rates in the author's cases were 71.9, 33.3, and 33.3 per cent preoperatively (n = 50), and 50.0, 62.5, and 55.6 per cent postoperatively (n = 36). Compared with Kurokawa and colleagues' natural course, the author's postoperative patients showed a higher rate of normal quotients.

Ishii and associates reported 10 of 20 patients with moyamoya disease after encephalomyosynangiosis showed a marked improvement in intelligence quotient postoperatively, although in 3 it remained unchanged and in 2 it declined.[20]

Special consideration should be directed to the patients who had the onset of the disease earlier than 5 years of age because these patients have been reported to have a poor prognosis.

According to Kikuchi and colleagues, among patients who had the onset of moyamoya disease at the age of 5 years or less, about half of those who had the onset at younger than 2 years of age presented with convulsive seizure and 80 per cent of them were admitted with completed stroke during the course.[27] Of those who had the onset at 2 to 5 years of age, 80 per cent had the onset with a transient ischemic attack and the disease progressed to completed stroke in about 60 per cent. The author's patients showed a similar tendency. Thus, in patients who have the onset of moyamoya disease at an age younger than 5 years, especially younger than 2 years, the incidence of infarction is high and the prognosis is expected to be poor.

Tagawa and colleagues reported that the intelligence quotient was low if the age of onset was low with a significant correlation between the two.[88]

Olds and associates operated on 15 children with moyamoya disease.[68] Ten of these children experienced the onset of the disease when younger than 5 years of age, and three of them had normal mental function. One of these three patients had the onset at 3 years of age and had been observed for 6 years after bilateral superficial temporal artery–middle cerebral artery anastomosis. The remaining two had been observed, one for 3 years and the other for 8 months, respectively, after encephaloduroarteriosynangiosis. Further development of these children is of profound interest. These results show the possibility that the mental outcome of moyamoya disease with early onset can be improved by surgical treatments.

Change in Postoperative Angiograms. Postoperative angiograms in Figure 49–11 show typical changes, after encephaloduroarteriosynangiosis, marked revascularization of the brain through the donor of the external carotid system, disappearance of preoperatively existing vault moyamoya vessels, and decrease in anterior and posterior basal moyamoya vessels.[58]

When followed by cerebral angiography after the operation within 1 to 3 months after the operation, dilatation of the dural arteries around the operated side is seen.[58] Subsequently, the donor scalp artery gradually becomes enlarged. Usually, angiographically visible brain revascularization is observed by 6 months after encephaloduroarteriosynangiosis. With the development of good revascularization, gradual withering and decrease in moyamoya vessels follows.

To evaluate the results of encephaloduroarteriosynangiosis, the author has measured the diameter of the superficial temporal artery and its branches and the size of the moyamoya vessels in preoperative and postoperative angiograms after an average postoperative period of 22 months.[52] The diameter of the posterior branch of the superficial temporal artery (the usual donor artery) increased to 152 per cent on the left side and 164 per cent on the right side. Therefore, the cross-sectional area of the vessels more than doubled in size. The anterior basal moyamoya area, which was preoperatively fed by the internal carotid artery, decreased in size and density; and the posterior basal moyamoya area, which was fed by the vertebral arterial system, tended to decrease in size and density. The ethmoidal moyamoya vessel areas sometimes increased postoperatively. Revascularized areas (expressed as an increase in the area of vault moyamoya here) newly produced by encephaloduroarteriosynangiosis were visualized in postoperative angiograms, showing the development of adequate anastomosis between the donor artery of the external carotid system and cerebral arteries.

The author believes that these two parameters, diameter change of the donor arteries and revascularized areas, make a good objective scale to compare the effectiveness of various bypass procedures.

Cerebral Blood Flow After Encephaloduroarteriosynangiosis. Since the cerebral blood flow in children changes markedly with age, it is difficult to compare the preoperative and postoperative cerebral blood flow without correcting the value with that of a normal child of the same age.[65] In the past, most researchers have not considered this aspect.[18, 20, 86] According to these reports, an increase in hemispheric and cortical flow after encephaloduroarteriosynangiosis was significant in patients with transient ischemic attacks but not in patients with infarction and hemorrhage.[18, 86] The increase in cortical flow at the site of operation was first noted after 2 weeks.[86] Interestingly, vascular reserve of not regional but the total hemisphere increased very much at this early postoperative stage, and this state eventually become well revascularized in follow-up angiograms. After encephalomyosynangiosis, according to Hosaka and colleagues, mean cerebral blood flow decreased slightly or remained unchanged within 3

Figure 49–11

Preoperative and postoperative selective external and internal carotid arteriograms. *A.* Preoperative external carotid arteriogram: marked transdural anastomoses (vault moyamoya) are observed at the vault. *B.* External carotid arteriogram at 9 postoperative months: transdural anastomoses observed in the preoperative angiogram are gone, and instead marked revascularization through the donor artery is demonstrated. *C.* Preoperative internal carotid arteriogram: marked basal moyamoya disease is observed associated with poor visualization of the anterior cerebral artery and no visualization of the middle cerebral artery. Ethmoidal moyamoya disease is also observed. *D.* Nine months postoperative internal carotid arteriogram: basal moyamoya disease is decreased in the preoperative angiogram. Distal visualization shows decreased ethmoidal moyamoya disease.

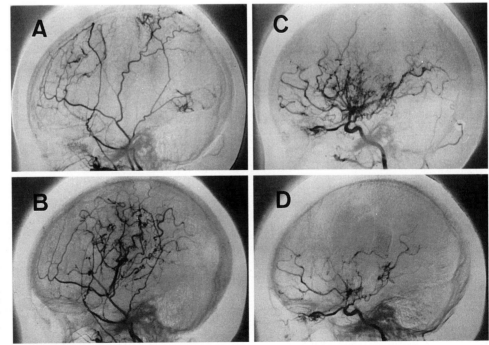

months after the operation in several patients and then increased gradually and became stationary 6 to 12 months later in most of the patients; and mean cerebral blood flow increased by an average of 11.4 per cent.[18] With encephaloduroarteriosynangiosis, the author has never experienced such a depression of cerebral blood flow in the early postoperative period.

Perioperative and Postoperative Complications of Encephaloduroarteriosynangiosis and Their Prevention. Possible perioperative complications and what has occurred after encephaloduroarteriosynangiosis are listed in Table 49–5.[54] Three of five patients who had perioperative infarctive episodes had their ischemic attacks just after crying. When performing operations on small children, it is important not to let them cry at the time of examinations, when being premedicated for anesthesia, or after operation. Postoperatively, changing dressings and laboratory examinations should be limited. The author prepares an oxygen tent with a cylinder of oxygen with 5 per cent carbon dioxide at bed side and lets the patient cry in the tent when crying is uncontrollable.

In one case, acidosis and myoglobinuria were observed during the operation and the operation was discontinued after the diagnosis of malignant hyperthermia.

In two cases, wound infection occurred. In moyamoya disease, a prolonged postoperative slight fever is sometimes present. In such a case, it is necessary to

Table 49–5

OPERATIVE COMPLICATIONS OF MOYAMOYA DISEASE

Complications	No. of Cases
Preoperative infarction	2
Intraoperative infarction	
Postoperative infarction	4
Postoperative mild fever	Many cases
Malignant hyperthermia	1
Wound infection	2
Hair loss around the wound	Most cases
Widening of operative scar	A few early cases
Subcutaneous hematoma	Many cases
Epidural hematoma	1
Subdural hematoma	0
Frontal facial nerve cutting	1
Donor laceration	7
Brain damage	0
Focal epilepsy	0
Difficulty in later operation	1
Neovascular tear	0
Increase in contralateral ischemic episodes	Possibly 2
Temporary appearance or aggravation of involuntary movements	5
Vascular headache	0
Dependence on donor artery	All successful cases

Reprinted by permission of the publisher from "Perioperative Complications of Encephalo-Duro-Arterio-Synangiosis: Prevention and Treatment," by Matsushima, Y., Aoyagi, M., et al., Surg. Neurol. vol. 36, pp. 343–353. Copyright 1991 by Elsevier Science Publishing Co., Inc.

observe the wound carefully because the wound infection may become apparent as time passes.

Vertical collateral communication is abundant in moyamoya disease. These communicating vessels can be injured in the operative field. Bleeding from these sites may cause subdural or epidural hematoma. In the author's experience, a small subdural hematoma, a layer of possibly inflowing blood from the operative field that is less than 1 mm thick, is sometimes recognized on routine computed tomography the next morning. The author has not yet met with a subdural hematoma acute enough to warrant an emergency operation but has experienced a case of acute epidural hematoma that required an emergency operation and resulted in permanent hemiparesis.

Patients with moyamoya disease typically are slow to awake from anesthesia. Therefore, the surgeon may have difficulty in checking the patient neurologically, especially when he or she is making an effort to keep the child from crying. It is necessary, however, to check the patient at intervals and to take immediate counter measures such as computed tomography or surgery as necessary.

The author's group has injured the donor arteries in 7 sides of 169 sides (4.14 per cent). All of the pediatric patients showed good revascularization despite these injuries.

One patient developed upper facial palsy by injuring the frontal branches of the facial nerve by excessive inferior elongation of the dermal excision.

Involuntary movements were temporarily aggravated in five cases after operation. They disappeared 1½ years after operation in the patient who had had involuntary movements the longest preoperatively.

There is a fear that the blood flow to the brain may be inhibited by mechanical pressure loaded by the frame of glasses or donor's trauma, for example, with an increase in dependency of the brain circulation to the donor artery. One patient needed to use contact lenses instead of framed glasses 8 years after the operation. It is necessary to take into consideration that the operative procedures might increase the chance of bleeding in head injury since the procedure artificially increases the so-called transdural anastomoses that bridge the dura mater and the brain. A case of acute subdural hematoma possibly due to the rupture of such an anastomosis has been reported.[92] Besides, future craniotomy may be difficult for new intracranial diseases, although the author has not yet met with such a case.

Long-Term Follow-Up. In 1979, the author and colleagues developed encephaloduroarteriosynangiosis to treat moyamoya disease. The procedure was performed on one side of a patient (case 1). Six months later, angiography revealed marked revascularization of the operated hemisphere. The operation was then performed on the other side of the same patient. Another patient (case 2) also underwent the operation.[47] With the cooperation of these first two patients, a full survey of them could be performed 11 years after the bilateral operations.[55]

Slight left-sided hemiparesis was observed preoperatively in the first patient, and this disappeared in about

1 month after the right side operation. In the second patient no motor dysfunction was seen except for episodic transient ischemic attacks, and this attack completely disappeared 3 months after the operation. Anticonvulsants were discontinued at the fourth postoperative year in case 1 and at the fifth postoperative year in case 2. Both patients have been free of ischemic or convulsive attacks for the past 11 years.

Remarkable progress in school achievement was observed in the first patient right after the operation. After that, no remarkable progress nor deterioration in school performance has been observed in either patient. Now, the first patient works as a clerk at a post office without any trouble and the second patient is studying law as a promising fourth-year university student. The intelligence quotient results by Wechsler Adult Intelligence Scale were TIQ 110, VIQ 110, and PIQ 96 for the first patient and TIQ 130, VIQ 128, and PIQ 122 for the second patient.

Angiography showed rapid increase in the diameter of transplanted donor arteries and dural arteries around the operated sites, remarkable revascularization of the brain through these arteries, and gradual decrease in moyamoya vessels at the base of the brain. The decrease in basal moyamoya vessels may cause decrease in the chance of intracranial bleeding as the patient gets older.

According to xenon-enhanced computed tomography, resting cerebral blood flow in the first patient is minimally low in total area but acetazolamide reaction is very good, especially at anterior circulation. The second patient shows a normal cerebral blood flow pattern at rest but the acetazolamide reaction is slightly decreased.

REFERENCES

1. Aihara, N., Nagai, H., Mase, M., et al.: Atypical moyamoya disease associated with brain tumor. Surg. Neurol., 37:46–50, 1992.
2. Aoyagi, M., Fukai, N., Matsushima, Y., et al.: Kinetics of ^{125}I-PDGF binding and down-regulation of PDGF receptor in arterial smooth muscle cells derived from patients with moyamoya disease. J. Cell Physiol., 154:281–288, 1993.
3. Aoyagi, M., Fukai, N., Sakamoto, H., et al.: Altered cellular response to serum mitogens, including platelet-derived growth factor, in cultured smooth muscle cells derived from arteries of patients with moyamoya disease. J. Cell Physiol., 147:191–198, 1991.
4. Arita, K., Uozumi, T., Oki, S., et al.: Moyamoya disease associated with pituitary adenoma: Report of two cases. Neurol. Med. Chir., 32:753–757, 1992.
5. Baquis, G. D., Pessin, M. S., and Scott, R. M.: Limb shaking: A carotid TIA. Stroke, 16:444–448, 1985.
6. Beyer, R. A., Paden, P., Sobel, D. F., et al.: Moyamoya pattern of vascular occlusion after radiotherapy for glioma of the optic chiasm. Neurology, 36:1173–1178, 1986.
7. Debrun, G., Sauvegrain, J., Aicardi, J., et al.: Moyamoya, a nonspecific radiological syndrome. Neuroradiology, 8:241–244, 1975.
8. Dillon, J. D., Stokes, H., and Meirowsky, A. M.: Moyamoya disease. Surg. Neurol., 3:233–236, 1975.
9. Ellison, P. H., Largent, J. A., and Popp A. J.: Moyamoya disease associated with renal artery stenosis. Arch. Neurol. 38:467, 1981.
10. Fukuyama, Y., Kanai, N., and Ohsawa, M.: Clinical genetic analysis on moyamoya disease. In Annual Report of the Research Committee on Spontaneous Occlusion of the Circle of Willis. Tokyo, Ministry of Health and Welfare of Japan, 1992, pp. 147–152 (in Japanese with English abstract).
11. Fukuyama, Y., Osawa, M., and Kanai, N.: Moyamoya disease (syndrome) and the Down syndrome. Brain Dev., 14:254–256, 1992.
12. Fukuyama, Y., and Umezu, R.: Clinical and cerebral angiographic evolutions of idiopathic progressive occlusive disease of the circle of Willis ("Moyamoya" disease) in children. Brain Dev., 7:21–37, 1985.
13. Garza-Mercado, R.: Pseudomoyamoya in sickle cell anemia. Surg. Neurol., 18:425–431, 1982.
14. Goto, Y., and Yonekawa, Y.: Worldwide distribution of moyamoya disease. Neurol. Med. Chir. (Tokyo), 32:883–886, 1992.
15. Halley S. E., White, W. B., Ramsby, G. R., et al.: Renovascular hypertension in moyamoya syndrome. Am. J. Hypertens., 1:348–352, 1988.
16. Harwood-Nash, D. C., McDonald, P., and Argent, W.: Cerebral arterial disease in children: An angiographic study of 40 cases. A.J.R., 111:672–686, 1971.
17. Hinshow, D. B., Thompson, J. R., and Hasso, A. N.: Adult arteriosclerotic moyamoya. Radiology, 118:633–636, 1976.
18. Hosaka, T., Horikoshi, S., Shibasaki, T., et al.: Hemodynamic evaluation by positron-emission CT after surgical treatment for children with moyamoya disease. Prog. Comput. Tomogr., 10:447–454, 1988 (in Japanese with English abstract).
19. Ikeda, E.: Systemic vascular changes in spontaneous occlusion of the circle of Willis. Stroke, 22:1358–1362, 1991.
20. Ishii, R., Takeuchi, S., Ibayashi, K., et al.: Intelligence in children with moyamoya disease: Evaluation after surgical treatments with special reference to changes in cerebral blood flow. Stroke, 15:873–877, 1984.
21. Jansen, J. N., Donker, J. M., Luth, W. J., et al.: Moyamoya disease associated with renovascular hypertension. Neuropediatrics, 21:44–47, 1990.
22. Kameyama, M., Shirane, R., Tsurumi, Y., et al.: Evaluation of cerebral blood flow and metabolism in childhood moyamoya disease: An investigation into "re-build-up" on EEG by positron CT. Child's Nerv. Syst., 2:130–133, 1986.
23. Kasusta, L., Daniels, O., and Renier, W. O.: Moya-moya syndrome and primary pulmonary hypertension. Neuropediatrics, 21:162–163, 1990.
24. Kawai, M.: A genetic study of idiopathic spontaneous multiple occlusion of the circle of Willis. Bull. Tokyo Women's Med. Coll., 55:427–441, 1985 (in Japanese with English abstract).
25. Kayama, T., Suzuki, S., Sakurai, Y., et al.: A case of moyamoya disease accompanied by an arteriovenous malformation. Neurosurgery, 18:465–468, 1986.
26. Kestle, J. R. W., Hoffman, H. J., and Mock, A. R.: Moyamoya phenomenon after radiation for optic glioma. J. Neurosurg., 79:32–35, 1993.
27. Kikuchi, H., Nagata, I., and Miyamoto, S.: Study on the children with moyamoya disease: I. Clinical course, cerebral angiography, and circulation. In Annual Report of Research Committee on the Cause and Treatment of Cerebrovascular Disorders in Developmental Age. Tokyo. Ministry of Health and Welfare of Japan, 1986, pp. 141–145 (in Japanese).
28. Kodama, N., Aoki, Y., Hiraga, H., et al.: Electroencephalographic findings in children with moyamoya disease. Arch. Neurol., 36:16–19, 1979.
29. Kodama, N., Fujiwara, S., Horie, Y., et al.: Transdural anastomosis in moyamoya disease: Vault moyamoya. Neurol. Surg., 8:729–737, 1080.
30. Kono, S., Oka, K., and Sueishi, K.: Histopathologic and morphometric studies of leptomeningeal vessels in moyamoya disease. Stroke, 21:1044–1050, 1990.
31. Krayenbuehl, H. A.: The moyamoya syndrome and neurosurgeon. Surg. Neurol., 4:353–361, 1975.
32. Kudo, T.: Occlusion of the internal carotid artery and the type of recovery of cerebral blood circulation. Clin. Neurol. (Tokyo), 1:199–200, 1960 (in Japanese).
33. Kudo, T.: General aspects. In Kudo, T., ed.: A Disease with Abnormal Intracranial Vascular Networks: Spontaneous Occlusion of the Circle of Willis. Tokyo, Igaku-Shoin, 1967.
34. Kudo, T.: Spontaneous occlusion of the circle of Willis: A disease apparently confined to Japanese. Neurology, 18:485–496, 1968.
35. Kudo, T., and Fukuda, S.: Spontaneous occlusion of the circle

of Willis. Shinkei-shimpo, 20:750–757, 1976 (in Japanese with English abstract).

36. Kurokawa, T., Chen, Y. J., Tomita, S., et al.: Cerebrovascular occlusive disease with and without the moyamoya vascular network in children. Neuropediatrics, 16:29–32, 1985.

37. Kurokawa, T., Tomita, S., Ueda, K., et al.: Prognosis of occlusive disease of the circle of Willis (moyamoya disease) in children. Pediatr. Neurol., 1:274–277, 1985.

38. Kurose, K., Kishi, H., and Sadatoh, T.: Moyamoya disease with persistent primitive hypoglossal artery: Case report. Neurol. Med. Chir. (Tokyo), 29:528–532, 1989.

39. Kwak, R., and Kadoya, S.: Moyamoya disease associated with persistent primitive trigeminal artery: Report of two cases. J. Neurosurg., 59:166–171, 1983.

40. Lamas, E., Lobato, R. D., Gabello, A., et al.: Multiple intracranial arterial occlusions (moyamoya disease) in patients with neurofibromatosis. Acta. Neurochir., 45:133–145, 1978.

41. Lecy, D. E.: Transient CNS deficits: A common benign syndrome in young adults. Neurology, 38:831–836, 1988.

42. Leiguarda, R., Berthier, M., Straekstein, S., et al.: Ischemic infarction in 25 children with tuberculous meningitis. Stroke, 19:200–204, 1988.

43. Lichtor, T., and Mullan, S.: Arteriovenous malformation in moyamoya syndrome: Report of three cases. J. Neurosurg., 67:603–608, 1987.

44. Mackenzie, C. A., Milner, R. D. G., Bergvall, U., et al.: Growth failure secondary to moyamoya syndrome. Arch. Dis. Child., 65:232–233, 1990.

45. Malley, R. A., and Frost, E. A. M.: Case report: Moyamoya disease: Pathophysiology and anesthetic management. J. Neurosurg. Anesthesiol., 2:110–114, 1989.

46. Mathew, N. T., Abraham, J., and Chandy, J.: Cerebral angiographic features in tuberculous meningitis. Neurology, 20:1015–1023, 1970.

47. Matsushima, Y.: An operation for Moyamoya disease, encephalo-duro-arterio-synangiosis. In Operative Neurosurgery 2. Tokyo, Neuron Publishing, 1989 (English version of the old edition is available through the author).

48. Matsushima, Y., and Inaba, Y.: Moyamoya disease in children and its surgical treatment. Child's Brain, 11:155–170, 1984.

49. Matsushima, Y., and Inaba, Y.: The specificity of the collaterals to the brain through the study and treatment of moyamoya disease. Stroke, 17:117–122, 1986.

50. Matsushima, Y., Aoyagi, M., Fukai, N., et al.: Angiographic demonstrations of cerebral revascularization after encephalo-duro-arterio-synangiosis (EDAS) performed on pediatric moyamoya patients. Bull. Tokyo Med. Dent. Univ., 29:7–17, 1982.

51. Matsushima, Y., Aoyagi, M., Koumo, Y., et al.: Effects of encephalo-duro-arterio-synangiosis on childhood moyamoya patients. Neurol. Med. Chir., 31:708–714, 1991.

52. Matsushima, Y., Aoyagi, M., Nariai, T., et al.: Angiographic evaluation of results of encephalo-duro-arterio-synangiosis in pediatric moyamoya patients. Child's Nerv. Syst. (Kobe), 17:353–358, 1992 (in Japanese with English abstract).

53. Matsushima, Y., Aoyagi, M., Niimi, Y., et al.: Symptoms and their pattern of progression in childhood moyamoya disease. Brain Dev., 12:784–789, 1990.

54. Matsushima, Y., Aoyagi, M., Suzuki, R., et al.: Perioperative complications of encephalo-duro-arterio-synangiosis: Prevention and treatment. Surg. Neurol., 36:343–353, 1991.

55. Matsushima, Y., Aoyagi, M., Tamaki, M., et al.: The first two post-EDAS pediatric moyamoya patients who have had EDAS for more than 10 years. Surg. Cerebral Stroke, 21:23–30, 1993 (in Japanese with English abstract).

56. Matsushima, Y., Fukai, N., Tanaka, K., et al.: A new operative method for "moya-moya" disease: A presentation of a case who underwent encephalo-duro-arterio (STA)-synangiosis. Child's Nerv. Syst. (Kobe), 5:249–255, 1980 (in Japanese with English abstract).

57. Matsushima, Y., Fukai, N., Tanaka, K., et al.: A new surgical treatment of moyamoya disease in children: A preliminary report. Surg. Neurol., 15:313–320, 1981.

58. Matsushima, Y., Suzuki, R., Ohno, K., et al.: Angiographic revascularization of the brain after EDAS: A case report. Neurosurgery, 21:928–934, 1987.

59. Matsushima, Y., Suzuki, R., Yamaguchi, T., et al.: Effects of indirect EC/IC bypass operations on adult moyamoya patients. Neurol. Surg., 14:1559–1566, 1986 (in Japanese with English abstract).

60. Matsushima, Y., Takasato, Y., Fukumoto, T., et al.: A case of internal carotid artery occlusion successfully treated by encephalo-duro-arterio-synangiosis (EDAS). Child's Nerv. Syst., 1:363–365, 1985.

61. Mawad, M. E., Hilal, S. K., Michelsen, W. J., et al.: Occlusive vascular disease associated with cerebral arteriovenous malformation. Radiology, 153:401–408, 1984.

62. Miyamoto, S., Kikuchi, H., Karasawa, J., et al.: Study of the posterior circulation in moymoya disease: Clinical and neuroradiological evaluation. J. Neurosurg., 61:1032–1037, 1984.

63. Nariai, T., Suzuki, R., Matsushima, Y., et al.: Indirect EC/IC bypass surgery as scavenger to cortex under chronic hemodynamic ischemia. J. Cereb. Blood Flow Metab., 13 (Suppl. 1):429, 1993.

64. Nishimoto, A., and Takeuchi, S.: Abnormal cerebrovascular network related to the internal carotid arteries. J. Neurosurg., 29:255–260, 1968.

65. Ogawa, A., Sakurai, Y., Kayama, T., et al.: Regional cerebral blood flow with age: Changes in rCBF in childhood. Neurol. Res., 11:173–176, 1989.

66. Okeda, R.: A moyamoya patient died of pulmonary cancer: A discussions on pathogenesis of arterial occlusion and abnormal basal networks. Shinkei-shimpo, 14:285–301, 1970 (in Japanese with English abstract).

67. Oku, S., Okumura, F., Kikuchi, H., et al.: The effects of arterial carbon dioxide on cerebral blood flow and on cerebral function in "Moyamoya" disease. J. Jpn. Soc. Clin. Anesth., 5:360–368, 1985 (in Japanese with English abstract).

68. Olds, M. V., Griebal, R. W., Hoffman, H. J., et al.: The surgical treatment of childhood moyamoya disease. J. Neurosurg., 66:675–680, 1987.

69. Outwater, E. K., Platenberg, R. C., and Wolpert, S. M.: Moyamoya disease in Down syndrome. A.J.N.R., 10:23–24, 1989.

70. Pavlakis, S. R., Schneider, S., Black, K., et al.: Steroid-responsive chorea in moyamoya disease. Movement Disord., 6:347–349, 1991.

71. Pracyk, J. B., and Massey, J. M.: Moyamoya disease associated with polycystic kidney disease and eosinophilic granuloma. Stroke, 20:1092–1094, 1989.

72. Rajakulasingam, K., Cerullo, L. J., and Raimondi, A. L.: Childhood moyamoya syndrome postradiation pathogenesis. Child's Brain, 5:467–475, 1979.

73. Satoh, S., Shibuya, H., Matsushima, Y., et al.: Analysis of the angiographic findings in cases of childhood moyamoya disease. Neuroradiology, 30:111–119, 1988.

74. Savir, A., Dickerman, Z., Karp, M., et al.: Moyamoya associated with peripheral vascular occlusive disease. Arch. Dis. Child., 49:964–966, 1974.

75. Seeler, R. A., Royal, J. E., Powe, L., et al.: Moyamoya in children with sickle cell anemia and cerebrovascular occlusion. J. Pediatr., 90:808–810, 1978.

76. Servo, A., and Puranen, M.: Moyamoya syndrome as a complication of radiation therapy: Case report. J. Neurosurg., 48:1026–1029, 1978.

77. Shields, W. D., Ziter, F. A., Osborn, A. G., et al.: Fibromuscular dysplasia as a cause of stroke in infancy and childhood. Pediatrics, 56:899–901, 1977.

78. Shimoji, T., Ito, M., and Sato, K.: Cerebral revascularization for Moyamoya disease: Usefulness of encephalo-duro-arterio-synangiosis. Child's Nerv. Syst. (Kobe), 15:161–168, 1990 (in Japanese with English abstract).

79. Subirana, A., and Subirana, M.: Malformations vasculaires du type de l'angiome arteriel racemeux. Rev. Neurol. (Paris), 107:545–550, 1962.

80. Sunder, T. R.: Moyamoya disease in a patient with type 1 glycogenosis. Arch. Neurol., 38:251–254, 1981.

81. Suzuki, J., and Kodama, N.: Cerebral vascular "moyamoya" disease: II. Collateral routes to forebrain via ethmoid sinus and superior nasal meatus. Angiology, 22:223–236, 1971.

82. Suzuki, J., and Kodama, N.: Moyamoya disease: A review. Stroke, 14:104–109, 1983.

83. Suzuki, J.: Moyamoya Disease. Berlin, Springer-Verlag, 1986.

84. Suzuki, J., and Takaku, A.: Cerebrovascular "moyamoya" disease: Disease showing abnormal net-like vessels in base of brain. Arch. Neurol., 20:288–299, 1969.

85. Suzuki, R., Matsushima, Y., Hiratsuka, H., et al.: A simplified method of xenon enhanced CT for regional cerebral blood flow (rCBF) measurement with reference to clinical experiences. Bull. Tokyo Med. Dent. Univ., 33:107–116, 1986.

86. Suzuki, R., Matsushima, Y., Takada, Y., et al.: Changes in cerebral hemodynamics following encephalo-duro-arterio-synangiosis in young patients with moyamoya disease. Surg. Neurol., 31:343–349, 1989.

87. Suzuki, R., Tsuruoka, S., Hiratsuka, H., et al.: Cerebral circulation in pediatric patients with moyamoya disease. Neuro. Med. Chir., 25:969–974, 1985 (in Japanese with English abstract).

88. Tagawa, T., Naritomi, H., Mimaki, T., et al.: Regional cerebral blood flow, clinical manifestations, and age in children with moyamoya disease. Stroke, 18:906–910, 1987.

89. Takasato, Y., Matsushima, Y., Nariai, T., et al.: A study of symptoms in ameliorated cases at an early post-EDAS period in moyamoya disease. Jpn. J. Stroke, 10:25–31, 1988 (in Japanese with English abstract).

90. Takeuchi, K.: Carotid artery obstruction. Shinkei-Shimpo, 5:511–543, 1961 (in Japanese).

91. Takeuchi, K., Hara, M., Yokota, H., et al.: Factors influencing the development of moyamoya phenomenon. Acta Neurochir., 59:79–86, 1981.

92. Takeuchi, K., Ichikawa, A., Koike, T., et al.: Acute subdural hematoma in young patient with moyamoya disease. Neurol. Med. Chir. (Tokyo), 32:80–83, 1992.

93. Tibbles J. A. R., and Brown, B. S. J.: Acute hemiplegia of childhood. Can. Med. Assoc. J., 113:309–314, 1975.

94. Tomsich, T. A., Lukin, R. R., Chambers, A. A., et al.: Neurofibromatosis and intracranial arterial occlusive disease. Neuroradiology, 11:229–234, 1976.

95. Waga, S., and Tochio, H.: Intracranial aneurysm associated with moyamoya disease in childhood. Surg. Neurol., 23:237–243, 1985.

96. Wanifuchi, H., Takeshita, M., Izawa, M., et al.: Management of adult moyamoya disease. Neurol. Med. Chir. (Tokyo), 33:300–305, 1993.

97. Ximin, L., Xuzhong, R., Zhuan, C., et al.: Moyamoya disease caused by leptospiral cerebral arteritis. Chin. Med. J., 93:599–604, 1980.

98. Yamada, H., Iwamura, M., Deguchi, K., et al.: Relationship between spontaneous occlusion of the circle of Willis (moyamoya disease) and bacterial infection. *In* Annual Report of the Research Committee on Spontaneous Occlusion of the Circle of Willis (Moyamoya Disease). Tokyo, Ministry of Health and Welfare of Japan, 1993, pp. 144–147 (in Japanese with English abstract).

99. Yamada, I., Matsushima, Y., and Suzuki, S.: Moyamoya disease: Diagnosis with three dimensional time-of-flight MR angiography. Radiology, 183:773–778, 1992.

100. Yamaguchi, T., Matsushima, Y., Takada, Y., et al.: Case-control study of moyamoya disease. Brain Nerve (Tokyo), 41:485–491, 1989 (in Japanese with English abstract).

101. Yamashiro, Y., Takahashi, H., and Takahashi, K.: Cerebrovascular moyamoya disease. Eur. J. Pediatr., 142:44–50, 1984.

102. Yamashita, M., Oka, K., and Tanaka, K.: Histopathology of the brain vascular network in moyamoya disease. Stroke, 14:50–58, 1983.

103. Yamashita, M., Tanaka, K., Kishikawa, T., et al.: Moyamoya disease associated with renovascular hypertension. Hum. Pathol., 15:191–193, 1984.

104. Yasutomo, Y., Hashimoto, T., Miyazaki, M., et al.: A moyamoya girl presented with periodical torticolis. Brain Dev., 24:391–393, 1992 (in Japanese).

105. Yonekawa, Y., ed.: Proceedings of open symposium on etiology of Moyamoya disease. In Annual Report (1991) of the Research Committee on Spontaneous Occlusion of the Circle of Willis (Moyamoya disease). Tokyo, Ministry of Health and Welfare of Japan, 1992.

Pathophysiology and Clinical Evaluation of Subarachnoid Hemorrhage

Bleeding into the subarachnoid space is termed "subarachnoid hemorrhage." It may be spontaneous or traumatic in onset and massive or trivial in volume and occur as the primary site of hemorrhage or secondary to rupture of parenchymal bleeding through the pia mater into the subarachnoid space. With trauma and subarachnoid hemorrhage secondary to intracerebral hemorrhage, the clinical features, pathophysiology, and treatment center around the primary disorder rather than the secondary subarachnoid hemorrhage. It is after rupture of an intracranial aneurysm, and sometimes an arteriovenous malformation, that the pathology, pathophysiology, and neurology are primarily a reflection of the effects of subarachnoid hemorrhage. Subarachnoid hemorrhage associated with these latter conditions is the subject of this chapter.

Etiology and Epidemiology

ETIOLOGY OF SUBARACHNOID HEMORRHAGE

The most common cause of blood in the subarachnoid space is head trauma, although the volume and distribution of subarachnoid bleeding after trauma differs from that due to, for example, rupture of a cerebral aneurysm.[78] Ruptured aneurysms and arteriovenous malformations are the most common causes of spontaneous subarachnoid hemorrhage.[60, 78] Of 5,836 patients reported in the first cooperative study, 57 per cent had subarachnoid hemorrhage from aneurysms or arteriovenous malformations.[60] Four-vessel angiography was not routine, and therefore that percentage might be higher today. In the remaining 43 per cent (2,530 cases), subarachnoid hemorrhage was due to hypertensive atherosclerotic disease in 15 per cent and miscellaneous

conditions, including neoplasm, blood dyscrasia, sickle cell anemia, endocarditis with emboli, and intracranial infections, in 6 per cent. Angiography and autopsy did not disclose a source of hemorrhage in 22 per cent. Most patients with fatal spontaneous subarachnoid hemorrhage had hypertensive atherosclerotic disease (52 per cent), and the usual cause of the hemorrhage in these cases was rupture of an intracerebral hemorrhage into the subarachnoid space or ventricular system (present in 85 per cent).[61] The cause of subarachnoid hemorrhage varies with age, with arteriovenous malformations presenting in younger patients and aneurysms and other causes predominating with increasing age (Fig. 50–1).[78]

With current diagnostic techniques, no cause for the

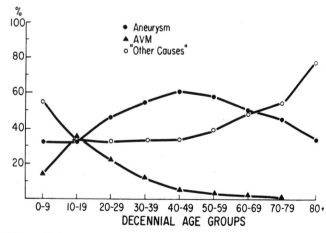

Figure 50–1

Relative probability of each major cause of subarachnoid hemorrhage by decade of life. (From Locksley, H. B.: Natural history of subarachnoid hemorrhage, intracranial aneurysms, and arteriovenous malformations: Based on 6368 cases in the cooperative study: I. *In* Sahs, A. L., Perret, G. E., Locksley, H. B., et al., eds.: Intracranial Aneurysms and Subarachnoid Hemorrhage. Philadelphia, J. B. Lippincott, 1969, p. 40. Reprinted by permission.)

R. L. Macdonald • B. Weir

hemorrhage is found in 9 to 30 per cent of cases. An incomplete list of the vast number of other diseases reported to be associated with subarachnoid hemorrhage is shown in Table 50–1.[118]

CLASSIFICATION AND ETIOLOGY OF ANEURYSMS

Aneurysms may be classified based on size, location, etiology, and pathology (Tables 50–2 and 50–3).[117] Aneurysms over 2.5 cm in diameter are considered giant. By far the most common aneurysm is the acquired saccular aneurysm. Among 1,092 patients admitted to the Cooperative Aneurysm Study between 1970 and 1977, the average maximum diameter of ruptured aneurysms was 8.2 ± 3.9 mm. Thirteen per cent of ruptured aneurysms were less than 5 mm in diameter. Unruptured, asymptomatic aneurysms were less than

Table 50–1
ETIOLOGY OF SUBARACHNOID HEMORRHAGE

Angiopathies
Aneurysms, arteriovenous malformations, atherosclerosis, hypertension, intra-arterial embolism, amyloid, systemic lupus erythematosus, giant cell arteritis, focal vascular necrosis, polyarteritis nodosa, telangiectasia, Sturge-Weber syndrome
Venous Thrombosis
Pregnancy, contraceptives, trauma, infection, coagulopathy, marasmus, volume depletion
Blood Diseases
Leukemia, Hodgkin's disease, hemophilia, sickle cell anemia, pernicious anemia, aplastic anemia, agranulocytosis, thrombocytopenic purpura, polycythemia vera, Waldenström's macroglobulinemia, lymphoma, myeloma, hereditary spherocytosis, afibrinogenemia, hypofibrinogenemia (liver disease), consumption coagulopathy, disseminated intravascular coagulation, anticoagulants
Allergic Diseases
Anaphylactoid purpura, hemorrhagic nephritis, Shwartzman phenomenon, Schönlein-Henoch syndrome
Infections
Bacterial meningitis, tuberculous meningitis, syphilitic meningoencephalitis, fungal meningitis, leptospirosis, *Listeria*, brucellosis, yellow fever, typhoid fever, dengue, malaria, anthrax, viral encephalitis, cytomegalic inclusion disease, parasites
Intoxications
Cocaine, epinephrine, monoamine oxidase inhibitors, amphetamines, alcohol, ether, carbon monoxide, morphine, nicotine, lead, quinine, phosphorus, Metraxol, hydrocyanic acid, insulin, snake venom
Neoplasms
Glioma, meningioma, hemangioblastoma, choroid plexus papilloma, chordoma, hemangioma, pituitary adenoma, sarcoma, osteochondroma, ependymoma, neurofibroma, bronchogenic carcinoma, choriocarcinoma, melanoma
Trauma
Blows, electrical injury, high altitude, caisson disease, radiation, uremia, strangulation, heat injury
Pediatric
Germinal matrix hemorrhage
Miscellaneous
Electroconvulsive therapy, sunstroke, scurvy, Valsalva maneuver, vitamin K deficiency, hyperbilirubinemia, electrolyte imbalance, eclampsia, intrathecal chymopapain

Modified from Weir, B.: Aneurysms Affecting the Nervous System. Baltimore, Williams & Wilkins, 1987, p 82. Reprinted by permission.

Table 50–2
CLASSIFICATION OF INTRACRANIAL ANEURYSMS

I. Size
  A. < 3 mm
  B. 4–6 mm (small)
  C. 7–10 mm (medium)
  D. 11–24 mm (large)
  E. > 25 mm (giant)
II. Location
  A. Anterior circulation
    1. Internal carotid artery
      a. Petrous
      b. Cavernous
      c. Paraclinoid (ophthalmic)
      d. Posterior communicating
      e. Anterior choroidal
      f. Carotid bifurcation
    2. Anterior cerebral artery
      a. Precommunicating
      b. Communicating artery complex
      c. Distal anterior cerebral artery
    3. Middle cerebral artery
      a. Sphenoidal segment (lenticulostriate)
      b. Bifurcation
      c. Distal
  B. Posterior circulation
    1. Vertebral artery
      a. Main trunk
      b. Posterior inferior cerebellar artery
    2. Basilar artery
      a. Trunk
      b. Anterior inferior cerebellar artery
      c. Superior cerebellar artery
      d. Basilar bifurcation
    3. Posterior cerebral artery
      a. Precommunicating segment
      b. Distal, postcommunicating segment
III. Pathology
  A. Saccular
  B. Dissecting
  C. Fusiform
  D. Microaneurysm (Charcot-Bouchard)

Modified from Weir, B.: Intracranial aneurysms and subarachnoid hemorrhage: An overview. *In* Wilkins, R. H., and Rengachary, S. S., eds.: Neurosurgery. New York, McGraw-Hill, 1985, p. 1309. Reprinted by permission.

10 mm in 94 per cent of cases, and the size of unruptured symptomatic aneurysms varied, with 70 per cent being from 3 to 10 mm in diameter and 13 per cent larger than 25 mm. Only 2 to 3 per cent of ruptured aneurysms were giant.[51]

The 2,349 single ruptured aneurysms entered into the Cooperative Aneurysm Study between 1958 and 1965 were located as shown in Table 50–4.[60] Only 24 per cent of patients had bilateral carotid and vertebral angiography. The incidence of aneurysms in the posterior circulation is probably higher when complete angiography is routinely done and ranges from 7 to 14 per cent.[118] Internal carotid artery aneurysms predominate in females (66 per cent versus 34 per cent in males), anterior cerebral artery aneurysms predominate in males (59 per cent versus 41 per cent in females), and middle cerebral artery aneurysms have no sex predilection.[118] Yasargil reported that 24 per cent of his 1,012 patients had more than one aneurysm, although this included aneurysms less than 3 mm ("microaneurysms"), which were only diagnosed intra-

Table 50–3

ETIOLOGY OF INTRACRANIAL ANEURYSMS

I. Saccular
  A. Hemodynamic
    1. Increased blood flow due to
      a. Arteriovenous malformation
      b. Aplasia, hypoplasia, or occlusion of contralateral artery normally present
      c. Persistent carotid-basilar anastomosis
    2. Increased blood pressure due to
      a. Coarctation of the aorta
      b. Polycystic kidney disease
      c. Fibromuscular dysplasia of renal arteries
  B. Structural
    1. Acquired, due to degeneration of internal elastic lamina
    2. Sickle cell anemia
  C. Genetic
    1. Familial intracranial aneurysms
    2. Type III collagen deficiency
    3. Other syndromes reported with aneurysms: Ehlers-Danlos syndrome, Marfan's syndrome, pseudoxanthoma elasticum, Rendu-Osler-Weber syndrome, Klippel-Trénaunay-Weber syndrome
  D. Inflammatory
    1. Infectious
      a. Bacterial
      b. Fungal
      c. Parasitic
    2. Inflammatory
      a. Systemic lupus erythematosus
  E. Traumatic
    1. Closed head injury
    2. Iatrogenic
    3. Penetrating head injury
  F. Neoplastic
    1. Primary brain neoplasm
    2. Metastatic brain neoplasms
      a. Choriocarcinoma
      b. Atrial myxoma
      c. Carcinoma
  G. Other vascular diseases
    1. Moyamoya disease
    2. Giant cell arteritis
II. Fusiform Aneurysms
  A. Atherosclerosis
  B. Genetic
  C. Structural
  D. Infectious
  E. Radiation
  F. Other vascular disorders
    1. Coarctation of the aorta
    2. Giant cell arteritis

Modified from Weir, B.: Intracranial aneurysms and subarachnoid hemorrhage: An overview. *In* Wilkins, R. H., and Rengachary, S. S., eds.: Neurosurgery. New York, McGraw-Hill, 1985, p. 1310. Reprinted by permission.

operatively.[123] A review of literature published between 1941 and 1979 indicated that multiple aneurysms were diagnosed at angiography in about 13 per cent (range: 4 to 33 per cent) of cases and at autopsy in 23 per cent.[123] All but one autopsy series found more than 20 per cent of patients had multiple aneurysms.[123] With current angiography techniques, the incidence of multiplicity is approaching that which is found at autopsy.

EPIDEMIOLOGY OF ANEURYSMAL SUBARACHNOID HEMORRHAGE

Inagawa and associates reviewed 13 studies of the average annual incidence of spontaneous subarachnoid hemorrhage per 100,000 population and found rates varying from 6.5 to 26.4.[45] For aneurysmal subarachnoid hemorrhage, the rates varied from 6 to 35.3. Rates are strongly affected by the age distribution of the studied population, so, for example, in Shimane Prefecture (Japan), for each decade rates per 100,000 population per year were as follows: (a) 0 to 9, 0; (b) 10 to 19, 0.2; (c) 20 to 29, 2.1; (d) 30 to 39, 3.9; (e) 40 to 49, 18.1; (f) 50 to 59, 30.4; (g) 60 to 69, 38.3; (h) 70 to 79, 26.2; and (i) 80 or more, 15.4.

Other studies show no great falloff at great age. About 56 per cent of aneurysm patients are female, so that rates of aneurysmal subarachnoid hemorrhage are slightly higher in females. Before age 50, aneurysm rupture is more common in males; and after age 50, females predominate.[117] The increasing number of females afflicted with aneurysms with increasing age is only partially explained by their greater longevity. There is probably some geographical variation in incidence of aneurysm rupture, with higher rates tending to be reported from Finland and possibly Japan. Whether the variation is due to racial (genetic), dietary, or environmental factors is unclear. Lower rates reported from Africa, China, India, and the Middle East may be due to a difference in health care or to a true difference in incidence rates.[118] Although the exact rates will vary depending on the age distribution of the population, on the standard of medical care, on racial and environmental factors, and possibly on the prevalence of hypertension and atherosclerosis, an overall approximation for the rate of aneurysmal subarachnoid hemorrhage is 10 per 100,000 population per year.

Table 50–4

LOCATION OF INTRACRANIAL SACCULAR ANEURYSMS BASED ON DATA FROM A COOPERATIVE ANEURYSM STUDY[58]

Location	No. of Cases	Percentage of Total
Internal carotid artery		
Proximal to posterior communicating	101	4.3
Posterior communicating artery	576	25.0
Posterior communicating to bifurcation	101	4.3
Internal carotid bifurcation	106	4.5
Anterior cerebral artery		
Proximal to anterior communicating	35	1.5
Anterior communicating complex	711	30.3
Distal to anterior communicating	66	2.8
Middle cerebral artery		
Proximal to bifurcation	91	3.9
Bifurcation region	307	13.1
Distal to bifurcation	32	1.4
Posterior circulation		
Basilar bifurcation	48	2.0
Basilar trunk	19	0.8
Posterior inferior cerebellar	11	0.5
Vertebral	20	0.9
Other, unspecified	104	4.4
Total	2,439	100

Data from Locksley, H. B.: Natural history of subarachnoid hemorrhage, intracranial aneurysms, and arteriovenous malformations: Based on 6,368 cases in the cooperative study: I. *In* Sahs, A. L., Perret, G. E., Locksley, H. B., et al., eds.: Intracranial Aneurysms and Subarachnoid Hemorrhage. Philadelphia, J. B. Lippincott, 1969, pp. 37–57. Reprinted by permission.

The overall incidence of intracranial saccular aneurysms in the general population was extensively studied by Stehbens.[99] In 14 autopsy series published between 1890 and 1966, between 0.2 and 9 per cent (average: 2.4 per cent) of the patients had aneurysms. Pathological series may be biased by having been performed mainly on older patients dying in general hospitals. The rate for children is close to zero. Data on angiography, also mainly from adults, suggest 1 to 2 per cent is a more reasonable approximation. Atkinson and colleagues reviewed 9,295 angiograms and selected 278 patients who were thought to be an unbiased representation of the general adult population. Three (1 per cent) had incidental aneurysms.[7] It is estimated that only about half of all aneurysms ever rupture.

Pathology

MENINGEAL RESPONSE TO SUBARACHNOID HEMORRHAGE

Saccular aneurysms arise from the major cerebral arteries as they course through the subarachnoid space. Therefore, rupture most commonly deposits blood in this space, which contains cerebrospinal fluid. The meningeal response was studied in 134 autopsied cases of subarachnoid hemorrhage.[4, 35] Within hours of the hemorrhage there was an influx of polymorphonuclear leukocytes into the subarachnoid space. Lymphocytes appeared later, accompanied by macrophages on the third day. The acute inflammatory response subsided after about 48 hours. Reticulin fibers (fine collagen) appeared as early as 3 days post hemorrhage, although definite fibrosis of the arachnoid spaces did not begin until 10 days after the hemorrhage. Most erythrocytes disappeared from the subarachnoid space by hemolysis, liberating hemoglobin and its breakdown products, other erythrocyte proteins, and membrane lipids. Intact red blood cells were observed trapped in the arachnoid trabeculae up to 35 days after hemorrhage. Experimental studies suggest that in addition to being cleared from the subarachnoid space by hemolysis and phagocytosis, erythrocytes depart directly into the bloodstream, possibly through the arachnoid villi.[32] The importance of this method of red blood cell removal, as well as of accessory outflow pathways for cerebrospinal fluid after subarachnoid hemorrhage in humans, is unknown.

PATHOLOGY OF ANEURYSMS

Rhoton summarized the pathological anatomy of common saccular cerebral aneurysms.[82] They arise at arterial bifurcations or at the origins of branches from the parent artery. Aneurysms usually arise where the parent artery curves, and the sac points in the direction that the blood would have flowed had it not been constrained by the curving of the branches of the bifurcation.

Small aneurysms are described as funnel-shaped outpouchings at bifurcations where the internal elastic lamina has undergone extensive fragmentation.[117, 118] With fully developed saccular aneurysms, the internal elastic lamina and tunica media end abruptly at the mouth of the aneurysm. A layer of endothelial cells may coat the intimal surface, although the endothelium is often deficient. The remainder of the aneurysm wall is collagen of variable thickness containing scattered fibroblasts and sometimes laminated thrombus. There are only fragments of degenerated internal elastic lamina. The aneurysm wall may show leukocyte infiltration, calcification, fibrin deposition, and hemosiderin-laden macrophages. Intimal cushions, or focal collections of myointimal cells and extracellular matrix within the tunica intima, are frequent at bifurcation points around the aneurysm orifice. Atherosclerotic change is common in the parent vessels and in the aneurysm wall. In giant aneurysms and in those that have previously ruptured, there may be infiltration of the aneurysm wall with capillaries from the arachnoid.[98]

Nystrom, in an autopsy study of 70 ruptured aneurysms, found hemorrhage emanated from the aneurysm neck in 10 per cent, from the middle of the aneurysm in 33 per cent, and from the dome in 57 per cent.[74] Others reported that 84 per cent of aneurysms ruptured from the dome and 2 per cent from the neck.[117] Daughter blebs and multiloculation of aneurysms may predispose to rupture since the wall tends to be greatly thinned in these areas.

VASCULAR PATHOLOGY ASSOCIATED WITH ANEURYSMS

A variety of congenital and acquired vascular lesions are associated with cerebral aneurysms.[117, 118] The most common anatomical variation is probably that associated with anterior communicating artery aneurysms. Yasargil and associates noted that among 375 aneurysms of the anterior communicating artery, the precommunicating segments of the anterior cerebral arteries were equal in size in only 19 per cent of cases and that with this relationship, the aneurysm arose from the middle of the communicating artery 67 per cent of the time.[123] In 81 per cent of patients, one precommunicating anterior cerebral artery was hypoplastic (more commonly the right) and aneurysms arose from the anterior communicating–anterior cerebral artery junction on the side of the large anterior cerebral artery in over 95 per cent of cases. The relationship between saccular aneurysms and hypoplasia of the posterior communicating artery is less obvious, although such aneurysms are probably more common if the communicating artery is large.

Infundibulae occur on about 7 per cent of normal angiograms, and their incidence increases with advancing age.[37] They are usually less than 3 mm in diameter, have small arteries arising from their domes, and are located at the junction of the internal carotid and posterior communicating arteries in 65 per cent of cases.

They are characterized histologically by areas of thinning or absence of the tunica media and occasionally of absence of the internal elastic membrane. In 132 patients with arteriovenous malformations, 17 per cent had associated aneurysms, 15 per cent had infundibula, and 8 per cent had both.[68] That infundibula are flow-related is suggested by their frequent occurrence on arteries feeding arteriovenous malformations and their disappearance after excision of the malformations. Infundibulae may very rarely develop into aneurysms. Subarachnoid hemorrhage from an infundibulum is extremely rare.

All of the persistent carotid-basilar anastomoses have been reported in association with aneurysms and subarachnoid hemorrhage, including the trigeminal, hypoglossal, otic, and proatlantal arteries.[118] Twenty-five per cent of patients with a trigeminal artery have a history of arteriovenous malformation or subarachnoid hemorrhage, and an aneurysm is found in 14 to 17 per cent.[2] The aneurysm is on the trigeminal artery in 13 per cent of cases. In contrast to trigeminal arteries, hypoglossal arteries are associated with a higher incidence of aneurysms on the persistent anastomotic artery itself, as well as in the posterior circulation in general.

Fenestrations were observed on 0.3 per cent of 3,841 angiograms reviewed by Nakajima and colleagues, although subsequent investigations suggest they are more common.[70, 118] About half the reported fenestrations of the internal carotid, anterior cerebral, anterior communicating, and vertebral arteries are associated with aneurysms. Basilar and middle cerebral artery fenestrations may also be associated with aneurysms.

Aneurysms may develop in association with the above anomalies due to alterations in cerebral blood flow patterns and rates, due to a common, underlying congenital or acquired vascular defect, or by coincidence. That blood flow is important is supported by reports of formation of aneurysms contralateral to carotid arteries that have thrombosed or have been surgically occluded. In a series of 205 patients with aneurysms, 1 per cent had arteriovenous malformations.[108] In seven series reported between 1956 and 1982 involving 1,112 patients with arteriovenous malformations, 8 per cent had aneurysms, which was judged to be higher than the incidence of aneurysms in the general population. Aneurysms associated with arteriovenous malformations are multiple in 28 per cent of cases and are on arteries feeding the malformations in about 50 per cent of cases.[75] These features, accompanied by reports of regression of aneurysms on feeding arteries following arteriovenous malformation obliteration, argue for a hemodynamic basis for aneurysm genesis.

Arterial wall pathology occurs after subarachnoid hemorrhage and is considered to be important in cerebral vasospasm.[118] The pathology includes changes typical of vasoconstriction (thickening of the arterial wall, folding of the internal elastic lamina, endothelial cell vacuolation, shortening and folding of smooth muscle cells), as well as endothelial cell loss, platelet adherence, smooth muscle cell necrosis and vacuolation, fibrosis, proliferation of myointimal cells, and periarterial fibrosis and inflammation. There is controversy about whether vasospasm represents smooth muscle contraction or whether other processes, including intimal proliferation, fibrosis, inflammation, and myofibroblasts, contribute to arterial narrowing after subarachnoid hemorrhage.[118, 122] Intimal proliferation is a late response to arterial injury and, although it occurs after the hemorrhage, it usually develops after the angiographic phase of vasospasm. It may be difficult to differentiate it from pre-existing atherosclerosis. The initial phase of vasospasm 3 to 7 days after subarachnoid hemorrhage is probably abnormal smooth muscle contraction, but, with time, the structural changes mentioned previously may be important in maintaining arterial narrowing, in making arteries relatively resistant to relaxation with vasodilators, and in inhibiting reconstruction after transluminal balloon angioplasty.[122]

PATHOLOGICAL SEQUELAE OF ANEURYSM RUPTURE

The pathological sequelae vary depending on the location of the aneurysm and how long it has been since the rupture (Table 50–5). In most reported pathological series, subarachnoid hemorrhage is almost universal, occurring in over 95 per cent of cases, intracerebral and intraventricular hemorrhages are common (about 50 per cent of cases having some component of one or the other), and subdural hemorrhage is uncommon (seen rarely in isolation, and in about 10 to 20 per cent of cases overall).[118] Cerebral infarction is more likely to be seen with increasing time from the subarachnoid hemorrhage. Among 83 autopsied cases of subarachnoid hemorrhage, cerebral edema was present

Table 50–5
PATHOLOGIC SEQUELAE OF ANEURYSM RUPTURE

I. Immediate
  A. Hemorrhage
    1. Subarachnoid
    2. Subdural
    3. Intracerebral
    4. Intraventricular
    5. Intra-aneurysmal
    6. Secondary brain stem Duret hemorrhages
  B. Brain herniation
    1. Subfalcine
    2. Transtentorial
    3. Foramen magnum
  C. Acute hydrocephalus
  D. Acute brain swelling
II. Delayed
  A. Aneurysmal rebleeding
  B. Cerebral edema
  C. Cerebral infarction
    1. Vasospasm
    2. Local pressure from intracerebral hematoma
    3. Arterial compressions from cerebral herniations
    4. Decreased cerebral perfusion due to systemic hypotension, intracranial hypertension, hypovolemia, hyponatremia, and hypoxia
  D. Chronic hydrocephalus

Modified from Weir, B.: Intracranial aneurysms and subarachnoid hemorrhage: An overview. *In* Wilkins, R. H., and Rengachary, S. S., eds.: Neurosurgery. New York, McGraw-Hill, 1985, p. 1315. Reprinted by permission.

in 96 per cent of those patients dying within 3 days of the hemorrhage and 74 per cent of those dying after 3 days. Evidence of herniation decreased with time, and cerebral infarction increased from 19 per cent in the first 3 days to 70 per cent of patients dying after 14 days.

Intracerebral Hemorrhage

Aneurysms arising from the distal anterior cerebral arteries are the most likely to produce an intracerebral hematoma. Because of the relative rarity of these aneurysms, however, intracerebral hematomas are more commonly seen with aneurysms of the middle and anterior communicating arteries; these aneurysms are associated with clots in autopsy series in about 67 and 62 per cent of cases, respectively. These percentages are lower in patients surviving their aneurysm ruptures. Intracerebral hematomas complicated 34 per cent of aneurysm cases reported by Pasqualin and associates.[80] The sites of hemorrhage vary depending on the location of the aneurysm and the direction of rupture of the aneurysm into the brain parenchyma. The pattern is usually distinctive but does not always differ sufficiently from that of hypertensive intracerebral hemorrhage to allow an accurate diagnosis based on computed tomography or magnetic resonance imaging. Indications for angiography must be based on clinical suspicion.

A retrospective review of patients from 11 medical centers identified 132 patients with intracerebral hematoma due to ruptured aneurysm.[11] Discriminant function analysis showed that, in order of importance, size and location of hematoma, aneurysm location, and size of midline shift were factors contributing to prediction of survival. Hematoma size was also a strong predictor of clinical grade. About 40 per cent of clots were frontal and 40 per cent were temporal. Patients with temporal lobe clots have the greatest capacity for clinical recovery.

Craniotomy for hematoma evacuation is generally indicated in patients with depressed or deteriorating level of consciousness, with or without signs of herniation. The aneurysm should be obliterated at the time of clot removal.

Intraventricular Hemorrhage

A major intraventricular hemorrhage complicates aneurysm rupture in 13 to 28 per cent of clinical series and 37 to 54 per cent of autopsy series.[69] It is common to see a small amount of blood layered out in the occipital horns after subarachnoid hemorrhage. In 91 cases of intraventricular hemorrhage, the aneurysm was located on the anterior cerebral artery in 40 per cent, the internal carotid artery in 25 per cent, and the middle cerebral artery in 21 per cent.[69] Anterior communicating and basilar termination aneurysms are the most likely aneurysms to cause large, primarily intraventricular hemorrhages. The pathogenesis of intraventricular bleeding probably depends on the location of the aneurysm. Anterior communicating artery and basilar aneurysms may rupture through the lamina terminalis or floor of the third ventricle and thence into the ventricular system. Intraventricular hemorrhage is associated with a periventricular intracerebral clot in about 50 per cent of cases; and in these situations, intraventricular blood is secondary to rupture of the parenchymal clot into the ventricular system. It is believed that repeated hemorrhages cause fibrosis and adherence of the arachnoid to the aneurysm dome, such that subsequent ruptures are more likely to penetrate into the brain parenchyma or ventricular system.[18] Blood may reflux from the subarachnoid cisterns into the outlets of the fourth ventricle and then the rest of the ventricular system, particularly with rupture of posterior inferior cerebellar artery aneurysms. Vasospasm is less common when blood is primarily intraventricular, as opposed to when it packs the basal cisterns. Over 50 per cent of patients with large intraventricular hemorrhage are admitted in poor clinical grades, and the mortality in most series exceeds 64 per cent. Ventricular size is a strong predictor of survival, in addition to age, clinical grade, hypertension, and other well-known prognostic factors.[69] If the ratio of the width of ventricles between the caudate nuclei to the width of the brain is over 0.25, the patient usually dies.[69]

Cerebral Infarction

An extensive study of pathology after subarachnoid hemorrhage was carried out by Crompton.[18] Of 159 consecutive patients with ruptured aneurysms who died after an initial survival of at least 24 hours, 75 per cent had cerebral infarcts. A review of literature to that time showed 42 per cent of patients with fatal hemorrhages had infarcts. Crompton found the following factors to be associated with cerebral infarction after aneurysm rupture: (1) cerebral arterial atherosclerosis, (2) bilateral hypoplasia or aplasia of the posterior communicating arteries, (3) bleeding into the perivascular sheaths of perforating ganglionic arteries, (4) large subarachnoid hematomas (particularly in the sylvian fissure), (5) hypotension, (6) vasospasm, (7) direct surgery on the aneurysm, and (8) carotid ligation. This study shows that infarction after subarachnoid hemorrhage may be produced by any of the pathophysiological processes that cause infarction under other circumstances. These include alterations in cardiovascular function, blood viscosity, and coagulation and in the cerebral vessels themselves. After subarachnoid hemorrhage, delayed cerebral ischemia is a major cause of morbidity and mortality and is most commonly due to vasospasm (see Chapter 61).

Hydrocephalus

Acute hydrocephalus may be defined as occurring within 3 days, subacute hydrocephalus between 4 and 29 days, and chronic ventricular dilation more than 29 days after subarachnoid hemorrhage. The frequency of acute ventricular dilation after subarachnoid hemorrhage approximates 20 per cent but will reflect whether the population studied includes all cases or a set of patients selected for surgery who will be in better clinical condition. Among 3,521 patients admitted within 3 days of the hemorrhage, an admission computed tomogram showed hydrocephalus in 15 per cent.[31] Clinical hydrocephalus, defined as ventricular enlargement developing at any time after the hemorrhage and that the surgeon thought was clinically important, was reported in 13 per cent of patients, 6 per cent of whom had had hydrocephalus shown by computed tomography on admission to the hospital. Factors predicting clinical hydrocephalus included increasing age, pre-existing or postoperative hypertension, intraventricular hemorrhage, diffuse or focal thick hemorrhage, posterior circulation aneurysm, focal ischemic deficit, use of antifibrinolytics, hyponatremia, admission level of consciousness, and score on the Glasgow Outcome Scale. These factors include many that adversely affect the overall outcome after subarachnoid hemorrhage and that predict development of other complications, highlighting the interdependence of a variety of factors that reflect the severity of the subarachnoid hemorrhage that has occurred.

The pathogenesis of hydrocephalus after subarachnoid hemorrhage is thought to be blockage of flow of cerebrospinal fluid through the basal subarachnoid cisterns, the outlets of the fourth ventricle, or the subarachnoid space around the tentorial incisura. The fluid accumulates because outflow resistance is increased in the absence of a decrease in production. Clogging of the arachnoid villi with erythrocytes and fibrin debris, particularly at the superior sagittal sinus, may also contribute to increasing resistance to outflow of the fluid. Elderly patients tend to have more pre-existing meningeal fibrosis and to have larger subarachnoid spaces that might fill with more blood, contributing to a higher risk of post–subarachnoid hemorrhage hydrocephalus. Van Gijn and co-workers attributed post–subarachnoid hemorrhage hyponatremia to hypothalamic dysfunction secondary to dilation of the third ventricle.[111] The pathophysiology of neurological deterioration with ventricular dilation includes increased intracranial pressure and decreased cerebral blood flow and metabolism, the latter occurring by mechanisms that are sometimes independent of the former.

The decision to insert a ventricular drain or cerebrospinal fluid shunt in patients shortly after subarachnoid hemorrhage should be made with the knowledge that it may increase the risk of rebleeding, infection, and chronic hydrocephalus. Despite these risks, the early and aggressive employment of ventricular drainage has been a major advance in the management of the initially poor-grade patient. Intracranial hypertension may not be associated with ventricular enlargement.[8] In another study, there was no obvious relationship between increasing ventricular size and decreased level of consciousness.[69] In other words, other factors often accounted for coma. Those authors used ventricular drainage for patients in poor clinical grades with a ventriculocranial ratio over 0.22. The ratio tends to increase with age in normal individuals. Rebleeding can be precipitated by acutely lowering intracranial

pressure, and Voldby and Enevoldsen recommend draining the cerebrospinal fluid only when the pressure is above 25 mm Hg.[114]

Chronic hydrocephalus develops in 10 per cent of patients surviving aneurysmal subarachnoid hemorrhage. Permanent diversion of the cerebrospinal fluid with a ventriculoperitoneal shunt is usually performed, although the indications remain subjective. The risks of shunting will usually be outweighed by the potential benefits in patients with dilated ventricles who have plateaued in their neurological recovery or deteriorated several weeks after the hemorrhage.

Pathophysiology of Subarachnoid Hemorrhage and Aneurysms

PATHOGENESIS OF ANEURYSMS

Normal cerebral arteries have a tunica intima composed of a single layer of endothelial cells lying on a basement membrane. Myointimal cells separate the endothelial cells from the thick internal elastic membrane, which is perforated by pores that are maximal at arterial bifurcations. The tunica media is composed of layers of smooth muscle and collagenous, elastic extracellular matrix. There is no external elastic lamina, and the adventitia, as well as the entire arterial wall, is thinner than a systemic artery of similar size.

Stehbens reviewed evidence against the theory that saccular aneurysms are congenital and noted that these aneurysms are extremely rare in children and that variations in the circle of Willis are generally no more common in patients with aneurysms than in those without.[98, 100] The major variation in the circle that is associated with aneurysms (imbalance in size between the two precommunicating anterior cerebral arteries) is more likely associated because of hemodynamic factors. This is also true with the variant having the highest rate of association with aneurysms—the azygous anterior cerebral artery. The incidence of deficiencies in the tunica media at major arterial branch points (about 80 per cent) is the same in patients with and without aneurysms, suggesting that some other factor is responsible for the genesis of aneurysms. The incidence of medial defects does, however, increase with age. Medial defects, which Stehbens believes are not areas deficient in smooth muscle but are raphes where smooth muscle cells interdigitate, are mainly congenital, whereas saccular aneurysms are acquired. There is no histological evidence to support the early theory that aneurysms develop from vestigial arteries that arise from the apex of arterial bifurcations.

It is now believed that hemodynamic factors create degenerative processes in the arterial wall, including atherosclerosis and breakdown of the internal elastic membrane, which contribute to formation and growth of aneurysms. Atherosclerosis in and around the aneurysm could be a coexisting development due to hemodynamic stress or play a pathogenetic role in the genesis of the saccular aneurysm. The Reynolds number for flow in the "normal" circle of Willis is 600 to 750, which suggests that biophysical factors responsible for arterial wall damage, such as axial stream impingement, shear stress, boundary layer separation, and turbulence, do not occur at normal bifurcations.[26] Under conditions of increased flow, however, these phenomena may damage the arterial wall, including the internal elastic membrane, and initiate aneurysm formation. Once an outpouching occurs, the hemodynamic factors create vibration and turbulence in the aneurysm, resulting in further degenerative change at the neck of the aneurysm and in the sac itself.[26, 101]

Rupture of aneurysms can be theoretically predicted by the law of Laplace, which states that wall stress is related to intra-aneurysm pressure and sac radius and inversely related to wall thickness. Bursting occurs when increased arterial pressure, larger aneurysm size, and reduced wall thickness surpass the tension that the stiff, collagenous wall can support. These factors would suggest that systemic hypertension should play a role in aneurysm formation, growth, and rupture. Evidence to support this hypothesis has not been conclusive.[117, 118] The increased prevalence of aneurysms in older females, and in certain families, as well as the failure for the incidence of aneurysmal subarachnoid hemorrhage to decline with the treatment of hypertension, argues for a role of other factors in the genesis of aneurysms. Aneurysm walls have decreased ability to withstand tension development.[101] The maximum stress that aneurysm walls can withstand is close to that imparted by the systolic blood pressure and is much lower than that which normal arteries can support. The pressure inside experimental aneurysms was similar to the prevailing blood pressure, and it was proposed, therefore, that aneurysm growth was passive yield to blood pressure, with reactive healing and thickening of the aneurysm wall as the diameter increased.[94, 101]

The formation of thrombus in aneurysms depends on the volume of the aneurysm, the size of the orifice, and probably other factors.[84] Small aneurysms rarely thrombose, but about half of giant aneurysms contain thrombus. Clot formation in an aneurysm might be accelerated by processes that decrease flow into the aneurysm, such as vasospasm. Thrombus inside the aneurysm may embolize into distal cerebral arteries. There are about 30 cases reported, mostly from giant aneurysms of the middle cerebral artery.[61, 102, 118] Criteria met in well-documented cases include presence of intra-aneurysmal thrombus, a transient ischemic attack or stroke in an arterial territory supplied by the parent vessel of the aneurysm, absence of subarachnoid hemorrhage, and cessation of attacks following obliteration of the aneurysm.

PATHOPHYSIOLOGY OF ANEURYSM RUPTURE

Intracranial Pressure Response

The volume of blood escaping during aneurysm rupture varies from negligible amounts, corresponding to a "warning leak," to massive volumes (more than 150 mL), resulting in immediate death. The pathophysiological changes probably depend principally on the volume of hemorrhage. During aneurysm rebleeding, intracranial pressure rises to diastolic blood pressure and cerebral blood flow occurs only during systole.[38, 73] This temporary circulatory arrest was thought to aid in stopping aneurysm bleeding by allowing blood to coagulate and to produce severe, transient global ischemia.[113] Coagulation without pressure tamponade may operate to stop bleeding in many cases, since consciousness is not lost.

Monitoring of intracranial pressure for a mean of 8 days after subarachnoid hemorrhage in 52 patients showed that mean intracranial pressure rose as clinical grade worsened.[54] Mean intracranial pressure was 10 mm Hg in grade 1 and 2 patients, 18 mm Hg in grade 2 and 3 patients, and 29 mm Hg in grade 3 to 5 patients. Vasospasm, which was more common in poor-grade patients with larger subarachnoid hemorrhage, was associated with a significant increase in intracranial pressure from a mean of 16 mm Hg in patients without vasospasm to 29 mm Hg in patients with vasospasm. Intracranial pressure is related to outcome; patients with pressures below 15 mm Hg do well in over 80 per cent of cases as opposed to good outcome in only 15 per cent of patients whose intracranial pressures exceed this.[118]

Cerebral Blood Flow, Volume, and Metabolism

Numerous studies of cerebral blood flow, blood volume, and metabolism have been conducted in patients with ruptured aneurysms. Almost all studies agree that cerebral blood flow is globally decreased after subarachnoid hemorrhage.[118] For example, among 30 patients with this type of hemorrhage, mean regional cerebral blood flow decreased from a mean of 54 mL per 100 g per minute in normal individuals to 42 mL in grade 1 to 2 patients without vasospasm, 35 mL in grade 3 to 4 patients without vasospasm, 36 mL in grade 1 to 2 patients with vasospasm, and 33 mL in grade 3 to 4 patients with vasospasm.[34] Cerebral metabolic rate for oxygen showed a similar pattern with progressive reductions associated with deteriorating clinical grade and worsening vasospasm. Cerebral blood volume was markedly increased in patients with severe neurological deficits associated with severe vasospasm. It was concluded that vasospasm was narrowing of the large, angiographically visible arteries at the base of the brain, accompanied by a compensatory dilation of distal, intracerebral arterioles. Few of the early studies examined the time course of blood flow and metabolism changes after subarachnoid hemorrhage, but once the importance of time from the hemorrhage was identified it could be demonstrated that mean cerebral blood flow tended to decrease with time, reaching a nadir about 10 to 14 days later, after which flows slowly increased toward normal.[66, 118] Immediately after the hemorrhage, there is relative hyperemia in relation to the reduced cerebral metabolic rate for oxygen.[16, 116] In poor-grade patients, blood flow and metabolism may remain depressed for weeks. In addition to global reductions in blood flow and metabolism, regional perfusion defects can develop after subarachnoid hemorrhage and can be correlated with areas of angiographically demonstrated severe vasospasm, intracerebral hematomas, and ventricular dilation. Regions of brain irrigated by vasospastic arteries have elevated oxygen extraction fractions. Positron emission tomography shows that as long as the area is only ischemic and infarction has not developed, the cerebral metabolic rate for oxygen remains normal, although flow is reduced. Development of infarction is heralded by a fall in the metabolism with relatively increased blood flow (relative hyperemia).[16] The degree to which reduced blood flow after the hemorrhage has been due to hypovolemia and hypotension is unclear, but there is some evidence that the alterations in flow can be at least partially prevented by maintenance of normovolemia or hypervolemia with or without hypertension.[76, 86]

There is little information on the pathogenesis of blood flow and metabolism changes after subarachnoid hemorrhage. In patients without vasospasm, intracerebral clots, or hydrocephalus studied in the first 4 days after hemorrhage, the metabolism for oxygen is decreased without accompanying changes in oxygen extraction fraction, suggesting that the primary alteration is a reduction in the metabolism and that blood flow falls due to decrease in demand.[16] There is usually a relative hyperemia, which probably is due to intracranial circulatory arrest, transient global cerebral ischemia, and lactic acidosis occurring at the time of rupture. Mitochondrial respiration, sodium-potassium adenosine triphosphatase activity, extracellular potassium, and calcium are altered in brain tissue of experimental animals exposed to subarachnoid blood, although the relationship of these changes to cerebral blood flow and the cerebral metabolic rate for oxygen is not fully known.[25, 42, 64]

The relationship of cerebral blood flow to blood pressure and arterial carbon dioxide tension ($PaCO_2$) is also altered after subarachnoid hemorrhage. The response of blood flow to changes in blood pressure at different times after the hemorrhage was studied in 38 patients.[115] Autoregulation was intact in good-grade patients but became progressively impaired in poor-grade patients and during the time of vasospasm. Autoregulation is not lost in an all-or-none fashion. The degree of impairment will tend to be worse as consciousness is more impaired, as vasospasm becomes more severe, and as the patient enters the 5- to 10-day post–subarachnoid hemorrhage interval. Loss of blood flow response to changes in $PaCO_2$ occurs with more severe brain damage than is required to disturb autoregulation, and the combined loss of autoregulation and variation of cerebral blood flow with changes in $PaCO_2$ is termed "vasomotor paralysis." After subarachnoid hemorrhage, this paralysis is relatively uncommon but may be observed in grade 4 and 5 patients, usually with severe vasospasm. Measurements of cerebral blood flow with intra-arterial xenon-133 in 38 cases of

aneurysmal subarachnoid hemorrhage found responses to alteration in $PaCO_2$ were generally preserved, although they were reduced.[115] Impaired carbon dioxide reactivity was associated with increased intracranial pressure and high lactate levels in the cerebrospinal fluid. Once again, poor clinical grade and vasospasm were associated with impaired carbon dioxide responsiveness. Transcranial Doppler studies have demonstrated impairment of carbon dioxide reactivity even in good-grade patients after subarachnoid hemorrhage.[21] The impairment tends to appear during vasospasm and then subsequently to resolve.

Clinical Features

SYMPTOMS AND SIGNS OF SUBARACHNOID HEMORRHAGE

Among 1,752 patients with aneurysm rupture from three series, 340 (20 per cent, range: 15 to 37 per cent) had a history of sudden, severe headache.[9, 39, 48] Such premonitory symptoms, usually an unusually severe headache of sudden onset, sometimes associated with nausea, vomiting, and dizziness, are usually attributed to minor subarachnoid bleeding from the aneurysm. Other possible pathogenetic mechanisms include hemorrhage into the aneurysm wall, acute expansion of the aneurysm sac, or ischemia. In poor-grade patients, it may be impossible to determine if a "warning leak" has occurred; and the true incidence of these events, therefore, may be higher. The importance of recognition of warning leaks has been repeatedly emphasized, since diagnosis may be delayed until a catastrophic hemorrhage occurs. Hauerberg and associates studied 99 patients who presented with major subarachnoid hemorrhage but who had had warning leaks that were misdiagnosed.[39] Outcome in these patients would have been significantly better had they been diagnosed at their initial presentation. Day and Raskin reported a patient with an aneurysm who presented with sudden severe headache, normal computed tomogram, and clear cerebrospinal fluid. The fluid may also be clear if rupture has been intraparenchymal.[20]

All patients with headaches that are unusually severe or sudden in onset, particularly if they are associated with vomiting, should be investigated for subarachnoid hemorrhage. Other ominous features include onset with exertion, alteration in level of consciousness, meningism, or any focal neurological deficit. Sudden severe headaches are relatively uncommon in the general population, although experience suggests they are not uncommon in patients coming to an emergency department. There are, however, few studies of how many patients with sudden severe headaches actually turn out to have a subarachnoid hemorrhage. Abbott and van Hille studied 49 patients presenting to an emergency department with sudden severe headache and found 35 had a subarachnoid hemorrhage (71 per cent).[1]

A variety of other symptoms and signs can develop

before aneurysm rupture. They depend on the site and size of the aneurysm and include hemiparesis, dysphasia, extraocular muscle impairment, visual loss, visual field defect, and localized headache.[118]

The hallmark of subarachnoid hemorrhage is sudden, severe headache. There is brief loss of consciousness in about 45 per cent. Fontanarosa retrospectively studied 109 patients with proven subarachnoid hemorrhage and found headache in 74 per cent, nausea or vomiting in 77 per cent, loss of consciousness in 53 per cent, and nuchal rigidity in 35 per cent.[28] Aneurysm rupture results in sudden death in about 15 per cent of patients.[78] In the most recent cooperative study on the timing of surgery, 41 per cent of patients admitted within 3 days of subarachnoid hemorrhage were alert, 67 per cent had normal speech, 52 per cent were oriented, 69 per cent had normal motor responses, 66 per cent had headache, 74 per cent had a stiff neck, 9 per cent had a third nerve palsy, and 4 per cent had another cranial nerve deficit.[52, 53]

Ruptured aneurysms at specific sites may produce distinct clinical features. Transient bilateral lower extremity weakness may be due to anterior cerebral artery aneurysm rupture. A subarachnoid hemorrhage from a middle cerebral artery aneurysm is more likely to produce hemiparesis, paresthesia, hemianopsia, and dysphasia. Sarner and Rose found that no particular aneurysm site had a higher propensity to produce coma.[90] Seizures occur more commonly with anterior circulation aneurysms, and probably with middle cerebral artery lesions. Third nerve palsy or unilateral retro-orbital pain suggests an aneurysm arising at the internal carotid—posterior communicating artery junction. Third nerve lesions also occur with aneurysms at the origin of the superior cerebellar artery. Carotid-ophthalmic artery aneurysms may produce unilateral visual loss or visual field defect. Focal neurological deficit after subarachnoid hemorrhage may be due to mass effect from the aneurysm, vasospasm, seizures, or hematomas in the brain or subdural spaces.

Terson reported vitreous hemorrhages and hemiparesis in association with subarachnoid hemorrhage.[118] Vitreous hemorrhage may occur immediately after the hemorrhage or days later, and opinions differ about the prognosis for visual recovery. Vitrectomy is sometimes performed after an observation period of several months.

Numerous exertional activities have been reported to be intimately associated with aneurysm rupture. In the first cooperative study, roughly a third of 2,288 aneurysm ruptures occurred during sleep, a third during unspecified circumstances, and a third during various exertional activities, including lifting, emotional strain, defecation, coitus, coughing, and parturition.[60] Schievink and associates found subarachnoid hemorrhage occurred during stressful events in 43 per cent of cases, during nonstressful events in 34 per cent, during rest or sleep in 12 per cent, and under uncertain circumstances in 11 per cent.[92] If one takes into account that such exertional activities probably occupy a small percentage of one's lifetime, then it seems likely that they do increase the risk of aneurysm rupture.

Cigarette smoking and alcohol consumption are risk factors for subarachnoid hemorrhage. A meta-analysis of 10 studies suggested that the relative risk of such a hemorrhage in current smokers was 2.9.[96] After adjusting for age and hypertension, smoking was associated with a relative risk of 3 in males and 4.7 in females in one study and relative risks of 2.7 and 3, respectively, in another series.[13, 50] Longstreth and associates reported that risk increased with amount smoked, was also elevated in former smokers, and was greatest within 3 hours of the last cigarette.[62] Cigarette smoking may increase the risk of aneurysm rupture by increasing the risk of developing an aneurysm, by increasing the risk of rupturing a pre-existing one, or by a combination of mechanisms. Smoking releases proteolytic enzymes into the circulation, which could promote aneurysm formation and growth through their destructive effects on vascular collagen and elastin. An influence on aneurysm formation is suggested by the persistent increased risk of subarachnoid hemorrhage in former smokers. Smoking accelerates atherosclerosis, although the causal relationship of the latter to aneurysm rupture remains unproven. Finally, smoking is associated with hypertension, particularly within 3 hours of intake, although the more long-term increased risk of subarachnoid hemorrhage that results, and the persistence of risk after adjusting for hypertension, suggests an independent effect of smoking.

Several investigations from Finland showed that recent alcohol intake is associated with an increased risk of aneurysm rupture in a dose-dependent fashion.[50, 118] Prolonged, heavy alcohol use (more than 2 drinks per day) was also associated with subarachnoid hemorrhage in King County, Washington.[62] It is believed that hemorrhages are related to blood pressure elevations during acute intoxication or withdrawal, although alcohol is also associated with chronic hypertension, coagulation abnormalities, and changes in cerebral blood flow.

Cocaine use causes sympathetic hyperactivity, acute hypertension, arteriopathy, and cerebral arterial constriction. These changes may precipitate aneurysm rupture, of which at least 53 cases have been reported, although many more probably go unreported or undetected.[77] If subarachnoid hemorrhage occurs after cocaine use, about 85 per cent of patients will harbor intracranial aneurysms. Cocaine-users with aneurysmal subarachnoid hemorrhage tend to be younger and to have smaller aneurysms than the average patient with a ruptured aneurysm.

GRADING SYSTEMS

Botterell and colleagues were the first to grade patients with subarachnoid hemorrhage to assess the operative risk (Table 50–6).[14] It is now apparent that clinical grading is important for estimating prognosis of these patients. There are numerous other grading systems, although most use headache, signs of meningeal irritation, level of consciousness, and focal neurological deficit to categorize patients.[43] Lindsay and colleagues

Table 50–6

CLINICAL GRADING SYSTEMS FOR PATIENTS WITH SUBARACHNOID HEMORRHAGE

Grade	Botterell, et al.[14]	Hunt and Hess[43]	World Federation of Neurologic Surgeons[105]	
			Glasgow Coma Score	*Motor Deficit*
1	Conscious with or without signs of blood in subarachnoid space	No symptoms or minimal headache and slight nuchal rigidity	15	No
2	Drowsy without significant neurological deficit	Moderate to severe headache, no neurological deficit other than cranial nerve palsy	13–14	No
3	Drowsy with neurological deficit and probably intracerebral clot	Drowsy, confusion, or mild focal deficit	13–14	Yes
4	Major neurological deficit and deteriorating due to intracerebral clot, or older patients with less severe neurological deficit but pre-existing cerebrovascular disease	Stupor, moderate to severe hemiparesis, possible early decerebrate rigidity and vegetative disturbances	7–12	Yes or no
5	Moribund with failing vital centers and extensor rigidity	Deep coma, decerebrate rigidity, moribund	3–6	Yes or no

found high interobserver variability when different surgeons graded the same patients on the Hunt and Hess, Botterell, or Nishioka grading systems.[59] There was less interobserver variability when level of consciousness was assessed using the Glasgow Coma Scale. Jagger and co-workers also noted that none of the grading scales had been derived using statistics.[46] With the use of data from the Cooperative Study on Timing of Aneurysm Surgery, clinical features that most accurately predicted outcome at 6 months were the eye opening scale of the Glasgow Coma Score, motor function (normal, hemiparesis, or posturing), and speech (normal, dysphasic, or none). These researchers developed a seven-point grading scale using eye opening and motor function that is similar to a universal subarachnoid hemorrhage scale reported by the World Federation of Neurosurgical Societies.[105] This scale may be more accurate and reproducible in classifying patients after the hemorrhage since it was derived based on statistical analysis of outcome in a large series of patients and since the clinical features used have been shown to be interpretable with less interobserver variability.

DIFFERENTIAL DIAGNOSIS OF SUBARACHNOID HEMORRHAGE

Sudden severe headache has a vast differential diagnosis, although a careful history, neurological examination, and sometimes computed tomography, lumbar puncture, and routine blood work, will usually lead to a diagnosis (Table 50–7). The causes of subarachnoid hemorrhage have been detailed (see Table 50–1), although in 9 to 30 per cent of cases no etiology will be found for the hemorrhage. Complete angiographic investigation is required, including four-vessel selective intracranial, bilateral external carotid, and sometimes spinal angiograms. It may be worthwhile having opinions from additional neuroradiologists. Potential causes of subarachnoid hemorrhage in these cases include missed aneurysms, partially or completely thrombosed aneurysms, bleeding diatheses, rupture of a small penetrating arteriole or venule, or bleeding from an occult vascular malformation. The most common missed aneurysm is also the most common aneurysm (anterior communicating artery aneurysm). Although no dogmatic statements can be made regarding repeat angiography in cases of unknown etiology, a high index of suspicion for aneurysm rupture must be

Table 50–7

DIFFERENTIAL DIAGNOSIS OF SUDDEN, SEVERE HEADACHE

I. Intracranial
  A. Vascular
    1. Subarachnoid hemorrhage
    2. Pituitary apoplexy
    3. Cerebral venous and dural sinus thrombosis
    4. Intracerebral hemorrhage
    5. Embolic stroke
  B. Infectious
    1. Meningitis
    2. Encephalitis
  C. Increased intracranial pressure due to neoplasms, intracranial hemorrhage, or brain abscess
II. Benign Headache
  A. Migraine
  B. Tension
  C. Cluster
  D. Benign exertional headache
  E. Headache associated with orgasm
III. Pain from Cranial Nerves
  A. Compression or inflammation of cranial nerves from neoplasm, aneurysm, Tolosa-Hunt syndrome, Raeder's paratrigeminal neuralgia, and Gradenigo's syndrome
  B. Neuralgias
    1. Trigeminal
    2. Glossopharyngeal
IV. Referred Cranial Pain
  A. Ocular
    1. Retrobulbar neuritis
    2. Glaucoma
  B. Sinusitis
  C. Dental abscess, temporomandibular joint pain
V. Systemic Diseases
  A. Malignant hypertension
  B. Viral illnesses

maintained in patients with typical aneurysmal sub-arachnoid hemorrhage patterns (e.g., blood in the anterior interhemispheric fissure or lateral sylvian fissure). There is a subgroup of cases in which angiography is negative and bleeding is confined to the perimesencephalic (interpeduncular, crural, ambient) cisterns. In one series, 20 (7 per cent) of 294 patients with subarachnoid hemorrhage fulfilled the criteria for this type of hemorrhage.[83] Follow-up of these cases and those from another center showed none had rebleeding, vasospasm was rare, and good outcome occurred in almost all cases. Results for this subtype of subarachnoid hemorrhage of unknown etiology are even better than the outcome in series of unselected patients with hemorrhage of unknown etiology. In a review of 15 of these latter series, Friedman noted that 80 per cent of patients were in good clinical grade, that vasospasm and other complications were rare, that rebleeding rates were generally low (4 per cent in the first 3 months, then 0.8 per cent per year), and that outcome was good.[29]

Natural History

UNRUPTURED ANEURYSMS

Unruptured aneurysms are usually seen in patients with subarachnoid hemorrhage and multiple aneurysms, with symptomatic but unruptured aneurysms (either small or giant), and with incidentally discovered aneurysms. The natural history may differ in each situation. Wiebers and co-workers followed 65 patients with 81 unruptured aneurysms until death or for at least 5 years.[119] Nineteen per cent were symptomatic and 71 per cent were asymptomatic. Discriminant function analysis demonstrated that aneurysm size was the most important determinant of eventual rupture. Of aneurysms under 10 mm in diameter, none ruptured and 2 per cent developed cranial nerve compression. In patients with aneurysms of 10 to 20 mm in diameter, 24 per cent had ruptured aneurysms, 18 per cent developed cranial nerve deficits, and 12 per cent experienced embolism from the aneurysm. These figures were even higher for aneurysms over 20 mm in diameter (33 per cent ruptured, 42 per cent cranial nerve compression, 25 per cent mass effect, 8 per cent embolism). Symptomatic aneurysms were not more dangerous than asymptomatic ones, although the numbers were small. It is also important to note that in virtually every published series, the average size of ruptured aneurysms is less than 10 mm, a fact that the authors noted and that seemed to be at variance with their observations. They suggested that after rupture, aneurysms might get smaller, a view not widely held. Others believe that aneurysms of any size are at risk of rupture. There are several reports of rupture of known incidental aneurysms that were less than 10 mm in diameter. The role of screening for aneurysms is currently unclear, although the authors believe it is indicated in families with a strong history of aneurysmal

subarachnoid hemorrhage and in patients with diseases associated with aneurysms, such as polycystic kidney disease.

The bleeding rate of 181 unruptured aneurysms in 142 patients observed for at least 10 years was 1.4 per cent per year.[49] Most of the aneurysms were in patients with multiple aneurysms who underwent clipping of the ruptured one. Rupture was predicted by younger patient age at diagnosis. Follow-up angiograms after 1 to 23 years in 31 patients showed 17 ruptured aneurysms increased in size a mean of 5 mm, whereas unruptured aneurysms had not changed in size. Sixty-seven per cent of the aneurysms that ruptured were initially less than 6 mm. Other investigators published a risk of rupture of unruptured aneurysms of 1 to 2 per cent per year.[47] Decision analysis was used to determine if an incidentally discovered aneurysm should be clipped.[109] The annual risk of rupture, patient age, and risk of surgical obliteration enter into consideration; and depending on the values used, benefit to the patient occurs at various ages, usually for patients younger than 60 or 65 years old. Most surgeons have the impression that aneurysms differ in their propensity to enlarge and rupture. The yearly risk of rupture, therefore, may be an artificial and static representation of the dynamic process of aneurysm growth and rupture. Magnetic resonance angiography may contribute to our understanding of which aneurysms are prone to rupture.[67]

RUPTURED ANEURYSMS

Pakarinen's study of patients with proven aneurysmal subarachnoid hemorrhage gives the best approximation of the natural history of ruptured aneurysms, although medical management was different from that currently employed.[78] Thirteen per cent of patients died before reaching the hospital. Overall only 25 per cent of patients underwent aneurysm surgery that was during the second week after hemorrhage in 7 per cent, the third week in 7 per cent, the fourth week in 14 per cent, and the first month in 73 per cent. Death from the initial hemorrhage occurred in 43 per cent, the majority of which were within the first 24 hours (74 per cent of the deaths). Among the 52 per cent of patients dying of rebleeding, the incidence of rerupture was highest during the second and fourth weeks after the initial hemorrhage. By the end of 2 months, the mortality rate from rebleeding was less than 1 per cent per month. Most other series reporting on the natural history of subarachnoid hemorrhage have had more extensive withdrawals of the patients because of their being operated on. In one series of 364 patients with anterior communicating artery aneurysms, surgery and conservative therapy were randomly allocated.[120] Mortality in conservatively treated patients was 41 per cent after 6 months and 48 per cent after 5 years. Preadmission deaths were not assessed.

The most important factors that contribute to estimating the prognosis for outcome and survival after aneurysmal subarachnoid hemorrhage include clinical grade, vasospasm, amount of blood on computed tomography, hypertension, mass lesion, general medical condition, age, and short interval from the hemorrhage to admission to the hospital.[52, 118] Numerous other factors have been suggested to be related to the prognosis of subarachnoid hemorrhage, although few have been shown to contribute additional prognostic value using multivariate statistical models. These factors include white blood cell count, blood glucose level, serum neuron-specific enolase levels, and cerebrospinal fluid levels of S-100 protein. Hypovolemia, hypotension, and, if early surgery is used, antifibrinolytic therapy, adversely affect the outcome of patients after rupture of the aneurysm.

Rebleeding rates after first aneurysm rupture were estimated by Jane and colleagues.[47] About 50 per cent of ruptured aneurysms rebleed in the first 6 months, and about 70 per cent of patients who experience rebleeding die. After 6 months the rebleeding rate was 3 per cent per year. Anterior or posterior communicating artery aneurysms treated by carotid ligation or intracranial proximal artery clipping rebled at a rate of 3 per cent per year. The peak of rebleeding is immediately after the first hemorrhage and falls off with time, in contrast to earlier studies that showed a higher rate of rebleeding during the second week after the initial hemorrhage. Seventeen patients having anterior cerebral artery ligation for anterior communicating artery aneurysm were followed a median of 16 years. One patient experienced rebleeding at 16 days, and there was one late hemorrhage proven and one possible. The expected number of deaths without treatment would have been five. From a review of 147 cases in the literature the number of expected rebleeding episodes was reduced by more than 80 per cent.[104] Sixty single anterior circulation aneurysms treated by wrapping were followed for 10 years, and the rebleeding rate within 6 months was 8.6 per cent. Rebleeding between 6 months and 10 years was at 1.5 per cent per year. The anticipated natural rebleeding rates were 35 and 3 per cent so that treatment was considered to offer some measure of protection.[106]

Surgical and medical treatments have improved the outcome of patients with ruptured aneurysms. For 3,521 patients with ruptured aneurysms admitted to hospital within 3 days of the ictus and managed between 1980 and 1984, 75 per cent were admitted in good neurological condition, 83 per cent were operated on, 58 per cent made a complete recovery, and 26 per cent died.[52, 53] The outcome could theoretically be better today since in that study, few patients were treated with hypervolemia, none received nimodipine, and many received antifibrinolytic agents.

Laboratory Investigations

COMPUTED TOMOGRAPHY

Nonenhanced cranial computed tomography is the first step in investigation of patients with suspected subarachnoid hemorrhage. The probability of detecting the hemorrhage is proportional to the clinical grade of the patient and the time after the hemorrhage. Three per cent of 1,553 patients had normal results of computed tomography within 24 hours of confirmed subarachnoid hemorrhage.[52] There was subarachnoid hemorrhage in 92 per cent, intraventricular hemorrhage in 20 per cent, intracerebral hematoma in 19 per cent, subdural hemorrhage in 2 per cent, hypodense areas in less than 1 per cent, mass effect in 8 per cent, hydrocephalus in 16 per cent, and an aneurysm in 5 per cent. With time, the incidence of normal computed tomography and of hypodense areas increased, whereas hydrocephalus and the hemorrhagic findings decreased. By 5 days post subarachnoid hemorrhage, 27 per cent of scans were normal and 58 per cent showed the hemorrhage. Intracerebral hemorrhages resolved more slowly than subarachnoid hemorrhage and were still seen in 18 per cent of cases scanned on day 5. Alert patients were significantly more likely than drowsy patients to have a normal scan or a thin, local collection of blood, and all other abnormalities evident on computed tomography were more common in sicker patients. The probability of detecting a subarachnoid hemorrhage at different times was analyzed based on computed tomography on 100 consecutive patients with aneurysmal hemorrhages.[110] Eighty-five per cent would be recognized after 5 days, 50 per cent after a week, and 30 per cent after 2 weeks. Abnormalities in the later times were mostly intracerebral hematomas, which did not begin to disappear substantially until after 2 weeks. Routine contrast medium infusion would increase the detection of aneurysms, although angiography will be performed before surgical intervention, and routine administration of another dose of contrast medium is generally unnecessary.

The volume and location of subarachnoid blood on computed tomography gives important prognostic information about vasospasm and outcome after the hemorrhage. A widely used system of grading subarachnoid hemorrhage on computed tomography is that of Fisher and associates (Table 50–8).[27, 55] In a prospective study, these authors reported a good correlation between the location and volume of the blood and the subsequent development of vasospasm. Regarding outcome, there is an association between worsening clinical grade, increasing subarachnoid hemorrhage on computed tomography, and poor outcome. In the Cooperative Timing Study, multivariate analysis showed that the degree of subarachnoid hemorrhage on computed tomography was a significant predictive factor, in addition to clinical condition, for death and disability.[52] In a smaller study of 471 patients with ruptured aneurysms, factors predicting delayed cerebral ischemia and outcome were analyzed.[15] Although it was related to outcome, the amount of blood on computed tomography added little to prediction of outcome in a multivariate analysis but much to prediction of delayed cerebral ischemia.

Computed tomography is also invaluable for detecting complications of subarachnoid hemorrhage and

Table 50–8

METHOD OF FISHER FOR GRADING AMOUNT OF SUBARACHNOID BLOOD ON COMPUTED TOMOGRAPHY AFTER SUBARACHNOID HEMORRHAGE

Grade	Features	Risk of Vasospasm
1	No detectable blood on computed tomography	Low
2	Diffuse blood that does not appear dense enough to represent a large, thick homogeneous clot	Low
3	Dense collection of blood that appears to represent a clot more than 1 mm thick in the vertical plane (interhemispheric fissure, insular cistern, or ambient cistern) or greater than 5×3 mm in longitudinal and transverse dimension in horizontal plane (stem of sylvian fissure, sylvian cistern, interpeduncular cistern)	High
4	Intracerebral or intraventricular clots but with only diffuse blood or no blood in basal cisterns	Low

Modified from Fisher, C. M., Kistler, J. P., and Davis, J. M.: Relation of cerebral vasospasm to subarachnoid hemorrhage visualized by computerized tomographic scanning. Neurosurgery, 6:1, 1980. Reprinted by permission.

surgery, including intracranial clots, low-density areas, infarcts, and hydrocephalus.

CEREBROSPINAL FLUID STUDIES

Lumbar puncture is indicated when computed tomography is normal in patients with sudden, severe headache suggestive of subarachnoid hemorrhage. Whether lumbar puncture is undertaken before or instead of performing computed tomography depends on how accessible the scan is and how likely infectious meningitis is considered to be. There is a risk of neurological deterioration or rebleeding after lumbar puncture; and in two studies involving 165 patients with subarachnoid hemorrhage, 17 (10 per cent) patients experienced deterioration in their conditions within 24 hours of lumbar puncture.[23, 81] The majority of patients who show deterioration after puncture have pre-existing depression in level of consciousness or a focal neurological deficit. Lumbar puncture has minimal risk in alert patients with no focal neurological deficit and no papilledema. A review of literature on lumbar puncture and meningitis concluded that there was no evidence to recommend computed tomography before spinal tapping in acute meningitis unless the patient shows atypical features or focal neurological findings.[6] The immediate and almost unlimited access to computed tomography in the United States makes these arguments somewhat irrelevant, but in areas where computed tomography is less available the risks of not diagnosing subarachnoid hemorrhage or meningitis may outweigh the risks of lumbar puncture.

The diagnosis of subarachnoid hemorrhage rests on the demonstration of erythrocytes or their breakdown products in cerebrospinal fluid. Lumbar fluid may remain clear for several hours after subarachnoid hemorrhage, and it has been advised to wait 2 hours after the ictus before lumbar puncture.[107] Traumatic lumbar puncture is differentiated from true subarachnoid hemorrhage by (1) diminishing number of erythrocytes in each successive tube, (2) clotting if the red blood cell count is over 250,000 per mL, (3) no xanthochromia on spectrophotometry, (4) normal ratio of red blood cells to white blood cells and approximately 1.5 mg per 100 mL protein per 1,000 erythrocytes, and (5) absence of macrophages containing erythrocytes or hemosiderin. The pressure is usually elevated after subarachnoid hemorrhage. Xanthochromia may be due to high cerebrospinal fluid protein or to blood breakdown products. The latter appear reliably more than 12 hours after subarachnoid hemorrhage. It is necessary to use spectrophotometry to accurately detect oxyhemoglobin and its breakdown products that are responsible for cerebrospinal fluid xanthochromia since small amounts may be missed if only visual inspection is performed.[112]

MAGNETIC RESONANCE IMAGING AND MAGNETIC RESONANCE ANGIOGRAPHY

Initial studies of subarachnoid hemorrhage with magnetic resonance imaging suggested that the signal characteristics of acute blood rendered it difficult to distinguish from brain tissue. More recent studies found magnetic resonance imaging to be as sensitive as computed tomography at detecting the hemorrhage. Satoh and Kadoya examined magnetic resonance imaging and computed tomography from 30 patients with ruptured aneurysms.[91] The findings were variable, and in one case, T2-weighted images showed the hemorrhage when the computed tomogram was normal. The T1-weighted images were not as sensitive. In another study, magnetic resonance imaging was at least as accurate as computed tomography and was particularly useful for detecting small hemorrhages in the posterior fossa and the ventricles and for detecting aneurysms.[65] Embolism from aneurysms and determining which aneurysm has ruptured in cases of multiple aneurysms may also be aided by magnetic resonance imaging. It is not clear whether the advantages will outweigh the additional cost and inconvenience of performing it on patients in intensive care units.

The use of magnetic resonance imaging in the postoperative evaluation of patients with ruptured aneurysms is also evolving. Any possibility of movement of aneurysm clips during the study would, however, preclude its use. Two groups investigated effects of magnetic resonance imaging on various aneurysm clips and found that clip movement was related to the content of martensitic or ferromagnetic stainless steel.[24, 85] Most modern clips are made from austenitic steel, resist corrosion, are nonferromagnetic, and do not move under experimental conditions in the magnetic field. Magnetic resonance imaging was performed without incident in 20 patients with aneurysm clips and was thought to be useful since abnormal areas were visualized that could not be seen on computed tomography.[41] The death related to magnetic resonance imaging of a patient with an aneurysm clip suggests caution should be exercised in performing the study on these patients.[57] Although documentation of this case is not yet available, the previous studies suggest that it was unlikely to have been one of the modern generation of clips.

Magnetic resonance angiography is a rapidly evolving technique. Of 21 aneurysms identified by intra-arterial digital subtraction angiography, magnetic resonance imaging showed 18 and the images were considered diagnostic in 16 cases. The sensitivity of the best technique was 86 per cent.[87] In another study, it detected 18 of 19 aneurysms, missing one that was 2 mm.[12] The anatomy of the neck was correctly shown in 17 cases.

CEREBRAL ANGIOGRAPHY AND PERIANGIOGRAPHIC RUPTURE

If a spontaneous subarachnoid hemorrhage is diagnosed, then cerebral angiography should be performed. The incidence of multiple aneurysms, as well as of coincident arteriovenous malformations, suggests that four-vessel angiography should generally be performed in all cases. Rapidly deteriorating neurological condition may preclude this, and even angiography at all, in patients with large intracerebral hematomas or acute ventricular dilation. Magnification, subtraction, and stereoscopic techniques delineate the cause of bleeding in most cases. When no lesion is immediately apparent, selective injection of the external carotid arteries may reveal a dural arteriovenous malformation. Views of the anterior communicating artery complex with cross-compression and injections of the vertebral artery with carotid compression may show aneurysms at the anterior or posterior communicating arteries, respectively.[17] If neck or back pain or lower extremity neurological deficit is prominent, then a search for a spinal arteriovenous malformation, aneurysm, or neoplasm may be indicated.

The risks of angiography were documented in a prospective study of 1,002 consecutive cerebral angiograms performed in 1983 and 1984.[22] Ischemic events occurred in 1.3 per cent (0.1 per cent permanent) in the first 24 hours after angiography. There was a statistically insignificant increase in these events to 2.5 per cent in patients investigated for cerebrovascular disease. Neurological deterioration occurred between 24 and 72 hours after angiography in 1.8 per cent (0.3 per cent permanent). Complications were related to increased volumes of contrast medium, increased serum creatinine level, when transient ischemic attacks or strokes were the indication for angiography, with increased numbers of catheters used, with longer duration of the procedure, and with increased patient age.

Rupture of an aneurysm during angiography is uncommon. In the first Cooperative Aneurysm Study 5,484 cases were studied by angiography. Seven patients (0.13 per cent) rebled during angiography, and 12 (0.22 per cent) rebled 10 minutes to 24 hours later.[60]

In another study, 3 per cent of patients showed dye extravasation when angiography was being performed for investigation of subarachnoid hemorrhage.[89] At least 104 cases have been reported in detail.* The average age was 47, and 66 per cent of patients were female. Angiography was performed within 24 hours of subarachnoid hemorrhage in 64 per cent and within 48 hours in 75 per cent. The aneurysms were located on the anterior communicating artery (24 per cent), on the middle cerebral artery (31 per cent), on the internal carotid artery (36 per cent), and in the posterior circulation (7 per cent). Only 7 per cent of patients were in clinical grade 1; 15 per cent were grade 2, 20 per cent were grade 3, 30 per cent were grade 4, and 28 per cent were grade 5. If dye extravasation was observed on an angiogram, then the patient died in 78 per cent of cases. Overall, therefore, there is probably an increased risk in poor-grade patients with internal carotid artery aneurysms undergoing angiography immediately after the subarachnoid hemorrhage. Some of these circumstances, however, are associated with an increased risk of rebleeding and, in some cases, bleeding during angiography may represent the natural history of the aneurysmal hemorrhage. Most cases have been reported in patients undergoing direct carotid puncture with hand injections for angiography, but in the absence of knowledge of the denominators for cases undergoing direct, or transfemoral, angiography, it is impossible to know if any particular technique is more associated with periangiographic aneurysm rupture. Rupture could be precipitated by factors that alter the transmural pressure gradient across the aneurysm or that decrease distal runoff, including systemic hypertension, intracranial pressure changes, pressure changes with injection, vasospasm, and during cross-compression studies.

How does one determine which lesion ruptured in patients with multiple aneurysms? A combination of clinical and radiological features led to the supposed correct diagnosis in 90 to 95 per cent of cases from five series in the literature (Table 50–9).[3, 63, 71, 88, 121] A review of 69 patients with multiple aneurysms generated the following algorithm to predict which aneurysm bled:[71]

1. Exclude extradural aneurysms.
2. Study computed tomography results for presence of focal subarachnoid hemorrhage.
3. Look for focal spasm or mass effect on angiogram.
4. Pick the larger or more irregularly shaped aneurysm.
5. Examine the patient for focal neurological signs.
6. Consider repeating the angiogram at a later date to look for change in aneurysm size or for focal angiographic signs.
7. Choose the aneurysm that has the highest chance of rupture (anterior communicating artery aneurysm).

Overall, the most proximal and largest aneurysm usually ruptures. In some cases, magnetic resonance imaging has provided additional evidence of localizing value. In about two thirds of patients with multiple

---

*See references 5, 10, 30, 40, 72, 79, and 89.

Table 50–9

CLINICAL AND RADIOLOGICAL CRITERIA USED TO DETERMINE WHICH ANEURYSM BLED
IN CASES OF MULTIPLE INTRACRANIAL ANEURYSMS

Author, Year	Population	Criteria for Identifying Ruptured Aneurysm	Percentage of Cases in Which Correct Aneurysm Identified
Wood, 1964[121]	105 patients with 248 aneurysms; site confirmed by autopsy in 83 and at surgery in 22	Angiography: vessel displacements, focal spasm, size, shape, and filling characteristics of aneurysm; no clinical criteria	Largest aneurysm bled in 87 per cent of cases; angiographic criteria localized site of bleed in 95 per cent
Marttila and Heiskanen, 1970[63]	101 patients with 211 aneurysms; site confirmed by autopsy in 14 and at surgery in 87	Clinical features: hemiparesis, dysphasia, hemianopsia, third nerve palsy Angiography: size, shape, local mass effect or spasm	Clinical features: localized site in 38 per cent, especially useful when aneurysms are on opposite sides Angiography: largest lesion bled in 96 per cent, all angiographic criteria identified responsible sac in 96 per cent; overall could identify the correct aneurysm in 97 per cent
Almaani and Richardson, 1978[3]	110 patients each with 2 or more aneurysms, computed tomography done in 58	Focal neurological signs (motor, sensory, or cranial nerve) or focal hematoma, spasm, aneurysm irregularity, and delayed emptying of aneurysm on angiogram or focal changes on electroencephalography or focal features on computed tomography	Focal signs localized the aneurysm in 30 per cent, angiogram in 53 per cent, electroencephalography in 31 of 50 (62 per cent), computed tomography in 29 of 58 (50 per cent)
Sakamoto, et al., 1978[88]	64 patients with multiple aneurysms	Angiographical criteria: size, location, sac length to width ratio, focal mass effect, or edema	Ruptured aneurysm was largest one in 85 per cent; aneurysms with greater length–width ratio, irregular wall, evidence of mass effect, or anterior communicating more likely to bleed; angiogram identified correct site in 90 per cent
Nehls, et al., 1985[71]	69 cases with 205 aneurysms; site of rupture identified from autopsy or surgery in 44 cases	Clinical signs, angiographic features (site, size, irregular shape, focal spasm or mass effect), computed tomography features	Clinical signs helpful in only 2 of 7 (29 per cent). Focal spasm (six cases), mass effect (two cases), size change (two cases) located aneurysm in 100 per cent, larger aneurysm in 83 per cent, more irregular in 93 per cent

aneurysms, all lesions will be clippable through a single craniotomy, and it may be advisable to do this depending on the age and condition of the patient and the location of the aneurysms. Under exceptional circumstances and despite the best diagnostic aids, it may not be possible to determine preoperatively which aneurysm bled. The literature contains cases in which recurrent subarachnoid hemorrhage occurred in patients with multiple aneurysms after the wrong one was clipped.

TRANSCRANIAL DOPPLER ULTRASOUND

Numerous investigators have used transcranial Doppler ultrasound to study changes in cerebral arterial flow velocity after subarachnoid hemorrhage.* Doppler

---

*See references 19, 33, 36, 44, 56, 58, 93, 95, 97, and 103.

flow velocity is proportional to the blood flow through the artery and inversely related to the cross-sectional area of the artery and, therefore, inversely proportional to the square of the radius. There is a rough correlation between angiographic vessel diameter and Doppler flow velocity.[36] Most of the major cerebral arteries of the circle of Willis can be insonated, but reliable, reproducible recordings are best obtained from the proximal portion of the middle cerebral artery. Anterior cerebral artery flow velocities vary depending on flow through the communicating artery, in addition to in relation to vessel diameter.

Seiler and colleagues followed 39 consecutive patients with subarachnoid hemorrhage with transcranial Doppler.[93] Normal middle cerebral artery flow velocity was 60 cm per second. All patients had abnormal flow velocities over 80 cm per second between 4 and 10 days post subarachnoid hemorrhage. Maximum flow velocities between 120 and 140 cm per second did not lead to ischemia, whereas patients with velocities over 200 cm per second sometimes developed ischemia. A steep, early increase in flow velocity seemed particularly likely to portend future ischemia. There was a correlation between higher flow velocities with steeper increases and more subarachnoid blood on computed tomography within 5 days of the hemorrhage. The time course of increased Doppler flow velocities is similar to angiographic vasospasm, although the onset of Doppler changes may be within 3 days of the hemorrhage and the elevations tend to persist for a longer time.[93] Mean middle cerebral artery flow velocity over 120 cm per second was 100 per cent specific but only 59 per cent sensitive for detection of vasospasm on angiography.[97]

Not all studies have found clear correlations between clinical vasospasm, Doppler flow velocities, and angiographic arterial diameters. A great number of variables that are altered by subarachnoid hemorrhage will affect interpretation of transcranial Doppler flow velocities, including overall cerebral blood flow, individual anatomical variations in vessel diameters and collateral flow, hemorheological values, and intracranial pressure. Changes in these factors may explain, in part, poor correlations between clinical vasospasm and Doppler flow velocities.[19, 33, 36, 58, 95] In general, flow velocities are only a rough guide to vasospasm and must take into account the clinical conditions and available radiological imaging. Practically, mean middle cerebral artery flow velocities below 100 cm per second are not associated with symptomatic vasospasm whereas velocities over 200 cm per second almost always occur in patients with severe vasospasm. High mean velocity may not occur in the presence of high intracranial pressure.[56]

Attempts have been made to identify transcranial Doppler parameters other than flow velocity that more accurately detect symptomatic vasospasm. Although peak velocity was significantly related to delayed ischemia in one study, the peak velocity often developed after the onset of the neurological deficit.[33] Flow velocities taken before neurological deterioration were not useful for predicting delayed ischemia. A rate of increase in flow velocity of more than 50 cm per second per 24 hours identified patients who later developed symptomatic vasospasm.

REFERENCES

1. Abbott, R. J., and van Hille, P.: Thunderclap headache and unruptured cerebral aneurysm. Lancet, 2:1459, 1986.
2. Agnoli, A. L.: Vascular anomalies and subarachnoid hemorrhage associated with persisting embryonic vessels. Acta. Neurochir., 60:183, 1982.
3. Almaani, W. S., and Richardson, A. E.: Multiple intracranial aneurysms: Identifying the ruptured lesion. Surg. Neurol., 9:303, 1978.
4. Alpers, B. J., and Forster, F. M.: The reparative processes in subarachnoid hemorrhage. J. Neuropathol. Exp. Neurol., 4:262, 1945.
5. Aoyagi, N., and Hayakawa, I.: Rerupture of intracranial aneurysms during angiography. Acta. Neurochir. (Wien), 98:141, 1989.
6. Archer, B. D.: Computed tomography before lumbar puncture in acute meningitis: A review of the risks and benefits. Can. Med. Assoc. J., 148:961, 1993.
7. Atkinson, J. L., Sundt, T. M., Jr., Houser, O. W., et al.: Angiographic frequency of anterior circulation intracranial aneurysms. J. Neurosurg., 70:551, 1989.
8. Bailes, J. E., Spetzler, R. F., Hadley, M. N., et al.: Management morbidity and mortality in poor-grade aneurysm patients. J. Neurosurg., 72:559, 1990.
9. Bassi, P., Bandera, R., Loiero, M., et al.: Warning signs in subarachnoid hemorrhage: A cooperative study. Acta. Neurol. Scand., 84:277, 1991.
10. Behr, R., Agnoli, A. L., and Zierski, J.: Rupture of giant cerebral aneurysms during angiography: Case report and review of literature. J. Neurol. Sci., 32:195, 1988.
11. Benoit, B. G., Cochrane, D. D., Durity, F., et al.: Clinical radiological correlates in intracerebral hematomas due to aneurysmal rupture. Can. J. Neurol. Sci., 9:409, 1982.
12. Blatter, D. D., Parker, D. L., Ahn, S. S., et al.: Cerebral MR angiography with multiple overlapping thin slab acquisition: II. Early clinical experience. Radiology, 183:379, 1992.
13. Bonita, R.: Cigarette smoking, hypertension and the risk of subarachnoid hemorrhage: A population-based case-control study. Stroke, 17:831, 1986.
14. Botterell, E. H., Lougheed, W. M., Scott, J. W., et al.: Hypothermia and interruption of carotid, or carotid and vertebral circulation, in the surgical management of intracranial aneurysms. J. Neurosurg., 13:1, 1956.
15. Brouwers, P. J. A. M., Dippel, D. W. J., Vermeulen, M., et al.: Amount of blood on computed tomography as an independent predictor after aneurysm rupture. Stroke, 24:809, 1993.
16. Carpenter, D. A., Grubb, R. L., Jr., Tempel, L. W., et al.: Cerebral oxygen metabolism after aneurysmal subarachnoid hemorrhage. J. Cereb. Blood Flow Metab., 11:837, 1991.
17. Chui, M., Muller, P., and Tucker, W.: Angiographic diagnosis of small aneurysms of the posterior communicating artery. A.J.N.R., 11:1165, 1990.
18. Crompton, M. R.: The pathogenesis of cerebral infarction following the rupture of cerebral berry aneurysms. Brain, 87:491, 1964.
19. Davis, S. M., Andrews, J. T., Lichtenstein, M., et al.: Correlations between cerebral arterial velocities, blood flow, and delayed ischemia after subarachnoid hemorrhage. Stroke, 23:492, 1992.
20. Day, J. W., and Raskin, N. H.: Thunderclap headache: Symptoms of unruptured cerebral aneurysm. Lancet, 2:1247, 1986.
21. Dernback, P. D., Little, J. R., Jones, S. C., et al.: Altered cerebral autoregulation and CO_2 reactivity after aneurysmal subarachnoid hemorrhage. Neurosurgery, 22:822, 1988.
22. Dion, J. E., Gates, P. C., Fox, A. J., et al.: Clinical events following neuroangiography: A prospective study. Stroke, 18:997, 1987.
23. Duffy, G. P.: Lumbar puncture in spontaneous subarachnoid haemorrhage. B.M.J., 285:1163, 1982.
24. Dujovny, M., Kossovsky, N., Kossowsky, R., et al.: Aneurysm clip motion during magnetic resonance imaging: In vivo experimental study with metallurgical factor analysis. Neurosurgery, 17:543, 1985.
25. Fein, J. M.: Brain energetics and circulatory control after subarachnoid hemorrhage. J. Neurosurg., 45:498, 1976.
26. Ferguson, G. G.: Physical factors in the initiation, growth, and rupture of human intracranial saccular aneurysms. J. Neurosurg., 37:666, 1972.
27. Fisher, C. M., Kistler, J. P., and Davis, J. M.: Relation of cerebral vasospasm to subarachnoid hemorrhage visualized by computerized tomographic scanning. Neurosurgery, 6:1, 1980.
28. Fontanarosa, P. B.: Recognition of subarachnoid hemorrhage. Ann. Emerg. Med., 18:1199, 1989.
29. Friedman, A. H.: Subarachnoid hemorrhage of unknown etiology. In Wilkins, R. H., and Rengachary, S. S., eds.: Neurosurgery Update II. New York, McGraw-Hill, 1991, pp. 73–77.
30. Gelmers, H. J., Simons, A. J., and Loew, F.: Rupture of intracranial aneurysms and ventricular opacification during carotid angiography. Acta. Neurochir., 70:43, 1984.
31. Graff-Radford, N. R., Torner, J., Adams, H. P., et al.: Factors associated with hydrocephalus after subarachnoid hemorrhage. Arch. Neurol., 46:744, 1989.

32. Griebel, R. W., Black, P. M., Pile-Spellman, J., et al.: The importance of "accessory" outflow pathways in hydrocephalus after experimental subarachnoid hemorrhage. Neurosurgery, 24:187, 1989.

33. Grosset, D. G., Straiton, J., McDonald, I., et al.: Use of transcranial Doppler sonography to predict development of a delayed ischemic deficit after subarachnoid hemorrhage. J. Neurosurg., 78:183, 1993.

34. Grubb, R. L., Raichle, M. E., Eichling, J. O., et al.: Effects of subarachnoid hemorrhage on cerebral blood volume, blood flow, and oxygen utilization in humans. J. Neurosurg., 46:446, 1977.

35. Hammes, E. M., Jr.: Reaction of the meninges to blood. Arch. Neurol., 52:505, 1944.

36. Harders, A. G., and Gilsbach, J. M.: Time course of blood velocity changes related to vasospasm in the circle of Willis measured by transcranial Doppler ultrasound. J. Neurosurg., 66:718, 1987.

37. Hassler, O., and Saltzman, G. F.: Angiographic and histologic changes in infundibular widening of the posterior communicating artery. Acta. Radiol., 1:321, 1963.

38. Hassler, W., Steinmetz, H., and Pirschel, J.: Transcranial Doppler study of intracranial circulatory arrest. J. Neurosurg., 71:195, 1989.

39. Hauerberg, J., Andersen, B. B., Eskesen, V., et al.: Importance of recognition of a warning leak as a sign of a ruptured intracranial aneurysm. Acta. Neurol. Scand., 83:61, 1991.

40. Henry, M. M. P., Guerin, J., Vallat, J. M., et al.: Extravasation per-angiographique du produit de contraste au cours des ruptures d'anéurysmes (à propos de 2 cas). Neurochirurgia, 14:121, 1971.

41. Holtas, S., Olsson, M., Romner, B., et al.: Comparison of MR imaging and CT in patients with intracranial aneurysm clips. A.J.N.R., 9:891, 1988.

42. Hubschmann, O. R., and Nathanson, D. C.: The role of calcium and cellular membrane dysfunction in experimental trauma and subarachnoid hemorrhage. J. Neurosurg., 62:698, 1985.

43. Hunt, W. E., and Hess, R. M.: Surgical risk as related to time of intervention in the repair of intracranial aneurysms. J. Neurosurg., 28:14, 1968.

44. Hutchinson, K., and Weir, B.: Transcranial Doppler studies in aneurysm patients. Can. J. Neurol. Sci., 16:411, 1989.

45. Inagawa, T., Ishikawa, S., Aoki, H., et al.: Aneurysmal subarachnoid hemorrhage in Izumo City and Shimane Prefecture of Japan: Incidence. Stroke, 19:170, 1988.

46. Jagger, J., Torner, J. C., and Kassell, N. F.: Neurologic assessment of subarachnoid hemorrhage in a large patient series. Surg. Neurol., 32:327, 1989.

47. Jane, J. A., Kassell, N. F., Torner, J. C., et al.: The natural history of aneurysms and arteriovenous malformations. J. Neurosurg., 62:321, 1985.

48. Juvela, S.: Minor leak before rupture of an intracranial aneurysm and subarachnoid hemorrhage of unknown etiology. Neurosurgery, 30:7, 1992.

49. Juvela, S., Porras, M., Heiskanen, O.: Natural history of unruptured intracranial aneurysms: A long-term follow-up study. J. Neurosurg., 79:174, 1993.

50. Juvela, S., Hillbom, M., Numminen, H., et al.: Cigarette smoking and alcohol consumption as risk factors for aneurysmal subarachnoid hemorrhage. Stroke, 24:639, 1993.

51. Kassell, N. F., and Torner, J. C.: Size of intracranial aneurysms. Neurosurgery, 12:291, 1983.

52. Kassell, N. F., Torner, J. C., Haley, E. C., Jr., et al.: The international cooperative study on the timing of aneurysm surgery: I. Overall management results. J. Neurosurg., 73:18, 1990.

53. Kassell, N. F., Torner, J. C., Haley, E. C., Jr., et al.: The international cooperative study on the timing of aneurysm surgery: II. Surgical results. J. Neurosurg., 73:37, 1990.

54. Kaye, A. H., and Brownbill, D.: Postoperative intracranial pressure in patients operated on for cerebral aneurysms following subarachnoid hemorrhage. J. Neurosurg., 54:726, 1981.

55. Kistler, J. P., Crowell, R. M., Davis, K. R., et al.: The relation of cerebral vasospasm to the extent and location of subarachnoid blood visualized by CT scan: A prospective study. Neurology, 33:424, 1983.

56. Klingelhofer, J., Sander, D., Holzgraffe, M., et al.: Cerebral vaso-

57. spasm evaluated by transcranial Doppler ultrasonography at different intracranial pressures. J. Neurosurg., 75:752, 1991.

57. Klucznik, R. P., Carrier, D. A., Pyka, R., et al.: Placement of a ferromagnetic intracerebral aneurysm clip in a magnetic field with a fatal outcome. Radiology, 187:855, 1993.

58. Laumer, R., Steinmeier, R., Gonner, F., et al.: Cerebral hemodynamics in subarachnoid hemorrhage evaluated by transcranial Doppler sonography: I. Reliability of flow velocities in clinical management. Neurosurgery, 33:1, 1993.

59. Lindsay, K. W., Teasdale, G. M., and Knill-Jones, R. P.: Observer variability in assessing the clinical features of subarachnoid hemorrhage. J. Neurosurg., 58:57, 1983.

60. Locksley, H. B.: Natural history of subarachnoid hemorrhage, intracranial aneurysms, and arteriovenous malformations: Based on 6368 cases in the cooperative study: I. In Sahs, A. L., Perret, G. E., Locksley, H. B., et al., eds.: Intracranial Aneurysms and Subarachnoid Hemorrhage. Philadelphia, J. B. Lippincott, 1969, pp. 37–57.

61. Locksley, H. B.: Natural history of subarachnoid hemorrhage, intracranial aneurysms, and arteriovenous malformations: Based on 6368 cases in the cooperative study: II. In Sahs, A. L., Perret, G. E., Locksley, H. B., et al., eds.: Intracranial Aneurysms and Subarachnoid Hemorrhage. Philadelphia, J. B. Lippincott, 1969, pp. 58–108.

62. Longstreth, W. T., Jr., Nelson, L. M., Koepsell, T. D., et al.: Cigarette smoking, alcohol use, and subarachnoid hemorrhage. Stroke, 23:1242, 1992.

63. Marttila, I., and Heiskanen, O.: Value of neurological and angiographic signs as indicators of the ruptured aneurysm in patients with multiple intracranial aneurysms. Acta. Neurochir., 23:95, 1970.

64. Marzatico, F., Gaetani, P., Rodriguez y Baena, R., et al.: Experimental subarachnoid hemorrhage. Lipid peroxidation and Na^+, K^+-ATPase in different rat brain areas. Molec. Chem. Neuropathol., 11:99, 1989.

65. Matsumura, K., Matsuda, M., Handa, J., et al.: Magnetic resonance imaging with aneurysmal subarachnoid hemorrhage: Comparison with computed tomography scan. Surg. Neurol., 34:71, 1990.

66. Meyer, C. H. A., Lowe, D., Meyer, M., et al.: Progressive change in cerebral blood flow during the first three weeks after subarachnoid hemorrhage. Neurosurgery, 12:58, 1983.

67. Meyer, F. B., Huston, J., III, and Riederer, S. S.: Pulsatile increases in aneurysm size determined by cine phase-contrast MR angiography. J. Neurosurg., 78:879, 1993.

68. Miyasaka, K., Wolpert, S. M., and Prager, R. J.: The association of cerebral aneurysms, infundibula, and intracranial arteriovenous malformations. Stroke, 13:196, 1982.

69. Mohr, G., Ferguson, G., Khan, M., et al.: Intraventricular hemorrhage from ruptured aneurysm. J. Neurosurg., 58:482, 1983.

70. Nakajima, K., Ito, Z., Hen, R., et al.: Congenital anomalies of cerebral artery and intracranial aneurysms. Brain Nerve, 28:197, 1976.

71. Nehls, D. G., Flom, R. A., Carter, L. P., et al.: Multiple intracranial aneurysms: Determining the site of rupture. J. Neurosurg., 63:342, 1985.

72. Noda, S., Tamaki, N., Yamaguchi, M., et al.: Giant suprasellar aneurysm with extravasation of contrast medium into the ventricular system. Surg. Neurol., 13:208, 1980.

73. Nornes, H.: The role of intracranial pressure in the arrest of hemorrhage in patients with ruptured intracranial aneurysm. J. Neurosurg., 39:226, 1973.

74. Nystrom, S. H. M.: On factors related to growth and rupture of intracranial aneurysms. Acta. Neuropathol., 16:64, 1970.

75. Okamoto, S., Handa, H., and Hashimoto, N.: Location of intracranial aneurysms associated with cerebral arteriovenous malformations. Surg. Neurol., 22:335, 1984.

76. Origitano, T. C., Wascher, T. M., Reichman, O. H., et al.: Sustained increased cerebral blood flow with prophylactic hypertensive hypervolemic hemodilution ("Triple-H" therapy) after subarachnoid hemorrhage. Neurosurgery, 27:729, 1990.

77. Oyesiku, N. M., Colohan, A. R. T., Barrow, D. L., et al.: Cocaine-induced aneurysmal rupture: An emergent negative factor in the natural history of intracranial aneurysms? Neurosurgery, 32:518, 1993.

78. Pakarinen, S.: Incidence, aetiology, and prognosis of primary subarachnoid haemorrhage. Acta. Neurol. Scand., *43*(Suppl. 29):1, 1967.

79. Palmieri, A., Liguori, R., and de Rosa, R.: A propos d'un cas de rupture d'anéurysme artériel sacculaire intracrânien au cours d'une artériographie. Ann. Radiol., *14*:943, 1971.

80. Pasqualin, A., Bazzan, A., Cavanazzi, P., et al.: Intracranial hematomas following aneurysmal rupture: Experience with 309 cases. Surg. Neurol., *25*:6, 1986.

81. Patel, M. K., and Clarke, M. A.: Lumbar puncture and subarachnoid haemorrhage. Postgrad. Med. J., *62*:1021, 1986.

82. Rhoton, A. L., Jr.: Microsurgical anatomy of saccular aneurysms. *In* Wilkins, R. H., and Rengachary, S., eds.: Neurosurgery. New York, McGraw-Hill, 1985, pp. 1330–1340.

83. Rinkel, G. J. E., Wijdicks, E. F. M., Hasan, D., et al.: Outcome in patients with subarachnoid haemorrhage and negative angiography according to pattern of haemorrhage on computed tomography. Lancet, *338*:964, 1991.

84. Roach, M. R.: A model study of why some intracranial aneurysms thrombose but others rupture. Stroke, *9*:583, 1978.

85. Romner, B., Olsson, M., Ljunggren, B., et al.: Magnetic resonance imaging and aneurysm clips: Magnetic properties and image artifacts. J. Neurosurg., *70*:426, 1989.

86. Rosenstein, J., Suzuki, M., Symon, L., et al.: Clinical use of a portable bedside cerebral flow machine in the management of aneurysmal subarachnoid hemorrhage. Neurosurgery, *15*:519, 1984.

87. Ross, J. S., Masaryk, T. J., and Modic, M. T.: Intracranial aneurysms: Evaluation by MR angiography. A.J.R., *155*:159, 1990.

88. Sakamoto, T., Kwad, R., Mizoi, K., et al.: Angiographical study of ruptured aneurysm in the multiple aneurysm patients. Neurol. Surg., *6*:549, 1978.

89. Sampei, T., Yasui, N., Mizuno, M., et al.: Contrast medium extravasation during cerebral angiography for ruptured intracranial aneurysm: Clinical analysis of 26 cases. Neurol. Med. Chir., *30*:1011, 1990.

90. Sarner, M., and Rose, F. C.: Clinical presentation of ruptured intracranial aneurysm. J. Neurol. Neurosurg. Psychiatry, *30*:67, 1967.

91. Satoh, S., and Kadoya, S.: Magnetic resonance imaging of subarachnoid hemorrhage. Neuroradiology, *30*:361, 1988.

92. Schievink, W. I., Karemaker, J. M., Hageman, L. M., et al.: Circumstances surrounding aneurysmal subarachnoid hemorrhage. Surg. Neurol., *32*:266, 1989.

93. Seiler, R. W., Grolimund, P., Aaslid, R., et al.: Cerebral vasospasm evaluated by transcranial ultrasound correlated with clinical grade and CT-visualized subarachnoid hemorrhage. J. Neurosurg., *64*:594, 1986.

94. Sekhar, L. N., Sclabassi, R. J., Sun, M., et al.: Intra-aneurysmal pressure measurement in experimental saccular aneurysms in dogs. Stroke, *19*:352, 1988.

95. Sekhar, L. N., Wechsler, L. R., Yonas, H., et al.: Value of transcranial Doppler examination in the diagnosis of cerebral vasospasm after subarachnoid hemorrhage. Neurosurgery, *22*:813, 1988.

96. Shinton, R., and Beevers, G.: Meta-analysis of relation between cigarette smoking and stroke. B.M.J., *298*:789, 1989.

97. Sloan, M. A., Haley, E. C., Jr., Kassell, N. F., et al.: Sensitivity and specificity of transcranial Doppler ultrasonography in the diagnosis of vasospasm following subarachnoid hemorrhage. Neurology, *39*:1514, 1989.

98. Stehbens, W. E.: Pathology of the Cerebral Blood Vessels. St. Louis, C. V. Mosby, 1972.

99. Stehbens, W. E.: The pathology of intracranial arterial aneurysms and their complications. *In* Fox, J. L., ed.: Intracranial Aneurysms. New York, Springer-Verlag, 1983, pp. 272–357.

100. Stehbens, W. E.: Etiology of intracranial berry aneurysms. J. Neurosurg., *70*:823, 1991.

101. Steiger, H.: Pathophysiology of development and rupture of cerebral aneurysms. Acta. Neurochir. Suppl., *48*:1, 1990.

102. Steinberger, A., Ganti, S. R., McMurtry, J. G., et al.: Transient neurological deficits secondary to saccular vertebrobasilar aneurysms. J. Neurosurg., *60*:410, 1984.

103. Steinmeier, R., Laumer, R., Bondar, L., et al.: Cerebral hemodynamics in subarachnoid hemorrhage evaluated by transcranial Doppler sonography: II. Pulsatility indices: Normal reference values and characteristics in subarachnoid hemorrhage. Neurosurgery, *33*:10, 1993.

104. Taylor, W., Miller, J. D., and Todd, N. V.: Long-term outcome following anterior cerebral artery ligation for ruptured anterior communicating artery aneurysms. J. Neurosurg., *74*:51, 1991.

105. Teasdale, G. M., Drake, C. G., Hunt, W., et al.: A universal subarachnoid haemorrhage scale: Report of a committee of the World Federation of Neurosurgical Societies. J. Neurol. Neurosurg. Psychiatry, *51*:1457, 1988.

106. Todd, N. V., Tocher, J. L., Jones, P. A., et al.: Outcome following aneurysm wrapping: A 10-year follow-up review of clipped and wrapped aneurysms. J. Neurosurg., *70*:841, 1989.

107. Tourtellotte, W. W., and Shorr, R. J.: Cerebrospinal fluid. In Youmans, J. R., ed.: Neurological Surgery: A Comprehensive Reference Guide to the Diagnosis and Management of Neurosurgical Problems. 3rd. ed. Philadelphia, W. B. Saunders, 1990, pp. 335–363.

108. Tran-Dinh, H., Williams, L. M., and Jayashinghe, L. S.: Association of intracranial aneurysm and arteriovenous malformation. Med. J. Aust., *l*:521, 1983.

109. van Crevel, H., Habbema, J. D. F., Braakman, R.: Decision analysis of the management of incidental intracranial saccular aneurysms. Neurology, *36*:1335, 1986.

110. van Gijn, J., and van Dongen, K. J.: The time course of aneurysmal haemorrhage on computed tomograms. Neuroradiology, *23*:153, 1982.

111. van Gijn, J., Hijdra, A., Wijdicks, E. F. M., et al.: Acute hydrocephalus after aneurysmal subarachnoid hemorrhage. J. Neurosurg., *63*:355, 1985.

112. Vermeulen, M., Hasan, D., Blijenberg, B. G., et al.: Xanthochromia after subarachnoid haemorrhage needs no revisitation. J. Neurol. Neurosurg. Psychiatry, *52*:826, 1989.

113. Voldby, B., and Enevoldsen, E. M.: Intracranial pressure changes following aneurysm rupture: Part 2. Associated cerebrospinal fluid lactacidosis. J. Neurosurg., *56*:197, 1982.

114. Voldby, B., and Enevoldsen, E. M.: Intracranial pressure changes following aneurysm rupture: Part 3. Recurrent hemorrhage. J. Neurosurg., *56*:784, 1982.

115. Voldby, B., Enevoldsen, E. M., and Jensen, F. T.: Cerebrovascular reactivity in patients with ruptured intracranial aneurysms. J. Neurosurg., *62*:59, 1985.

116. Voldby, B., Enevoldsen, E. M., and Jensen, F. T.: Regional CBF, intraventricular pressure and cerebral metabolism in patients with ruptured intracranial aneurysms. J. Neurosurg., *62*:48, 1985.

117. Weir, B.: Intracranial aneurysms and subarachnoid hemorrhage: An overview. *In* Wilkins, R. H., and Rengachary, S. S., eds.: Neurosurgery. New York, McGraw-Hill, 1985, pp. 1308–1329.

118. Weir, B.: Aneurysms Affecting the Nervous System. Baltimore, Williams & Wilkins, 1987.

119. Wiebers, D. O., Whisnant, J. P., and O'Fallon, W. M.: The natural history of unruptured intracranial aneurysms. N. Engl. J. Med., *304*:696, 1981.

120. Winn, H. R., Richardson, A. E., and Jane, J. A.: The assessment of the natural history of single cerebral aneurysms that have ruptured. *In* Hopkins, L. N., and Long, D. M., eds.: Clinical Management of Intracranial Aneurysms. New York, Raven Press, 1982, pp. 1–10.

121. Wood, E. H.: Angiographic identification of the ruptured lesion in patients with multiple cerebral aneurysms. J. Neurosurg., *21*:182, 1964.

122. Yamamoto, Y., Smith, R. R., and Bernanke, D. H.: Accelerated nonmuscle contraction after subarachnoid hemorrhage: Culture and characterization of myofibroblasts from human cerebral arteries in vasospasm. Neurosurgery, *30*:337, 1992.

123. Yasargil, M. G.: Microneurosurgery. Vol. II: Clinical Considerations, Surgery of the Intracranial Aneurysms and Results. Stuttgart, Georg Thieme Verlag, 1984.

Cerebrovascular Diseases in Children

erebrovascular disease in children encompasses a variety of disorders that together constitute about 10 per cent of a pediatric neurosurgical practice. The data in Tables 51–1 and 51–2 are typical of a year's practice in pediatric neurosurgery at Shands Hospital of the University of Florida. In addition, the pediatric neurosurgeon is frequently asked to consult on cases that are primarily addressed with medical management. Several cerebrovascular diseases occur almost exclusively in childhood, whereas other diseases present in children or adults. Frequently, the presentation is quite different in the child than in the adult. Although some of these processes present in a classical fashion, such as an acute ictal event, the presentation of some of these entities can be more subtle and must be included in the differential diagnosis.

The most common vascular disorders treated by the pediatric neurosurgeon are the vascular anomalies. This group of diseases includes arteriovenous malformations, aneurysms, moyamoya disease, vein of Galen malformations, carotid cavernous fistulae, Sturge-Weber syndrome, and dural arteriovenous malformations. Other vascular disorders of the central nervous system in children are diagnosed after embolic, thrombotic, hemorrhagic, or epileptic events but are principally treated with nonoperative measures. This group includes infarctions, vasculitis, intracerebral hemorrhage without a structural lesion, and neonatal intraventricular hemorrhage.

Although the sequelae of cerebrovascular disease in children can be devastating, this is not universally the case. The plasticity of the infant's and child's brain allows for optimism in its potential for recovery. Because of this forgiving aspect of the pediatric central nervous system, aggressive therapy often proves rewarding.

The diagnosis and management of cerebral vascular diseases in childhood has changed dramatically in recent years as a result of new technologies. Newer imaging techniques such as magnetic resonance imaging, magnetic resonance angiography, and intraoperative angiography are more readily available, and therefore earlier, more accurate diagnoses are being made. Interventional neuroradiological techniques are being applied to many vascular disorders of childhood that previously could not be treated or had dismal outcomes with standard surgical intervention. Stereotactic radiosurgery is another nonoperative advance in neurosurgical practice that is being used to treat childhood cerebrovascular diseases. The approach to this group of disorders has significantly been altered by these newer technologies. The purposes of this chapter are to briefly discuss the cerebrovascular diseases of childhood that are managed nonoperatively and, in a more detailed fashion, to delineate the neurosurgical approach to the more common vascular anomalies.

Interventional Neurosurgery

The rapid development of steerable and directed catheters and guide wires allows access to almost every intracranial vessel. The functional testing developed in this area (e.g., intra-arterial methohexital) has allowed for thorough understanding of vascular territories and the consequences of eliminating these therapeutically. The use of interventional embolization in the treatment

Table 51–1

PERCENTAGE OF VASCULAR/INTERVENTIONAL CASES (APPROX. 10%) AT UNIVERSITY OF FLORIDA PEDIATRIC NEUROSURGICAL PRACTICE, 1991–1992

No. of cases: 378
No. of vascular/interventional cases: 31

J. P. Mickle • R. S. Glasser

Table 51-2
LESIONS CONSTITUTING
VASCULAR/INTERVENTIONAL
CASES AT THE UNIVERSITY OF FLORIDA, 1991–1992

Lesion Type	Number
AVM	12
VGA	7
Tumors	4
DAVM	2
Aneurysms	2
CCF	2
VVF	2

AVM, arteriovenous malformation; VGA, vein of Galen aneurysm; DAVM, dural arteriovenous malformation; CCF, carotid-cavernous fistula; VVF, vertebrovertebral fistula.

of arteriovenous malformations has brought about a dramatic change in the surgical approach to these lesions. At the authors' institution, all arteriovenous malformations of the brain and spinal cord are embolized before surgery. The surgeries become safer, more rapid, and far easier to perform after embolization. The authors have had no incidences of normal perfusion breakthrough since the policy of aggressive preoperative embolization was adopted. Anatomical features of lesions are often discovered at the time of flow reduction and embolization, which makes the surgery safer and easier. Interventional technologies are now also a major part of the treatment of congenital vascular malformations such as vein of Galen aneurysms. Not only has treatment of these high-flow lesions been improved with these technologies, but understanding of the basic science of cerebrovascular disease also has improved dramatically as a result of the information obtained during investigation of these lesions.

Vascular Disorders Without Structural Lesions

Cerebrovascular disease in the pediatric population that is not secondary to an intracranial vascular anomaly is frequently heralded by an ischemic or hemorrhagic event. The preponderance of ischemic strokes that occur in childhood are not related to intracranial lesions, but most hemorrhages are secondary to an intracranial structural abnormality (Table 51–3).[71, 75] Excluding trauma and intracranial hemorrhage associated with prematurity, the overall incidence of childhood stroke has been estimated to be 2.5 to 2.7 cases per 100,000 per year.[13, 81] In most series, hemorrhages outnumber ischemic insults by a ratio of three to one.[13] The causes of childhood stroke are varied, and 30 to 50 per cent have no identifiable cause.

Ischemic strokes can almost always be managed without surgery acutely; however, some diseases, such as moyamoya disease, require revascularization procedures to minimize the risk of future ischemic events. Hemorrhagic strokes in children are approached simi-

larly to those in adults; they are evaluated on a case-by-case basis, and treatment is directed at the source of the hemorrhage.

ETIOLOGY

Whether a cerebral infarction is ischemic or hemorrhagic in nature, the cause of the stroke should be determined. In series that include all radiographically diagnosed infarctions, the neonatal predominant causes are trauma and hemorrhagic and anoxic injuries.[20] Thereafter, the causes for hemorrhagic and ischemic cerebrovascular disease that are not associated with a vascular anomaly are protean; these are listed in Table 51–4.[16, 20, 73, 74]

Vascular disease without a structural lesion typically occurs secondary to a systemic illness or is classified as idiopathic. Many systemic diseases predispose the pediatric patient to cerebrovascular insult (see Table 51–3). These disorders most commonly present with either transient or permanent deficits of an ischemic nature, but they can predispose to an intracranial hemorrhage. Furthermore, some diseases produce strokes secondary to the primary disease but also are associated with a higher incidence of vascular anomalies. For example, sickle cell anemia has been shown to be a risk factor for cerebral aneurysms, but it also predisposes to ischemic infarctions.[57]

In the pediatric population, in contrast to that of adults, intraparenchymal hemorrhages are more common than ischemic cerebral infarctions.[13, 53, 81] Reviews suggest that most intraparenchymal hemorrhages are caused by vascular anomalies, with arteriovenous malformations and aneurysms being the most common.[13] However, Mazza and colleagues, in an analysis of 66 cases of hemorrhagic stroke, found 16 cases to be spontaneous hemorrhages without identifiable cause.[53] Most series find that ischemic strokes are more likely than hemorrhages if the patients harboring vascular structural lesions are excluded.[13, 81] Up to 25 per cent of pediatric intraparenchymal hemorrhages remain idiopathic.[82] Common causes that are identified include

Table 51-3
PEDIATRIC CEREBROVASCULAR DISEASE RESULTING FROM STRUCTURAL LESIONS

Vascular Anomalies	Vasculitis
Aneurysms	Unknown cause
Arteriovenous malformations	AIDS (acquired immune deficiency syndrome)
Moyamoya disease	Drug abuse (amphetamines, cocaine, LSD)
Vein of Galen malformations	Wegener's granulomatosis
Sturge-Weber syndrome	Immune-related diseases (polyarteritis nodosa, systemic lupus erythematosus, juvenile onset rheumatoid arthritis)
Fibromuscular dysplasia	Crohn's disease–related
Carotid dissections	Granulomatous angiitis
Vertebral dissections	Antiphospholipid antibody syndrome

Table 51–4

PEDIATRIC CEREBROVASCULAR DISEASE WITHOUT STRUCTURAL LESIONS

Heart Disease	**Hematologic Disorders**
Cyanotic heart defects	Sickle cell disease
Valvular diseases (including prosthetic)	Disseminated intravascular coagulopathy
Endocarditis	Polycythemia
Patent ductus arteriosus	Idiopathic thrombocytopenic purpura
Septal defects	Thrombotic thrombocytopenic purpura
Patent foramen ovale	Leukemia
Rhabdomyoma	Pregnancy-related
Atrial myxoma	Vitamin K deficiency
Acute cardiogenic hypotension	Contraceptive use–related
Surgical complications	Hemophilia
Angiographic complications	Leukemia-related
Emboli from other cardiac sources (i.e., arrhythmias)	**Infections**
Hypertension (usually associated with coarctation of aorta)	Meningitis
Metabolic Disorders	Mucormycosis
Homocystinuria	Tonsillitis
Diabetes	Cavernous sinus thrombophlebitis
Fabry's disease	Malaria
Hypercholesterolemia	Herpes ophthalmicus
Kinky-hair syndrome	Systemic infections
	Other
	Migraine
	Periventricular/intraventricular hemorrhage
	Venous/sinus thrombosis
	Pulmonary arteriovenous fistula
	MELAS syndrome (mitochondrial encephalopathy, lactic acidosis and strokes)

hemorrhage into an ischemic infarct, hemophilia or other coagulopathy, and occult arteriovenous malformation.

Cerebral infarctions in childhood are rarely caused by atherosclerosis, as is the case in adults, but typically are related to a systemic process or an intracranial structural lesion. Intraventricular or periventricular hemorrhage associated with prematurity is a common event that is manifested as neonatal distress. These hemorrhages almost never require surgical intervention and are managed by the neonatologist. The most common cause of ischemic stroke in children is cardiac disease, which accounts for approximately one third of all ischemic insults.[75] Typically, the infarction is a result of an embolic phenomenon, but it may be caused by cerebral anoxia associated with severe heart failure or by a complication of cardiovascular surgery (Fig. 51–1). Infection can be the cause of cerebral infarctions in older children, usually as a result of a local invasion of the infectious process with subsequent arterial occlusion (Fig. 51–2) or from a septic embolus. Up to 50 per cent of ischemic infarctions in pediatrics elude etiological diagnosis and are classified as idiopathic.[74] Broderick and colleagues noted recurrent migraine attacks in two of their patients who had ischemic infarctions of unknown origin.[13] Establishing a cause for pediatric strokes is important if attempts at preventing recurrent hemorrhagic or ischemic events are to be successful.

CLINICAL PRESENTATION AND DIAGNOSIS

Cerebral infarction in children, both hemorrhagic and ischemic, is manifested most commonly by an acute event that causes a focal deficit, as it is in adults. Pediatric patients without a structural lesion do not have different symptoms than those patients with a lesion unless a sign or symptom of their underlying disease is evident. In infants and younger children, a focal deficit may not be appreciated, but rather a stroke may be heralded by the acute or subacute onset of lethargy. A large intraparenchymal or intraventricular hemorrhage frequently is accompanied by an altered level of consciousness in all age groups.

Seizures are more frequent after a hemorrhage than after an ischemic stroke.[33] The patient who presents with a seizure may be so obtunded in the postictal state that a focal deficit such as a hemiparesis may be masked. Nevertheless, hemiparesis is the most common presenting symptom in childhood stroke. It is uncommon for patients with an ischemic stroke not to be hemiparetic at presentation.[81] Transient ischemic attacks initially presenting in childhood are most frequently associated with an identifiable underlying disorder. Moyamoya disease, fibromuscular dysplasia, and migraines can present with recurrent, transient ischemic events. Other than these disorders, however, recurrent symptoms are unusual in pediatric cerebrovascular disease.

The diagnosis of an acute cerebrovascular event should be suspected by its characteristic clinical presentation. If signs of increased intracranial pressure or significant mass effect (decreased level of consciousness) are present, a computed tomography scan should be done immediately. This test reliably evaluates for an intracranial hemorrhage as the cause of the acute neurological deterioration. However, usually it is normal in the acute stages of ischemic cerebral infarction. By 24 to 48 hours after an ischemic infarction, vaso-

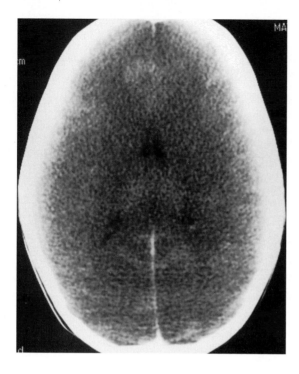

Figure 51–1

A 6-year-old girl suffered from acute cardiogenic hypotension during cardiovascular surgery. She suffered a severe anoxic injury and subsequently died from this injury. Computed tomography of the head without the use of contrast medium depicts diffuse cerebral edema. The gray-white matter definition is lost. The sulci are effaced, and the ventricles are small, all secondary to diffuse cerebral edema of an anoxic origin.

genic edema is evident on the scan as a hypodense lesion that corresponds to an arterial distribution. A venous infarction, such as would result from a sagittal sinus thrombosis, covers a large area and frequently becomes hemorrhagic.[4] By 2 weeks after the infarction, the hypodense lesion becomes more discrete and displays no evidence of mass effect. Coagulative necrosis is responsible for this radiographic finding.[74] Computed tomography may provide evidence of the underlying cause in the patient with a hemorrhagic lesion resulting from a vascular malformation. However, it usually is not helpful in patients with hemorrhagic and ischemic lesions occurring without a structural lesion.

Angiography is not recommended in the acute evaluation of an ischemic infarction. However, arteriography should be performed on every child, excluding premature neonates, with an intraparenchymal or intraventricular hemorrhage. In the pediatric population, an underlying vascular malformation or tumor is found in 75 to 90 per cent of the cases.[45, 82]

The use of magnetic resonance imaging and magnetic resonance angiography has been instrumental in

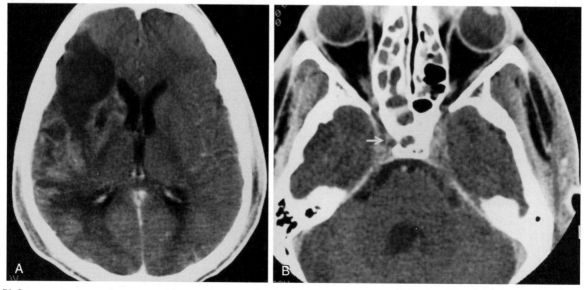

Figure 51–2

A 15-year-old diabetic boy presented with left hemiparesis and right ophthalmoplegia. *A.* Contrast medium–enhanced computed tomography demonstrates a hypodensity in the territory of the right middle cerebral artery, with gyriform enhancement that is typical of an ischemic infarction. *B.* Hypodensity within the region of the right cavernous sinus represents an intracavernous carotid artery thrombosis *(arrow)*. The cause of this patient's ischemic infarction proved to be a mucormycosis infection that spread to the cavernous sinus region.

further defining cerebrovascular disease in children. Magnetic resonance imaging, in particular, identifies infarctions with a high degree of sensitivity. Also, angiographically occult arteriovenous malformations are diagnosed with increased frequency with magnetic resonance imaging. Magnetic resonance angiography is a newer technology that has not been extensively utilized in the pediatric population. However, Kurlemann and colleagues have described the use of magnetic resonance angiography in moyamoya disease.[49] As it becomes more available, it may prove useful in other diseases such as arteriovenous malformations, in traumatic dissections (magnetic resonance imaging is an excellent imaging modality in this disease), and in aneurysms.

MANAGEMENT

The evaluation of the child with acute onset of a focal neurological deficit from a vascular cause centers initially on determining whether a hemorrhagic or ischemic lesion exists. Pediatric patients usually fall into one of several categories: (1) ischemic infarction without mass effect, (2) ischemic infarction with global or focal mass effect, (3) hemorrhage with little or no mass effect, (4) hemorrhage with mass effect, (5) hemorrhage in deep or eloquent cortex. The acute management of the child with an ischemic infarction centers primarily on establishing the diagnosis and subsequently on establishing the cause. Otherwise, the pediatric patient is managed acutely with hydration and conservative treatment, as is the adult. Uncommonly, edema caused by the infarction produces a local or diffuse increase in the intracranial pressure. Again, as in the adult, medical measures such as hyperventilation and the use of osmotic diuretics and barbiturates are the treatments applied in this situation.[92]

The management of the infant or child with a spontaneous intracerebral hemorrhage of unknown cause has been the source of some controversy. Wakai and colleagues suggest that angiographically occult arteriovenous malformations are found in a high percentage of young patients with angiographically negative lobar hematomas, ranging from 27 to 53 per cent.[93, 95] For that reason, they propose operative exploration in most cases. However, the authors agree with Shah and Heros, who advocate that conservative management be applied to angiographically negative lobar hematomas without neuroimaging evidence of an occult lesion and without mass effect or neurological deterioration.[83] As they point out, however, a superficially located hematoma in noneloquent cortex may be safely approached surgically in 3 to 4 weeks, after the hematoma has liquefied.

The patient with a life-threatening mass (hemorrhage) obviously requires emergent surgical evacuation. In this setting, there probably will not be time for a preoperative angiogram. Given the high likelihood that the hemorrhage is secondary to a structural lesion in this age group, an intraoperative search for a possible source should be thorough after the hematoma

has been evacuated. If a cause is not found, then an arteriogram should be performed intraoperatively or postoperatively. In the patient with a negative angiogram, a magnetic resonance image scan should be performed to evaluate for a possible occult vascular malformation. Not uncommonly, however, this radiographic evaluation also fails to yield the cause.

The patient with an intracranial hemorrhage and a coexisting coagulation defect represents a special circumstance that requires the collaboration of the neurosurgeon and the hematologist. Normal hemostasis can be expected in those children with hemophilia, in whom factor replacement is usually effective, but it must be continued for 2 weeks after surgery.[70] However, a normal coagulation environment in the patient with disseminated intravascular coagulopathy, although frequently difficult to achieve, is required before intracranial surgery is attempted. In this situation, the source underlying the coagulopathy must be addressed, if possible, and every attempt must be made to correct it before surgical intervention.

Vascular Anomalies

ANEURYSMS

Intracranial aneurysms are rare in the pediatric population, representing only 2 to 3 per cent of all aneurysms diagnosed.[58, 66, 68] The characteristics of these lesions can be quite different from those seen in the adult population. The solitary saccular aneurysm without identifiable cause is seen in childhood, but up to 55 per cent of pediatric patients with aneurysms have an underlying disorder or unusual characteristic associated with the aneurysm formation.[37] Giant, mycotic, and traumatic aneurysms account for a much higher proportion of childhood aneurysms than do those that present in adulthood.

The clinical presentation of most childhood aneurysms is that of subarachnoid hemorrhage, as it is in adults. However, giant aneurysms typically present with neurocompressive symptoms; only 35 per cent of giant aneurysms present with subarachnoid hemorrhage.[36, 39] Compared with adults, pediatric patients with aneurysmal subarachnoid hemorrhage tend to have higher Hunt-Hess grades on presentation. Primarily because of the unique characteristics of aneurysms that arise in the pediatric age group, alternative techniques that are not often required in adults must be employed in some situations.

Saccular Aneurysms

Characteristics

In children, saccular or berry aneurysms most closely approximate the aneurysmal disease that is seen in adults. However, several features serve to distinguish pediatric saccular aneurysms from those of their adult counterparts. The gender, the topography, associated systemic diseases, and possibly the cause all differ between the two age groups.

Although females predominate in adult series, particularly in aneurysmal disease located on the internal carotid artery, the reverse is true in children.[37, 65] Male predominance is most evident in the patients with berry aneurysms. This is partly because of the higher proportion of males affected by those diseases associated with saccular aneurysm formation. In a series of 20 patients with coarctation of the aorta and an intracranial aneurysm, 80 per cent were males.[37]

The location of saccular aneurysms differs in infants and children compared with adults. Although internal carotid aneurysms are most frequently seen in both groups, bifurcation aneurysms account for almost half of occurrences in children.[37, 47] Other common locations in children are the middle cerebral and anterior communicating arteries. Posterior circulation aneurysms in pediatric patients account for a higher proportion of cases than they do in adults. Of these, however, most are giant aneurysms.[58]

The percentage of patients with multiple aneurysms is lower in children than it is in adults. In one study, multiple aneurysms were found in only 6.4 per cent of pediatric cases.[37] The most likely type of aneurysm in childhood to present with multiple lesions (20 per cent of cases) is that caused by infection.[37]

Although the cause of aneurysms in adults is thought to be degenerative, the pathogenesis in children is not so clear. Several findings support the contention that the etiological process is multifactorial. Disease processes that are associated with hypertension predispose to intracranial aneurysm formation. These include polycystic kidneys and coarctation of the aorta.[37, 69] Likewise, fibromuscular dysplasia, a disorder of both intima and media, predisposes to the development of intracranial aneurysms.[37, 69] Type III collagen deficiency has been identified in association with intracranial aneurysm formation and may prove to be important in childhood aneurysms.[64]

In addition to these diseases that predispose to aneurysms, the incidence of aneurysms is higher in the older child than in the infant, suggesting that time for formation may be essential for intracranial aneurysms. Although aneurysms have been reported in very young infants,[51] they are rare, and no convincing evidence exists to substantiate the congenital nature of aneurysms.[87] Hemodynamic factors are thought to be important in both pediatric and adult aneurysmal disease. This appears to be the most likely explanation for the formation of aneurysms associated with arteriovenous malformations or with moyamoya disease.[62, 64]

Management

The management of saccular aneurysms in most cases is similar in adults and in children. Because of the life expectancy of the child and the likelihood of aneurysm rupture, the rare aneurysm that presents before hemorrhage should be treated by clipping. The pediatric patient with a subarachnoid hemorrhage caused by a saccular aneurysm, however, is managed by early surgical treatment to prevent the risk of re-

bleeding. Fortunately, pediatric patients with aneurysmal subarachnoid hemorrhage appear to be at lower risk for vasospasm than their adult counterparts.[42, 46] Prognosis for the patient who presents with a grade I to grade III subarachnoid hemorrhage is good, whereas those who present comatose do poorly, as is the case with adults.[42]

Traumatic Aneurysms

Characteristics

Aneurysm formation after trauma is unusual, but it does account for 10 to 12 per cent of all pediatric aneurysms.[19, 42] The type of trauma necessary to produce an intracranial aneurysm is varied; closed head injuries with or without skull fracture and, more commonly, penetrating injuries account for most cases. The topographical distribution of traumatic aneurysms lends some insight as to their formation. The anterior cerebral artery and middle cerebral artery, often distally, are the most common sites for traumatic aneurysms. It is theorized that the edge of the falx injures the anterior cerebral artery in the setting of closed head injury, with resultant aneurysm formation, whereas superficial vessels are more susceptible in cases of penetrating injuries.[85, 86] Males outnumber females in traumatic aneurysms, as they do in most head injury series.

Aneurysm formation may be associated with an underlying head injury. Acute subdural, epidural, or intraparenchymal hemorrhages are commonly present. If the arterial injury is not appreciated at the time of surgical evacuation of the intracranial clot (if performed), then an aneurysm may subsequently develop. The average time from traumatic event to diagnosis of an aneurysm is 14 to 21 days.[6, 8]

The presentation is varied and is related both to the extent of the associated injury and to the location. Subarachnoid hemorrhage occurs in almost half of patients, but frequently traumatic aneurysms are found incidentally. Traumatic aneurysms may be identified during surgical evacuation of an intraparenchymal hematoma or, in severe cases of head injury, at autopsy. Presentations unique to aneurysms of the cavernous segment of the carotid artery are epistaxis, proptosis, chemosis, and ophthalmoplegia caused by a carotid cavernous fistula. Overall, the best prognostic indicator for patients with traumatic aneurysms is the extent of the underlying brain injury.

Management

Although case reports documenting spontaneous resolution of traumatic aneurysms exist, this course is distinctly unusual.[8, 80] Of the patients who survive their brain injury, aneurysmal rupture is likely if no intervention is undertaken. Therefore, an angiogram should be performed in any case of delayed hemorrhage after penetrating or closed head trauma. Likewise, treatment should be instituted early after the diagnosis has been established.

Because most traumatic aneurysms are located peripherally, surgical obliteration is the preferred treatment. Most traumatic aneurysms are actually pseudoaneurysms, the wall being composed of fibrous, reactive tissue. In these cases, clipping of the neck often can not be achieved. Rather, removal of the aneurysmal portion of the vessel effectively cures these lesions.

Because laceration of the vessel wall is the most common finding, arterial repair can sometimes be achieved while vessel patency is maintained,[86] although this is not invariably the case. If obliteration is required, the need for augmentation of blood flow in the distribution of the parent vessel must be determined.

The authors recently encountered a situation in which blood flow augmentation was deemed necessary because of the proximal nature of the vessel injury. A 12-year-old patient sustained a BB gunshot wound to the head with resultant intracerebral and predominant subarachnoid hemorrhage (Fig. 51–3). Because there was a preponderance of subarachnoid blood located in the basilar cisterns and extending into the right sylvian fissure, a traumatic aneurysm was suspected. The arteriogram verified the presence of a proximal middle cerebral artery aneurysm. At operation, the middle cerebral artery had essentially been transected, precluding primary repair. The patient was treated with clipping of the middle cerebral artery and a superficial bypass from the temporal to the middle cerebral artery (see Fig. 51–3).

The treatment of intracavernous traumatic aneurysms is approached similarly to treatment of carotid cavernous fistulae without associated aneurysms. Endovascular obliteration of the aneurysm is the therapeutic goal. This result is best achieved through the use of detachable balloons (Fig. 51–4).

The outcome is good when surgical or endovascular treatments are used for traumatic aneurysms. Neurological recovery typically depends on the nature of the initial trauma and recovery from that event, but it is clearly worsened if a delayed hemorrhage from an undiagnosed traumatic aneurysm occurs.

Mycotic Aneurysms

Characteristics

Mycotic or infectious aneurysms are most commonly caused by a bacterial infection and only occasionally by a fungal infection, and they account for 2.5 to 10 per cent of pediatric aneurysms.[37] These lesions occur equally among boys and girls and are most commonly associated with bacterial endocarditis. Because of its rate of blood flow, the middle cerebral artery is most commonly affected, being the site of aneurysm formation in up to 60 per cent of cases.[14, 37] Other than by embolus, mycotic aneurysms occasionally arise as a result of direct extension of an infection, such as with intracavernous aneurysms associated with cavernous sinus thrombophlebitis. Subarachnoid hemorrhage is the mode of presentation in 91 per cent of cases.[37] In addition, mycotic aneurysms are multiple in 20 per cent of cases.[5, 11, 28]

As in cases of infective endocarditis, alpha- and beta-hemolytic Streptococci and *Staphylococcus aureus* predominate.[5, 11] Regardless of whether surgical obliteration of the aneurysm is undertaken early, antibiotic treatment remains an essential component of therapy. Also, on occasion, surgical treatment of the valvular lesion is required; this must be considered when the therapy for mycotic aneurysms is planned.

Management

Historically, mycotic aneurysms have been managed primarily with long-term antibiotic therapy. However, mortality has been reported to be as high as 90 per cent with this treatment if the aneurysm has ruptured.[15, 21] Despite this, treatment with antibiotics alone or surgery plus antibiotic therapy has been advocated, but patient selection for nonsurgical management remains controversial.[5, 10, 14, 21] Bingham recommends initially treating patients with antibiotics plus serial angiography. He does advise surgical treatment for those patients with documented enlargement of the aneurysm while on therapy or the persistence of an aneurysm after 6 weeks of antibiotic treatment.[10] Conversely, Frazee and colleagues support early surgical intervention for mycotic aneurysms. They reviewed 13 patients; the 5 treated surgically all survived, but 6 of 8 treated with antibiotics alone died.[28] Still others advocate early treatment of all peripherally located aneurysms but antibiotic therapy initially for proximal, more difficult aneurysms.[21] The authors agree with this approach and advocate surgical intervention for any patient who demonstrates aneurysm enlargement during antibiotic treatment or persistence after treatment. Unfortunately, most mycotic aneurysms are not diagnosed until they have hemorrhaged and therefore have shown their propensity to bleed.

Because of the friable and fusiform nature of mycotic aneurysms, clipping of these lesions is usually not possible. Rather, excision of the aneurysm and debridement of surrounding reactive tissue or abscess is required. This is readily achieved with peripheral cerebral vessels and is well tolerated by the pediatric patient. However, in more proximal lesions, in which vessel patency is essential, aneurysm excision may need to be supplemented by an extracranial-intracranial bypass.[22, 38]

Cavernous sinus mycotic aneurysms, typically caused by adjacent cavernous sinus thrombophlebitis, are different from the more common peripheral aneurysms secondary to septic embolus. These lesions rarely produce catastrophic subarachnoid hemorrhage but rather can produce symptoms of neurocompression or carotid cavernous syndrome or fistula. Intracavernous aneurysms can be managed with antibiotic treatment alone. If ophthalmoplegia persists or aneurysmal enlargement on therapy is observed, then endovascular treatment should be initiated. Using detachable balloons, exclusion of the aneurysm from the parent vessel with maintenance of internal carotid patency may be possible. Not infrequently, internal carotid occlusion is required, but this is usually well tolerated in the pediatric population.

Occasionally a situation arises, peculiar to this dis-

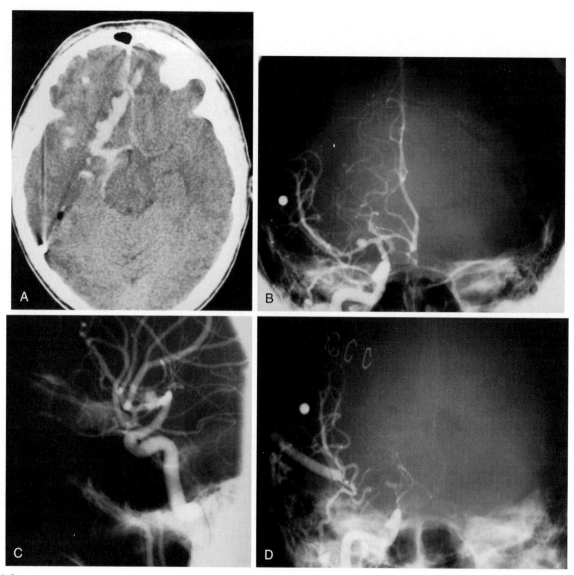

Figure 51–3

A. A nonenhanced computed tomography scan depicts the trajectory of a BB with subarachnoid blood in its path. Also note the subarachnoid blood layering in the right sylvian fissure and basilar cisterns. *B* and *C.* Anteroposterior and oblique arteriograms reveal a proximal right middle cerebral artery traumatic aneurysm. Note that this aneurysm does not have a well-defined neck. *D.* This postoperative anteroposterior arteriogram, common carotid injection, demonstrates good flow through the superficial temporal artery filling the distal middle cerebral artery branches. (Courtesy of Arthur Day, M.D.)

ease, in which both cardiac surgery for valvular replacement and intracranial surgery are required. In addition to the anticoagulation necessary to perform the cardiac surgery, patients frequently require long-term anticoagulation. Morawetz and Karp, however, do not believe that the anticoagulation with cardiac bypass is associated with a higher incidence of intracranial hemorrhage in this setting. They point out that removing the septic focus and improving cardiac function take precedence and therefore should be performed first.[61]

Giant Aneurysms

Characteristics

"Giant" aneurysms may be defined as all aneurysms greater than 2.5 cm in diameter. They can be fusiform or saccular; in pediatric cases, 24 per cent are fusiform in shape.[70] Giant aneurysms account for 20 per cent of all aneurysms seen in childhood[36, 37] and present a challenge to the pediatric cerebrovascular surgeon.

A high percentage (45 to 50 per cent) of giant aneurysms are found in the posterior circulation, with basilar artery aneurysms making up one half of this group.[37, 58] Of the anterior circulation giant aneurysms, the internal carotid artery is the vessel most commonly involved. Among the internal carotid artery aneurysms, a strong predilection for the cavernous segment exists.

Because of the large size of these lesions, they often present with focal neurological deficit secondary to mass effect. Some 57 to 64 per cent of initial symptoms are from neural compression.[37, 70] In contrast to the 90 per cent rate of subarachnoid hemorrhage for all

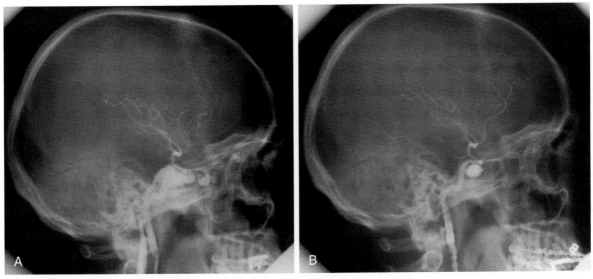

Figure 51–4

A carotid cavernous fistula developed in this 14-year-old after trauma. *A.* A lateral arteriogram, internal carotid artery injection, reveals rapid flow into the cavernous sinus from the cavernous segment of the carotid artery. Also note filling of the ophthalmic veins. *B.* A lateral arteriogram after endovascular balloon occlusion of this lesion demonstrates patency of the internal carotid artery with a balloon located in the cavernous sinus.

aneurysm types, giant aneurysms bleed only in 35 per cent of cases.[37, 70] These two presentations are seen in almost all of the giant aneurysms of childhood, but hydrocephalus is not an uncommon associated finding.

Giant aneurysms represent a type of lesion with which infectious or traumatic causes (possibly unrecognized or forgotten) may be associated. In addition, presentation in infancy represents 20 per cent of pediatric giant aneurysms.[19] Most infant patients with giant aneurysms do suffer from a subarachnoid hemorrhage; in contrast, in the older child, aneurysms are most commonly diagnosed after signs from neural compression are recognized.

Management

The fact that multiple surgical procedures are applied to giant aneurysms both in adults and in children underscores the need to approach these lesions on an individualized basis. The principal goal of surgery remains to prevent hemorrhage or rehemorrhage. However, because of the frequent signs of neural compression associated with giant aneurysm, decompression and exclusion of the aneurysm from the circulation are often required. The treatment options are clipping, trapping, proximal vessel occlusion, excision or occlusion with a bypass, and wrapping.

Primary clipping achieves exclusion of the aneurysm from the parent vessel while maintaining patency of the parent vessel, and it is the treatment of choice if it is applicable. This approach not infrequently can be used to treat anterior circulation and basilar apex aneurysms. Hypothermic cardiac standstill, however, may be a necessary adjunct, particularly with basilar apex aneurysms. In addition, as detailed by Sundt and colleagues, leaving a small cuff at the base of the aneurysm is sometimes required; because of the thick-

walled nature of these giant aneurysms, the risk of hemorrhage is very low.[89] After successful clipping, opening of the aneurysm and thrombectomy are required to alleviate neural compressive symptoms.

Trapping or proximal occlusion can frequently be applied to proximal internal carotid artery and vertebral artery aneurysms. Children typically tolerate internal carotid artery occlusion well.[91] Performing the internal carotid artery occlusion through percutaneous transluminal placement of balloons allows for a neurological examination during a trial occlusion. In addition, single photon emission computed tomography has been shown to be useful in evaluation of the adequacy of collateral cerebral blood flow when an extracranial-intracranial bypass is considered.[12] As with the internal carotid artery, vertebral artery occlusion usually can be undertaken in the child without neurological deficit. In both cases, however, if significant mass effect exists from the aneurysm, the patient may be better served by a trapping procedure with thrombectomy. Also, if excellent cross-filling of the contralateral vertebral artery is present, proximal occlusion may not successfully affect aneurysm thrombosis.

The authors treated a 10-year-old boy with a giant left vertebral artery aneurysm (Fig. 51–5). This patient had both mass effect from the aneurysm and excellent cross-filling. Intraoperative arteriography demonstrated persistent filling of the aneurysm from the right vertebral artery despite proximal vertebral artery clipping. This patient recovered nicely from a trapping procedure.

Most of the cases of giant aneurysm in children can be successfully managed with one of these procedures. If the child does not have adequate collateral flow with parent vessel ligation, then an extracranial-intracranial bypass should be planned to augment blood flow. Wrapping is reserved for the patient whose aneurysm

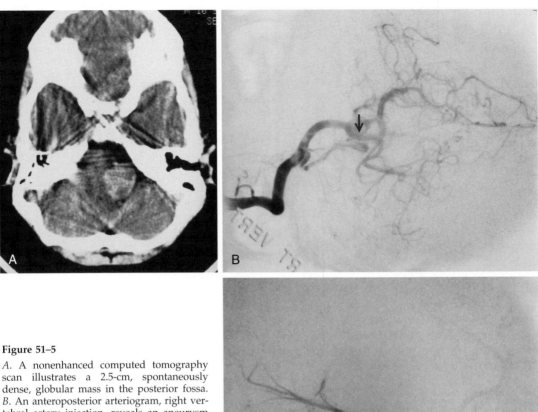

Figure 51–5

A. A nonenhanced computed tomography scan illustrates a 2.5-cm, spontaneously dense, globular mass in the posterior fossa. *B.* An anteroposterior arteriogram, right vertebral artery injection, reveals an aneurysm located at the left vertebrobasilar junction *(arrow)*. *C.* A lateral arteriogram, left vertebral artery injection, demonstrates the fusiform nature of this aneurysm and its proximal extension, which begins just distal to the origin of the posterior inferior cerebellar artery. (Courtesy of Arthur Day, M.D.)

cannot be excluded from the circulation by any other means.

ARTERIOVENOUS MALFORMATIONS

A variety of congenital arteriovenous malformations occur in childhood and come to the attention of the pediatric neurosurgeon because of an acute hemorrhage, a seizure, a mass effect, or as an incidental finding. The group of lesions known as arteriovenous malformations actually comprises the classic arteriovenous malformation, the cavernous malformation, the venous angioma, and the capillary telangiectasia. Transitional forms with features of two of these types have also been described.[55]

Vascular malformations represent the most common cause of spontaneous intracranial hemorrhage in children.[13, 81] Arteriovenous malformations in children younger than 15 years of age are about four times more frequent as a cause of subarachnoid hemorrhage than are aneurysms.[30] The rate of hemorrhage in the pediatric population for the classical arteriovenous malformation has been estimated to be 1 per 100,000 children per year.[46, 81] Although in autopsy series venous angiomas are the most common vascular malformation discovered, followed by the capillary telangiectasias,[55] the less common arteriovenous malformation and cavernous malformation are by far the more clinically important lesions.

All of the vascular malformations result from an abnormal development of the cerebral vasculature. They may remain silent throughout life, as is true of capillary telangiectasias, or become clinically apparent any time from infancy through adulthood. With modern imaging techniques being used much more commonly, the rate of diagnosis of these lesions in childhood will undoubtedly continue to increase.

Characteristics

Arteriovenous malformations are typically tightly coiled vessels that are maldeveloped without the normal intervening capillary bed.[54, 88] A high-flow system results in enlarged, tortuous, often multiple arterial feeders and dilated venous drainage. Intervening parenchyma may be found with these lesions but is characteristically gliottic. Arterial aneurysms, usually considered "flow-related," and thin-walled venous aneurysms may be found in relation to arteriovenous malformations.

The arteriovenous malformations diagnosed in children are similar to those seen in adults. However, a maturing process or evolution of these vascular malformations is possible. Luessenhop commented that such malformations in young children may not demonstrate the enlarged, high-flow arterial feeder or engorged venous drainage but consist only of an abnormal arteriovenous connection.[51] This "fluffy" or diffuse vascular malformation may represent an early stage of development (Fig. 51–6).

The natural history of arteriovenous malformations suggests that, if they are left untreated in the long life expectancy of a child, there is a high risk of hemorrhage. The rate of bleeding for an unruptured malformation has been estimated to be about 2 per cent per year.[34, 63, 90] The incidence of hemorrhage in ruptured malformations is about 6 to 7 per cent in the first year after the bleed and then 2 to 3 per cent per year thereafter.[31, 34] However, there is a progressive increase in mortality with each hemorrhage.

Besides subarachnoid or intraparenchymal hemorrhage, arteriovenous malformations may present with seizures, headache, or progressive neurological deficit. Drake suggested that small malformations tend to present with hemorrhage, whereas large ones are less likely to hemorrhage.[26] Large malformations typically are diagnosed after seizures or progressive neurological deficit have occurred.

Management

The natural history of arteriovenous malformations dictates that the pediatric neurosurgeon should offer

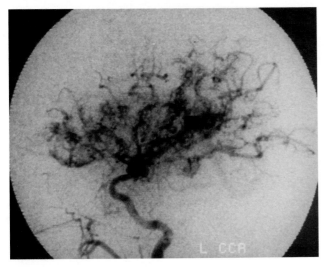

Figure 51–6

A lateral arteriogram, left common carotid artery injection, illustrates a huge arteriovenous malformation that involves essentially the entire left hemisphere. Also note the "fluffy" nature of this lesion, which may represent an immature stage in its formation.

some form of treatment in most of these cases. Whether the malformation is diagnosed before or after hemorrhage, the potential exists for devastating sequelae. Treatment options are similar for adults and children. Microsurgical resection, endovascular embolization, and radiosurgical treatment are the primary therapies. An extensive radiological evaluation of the malformation should be performed before selecting the appropriate treatment regimen.

Computed tomography is the initial study of choice in the child who has suffered an ictal event. The location and extent of the hemorrhage and the ventricular size can all be assessed. It is not uncommon for the hemorrhage to rupture into the ventricles, with attendant acute hydrocephalus. In such a situation, a ventriculostomy may be indicated before arteriography is performed. Most patients with subarachnoid or intraparenchymal hemorrhage from an arteriovenous malformation do not require emergent surgery except possibly for placement of a ventricular drain. Most surgeons advocate delayed surgery to allow for the cerebral edema to subside, thereby making the resection easier and safer. The authors recommend proceeding with surgery as soon as the patient shows clinical improvement, typically in about a week, because the child remains at risk of rehemorrhage, although less so than after aneurysmal subarachnoid hemorrhage.

Four-vessel angiography is required and should be coordinated with a neuroradiologist so that embolization may also be undertaken. Preoperative embolization has been shown to decrease blood loss and make extirpation of the malformation easier and less time-consuming.[23] It is unusual for embolization to cure intracranial lesions, but markedly decreased flow in the nidus greatly facilitates surgical resection. Because embolization changes the flow characteristics of the malformation in the context of an already perturbed state of autoregulation, the child may be at increased risk of hemorrhage after embolization. Handa and colleagues showed that the pressure in the arterial feeder increases after embolization.[39] For these reasons, surgical or radiosurgical treatment should follow embolization. The size, shape, location, and hemorrhage status all help determine the best mode of therapy.

The authors treated a 7-year-old boy with a combined treatment regimen after he suffered a subarachnoid hemorrhage from a malformation in the corpus callosal region (Fig. 51–7). This case demonstrated the multimodality therapy needed in some of these lesions. The lesion extended from the rostrum to the splenium and probably was too long to be treated by radiosurgery alone. In addition, after a recent hemorrhage, direct surgical resection is preferable to radiosurgery. This patient was, therefore, treated with preoperative embolization using polyvinyl alcohol and silk, followed by surgical excision through a transcallosal approach. Figure 51–7 demonstrates that the most posterior aspect of the malformation remained. Intraoperative angiography possibly would have permitted total excision, but it was not available at the time of this patient's surgery. Because subtotal resection does not decrease the risk of hemorrhage, this patient required

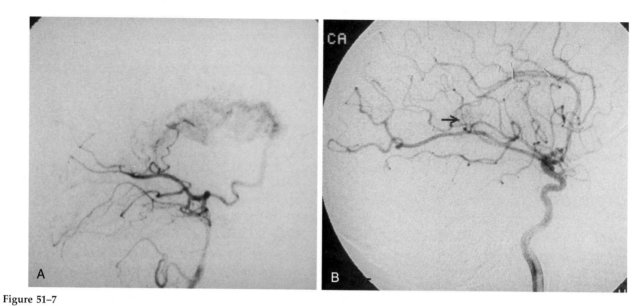

Figure 51–7

A. A lateral arteriogram, left vertebral artery injection, shows a large arteriovenous malformation outlining the corpus callosum. Note the multiple feeders to this lesion. *B.* Postoperative lateral arteriogram, right internal carotid artery injection, demonstrates almost total resection of the malformation. However, the most posterior aspect of the malformation fills, as illustrated by a diffuse vascular blush *(arrow).*

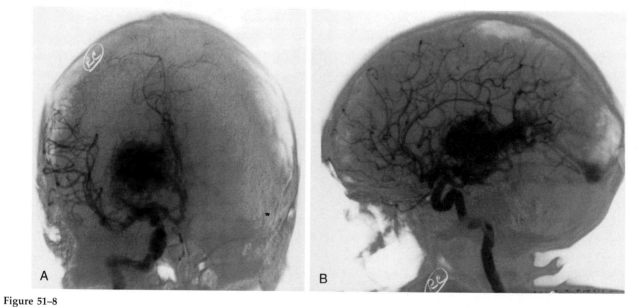

Figure 51–8

A and *B.* Anteroposterior and lateral arteriograms, right internal carotid artery injection, illustrate a large, right thalamic arteriovenous malformation. This lesion was treated with endovascular embolization followed by radiosurgery. However, several months after radiosurgery, the patient suffered a subarachnoid hemorrhage. (Courtesy of William Friedman, M.D.)

further treatment. Owing to its small size and deep location, the residual malformation was treated with stereotactic radiosurgery (see Fig. 51–7).

Stereotactic radiosurgery has been used extensively in cases of arteriovenous malformations in adults, and it has also been shown to be safe and effective in such cases in children. Yamamoto and colleagues reported no radiation-associated side effects and two-thirds complete obliteration rate in a pediatric series.[96] Complete thrombosis, and therefore protection from hemorrhage, typically takes 2 years to occur (Fig. 51–8). Friedman and Bova reported an 81 per cent 2-year occlusion rate in a large adult series.[29] Stereotactic radiosurgery is an excellent form of treatment for deep-seated lesions such as brain stem malformations (Fig. 51–9).

For almost all lobar malformations, preoperative embolization with surgical excision remains the treatment of choice, as it effectively cures these lesions with a low morbidity. Rarely, malformations can become massive, involving the majority of a hemisphere (see Fig. 51–6). Unfortunately, no good treatment options exist for

management of these lesions, aside from embolization and perhaps hemispherectomy.

Cavernous Malformations

Characteristics

Cavernous malformations, or cavernous angiomas, typically present in early adulthood but may be found in children. Because of the widespread use of magnetic resonance imaging and computed tomography, these angiomas are being diagnosed with increased frequency in all age groups.[76] Cavernous malformations account for 5 to 13 per cent of vascular malformations in clinical series.[84] These lesions typically occur sporadically and are usually solitary, but they may be multiple. Familial occurrences, however, have been reported.[9, 40]

Pathologically, cavernous malformations are composed of sinusoidal vessels that are compact and discrete from the surrounding brain.[55] No intervening brain tissue is present, and hemosiderin-stained paren-

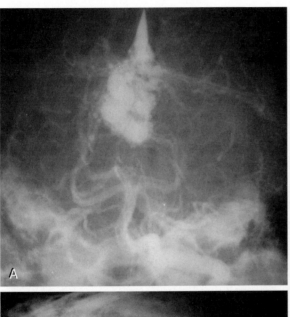

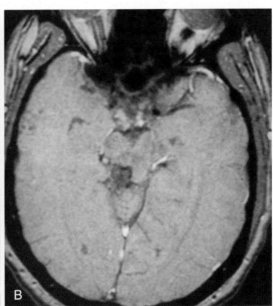

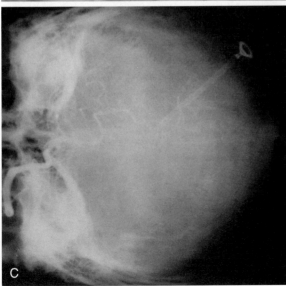

Figure 51–9

A. A left vertebral arteriogram, anteroposterior view, depicts an arteriovenous malformation fed primarily by the superior cerebellar arteries in a 17-year-old patient. Note the large, dilated venous structures visualized on this arterial phase. *B.* A T1-weighted magnetic resonance image was obtained 2 years after radiosurgery of this arteriovenous malformation. This study shows no filling of the malformation but apparent thrombosis. *C.* An anteroposterior vertebral arteriogram verifies its complete obliteration. (Courtesy of William Friedman, M.D.)

chyma surrounds the lesion. Almost all cavernous malformations show pathological evidence of previous hemorrhage.[84] Cavernous angiomas tend to hemorrhage, but symptomatic hemorrhage is not common and probably accounts for fewer than 15 per cent of cases.[27] Seizures are the most common presenting symptom in most patients and in the remaining patients present with a neurological deficit or headaches or as an incidental finding.

An increasing number of cavernous malformations are being diagnosed, and their radiographic characteristics have been well defined.[35] Their appearance on computed tomography is fairly characteristic. The cavernous angioma is typically hyperdense and discrete and has only slight contrast enhancement (Fig. 51–10). Although they are evident on computed tomography, magnetic resonance imaging better displays the surrounding hemosiderin deposition that is characteristic of these lesions. The hemosiderin is seen as low signal density around the high signal density of the angioma.[35] Angiographically, cavernous malformations do not fill because they lack arterial feeders. This fact places cavernous malformations in the differential diagnosis of angiographically occult arteriovenous malformations. Cavernous malformations account for approximately one third of angiographically occult arteriovenous malformations in children.[27]

Management

The exact risk of clinically symptomatic hemorrhage of cavernous malformations is not known. Because of this uncertainty and the relatively good seizure control achieved with excision, surgical treatment should be recommended for most patients with these lesions. Radiosurgical treatment is not indicated for cavernous

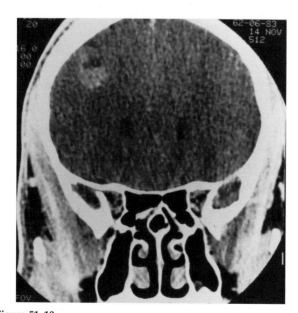

Figure 51–10

A reformatted computed tomography scan, coronal section, shows a spontaneously dense, fairly well-circumscribed lesion in the right frontal lobe. This appearance is fairly characteristic of a cavernous angioma.

angiomas at this time. Supratentorial cavernous malformations are almost always surgically accessible. The surrounding hemosiderin-stained, gliottic tissue allows the surgeon to readily develop a plane surrounding the angioma, permitting complete extirpation. Surgical excision typically cures cavernous malformations, although recurrence has been reported.[50] If cavernous angiomas are located in the brain stem, they may be more difficult to remove. Frequently, however, the lesion projects to a pial surface; this allows safer resection.

Venous Angiomas

Venous angiomas represent by far the most common vascular malformation found in autopsy specimens.[17, 55, 56] This malformation is composed entirely of anomalous veins without arterial or capillary contributions. In addition, venous angiomas drain normal brain and contain intervening areas of normal brain.

It is unclear what symptoms, if any, are caused by venous angiomas. They are frequently diagnosed during evaluation of headaches or unrelated minor trauma. The natural history of these angiomas is thought to be benign. However, hemorrhage has been reported with venous angiomas, particularly if they are located in the posterior fossa.[79]

Because excision of venous angiomas may produce venous infarction, they should be managed nonoperatively.[77] In the unusual circumstance in which a hemorrhage is caused by a venous angioma, surgical excision may be considered.

Capillary Telangiectasia

The capillary telangiectasia is of much greater interest to the pathologist than to the neurosurgeon. These lesions are common in autopsy series but rarely are clinically relevant.[55] Pathologically, telangiectasias are formed of dilated capillaries with normal intervening parenchyma.[55, 56] Most commonly found in the pons, they also may be located in the cerebral hemispheres. These lesions may be multiple, as in the Osler-Weber-Rendu syndrome.

The capillary telangiectasia is not visualized on angiography but may be visualized by magnetic resonance imaging and labeled an occult malformation.[35] Although this malformation rarely causes hemorrhage, it has been reported as the pathological entity responsible for a brain stem hematoma in a 3-year-old patient.[27] No treatment is indicated for the incidental finding of a capillary telangiectasia.

DURAL ARTERIOVENOUS MALFORMATIONS

Dural arteriovenous malformations are rare in childhood, but if clinically apparent, the presentation tends to be during infancy. The dural malformation that occurs in adulthood is thought to be acquired after a region within a sinus becomes thrombosed with subsequent recanalization and fistula formation.[18] In children, the dural lesions may occasionally be congenital, resulting from the persistence of an abnormal arteriovenous connection within the dura mater.[1] Most, however, are probably acquired, particularly those that present later in life.

These lesions are of the high-flow type and typically are supplied by branches of the external carotid, vertebral, and internal carotid arteries. Dural malformations can involve any of the major venous sinuses and most commonly drain into the transverse sinus, the sagittal sinus, or the torcula. They have, in addition, been described as multifocal, with shunts located in the sphenoparietal sinus, cavernous sinus, petrosal sinus, and posterior fossa dural sleeves.[32] Some also drain transcortically and then probably carry a risk of subarachnoid hemorrhage similar to that for pial arteriovenous malformations.

Because of the high-flow nature of these lesions, the infant typically presents with cardiac failure but may also develop hydrocephalus, neurological deficits, or intracranial hemorrhage.[78] The presentation in the neonate, in particular, represents a formidable challenge to the pediatric neurosurgeon. The heart failure experienced by these neonates is resistant to medical therapy, and unless an aggressive approach is taken to eliminate or reduce the shunt, the child will die from high-output cardiac failure.

A neonate with cardiac failure was treated at the authors' institution. Because of the presence of a cranial bruit, the diagnosis of a dural arteriovenous malformation was made. As is common in the neonate, the shunt was located posteriorly (Fig. 51–11). It was elected to treat this lesion with endovascular embolization using a combination of coils, polyvinyl alcohol, and silk; this proved successful in eradicating the malformation. The patient did not require multiple embolizations, which is not uncommon for these lesions. More complex lesions are usually not successfully treated with emboli-

zation alone; in this situation, staged embolization followed by surgical resection of the involved segment of sinus is required.

The prognosis for dural arteriovenous malformations of childhood is poor if the heart failure is not cured by treating the shunt. A good outcome can be expected, however, with the smaller lesions and in those patients who experience resolution of the heart failure after treatment.

VEIN OF GALEN MALFORMATIONS

The direct surgical approach to vein of Galen malformations has been almost totally supplanted by the newer transvenous and transarterial interventional technologies. The extremely dangerous type II lesions and true arteriovenous malformations in and around the brain stem with egress through an enlarged vein of Galen defy surgical intervention (Fig. 51–12). In the type I lesions involving one or two feeders directly into a dilated vein of Galen, interventional technologies are so much simpler than the direct surgical approach that neurosurgery is reserved principally for access and for the treatment of hydrocephalus. If the microneurosurgical approach to vein of Galen malformations is required, this can be accomplished through a standard craniotomy using a supratentorial paraoccipital approach.

The vein of Galen malformations are conveniently categorized into age-dependent groups: neonate, infant, and older child.[60] The neonate symptomatic with a vein of Galen malformation has high-output heart failure, which becomes apparent very early, often 1 to 2 hours after birth. Transvaginal ultrasound is very helpful in defining these lesions prenatally.[48] Those patients with prenatal cardiomegaly have a much worse prognosis. The babies are born with very hyperactive precordia; a pan–cardiac cycle bruit involving the chest,

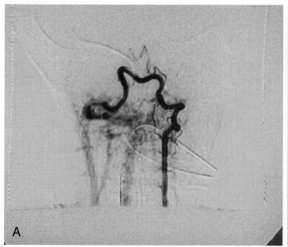
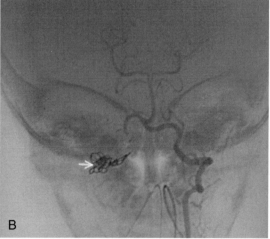

Figure 51–11

A. A left vertebral arteriogram, anteroposterior view, depicts a posterior fossa, dura-based arteriovenous malformation. This lesion is primarily a fistula and does not have multiple arterial feeders. *B.* A post-therapy vertebral arteriogram, anteroposterior view, demonstrates the complete obliteration of the malformation. Note the visualization of coils *(arrow)* that were placed during endovascular treatment.

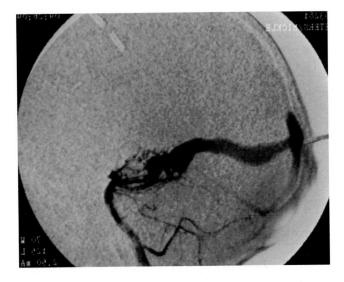

Figure 51–12

A lateral arteriogram, vertebral artery injection, shows a type II vein of Galen malformation. Note the multiple arterial feeders as well as a dilated vein of Galen.

neck, and head; and an enlarged liver and spleen—all signs and symptoms of progressive heart failure. These symptoms are resistant to standard medical therapies but respond quickly to adequate interruption of the fistula's flow, either interventionally or surgically. The neonate can have intracranial hemorrhage as well as hydrocephalus, and virtually all patients have compensated heart failure. The infant harboring a vein of Galen malformation has a lesion with higher resistance and therefore relatively lower flow than that of the neonate. Such a child usually has a mildly enlarged heart, an enlarged head, and moderate ventriculomegaly. Older children and young adults can present with progressive neurological deficits, subarachnoid hemorrhage, hydrocephalus, or mass effect.[2] Although these groups are relatively well defined, these lesions represent a continuum of compensated and uncompensated cardiac failure.

It is believed that the vein of Galen malformations represent a high-flow fistulous state that tends to be progressive even in its most benign forms. The asymptomatic lesion should be observed expectantly, because the true natural history of these lesions is not known. These lesions should be investigated early with angiography, especially in the neonate. This can be accomplished through an indwelling umbilical artery catheter, which also permits transarterial embolization, if necessary.

The transvenous approach to the malformation should be applied early in the therapy of the neonate to measure pressures and flow and to deposit an indwelling wire basket onto which future therapies can be designed.[59, 60] The transvenous approach can be accomplished either transtorcularly, directly with craniotomy, or transfemorally. In the neonate, it is essential to reduce the flow in the fistula substantially with a transvenous or transarterial approach to effect a cardiac survivor (Fig. 51–13). This may require two to four treatments during the first several days of life. All depositions of wires must be done extremely carefully because the most ventral part of the malformation is paper-thin. Any forcing of a wire can produce perfora-

tion of the complex with hemorrhage. After the flow has been substantially reduced with this therapy, cardiac failure rapidly resolves. All patients with hydrocephalus must receive a ventriculoperitoneal shunt early in therapy. The shunting procedure must be done carefully because many of the subependymal veins are dilated as a result of the abnormal flow patterns around the vein of Galen complex.

The infant, older child, and young adult are treated in a similar fashion, but somewhat less aggressively, in order to reduce the major risk to this procedure, which is venous outlet occlusion with thrombosis and hemorrhage (Fig. 51–14). Results with these therapies in 40 cases are shown in Tables 51–5 and 51–6.

MOYAMOYA DISEASE

Moyamoya disease is discussed in Chapter 49.

STURGE-WEBER SYNDROME

The Sturge-Weber syndrome is a rare cerebrovascular disease that may come to the physician's attention in infancy or childhood as a result of mental impairment and epilepsy that is often medically intractable. Also known as encephalotrigeminal angiomatosis, this syndrome is characterized by a facial nevus flammeus and extensive angiomatous changes involving the leptomeninges, the dura, and the vessels of the gray and white matter.[24] The pediatric neurosurgeon greatly improves the prognosis of this disease by performing a hemispheric resection on the appropriately selected patient. This procedure has been shown to decrease or alleviate seizures and possibly improve intellectual capacity.[41, 44]

Pathogenesis

Sturge-Weber syndrome, classified with the neurocutaneous syndromes, is often recognized by its cutane-

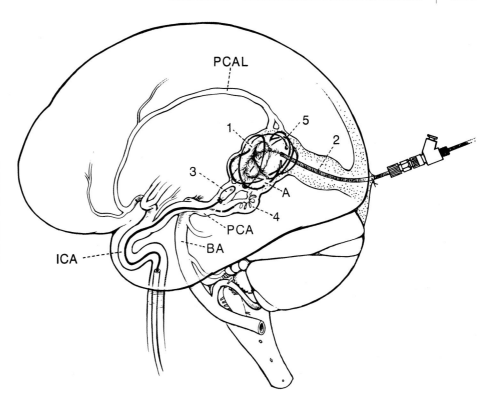

Figure 51–13

This semidiagram of a vein of Galen malformation depicts the various interventional treatment modalities available. ICA, internal carotid artery; BA, basilar artery; PCA, posterior cerebral artery; PCAL, pericallosal artery; A, aneurysm; 1, Gianturco coil; 2, short angiography catheter; 3, detachable balloon; 4, microcoil; 5, wire basket within vein of Galen aneurysm.

ous manifestations but becomes clinically important because of its cerebral vascular pathology. An abnormal development of the embryonal vasculature is probably responsible for the vascular malformation in this disease.[24] Angiomatous formation occurs in the pial and dural veins and capillaries overlying the cerebral cortex but spares the cerebral arteries. This hypervascularity is evident both grossly and microscopically.

The vascular malformation most commonly affects the parieto-occipital region but may also affect the frontal or temporal lobes. Unihemispheric involvement is most frequent, but in one series, bihemispheric lesions were identified in 14 per cent of cases.[7] Much of the interest in this syndrome stems from the roentgenographic findings of intracranial calcifications. These calcifications are located in the second and third layers of the cortex but also in the vessel wall, in the perivascular space, in the white matter, and, rarely, within the neuron.[79] Many authors have proposed that the deposition of calcium is a secondary phenomenon related to cerebral anoxic injuries.[69] However, others suggest that altered vascular permeability or a primary vascular factor is responsible. Di Trapani and colleagues found that a mucopolysaccharide provides a matrix for calcium deposition centered within the wall of the vessel, with progressive migration of the calcium deposits

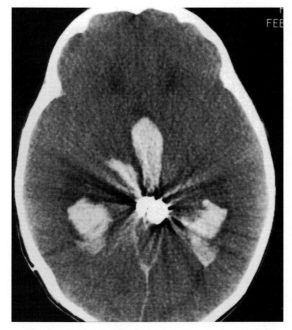

Figure 51–14

A neonate with a large vein of Galen malformation underwent transvenous occlusive therapy, which was complicated by hemorrhage. Nonenhanced computed tomography reveals extensive hemorrhage extending into the ventricular system. Note the coils in place in the vein of Galen.

Table 51–5

CASES OF VEIN OF GALEN MALFORMATIONS TREATED WITH TRANSVENOUS THERAPY AT THE UNIVERSITY OF FLORIDA, 1984–1992

Number of cases:	40
Number of neonates:	16
Infants/children:	24
Deaths:	10

Table 51–6

RESULTS WITH 40 CASES OF VEIN OF GALEN MALFORMATIONS

Died:	10 (8 neonates)
Cured:	21
Persistent fistula:	9

around the blood vessels.[25] In addition to the calcifications, extensive gliosis, atrophy, and loss of neurons may be found in the involved regions. The disease may be progressive and frequently correlated clinically with worsening intellectual development and poor seizure control.

Diagnosis and Clinical Course

The characteristic port-wine stain, which is evident at birth, usually involves the distribution of the first and second divisions of the trigeminal nerve to varying degrees, with nevus present in the supraorbital region being essential for diagnosis. The nevus is typically unilateral and corresponds to the side of angiomatosis, but it may extend bilaterally in 10 to 20 per cent of cases.[72] Although they are less common, variants have been described in which the leptomeningeal angiomatosis is present in the absence of facial nevus.[3, 72]

Focal or generalized seizures occur in 75 to 89 per cent of cases and are more likely and begin earlier in those patients with bilateral involvement.[7, 72] The onset of seizure activity usually begins in infancy but sometimes not until childhood. An earlier onset of seizures appears to be associated with a worse prognosis for mental development. Mental retardation can be severe, but it is not an invariable feature of this syndrome. Mental retardation is seen in more than half of patients with unilateral involvement and in up to 92 per cent of patients afflicted bihemispherically.[7] Other features of the disease, which are present in some but not all patients, include hemiparesis, buphthalmos, and homonymous hemianopsia.

The diagnosis is made based on clinical manifestations. However, radiological studies have helped characterize the extent of the cortical involvement. The characteristic tramline calcifications and asymmetric cranial vault are usually evident on skull x-ray films by the age of 20 but are rarely visible in early infancy. Computed tomography, particularly with the use of contrast medium, and magnetic resonance imaging have allowed evaluation of this disease at an early age (Fig. 51–15).

Angiography, which was often used before the advent of computed tomography, demonstrates a diffuse capillary "blush" and abnormal venous drainage. Surgical planning, however, can easily be achieved using neuroimaging and without angiography. Current imaging techniques permit the surgeon to evaluate the extent of the angiomatosis in the first years of life, when surgical intervention has been shown to have the most beneficial effect.

Management

The treatment goals in this syndrome are to minimize or eliminate seizures and to maximize intellectual

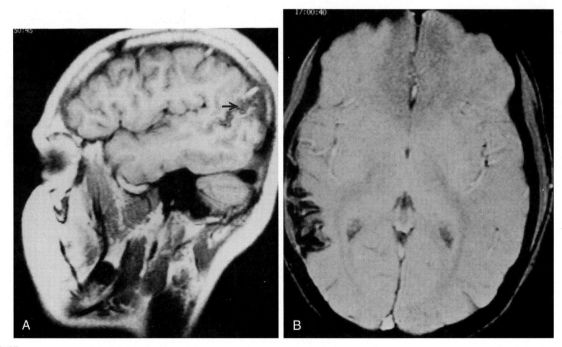

Figure 51–15

This 12-year-old boy with a focal seizure disorder was found to have Sturge-Weber disease. *A.* T1-weighted parasagittal section illustrates the angiomatous lesion in the parieto-occipital region *(arrow)*. *B.* T1-weighted spin echo axial section illustrates the serpentine nature of the angioma that extends into the sulci.

potential. Therefore, the patient with medically intractable seizures and the child at risk for mental deterioration should be selected for early surgical intervention. Surgical options for this disease include anatomical and functional hemispherectomy, localized cortical resection, and corpus callosotomy.

Several authors have proposed that if seizure onset occurs in early infancy, then progressive, severe mental retardation and worsening of seizures is likely.[41, 43] An infant with this type of presentation should undergo hemispherectomy before the age of 1 year for best results.

In the past, anatomical hemispherectomy has been carried out with excellent seizure control and good intellectual development.[41, 43, 44] Anatomical hemispherectomy is performed as an en bloc resection conforming to certain technical considerations. First, the bone flap should be fashioned to permit adequate midline as well as temporal exposure. Second, the middle and anterior cerebral arteries should be ligated at the bifurcation early in the procedure. Third, the ipsilateral choroid plexus should be removed up to the foramen of Monro, with the foramen being left patent. Last, the corpus callosum should be completely divided and the basal ganglia and thalamus left intact.

Operative morbidity and mortality are low if fluid management and blood replacement are carefully monitored. However, delayed complications of hydrocephalus and superficial cerebral hemosiderosis are not uncommon. In an effort to diminish these complications, Villemure and Rasmussen have advocated functional hemispherectomy instead of complete anatomical hemispherectomy.[94] Technically, the functional hemispherectomy differs in that the frontal and parieto-occipital regions are left intact but disconnected. All fibers going to the corpus callosum are divided. A large temporal lobectomy and resection of posterior frontal and anterior parietal cortex are also performed. Villemure and Rasmussen reported complete eradication of seizures in three infants with Sturge-Weber syndrome after functional hemispherectomy.[94]

Surgical decisions concerning the patient with onset of seizures in late infancy or childhood or with form fruste disease are more difficult; some of these patients may benefit from surgery. For example, anatomical or functional hemispherectomy offers the best results for the child with hemiplegia and uncontrollable epilepsy. However, in the patient without hemiplegia but with focal disease, as identified by intensive electroencephalographic monitoring and imaging studies, a cortical resection yields good results and less morbidity. Finally, for the patient with intractable generalized seizures and rare or controlled focal seizures, corpus callosotomy can decrease or eliminate that subtype of epilepsy.[73]

In summary, the best results in the management of Sturge-Weber syndrome have been obtained with hemispherectomy procedures. Treatment of children with later onset and less severe courses should be directed at treating the seizures with local cortical resection, if possible, and hemispherectomy should be reserved for the patient with extensive disease and hemiplegia.

REFERENCES

1. Albright, A. L., Latchaw, R. E., and Price, R. A.: Posterior dural arteriovenous malformation in infancy. J. Neurosurg., 13:129–135, 1983.
2. Amacher, A. L., and Shillito, J., Jr.: The syndromes and surgical treatment of aneurysms of the great vein of Galen. J. Neurosurg., 64:731–735, 1986.
3. Ambrosetto, P., Ambrosetto, G., Michelucci, R., et al.: Sturge-Weber syndrome without port-wine facial nerves: Report of two cases studied by CT. Child's Brain, 10:387–392, 1983.
4. Anderson, S. C., Shah, C. P., and Murtaugh, F. R.: Congested deep subcortical veins as a sign of dural venous sinus thrombosis: MR and CT correlation. J. Comput. Assist. Tomogr., 11:1059–1061, 1987.
5. Andrews, B. T., Hudgins, R. J., and Edwards, M. S. B.: Mycotic aneurysms in children. In Edwards, M. S. B., and Hoffman, H. J., eds.: Cerebral Vascular Diseases in Children and Adolescents. Baltimore, Williams & Wilkins, 1989, pp. 275–282.
6. Asari, S., Nakamura, S., Yamada, O., et al.: Traumatic aneurysms of peripheral cerebral arteries: Report of two cases. J. Neurosurg., 46:795–803, 1977.
7. Bebin, E. M., and Gomez, M. R.: Prognosis in Sturge-Weber disease: Comparison of unihemispheric and bihemispheric involvement. J. Child. Neurol., 3:181–184, 1988.
8. Benoit, B. G., and Wortzman, G.: Traumatic cerebral aneurysm: Clinical features and natural history. J. Neurol. Neurosurg. Psychiatry, 36:127–138, 1973.
9. Bicknell, J. M., Carlow, T. J., Kornfield, M., et al.: Familial cavernous angiomas. Arch. Neurol., 35:746–749, 1978.
10. Bingham, W. F.: Treatment of mycotic intracranial aneurysms. J. Neurosurg., 46:428–437, 1977.
11. Bohmfalk, G. L., Story, J. L., Wissinger, J. P., et al.: Bacterial intracranial aneurysm. J. Neurosurg., 48:369–382, 1978.
12. Boyko, O. B., Rark, H. M., Edwards, M. K., et al.: I-123 HIPDM SPECT imaging and cerebral angiography for EC-IC bypass evaluation. Radiographics, 7:563–577, 1987.
13. Broderick, J., Talbot, G. T., Prenger, E., et al.: Stroke in children within a major metropolitan area: The surprising importance of intracerebral hemorrhage. J. Child Neurol., 8:250–255, 1993.
14. Brust, J. C. M., Dickinson, P. C. T., Hughes, J. E. O., et al.: The diagnosis and treatment of cerebral mycotic aneurysms. Ann. Neurol., 27:238–246, 1990.
15. Bullock, R., and van Dellen, J. R.: Rupture of bacterial intracranial aneurysms following replacement of cardiac valves. Surg. Neurol., 17:9–11, 1982.
16. Butler, I. J.: Cerebrovascular disorders of childhood. J. Child Neurol., 8:197–200, 1993.
17. Cabanes, J., Blasco, R., Garcia, M., et al.: Cerebral venous angiomas. Surg. Neurol., 11:385–389, 1979.
18. Chaudhary, M., Sachved, V., Cho, S., et al.: Dural arteriovenous malformations of the major venous sinuses: An acquired lesion. A.J.N.R., 3:13–19, 1982.
19. Choux, M., Lena, G., and Genitori, L.: Intracranial aneurysms in children. In Raimondi, A. J., Choux, M., et al., eds.: Cerebrovascular Diseases in Children. New York, Springer-Verlag, 1992, pp. 123–131.
20. Chuang, S.: Vascular diseases of the brain in children. In Edwards, M. S. B., and Hoffman, H. J., eds.: Cerebral Vascular Diseases in Children and Adolescents. Baltimore, Williams & Wilkins, 1989, pp. 69–94.
21. Clare, C. E., and Barrow, D. L.: Infectious intracranial aneurysms following replacement of cardiac valves. Neurosurg. Clin., North Am., 3:551–566, 1992.
22. Day, A. L.: Extracranial-intracranial bypass grafting in the surgical treatment of bacterial aneurysms: Report of two cases. Neurosurgery, 9:583–588, 1981.
23. Debrun, G., Vinuela, F., Fox, A. J., et al.: Embolization of cerebral arteriovenous malformations with bucrylate: Experience of 46 cases. J. Neurosurg., 56:615–627, 1982.
24. Di Rocco, C.: Sturge-Weber disease. In Raimondi, A. J., Choux, M., and Di Rocco, C., eds.: Cerebrovascular Disease in Children. New York, Springer-Verlag, 1992, pp. 168–187.
25. Di Trapani, G., Di Rocco, C., Abbamond, A. L., et al.: Light microscopy and ultrastructural studies of Sturge-Weber disease. Child's Brain, 9:23–26, 1982.

26. Drake, C. G.: Cerebral arteriovenous malformations: Considerations for and experience with surgical treatment in 166 cases. Clin. Neurosurg., 26:145–208, 1979.

27. El-Gohary, M. E., Tomita, T., Gutierrez, F. A., et al.: Angiographically occult vascular malformations in childhood. Neurosurgery, 20:759–766, 1987.

28. Frazee, J. G., Cahan, L. D., and Winter, J.: Bacterial intracranial aneurysms. J. Neurosurg., 48:369–382, 1978.

29. Friedman, W. A., and Bova, F. J.: Linear accelerator radiosurgery for arteriovenous malformations. J. Neurosurg., 77:832–841, 1992.

30. Fujita, K., Ehara, K., Kimuro, M., et al.: Nationwide investigation of intracranial malformations in children. Child's Nerv. Syst., 13:229–236, 1988.

31. Fults, D., and Kelly, O. L., Jr.: Natural history of arteriovenous malformations of the brain: A clinical study. Neurosurgery, 15:658–662, 1984.

32. Garcia-Monaco, R., Rodesch, G., Terbrugge, K., et al.: Multifocal dural arteriovenous shunts in children. Child's Nerv. Syst., 7:425–431, 1991.

33. Gastaut, H., Pinsard, N., Gastaut, J. L., et al.: Acute hemiplegia in children. Adv. Neurol., 25:329–337, 1979.

34. Graf, C. J., Perret, G. E., and Roner, J. C.: Bleeding from cerebral arteriovenous malformations as part of natural history. J. Neurosurg., 58:331–337, 1983.

35. Gray, L., Blinder, R. A., and Djang, W. T.: Magnetic resonance imaging of cerebrovascular diseases. In Wilkins, R. H., and Rengachary, S. S., eds.: Neurosurgery Update I. New York, McGraw-Hill, 1990, pp. 69–87.

36. Hacker, R. J.: Intracranial aneurysms of childhood: A statistical analysis of 500 cases from the world literature. (abstr.). Neurosurgery, 10:775, 1982.

37. Hacker, R. J., Krall, J. M., and Fox, J. C.: Intracranial aneurysm occurring in children. In Fox, J. C., ed.: Intracranial Aneurysms. Vol. 1. New York, Springer-Verlag, 1983, pp. 43–52.

38. Hadley, M. N., Petzler, R. F., Martin, I. V. A., et al.: Middle cerebral artery aneurysm due to Nocardia asteroides: Case report of aneurysm excision and extracranial-intracranial bypass. Neurosurgery, 22:923–928, 1988.

39. Handa, T., Negoro, M., Miyachi, S., et al.: Evaluation of pressure changes in feeding arteries during embolization of intracerebral arteriovenous malformations. J. Neurosurg., 79:383–389, 1993.

40. Hayman, L. A., Evans, R. A., Ferrell, R. E., et al.: Familial cavernous angiomas: Natural history and genetic study over a 5-year period. Am. J. Med. Genet., 11:147–160, 1982.

41. Hendrick, E. B., Hoffman, H. J., and Hudson, A. R.: Hemispherectomy in children. Clin. Neurosurg., 16:315–327, 1969.

42. Herman, J. M., Rekate, H. L., and Spetzler, R. F.: Pediatric intracranial aneurysms: Simple and complex cases. Pediatr. Neurosurg., 17:66–73, 1991–1992.

43. Hoffman, H. J., and Griebel, R. W.: Moyamoya syndrome in children. In Edwards, M. S. B., and Hoffman, H. J., eds.: Cerebral Vascular Diseases in Children and Adolescents. Baltimore, Williams & Wilkins, 1989, pp. 229–237.

44. Hoffman, H. J., Hendrick, E. B., Dennis, M., et al.: Hemispehrectomy for Sturge-Weber syndrome. Childs' Brain, 5:233–248, 1979.

45. Hourihan, M. D., Dates, P. C., and McAllister, V. L.: Subarachnoid hemorrhage in childhood and adolescence. J. Neurosurg., 60:1163–1166, 1984.

46. Humphreys, R. P.: Arteriovenous malformations of the brain. In McLaurin, R. L., Schut, L., Venes, J. L., et al., eds.: Pediatric Neurosurgery. Philadelphia, W. B. Saunders, 1989, pp. 508–516.

47. Humphreys, R. P., Hendrick, E. B., Hoffman, H. J., et al.: Childhood aneurysms: Atypical features, atypical management. Concepts Ped. Neurosurg., 6:213–229, 1985.

48. Jeanty, P., Kepple, D., Rousis, P.: In utero detection of cardiac failure from an aneurysm of the vein of Galen. Am. J. Obstet. Gynecol., 163:50–51, 1990.

49. Kurlemann, G., Bongartz, G., Krings, W., et al.: Asymptomatic moyamoya syndrome: Diagnosis by EEG and magnetic resonance angiography. (abstr.) Monatsschr-Kinderheilkd., 39:235–238, 1991.

50. Lee, K. S., and Rekate, H. L.: Cavernous malformations of the central nervous system. In Raimondi, A. J., Choux, M., and Di Rocco, C., eds.: Cerebrovascular Disease in Children. New York, Springer-Verlag, 1992, pp. 59–74.

51. Lipper, S., Morgan, D., Krigman, M. R., et al.: Congential saccular aneurysm in a 19-day-old neonate: Case report and review of the literature. Surg. Neurol., 10:161–165, 1978.

52. Luessenhop, A. J.: Natural history of cerebral arteriovenous malformations. In Wilson, C. B., and Stein, B. M., eds.: Intracranial Arteriovenous Malformations. Baltimore, Williams & Wilkins, 1984, pp. 12–23.

53. Mazza, C., Pasqualin, A., Cavazzani, P., et al.: Childhood cerebrovascular diseases not associated with vascular malformations. Child's Nerv. Syst., 1:268–271, 1985.

54. McCormick, W. F.: Pathology of vascular malformations of the brain. In Wilson, C. B., and Stein, B. M., eds.: Intracranial Arteriovenous Malformations: Current Neurosurgical Practice. Baltimore, Williams & Wilkins, 1984.

55. McCormick, W. F.: The pathology of angiomas. In Fein, J. M., and Flamm, E. S., eds.: Cerebrovascular Surgery. Vol. 4. New York, Springer-Verlag, 1985, pp. 1073–1095.

56. McCormick, W. F., and Schochett, S. S., Jr.: Atlas of cerebrovascular disease. Philadelphia, W. B. Saunders Co., 1976, pp. 72–105.

57. Merkel, R. H. H., Gilsberg, P. L., Parker, J. C., et al.: Cerebrovascular diseases in sickle cell anemia: A clinical, pathological and radiological correlation. Stroke, 9:45–52, 1978.

58. Meyer, F. B., Sundt, T. M., Fode, N. C., et al.: Cerebral aneurysms in childhood and adolescence. J. Neurosurg., 70:420–425, 1989.

59. Mickle, J. P., and Quisling, R. G.: The transtorcular embolization of vein of Galen aneurysms. J. Neurosurg., 64:731–735, 1986.

60. Mickle, J. P., and Quisling, R. G.: Vein of Galen fistulae. Neurosurg. Clin. North Am., 5(3):529–540, 1994.

61. Morawetz, R. B., and Karp, R. B.: Evolution and resolution of intracranial bacterial (mycotic) aneurysms. Neurosurgery, 15:43–49, 1984.

62. Nagamine, Y., Takahashi, S., and Sonobe, M.: Multiple intracranial aneurysms associated with moyamoya disease. J. Neurosurg., 54:673–676, 1981.

63. Ondra, S. L., Troupp, H., George, E. D., et al.: The natural history of symptomatic arteriovenous malformations of the brain: A 24-year follow-up assessment. J. Neurosurg., 73:387–391, 1990.

64. Ostergaard, J. R.: Association of intracranial aneurysm and arteriovenous malformation in childhood. Neurosurgery, 14:358–362, 1984.

65. Ostergaard, J. R.: Aetiology of intracranial saccular aneurysms in childhood. Br. J. Neurosurg., 5:575–580, 1991.

66. Ostergaard, J. R., and Voldby, B.: Intracranial aneurysms in children and adolescents. J. Neurosurg., 58:832–837, 1983.

67. Pagni, C. A., and Wild, E.: Pathogenetic hypothesis of intracortical calcifications in Sturge-Weber disease: Case report following lobectomy. Mod. Probl. Paediatr., 18:250–257, 1977.

68. Pasqualin, A., Mazza, C., Cavazzani, P., et al.: Intracranial aneurysms and subarachnoid hemorrhage in children and adolescents. Child's Nerv. Syst., 2:185–190, 1986.

69. Patel, A. N., and Richardson, A. E.: Ruptured intracranial aneurysms in the first two decades of life. J. Neurosurg., 35:517–526, 1971.

70. Peerless, S. J., Nemoto, S., and Drake, C. G.: Giant intracranial aneurysms in children and adolescents. In Edwards, M. S. B., and Hoffman, H. J., eds.: Cerebral Vascular Disease in Children and Adolescents. Baltimore, Williams & Wilkins, 1989, pp. 255–273.

71. Pelligrino, P. A., Zanesco, L., and Battistelle, P. A.: Coagulopathies and vasculopathies. In Raimondi, A. J., Choux, M., Di Rocco, C., eds.: Cerebrovascular Diseases in Children. New York, Springer-Verlag, 1992, pp. 188–205.

72. Peterman, A. F., Hayles, A. B., Dockerty, M. B., et al.: Encephalotrigeminal angrinatosis (Sturge-Weber disease): Clinical study of 35 cases. J.A.M.A., 167:2169–2176, 1958.

73. Rappaport, Z. H.: Corpus collosum section in the treatment of intractable seizures in the Sturge-Weber syndrome. Child's Nerv. Syst., 4:231–232, 1988.

74. Raybaud, C. A., Livet, M. O., Jiddane, M., et al.: Radiology of ischemic strokes in children. Neuroradiology, 27:567–578, 1985.

75. Riela, A. R., and Roach, E. S.: Etiology of stroke in children. J. Child Neurol., 8:201–220, 1993.

76. Rigamonti, D., Hadley, M. N., Drayer, B. P., et al.: Cerebral arteriovenous malformations: Incidence and familial occurrence. N. Engl. J. Med., 319:343–347, 1988.

77. Rigamonti, D., and Spetzler, R. F.: The association of venous and cavernous malformations: Report of four cases and discussion of

the pathophysiological, diagnostic, and therapeutic implications. Acta Neurochir. (Wien), *92*:100–105, 1988.

78. Rosenbloom, S. A., and Edwards, M. S. B.: Dural arteriovenous malformations. *In* Edwards, M. S. B., and Hoffman, H. J., eds.: Cerebral Vascular Disease in Children and Adolescents. Baltimore, Williams & Wilkins, 1989, pp. 343–366.

79. Rothfus, W. E., Albright, A. L., Casey, K. F., et al.: Cerebellar venous angioma: "Benign" entity? A.J.N.R., *5*:61–66, 1984.

80. Rumbaugh, C. L., Bergeroa, R. T., Talalla, A., et al.: Traumatic aneurysms of the cortical cerebral arteries: Radiographic aspects. Radiology, *96*:49–54, 1970.

81. Schoenberg, B. S., Mellinger, J. F., and Schoenberg, D. G.: Cerebrovascular disease in infants and children: A study of incidence, clinical features, and survival. Neurology, *28*:763–768, 1978.

82. Sedzimir, C. B., and Robinson, J.: Intracranial hemorrhage in children and adolescents. J. Neurosurg., *38*:269–281, 1973.

83. Shah, M. V., and Heros, R. C.: Intracerebral hemorrhage due to cerebral arteriovenous malformations. Neurosurg. Clin. North Am., *3*:567–576, 1992.

84. Simard, J. M., Garcia-Bengochea, F., Ballinger, W. E., et al.: Cavernous angiomas: A review of 126 collected and 12 new clinical cases. Neurosurgery, *18*:162–167, 1986.

85. Smith, D. R., and Bardenhier, J. A., III: Aneurysm of the pericallosal artery caused by closed cranial trauma: Case report. J. Neurosurg., *29*:551–554, 1968.

86. Soria, E. D., Paroski, M. W., and Schamann, M. E.: Traumatic aneurysms of cerebral vessels: A case study and review of the literature. Angiology, *39*:609–615, 1988.

87. Stehbens, W. E.: Intracranial berry aneurysms in infancy. Surg. Neurol., *18*:58–60, 1982.

88. Stein, B. M., and Wolpert, S. M.: Arteriovenous malformations of the brain: I. Current concepts and treatment. Arch. Neurol., *37*:1–5, 1980.

89. Sundt, T. M., Piepgras, D. G., Fode, N. C., et al.: Giant intracranial aneurysms. Clin. Neurosurg., *54*:681–684, 1981.

90. Tamaki, N., and Ehara, K.: Arteriovenous malformations: Indications and strategies for surgery. *In* Raimondi, A. J., Choux, M., and Di Rocco, C., eds.: Cerebrovascular Diseases in Children. New York, Springer-Verlag, 1992, pp. 59–74.

91. Tomita, T., McLone, D. G., and Naidich, T. P.: Mycotic aneurysm of the intracavernous portions of the carotid artery in childhood. J. Neurosurg., *54*:681–684, 1981.

92. Traumer, B. I., Kindt, G. W., and Gross, C. E.: Medical management of acute cerebral ischemia. *In* Youmans, J. R., ed.: Neurological Surgery. Vol. 3. Philadelphia, W. B. Saunders, 1990, pp. 1516–1533.

93. Vander Ark, G. D., and Kahn, E. A.: Spontaneous intracerebral hematoma. J. Neurosurg., *28*:256, 1968.

94. Villemure, J. G., and Rasmussen, T. H.: Functional hemispherectomy in children. Neuropediatrics *24*:53–55, 1993.

95. Wakai, S., Ueda, Y., Inoh, S., et al.: Angiographically occult angiomas: A report of thirteen cases with analysis of the cases documented in the literature. Neurosurgery, *17*:549–556, 1985.

96. Yamamoto, M., Jimbo, M., Ide, M., et al.: Long-term follow-up of radiosurgically treated arteriovenous malformations in children: Report of nine cases. Surg. Neurol., *38*:95–100, 1992.

CHAPTER 52

Nonoperative Treatment of Aneurysmal Subarachnoid Hemorrhage

An estimated 5 million North Americans harbor intracranial aneurysms; of these, approximately 28,000 will suffer aneurysmal rupture in a given year.[36] Although a majority of patients survive initial subarachnoid hemorrhage in good health, only one of three patients make a full recovery to their pre-existing condition.[35] Clearly, there is still enormous potential for improvements in both the medical and the surgical management of aneurysmal subarachnoid hemorrhage.

Outcome after aneurysmal subarachnoid hemorrhage depends on a myriad of interrelated factors, including the severity of the initial ictus, rebleeding, perioperative medical management, and the timing and technical success of surgery. Surgical obliteration of the ruptured aneurysm is the primary concern in all patients after subarachnoid hemorrhage, but the contribution of perioperative medical management can be considerable. The first 14 days after aneurysmal rupture is the peak period for morbidity and mortality, principally because of the initial effects of hemorrhage, vasospasm, and rebleeding, in decreasing order of incidence.[60] In theory, optimization of the medical management of rebleeding and vasospasm can result in substantial benefit to the patient.

Appropriate surgical treatment of ruptured aneurysm is contingent on both the technical components and the timing of the procedure. Improvements in microsurgical techniques during the past two decades have made most aneurysms approachable. However, in the future, it is doubtful that further technical advances in microsurgery will significantly alter outcome after aneurysmal subarachnoid hemorrhage. It is much more likely that such vital progress will occur in perioperative medical management of the neurological and systemic effects of subarachnoid hemorrhage, including vasospasm, rebleeding, hydrocephalus, electrolyte disturbances, hyperglycemia, cardiac abnormalities, and pulmonary complications. A multidisciplinary approach to the medical and surgical treatment of subarachnoid hemorrhage is a necessity. A special collaborative relation must exist among the neurosurgeon, the neuroanesthetist, and the neurointensivist in the intensive care unit, in the operating theater, and in the laboratory.

Indications for Operative and Nonoperative Treatment

If it is technically feasible, surgical obliteration of a ruptured intracranial aneurysm is the procedure of choice for any grade of patient.[3, 77] For cases in which direct surgical obliteration is not possible because of medical instability or location of the aneurysm, the surgeon should consider endovascular procedures such as thrombosis by platinum microcoils, balloon embolization, aneurysm trapping, and intracranial vessel occlusion.* Direct surgical obliteration should be performed in most cases, and improvements in microsurgical techniques have permitted most aneurysms to be approached with low operative morbidity and mortality.[39, 50, 66] Supportive care with no planned intervention is usually indicated in cases with evidence of irreversible massive brain injury on neurological examination and imaging studies and in cases of severe intracranial hypertension in which there has been no evidence of improvement despite attempted stabilization of the patient's condition.[3, 47] Treatment with ventriculostomy, early surgery, and aggressive postoperative management has markedly reduced the mortality in high-grade patients and has resulted in good outcomes in as many as half of patients treated in this manner.[3, 47]

Aggressive treatment is also indicated in most elderly patients with aneurysmal subarachnoid hemorrhage, although overall results may not be as good

*See references 6, 15, 22, 38, 63, and 68.

M. E. Shaffrey • *C. I. Shaffrey* • *G. Lanzino* • *N. F. Kassell*

as in younger patients, especially for poorer grades.* Concomitant diseases may affect overall outcome, but in most patients, the risks associated with rebleeding from an unsecured aneurysm are greater than those of intervention despite medical conditions that would normally preclude elective surgery.[42] The goals of treatment for good-grade elderly aneurysmal subarachnoid hemorrhage patients should be similar to those for younger patients. Treatment of unruptured aneurysm in the elderly depends on aneurysm size, location, and number. The physiological age, pre-existing medical conditions, and patient preference should also be considered when weighing therapeutic options. The risk of death and neurological deficit from surgery must be less than the natural risk from ruptured aneurysm for the procedure to be considered. Surgery can be performed with relative safety in this age group, but the lifetime risk of hemorrhage of an unruptured intracranial aneurysm discovered at 60 years of age is estimated at only 4.7 per cent.[7, 24] At the authors' institution, most patients with a physiological age of 70 years or less are offered surgical obliteration if the aneurysm is in a readily approachable location. However, conservative management at bed rest remains an option for subarachnoid hemorrhage patients of advanced age with prohibitive medical problems and for any patient who has an unclippable aneurysm or is in devastated neurological condition. A schema for conservative management (monitored bed rest) is quite similar to preoperative medical management except that the treatment period is extended at least through the high-risk period for vasospasm (Table 52–1).

Complications After Subarachnoid Hemorrhage

Complications after subarachnoid hemorrhage can be divided into medical and neurological subsets. Although the largest proportion of major morbidity and mortality after aneurysmal subarachnoid hemorrhage has been attributed to neurological complications (i.e., direct effects of the bleed, aneurysmal rebleeding, and vasospasm), medical complications are now recognized to contribute significantly.[62] In fact, severe medical complications are responsible for about 23 per cent of deaths registered after subarachnoid hemorrhage, a proportion comparable to that of patients dying directly from neurological complications.[62] Medical complications occur more frequently in patients with poor clinical grade on admission and in patients with diffuse, thick clot deposition on admission computed tomography studies.[62] Admission to an intensive care unit where there is continuous close monitoring is mandatory, however, even for patients in good clinical condition. Thus, in addition to the prevention and treatment of the neurological complications of subarachnoid hemorrhage, the goal of conservative or preoperative management is also to prevent and treat the numerous possible medical dilemmas.[29, 72]

---

*See references 1, 10, 11, 25, 57, and 67.

Table 52–1

CONSERVATIVE MANAGEMENT OF ANEURYSMAL SUBARACHNOID HEMORRHAGE

General Care
Bed rest for 14–21 days
Restrict excessive stimulation
Sedation, analgesia
Nothing by mouth except medications
Recording of vital signs, intake, output, and daily weight
Obtain intravenous access
Isotonic intravenous fluids; titrate according to physiological parameters
Indwelling bladder catheter
Automated intermittent leg compression apparatus
Orotracheal intubation if indicated

Physiological Monitoring
Mean arterial blood pressure
Continuous electrocardiography monitoring
Oxygen saturation
Central venous pressure, pulmonary wedge pressure as needed

Laboratory Investigations
Hematology and biochemistry profiles × 7–10 days
Urinalysis at admission

Routinely Prescribed Medications
Steroids
Dexamethasone sodium phosphate (Decadron) intravenous injection 6 mg every 6 hr
Anticonvulsants
Phenytoin sodium (Dilantin), 10–15 mg/kg intravenous injection loading dose, followed by maintenance dose of 100 mg every 8 hr
Phenobarbital sodium (Luminal), 30–60 mg every 6–8 hr
Gastric protectors
Ranitidine (Zantac), 50 mg intravenous injection over 30 min every 8 hr
Cimetidine (Tagamet), 300 mg intravenous injection every 6 hr
Aluminum hydroxide (Maalox), 10–20 mL every 4 hr
Famotidine (Pepcid), 20 mg intravenous injection every 12 hr
Stool softeners
Docusate sodium (Colace), 100 mg by mouth every 12 hr

Medications Given As Needed
Analgesic-sedatives
Fentanyl citrate (Sublimaze), 100–150 μg every 1–2 hr
Midazolam hydrochloride (Versed), 1–2 mg every 1–2 hr
Morphine, 2–10 mg every 2–4 hr
Antiemetics
Trimethobenzamide hydrochloride (Tigan), 200 mg every 6–8 hr by intramuscular injection
Agents for refractory elevation in intracranial pressure
Mannitol, 0.5–2 g/kg intravenous injection over 20 min, then 0.5 g/kg every 6 hr if needed
Thiopental (Pentothal), 3–10 mg/kg, then adjust as needed
Antihypertensive agents
Hydralazine hydrochloride, 10–20 mg every 2–4 hr if systolic blood pressure >160 or diastolic >90 or pulse <90/min
Labetalol, 10 mg intravenous injection every 30 min if systolic blood pressure >160 or diastolic >90 or pulse >90/min
Antifibrinolytic agents
Epsilon-aminocaproic acid, 32–48 g/24 hr intravenous injection for 2–3 wk
Tranexamic acid, 6–12 g/24 hr intravenous injection for 2–3 wk

---

Medical Complications

ELECTROLYTE ABNORMALITIES

Fluid and electrolyte abnormalities are relatively common in the perioperative period after aneurysmal rupture. The most common abnormality is hyponatremia. Decreased plasma sodium may be present in as many as 35 per cent of subarachnoid hemorrhage patients, and it is most common between the second and tenth days after initial ictus.[75, 76] Alterations in level of consciousness, seizure activity, and cerebral edema may be exacerbated by hyponatremia. The exact nature of low plasma sodium levels after subarachnoid hemorrhage is unclear, but possible explanations include cerebral salt-wasting syndrome and the syndrome of inappropriate antidiuretic hormone secretion.

Although serum vasopressin levels are usually normal or elevated on admission after subarachnoid hemorrhage, levels decrease at the time that hyponatremia occurs.[70] In addition, the circulating plasma volume decreases in some patients with normal sodium levels, usually as a result of natriuresis.[70] Natriuresis may result from secretion of atrial natriuretic factor, but a causative role has yet to be proved. Clinical differentiation of natriuresis from the syndrome of inappropriate antidiuretic hormone secretion is important because in the former the patients are hypovolemic and sodium-depleted and require volume replacement and salt, but in the latter the patients require fluid restriction. Fluid restriction of a patient with incipient hyponatremia and hypovolemia secondary to natriuresis could be detrimental, particularly in the setting of cerebral vasospasm.

HYPERGLYCEMIA

Significant hyperglycemia can result from the stress of aneurysmal subarachnoid hemorrhage. Elderly patients with undiagnosed diabetes mellitus are particularly at risk. Oral or intravenous corticosteroids can further exacerbate hyperglycemia related to stress or predilection. Extreme hyperglycemia can contribute to a depressed level of consciousness, but it more frequently results in focal or generalized seizure activity.[14, 71] Furthermore, hyperglycemia in the setting of ischemia from cerebral vasospasm is theoretically disadvantageous, since detrimental effects have been seen on neurological recovery after other forms of central nervous system ischemia.[53, 61, 74] Although avoidance and correction of dehydration remain the mainstays of treatment for nonketotic hyperglycemia, the use of insulin remains somewhat controversial because of implications in the exacerbation of cerebral edema.[70] However, insulin has been used in experimental studies to lower blood glucose concentration and alleviate the severity of both cerebral and spinal cord infarction.[41, 55, 65]

HYPERTENSION

The rise in blood pressure after subarachnoid hemorrhage is in many cases a compensatory response to a reduction in cerebral perfusion pressure (Cushing's phenomenon). Several coexisting conditions such as agitation, pain, and hypoxia may aggravate the systemic hypertensive response to the neurological insult.

Adequate control of mean arterial pressure in the early phase after aneurysmal rupture is important to reduce the chances of rebleeding. Elevated arterial pressure, in fact, causes an increase in transmural pressure. Elevation in transmural pressure is more likely if measures to decrease intracranial pressure (e.g., administration of osmotic diuretics, corticosteroids, controlled ventilation) are undertaken without concomitant reduction in mean arterial pressure. Sedation and correction of the underlying coexisting conditions can be sufficient to reduce mean arterial pressure. If these measurements are insufficient, antihypertensive medications are used (see Table 52–1). The goal of therapy in these cases is to lower arterial pressure to a level consistent with maintenance of organ perfusion, including cerebral perfusion, while minimizing the immediate risks associated with the hypertensive state.

CARDIAC COMPLICATIONS

Abnormalities and frank rhythm disorders are often observed on electrocardiography after subarachnoid hemorrhage.[2, 9, 40] These abnormalities tend to be more common immediately after the hemorrhage and are likely to contribute to the initial loss of consciousness and to the sudden death that can occur after subarachnoid hemorrhage.[2, 9] Arrhythmias have been recorded in 91 per cent of patients followed by Holter monitoring after the onset of subarachnoid hemorrhage. These arrhythmias are usually benign, but in some cases they can take the form of life-threatening arrhythmias such as ventricular tachycardia, ventricular flutter, ventricular fibrillation, and torsades de pointes.[2, 9, 40] Serious arrhythmias are more likely to occur if factors such as advanced age, hypokalemia, and prolonged QT interval are present.[2, 9] Continuous electrocardiography monitoring is suggested after subarachnoid hemorrhage in view of its potential role in alerting clinicians to the need for treatment.[9]

Therapy for the rhythm disorders encountered after subarachnoid hemorrhage is indicated only in the presence of serious arrhythmias that may interfere with normal cardiac function or significantly impair organ perfusion. In these cases, the treatment is not different from the treatment of arrhythmias observed in other situations. In complicated cases, involvement of a cardiologist is warranted. In patients with severe, sustained bradycardia, an external pacemaker may be indicated.[27] A marked rate reduction significantly decreases end-organ perfusion and may aggravate the ischemic consequences of vasospasm.[27]

DEEP VENOUS THROMBOSIS

Approximately 2 per cent of patients suffer deep vein thrombosis after aneurysmal rupture.[29] As many as one half of these patients develop pulmonary emboli.[29] The likelihood of deep venous thrombosis is increased if a neurological deficit is present. Heparinization is contraindicated in patients with an unsecured aneurysm; therefore, the introduction of a vena cava umbrella should be considered in those patients with established deep vein thrombosis. An automated intermittent leg compression apparatus and passive exercise are useful in the prophylaxis of this complication.

PULMONARY COMPLICATIONS

Pulmonary complications remain a significant contributor to mortality after subarachnoid hemorrhage; they are responsible for 50 per cent of all deaths from medical complications.[62] Pneumonia, adult respiratory distress syndrome, and pulmonary emboli are the most common causes of respiratory morbidity and mortality after subarachnoid hemorrhage.[62]

GASTROINTESTINAL BLEEDING

Gastrointestinal bleeding can occur after subarachnoid hemorrhage.[29] The gastroduodenal ulcerations observed in association with intracranial diseases are termed Cushing's ulcers. It has been reported that 83 per cent of patients with fatal ruptured anterior communicating artery aneurysms showed significant gastroduodenal hemorrhagic and ulcerative lesions at autopsy.[54] Indeed, clinically significant gastrointestinal bleeding occurs in approximately 4 per cent of patients after aneurysmal rupture.[29] Treatment of acute gastrointestinal bleeding includes nasogastric intubation and lavage with saline, fluid resuscitation, and transfusions. If uncontrollable bleeding is present, partial gastrectomy and vagotomy may be indicated. Histamine$_2$ blockers and antacids are routinely used to prevent these complications, although no convincing study showing their efficacy in these conditions has been conducted.

Neurological Complications

HYDROCEPHALUS

The frequency of acute hydrocephalus during the first 3 days after aneurysmal subarachnoid hemorrhage is about 20 per cent.[19, 43] Although hydrocephalus may impair the level of consciousness at the time of initial evaluation, those patients who are initially alert and become progressively more drowsy have a more classic presentation. The proportion of patients who have acute hydrocephalus concurrent with intraventricular hemorrhage varies from 35 to 65 per cent.[70] Therefore, a significant number of patients develop acute hydrocephalus not specifically related to cerebrospinal fluid outflow obstruction.

Treatment options for subarachnoid hemorrhage patients with acute hydrocephalus include observation and lumbar drainage or ventricular drainage (internal or external). In patients who are asymptomatic in the early postbleed period, observation in the presence of ventricular dilatation appears justified because about one in three will develop neurological symptoms over the ensuing few days. In addition, alterations in intracranial pressures related to lumbar puncture or ventricular drainage may precipitate aneurysmal rebleeding because of changes in forces that are sealing the original site of rupture.[49] Lumbar drainage is unwise in the presence of noncommunicating hydrocephalus because of the possible precipitation of focal brain herniation. Prolonged ventricular drainage from a single site runs an ever-increasing risk of infection as this treatment continues.

REBLEEDING

Aneurysmal rebleeding continues to be the most disastrous and disabling event after initial subarachnoid hemorrhage. Mortality rates from rebleeding are as high as 70 to 90 per cent, with the peak incidence of rebleeding occurring within the first 48 hours.[56, 60] Without exclusion of the aneurysm from arterial circulation, there is a 20 to 30 per cent incidence of rebleeding within 2 weeks of the initial hemorrhage.[59] As many as one in six patients with aneurysmal subarachnoid hemorrhage suffer death or severe disability from rebleeding.[30] Early surgical treatment of the aneurysm eliminates the rebleeding potential during the highest risk period.

To prevent aneurysmal rebleeding for a delayed surgical approach, there is a significant theoretical advantage in impeding the lysis of the blood clot that seals the site of initial aneurysmal rupture by the use of pharmacological agents. The two most commonly prescribed antifibrinolytic drugs, epsilon-aminocaproic acid and tranexamic acid, affect antifibrinolysis by competitive inhibition of plasminogen activation.[59] However, the theoretical advantages of antifibrinolytic therapy have not been fully realized in clinical practice. Antifibrinolytic agents reduce the rate of rebleeding by almost 50 per cent, but there is a concurrent increase in ischemic neurological deficits.[32] Therefore, rebleeding rates are diminished at the expense of increased ischemic neurological complications.

The nature of the exacerbation of ischemic neurological complications with antifibrinolytic therapy is uncertain. Theories include an increase in the propensity for cerebrovascular thrombotic events directly related to these medications and a reduction in the clearance of the subarachnoid clot, which prolongs the influence of the factors that cause vasospasm. It may be that the incidence of ischemia is not increased per se but that the drugs reduce the mortality related to rebleeding so that more patients survive to suffer the ischemic complications of vasospasm.[59]

Irrespective of the cause of the ischemic complications, there appears to be no definite role for antifibrinolytic therapy if early surgery is anticipated. If surgical treatment is to be delayed or not performed, it may be reasonable to employ these agents despite the potential to develop focal ischemic neurological deficits. Contraindications to antifibrinolytic therapy include pregnancy, deep venous thrombosis, pulmonary embolism, and coagulopathy.[73]

VASOSPASM

Angiographic vasospasm may occur in as many as 70 to 90 per cent of patients at some time during the first 14 days after aneurysmal subarachnoid hemorrhage.[37] Ischemic neurological deficits from clinical vasospasm occur in approximately one half of patients demonstrating vasospasm on angiography.[37] Although rebleeding is the most feared complication of aneurysmal rupture, vasospasm is still the leading treatable cause of death and disability in patients with aneurysmal subarachnoid hemorrhage.[36] The impact of improvements in medical management of patients in clinical vasospasm must be partially responsible for the reduction in related mortality from more than 40 per cent in the 1960's to 8 per cent or less currently.[37]

Diagnosis. The clinical diagnosis of vasospasm is contingent on recognition of a syndrome that may consist of alteration in the level of consciousness and focal neurological deficits.[36] Changes in the results of neurological examination may be accompanied by gradually increasing blood pressure, headache, fever, and a tendency toward hyponatremia.[37] To make the diagnosis of clinical vasospasm, other causes for neurological deterioration must be excluded, such as intracranial hematomas, hydrocephalus, and metabolic disturbances. However, cerebral vasospasm must always be suspected in the setting of neurological deterioration after subarachnoid hemorrhage because it is such a common and serious contributing factor.

Although angiography remains the standard for the diagnosis of vasospasm, its necessity has been diminished with the advent of transcranial Doppler ultrasound.[37] This technique has proved to be a reliable adjunct for demonstration of arterial narrowing on angiography. The medical management of vasospasm has been greatly facilitated by this noninvasive technique, which can be performed as often as necessary to diagnose the arterial narrowing in advance of the development of ischemic signs and symptoms. Patients with a mean middle cerebral artery velocity greater than or equal to 200 cm per second are considered at risk for clinical vasospasm.[23, 58] The sensitivity of transcranial Doppler ultrasound does not appear to be adversely affected by a high incidence of distal vasospasm.[45]

From a practical standpoint, the diagnosis of arterial narrowing in the author's institution is based primarily on the transcranial Doppler examination. Doppler examinations are obtained at least every other day during the first 14 days after subarachnoid hemorrhage. The frequency of Doppler examination is increased in response to changes in the patient's neurological status or increase in the mean arterial velocity. Most patients receive routine postoperative angiography between the seventh and tenth days after subarachnoid hemorrhage, the peak period of vasospasm. Angiography continues to be the most important diagnostic tool if discrepancies develop between the clinical condition and the Doppler ultrasound results.

Management. There are five theoretical approaches to the management of vasospasm: prevention of arterial narrowing; reversal of arterial narrowing; prevention of ischemic consequences related to arterial narrowing; reversal of ischemic consequences related to arterial narrowing; and protection of the brain from infarction.[37]

Prevention of Arterial Narrowing. Theoretically, prevention of arterial narrowing can be accomplished by the removal or inactivation of spasmogenic substances within the subarachnoid space. This may be achieved by removal of blood and spasmogenic substances from the basal cisterns or by the use of cerebral vasodilating agents. Some of the agents that have been used in clinical and preclinical settings including vitamin E, ticlopidine, cyclosporine, thromboxane synthetase inhibitors, and nicardipine.[37]

Potential benefits of cyclosporin A have been ascribed to its role as an immunosuppressant and as a calmodulin antagonist.[51] High-dose, continuous intravenous infusions of the calcium antagonist, nicardipine, can prevent arterial narrowing. Nicardipine decreases the incidence of moderate or severe angiographic vasospasm during days 7 through 11 by almost 40 per cent and decreases the incidence of clinical vasospasm by approximately 30 per cent.[16]

Blood and spasmogenic substances from the subarachnoid spaces can be removed during aneurysm surgery. This usually results in only partial removal of the subarachnoid hematoma and carries a risk of damage to pial banks and small vessels. Clinical studies cast some doubt on the significance of clot removal in the amelioration of vasospasm despite encouraging preclinical studies.[26, 46]

Removal of subarachnoid clot may be enhanced through the use of thrombolytic therapy.[64] This treatment consists of the irrigation of the subarachnoid space with recombinant tissue plasminogen activator or urokinase at the time of surgery or postoperatively.[64] Preclinical data have demonstrated dramatic clearing of thick subarachnoid blood clots and are suggestive for the prevention of arterial narrowing and ischemic neurological deficits.[12, 13] The major concern about the use of perioperative thrombolytic therapy is the possible precipitation of intracranial bleeding, especially in patients who have significant cortical disruption related to surgery or initial hemorrhage. Results of rigorous multicenter clinical trials are now nearing completion.

At the authors' institution, all patients are operated on at the earliest convenient time after admission. The basal cisterns are opened widely, and only subarachnoid blood that can be removed with gentle suction and irrigation is pursued. Our unsubstantiated impression is that clot removal may be facilitated in those patients with thick subarachnoid hematomas by cisternal installation of recombinant tissue plasminogen activator at the time of surgery. This therapy is most likely to curtail vasospasm in those patients at maximal risk, but it should be used in the first 2 to 3 days after bleeding to be effective.[13]

Reversal of Arterial Narrowing. Theoretically, reversal of arterial narrowing can be accomplished through inactivation or blockade of spasmogenic substances by the use of cerebral vasodilators or by mechanical dilation of the lumina of narrowed arteries. Once arterial narrowing has been established, no agent has been identified that can specifically inactivate or block the spasmogenic substances.[37] Potent vasodilating agents administered intravenously to reverse vasospasm have failed. However, in selected patients, intra-arterial and intracisternal administration of papaverine is capable of dilating narrowed arteries and reversing clinical vasospasm.[20, 37]

Transluminal balloon angioplasty is a relatively new technique for the treatment of vasospasm. In some patients, it has been effective in reversing arterial narrowing and corresponding neurological deficits.[5, 8, 21, 44, 78] Complications of this procedure include delayed arterial occlusion, arterial rupture, conversion to hemorrhagic infarction, and displacement of surgical clips from aneurysm necks.[8, 21, 44] The safety and efficacy of balloon angioplasty has yet to be proved, although preliminary results reveal that patients who demonstrate clinical deterioration from vasospasm may benefit from this procedure.[44]

Prevention and Reversal of Ischemic Deficits. Of the cytoprotective agents that are not involved with blockade of the final common pathway of neuronal death (i.e., calcium influx), the most promising appears to be the 21-aminosteroid, tirilazad. This agent is attractive because of its potential to reduce cerebral vasospasm and its cytoprotective effects in focal ischemia, possibly related to free radical–scavenging or anti-inflammatory properties.[17, 18, 79] Recent release of data from a European phase III trial has confirmed significant reductions in clinical vasospasm and improvements in favorable outcomes at dosages of 2.0 and 6.0 mg per kg per day.[31] Results of the North American phase III trial will be available soon.

Prevention or reversal of ischemic deficits may be achieved through optimization of the patient's hemodynamic and rheological status, often referred to as hypervolemic, hypertensive, hemodilution (or "triple H") therapy.[34] Cerebral perfusion pressure can be escalated through augmentation of mean arterial pressure or reduction of intracranial pressure. Cardiac output can be increased through the use of cardiac inotropes or by increasing the intravascular volume. Collateral circulation to potentially ischemic zones can be improved by dilation of leptomeningeal collaterals. Blood viscosity can be effectively lowered by decreasing the hematocrit, either through hemodilution or through the disaggregating properties of colloid solutions, thereby decreasing cerebrovascular resistance and increasing cerebral blood flow.[37]

There is no doubt that hypertensive, hypervolemic, hemodilution therapy is a poor substitute for definitive measures for preventing or reversing arterial narrowing. Although proof of the effectiveness of "triple H" therapy has been largely anecdotal, these reports have been sufficiently convincing to result in prevalent application.

Negative features of "triple H" therapy include the expense of intensive critical care, medications, and intravenous fluids and the morbidity associated with invasive hemodynamic monitoring. Increasing the arterial pressure can result in rebleeding of previously unruptured aneurysms, new bleeding from incidental but unsecured aneurysms, intracerebral hemorrhage from ruptured small vessels, conversion to hemorrhagic infarctions, exacerbation of cerebral edema and increased intracranial pressure, and a high incidence of pulmonary edema.[33, 37] However, "triple H" therapy will continue to be an important feature of the treatment regimen of cerebral vasospasm until more specific therapy is discovered.

At the authors' institution, asymptomatic patients are treated with mild volume expansion by means of an intravenous intake of approximately 3,000 mL per day, of which approximately one third is colloid and two thirds is crystalloid. Induced hypertension is avoided at this stage. The authors do not raise arterial pressure in asymptomatic patients unless they are significantly hypotensive after clipping of the aneurysm.

In asymptomatic patients with vasospasm diagnosed by transcranial Doppler ultrasound or angiography, an intake of approximately 3,000 mL per day is continued, but the amount of colloid is increased to two thirds of the total volume. Hemodilution consists of maintaining the hematocrit at approximately 35 to 40 per cent. Induced hypertension is not used, but antihypertensive medications are discontinued.

In patients with clinically symptomatic vasospasm, hypervolemia is induced to optimize cardiac output (determined by Swan-Ganz catheter). This is accomplished through infusion of colloid, crystalloid, and red blood cells in whatever proportions and volumes are necessary to maintain normal plasma electrolytes and a hematocrit between 30 and 35 per cent. Pulmonary function is closely monitored. Mannitol is infused for its rheological effect on the microcirculation as well as its antioxidant properties. Hypertension is induced with inotropic agents and titrated to the neurological deficit. In certain patients, it may be necessary to decrease the dosage of calcium antagonists in order to reduce their antihypertensive effects, which are counterproductive at this time. If there is no improvement after 1 hour of hypertensive therapy, the patient is taken for balloon angioplasty.

Prevention of Cerebral Infarction. The mechanism for neurological deficits related to clinical vasospasm is neuronal ischemia. Because of the lack of reliable methods of preventing or reversing vasospasm, cytoprotective agents are needed to reduce the impact of neuronal hypoxia. The efficacies of cytoprotective agents, including nimodipine, naloxone, and monosialoganglioside, are reported in some clinical trials.[4, 48, 69] Monosialoganglioside, a natural component of neuronal membranes, is reported to improve level of consciousness over short periods, but more rigorous studies are necessary to determine the possibility of long-term benefits.[48]

The role of oral nimodipine in prevention or treatment of delayed ischemic events has been exhaustively reviewed.[69] Most reports confirm that the incidence of severe neurological deficits is reduced, despite evidence that there is little effect on the incidence and severity of angiographic vasospasm.[52] Nonvascular, anti-ischemic effects of nimodipine and nicardipine may occur by limitation of excess neuronal calcium entry, which reduces cell damage caused by ischemia.[52, 69] Nimodipine and nicardipine are pharmacologically equivalent dihydropyridines, but an equivalent intravenous dose of nicardipine at 10 mg per hour has approximately 10 times the biological equivalency of an oral dose of nimodipine at 60 mg every 4 hours.[28]

At the authors' institution, calcium channel blocking agents are used in all aneurysmal subarachnoid hemorrhage patients. Nimodipine, in a dosage of 60 mg orally every 4 hours, has no effect on angiographic vasospasm but does appear to reduce clinical vasospasm; nicardipine, in a dose of approximately 10 mg per hour by continuous intravenous infusion, reduces both angiographic and clinical vasospasm.[37] The intravenous formulation of nimodipine is still unavailable in the United States.

If all of the aforementioned approaches fail, additional measures can be undertaken to prevent infarction from developing until the arterial narrowing resolves spontaneously and an adequate blood flow has been restored. Along with the use of cytoprotective agents such as the calcium antagonists and mannitol, other measures include maintenance of blood glucose below 100 mg per dL and prevention of seizures. Barbiturate coma has been tried in patients who are desperately ill from vasospasm, but with unsatisfactory results.[33]

REFERENCES

1. Amacher, A. L., Ferguson, G. G., Drake, C. G., et al.: How old people tolerate intracranial surgery for aneurysm. Neurosurgery, 1:242–244, 1977.
2. Andreoli, A., Di Pasquale, G., Pinelli, G., et al.: Subarachnoid hemorrhage: Frequency and severity of cardiac arrhythmias. Stroke, 18:558–564, 1987.
3. Bailes, J. E., Spetzler, R. F., Hadley, M. N., et al.: Management morbidity and mortality of poor-grade aneurysm patients. J. Neurosurg., 72:559–566, 1990.
4. Bell, B. A., Miller, J. D., Neto, N. G. F., et al.: Effect of naloxone on deficits after aneurysmal subarachnoid hemorrhage. Neurosurgery, 16:498–500, 1985.
5. Brothers, M. F., and Holgate, R. C.: Intracranial angioplasty for treatment of vasospasm after subarachnoid hemorrhage: Technique and modifications to improve branch access. A. J. N. R., 11:239–247, 1990.
6. Casasco, A. E., Aymard, A., Gobin, Y. P., et al.: Selective endovascular treatment of 71 intracranial aneurysms with platinum coils. J. Neurosurg., 79:3–10, 1993.
7. Dell, S.: Asymptomatic cerebral aneurysm: Assessment of its risk of rupture. Neurosurgery, 10:162–166, 1982.
8. Dion, J. E., Duckwiler, G. R., Vinuela, F., et al.: Pre-operative microangioplasty of refractory vasospasm secondary to subarachnoid hemorrhage. Neuroradiology, 32:232–236, 1990.
9. Di Pasquale, G., Pinelli, G., Andreoli, A., et al.: Holter detection of cardiac arrhythmias in intracranial subarachnoid hemorrhage. Am. J. Cardiol., 59:596–600, 1987.
10. Disney, L., Weir, B., and Grace, M.: Factors influencing the out-
come of aneurysm rupture in poor-grade patients: A prospective series. Neurosurgery, 23:1–9, 1988.
11. Drake, C. G., Slosberg, P. S., and Simeone, F. A.: Senior citizen with ruptured aneurysm. Neurosurgery, 6:605–606, 1980.
12. Findlay, J. M., Weir, B. K. A., Kanamaru, K., et al.: Intrathecal fibrinolytic therapy after subarachnoid hemorrhage: Dosage study in a primate model and review of the literature. Can. J. Neurol. Sci., 16:28–40, 1989.
13. Findlay, J. M., Weir, B. K. A., Kanamaru, K., et al.: The effect of timing of intrathecal fibrinolytic therapy on cerebral vasospasm in a primate model of subarachnoid hemorrhage. Neurosurgery, 26:201–206, 1990.
14. Grant, C., and Warlow, C.: Focal epilepsy in diabetic nonketotic hyperglycemia. B.M.J., 290:1204–1205, 1985.
15. Guglielmi, G., Vinuela, F., Dion, J., et al.: Electrothrombosis of saccular aneurysms via endovascular approach: Part 2. Preliminary clinical experience. J. Neurosurg., 75:8–14, 1991.
16. Haley, E. C., Kassell, N. F., and Torner, J. C.: A randomized trial of nicardipine in subarachnoid hemorrhage: Angiographic and transcranial Doppler ultrasound results. J. Neurosurg., 78:548–553, 1993.
17. Hall, A. D., and Travis, M. A.: Effects of the nonglucocorticoid U74006F on progressive brain hypoperfusion following experimental subarachnoid hemorrhage. Exp. Neurol., 102:244–248, 1988.
18. Hall, A. D., and Travis, M. A.: Inhibition of arachidonic acid–induced brain edema by the nonglucocorticoid 21-aminosteroid U74006F. Brain Res., 451:350–352, 1988.
19. Hasan, D., Lindsay, K. W., and Vermeulen, M.: Treatment of acute hydrocephalus after subarachnoid hemorrhage with serial lumbar puncture. Stroke, 22:190–194, 1991.
20. Helm, G. A., and Kassell, N. F.: Intra-arterial papaverine for the treatment of cerebral vasospasm. Annual Meeting of the Congress of Neurological Surgeons. Orlando, October 1991 [Abstract].
21. Higashida, R. T., Halbach, V. V., Dormandy, B., et al.: New microballoon device for transluminal angioplasty of intracranial arterial vasospasm. A. J. N. R., 11:233–238, 1990.
22. Higashida, R. T., Halbach, V. V., Dowd, C., et al.: Endovascular detachable balloon embolization therapy of cavernous carotid artery aneurysms: Results in 87 cases. J. Neurosurg., 72:857–863, 1990.
23. Hutchison, K., and Weir, B.: Transcranial Doppler studies in aneurysm patients. Can. J. Neurol. Sci., 16:411–416, 1989.
24. Inagawa, T., Hada, H., and Katoh, Y.: Unruptured aneurysms in elderly patients. Surg. Neurol., 38:364–370, 1992.
25. Inagawa, T., Yamamoto, M., Kamiya, K., et al.: Management of elderly patients with aneurysmal subarachnoid hemorrhage. J. Neurosurg., 69:332–339, 1988.
26. Inagawa, T., Yamamoto, M., Kazuko, K., et al.: Effect of clot removal on cerebral vasospasm. J. Neurosurg., 72:224–230, 1990.
27. Kamiya, K., Inagawa, T., Ohta, K., et al.: Effect of temporary pacing on patients with bradycardia in the acute stage following subarachnoid hemorrhage. Surg. Neurol., 37:261–263, 1992.
28. Kassell, N. F.: Nicardipine and angiographic vasospasm. Fifty-ninth Annual Meeting of the American Association of Neurological Surgeons. New Orleans, April 1991 [Presentation].
29. Kassell, N. F., and Boarini, D. J.: Perioperative care of the aneurysm patient. Contemp. Neurosurg., 6:1–6, 1984.
30. Kassell, N. F., and Drake, C. G.: Timing of aneurysm surgery. Neurosurgery, 10:514–519, 1982.
31. Kassell, N. F., Haley, E. C., Alves, W., et al.: Phase III trial of tirilazad in aneurysmal subarachnoid hemorrhage. Sixty-second Annual Meeting of the AANS. San Diego, April, 1994 [Presentation].
32. Kassell, N. F., Haley, E. C., and Torner, J. C.: Antifibrinolytic therapy in the treatment of aneurysmal subarachnoid hemorrhage. Clin. Neurosurg., 33:137–145, 1986.
33. Kassell, N. F., Peerless, S. J., Drake, C. G., et al.: Treatment of ischemic deficits from cerebral vasospasm with high-dose barbiturate therapy. Neurosurgery, 7:593–597, 1980.
34. Kassell, N. F., Peerless, S. J., Durward, Q. J., et al.: Treatment of ischemic deficits from vasospasm with intravascular volume expansion and induced arterial hypertension. Neurosurgery, 11:337–343, 1982.

35. Kassell, N. F., Sasaki, T., Colohan, A. R. T., et al.: Cerebral vasospasm following aneurysmal subarachnoid hemorrhage. Stroke, 16:562–572, 1985.
36. Kassell, N. F., Shaffrey, C. I., and Shaffrey, M. E.: Timing of aneurysm surgery. In Wilkins, R. H., and Rengachary, S. S., eds.: Neurosurgery Update. Vol 2. New York, McGraw-Hill, 1990, pp. 95–99.
37. Kassell, N. F., Shaffrey, M. E., and Shaffrey, C. I.: Cerebral vasospasm following aneurysmal subarachnoid hemorrhage. In Apuzzo, M. L. J., ed.: Brain Surgery: Complication Avoidance and Management. New York, Churchill Livingstone, 1992, pp. 847–856.
38. Knuckey, N. W., Haas, R., Jenkins, R., et al.: Thrombosis of difficult intracranial aneurysm by the endovascular placement of platinum-Dacron microcoils. J. Neurosurg., 77:43–50, 1992.
39. Lang, D. A., and Galbraith, S. L.: The management outcome of patients with a ruptured posterior circulation aneurysm. Acta Neurochir. (Wien), 125:9–14, 1993.
40. Lanzino, G., Kongable, G. L., and Kassell, N. F.: Electrocardiographic abnormalities after nontraumatic subarachnoid hemorrhage. J. Neurosurg. Anesthesiol., 6:156–162, 1994.
41. Lemay, D. R., Gehua, L., Zelenock, G. B., et al.: Insulin administration protects neurologic function in cerebral ischemia in rats. Stroke, 19:1411–1419, 1988.
42. McNutt, R. A., and Pauker, S. G.: Competing rates of risk in a patient with subarachnoid hemorrhage and myocardial infarction: It's now or never. Med. Decis. Making, 7:250–259, 1987.
43. Milhorat, T. H.: Acute hydrocephalus after aneurysmal subarachnoid hemorrhage. Neurosurgery, 20:15–20, 1987.
44. Newell, D. W., Eskridge, J. M., Mayberg, M. R., et al.: Angioplasty for the treatment of symptomatic vasospasm following subarachnoid hemorrhage. J. Neurosurg., 71:654–660, 1989.
45. Newell, D. W., Grady, M. S., Eskridge, J. M., et al.: Distribution of angiographic vasospasm after subarachnoid hemorrhage: Implications for diagnosis by transcranial Doppler ultrasound. Neurosurgery, 27:574–577, 1990.
46. Nosko, M., Weir, B. K. A., Lunt, A., et al.: Effect of clot removal at 24 hours on chronic vasospasm after SAH in the primate model. J. Neurosurg., 66:416–422, 1987.
47. Nowak, G., Schwachenwald, R., and Arnold, H.: Early management in poor-grade aneurysm patients. Acta Neurochir. (Wien), 126:33–37, 1994.
48. Papo, I., Benedetti, A., Carteri, A., et al.: Monosialoganglioside in subarachnoid hemorrhage. Stroke, 22:22–26, 1991.
49. Pare, L., Delfino, R., and Leblanc, R.: The relationship of ventricular drainage to aneurysmal rebleeding. J. Neurosurg., 76:422–427, 1992.
50. Peerless, S., and Drake, C. G.: Surgical techniques of posterior cerebral aneurysms. In Schmidek, H. N., and Sweet, W. H., eds.: Operative Neurosurgical Techniques: Indications, Methods and Results. 2nd ed. Vol. 2. Orlando, Grune & Stratton, 1988, pp. 973–995.
51. Peterson, J. W., Nishizawa, S., Hackett, J. D., et al.: Cyclosporin A reduces cerebral vasospasm after subarachnoid hemorrhage in dogs. Stroke, 21:133–137, 1990.
52. Pickard, J. D., Murray, G. D., and Illingworth, R.: Effect of oral nimodipine on cerebral infarction and outcome after subarachnoid hemorrhage: British aneurysm nimodipine trial. B. M. J., 298:636–642, 1989.
53. Pulsinelli, W. A., Waldman, S., Rawlinson, D., et al.: Moderate hyperglycemia augments ischemic brain damage. Neurology, 32:1239–1246, 1982.
54. Redondo, A., Hanau, J., Creissard, P., et al.: Complications gastroduodenales des rupture aneurismales du systeme communicant anterieur. Neurochirurgie, 16:471–488, 1970.
55. Robertson, C. S., and Grossman, R. G.: Protection during spinal cord ischemia with insulin-induced hypoglycemia. J. Neurosurg., 67:739–744, 1988.
56. Rosenorn, J., Eskesen, V., Schmidt, K., et al.: The risk of rebleeding from ruptured intracranial aneurysms. J. Neurosurg., 67:329–332, 1987.
57. Sakaki, S., Ohta, S., Ohue, S., et al.: Outcome in elderly patients with ruptured intracranial aneurysm. Clin. Neurol. Neurosurg., 91:21–27, 1989.
58. Sekhar, L. N., Wechsler, L. R., Yonas, H., et al.: Value of transcranial Doppler examination in the diagnosis of cerebral vasospasm after subarachnoid hemorrhage. Neurosurgery, 22:813–821, 1988.
59. Shaffrey, M. E., Shaffrey, C. I., and Kassell, N. F.: Early versus delayed surgery for ruptured aneurysms. In Awad, I. A., ed.: Current Management of Cerebral Aneurysms. Park Ridge, IL, American Association of Neurological Surgeons Publications, 1993, pp. 119–124.
60. Shaffrey, M. E., Shaffrey, C. I., and Kassell, N. F.: Surgical management of ruptured aneurysms. In Adams, H. P., ed.: Handbook of Cerebrovascular Diseases. New York, Marcel Dekker, 1993, pp. 509–518.
61. Siemkowicz, E., and Hansen, A. J.: Clinical restitution following cerebral ischemia in hypo-, normo-, and hyperglycemic rats. Acta Neurol. Scand., 58:1–8, 1978.
62. Solenski, N. J., Haley, C. E., Kassell, N. F., et al.: Medical complications of aneurysmal subarachnoid hemorrhage: A report of the cooperative study. Crit. Care Med., 6:1007–1017, 1995.
63. Steinburg, G. K., Drake, C. G., and Peerless, S. J.: Deliberate basilar or vertebral artery occlusion in the treatment of intracranial aneurysms: Immediate results and long-term outcome in 201 patients. J. Neurosurg., 79:161–173, 1993.
64. Stolke, D., and Seifert, V.: Single intracisternal bolus of recombinant tissue plasminogen activator in patients with aneurysmal subarachnoid hemorrhage: Preliminary assessment of efficacy and safety in an open clinical study. Neurosurgery, 30:877–881, 1992.
65. Strong, A. J., Miller, S. A., and West, I. C.: Protection of respiration of a crude mitochondrial preparation in cerebral ischemia by control of blood glucose. J. Neurol. Neurosurg. Psychiatry, 48:450–454, 1985.
66. Sugita, K., Kobayashi, S., Shintani, A., et al.: Microneurosurgery for aneurysms of the basilar artery. J. Neurosurg., 51:615–620, 1979.
67. Takeuchi, J.: Aneurysm surgery in patients over the age of 80 years. Br. J. Neurosurg., 7:307–309, 1993.
68. Taki, W., Nishi, S., Yamashita, K., et al.: Selection and combination of various endovascular techniques in the treatment of giant aneurysms. J. Neurosurg., 77:37–42, 1992.
69. Tettenborn, D., and Dycka, J.: Prevention and treatment of delayed ischemic dysfunction in patients with aneurysmal subarachnoid hemorrhage. Stroke, 21(Suppl. 4):85–89, 1990.
70. Van Gijn, J., and Wijdicks, E. F. M.: Medical management of subarachnoid hemorrhage. In Adams, H. P., ed.: Handbook of Cerebrovascular Diseases. New York, Marcel Dekker, 1993, pp. 467–508.
71. Venna, N., and Sabin, T. D.: Tonic focal seizures in nonketotic hyperglycemia of diabetes mellitus. Arch. Neurol., 38:512–514, 1981.
72. Weir, B.: Medical aspects of the preoperative management of aneurysms: A review. Can. J. Neurol. Sci., 6:441–450, 1979.
73. Weir, B.: Aneurysms Affecting the Nervous System. Baltimore, Williams & Wilkins, 1987, pp. 88–93, 429–432, 625–629.
74. Welsh, F. A., Ginsberg, M. D., Rieder, W., et al.: Deleterious effect of glucose pretreatment on recovery from diffuse cerebral ischemia in the cat: II. Regional metabolic levels. Stroke, 11:355–363, 1980.
75. Whiting, D. M., Barnett, G. H., and Little, J. R.: Management of subarachnoid hemorrhage in the critical care unit. Cleve. Clin. Med., 56:775–785, 1989.
76. Wijdicks, E. F. M., Vermeulen, M., Hijdra, A., et al.: Hyponatremia and cerebral infarction in patients with ruptured intracranial aneurysms: Is fluid restriction harmful? Ann. Neurol., 17:137–140, 1985.
77. Winn, H. R., Newell, D. W., Mayberg, M. R., et al.: Early surgical management of poor-grade patients with intracranial aneurysms. Clin. Neurosurg., 36:289–298, 1990.
78. Zubkov, Y. N., Nikiforov, B. M., and Shustin, V. A.: Balloon catheter technique for dilatation of constricted cerebral arteries after aneurysmal SAH. Acta Neurochir. (Wien), 70:665–679, 1984.
79. Zuccarello, M., Marsch, J. T., Schmitt, G., et al.: Effect of the 21-aminosteroid U-74006F on cerebral vasospasm following subarachnoid hemorrhage. J. Neurosurg., 71:98–104, 1989.

Management of Aneurysms of the Anterior Circulation

Intracranial aneurysms can be divided into those that arise from the anterior (carotid) circulation and those from the posterior (vertebrobasilar) circulation. Anterior circulation aneurysms include those that arise from the internal carotid artery or its two terminal branches, the anterior cerebral and middle cerebral arteries. Intracranial aneurysms have also been classified according to shape and etiology into saccular (berry) and nonsaccular types (Table 53–1). Collier coined the term "berry aneurysms" in 1931, in an attempt to portray "their shiny coats and rounded outlines; they hang like berries on the arterial stalks. . . . "[23] Although vivid, this characterization is somewhat inaccurate, because rarely can any intracranial aneurysm be said to possess a long, narrow pedicle with a bulbous, rounded head.

This chapter addresses the general and specific clinical features and management of small and large anterior circulation saccular aneurysms. Because of their unique pathophysiology and technical challenges, giant or nonsaccular anterior circulation aneurysms receive special emphasis in Chapter 54. Internal carotid artery aneurysms that originate proximal to where the vessel penetrates into the subarachnoid space have also been omitted for similar reasons.

Pathogenesis and General Characteristics

In 1887, Eppinger was the first to implicate a defect in the internal elastic lamina of arterial walls in the pathophysiology of saccular intracranial aneurysm formation.[46] Later, Forbus described gap defects, termed "loci minoris resistentiae," that were commonly found in the media of normal arteries and surmised their probable etiological role in aneurysm formation.[54] However, it is now Stehben's belief, based on numerous histological and experimental studies, that there is little or no evidence for a congenital or developmental vessel wall weakness, and that the overwhelming pathogenetic factor in aneurysmal formation and growth is mural degeneration at apices of arterial forks, where sustained hemodynamic stresses are maximal.[205, 208] Polycystic kidney disease, coarctation of the aorta, hypertension, arteriovenous malformations, anomalies of the circle of Willis, female sex, heredity, and connective tissue diseases all can be viewed as aggravating but nonessential pathogenetic factors.*

Because of their shape and relationship to their artery of origin, saccular or berry aneurysms display several anatomical characteristics that distinguish them from other types of intracranial aneurysms (Fig. 53–1).[173, 174] Saccular aneurysms typically (1) arise at bifurcations, usually just distal to a branch from a large parent vessel (e.g., internal carotid–posterior communi-

Table 53–1
TYPES OF ANEURYSMS

Saccular (Berry)
Small (less than 1 cm)
Large or globoid (1.0–2.4 cm)
Giant (2.5 cm or greater)

Nonsaccular
Dissecting
Fusiform
Serpentine
Arteriosclerotic
Traumatic
Infectious (mycotic)
Inflammatory
Neoplastic

---

*See references 17, 27, 36, 37, 38, 55, 94, 101, 103, 104, 118, 123, 125, 135, 147, 154, 155, 156, 162, 169, 171, 179, 187, 188, 189, 208, 218, 227, and 255.

A. L. Day • J. J. Morcos • F. Revilla

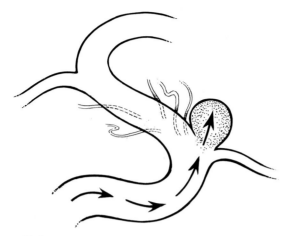

Figure 53–1

Typical anatomical features of saccular aneurysms. Intracranial saccular aneurysms generally (1) arise at a branching site along the parent artery, (2) arise along the outside (convex) surface of a bend in the parent artery, (3) project in the direction of flow *(arrows)* that the parent artery would have if the bend had not been present, and (4) are associated with a specific set of perforators. Aneurysms at specific sites are usually best obliterated with a specific clip type that conforms to the lesion's shape, size, and anatomical relationships to the parent vessel, its branches, and adjacent structures.

cating artery junction); (2) arise along a curve of the parent vessel; (3) point in the direction that flow would have proceeded had the curve not been present; (4) are associated with a specific set of perforators; and (5) are often best managed surgically with a specific clip type.

Incidence and Distribution

The incidence and prevalence of saccular intracranial aneurysms vary, depending on referral patterns and whether the data are derived from clinical, radiological, or pathological (autopsy) sources (Table 53–2). More than 90 per cent of all intracranial aneurysms are found in the vicinity of the circle of Willis, most of which arise from the anterior circulation (Fig. 53–2).[55] Summarizing data from several large clinical series, Table 53–3 outlines the anatomical distribution of aneurysms according to their major trunks of origin. Overall, there is a slight preponderance on the anterior cerebral artery complex, followed closely by the internal carotid artery. In routine autopsy studies, however, which naturally include larger numbers of asymptomatic incidental aneurysms, the middle cerebral artery is the most prevalent location (30 to 36 per cent).[55, 83, 134] Giant aneurysms or incidental lesions discovered prior to rupture have distributions different from those diagnosed following hemorrhage.[32] This diversity of autopsy incidence versus clinical significance underscores the fact that the factors involved in aneurysmal formation may be quite distinct from those that promote rupture.

Aneurysms, particularly those found in the anterior circulation, are more common in women, with a female predominance ranging from 54 to 62 per cent.[55, 102, 243] In surgical series, the male-to-female ratio at the time of presentation is three to two in children, one to one in young adults, and two to three in older adults. This later female dominance may indicate possible hormonal influences in the pathogenesis of intracranial aneurysms.[207] Gender also influences the prevalence of aneurysms at certain anatomical locations. In females, the most common location of aneurysms (ruptured or unruptured) is the supraclinoid carotid (40 per cent ruptured, 66 per cent unruptured). In males, the most common site of ruptured aneurysms is the anterior communicating complex (40 per cent); for unruptured aneurysms, it is the supraclinoid carotid (34 per cent). Females are much more prone than males to developing aneurysms of the ophthalmic segment (3.3 to 1), cavernous segment (2.4 to 1), and posterior communicating artery (2.1 to 1). Males are more prone than females to harboring anterior communicating artery aneurysms (1.4 to 1).

Intracranial aneurysms are more common during middle life, but no age is spared completely. Among symptomatic aneurysms, Fox documented a peak incidence between the ages of 40 and 49 years, while the two Cooperative Studies and Suzuki's report showed an age peak between ages 50 and 59 years.[55, 102, 190, 215] When childhood aneurysms do occur, they are more likely to be associated with vascular anomalies, trauma, infection, or some systemic disease and have a peculiar predilection for the carotid bifurcation.[2, 55]

The prevalence of aneurysm multiplicity is generally higher in autopsy series (25 to 31 per cent) than in large clinical series (15 to 24 per cent).* Females make up between 60 and 81 per cent of cases in which multiple aneurysms are discovered.[3, 55, 134, 140] The internal carotid and middle cerebral segments are particularly prone to multiplicity of aneurysms.†

Natural History: Growth, Size, and Rupture

Whether intracranial aneurysms are present at birth or develop de novo in adulthood, they generally grow. Juvela and colleagues recently followed 142 patients with 181 unruptured aneurysms with an initial median diameter of 4 mm.[93] Of the 27 patients who hemorrhaged over a median follow-up period of 13.9 years, 17 showed clear enlargement over time. Symptomatic aneurysms also tend to be larger at older ages; in one such study, the percentage of aneurysms larger than 8 mm was 16 per cent below age 50 years, 30 per cent between ages 50 and 60 years, and 44 per cent above age 60 years.[213]

The greater prevalence of small aneurysms among the unruptured asymptomatic population, and of larger ones among the ruptured group, has led to the notion that aneurysms reach a certain "critical size" beyond which hemorrhage becomes increasingly probable. Based on autopsy studies, the critical size is believed to be 4 to 5 mm.[26, 70, 206] From clinical experience, critical

---

*References 26, 101, 132, 189, 206, 219, and 255.
†See references 57, 71, 140, 189, 191, and 255.

Table 53–2
ANEURYSM PREVALENCE AND INCIDENCE

Autopsy Series	Year	No. Studied	Prevalence (%)
Multiple routine series*	1928–1990	>130,000	0.3–1.4
Pakarinen[158]	1967	Review	2.0–4.7†
Stehbens[206]	1963	1364	5.6‡
McCormick[130]	1970	1587	7.9‡

Radiological Series, Cerebral Arteriography	Year	No. Studied	Prevalence (%)
Pia et al.[167]	1972	23,876	0.5
Multiple small series[4, 229, 237]	1979–1993	>2,000	1.1–2.7

Clinical Series, Incidence of Aneurysmal Subarachnoid Hemorrhage	Year	Population Base	Incidence (per 100,000)
Pakarinen[158]	1967	439,751	10.3
Fogelholm[53]	1981	241,000	19.4
Bonita et al.[18]	1983	829,464	14.6
Ljunggren et al.[121]	1985	1,460,000	5.7

*See references 24, 124, 130, 132, 158, and 206.
†Forensic series; higher incidence of sudden death.
‡Pathologist specifically searching for incidental aneurysms; little more than a "fullness" at an apical angle could be considered an aneurysm.

size is thought to be between 5 and 10 mm, with an average angiographic diameter reproducibly close to 8 mm.* Although the notion of critical size for saccular aneurysm rupture exists, there is no absolute safe limit below which they do not rupture. In addition, their natural history is far from homogeneous, and the commonly held estimate of rupture risk at 2 per cent per year is undoubtedly in need of further refinement. The current International Study of Unruptured Intracranial Aneurysms, initiated in 1991, is examining these natural

*See references 50, 70, 99, 183, 215, 243, and 245.

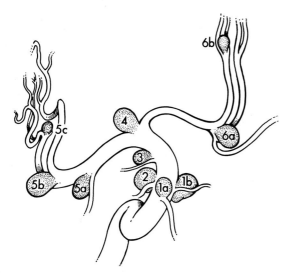

Figure 53–2

Common sites of saccular aneurysms. (1) Ophthalmic segment–internal carotid artery (1a, ophthalmic artery variant; 1b, superior hypophyseal artery variant); (2) posterior communicating–internal carotid artery; (3) anterior choroidal–internal carotid arteries; (4) internal carotid artery bifurcation; (5) middle cerebral artery (5a, proximal to genu; 5b, typical bifurcation at genu; 5c, distal to genu); and (6) anterior cerebral artery (6a, anterior communicating artery; 6b, distal anterior cerebral artery).

history issues as well as the morbidity and mortality of endovascular and microsurgical intervention and, hopefully, will clarify some of these complexities (D. O. Wiebers, personal communication).

Clinical Presentation

In a review of the world literature, Fox noted that 89 per cent of saccular intracranial aneurysms presented with subarachnoid hemorrhage, 7 per cent presented with mass effect, and 4 per cent were incidental, confirming Dandy's statement, in 1941, that "until a sudden rupture, aneurysms are usually silent."[29, 55] In the hope of preempting the catastrophic hemorrhage, numerous studies have searched for possible "warning" symptoms, with an incidence prior to a clear hemorrhage variably quoted between 15 and 60 per cent.* These warning symptoms and signs have been classified on the basis of their presumed pathophysiology into three categories: minor bleed (or "sentinel leak"), aneurysmal expansion, and ischemia.[153] Half of warning events occur within a week of the hemorrhage, and 90 per cent within 6 weeks.[116, 153] The time interval between warning and frank hemorrhage varies widely, probably reflecting individual characteristics between aneurysms. The obvious implication of missing the warning event is a lost opportunity to prevent a devastating hemorrhage.[45, 68]

The classic description of subarachnoid hemorrhage from a ruptured saccular intracranial aneurysm is a sudden and explosive "worst headache of one's life." The resultant clinical picture, regardless of aneurysm location, is usually dominated by the dramatic effects of flooding of the subarachnoid space with blood under arterial pressure.[72, 121, 128] Most patients experience at least a temporary state of altered mentation that is often initially mistaken for a seizure, heart attack, or

*See references 12, 23, 68, 106, 153, 222, 234, and 236.

Table 53–3
ANEURYSM DISTRIBUTION BY LOCATION

Parent Vessel	Percentage at Each Site, Clinical Series*						
	Cooperative Study, 1969 (n = 2,630)	Yoshimoto et al., 1979 (n = 1,000)	Fox, 1983 (n = 3,110)	Rosenorn et al., 1987 (n = 1,076)	Yasargil, 1987 (n = 1,012)	Cooperative Study, 1990 (n = 3,521)	Weighted Averages (n = 12,349)
ICA	41	25	37	26	31.5	30	33.5
ACA	34	39	30.7	36	40.7	39	35.7
MCA	20	17	13.4	27	18.2	22	19.1
BA/VA	3.8	2.3	13.5	8	9.6	7	7.9

*See references 55, 101, 102, 183, 191, 255, and 260.

ICA, internal carotid artery; ACA, anterior cerebral artery complex; MCA, middle cerebral artery; BA/VA, basilar and vertebral artery complex.

ischemic stroke.[51, 55, 239] The "catecholamine surge" of subarachnoid hemorrhage induces electrocardiographic and myocardial changes that may create diagnostic confusion and can cause lethal arrhythmias, pulmonary edema, or heart failure.[1, 11, 127, 223]

The clinical findings in survivors of aneurysm rupture vary, depending on the origin, location, and severity of the hemorrhage and any concomitant increase in intracranial pressure from acute hydrocephalus or intraparenchymal clot. Traditionally, physicians assign a clinical grade to patients harboring ruptured saccular aneurysms, using a system that has been very useful in predicting surgical outcomes but does not differentiate between altered states of consciousness due to systemic derangements, hydrocephalus, or hemorrhage extent (Table 53–4).[81]

Bleeding confined to the subarachnoid space usually produces nonfocal symptoms and signs of increased intracranial pressure and meningeal irritation, including headache, confusion, photophobia, nausea, vomiting, blurred vision, nuchal rigidity, radicular pains, and abducens nerve palsies.[5] A detailed bedside neuro-ophthalmological exam, including funduscopy, allows the detection of retinal, preretinal (subhyaloid), or intravitreous (Terson's sign) hemorrhage or other findings that aid in confirming the clinical diagnosis.[32, 141, 225]

Focal neurological deficits are often indicative of mass effect from an intracranial hematoma, especially when they appear early in the clinical course. The type of deficit subsequently produced differs, depending on the lobe affected and the size of the clot, and may include cranial neuropathies (especially optic and oculomotor nerves) or sensorimotor, visual field, or speech deficits (Table 53–5).

Diagnostic Evaluation

A strong clinical suspicion of an aneurysm can be validated by several diagnostic studies, including computed tomography, lumbar puncture, magnetic resonance imaging, and arteriography. Computed tomography has become indispensable in the evaluation of subarachnoid hemorrhage and is, in general, the first diagnostic test to be ordered in cases in which bleeding is suspected. An unenhanced scan confirms subarachnoid blood in 90 per cent of acute cases and also clarifies associated conditions such as intracranial hematomas, edema, and hydrocephalus. The pattern of hemorrhage suggests the aneurysm site in most instances and allows accurate predictions of the risk of subsequent vasospasm (Table 53–6).[110, 129, 177, 230, 253] Clinical deterioration from rebleeding can be clarified, and the evolution of vasospasm-related edema and ischemia can be followed to resolution or infarction. Computed tomography can also be extremely useful in clarifying the exact anatomical relation of the aneurysm to the skull base, or the presence of thrombosis or calcification within the aneurysm or its walls. This study has limited value as a screening tool, however, because it can reliably visualize aneurysms that are 7 mm or larger. Lumbar puncture is generally reserved for screening patients with potential sentinel bleeds or for confirming bleeding in patients who have a suggestive clinical history but a negative computed tomographic scan.[111]

Compared with computed tomography, magnetic resonance imaging can provide superior detail about regional anatomy and the size, shape, and content of an aneurysm, but it does not visualize acute blood as well. It can, however, detect small amounts of parenchymal blood surrounding aneurysms and thus suggest which one among multiple aneurysms actually

Table 53–4
CLINICAL GRADING OF SUBARACHNOID HEMORRHAGE*

Grade	Condition
I	Asymptomatic or with mild headache
II	Moderate or severe headache, nuchal rigidity
III	Confusion, drowsiness, or mild focal deficit (discounting third nerve palsy)
IV	Stupor or hemiparesis, early decerebrate rigidity
V	Deep coma, extensor posturing

*According to Hunt and Hess scale.[81]

Table 53–5
SPECIFIC ANEURYSM SYNDROMES, ANTERIOR CIRCULATION (SUBARACHNOID ORIGIN)

Characteristic	Percentage with SAH Presentation	Specific Features (Ruptured or Unruptured)
Ophthalmic[32, 180]	22–47	Ipsilateral optic nerve or junctional visual field defect
Superior hypophyseal[32]	33.33	Hypopituitarism; chiasmal or optic tract visual field defect
Posterior communicating[55, 180, 243]	88	Oculomotor nerve palsy affecting pupil (posterior projection); temporal lobe hematoma (lateral projection); retro-orbital pain
Anterior choroidal[55]	100	None (may rarely resemble posterior communicating aneurysm)
Carotid bifurcation[55, 180]	94	Aphasia, contralateral sensorimotor deficit, optic tract syndromes
Middle cerebral[55, 180, 243]	90	Aphasia, contralateral sensory, motor, or visual deficit, seizures
Anterior communicating and distal anterior cerebral[55, 180]	97	Paraparesis, incontinence, amnesia, frontal lobe syndromes, chiasmal syndromes, hypothalamic dysfunction

SAH, subarachnoid hemorrhage.

bled. This study is also superior in demonstrating small infarcts. Recent reports indicate that magnetic resonance angiography can be quite useful in the screening and detection of incidental aneurysms.[16, 63, 195] Despite a 90 per cent sensitivity, however, the low spatial resolution and misleading imaging of low flow and thrombosed lesions can result in suboptimal information for surgical planning.[8]

Cerebral arteriography is currently unsurpassed in its ability to convey the anatomy, physiology, and pathology of the vascular tree. This study remains the gold standard in accurately clarifying aneurysm location and shape and the technical obstacles that face the treating physician. Arteriography is also useful in the detection and evaluation of multiplicity or other associated vascular diseases, the assessment of collateral circulation, the identification of congenital anomalies, and

the diagnosis and treatment of vasospasm.[56] In patients with multiple aneurysms and subarachnoid hemorrhage, the largest aneurysm is generally the offending lesion. Further angiographic clues to the bleeding source include vessel displacements from adjacent hematomas, local vasospasm, irregular aneurysm contour or nipple-like protrusion on the aneurysm, and the escape of contrast agent during the study.

Preoperative Assessment and Management

UNRUPTURED ANEURYSMS

Once an intracranial aneurysm is suspected, the type and timing of diagnostic evaluation and treatment de-

Table 53–6
HEMORRHAGE PATTERNS FROM ANTERIOR CIRCULATION ANEURYSMS[129]

Site	SAH (Cistern)	ICH	IVH (Ventricle)	SDH
Internal Carotid Artery				
Ophthalmic segment	Anterior suprasellar	Medial inferior frontal	Rare	Rare
Posterior communicating artery	Lateral suprasellar, ambient	Medial temporal (near uncus)	Temporal	Inferior lateral convexity
Anterior choroidal artery	Lateral suprasellar, ambient	Rare	Temporal	Rare
Internal carotid artery bifurcation	Lateral suprasellar, proximal sylvian	Basal ganglia	Lateral ventricle	Rare
Middle Cerebral Artery				
Typical bifurcation	Sylvian	Temporal	Temporal	Convexity
Proximal	Lateral suprasellar, proximal sylvian	Temporal, lateral basal ganglia	Temporal or frontal	Rare
Distal	Distal sylvian	Frontal or temporal	Rare	Convexity
Anterior Cerebral Artery				
Anterior communicating artery	Interhemispheric, septal, anterior suprasellar	Inferior frontal (gyrus rectus), often opposite to lesion origin	Anterior third ventricle	Rare
Pericallosal	Interhemispheric	Medial frontal	Rare	Falcine

SAH, subarachnoid hemorrhage; ICH, intracerebral hemorrhage; IVH, intraventricular hemorrhage; SDH, subdural hemorrhage.

pend on whether the lesion is ruptured or unruptured (Table 53–7). Unruptured aneurysms are either *incidental* (discovered during the investigation of unrelated events, such as headache, head trauma, and cerebral ischemia) or *symptomatic* (by virtue of mass effect or thromboembolism). The incidental category may be subdivided into aneurysms that are truly incidental, those that coexist with a ruptured aneurysm, and those associated with other factors (family history or associated genetic diseases). As a group, previously unruptured aneurysms have a 1 to 2 per cent risk of rupture per year.[249] The recently symptomatic aneurysm should be regarded as a much more urgent clinical entity, although no specific natural history data clearly demonstrate this.

The decision to treat unruptured aneurysms rests on an analysis that primarily includes the natural history of the lesion in question, the risks of the proposed treatment, and the benefits derived from that procedure. The natural history of an individual aneurysm is dependent principally on the patient's age and general health, which directly determine life expectancy and cumulative lifetime risk from hemorrhage. Increasing aneurysm size may negatively affect this risk, assuming that larger aneurysms are more rupture-prone. Aneurysms in certain locations (proximal subarachnoid portions of the internal carotid artery) may be less likely to rupture than others.[32] Coexisting intracranial pathologies (ruptured second aneurysm, arteriovenous malformation) also have negative effects on long-term survival of patients.

Surgical risks are also greatly influenced by the patient's age and general medical state. Advanced age, especially when associated with a poor prediscovery neurological state or significant cardiovascular, respiratory, or other systemic disease, increases the likelihood of perioperative complications and reduces the patient's ability to recover from surgically related neurological and systemic injury. Operative risks are also influenced by the aneurysm's size and location, associated arteriosclerosis or calcification, the expertise of the surgical team, and the presence or absence of prior hemorrhage.

The psychological impact of harboring an unclipped intracranial aneurysm is also not an insignificant factor in the decision process. Once an aneurysm has been identified, many patients become quite apprehensive about the "time bomb" in their head and actively seek repair so that future activities will be unencumbered by worry. Since an uncomplicated and unruptured small (5 mm or greater) or large anterior circulation saccular aneurysm can usually be repaired by an experienced microvascular surgeon with a low combined perioperative morbidity and mortality (Table 53–8), surgical treatment is generally advised for patients in good health and who have reasonable life expectancies (5 years or more). In the presence of added risk factors, however, aggressive intervention should be carefully weighed against the symptoms produced by the lesion and the patient's quality life expectancy.

RUPTURED ANEURYSMS

Unlike the unruptured lesion, for which acute risks are generally low and decisions are usually elective, the ruptured saccular intracranial aneurysm is a dramatic intracranial catastrophe, associated with very high morbidity and mortality.* Many patients do not survive to reach the hospital, or die soon thereafter. If untreated surgically, 4.1 per cent of aneurysms would rebleed on the first day and 1.5 per cent would rebleed daily thereafter for 2 weeks.[97, 98, 101, 102] By 6 months, 50 per cent would have rebled at least once. The rebleeding risk stabilizes thereafter at about 3 per cent per year.[89, 90] Without surgical treatment, 18 per cent of patients would be functional survivors at 10 years, 8 per cent would be disabled, and 74 per cent would die.[91] Even with aggressive modern treatment, only about one third of all afflicted patients achieve good functional neurological outcomes.[120] These greatly increased risks, compared with those for unruptured lesions, mandate urgent and occasionally emergent intervention if the natural history is to be substantially altered.

The authors' algorithm for the perioperative management of small or large ruptured anterior circulation aneurysms is outlined in Figure 53–3. Initial management should be directed toward the conditions that could be acutely life-threatening, including common systemic problems such as hypoxia from seizures, respiratory depression, and cardiovascular dysfunction (Table 53–9). Non–contrast-enhanced computed cranial tomography should be done as soon as possible thereafter, especially in the declining or obtunded patient. The pattern and extent of the hemorrhage, the ventricular size, and an evaluation of overall brain "tightness" on the scan should be carefully correlated with the patient's clinical state. Large intraparenchymal clots, alone or combined with acute hydrocephalus, may produce transtentorial herniation early after the onset of

Table 53–7
PREOPERATIVE ASSESSMENT

Ruptured or unruptured?
    Time interval since last bleed
    Clinical grade and dynamic trend (stable, improving, declining)
    Computed tomography findings
        Extent of hemorrhage
        Increased intracranial pressure (edema, hydrocephalus)
        Infarction
General medical status
    Age
    General health
        Prediscovery neurological status
        Cardiovascular and respiratory status
        Other systemic illnesses
Site, size, configuration, number of aneurysms
Surgeon's experience
Modern ancillary support
    Neuroradiology
    Neuroanesthesia
    Nursing

---

*See references 72, 98, 101, 102, 121, and 128.

Table 53–8

SURGICAL MORBIDITY AND MORTALITY FOR UNRUPTURED ANEURYSMS

Series	Year	No. of Patients		No. of Aneurysms		Morbidity (%)			Mortality (%)
Salazar[193]	1980		29		38	3.3			0
Wirth et al.[251]	1983		107		119	6.5			0
Eskesen et al.[47]	1987	Sympt: 27 Incid: 21		Sympt: 30 Incid: 23		15			4
Inagawa et al.[82]	1992		52		52	6			0
Solomon et al.[202]	1994		202	Sympt: 113 Incid: 34 Other: 55		*Size* <7 7–10 11–25 >25	*Early* 3 7 8 16	*Late* 0 2 3 10	0 0 3 10
Nakagawa and Hashi[142]	1994		20		20	0			0

ACA, anterior cerebral artery; MCA, middle cerebral artery; ICA, internal carotid artery; Sympt, symptomatic; Incid, incidental; Other, coexisting with previously ruptured aneurysm; Early, transient morbidity; Late, permanent morbidity; N/A, not available.

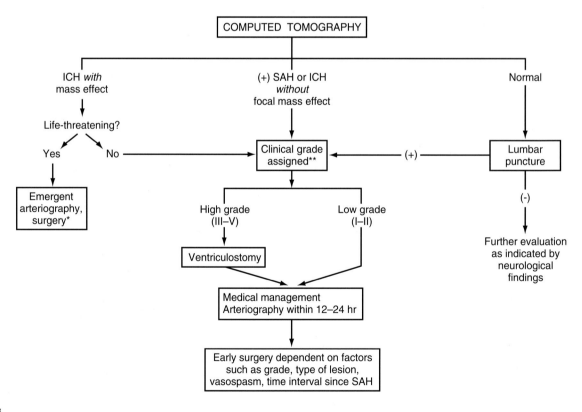

Figure 53–3

Algorithm for the evaluation and management of anterior circulation aneurysms. Asterisk (*) indicates that the surgeon should consider direct surgery without arteriography in rapidly declining patients with classic hematoma patterns. Two asterisks (**) indicate Hunt-Hess clinical grading system (see Table 53–4). CT, computed tomography scan; ICH, intracerebral hematoma; SAH, subarachnoid hemorrhage.

Table 53–9
CAUSES OF POOR OUTCOME

Effects of initial bleed
Vasospasm
Rebleeding
Hydrocephalus
Medical complications
    Cardiac abnormalities
    Electrolyte disturbances
    Thrombophlebitis and pulmonary embolism
    Systemic infection
    Seizures
Surgical complications
    Intraoperative
        Rupture
        Arterial occlusion
        Perforator injury
        Distal embolization
        Direct neural injury
    Postoperative
        Intracranial hemorrhage
        Delayed ischemic deficits
        Systemic complications
        Incomplete clipping

bleeding. Careful scan interpretation usually allows diagnosis of the ruptured aneurysm causing the hematoma with an accuracy rate up to 90 per cent, a factor that may be critical to a patient who is rapidly deteriorating and who cannot afford the time for arteriography.[9, 14, 113, 185]

More severe hemorrhages are often associated with some element of acute hydrocephalus, which may further depress consciousness, producing lethargy that potentially can progress to coma or death. Normal cerebrospinal fluid flow and absorption are impeded by the subarachnoid blood, and bloody cerebrospinal fluid accumulates within the sulci over the convexities to produce a "swollen, angry brain" that represents an acute "external" hydrocephalus. Because the ventricles may then be less able to expand, especially in younger patients with higher ependymal resistance and less cortical atrophy, they remain smaller than expected, and the contribution of acute hydrocephalus and increased intracranial pressure to the depressed level of consciousness can be overlooked or underestimated. This state is often reflected on the scan by smaller but "tight" ventricles combined with prominently delineated convexity gyri highlighted by subarachnoid blood within the sulci. In the context of a drowsy or deteriorating patient, immediate cerebrospinal fluid diversion through a ventriculostomy can be life-saving. The danger of increasing the transmural pressure across the aneurysm wall and promoting rebleeding can be minimized by controlled spinal fluid removal, maintaining higher intraventricular pressures until the aneurysm has been obliterated surgically.

Timing of Surgery

The currently used grading system (see Table 53–4), devised prior to the advent of computed tomography,

is entirely dependent on the neurological state of the patient at the time of assessment. As this system is currently applied, many surgeons delay operative intervention in high-grade patients, a practice that automatically confers a worse prognosis from the complications of rebleeding and vasospasm. The contributions of untreated acute hydrocephalus and increased intracranial pressure to poorer outcomes in high-grade subarachnoid hemorrhage patients are not reflected in this system, and, in the authors' opinion, their impact is greatly underestimated.[10] The ideal grading system should not "prelabel" patients as likely to have poor surgical outcomes until reversible factors (i.e., hydrocephalus) are separated from those that are not, which would allow a more accurate prediction of outcome. Early ventriculostomy placement in patients with altered levels of consciousness and higher clinical grades often improves the neurological state within a few hours, thereby making the patient a more obviously viable surgical candidate.[10, 114, 250]

At the authors' institution, all patients evaluated as grade III or higher have a ventriculostomy placed on arrival, followed by early (within 24 hours) operative obliteration of the aneurysm, unless a life-threatening clot requires emergent intervention. The authors' general exceptions to early surgical intervention for small or large anterior circulation aneurysms include (1) severe fixed neurological deficits, (2) very advanced age or medical debilitation, (3) long-standing grade V clinical state (>4 hours) despite focal clot, and (4) persistent grade IV or V clinical state despite ventriculostomy, especially in older patients. In the past, it was generally accepted dogma to delay surgical intervention in patients with severe angiographic vasospasm, especially if this was combined with an unstable or a declining clinical grade. Now that angioplasty techniques are available, some of these patients may be considered for urgent aneurysm obliteration to eliminate the risk of aneurysm rupture and facilitate aggressive interventional treatment of the vasospasm.[115] Patients at high risk for cerebral vasospasm (as judged by the amount of blood on the admission computed tomography scan) are prophylactically kept well hydrated during the interval of maximal risks.

The authors' approach, combining early ventricular decompression, early surgery, and aggressive fluid volume maintenance in patients at high risk for vasospasm, minimizes the risks of rebleeding, reduces the interval that the brain is subjected to increased intracranial pressure (and thereby reduced perfusion pressure), relaxes the brain during surgery, and greatly facilitates the aggressive treatment of cerebral vasospasm with fluids, medications, and interventional neuroradiological techniques postoperatively. The recent Cooperative Study indicated that in the overall management of 3,521 patients with subarachnoid hemorrhage, 18 per cent and 8 per cent required temporary and permanent cerebrospinal fluid diversion, respectively.[101, 102] The liberal use of preoperative ventriculostomy and the inclusion of more higher-grade patients may increase the need for postoperative shunting but, when combined with early surgery, have not been accompanied by simultaneously increasing rebleeding rates.

The management and surgical outcomes for several recent large clinical series are included in Table 53–10. These results include patients of all clinical grades presenting at random time intervals after hemorrhage. Good outcome rates (and mortality) generally parallel the preoperative clinical grade, averaging 79 per cent (9 per cent) in grades I and II patients, 58 per cent (19 per cent) in grade III patients, 33 per cent (35 per cent) in grade IV patients, and 14 per cent (45 per cent) in grade V patients.[101, 102] Early aggressive intervention has clearly improved the outcome in grade IV and V patients.[10, 114]

General Operative Techniques

INSTRUMENTATION

While a modern operating room is stocked with the most sophisticated and complicated instruments, there is still a place for simplicity, particularly in aneurysm surgery. Whenever possible, the surgeon should establish a routine so that all aspects of the procedure are widely understood by all members of the operating team.

Success begins with a surgeon who has an intimate knowledge of the anatomy of the skull base and the circle of Willis and who uses a delicate operative technique without undue force or pressure. A binocular surgical dissecting microscope is also indispensable.

The basic principles behind the microscope (improved magnification, improved lighting in deep fields, and a stereoscopic perspective for the operating surgeon) allow most procedures to take place in a narrower gap at the skull base, without excessive brain retraction. The authors' current microscope system incorporates a floor-mounted Contravis stand, carefully balanced for each individual case after all ancillary equipment is added and before the scope is sterilely draped. A floor pedal allows the surgeon to adjust focus and field size while leaving the hands free and also provides a switch for intraoperative still photography. The microscope is equipped with a beam splitter, which provides two lateral portals: on one side a binocular eyepiece for the surgical assistant, on the other the video system. Attached television and still cameras not only are excellent teaching tools but also provide essential feedback to the anesthesiologist and nursing staff to improve communications and efficiency of the procedure.

A self-retaining retraction system is mandatory for exposure and dissection of deep brain areas. The blades of these instruments should be applied parallel to the desired plane of exposure and are ideally used to gently hold the bulk of the brain back rather than to forcibly retract it. These retractors should enter the field with a low profile, so as not to disturb the surgeon's ability to place the hands in a comfortable and steady position within the operative field.

A generous array of Yasargil or Sugita clips will take care of virtually all saccular aneurysms of the anterior circulation. Atraumatic clips should also be available in case temporary vascular occlusion is needed. The authors prefer to begin the dissection with a simple set

Table 53–10
MANAGEMENT AND SURGICAL RESULTS FOR RUPTURED ANEURYSMS

Clinical Series	No. of Patients	Management		Surgical	
		Morbidity (%)	*Mortality (%)*	*Morbidity (%)*	*Mortality (%)*
Yoshimoto et al.[260] (1979)	1,000	N/A	N/A	8.4	6.4
Sundt et al.[214] (1982)	722	All grades: 10	17	12	4
		†G1: 3	6	2	2
		G2: 16	11	7	4
Ropper et al.[181] (1984)	112	20	11	N/A	N/A
Ljunggren et al.[121] (1985)	251	19	39	20	5
Rosenorn et al.[183] (1987)	1,076	27	45.5	36	23
Disney et al.[39] (1987)	437	1968–1977: 24	47	18	19
		1978–1985: 23	38	14	11
Chyatte et al.[22] (1988)	244	13	23	14	15
Ohman et al.[151] (1989)	216	AS: 3	6	3	6
		IS: 16	6	16	1.5
		LS: 7	13	8	4.7
Kassell et al.[101, 102] (1990)	3,521	16	26	18	14
Lee (1991)[117]	780	N/A	N/A	2.7	4
Saveland et al.[194] (1992)	325	23	21	24	10.5
Krupp et al.[109] (1994)	131	All grades: 25	13	27.5	5
		G1,2: 10	N/A	11	N/A
		G3: 26	N/A	28	N/A
		G4,5: 63	43	69	14

*Almost all the listed series are restricted to patients with *ruptured aneurysms* of *all clinical grades* being admitted at *random times* after their subarachnoid hemorrhage.
†Only this series uses the Botterell grading system. All others use the Hunt and Hess scale.
‡AS, acute surgery (0–3 days); IS, intermediate surgery (4–7 days); LS, late surgery (>7 days).
G, clinical grade (Hunt and Hess Scale); N/A, not available in article.

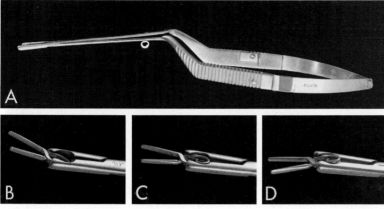

Figure 53–4

Clips and appliers, typical set-up. *A through D.* The most commonly used clip appliers are ones that project the clip either straight ahead or slightly upward or downward, with other variations available if necessary. The authors prefer low-profile clips and appliers so that the view of the operative field will be less obstructed during and after clip placement. *E.* The basic clips for small or large anterior circulation aneurysms include straight, gently curved, and side-angled permanent varieties (both standard and miniature sizes) and straight and gently curved temporary clips. Fenestrated (aperture) clips are added for superior hypophyseal (right-angle large fenestration) or superiorly projecting anterior communicating artery aneurysms (short, straight, small fenestration). The clips are selected early in the procedure, and the numbers and types are further amplified as more of the aneurysm becomes exposed. Temporary clips *(not shown)* are reserved for lesions at high risk for intraoperative rupture before the exposure is completed. To minimize the duration and severity of ischemia, these clips are applied only during the final stages of dissection, after barbiturate-induced burst suppression and mild hypertension have been established. Once the aneurysm has been clipped, the temporary clips should be removed rapidly, and the remaining parts of the aneurysm exposed and collapsed to ensure that the lesion is clipped completely and that all branches and perforators are spared.

that includes straight, gently curved, and side-angled permanent clips, and a straight and curved temporary clip (Fig. 53–4). As the dissection proceeds, further clips are added as the true projection of the aneurysm appears. In general, the shortest clip that will completely obliterate the aneurysm neck is best, and a direct clip is superior to a fenestrated one.

Clip appliers also come in a variety of shapes, sizes, and lengths. In general, a short clip applier is better for peripheral or "typical bifurcation" middle cerebral bifurcation aneurysms, while longer appliers are more useful for deeper portions of the circle of Willis. The authors currently prefer a low-profile applier system, with clip angles varied between 10 degrees up, straight, 15 degrees down, right or left. A variable angle clip applier is useful when more extreme clip application angles are required. Before the aneurysm dissection is begun, the nomenclature should be carefully reviewed with the nursing personnel so that there is no confusion about which clip or applier is desired during critical moments.

Skull fixation, also beneficial for microsurgical procedures, is generally obtained using a three-point fixation apparatus. Radiolucent skull clamps have recently become available, and at the authors' institution, they are utilized for all aneurysm cases or any other type of vascular procedure in which intraoperative arteriography could be of potential value. In cases in which operative difficulty will probably be high (e.g., complex shape, calcifications or thrombus within aneurysm, giant size), an arterial sheath is placed in the femoral artery before the procedure is begun, unless the cervical carotid artery is to be exposed during the procedure. When intraoperative arteriography is thought to be unlikely, the groin is left unobstructed and available to the neuroradiologist should the need arise.

Evoked potential and electroencephalographic monitoring also have significant value in the intraoperative management of anterior circulation aneurysms. Evoked potentials are reliable indicators of perfusion abnormalities through a parent vessel whose lumen may be obstructed during clipping; they are also useful estimators of the adequacy of collateral circulation. Electroencephalographic monitoring is useful primarily in defining burst suppression from etomidate or barbiturates during temporary clipping intervals.[21, 58, 137]

HEAD POSITION AND FIXATION

After induction of satisfactory general anesthesia, the patient is positioned supine on a standard operating table. As the fixation apparatus is applied to the head, the blood pressure is carefully monitored to avoid significant elevations that may precipitate aneurysm rupture. The ipsilateral anterior prong of the clamp should be placed behind the ear, just above the ipsilateral mastoid region, and the other prongs should be placed high enough on the posterior and contralateral skull to provide secure fixation without interfering with the operative field. The head is then gently directed vertex down, to facilitate gravitational retraction on the frontal and temporal lobes; elevated slightly higher than the heart, to facilitate venous drainage; and turned between 30 and 60 degrees, depending on the location of the lesion to be approached. A shoulder roll beneath the ipsilateral shoulder is often useful in allowing gentle neck turning without excessive torque on the airway or cervical vascular structures (Fig. 53–5).

CRANIOTOMY

After the placement of appropriate electrodes for evoked potential monitoring, the scalp is then prepped and draped. As a general rule, the scalp incision begins at the midline, curves backward just behind the hairline, and then extends downward to end at the zygoma 1 cm anterior to the ear (see Fig. 53–5). Almost all anterior circulation aneurysms can be secured through the pterional approach, with the surgeon taking advantage of natural planes and portals that allow exposure of the basal brain surface and circle of Willis without significant brain retraction. A free bone flap is generally preferred, and to provide unimpeded visualization of the desired area, the temporalis muscle must be incised and retracted. Ideally, the muscle should be maximally mobilized while the surgeon avoids injuring the frontalis nerve or anterior branch of the superficial temporal artery. Turning a combined skin and muscle flap (muscle-splitting technique) minimizes risks to these structures, but the bulk of temporalis muscle reflected anteriorly and inferiorly may limit exposure of the skull base (Fig. 53–6A). Posterior and inferior reflection of the temporalis muscle and fascia separate from the scalp flap (interfascial technique) carries a significant risk of frontalis nerve palsy, but the greatly enhanced basal visualization makes this approach preferable in many instances (see Fig. 53–6B).[55, 204, 255, 258] The scalp flap and temporalis muscles are maintained in the desired position with the liberal use of low profile fishhook retractors.

After a bolus of mannitol, 0.5 mg per kg, is administered, a frontal burr hole is placed just superior to the frontal-zygomatic suture and just behind the temporalis line. A second hole is placed in the temporalis squama low and 3 cm posterior to the initial opening. The dura is stripped away from the burr hole edges with the use of a small angled curet, wide enough to allow a good initial purchase of the footplate attachment of the craniotome. The burr holes are then connected with the craniotome in the desired shape of the free bone flap perimeter. Slight variations in the degree of bone removal depend on the specific lesion to be approached. The bone between the two burr holes overlying the lateral sphenoid ridge is thinned with the combined use of the drill and rongeur, and the bone flap is elevated by a final gentle controlled "fracture" across the thinned residual isthmus.

The remaining portions of the lateral sphenoid wing and the anterior-inferior temporal squama are removed with the rongeur, applying bone wax as needed to control osseous bleeding. Holes are drilled in the skull for dural tack-up sutures and later reapproximation of the bone flap. The dura is separated from the medial extension of the sphenoid ridge, and bone is removed to leave only a thin rim of superior and lateral posterior orbital wall down to the base of the anterior clinoid

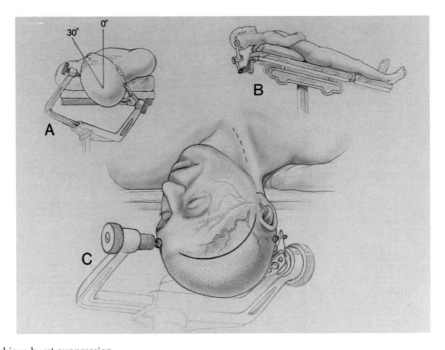

Figure 53–5

Operative position, skull fixation, and scalp incision. After the incision has been outlined, the scalp is fixated in a three- or four-pronged skull clamp, positioned so that the surgical field and the position of the surgeon's hands are not obstructed by the superiormost pins on each side. The third and fourth pins should be positioned securely beneath the head so that downward pressure on the surgical field from above does not result in slippage. At the authors' institution, a radiolucent headholder is used in all aneurysm procedures to allow intraoperative arteriography if needed. A femoral catheter is placed beforehand for complex aneurysms, while for simpler lesions, the groin is left unimpeded should an intraoperative arteriogram become necessary.

A. After fixation, the head is placed slightly higher than the level of the heart and turned the appropriate degrees to place the operative field into ideal position (see Figs. 53–11, 53–12, 53–17, 53–19, and 53–21). *B.* For a pterional approach, the vertex of the skull is dropped slightly to allow gravitational distraction of the frontal and temporal lobes. Evoked potential electrodes are applied in almost all cases, both to monitor ischemic changes during the procedure and to regulate the amount of barbiturates needed to achieve burst suppression.

C. The scalp incision *(solid line)* extends from the midline to the zygoma and is gently curved to stay approximately 1 cm behind the hairline. The inferior part of the incision stays within 1 cm of the tragus, to avoid injury to the frontalis branch of the facial nerve and to spare the anterior branch of the superficial temporal artery. The cervical carotid bifurcation region is marked *(dotted line)*, prepped, and draped into the field in cases where a need for proximal control is anticipated.

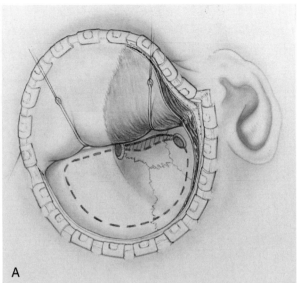 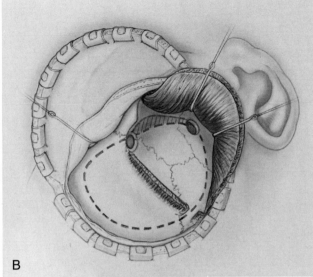

Figure 53–6

Types of temporalis muscle incisions and craniotomy. *A.* Muscle-splitting technique. The scalp and temporalis fascia are reflected as a single unit anteriorly and inferiorly. Two burr holes are placed on each side of the sphenoid wing, and connected with a rongeur *(stripped area)* and a high-speed drill *(dotted line)*. This method carries little risk to the frontalis nerve, but the muscle bulk over the pterion inhibits basal exposure, a particular disadvantage for some aneurysms. *B.* Interfascial technique. The scalp is reflected anteriorly independent of the temporalis muscle until the fat pad carrying the frontalis nerve is encountered. The fat pad and its investing fascia are then swept forward, and the temporalis muscle is detached and retracted posteriorly and inferiorly. The bone flap is then turned in a fashion similar to that for the muscle-splitting technique, with a small cuff of temporalis muscle and fascia left on the flap for closure. The skull base, orbital roof, and sphenoidal compartment of the deep sylvian fissure can now be seen more easily with less brain retraction.

process (Fig. 53–7). The meningo-orbital artery is isolated, coagulated, and sectioned to facilitate further medial ridge flattening. For proximal carotid aneurysms, the remaining thinned orbital walls are removed to expose the periorbita and then followed medially until the edge of the optic nerve at the posterior orbital margin is encountered. The remainder of the anterior clinoid process is then removed intradurally, while the surgeon simultaneously views any disturbances to the aneurysm or other structures (Fig. 53–8).[31, 33, 41, 149]

The dura is then opened in a semicircular fashion over the sylvian fissure, with its base on the drilled-down portion of the sphenoid ridge. The dural flap is tightly elevated anteroinferiorly to secure an unobstructed view to the skull base along the sphenoid ridge medially. If the brain is tight despite mannitol, cerebrospinal fluid may be released by opening the ventriculostomy, if present, or by gently retracting the frontal lobe to open the basal cisterns (for anterior circulation aneurysms approached pterionally, the authors do not routinely employ intraoperative spinal drainage). Patience will usually be rewarded, and as more of the bloody cerebrospinal fluid is removed, the swollen and angry brain will gradually "relax." Hyperventilation or partial hematoma evacuation can be added as indicated.

The real key to a successful anterior circulation aneurysm operation is the arachnoid dissection, beginning with a liberal opening of the sylvian fissure (see Fig. 53–7). The authors prefer to initiate this process in a lateral-to-medial direction, regardless of the location of the aneurysm or presence of prior rupture. Using a round arachnoid knife, the surgeon separates the su-

perficial adhesions between the frontal and the temporal lobes, beginning approximately 2 to 3 cm posterior to the sphenoid ridge on the frontal lobe side of the sylvian veins. This path is continued medially with gentle forceps spreading until the M_2 branches of the middle cerebral artery are encountered within the insular compartment of the sylvian fissure. The M_2 branches are then followed proximally to the genu, and the fissure opened further in an "inside-to-outside" direction. The frontotemporal adhesions are most problematic anteromedially but can usually be separated without significant parenchymal injury. The basal cisterns surrounding the internal carotid artery and optic nerves are then opened to further relax and broaden the operative exposure. When the procedure is completed, the frontal and temporal lobes fall apart away from the sphenoid ridge and orbital roof and are gently held apart by retractors placed parallel to the brain surface. Thus, a broad view of basal structures is provided, without sacrifice of the sphenoparietal veins.

Specific Aneurysm Sites

Anterior circulation saccular aneurysms are broadly divided into three groups, depending on their origin from the internal carotid, middle cerebral, or anterior cerebral arteries. Each group contains several common sites that produce special clinical problems and require different operative considerations. The subarachnoid portion of the internal carotid artery contains four sites of aneurysm development, each of which have an ori-

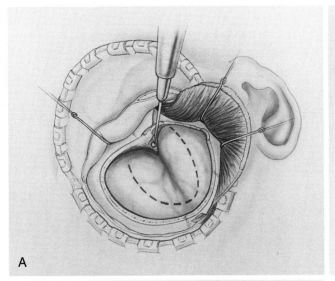

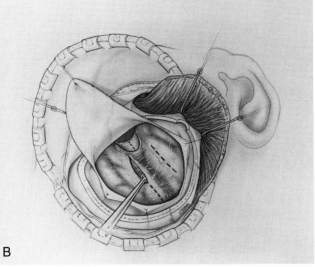

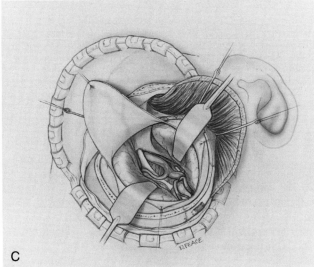

Figure 53–7

Dural incision, sylvian fissure splitting. *A.* The sphenoid ridge and bony indentations of the orbital roof are removed with a rongeur and a high-speed drill to produce a smooth, flat sphenoid surface down to the orbitomeningeal artery. This vessel is coagulated and sectioned if more medial bone removal is required (see Fig. 53–8). The dura is incised in a semicircle *(dotted line)* based on the sphenoid ridge. *B.* The sylvian fissure is generally opened from lateral to medial, on the frontal side of the superficial sylvian veins, with a round arachnoid knife. When the brain is excessively tight, the frontal lobe may be gently retracted to open the carotid and interpeduncular cisterns *(short dotted line)*. For typical bifurcation middle cerebral artery aneurysms (see Fig. 53–15), a superior temporal gyrus approach may be useful *(long dotted line)*, especially when associated with a temporal lobe clot. *C.* At the end of a broad fissure splitting, the entire course of the internal carotid and middle cerebral arteries can be inspected from the anterior clinoid process to just beyond the genu. Whenever possible, the veins of the sylvian fissure and sphenoparietal sinus are preserved to minimize venous congestion.

gin and intimate association with named internal carotid artery branches or perforators, including (1) the ophthalmic segment, which produces two distinct variants, the ophthalmic and superior hypophyseal types; (2) the communicating segment; (3) the choroidal segment; and (4) the terminal carotid bifurcation. The middle cerebral artery harbors two common aneurysm sites, including (5) the typical bifurcation and (6) the proximal varieties. Finally, the anterior cerebral artery gives rise to two common types of aneurysms: (7) the anterior communicating type and (8) the distal (pericallosal) lesion. A schematic representation of the various anterior circulation aneurysm types is presented in Figure 53–2.*

OPHTHALMIC SEGMENT (INTERNAL CAROTID ARTERY) ANEURYSMS

Anatomy and Terminology

The ophthalmic segment is typically the longest subarachnoid segment of the internal carotid artery, begin-

*See references 55, 166, 173, 174, 243, and 255.

ning at the dural ring and ending at the origin of the posterior communicating artery.[61] There are two major arterial bends in the ophthalmic segment that create hemodynamic stresses on flow that predispose to aneurysm formation. The first bend, best seen on lateral views, occurs as the carotid artery ascends and then bends sharply posteriorly after penetrating the dura. The second bend, best appreciated on a dorsal view, is a gentler, medial-to-lateral curve as the artery exits from the clinoidal segment medial to the anterior clinoid process and then arcs laterally as it ascends toward its terminal bifurcation.

The ophthalmic segment also has two major branches, both of which typically originate just above the dural ring. The first, largest, and best known is the ophthalmic artery. This vessel usually arises at the base of the first bend, from the dorsal or dorsomedial surface of the internal carotid artery immediately beneath the lateral aspect of the overlying optic nerve. Several large perforating vessels also arise from the ophthalmic segment, the largest of which has been named the superior hypophyseal artery.[30, 184] These perforators supply the dura around the cavernous sinus, the supe-

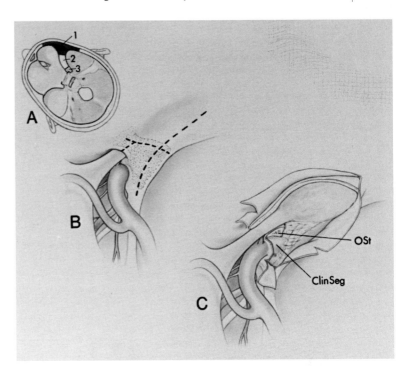

Figure 53–8

Intradural clinoid removal. *A.* The extradural bone removal is shown, including the craniotomy (1, *darkened area*) and most of the sphenoid ridge and posterior orbital roof until the optic nerve is encountered at the back of the orbit (2, *clear area*). The dura is then opened, and the remaining bone of the anterior clinoid process, optic strut, and optic canal (3, *stippled area*) is removed while the aneurysm is directly visualized. *B.* The dotted lines mark the dural incision overlying the clinoid and include a limb to section the falciform ligament to untether the optic nerve. *C.* Drilling down the optic strut (OSt) allows isolation of the clinoid segment (ClinSeg) of the internal carotid artery, which may then be used for proximal control as necessary.

rior aspect of the pituitary gland and stalk, and the optic nerves and chiasm. They typically arise from the medial or ventromedial surface of this segment, usually along the second medial-to-lateral bend of the internal carotid artery prior to the origin of the posterior communicating artery. This ventral origin, together with the gentle downward slope of the dural ring posteriorly, often places the origin of the superior hypophyseal artery on a horizontal plane below the level of both the anterior clinoid process and the ophthalmic artery.

Ophthalmic segment aneurysms are divided herein into two large categories, depending on an association of the aneurysm neck with the arterial branches of the segment.[32] Ophthalmic artery aneurysms typically arise along the first bend of the internal carotid artery just distal to the origin of the ophthalmic artery, and initially project dorsally or dorsomedially toward the optic nerve (Fig. 53–9). Superior hypophyseal artery aneurysms have no association with the ophthalmic artery and, instead, incorporate the perforating branches to the hypophysis in their origins. Small superior hypophyseal artery aneurysms usually arise from the inferior or inferomedial surface of the internal carotid artery just opposite and slightly distal to the origin of the ophthalmic artery, lateral to the sella and medial to the internal carotid artery and anterior clinoid process (Fig. 53–10). Because the space medial to the internal carotid artery is limited, most larger lesions eventually expand medially or superomedially above the diaphragma sellae into the suprasellar space.

Clinical and Radiographic Features

The clinical presentation of ophthalmic segment aneurysms includes roughly equal proportions between visual symptoms, hemorrhage, and incidental discov-

ery (see Table 53–5).* Most ophthalmic segment aneurysms arise in women, and their incidence is probably greatly underestimated because of the apparently lower hemorrhage rates. Approximately one half of symptomatic ophthalmic segment aneurysms present with visual loss, almost all of which are giant lesions (more than 2.5 cm in external diameter). Smaller lesions may produce acute blindness if they rupture and bleed directly into the overlying optic nerve. Otherwise, the visual loss from ophthalmic artery aneurysms occurs gradually as the lesion progressively elevates the lateral portion of the optic nerve superiorly and medially, angulating the nerve against the sharp edge of the falciform ligament (see Fig. 53–9) to produce a unilateral visual loss typically initially noted in the ipsilateral inferior nasal field. When suprasellar extension of superior hypophyseal artery aneurysms occurs, the entire optic apparatus is elevated, with the accompanying pressure directed more toward the chiasm than toward the optic nerve (see Fig. 53–10). Sharp angulation against the falciform ligament is not typical, and visual field deficits are more closely akin to those seen with pituitary tumors.

The high frequency of ophthalmic segment lesions reaching large or giant proportions without bleeding is probably explained by their reinforcement by adjacent structures. The fundus of an ophthalmic artery aneurysm expands upward and medially into the optic nerve, while superior hypophyseal artery aneurysms initially are reinforced by the dura of the lateral sellar wall and roof of the cavernous sinus.

Small ophthalmic segment aneurysms are frequently not well seen on computed tomography because of their close approximation to the skull base. Small or large

---

*See references 32, 48, 49, 55, 243, and 255.

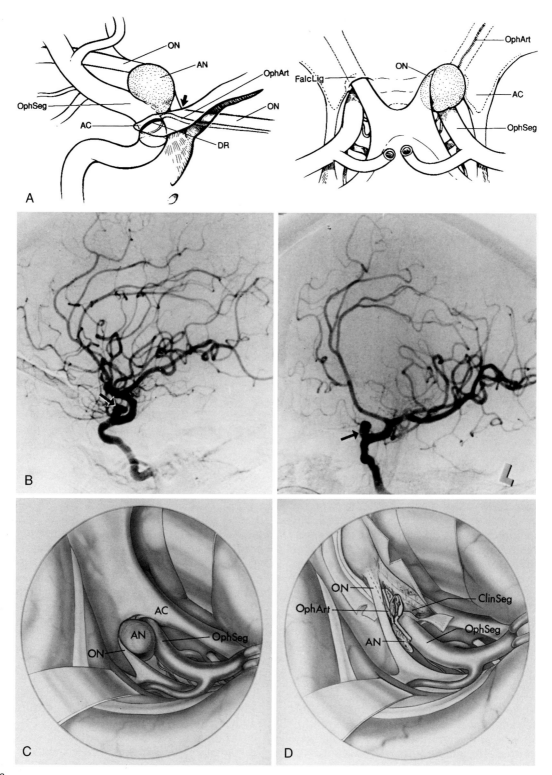

Figure 53–9

Ophthalmic artery aneurysm. *A.* Lateral *(left)* and dorsal *(right)* schematic views, anterior clinoid intact. As the aneurysm enlarges, the optic nerve is elevated, displaced medially, and sharply angulated against the falciform ligament. The anterior clinoid process inhibits the view of the proximal aneurysm neck and ophthalmic artery origin. *B.* Arteriogram, lateral and oblique views. The aneurysm *(arrow)* originates just beyond the ophthalmic artery takeoff and projects largely superiorly and slightly medially, above the posterior bend of the internal carotid artery. *C.* Initial operative view, right pterional approach. The cervical carotid artery has been draped into the field, to be available if needed. Note that the ophthalmic artery is obscured from view by the aneurysm and the anterior clinoid process. *D.* Final operative view, clipping. The anterior clinoid process has been extensively removed to expose the clinoidal segment (see Fig. 53–8). The deep blade of a side-angled clip is placed into the ophthalmic artery–aneurysm junction, then rotated medial to the aneurysm, ending in a plane parallel to the long axis of the internal carotid artery. The aneurysm is then aspirated, and the parent vessel inspected for patency. ON, optic nerve; OphSeg, ophthalmic segment; ClinSeg, clinoidal segment; OphArt, ophthalmic artery; AC, anterior clinoid process; DR, dural ring; FalcLig, falciform ligament; arrow, point of optic nerve compression; AN, aneurysm.

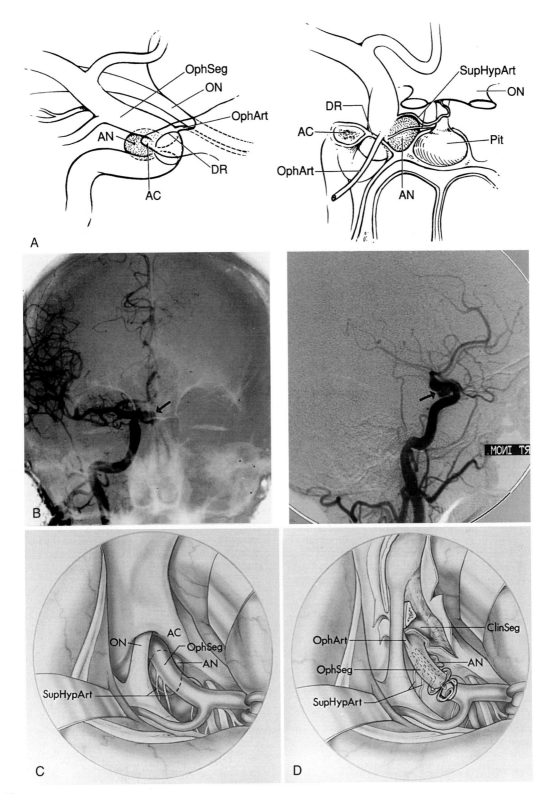

Figure 53–10

Superior hypophyseal artery aneurysm. *A.* Lateral *(left)* and anterior *(right)* schematic views, anterior clinoid intact. Note the ventromedial origin of the aneurysm (independent of the ophthalmic artery origin) and its initial projection against the lateral sella wall. Also note that the anterior clinoid process inhibits the view of the proximal aneurysm neck, but in a region different from that seen with ophthalmic artery lesions (see Fig. 53–9A). *B.* Arteriogram, anteroposterior and lateral views. The aneurysm *(arrow)* balloons ventrally and medially into the suprasellar space (anteroposterior view) and appears to project toward or into the cavernous sinus on the lateral view. Note that the aneurysm origin has no relationship to the ophthalmic artery origin. *C.* Initial operative view, right pterional approach. Note the aneurysm's medial position, and the multiple perforators (superior hypophyseal arteries) near its origin. *D.* Final operative view, clipping. The anterior clinoid process has been extensively removed in a fashion similar to that for ophthalmic artery aneurysms. A fenestrated clip is placed parallel to the internal carotid artery to reconstruct the carotid lumen. The butt of the clip must spare the posterior communicating artery, while the tips are advanced to the border of the dural ring. The aneurysm is then aspirated, and the internal carotid artery inspected for patency. The superior hypophyseal arteries should be spared, if possible, to reduce ischemic damage to the optic nerves or chiasm. ON, optic nerve; OphSeg, ophthalmic segment; ClinSeg, clinoidal segment; OphArt, ophthalmic artery; SupHypArt, superior hypophyseal arteries; AC, anterior clinoid process; DR, dural ring; Pit, pituitary gland; AN, aneurysm.

ophthalmic segment aneurysms do not erode the skull base enough to be detectable on the bone sections of computed tomography, and if clinoidal erosion is noted, an aneurysm originating more proximally from the clinoidal segment should be strongly suspected.[34, 35] Magnetic resonance imaging (scans and angiography) can identify these lesions more easily. However, the curves of the carotid artery in this region may still create some diagnostic uncertainty, and cerebral arteriography remains the definitive diagnostic test. Ophthalmic artery aneurysms are easiest to diagnose on the lateral view, as they always arise just distal to the ophthalmic artery and project superiorly or superomedially (see Fig. 53–9). Superior hypophyseal artery aneurysms have no clear association with the ophthalmic artery origin but can be clearly seen to arise proximal to the posterior communicating artery, projecting medially or inferomedially to often produce an erroneous arteriographic interpretation that they are extending "into" the cavernous sinus (see Fig. 53–10).[108, 148]

On rare occasions, aneurysms arise more distally from the ophthalmic segment and have no clear association with the ophthalmic or superior hypophyseal arteries. These lesions, termed "dorsal" carotid artery aneurysms, appear to be pure hemodynamically induced lesions originating at the dorsal carotid surface several millimeters distal to the ophthalmic artery takeoff.[142]

Surgical Approaches

With proper lesion exposure and a firm understanding of parasellar and vascular anatomy, the surgeon should be able to clip most ophthalmic segment aneurysms with low risks to the brain or visual apparatus.* Carotid ligation or endovascular treatments should be considered secondary alternatives, as the risks of stroke are higher from parent vessel sacrifice, the visual system is not as effectively decompressed, and complete thrombosis of the aneurysm is not ensured.[57, 65]

The head position, craniotomy flap, and amount of basal bone removed during surgery for ophthalmic segment aneurysms are outlined in Figures 53–8 and 53–11. Although the neck should always be prepped into the operative field, proximal control can be gained either within the clinoidal segment intracranially or via a cervical carotid exposure. Regardless of the method chosen, excellent visualization of the internal carotid artery and its branches is mandatory for both aneurysm types. Extensive clinoidal removal is frequently required for safe and accurate clipping, especially for larger lesions.[41] With unruptured aneurysms, extradural clinoidal removal can be done safely. Following subarachnoid hemorrhage, or with fusion between the clinoid processes, the authors strongly believe that the clinoid tip should be removed intradurally while the aneurysm is simultaneously visualized.[13, 33, 34, 87, 149]

Because some optic nerve displacement is usually necessary for visualizing the proximal neck, the falciform ligament should be sectioned before the aneurysm is manipulated. The proximal neck of the ophthalmic artery originates just distal to the ophthalmic artery, while the distal neck is usually unencumbered by major branch attachments (see Fig. 53–9). Any perforators to the optic nerves, chiasm, or hypophysis should be dissected free and spared. Straight or side-angled clips, closed down parallel to the course of the internal carotid artery and sparing the ophthalmic artery, satisfactorily secure most ophthalmic artery lesions. "Dorsal" carotid artery aneurysms are handled in a similar fashion.[142] Small ophthalmic artery aneurysms can often be clipped from a contralateral approach between or behind the optic nerves.[146]

Small superior hypophyseal artery aneurysms may be initially hidden from the surgeon by the overlying internal carotid artery and anterior clinoid process.[108] In large and giant varieties, the internal carotid artery is displaced slightly laterally and superiorly, and the aneurysm neck is often so wide and long that the entire carotid wall appears to be incorporated. By carefully adhering to the dural ring surface, the surgeon can separate the parasellar origin of the aneurysm from the clinoidal dura, thus freeing up the proximal neck. The posterior communicating artery or its thalamoperforating branches are often draped over the distal end of the aneurysm, and these vessels must be carefully identified, separated, and preserved (see Fig. 53–10). Superior hypophyseal artery lesions are usually best obliterated with a fenestrated clip whose blades pass over and then run parallel to the internal carotid artery, spanning the distance between the posterior communicating artery and the dural ring. Although the superior hypophyseal arteries do not generally supply brain parenchyma, some reach the optic chiasm, and every attempt should be made to spare them from the surgical clip.

POSTERIOR COMMUNICATING ARTERY (INTERNAL CAROTID ARTERY) ANEURYSMS

Anatomy and Terminology

The communicating segment of the internal carotid artery begins with the takeoff of the posterior communicating artery and ends at the origin of the anterior choroidal artery.[61] Because of its short length, only one aneurysm develops from this segment, traditionally termed a posterior communicating artery aneurysm.[67] This segment has two major bends and one major named branch, the posterior communicating artery. The first bend, best appreciated on a lateral view, begins at the end of the ophthalmic segment, where the artery begins an upward curve as it nears its terminal bifurcation. The hemodynamic flow from this change in direction creates a potential aneurysm site that projects posteriorly and sometimes slightly inferiorly. The second bend represents a continuance of the medial-to-lateral curve that originated in the clinoidal segment and continues to the carotid artery termination.

The posterior communicating artery originates from

---

*See references 13, 32, 42, 74, 107, and 259.

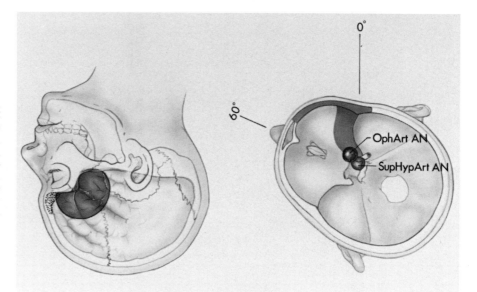

Figure 53–11

Operative position and bone removal *(darkened area)*, ophthalmic segment aneurysm. The head is generally turned 60 degrees, and the craniotomy includes a low frontal extension and an interfascial temporalis muscle incision (see Fig. 53–6*B*) to allow access to the orbital roof and anterior clinoid process without undue frontal lobe retraction. OphArt AN, ophthalmic artery aneurysm; SupHypArt AN, superior hypophyseal artery aneurysm.

the posteromedial surface of the internal carotid artery, courses medially and inferiorly, penetrates the membrane of Liliequist, and joins the posterior cerebral artery just lateral to the terminal basilar artery bifurcation. Several large perforators also originate from the communicating segment (unnamed) or posterior communicating artery (collectively called the anterior thalamoperforating arteries), which must be visualized and preserved at surgery.[184] These small vessels often run near the posterior communicating artery through much of its course and may be adherent to the aneurysm wall.

The typical posterior communicating artery aneurysm arises just beyond the origin of the posterior communicating artery, and points posteriorly, slightly inferiorly, and slightly laterally. Depending on the degree of inferior or lateral projection, two distinct variants arise: (1) posterior, and often inferior, lesions extend medial to the tentorial incisura and may compress the oculomotor nerve at the point where that nerve enters the dura lateral to the posterior clinoid process; and (2) lateral lesions enlarge above the tentorium, often densely adherent to the medial temporal lobe surface.[28] Neither type primarily projects toward the sella, because the posterior communicating artery, together with the lateral curve of the internal carotid artery as it nears its terminal bifurcation, prevents medial extension.

Clinical and Radiographic Features

Posterior communicating artery aneurysms represent the most common type of internal carotid artery aneurysm in adults and are the most common specific type of aneurysm found in females.* These lesions frequently present when small, less than 1 cm, producing retro-orbital headaches, oculomotor nerve deficits, invariably involving the pupil, or subarachnoid hemorrhage. The distinct clinical features and patterns of

hemorrhage are outlined in Tables 53–5 and 53–6. This aneurysm and other distal internal carotid artery lesions have a risk of rupture higher than that of ophthalmic segment aneurysms, as their walls and fundus are not secondarily reinforced by adjacent structures to the degree seen with more proximal lesions. Visual loss from optic tract compression is rare, and cranial neuropathies (other than oculomotor nerve dysfunction) do not occur.

Surgical Approaches

The operative position and extent of bone removal to expose this lesion are similar to that required for anterior choroidal, internal carotid bifurcation, and proximal middle cerebral artery aneurysms (Fig. 53–12).[159, 216] A muscle-splitting temporalis incision is generally chosen for its safety and simplicity, unless other coexisting lesions warrant a different view of the skull base (see Fig. 53–6*B*). The sylvian fissure is split from lateral to medial, as described in Figure 53–7, until the entire course of the internal carotid artery and the M_1 segment of the middle cerebral artery is delineated. Wide opening of the sylvian fissure greatly facilitates the safety of clipping but must be done with caution in laterally projecting cases to avoid avulsion of the fundus from its temporal lobe attachments. In such cases, a more frontal approach is warranted until the aneurysm neck is visualized, but the wider separation between the neck and the posterior communicating artery makes the clipping very straightforward.

With the posteriorly projecting type, part of the fundus, especially in patients presenting with oculomotor nerve deficits, is hidden by the basal dura of the tentorial incisura (Fig. 53–13). When the ophthalmic segment is shortened, or when the anterior clinoid process is elongated, the clinoid may have to be partially removed to secure adequate exposure and proximal control of the internal carotid artery. Posterior communicating artery aneurysms always arise distal to the origin of the posterior communicating artery. Even

___

See references 55, 112, 133, 176, 243, and 255.

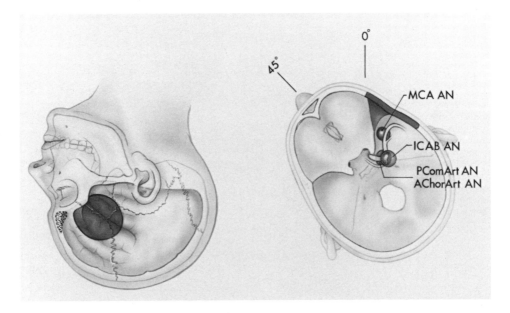

Figure 53–12

Operative position and bone removal *(darkened area)*, posterior communicating, anterior choroidal, internal carotid bifurcation, and proximal middle cerebral aneurysms. The head is generally turned 45 degrees, and the amount of bone removal is similar for each of these aneurysms. The muscle-splitting temporalis incision (see Fig. 53–6*A*) is quite satisfactory for posterior communicating and anterior choroidal lesions. The deeper position of the carotid bifurcation or proximal middle cerebral arteries requires a more basal angle of view, making the interfascial temporalis incision (see Fig. 53–6*B*) preferable for these types of aneurysms. MCA AN, proximal middle cerebral artery aneurysm; PComArt AN, AChorArt AN, posterior communicating or anterior choroidal artery aneurysm; ICAB AN, internal carotid artery bifurcation aneurysm.

when this vessel's course is obscured from view by the aneurysm, its origin is represented as a "flattened" spot at the proximal base of the aneurysm at its seeming junction with the internal carotid artery. Gently elevating the aneurysm base away from the dura allows visualization of two "indentations," the first and most proximal representing the internal carotid artery–posterior communicating artery junction, and the second and more distal representing the posterior communicating artery–aneurysm junction. With care, the posterior communicating artery can be gently dissected away from the anterior wall of the aneurysm, allowing the proximal clip blade to be clearly placed into the more distal indentation so as to spare the origin of this vessel from its jaws. The surgeon places the other clip blade distal to the aneurysm, carefully sparing the anterior choroidal artery or other perforators while gently hugging the internal carotid wall.

Many posterior communicating aneurysms, especially those presenting with oculomotor nerve palsies, are bilobed, with the terminal lobe partially hidden from view by the incisura. This distal "bubble" usually lodges in the oculomotor trigone, where the aneurysm fundus becomes intimately adherent to the oculomotor nerve and dura. Closure of the clip frequently disrupts these adhesions, leading to arterial bleeding that ceases when the clip is allowed to close completely. The authors prefer a gently curved clip that incorporates the entire medial extent of the aneurysmal bulge, as the incidence of delayed recurrence can be significant and difficult to manage if the aneurysm is not properly obliterated initially.[192] The surgeon should advance the clip just beyond the course of the posterior communicating artery, without compromising its patency or

that of the anterior thalamoperforators, internal carotid perforators, or anterior choroidal artery. After the clip is properly situated, the aneurysm should be punctured and detached from its dural adhesions, both to decompress the oculomotor nerve and to facilitate further inspection. The membrane of Liliequist is opened widely to display and free up any tethering or compromise of the posterior communicating artery and its accompanying thalamoperforating vessels. These vessels should also be inspected from the medial side of the carotid artery through the opticocarotid interval, a path that often provides the best view of these channels.

ANTERIOR CHOROIDAL ARTERY (INTERNAL CAROTID ARTERY) ANEURYSMS

Anatomy and Terminology

The choroidal segment of the internal carotid artery begins with the takeoff of the anterior choroidal artery and ends at the base of the terminal carotid bifurcation into the anterior and middle cerebral arteries.[61] This short segment lies superior and slightly lateral to the communicating segment and has similar hemodynamic vectors. The single named branch from this segment, the anterior choroidal artery, typically arises several millimeters distal and lateral to the posterior communicating artery.[157] The artery initially swings laterally and then posteriorly following the optic tract, often giving off branches or a separate trunk to the uncus and portions of the amygdala and anterior hippocampus.[184]

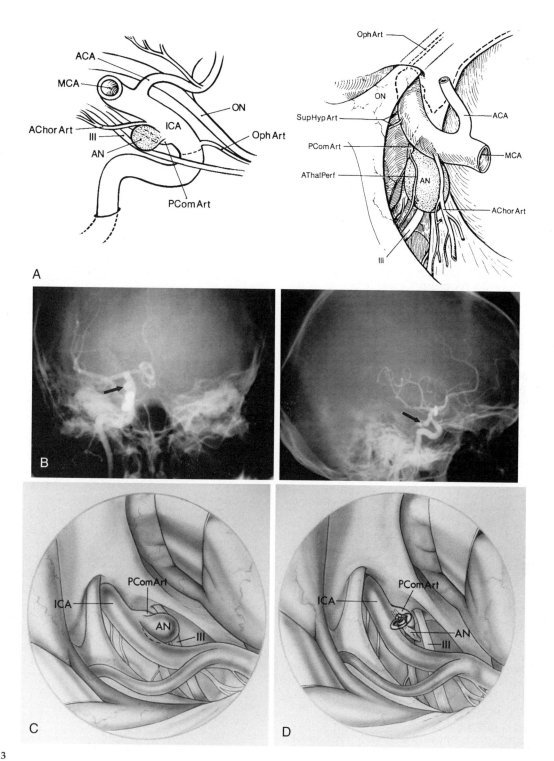

Figure 53–13

Posterior communicating artery aneurysm. *A.* Lateral *(left)* and dorsal *(right)* schematic views. The aneurysm originates just beyond the posterior communicating artery and typically projects posteriorly and slightly laterally and inferiorly, toward the oculomotor nerve. The posterior communicating artery courses medial to the aneurysm ("tethering" the aneurysm from medial expansion) and gives off small branches (the anterior thallamoperforating arteries) that may adhere to the medial aneurysm surface. *B.* Arteriogram, anteroposterior and lateral views. Note the typical bilobed posterior communicating artery aneurysm *(arrow)* pointing posteriorly and slightly laterally and inferiorly off the posterior carotid artery wall. The dent separating the proximal from distal lobe invariably marks the compressed oculomotor nerve. *C.* Initial operative view, right pterional approach. The sylvian fissure has been broadly split to expose the entire subarachnoid course of the internal carotid artery. With laterally projecting lesions, the aneurysm's fundus may have dense attachments to the temporal lobe. In cases with a shortened ophthalmic segment, the tip of the anterior clinoid process may need to be removed to ensure adequate exposure. Note that the surgical view allows only a glimpse of the posterior communicating artery origin. *D.* Final operative view, clipping. The surgeon must pass the proximal blade of a gently curved clip in the interval between the posterior communicating artery and the aneurysm, making sure to preserve posterior communicating and thalamoperforating artery patency. The distal blade must spare the anterior choroidal artery and any other carotid perforators that arise immediately distal to the aneurysm. After clipping, the aneurysm should be collapsed and the membrane of Liliequist widely opened to facilitate visualization of all branches and to eliminate continued pressure on the oculomotor nerve. ICA, internal carotid artery; MCA, middle cerebral artery; ACA, anterior cerebral artery; OphArt, ophthalmic artery; SupHypArt, superior hypophyseal arteries; PComArt, posterior communicating artery; AChorArt, anterior choroidal artery; AThalPerf, anterior thallamoperforating arteries; III, oculomotor nerve; AN, aneurysm.

The main trunk continues posteriorly, inferior to the optic tract, to enter the choroidal fissure. Variability in size is considerable, and the artery is duplicated in as many as 30 per cent of cases.[255]

Clinical and Radiographic Features

The distinctive hemorrhage patterns and clinical features of anterior choroidal aneurysms are outlined in Tables 53–5 and 53–6. This aneurysm type is extremely difficult to radiographically distinguish from the posterior communicating variety, and surgical confirmation is required in most instances. Because the choroidal segment is more lateral and distal than the communicating segment, however, anterior choroidal aneurysms invariably lie above the tentorium, away from the oculomotor nerve, and palsy of this nerve is rare. The typical anterior choroidal aneurysm has an intimate relationship with the mesial temporal lobe and is not infrequently buried within the uncus, in a fashion quite similar to that of the lateral variant posterior communicating aneurysm.

Surgical Approaches

The surgical approach to anterior choroidal artery aneurysms is identical to that of posterior communicating artery aneurysms (see Fig. 53–12) for the temporalis muscle incision, the size of the craniotomy, the degree of basal bone removal, and the method of splitting the sylvian fissure. Aneurysms associated with the anterior choroidal artery are usually small and thinly walled, accounting for 3 to 5 per cent of all intracranial saccular aneurysms.[55, 164, 235, 243, 255] During the initial exposure, the surgeon must remember the aneurysm's possible adherence to the temporal lobe, and direct the approach more frontally until this relationship can be visually clarified. A small amount of subpial resection of the uncus surrounding the aneurysm's attachment may facilitate completion of the fissure splitting and dissection of the subarachnoid cisterns. Once proximal control has been obtained, the number and course of the anterior choroidal artery (or arteries) must be ascertained, and the artery separated from the aneurysm neck. Unlike the posterior communicating artery, this artery is vital and unforgiving, and temporary clipping with flow interruption is not well tolerated. This artery must be spared from the clip, as its loss can result in a capsular infarct often accompanied by a severe neurological deficit (hemiparesis, hemianesthesia, and hemianopsia).

INTERNAL CAROTID ARTERY BIFURCATION ANEURYSMS

Anatomy and Terminology

Internal carotid bifurcation aneurysms (Fig. 53–14) arise at the distal end of the artery and project as a direct extension of the terminal carotid flow toward and into the anterior perforated substance.[61, 64] De-

pending on the tortuosity of the vessel at this site, these aneurysms may point anterosuperiorly, directly superiorly, or posterosuperiorly and may also be based more toward the anterior cerebral artery medially or the middle cerebral artery laterally. The lenticulostriate perforators, usually arising independent of the aneurysm neck, are invariably displaced posteriorly and are frequently adherent to the expanding sac.

Clinical and Radiographic Features

Carotid bifurcation aneurysms account for about 3 to 5 per cent of all saccular intracranial aneurysms, the great majority of which present with hemorrhage.[55, 163, 198, 243, 255] This site accounts for nearly 50 per cent of saccular lesions identified in childhood. There is a high incidence of hemiplegia associated with hemorrhage in this location, and the pattern of intracerebral hematoma can closely resemble that seen with hypertensive medial ganglionic bleeds (see Tables 53–5 and 53–6).[129]

Surgical Approaches

The craniotomy and basal bone removal for carotid bifurcation aneuryms are quite similar to those required for posterior communicating and anterior choroidal aneurysms (see Fig. 53–12).[256] The interfascial temporalis muscle incision (see Fig. 53–6B), however, is preferable for these lesions to minimize the amount of retraction needed to see this region well. The surgeon splits the sylvian fissure from medial to lateral, carefully staying on the anteroinferior surface of the middle cerebral artery until the carotid is encountered to avoid disturbance of the aneurysm. The basal cisterns should be broadly opened to obtain proximal control (ideally just distal to the anterior choroidal artery) and to further relieve any tension on the retracted brain. The anterior cerebral and middle cerebral arteries should then be dissected several millimeters distal to the aneurysm origin to allow temporary clips on these trunks, if needed. Finally, the aneurysm base is gradually approached from both sides until its neck is completely clarified and separated from the posteriorly displaced lenticulostriate vessels. The recurrent artery of Heubner frequently runs from medial to lateral with these perforators on the back surface of the aneurysm, and the anterior choroidal artery is also nearby, running from anterior to posterior behind the lesion's base. A straight or gently curved clip, placed parallel to the axis of the anterior cerebral–middle cerebral plane while the perforators are gently displaced posteriorly, is most ideal.

MIDDLE CEREBRAL ARTERY ANEURYSMS (PROXIMAL, TYPICAL BIFURCATION, AND DISTAL)

Anatomy and Terminology

The middle cerebral artery begins at the terminal bifurcation of the internal carotid artery and supplies

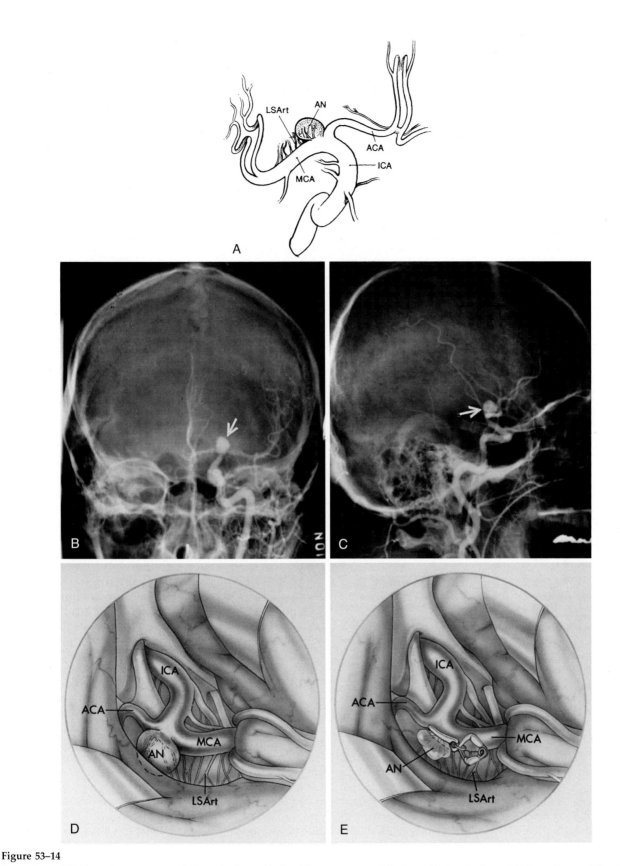

Figure 53–14

Internal carotid bifurcation aneurysm. *A.* Frontal schematic view. The aneurysm originates at the terminal carotid bifurcation, and the direction of flow generally projects the lesion superiorly toward the anterior perforated substance. *B and C.* Arteriograms, anteroposterior and lateral views. Note the superior projection of the aneurysm *(arrow)* as a direct extension of the termination of the internal carotid artery. *D.* Initial operative view, right pterional approach. The lenticulostriate arteries typically originate from the posterosuperior surface of the parent vessels, and the aneurysm arises more anteriorly. These perforating vessels are frequently adherent to the posterior or lateral aneurysm wall and must be separated from the aneurysm's base. *E.* Final operative view, clipping. A gently curved clip has been placed parallel to the anterior cerebral artery–middle cerebral artery axis, with the deep (posterior) blade passed closely applied to the posterior neck of the aneurysm to spare the lenticulostriate vessels. ICA, internal carotid artery; MCA, middle cerebral artery; ACA, anterior cerebral artery; LSArt, lenticulostriate arteries; AN, aneurysm.

the lateral two thirds of the cerebral hemisphere centered around the sylvian fissure.[60, 64] The vessel initially runs laterally, paralleling the sphenoid ridge, within the sphenoidal compartment of the deep sylvian fissure. At the level of the limen insulae, it makes an abrupt turn (genu) posteriorly and superiorly to enter the insular compartment of the deep fissure. The middle cerebral artery can be divided into four segments, including (1) M_1, the segment between the carotid bifurcation and the genu; (2) M_2, the segments that run over the deep insular surface; (3) M_3, the segments that traverse the opercular surface of the sylvian fissure to reach the cortical surface; and (4) M_4, cortical branches. The M_1 segment typically divides into two trunks just proximal to the genu, creating a long prebifurcation (main trunk) and short postbifurcation portion (superior and inferior trunks). The prebifurcation segment gives rise to lenticulostriate vessels from its posterosuperior surface and often contributes an early or anterior temporal branch off its anteroinferior surface. Recurrent lateral lenticulostriate branches occasionally originate from the postbifurcation M_1 segment or from proximal portions of the M_2 trunks.[184]

Approximately 20 per cent of all clinically significant saccular intracranial aneurysms originate from the middle cerebral artery.[55, 243, 255] These lesions may be divided into three types: (1) proximal, (2) typical bifurcation, and (3) distal. The majority are typical bifurcation aneurysms that originate as a direct extension of the main trunk to project laterally, anteriorly, and slightly inferiorly between and beyond its two branches and the genu toward the temporal lobe (Fig. 53–15). A smaller number originate proximal to the genu and include lesions associated with the main trunk–anterior temporal artery bifurcation, a shortened prebifurcation M_1 portion (with correspondingly long postbifurcation trunks straddling the aneurysm), and a lenticulostriate origin (Fig. 53–16). A few arise distally, usually from a delayed bifurcation of the main trunk beyond the genu, or from a second- or third-order bifurcation thereafter. Whenever distal lesions arise significantly beyond the genu, an infectious or traumatic etiology should at least be considered.

Clinical and Radiographic Features

Unruptured middle cerebral artery aneurysms are generally asymptomatic, although when larger they may occasionally present with temporal lobe seizures or intra-aneurysmal thrombosis and embolism.[77] Rupture and subarachnoid hemorrhage usually result in a syndrome indistinguishable from that seen with aneurysms at other sites. Certain clinical characteristics, however, favor a middle cerebral origin of the bleed, including a unilateral temporal region headache or a focal neurological deficit including dysphasia or weakness of the contralateral arm or face (see Table 53–5). These focal signs and symptoms are presumably related to the tendency of typical bifurcation middle cerebral aneurysms to project into the temporal lobe, resulting in a higher incidence of intracerebral hemorrhage (30 to 50 per cent) than that with saccular intracranial aneurysms at other locations.

The common hemorrhage patterns for proximal, typical bifurcation, and distal middle cerebral aneurysms are outlined in Table 53–6. In an acutely deteriorating patient with a classically located temporal lobe clot, computed tomography may be the only study required prior to emergent surgical intervention. The arteriogram should be carefully inspected for the aneurysm's position relative to the genu and for its direction of projection, because subtle differences may alter the choice of temporalis muscle incisions and the method of sylvian fissure dissection.

Surgical Approaches

Most middle cerebral artery aneurysms are best approached via a pterional craniotomy, with slight bone flap alterations to broaden the length of sylvian fissure exposure (Fig. 53–17).[217, 220] The initial scalp incision should ideally preserve the dominant branch of the superficial temporal artery for its potential future use as a bypass donor vessel. The aneurysm may thereafter be exposed by three basic methods (see Fig. 53–7), including (1) transcortical, through the superior temporal gyrus; (2) medial-to-lateral trans-sylvian, opening the sylvian fissure medially at the internal carotid artery and following the main trunk laterally until the aneurysm is encountered; and (3) lateral-to-medial trans-sylvian, opening the fissure laterally and following an M_2 trunk proximally to the aneurysm.[75, 170] Regardless of the method chosen, the sylvian and sphenoparietal veins should be preserved whenever possible to minimize venous congestion and swelling in the frontal and temporal operculum.

The superior temporal gyrus approach requires little brain retraction and can be performed quite rapidly, making it especially useful for typical bifurcation aneurysms with significant temporal lobe hematomas. When the brain is tight, the surgeon should enter the hematoma early and evacuate it peripherally with gentle suction, taking care not to disturb the clot adjacent to the aneurysm. Once the brain has been decompressed, the sylvian fissure should be entered, and the anatomy further clarified from within the subarachnoid space. The disadvantages of a transcortical approach include the production of trauma to otherwise normal temporal lobe structures (which may increase the risk of postoperative epilepsy) and premature disturbance of the clot adjacent to the aneurysm (which may precipitate rebleeding). This approach is contraindicated for proximal aneurysms and for distal lesions projecting into more posterior portions of the temporal lobe (i.e., Heschl's gyrus).

The trans-sylvian fissure methods are more esthetically appealing because they respect the brain's natural pial barriers. The medial-to-lateral sylvian fissure–splitting approach has the advantage of proximal M_1 control before the aneurysm comes into view, while the lateral-to-medial trans-sylvian approach requires less retraction and reduces the risks of perforator vessel injury. In general, the authors prefer the lateral-to-me-

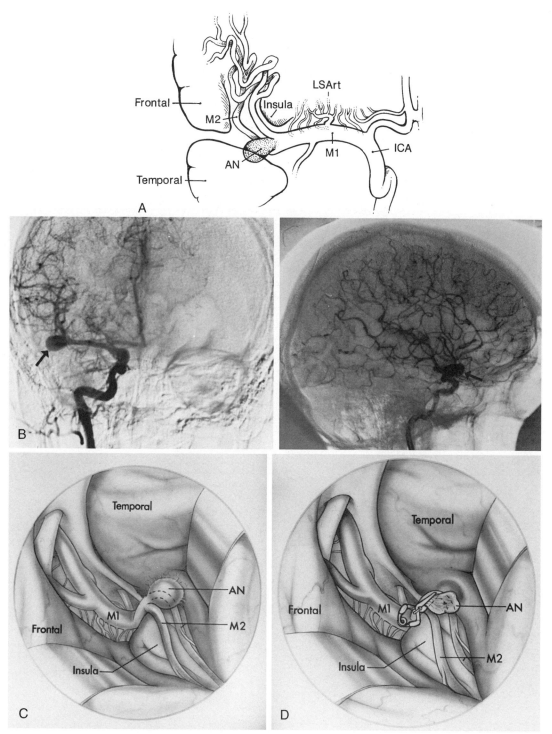

Figure 53–15

Middle cerebral artery aneurysm, typical bifurcation. *A.* Frontal schematic view. The aneurysm arises at the terminal end of the M_1 segment and continues laterally toward and often into the temporal lobe. The M_2 branches, beginning at the genu, sharply angle posteriorly and superiorly to enter the insular compartment of the sylvian fissure. *B.* Arteriogram, anteroposterior and lateral views. Note the aneurysm *(arrow)* projecting as a direct extension of the middle cerebral artery laterally toward the superior portion of the temporal lobe (patient also has an ophthalmic artery aneurysm). The study should be carefully inspected for the aneurysm's exact point of origin relative to the genu, and its direction of projection within the sylvian fissure (frontal versus temporal). *C.* Initial operative view, right pterional approach. The sylvian fissure has been broadly opened from lateral to medial, beginning more posteriorly in the fissure to avoid premature disturbance of the aneurysm. Once an M_2 branch is identified within the fissure, it is followed proximally, generally on its frontal lobe surface (most typical bifurcation middle cerebral aneurysms project toward the temporal lobe), until the aneurysm is identified and proximal control is secured. *D.* Final operative view, clipping. A straight or gently curved clip is ideally placed parallel to the axis of the two exiting M_2 trunks. Significant atheroma in the bifurcation should prompt the leaving of some residual neck to ensure that both branches remain widely patent. Frontal, frontal lobe; Temporal, temporal lobe; ICA, internal carotid artery; LSArt, lenticulostriate arteries; AN, aneurysm.

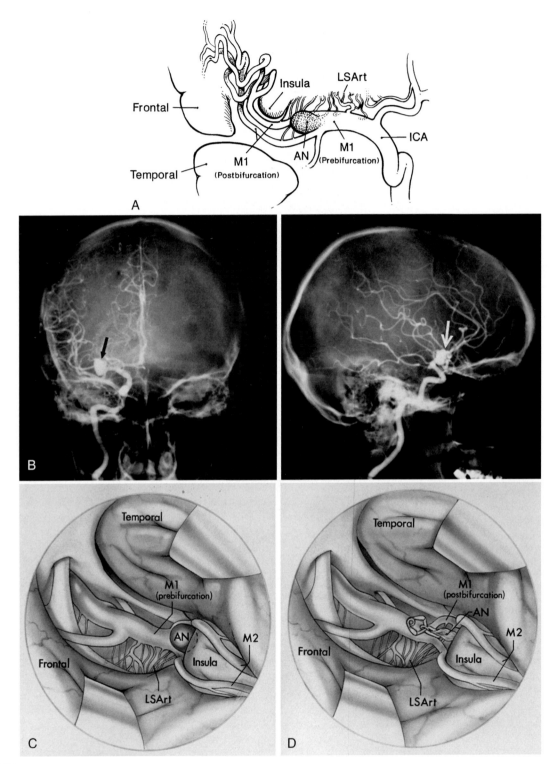

Figure 53–16

Middle cerebral artery aneurysm, proximal bifurcation. *A.* Frontal schematic view. The aneurysm arises well proximal to the genu, in association with a shortened M₁ prebifurcation segment *(shown here),* an early temporal branch, or a lenticulostriate vessel. Depending on the exact site of origin, proximal middle cerebral artery aneurysms may project into the anterior perforating substance, insula, or base of the temporal lobe. *B.* Arteriogram, anteroposterior and lateral views. Note the short prebifurcation M₁ segment, and the aneurysm *(arrow)* projecting between the two postbifurcation M₁ segments. The studies should be carefully inspected for the aneurysm's exact point of origin relative to the bifurcation and its direction of projection relative to the lenticulostriate vessels (superiorly versus inferiorly). *C.* Initial operative view, right pterional approach. The sylvian fissure has been broadly opened from lateral to medial, in a standard fashion down to the insular surface. Exposure of these lesions is more hazardous than that of the typical bifurcation aneurysms, as the aneurysm neck is hidden beneath the insula and the lenticulostriate arteries are more intimately involved. Proximal control is obtained by following the postbifurcation M₁ vessels on their outer surface (the aneurysm will arise between the two branches) until the main trunk of the middle cerebral artery (prebifurcation segment) is identified. *D.* Final operative view, clipping. A gently curved clip is placed between the two exiting M₁ trunks. The aneurysm is collapsed and dissected free from its bed to ensure patency of all lenticulostriate vessels. Frontal, frontal lobe; Temporal, temporal lobe; ICA, internal carotid artery; LSArt, lenticulostriate arteries; AN, aneurysm.

Figure 53–17

Operative position and bone removal *(darkened area),* typical middle cerebral bifurcation aneurysm. The head is generally turned 45 degrees, and a muscle-splitting temporalis incision is sufficient, as the aneurysm projects superficial to the insula. The craniotomy includes more temporal and posterior bone removal so that the sylvian fissure can be entered distal to the aneurysm. MCA AN, middle cerebral artery aneurysm.

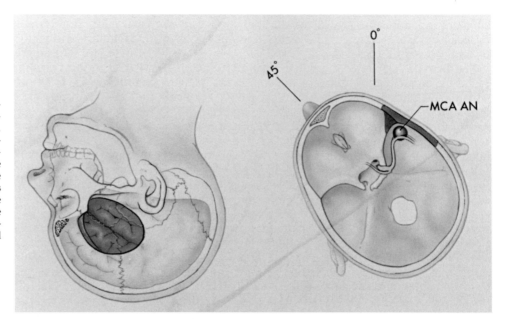

dial approach in most instances. For typical bifurcation middle cerebral artery aneurysms, the sylvian fissure is entered slightly more posteriorly (3 to 4 cm behind the sphenoid ridge) than for other aneurysms. When an M_2 branch has been encountered, it is followed proximally on the side opposite the aneurysm's projection (e.g., if the aneurysm is projecting temporally, the trunk is followed on the frontal lobe side) until the genu and bifurcation are encountered. When proximal control has been established, the fissure can be more broadly opened, as needed, to obtain good exposure without undue retraction. The subarachnoid plane between the frontal and the temporal lobes may be difficult to preserve, especially in younger patients or in patients with hemorrhage; if this plane is lost during the dissection, it is far better to veer inferiorly toward the superior temporal gyrus rather than risk injury to the frontal lobe operculum, especially in the dominant hemisphere.

The type of temporalis muscle incision and the methods of sylvian fissure dissection vary according to the clinical and radiographic features of the individual aneurysm. The muscle-splitting technique (see Fig. 53–6A), combined with a lateral-to-medial sylvian fissure dissection, is quite adequate for typical bifurcation and distally located lesions. The interfascial temporalis muscle technique (see Fig. 53–6B) is more ideal for proximal middle cerebral artery aneurysms because it allows better inferior and anterior trajectories of vision and access to the proximal fissure and middle cerebral artery with less retraction on the brain or undissected aneurysm (see Fig. 53–16).

Once the fissure has been widely opened, typical bifurcation lesions are usually best controlled with a curved or straight clip running parallel to the axis between the two exiting trunks (see Fig. 53–15). The aneurysm neck is often bulbous and arteriosclerotic at this location, making "perfect" clip placement difficult in some instances. Most of the lenticulostriate vessels

exit prior to the aneurysm origin, but some arise more distally, and in their recurrent course they may be adherent to the aneurysm and inadvertently included in the clip. After the lesion has been satisfactorily secured, it should be punctured and collapsed, and the dissection continued until all significant sylvian and intracerebral clot is removed. The safe passage of all nearby vessels must be visually ascertained, with the use of intraoperative arteriography in questionable cases.

Proximal middle cerebral artery aneurysms are somewhat buried beneath the insula and have a much more intimate association with the lenticulostriate vessel origins, making exposure and clipping more difficult (see Fig. 53–16).[79] Temporary clipping under barbiturate and mild hypothermic protection is particularly useful in treating these aneurysms, as premature rupture risks disastrous perforator injury. Clips of excessive length are particularly hazardous in this region, and all perforators must be spared from the blades. Any neurological deficit appearing immediately after the operation cannot be attributed to delayed cerebral vasospasm and, if unexplained by intraoperative events, should prompt a re-exploration that inspects for a clipped or kinked perforator.

Distal middle cerebral artery aneurysms generally lie entirely within the insular compartment of the sylvian fissure, with little or no association with the lenticulostriate vessels. In this position, the aneurysm often has a projection that is more superiorly oriented, making any intracerebral hemorrhage more likely to be in the frontal lobe than hemorrhage from lesions that originate from the typical bifurcation site (which invariably produces a temporal lobe hematoma). When exposing these lesions, the surgeon must take care to notice which trunk harbors the aneurysm, staying on the "safe" side of the fissure away from the aneurysm until proximal control is obtained. More peripheral middle cerebral branches and their aneurysms are generally smaller, and miniclips are correspondingly more appropriate so that the weight of the clip does not torque or kink the parent vessel.

The hemorrhage from middle cerebral artery aneurysms is frequently confined to the ipsilateral hemisphere, and the risks of generalized secondary events following the bleed may be reduced, compared with more centrally located lesions. The incidence of hydrocephalus and the need for ventricular drainage and later shunting appear lower, presumably because the basal cisterns are less often filled with fresh clot and the contralateral convexity can still conduct and absorb cerebrospinal fluid. Vasospasm is more often confined to the ipsilateral hemisphere, and the incidence of electrolyte disturbances (i.e., hyponatremia) appears reduced, especially compared with anterior communicating artery aneurysms. The surgical approaches to middle cerebral artery aneurysms require the least brain retraction, and when this fact is combined with the increased facility with which vasospasm affecting the middle cerebral artery can be treated (with papaverine or angioplasty), early surgery should be performed in all good-grade patients. In addition, early intervention should at least be considered in poorer-grade patients who are younger or harbor large hematomas, especially if the lesion is diagnosed soon after the bleeding.

ANTERIOR COMMUNICATING ARTERY (ANTERIOR CEREBRAL ARTERY) ANEURYSMS

Anatomy and Terminology

The proximal anterior cerebral artery (A_1 segment) begins at the terminal internal carotid artery bifurcation, proceeds medially and somewhat anteriorly above the optic chiasm and nerves to the interhemispherical fissure, and ends where it joins its contralateral counterpart at the anterior communicating artery.[44, 160] Inequality in the sizes of the two A_1 segments occurs in approximately 40 per cent of unselected cases (with severe hypoplasia or aplasia in 5 per cent) and in 85 per cent of patients harboring an anterior communicating artery aneurysm.[55, 243, 248, 255] Several small perforators arise from the A_1 segment that supply the fornix, optic chiasm, anterior hypothalamus, anterior limb of the internal capsule, and other septal region structures.[44, 184]

The anterior communicating artery usually exists as a single channel, but variations such as duplications, triplications, and fenestrations are encountered in as many as 25 per cent of cases.[150, 255] Anterior communicating artery aneurysms usually arise as a direct extension of a dominant A_1 segment that delivers blood to both distal anterior cerebral arteries, with the aneurysm attributed to the increased hemodynamic stress placed on the communicating channel, and the direction of aneurysm projection determined by the angle at which the dominant A_1 approaches the communicating region (Fig. 53–18). The posteroinferior surface of the anterior communicating artery typically gives rise to at least one perforator supplying the anterior hypothalamic region.

The distal (A_2) anterior cerebral artery begins at the anterior communicating artery and runs within the interhemispheric fissure to supply the medial third of the cerebral hemispheres and the corpus callosum. In most cases, the A_2 segments are equal in size, and each supplies only the ipsilateral hemisphere. Common variations in this pattern and their incidence include an unpaired (azygous) A_2, also known as the "arteria termatica" (2 per cent of cases), and a median callosal artery, or third A_2 (10 per cent of cases).[255] The first branch of the distal anterior cerebral artery is usually the recurrent artery of Heubner, which typically originates from the lateral surface of the A_2 segment just beyond the communicating artery and proceeds laterally, paralleling the course of the ipsilateral A_1 segment, to supply anterior portions of the caudate nucleus, putamen, globus pallidus, and internal capsule.[44, 160, 161]

Clinical and Radiographic Features

Anterior communicating artery aneurysms represent the single most common type identified in adult clinical series and account for 40 to 50 per cent of those found in males.* Most lesions are identified following subarachnoid hemorrhage; on rare occasions, they reach giant proportions and cause compression of the visual system. Their distinctive clinical features and hemorrhage patterns are outlined in Tables 53–5 and 53–6. Following severe subarachnoid hemorrhage, these lesions are particularly prone to developing electrolyte imbalances (hyponatremia), and a dropping serum sodium level is invariably a reflection of hypothalamic ischemia caused by vasospasm.

Most anterior communicating artery aneurysms arise in association with a dominant A_1 segment and, as direct extensions of that vessel, are often somewhat directed toward the contralateral hemisphere (see Fig. 53–18).[248] These aneurysms have been classified, according to their direction of projection relative to the planum sphenoidale, into inferior (toward the planum), anterior (toward the nose parallel to the planum), superior (toward the vertex), and posterior (toward the occiput).[231, 255] Combinations of these projections are commonplace.

The authors use a simpler system that is quite useful in choosing the direction of surgical approach (dominant A_1 versus nondominant hemisphere). This system basically divides anterior communicating artery aneurysms into two categories. The first type, aneurysms that project anteriorly or inferiorly, extend below the plane of the ascending A_2 vessels (as seen on lateral view), are often adherent to the top of the visual system, and produce hemorrhage patterns confined to the basal subarachnoid space or contralateral inferior frontal lobe and gyrus rectus (see Fig. 53–18). The inferior projection of this type makes early visualization of the contralateral A_1 segment more difficult, and

---

*See references 55, 66, 78, 105, 221, 243, and 255.

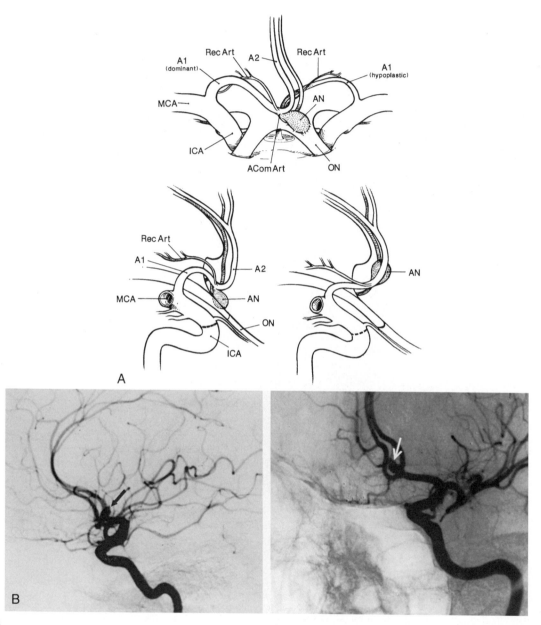

Figure 53–18

Anterior communicating artery aneurysm. *A.* Frontal *(top)* and lateral *(lower left and right)* schematic views. Many anterior communicating aneurysms arise in association with a hypoplastic A_1 segment and project as a direct extension of the dominant A_1 toward the contralateral frontal lobe *(top).* If the aneurysm is also directed inferiorly, the fundus is often attached to the contralateral optic nerve, an attachment that makes exposure from the nondominant (hypoplastic) A_1 side hazardous for premature rupture as the frontal lobe is elevated (lower left). If the lesion projects more superiorly, expansion occurs between the two frontal lobes within the interhemispheric fissure, and the aneurysm will not be visible at the initial subfrontal exposure without removal of some gyrus rectus (lower right). *B.* Arteriogram, lateral and oblique views. Note the aneurysm *(arrow)* arising as a direct extension of a dominant A_1 segment, projecting superiorly and to the contralateral side. The studies should be carefully inspected for the side of A_1 dominance and the aneurysm's direction of projection relative to the frontal fossa floor (superiorly versus inferiorly). The computed tomography scan should also be inspected for significant intraparenchymal clots that may alter the operative laterality.

Illustration continued on following page

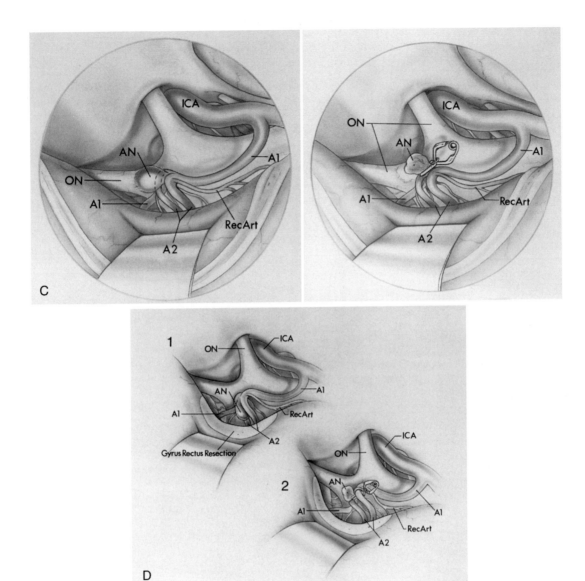

Figure 53–18 *Continued*

C. Inferiorly projecting aneurysm. *Left.* Initial operative view, right pterional approach. The sylvian fissure has been broadly opened, so that the temporal lobe remains in place when the frontal lobe is elevated, allowing a more complete view of the entire A_1 segment from a more posterior path to the aneurysm neck without interference from the temporal lobe. Because of the anteroinferior projection of the aneurysm, it has been approached on the side of the dominant A_1 segment. Less gyrus rectus removal is necessary to delineate this type of aneurysm, and the contralateral A_1 segment is not seen well initially. Note the adherence of the aneurysm fundus to the contralateral optic nerve, and that the aneurysm neck can be completely dissected without disturbance of this attachment. *Right.* Final operative view, clipping. A straight or gently curved clip is placed across the aneurysm neck, parallel to the anterior surface of the anterior communicating artery. The aneurysm is collapsed and dissected free from its attachments to ensure that the contralateral A_1 segment and Heubner's artery are patent. *D.* Superiorly projecting aneurysm. *Top Left.* Initial operative view, right pterional approach. Because of the superior projection of the aneurysm, approach from the side of the dominant A_1 segment is less advantageous for the initial exposure. More removal of gyrus rectus is necessary for aneurysm delineation, and the contralateral A_2 segment is not seen well initially. This type of lesion projects between the two A_2 vessels and has an intimate association with the septal perforators off the posterior inferior anterior communicating artery wall. *Bottom Right.* Final operative view, clipping. A short fenestrated clip is placed across the aneurysm neck, parallel to the posterosuperior surface of the anterior communicating artery. The aneurysm is collapsed and inspected to make sure that the septal perforators are free, and that the contralateral A_2 segment is not compromised. ICA, internal carotid artery; MCA, middle cerebral artery; AComArt, anterior communicating artery; RecArt, recurrent artery of Heubner; ON, optic nerve; AN, aneurysm.

this type of aneurysm is invariably best approached from the side of the dominant A_1.

The second type of anterior communicating artery aneurysm includes those that project between or behind the two A_2 vessels in a superior or posterior direction. Visualization of small aneurysms of this type can be limited by the overlying A_2 vessels, especially on lateral view, and this lesion, in the authors' experience, is the most common anterior circulation aneurysm to escape detection on a good-quality initial arteriogram.[88] Detailed oblique and magnified films of the communicating region, with and without cross-compression of the contralateral internal carotid artery, or repeat arteriography in suspicious cases may be required to demonstrate the offending lesion. Because this type of aneurysm projects more into the interhemispheric fissure and is completely hidden by the overlying gyrus rectus on initial frontal lobe elevation, proximal control of the two A_1 vessels is easily obtained before the aneurysm dissection is begun, making a surgical approach from the side of the dominant A_1 segment less advantageous.

Surgical Approaches

The operative position and extent of bone removal used by the authors to expose aneurysms of the anterior communicating artery region are delineated in Figure 53–19.[105] Because the aneurysm location and direction of view is more anterior than for other anterior circulation lesions, the frontal portion of the craniotomy must be low and more extensive to minimize the amount of frontal lobe retraction necessary for exposure. An interfascial temporalis muscle incision further facilitates a low subfrontal angle of approach (see Fig. 53–6B).

The decision for the laterality of approach is based on the presence or absence of A_1 dominance, the direction of projection of the aneurysm fundus, and the presence or absence of a significant intraparenchymal hematoma or other anterior circulation aneurysm. Approaching an anterior communicating artery aneurysm from the side of the dominant A_1 segment is both technically easier and safer, especially when the aneurysm is pointing somewhat inferiorly toward the contralateral optic nerve. The surgeon enters the region of the aneurysm in control of the dominant A_1 segment and encounters the aneurysm at its base, with the fundus (and site of rupture) pointing toward the contralateral side. If such cases are approached from the nondominant A_1 side, the aneurysm's adhesions to the visual system may be disrupted during elevation of the frontal lobe and may limit access to the contralateral A_1 segment should temporary clipping be necessary.

In the authors' opinion, these technical advantages more than compensate for any perceived increased risks associated with dominant hemisphere (left-sided) approaches, especially when a skull base style of exposure minimizes frontal lobe retraction. The indications for approaching an anterior communicating artery aneurysm from the side of the nondominant A_1 segment include the presence of another aneurysm or a large hematoma on that side. Aneurysms not associated with significant A_1 asymmetry, especially those that fill arteriographically from both sides or that project superiorly, are approached from the side of the nondominant (right) hemisphere.

When the craniotomy has been completed, the sylvian fissure is split in a lateral-to-medial direction to expose the middle cerebral and internal carotid arteries, and to detach the temporal lobe from its sylvian arachnoid adhesions. While seemingly superfluous for this aneurysm type, wide fissure splitting allows the frontal lobe to be independently elevated, without the

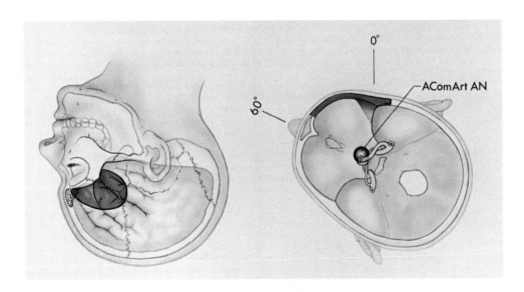

Figure 53–19

Operative position and bone removal *(darkened area)*, anterior communicating artery aneurysm. The head is generally turned 60 degrees, and an interfascial temporalis muscle incision (see Fig. 53–6B) is used to provide a good subfrontal view with minimal frontal lobe retraction. The craniotomy includes more anterior frontal bone removal because of the aneurysm's relatively anterior position. Enough temporal and sphenoid bone is removed so that the sylvian fissure can be easily split. AComArt AN, anterior communicating artery aneurysm.

temporal lobe crowding into the operative field, and also permits a more posterior trajectory of approach to the aneurysm base rather than a more anterior one toward the fundus of the aneurysm.

The surgeon identifies the ipsilateral A_1 segment and follows it to the communicating region, carefully avoiding injury to any perforators or to the recurrent artery of Heubner. A short segment of the ipsilateral (and usually dominant) A_1 vessel is prepared to receive a temporary clip, if needed. The subsequent stages of dissection then differ, dependent on the direction of aneurysm projection. With the anteroinferiorly projecting lesion, the aneurysm fundus may be stuck to the visual system, making visualization and control of the contralateral A_1 segment hazardous. The two A_2 vessels and the origins of their branches, especially the recurrent arteries, are less problematic, and they can be more easily identified and dissected, often with little gyrus rectus removal adjacent to the communicating artery. After both A_2 vessels have been clarified, the final dissection of the aneurysm neck is completed, including identification of the contralateral A_1 segment. For very thinly walled or bulbous aneurysms, the surgeon can perform the last stages of dissection and clipping using barbiturate-induced burst suppression, mild hypertension and hypothermia (33° C), and temporary clips on at least the dominant A_1 segment. If the aneurysm prematurely ruptures, it may be necessary to also clip both A_2 vessels until control is re-established. This type of aneurysm usually projects away from critical septal and hypothalamic perforators and is usually best clipped with a straight or gently curved clip paralleling the anterior surface of the anterior communicating artery (see Fig. 53–18).

For the more superiorly projecting type of lesion, the aneurysm fundus is embedded entirely within the interhemispheric fissure, and the ipsilateral frontal lobe can be gently elevated and detached from the visual system with much more safety. The contralateral A_1 vessel is easily seen, and both A_1 vessels are prepared to receive a temporary clip, as required. The region of the communicating artery is clarified, and a subpial resection of the gyrus rectus (about 1 cm) allows visualization of the ipsilateral A_2 segment and its branches.[232] The contralateral A_2 vessel is the problematic one, usually being obstructed from view by the intervening aneurysm. After the location of both A_1 segments and the ipsilateral A_2 vessel (and Heubner's artery) has been ascertained, the surgeon begins the final neck dissection, using the same methods of cerebral protection as those outlined previously. This type of aneurysm has a much more intimate association with the septal area perforators and is often best managed with a short fenestrated clip that encircles the ipsilateral A_2 segment and parallels the posterior and superior surface of the anterior communicating artery, carefully avoiding compromise of the contralateral A_2 and penetrating vessels (see Fig. 53–18).

At the completion of apparently satisfactory clipping, the aneurysm should be punctured and collapsed, and all branches carefully inspected for patency, including both A_1 segments and A_2 vessels,

recurrent arteries of Heubner, perforators, and the anterior communicating artery itself.

DISTAL ANTERIOR CEREBRAL (PERICALLOSAL) ARTERY ANEURYSMS

Anatomy and Terminology

In the typical situation, two distal anterior cerebral arteries (also known as the A_2, postcommunicating, or pericallosal arteries) initially run dorsally and then arch posteriorly within the midline pericallosal sulcus deep within the interhemispheric fissure, parallel and closely applied to the genu and body of the corpus callosum (Fig. 53–20).[161] The callosomarginal artery arises from the pericallosal artery near the genu and runs within the cingulate sulcus, giving off several major cortical branches to the mesial cerebral hemisphere.

Clinical and Radiographic Features

Distal anterior cerebral aneurysms account for 2 to 4 per cent of all intracranial aneurysms.* Almost all are saccular, but those that originate near the falx cerebri may be traumatic, and those that arise distal to the pericallosal-callosomarginal bifurcation may have infectious origins.[126] The typical distal anterior cerebral artery aneurysm presents with subarachnoid hemorrhage, usually confined to the interhemispheric fissure distal to the anterior communicating artery region, but occasionally extending into the cingulate gyrus or subdural space (see Tables 53–5 and 53–6). Most arise from the pericallosal artery, usually at the branching point between the pericallosal and the callosomarginal arteries. Less commonly, distal aneurysms arise at the bifurcation of an azygous A_2 segment, where it divides to form two pericallosal arteries.

Surgical Approaches

The operative position, scalp incision, and craniotomy flap for the typical distal anterior cerebral artery aneurysm is shown in Figure 53–21. The bicoronal incision is placed behind the hairline and is extended farther laterally on the side of the bone flap. The medial part of the bone flap runs parallel to the superior sagittal sinus for 5 to 6 cm and extends across the midline so that the dura can be retracted medially to expose the interhemispheric fissure without excessive lateral frontal lobe retraction. In most instances, the bone flap should extend well anterior to the coronal suture to allow dissection of the pericallosal artery around the genu of the corpus callosum. The posterior limit of the flap should be placed so that the surgeon can enter the interhemispheric fissure (sparing as many veins as possible) and identify the pericallosal artery distal to the aneurysm without the retraction disturbing the aneurysm. The pericallosal artery is then followed anteriorly until the aneurysm is encountered,

---

*See references 55, 73, 152, 243, 255, 257, and 261.

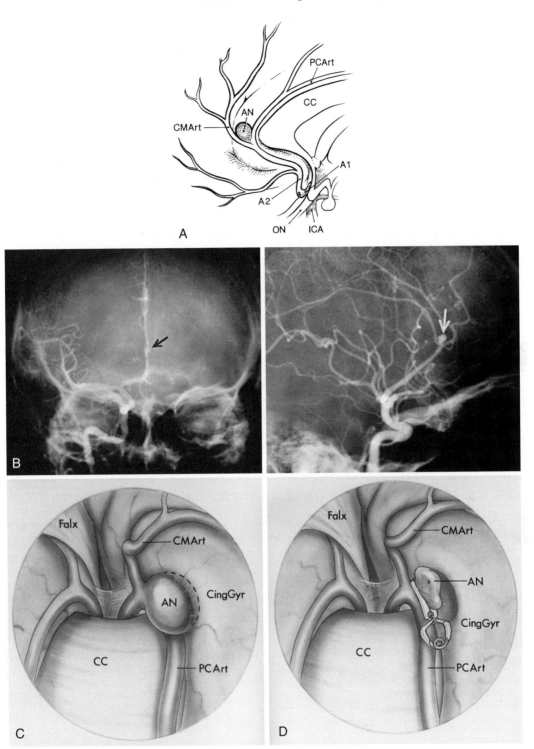

Figure 53–20

Anterior cerebral artery aneurysm, distal. *A.* Lateral schematic view. Many distal anterior cerebral artery aneurysms arise at the bifurcation between the pericallosal and the callosomarginal arteries, a point that is variable but often occurs near the genu of the corpus callosum. *B.* Arteriogram, anteroposterior and lateral views. Note the origin of the aneurysm *(arrow)* at the bifurcation of the pericallosal and callosomarginal arteries. The studies should be carefully inspected for the exact site of aneurysm origin relative to the genu of the corpus callosum and its relationship to the coronal suture. *C.* Initial operative view. The interhemispheric fissure is opened down to the corpus callosum, behind the plane of the aneurysm, until the appropriate pericallosal artery is identified. The surgeon then follows the vessel anteriorly until the aneurysm is encountered, carefully avoiding undue anterior and superior frontal lobe retraction until proximal control is secured. *D.* Final operative view, clipping. Without disturbing the aneurysm's attachment to the falx or medial frontal lobe *(dotted line),* a straight or gently curved clip is placed across the aneurysm neck parallel to the superior surface of the pericallosal artery. ICA, internal carotid artery; CMArt, callosomarginal artery; PCArt, pericallosal artery; CC, corpus callosum; Falx, falx cerebri; ON, optic nerve; CingGyr, cingulate gyrus; AN, aneurysm.

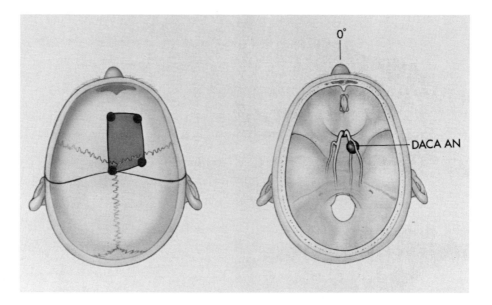

Figure 53–21

Operative position and bone removal *(darkened area)*, distal anterior cerebral artery aneurysm. The surgeon should approach almost all distal anterior cerebral artery aneurysms from the right side, using a bicoronal incision extended into the right temporalis muscle. The patient's head is generally placed straight up or turned slightly toward the operative side to facilitate gravitational retraction of the frontal lobe away from the midline. The medial margin of the free bone flap extends just across the midline, so that the dura can be retracted to the superior sagittal sinus and less lateral frontal lobe retraction will be needed. The front-to-back extent of the flap is chosen, depending on the exact site of the aneurysm's origin along the distal anterior cerebral artery, and is made longer so that the surgeon can choose the direction of approach without sacrificing significant bridging veins. DACA AN, distal anterior cerebral artery aneurysm.

proximal control is obtained, and the aneurysm is clipped.

REFERENCES

1. Adams, H., Jr., Jergenson, D. D., Kassell, N. F., et al: Pitfalls in the recognition of subarachnoid hemorrhage. J.A.M.A., *244*(8): 794–796, 1980.
2. Almeida, G. M., Pindaro, J., Plese, P., et al.: Intracranial arterial aneurysms in infancy and childhood. Child's Brain, *3*:193–199, 1977.
3. Andrews, R. J., and Spiegel, P. K.: Intracranial aneurysms: Age, sex, blood pressure, and multiplicity in an unselected series of patients. J. Neurosurg., *51*:27–32, 1979.
4. Atkinson, J. L., Sundt, T., Jr., Houser, O. W., et al: Angiographic frequency of anterior circulation intracranial aneurysms. J. Neurosurg., *70*:551–555, 1989.
5. Austin, D. C.: A review of intracranial aneurysms. Henry Ford Hosp. Med. Bull., *12*:251–271, 1964.
6. Austin, G. M., Schievink, W., and Williams, R.: Controlled pressure-volume factors in the enlargement of intracranial aneurysms. Neurosurgery, *24*:722–730, 1989.
7. Awad, I. A., Carter, I. P., and Spetzler, R. F., et al: Clinical vasospasm after subarachnoid hemorrhage: Response to hypervolemic hemodilution and arterial hypertension. Stroke, *18*:365–372, 1987.
8. Awad, I. A., Mckenzie, R., Magdinec, M., et al: Application of magnetic resonance angiography to neurosurgical practice: A critical review of 150 cases. Neurol. Res., *14*:360–368, 1992.
9. Ayuzawa, S., Matsumura, A., and Nose, T.: Emergent aneurysmal surgery without preoperative angiography: Usefulness of the intraoperative portable digital subtraction angiography. Surg. Neurol., *40*:251–254, 1993.
10. Bailes, J. E., Spetzler, R. F., Hadley, M. N., et al: Management morbidity and mortality of poor-grade aneurysm patients. J. Neurosurg., *72*:559–566, 1990.
11. Barton, C. W.: Subarachnoid hemorrhage presenting as acute chest pain: A variant of le coup de poignard. Ann. Emerg. Med., *17*:977–978, 1988.
12. Bassi, P., Bandera, R., Loiero, M., et al.: Warning signs in subarachnoid hemorrhage: A cooperative study. Acta Neurol. Scand., *84*:277–281, 1991.
13. Batjer, H. H., Kopitnik, T. A., Giller, C. A., et al.: Surgery for paraclinoidal carotid artery aneurysms. J. Neurosurg., *80*:650–658, 1994.
14. Batjer, H. H., and Samson, D. S.: Emergent aneurysm surgery without cerebral angiography for the comatose patient [see comments]. Neurosurgery, *28*:283–287, 1991.
15. Benoit, B. G., Cochrane, D. D., Durity, F., et al.: Clinical-radiological correlates in intracerebral hematomas due to aneurysmal rupture. Can. J. Neurol. Sci., *9*:409–14, 1982.
16. Blatter, D. D., Parker, D. L., Ahn, S. S., et al: Cerebral MR angiography with multiple overlapping thin slab acquisition. Part II: Early clinical experience. Radiology, *183*:379–389, 1992.
17. Bonita, R.: Cigarette smoking, hypertension and the risk of subarachnoid hemorrhage: A population-based case-control study. Stroke, *16*:591–594, 1986.
18. Bonita, R., Beaglehole, R., and North, J. D. K.: Subarachnoid hemorrhage in New Zealand: An epidemiological study. Stroke, *14*:342–346, 1983.
19. Canham, P. B., and Ferguson, G. G.: A mathematical model for the mechanics of saccular aneurysms. Neurosurgery, *17*:291–295, 1985.
20. Carmichael, R.: Gross defects in the muscular and elastic coats of the larger cerebral arteries. J. Pathol. Bacteriol., *57*:345–351, 1945.
21. Charbel, F. T., Ausman, J. I., Diaz, F. G., et al.: Temporary clipping in aneurysm surgery: Technique and results. Surg. Neurol., *36*:83–90, 1991.
22. Chyatte, D., Fode, N. C., and Sundt, T., Jr.: Early versus late intracranial aneurysm surgery in subarachnoid hemorrhage. J. Neurosurg., *69*:326–331, 1988.
23. Collier, J.: Observations on cerebral haemorrhage due to causes other than arteriosclerosis. B.M.J., *2*:519–521, 1931.
24. Courville, C. B.: Vascular anomalies of the brain. *In* Courville, C. B., eds.: Pathology of the Central Nervous System. Mountain View, CA, Pacific Press, 1950, pp. 142–152.
25. Crompton, M. R.: Intracerebral haematoma complicating ruptured cerebral berry aneurysm. J. Neurol. Neurosurg. Psychiatry, *25*:378–386, 1962.

26. Crompton, M. R.: Mechanism of growth and rupture in cerebral berry aneurysms. B.M.J., *5496:*1138–1142, 1966.
27. Crompton, M. R.: The pathogenesis of cerebral aneurysms. Brain, *89:*797–814, 1966.
28. Dailey, E. J., Holloway, J. A., Murto, R. E., et al.: Evaluation of ocular signs and symptoms in cerebral aneurysms. Arch. Ophthalmol., *71:*463–474, 1964.
29. Dandy, W. E.: The surgical treatment of intracranial aneurysms of the internal carotid artery. Ann. Surg., *114:*336–340, 1941.
30. Dawson, B. H.: The blood vessels of the human optic chiasma and their relation to those of hypophysis and hypothalamus. Brain, *81:*207–217, 1958.
31. Day, A. L.: Clinico-anatomic features of supraclinoid aneurysms. Clin Neurosurg., *36:*256–274, 1989.
32. Day, A. L.: Aneurysms of the ophthalmic segment: A clinical and anatomical analysis. J. Neurosurg., *72:*677–691, 1990.
33. Day, A. L.: Ophthalmic segment aneurysms. *In* Neurosurgical Operative Atlas. Vol. 2. Baltimore, Williams & Wilkins, 1992, pp. 25–41.
34. Day, A. L., Dickinson, L., Knego, R. S., et al.: Aneurysms of the Clinoidal Segment: A Clinicoanatomic Study. Presented at the American Association of Neurological Surgeons Annual Meeting, Boston, Mass, April 1993 (manuscript in preparation).
35. Day, A. L., Masson, R. L., Knego, R. S.: Surgical management of aneurysms and fistulas involving the cavernous sinus. *In* Schmidek, H. H., and Sweet, W. H., eds.: Operative Neurosurgical Techniques. 3rd ed. Philadelphia, W. B. Saunders, 1995.
36. de-la-Monte, S. M., Moore, G. W., Monk, M. A., et al: Risk factors for the development and rupture of intracranial berry aneurysms. Am. J. Med., *78*(6 Pt. 1):957–964, 1985.
37. Deruty, R., Mottolese, C., Soustiel, J. F., et al.: Association of cerebral arteriovenous malformation and cerebral aneurysm: Diagnosis and management. Acta Neurochir. (Wien), *107:*133–139, 1990.
38. Diggs, I. W., and Brookoff, D.: Multiple cerebral aneurysms in patients with sickle cell disease [see comments]. South. Med. J., *86:*377–379, 1993.
39. Disney, L., Weir, B., and Petruk, K.: Effect on management mortality of a deliberate policy of early operation on supratentorial aneurysms. Neurosurgery, *20:*695–701, 1987.
40. Doczi, T., Bende, J., Huszka, E., et al.: Syndrome of inappropriate secretion of antidiuretic hormone after subarachnoid hemorrhage. Neurosurgery, *9:*394–397, 1981.
41. Dolenc, V. V.: A combined epi- and subdural direct approach to carotid-ophthalmic artery aneurysms. J. Neurosurg., *62:*667–672, 1985.
42. Drake, C. G., Vanderlinden, R. G., and Amacher, A. L.: Carotid-ophthalmic aneurysms. J. Neurosurg., *29:*24–36, 1968.
43. Drake, C. G., et al.: Report of World Federation of Neurological Surgeons Committee on a Universal Subarachnoid Hemorrhage Grading Scale [see comments]. J. Neurosurg., *68:*985–986, 1988.
44. Dunker, R. O., and Harris, A. B.: Surgical anatomy of the proximal anterior cerebral artery. J. Neurosurg., *44:*359–367, 1976.
45. Edner, G., and Ronne-Engstrom, E.: Can early admission reduce aneurysmal rebleeds? A prospective study on aneurysmal incidence, aneurysmal rebleeds, admission and treatment delays in a defined region. Br. J. Neurosurg., *5:*601–608, 1991.
46. Eppinger, H.: Pathogenesis (Histogenesis und Aetiologie) der Aneurysmen einschliesslich des Aneurysma Equi Verminosum: Pathologisch-anatomische Studien. Arch. Klin. Chir., *35*(Suppl. 1):1–563, 1887.
47. Eskesen, V., Rosenorn, J., Schmidt, K., et al.: Clinical features and outcome in 48 patients with unruptured intracranial saccular aneurysms: A prospective consecutive study. Br. J. Neurosurg., *1:*47–52, 1987.
48. Ferguson, G. G., and Drake, C. G.: Carotid-ophthalmic aneurysms: The surgical management of those cases presenting with compression of the optic nerves and chiasm alone. Clin. Neurosurg., *27:*263–308, 1980.
49. Ferguson, G. G., and Drake, C. G.: Carotid-ophthalmic aneurysms: Visual abnormalities in 32 patients and the results of treatment. Surg. Neurol., *16:*1–8, 1981.
50. Ferguson, G. G., Peerless, S. J., and Drake, C. G.: Natural history of intracranial aneurysms [letter]. N. Engl. J. Med., *305*(2):99, 1981.
51. Fisher, C. M.: Clinical syndromes in cerebral thrombosis, hypertensive hemorrhage, and ruptured saccular aneurysm. Clin. Neurosurg., *22:*117–147, 1975.
52. Fisher, C. M., Kistler, J. P., and Davis, J. M.: Relation of cerebral vasospasm to subarachnoid hemorrhage visualized by computerized tomographic scanning. Neurosurgery, *6:*1–9, 1980.
53. Fogelholm, R.: Subarachnoid hemorrhage in middle-Finland: Incidence, early prognosis and indications for neurosurgical treatment. Stroke, *12:*296–301, 1981.
54. Forbus, W. D.: On the origin of miliary aneurysms of the superficial cerebral arteries. Bull. Johns Hopkins Hosp., *47:*239–284, 1930.
55. Fox, J. L.: Intracranial Aneurysms. Vol. I. New York, Springer-Verlag, 1983.
56. Fox, J. L.: Management of aneurysms of anterior circulation by intracranial procedures. *In* Youmans, J. R., eds.: Neurological Surgery. 3rd ed. Philadelphia, W. B. Saunders, 1990, pp. 1689–1732.
57. Fox, A. J., Viñuela, F., Pelz, D. M., et al.: Use of detachable balloons for proximal artery occlusion in the treatment of unclippable cerebral aneurysms. J. Neurosurg., *66:*40–46, 1987.
58. Friedman, W. A., Kaplan, B. L., Day, A. L., et al.: Evoked potential monitoring during aneurysm operation: Observations after fifty cases. Neurosurgery, *20:*678–687, 1987.
59. Gao, Y. Z., and van-Alphen, H. A.: Pathogenesis and histopathology of saccular aneurysms: Review of the literature. Neurol. Res., *12:*249–255, 1990.
60. Gibo, H., Carver, C. C., Rhoton, A. L., Jr., et al.: Microsurgical anatomy of the middle cerebral artery. J. Neurosurg., *54:*151–169, 1981.
61. Gibo, H., Lenkey, C., and Rhoton, A. L., Jr.: Microsurgical anatomy of the supraclinoid portion of the internal carotid artery. J. Neurosurg., *55:*560–574, 1981.
62. Glynn, L. E.: Medial defects in the circle of Willis and their relation to aneurysm formation. J. Pathol., *51:*213–222, 1940.
63. Gouliamos, A., Gotsis, E., Vlahos, L., et al.: Magnetic resonance angiography compared to intra-arterial digital subtraction angiography in patients with subarachnoid haemorrhage. Neuroradiology, *35:*46–49, 1992.
64. Grand, W.: Microsurgical anatomy of the proximal middle cerebral artery and the internal carotid artery bifurcation. Neurosurgery, *7:*215–218, 1980.
65. Guglielmi, G., Viñuela, F., Dion, J., et al.: Electrothrombosis of saccular aneurysms via endovascular approach: Part 2. Preliminary clinical experiences. J. Neurosurg., *75:*8–14, 1991.
66. Handa, J., Nakasu, Y., Matsuda, M., et al.: Aneurysms of the proximal anterior cerebral artery. Surg. Neurol., *22:*486–490, 1984.
67. Harris, P., and Udvarhelyi, G. B.: Aneurysms arising at the internal carotid-posterior communicating artery junction. J Neurosurg., *14:*180–191, 1957.
68. Hauerberg, J., Andersen, B. B., Eskesen, V., et al.: Importance of the recognition of a warning leak as a sign of a ruptured intracranial aneurysm. Acta Neurol. Scand., *83:*61–64, 1991.
69. Hayashi, M., Handa, Y., Kobayashi, H., et al.: Prognosis of intraventricular hemorrhage due to rupture of intracranial aneurysm. Zentralbl. Neurochir., *50:*132–137, 1989.
70. Heiskanen, O.: Risk of bleeding from unruptured aneurysm in cases with multiple intracranial aneurysms. J. Neurosurg., *55:*524–526, 1981.
71. Heiskanen, O., and Marttila, I.: Risk of rupture of a second aneurysm in patients with multiple aneurysms. J. Neurosurg., *32:*295–299, 1970.
72. Helpern, M., and Rabson, S. M.: Sudden and unexpected natural death: III. Spontaneous subarachnoid hemorrhage. Am. J. Med. Sci., *220:*262–271, 1950.
73. Hernesniemi, J., Tapaninaho, A., Vapalahti, M., et al.: Saccular aneurysms of the distal anterior cerebral artery and its branches. Neurosurgery, *31:*994–999, 1992.
74. Heros, R. C., Nelson, P. B., Ojemann, R. G., et al.: Large and giant paraclinoid aneurysms: Surgical techniques, complications, and results. Neurosurgery, *12:*153–163, 1983.
75. Heros, R. C., Ojemann, R. G., and Crowell, R. M.: Superior temporal gyrus approach to middle cerebral aneurysms: Technique and results. Neurosurgery, *10:*308–313, 1982.

76. Hoff, J. T., and Potts, D. G.: Angiographic demonstration of hemorrhage into the fourth ventricle: Case report. J. Neurosurg., 30:732–735, 1969.

77. Hook, O., and Norlen, G.: Aneurysms of the middle cerebral artery. Acta Chir. Scand. [Suppl.], 235:1–39, 1958.

78. Hori, S., and Suzuki, J.: Early and late results in intracranial direct surgery of anterior communicating artery aneurysms. J. Neurosurg., 50:433–440, 1979.

79. Hosoda, K., Fujita, S., Kawaguchi, T., et al.: Saccular aneurysms of the proximal (M₁) segment of the middle cerebral artery. Neurosurgery, 36:441–446, 1995.

80. Housepian, E. M., and Pool, J. L.: A systematic analysis of intracranial aneurysms from the autopsy file of the Presbyterian Hospital 1914 to 1956. J. Neuropathol. Exp. Neurol., 17:409–423, 1958.

81. Hunt, W. E., and Hess, R. M.: Surgical risk as related to time of intervention in the repair of intracranial aneurysms. J. Neurosurg., 28:14–20, 1968.

82. Inagawa, T., Hada, H., and Katoh, Y.: Unruptured intracranial aneurysms in elderly patients. Surg. Neurol., 38:364–370, 1992.

83. Inagawa, T., and Hirano, A.: Autopsy study of unruptured incidental intracranial aneurysms [see comments]. Surg. Neurol., 34:361–365, 1990.

84. Inagawa, T., and Hirano, A.: Ruptured intracranial aneurysms: An autopsy study of 133 patients. Surg. Neurol., 33:117–123, 1990.

85. Inagawa, T., Matsuda, Y., Kamiya, K., et al.: Saccular aneurysm of the distal anterior choroidal artery: Case report. Neurol. Med. Chir. (Tokyo), 30:498–502, 1990.

86. Ingall, T. J., Whisnant, J. P., Wiebers, D. O., et al.: Has there been a decline in subarachnoid hemorrhage mortality? Stroke, 20:718–724, 1989.

87. Inoue, T., Rhoton, A. L., Jr., Theel, D., et al.: Surgical approaches to the cavernous sinus: A microsurgical study. Neurosurgery, 26:903–932, 1990.

88. Iwanaga, H., Wakai, S., Ochiai, C., et al.: Ruptured cerebral aneurysms missed by initial angiographic study. Neurosurgery, 27:45–51, 1990.

89. Jane, J. A., Kassell, N. F., Torner, J. C., et al.: The natural history of aneurysms and arteriovenous malformations. J. Neurosurg., 62:321–323, 1985.

90. Jane, J. A., Winn, H. R., and Richardson, A. E.: The natural history of intracranial aneurysms: Rebleeding rates during the acute and long-term period and implication for surgical management. Clin. Neurosurg., 24:176–184, 1977.

91. Jennett, B., and Galbraith, S.: An Introduction to Neurosurgery. 4th ed. Chicago, Year Book, 1983.

92. Joensen, P.: Subarachnoid hemorrhage in an isolated population: Incidence on the Faroes during the period 1962–1975. Stroke, 15:438–440, 1984.

93. Juvela, S., Porras, M., and Heiskanen, O.: Natural history of unruptured intracranial aneurysms: A long-term follow-up study. J. Neurosurg., 79:174–182, 1993.

94. Kahn, E., Markowitz, J., Duffy, L., et al.: Berry aneurysms, cirrhosis, pulmonary emphysema, and bilateral symmetrical cerebral calcifications: A new syndrome. Am. J. Med. Genet. Suppl., 3:343–356, 1987.

95. Kamiya, K., Inagawa, T., Yamamoto, M., et al.: Subdural hematoma due to ruptured intracranial aneurysm. Neurol. Med. Chir. (Tokyo), 31:82–86, 1991.

96. Kassell, N. F., Sasaki, T., Colohan, A. R., et al.: Cerebral vasospasm following aneurysmal subarachnoid hemorrhage. Stroke, 16:562–572, 1985.

97. Kassell, N. F., and Torner, J. C.: Epidemiology of intracranial aneurysms. Int. Anesthesiol. Clin., 20:13–17, 1982.

98. Kassell, N. F., and Torner, J. C.: Aneurysmal rebleeding: A preliminary report from the Cooperative Aneurysm Study. Neurosurgery, 13:479–481, 1983.

99. Kassell, N. F., and Torner, J. C.: Size of intracranial aneurysms. Neurosurgery, 12:291–297, 1983.

100. Kassell, N. F., Torner, J. C., and Adams, H., Jr.: Antifibrinolytic therapy in the acute period following aneurysmal subarachnoid hemorrhage: Preliminary observations from the Cooperative Aneurysm Study. J. Neurosurg., 61:225–230, 1984.

101. Kassell, N. F., Torner, J. C., Haley, E., Jr., et al.: The International

Cooperative Study on the Timing of Aneurysm Surgery: Part 1. Overall management results. J. Neurosurg., 73:18–36, 1990.

102. Kassell, N. F., Torner, J. C., Jane, J. A., et al.: The International Cooperative Study on the Timing of Aneurysm Surgery: Part 2. Surgical results. J. Neurosurg., 73:37–47, 1990.

103. Kaufmann, A. M., Reddy, K. K., West, M., et al.: Alkaptonuric ochronosis and multiple intracranial aneurysms. Surg. Neurol., 33:213–216, 1990.

104. Kayembe, K. N., Sasahara, M. and Hazama, F.: Cerebral aneurysms and variations in the circle of Willis. Stroke, 15:846–850, 1984.

105. Keogh, A. J., Sharma, R. R., and Vanner, G. K.: The anterior interhemispheric trephine approach to anterior midline aneurysms: Results of treatment in 72 consecutive patients. Br. J. Neurosurg., 7:5–12, 1993.

106. King, R. B., and Saba, M. I.: Forewarnings of major subarachnoid hemorrhage due to congenital berry aneurysm. N. Y. State J. Med., 74:638–639, 1974.

107. Knosp, E., Muller, G., and Perneczky, A.: The paraclinoid carotid artery: Anatomical aspects of a microsurgical approach. Neurosurgery, 22:896–901, 1988.

108. Kobayashi, S., Kyoshima, K., Gibo, H., et al.: Carotid cave aneurysms of the internal carotid artery. J. Neurosurg., 70:216–221, 1989.

109. Krupp, W.: Management results attained by predominantly late surgery for intracranial aneurysms. Neurosurgery, 34:227–234, 1994.

110. Laissy, J. P., Normand, G., Monroc, M., et al.: Spontaneous intracerebral hematomas from vascular causes: Predictive value of CT compared with angiography. Neuroradiology, 33:291–295, 1991.

111. Lang, D. T., Berberian, L. B., and Lee, S., et al.: Rapid differentiation of subarachnoid hemorrhage from traumatic lumbar puncture using the D-dimer assay. Am. J. Clin. Pathol., 93:403–405, 1990.

112. Lanzino, G., Andreoli, A., Tognetti, F., et al.: Orbital pain and unruptured carotid-posterior communicating artery aneurysms: The role of sensory fibers of the third cranial nerve. Acta Neurochir. (Wien), 120:7–11, 1993.

113. Le-Roux, P. D., Dailey, A. T., Newell, D. W., et al.: Emergent aneurysm clipping without angiography in the moribund patient with intracerebral hemorrhage: The use of infusion computed tomography scans. Neurosurgery, 33:189–197, 1993.

114. Le-Roux, P. D., Elliott, J. P., Grady, M. S., et al.: Anterior circulation aneurysms: Improvement in outcome in good-grade patients 1983–1993. Clin. Neurosurg., 41:325–333, 1993.

115. Le-Roux, P. D., Newell, D. W., Eskridge, J., et al.: Severe symptomatic vasospasm: The role of immediate postoperative angioplasty. J. Neurosurg., 80:224–229, 1994.

116. Leblanc, R.: The minor leak preceding subarachnoid hemorrhage. J. Neurosurg., 66:35–39, 1987.

117. Lee, K. C.: Surgery of intracranial aneurysms at Yonsei University: 780 cases. Keio J. Med., 40:1–5, 1991.

118. Levey, A. S., Pauker, S. G., and Kassirer, J. P.: Occult intracranial aneurysms in polycystic kidney disease: When is cerebral arteriography indicated? N. Engl. J. Med., 308:986–994, 1983.

119. Little, J. R., Blomquist, G., Jr., and Ethier, R.: Intraventricular hemorrhage in adults. Surg. Neurol., 8:143–149, 1977.

120. Ljunggren, B., Brandt, L., Saveland, H., et al.: Management of ruptured intracranial aneurysm: A review. Br. J. Neurosurg., 1:9–32, 1987.

121. Ljunggren, B., Saveland, H., Brandt, L., et al.: Early operation and overall outcome in aneurysmal subarachnoid hemorrhage. J. Neurosurg., 62:547–551, 1985.

122. Locksley, H. B.: Natural history of subarachnoid hemorrhage, intracranial aneurysms and arteriovenous malformations. J. Neurosurg., 25:321–368, 1966.

123. Lye, R. H., and Dyer, P. A.: Intracranial aneurysm and HLA-DR2 [letter]. J. Neurol. Neurosurg. Psychiatry, 52:291, 1989.

124. Magner, W.: Multiple intracranial aneurysms. Can. Med. Assoc. J., 33:401–403, 1935.

125. Majamaa, K., and Myllyla, V. V.: A disorder of collagen biosynthesis in patients with cerebral artery aneurysm. Biochim. Biophys. Acta, 1225:48–52, 1993.

126. Mann, K. S., Yue, C. P., and Wong, G.: Aneurysms of the

pericallosal-callosal marginal junction. Surg. Neurol., *21*:261–266, 1984.

127. Marion, D. W., Segal, R., and Thompson, M. E.: Subarachnoid hemorrhage and the heart. Neurosurgery, *18*:101–106, 1986.

128. Martland, H. S.: Spontaneous subarachnoid hemorrhage and congenital "berry aneurysms" of the circle of Willis. Am. J. Surg., *43*:10–19, 1939.

129. Masson, R. L., Jr., and Day, A. L.: Aneurysmal intracerebral hemorrhage. Neurosurg. Clin. North Am., *3*:539–550, 1992.

130. McCormick, W. F.: Problems and pathogenesis of intracranial arterial aneurysms. *In* Toole, J. F., Moossy, J., and Janeway, R., eds.: Cerebral Vascular Diseases. New York, Grune & Stratton, 1971, pp. 219–231.

131. McCormick, W. F., and Acosta-Rua, G. J.: The size of intracranial saccular aneurysms: An autopsy study. J. Neurosurg. *33*:422–427, 1970.

132. McCormick, W. F., and Nofzinger, J. D.: Saccular intracranial aneurysms: An autopsy study. J. Neurosurg., *22*:155–159, 1965.

133. McKissock, W., Richardson, A., and Walsh, L.: Posterior communicating artery aneurysms: A controlled trial of the conservative and surgical treatment of ruptured aneurysms of the internal carotid artery at or near the point of origin of the posterior communicating artery. Lancet, *1*:1203–1206, 1960.

134. McKissock, W., Richardson, A., and Walsh, L., et al.: Multiple intracranial aneurysms. Lancet *1*:623–626, 1964.

135. Mellergard, P., Ljunggren, B., Brandt, L., et al.: HLA-typing in a family with six intracranial aneurysms. Br. J. Neurosurg., *3*:479–485, 1989.

136. Meyer, F. B., Huston, J. 3d, and Riederer, S. S.: Pulsatile increases in aneurysm size determined by cine phase-contrast MR angiography. J. Neurosurg., *78*:879–883, 1993.

137. Mizoi, K., and Yoshimoto, T.: Permissible temporary occlusion time in aneurysm surgery as evaluated by evoked potential monitoring. Neurosurgery, *33*:434–440, 1993.

138. Mohr, G., Ferguson, G., Khan, M., et al.: Intraventricular hemorrhage from ruptured aneurysm: Retrospective analysis of 91 cases. J. Neurosurg., *58*:482–487, 1983.

139. Morcos, J. J., and Heros, R. C.: Results and complications of the surgical management of intracranial aneurysms. *In* Awad, I., ed.: Neurosurgical Topics: Current Management of Cerebral Aneurysms. Park Ridge, IL, American Association of Neurological Surgeons, 1993, pp. 297–316.

140. Moyes, P. D.: Surgical treatment of multiple aneurysms and of incidentally discovered unruptured aneurysms. J. Neurosurg., *35*:291–295, 1971.

141. Muller, P. J., and Deck, J. H.: Intraocular and optic nerve sheath hemorrhage in cases of sudden intracranial hypertension. J. Neurosurg., *41*:160–166, 1974.

142. Nakagawa, F., Kobayashi, S., Takamae, T., et al.: Aneurysms protruding from the dorsal wall of the internal carotid artery. J. Neurosurg., *65*:303–308, 1986.

143. Nakagawa, F., and Hashi, K.: The incidence and treatment of asymptomatic, unruptured cerebral aneurysms. J. Neurosurg., *80*:217–223, 1994.

144. Nelson, P. B., Seif, S. M., and Maroon, J. C., et al.: Hyponatremia in intracranial disease: Perhaps not the syndrome of inappropriate secretion of antidiuretic hormone (SIADH). J. Neurosurg., *65*:938–941, 1981.

145. Nishihara, J., Kumon, Y., Matsuo, Y., et al.: A case of distal anterior choroidal artery aneurysm: Case report and review of the literature. Neurosurgery, *32*:834–837, 1993.

146. Nishio, S., Matsushima, T., Fukui, M., et al.: Microsurgical anatomy around the origin of the ophthalmic artery with reference to contralateral pterional surgical approach to the carotid-ophthalmic aneurysm. Acta Neurochir. (Wien), *76*:82–89, 1985.

147. Norrgard, O., Angquist, K. A., Fodstad, H., et al.: Intracranial aneurysms and heredity. Neurosurgery, *20*:236–239, 1987.

148. Nutik, S. L.: Carotid paraclinoid aneurysms with intradural origin and intracavernous location. J. Neurosurg., *48*:526–533, 1978.

149. Nutik, S. L.: Removal of the anterior clinoid process for exposure of the proximal intracranial carotid artery. J. Neurosurg., *69*:529–534, 1988.

150. Ogawa, A., Suzuki, M., Sakurai, Y., et al.: Vascular anomalies associated with aneurysms of the anterior communicating ar-

tery: Microsurgical observations. J. Neurosurg., *72*:706–709, 1990.

151. Ohman, J., and Heiskanen, O.: Timing of operation for ruptured supratentorial aneurysms: A prospective randomized study [see comments]. J. Neurosurg., *70*:55–60, 1989.

152. Ohno, K., Monma, S., Suzuki, R., et al.: Saccular aneurysms of the distal anterior cerebral artery. Neurosurgery, *27*:907–913, 1990.

153. Okawara, S. H.: Warning signs prior to rupture of an intracranial aneurysm. J. Neurosurg., *38*:575–580, 1973.

154. Oken, B. S.: Intracranial aneurysms in polycystic kidney disease [letter]. N. Engl. J. Med., *309*:927–928, 1983.

155. Ostergaard, J. R., Bruun-Petersen, G., and Kristensen, B. O.: The C3-F gene in patients with intracranial saccular aneurysms. Acta Neurol. Scand., *74*:356–359, 1986.

156. Ostergaard, J. R., and Hog, E.: Incidence of multiple intracranial aneurysms: Influence of arterial hypertension and gender. J. Neurosurg., *63*:49–55, 1985.

157. Otomo, E.: The anterior choroidal artery. Arch. Neurol., *13*:656–658, 1965.

158. Pakarinen, S.: Incidence, aetiology, and prognosis of primary subarachnoid haemorrhage: A study based on 589 cases diagnosed in a defined urban population during a defined period. Acta Neurol. Scand., *29*:1–28, 1967.

159. Peerless, S. J.: The surgical approach to middle cerebral and posterior communicating aneurysms. Clin. Neurosurg., *21*:151–165, 1974.

160. Perlmutter, D., and Rhoton, A. L., Jr.: Microsurgical anatomy of the anterior cerebral–anterior communicating–recurrent artery complex. J. Neurosurg., *45*:259–272, 1976.

161. Perlmutter, D., and Rhoton, A. L., Jr.: Microsurgical anatomy of the distal anterior cerebral artery. J. Neurosurg., *49*:204–228, 1978.

162. Perret, G., and Nishioka, H.: Arteriovenous malformations: An analysis of 545 cases of craniocerebral arteriovenous malformations and fistula reported to the cooperative study. *In* Sahs, A. L., Perret, G. E., Locksley, H. B., et al., eds.: Intracranial Aneurysms and Subarachnoid Hemorrhage: A Cooperative Study. Philadelphia, J. B. Lippincott, 1969, pp. 200–222.

163. Perria, L., Rivano, C., Rossi, G. F., et al.: Aneurysms of the bifurcation of the internal carotid artery. Acta Neurochir. (Wien), *19*:51–68, 1968.

164. Perria, L., Viale, G. L., and Rivano, C.: Further remarks on the surgical treatment of carotid-choroidal aneurysms. Acta Neurochir. (Wien), *24*:253–262, 1971.

165. Petruk, K. C., West, M., Mohr, G., et al.: Nimodipine treatment in poor-grade aneurysm patients: Results of a multicenter, double-blind, placebo-controlled trial. J. Neurosurg., *68*:505–517, 1988.

166. Pia, H. W.: Classification of aneurysms of the internal carotid system. Acta Neurochir. (Wien), *40*:5–31, 1978.

167. Pia, H. W., Obrador, S., and Martin, J. G.: Association of brain tumours and arterial intracranial aneurysms. Acta Neurochir. (Wien), *27*:189–204, 1972.

168. Pickard, J. D., Murray, J. D., and Illingworth, R., et al.: Effect of oral nimodipine on cerebral infarction and outcome after subarachnoid hemorrhage. B. M. J., *298*:636–642, 1989.

169. Pope, F. M., Kendall, B. E., Slapak, G. I., et al.: Type III collagen mutations cause fragile cerebral arteries. Br. J. Neurosurg., *5*:551–574, 1991.

170. Pritz, M. B., and Chandler, W. F.: The transsylvian approach to middle cerebral artery bifurcation-trifurcation aneurysms. Surg. Neurol., *41*:217–220, 1994.

171. Reifenstein, G. H., Levine, S. A., and Gross, R. E.: Coarctation of the aorta: A review of 104 autopsied cases of the "adult type," 2 years of age or older. Am. Heart J., *33*:146–168, 1947.

172. Reynolds, A. F., and Shaw, C. M.: Bleeding patterns from ruptured intracranial aneurysms: An autopsy series of 205 patients. Surg. Neurol., *15*:232–235, 1981.

173. Rhoton, A., Jr.: Anatomy of saccular aneurysms. Surg. Neurol., *14*:59–66, 1980.

174. Rhoton, A. L., Jr.: Anatomic foundations of aneurysm surgery. Clin. Neurosurg., *41*:289–324, 1993.

175. Richardson, J. C., and Hyland, H. H.: Intracranial aneurysms: A clinical and pathological study of subarachnoid and intracerebral hemorrhage caused by berry aneurysms. Medicine, *20*:1–83, 1941.

176. Riise, R.: Ocular symptoms in saccular aneurysms of the internal carotid artery: A survey of 100 cases. Acta Ophthalmol., 47:1012–1020, 1969.

177. Rinkel, G. J., Wijdicks, E. F., Vermeulen, M., et al.: Nonaneurysmal perimesencephalic subarachnoid hemorrhage: CT and MR patterns that differ from aneurysmal rupture. A.J.N.R., 12:829–834, 1991.

178. Robertson, E. G.: Cerebral lesions due to intracranial aneurysms. Brain, 72:150–185, 1949.

179. Robinson, R. G.: Coarctation of the aorta and cerebral aneurysm: Report of two cases. J. Neurosurg., 26:527–531, 1967.

180. Rodman, K. D., and Awad, I. A.: Clinical presentation. In Awad, I., eds: Neurosurgical Topics: Current Management of Cerebral Aneurysms. Park Ridge, IL, American Association of Neurological Surgeons, 1993, pp. 21–41.

181. Ropper, A. H., and Zervas, N. T.: Outcome 1 year after SAH from cerebral aneurysm: Management morbidity, mortality, and functional status in 112 consecutive good-risk patients. J. Neurosurg., 60:909–915, 1984.

182. Rosenorn, J., and Eskesen, V.: Does a safe size-limit exist for unruptured intracranial aneurysms? Acta Neurochir. (Wien), 121:113–118, 1993.

183. Rosenorn, J., Eskesen, V., Schmidt, K., et al.: Clinical features and outcome in 1076 patients with ruptured intracranial saccular aneurysms: A prospective consecutive study. Br. J. Neurosurg., 1:33–45, 1987.

184. Rosner, S. S., Rhoton, A. L., Ono, M., et al.: Microsurgical anatomy of the anterior perforating arteries. J. Neurosurg., 61:468–485, 1984.

185. Russegger, L., and Twerdy, K.: Peracute surgery of aneurysms with intracerebral hematomas. Neurochirurgia (Stuttg.), 36:37–43, 1993.

186. Rusyniak, W. G., Peterson, P. C., Okawara, S. H., et al.: Acute subdural hematoma after aneurysmal rupture; evacuation with aneurysmal clipping after emergent infusion computed tomography: Case report. Neurosurgery, 31:129–131, 1992.

187. Sacco, R. L., Wolf, P. A. and Bharucha, N. E., et al.: Subarachnoid and intracerebral hemorrhage: Natural history, prognosis, and precursive factors in the Framingham study. Neurology, 34:847–854, 1984.

188. Sahs, A. L.: Intracranial aneurysms and polycystic kidney. Arch. Neurol. Psychiatry, 63:524, 1950.

189. Sahs, A. L.: Report on the cooperative study of intracranial aneurysms and subarachnoid hemorrhage. Section VII. 2. Hypotension and hypothermia in the treatment of intracranial aneurysms. J. Neurosurg., 25:593–600, 1966.

190. Sahs, A. L., Perret, G., Locksley, H. B., et al.: Preliminary remarks on subarachnoid hemorrhage. J. Neurosurg., 24:782–788, 1966.

191. Sahs, A. L., Perret, G. E., Locksley, H. B., et al.: Intracranial Aneurysms and Subarachnoid Hemorrhage: A Cooperative Study. Philadelphia, J. B. Lippincott, 1969.

192. Sakaki, T., Takeshima, T., Tominaga, M., et al.: Recurrence of ICA-PCoA aneurysms after neck clipping. J. Neurosurg., 80:58–63, 1994.

193. Salazar, J. L.: Surgical treatment of asymptomatic and incidental intracranial aneurysms. J. Neurosurg., 53:20–21, 1980.

194. Saveland, H., Hillman, J., Brandt, L., et al.: Overall outcome in aneurysmal subarachnoid hemorrhage: A prospective study from neurosurgical units in Sweden during a 1-year period. J. Neurosurg., 76:729–734, 1992.

195. Schuierer, G., Huk, W. J., and Laub, G.: Magnetic resonance angiography of intracranial aneurysms: Comparison with intra-arterial digital subtraction angiography. Neuroradiology, 35:50–54, 1992.

196. Schurmann, K., Brock, M., and Samii, M.: Circumscribed hematoma of the lateral ventricle following rupture of an intraventricular saccular arterial aneurysm: Case report. J. Neurosurg., 29:195–198, 1968.

197. Sekhar, L. N., and Heros, R. C.: Origin, growth, and rupture of saccular aneurysms: A review. Neurosurgery, 8:248–260, 1981.

198. Sengupta, R. P., Lassman, L. P., de Moraes, A. A., et al.: Treatment of internal carotid bifurcation aneurysms by direct surgery. J. Neurosurg., 43:343–351, 1975.

199. Simkins, Y. E., and Stehbens, W. E.: Vibrations recorded from the adventitial surface of aneurysms and arteriovenous fistulas. Vasc. Surg., 8:153–165, 1974.

200. Solomon, R. A., Fink, M. E., and Lennihan, L.: Early aneurysm surgery and prophylactic hypervolemic hypertensive therapy for the treatment of aneurysmal subarachnoid hemorrhage. Neurosurgery, 23:699–704, 1988.

201. Solomon, R. A., Fink, M. E., and Lennihan, L.: Prophylactic volume expansion therapy for the prevention of delayed cerebral ischemia after early aneurysm surgery: Results of a preliminary trial. Arch. Neurol., 45:325–332, 1988.

202. Solomon, R. A., Fink, M. E., and Pile-Spellman, J.: Surgical management of unruptured intracranial aneurysms. J. Neurosurg., 80:440–446, 1994.

203. Solomon, R. A., Onesti, S. T., and Klebanoff, L.: Relationship between the timing of aneurysm surgery and the development of delayed cerebral ischemia. J. Neurosurg., 75:56–61, 1991.

204. Spetzler, R. F., and Lee, K. S.: Reconstruction of the temporalis muscle for the pterional craniotomy. J. Neurosurg., 73:636–637, 1990.

205. Stehbens, W. E.: Hypertension and cerebral aneurysms. Med. J. Aust., 2:8–10, 1962.

206. Stehbens, W. E.: Aneurysms and anatomical variation of cerebral aneurysms. Arch. Pathol., 75:45–64, 1963.

207. Stehbens, W. E.: Pathology of the Cerebral Blood Vessels. St. Louis, C. V. Mosby, 1972.

208. Stehbens, W. E.: Etiology of intracranial berry aneurysms. J. Neurosurg., 70:823–831, 1989.

209. Steiger, H. J., Liepsch, D. W., Poll, A., et al.: Hemodynamic stress in terminal saccular aneurysms: A laser-Doppler study. Heart Vessels, 4:162–169, 1988.

210. Steiger, H. J., and Reulen, H. J.: Low-frequency flow fluctuations in saccular aneurysms. Acta Neurochir. (Wien), 83:131–137, 1986.

211. Strang, R. R., Tovi, D., and Hugosson, R.: Subdural hematomas resulting from the rupture of intracranial arterial aneurysms. Acta Chir. Scand., 121:345–350, 1961.

212. Strother, C. M., Graves, V. B., and Rappe, A.: Aneurysm hemodynamics: An experimental study. A.J.N.R. 13:1089–1095, 1992.

213. Sugai, M., and Shoji, M.: Pathogenesis of so-called congenital aneurysms of the brain. Acta Pathol. Jpn., 18:139–160, 1968.

214. Sundt, T., Jr., Kobayashi, S., Fode, N. C., et al.: Results and complications of surgical management of 809 intracranial aneurysms in 722 cases: Related and unrelated to grade of patient, type of aneurysm, and timing of surgery. J. Neurosurg., 56:753–765, 1982.

215. Suzuki, J.: Cerebral Aneurysms: Experience with 1000 Directly Operated Cases. Tokyo, Neuron Publishing, 1979.

216. Suzuki, J., Kodama, N., and Fujiwara, S.: Surgical treatment of internal carotid–posterior communicating aneurysms: From the experience of 213 cases. In Suzuki, J., ed.: Cerebral Aneurysms. Tokyo, Neuron Publishing, 1979.

217. Suzuki, J., Kodama, N., Fujiwara, S., et al.: Surgical treatment of middle cerebral aneurysms: From the experience of 174 cases. In Suzuki, J., ed.: Cerebral Aneurysms. Tokyo, Neuron Publishing, 1979.

218. Suzuki, J., and Onuma, T.: Intracranial aneurysms associated with arteriovenous malformations. J. Neurosurg., 50:742–746, 1979.

219. Suzuki, J., and Yoshimoto, T.: Distribution of cerebral aneurysms. In Pia, H. W., Langmaid, C., and Ziersky, Z., eds.: Cerebral Aneurysms. Berlin, Springer-Verlag, 1979, pp. 127–133.

220. Suzuki, J., Yoshimoto, T., and Takamasa, K.: Surgical treatment of middle cerebral aneurysms. J. Neurosurg., 61:17–23, 1984.

221. Suzuki, M., Onuma, T., Sakurai, Y., et al.: Aneurysms arising from the proximal (A_1) segment of the anterior cerebral artery: A study of 38 cases. J. Neurosurg., 76:455–458, 1992.

222. Symonds, C. P.: Contributions to the clinical study of intracranial aneurysms. Guy's Hosp. Rep. (Lond.) 72:139–158, 1923.

223. Tabbaa, M. A., Ramirez-Lassepas, M., and Snyder, B. D.: Aneurysmal subarachnoid hemorrhage presenting as cardiorespiratory arrest. Arch. Intern. Med., 147:1661–1662, 1987.

224. Taylor, B., Harries, P., and Bullock, R.: Factors affecting outcome after surgery for intracranial aneurysm in Glasgow. Br. J. Neurosurg., 5:591–600, 1991.

225. Terson, A.: Le syndrome de l'hematome du corps vitre et de

l'hemorrhagie intracranienne spontanes. Ann. Ocul., *163*:666–673, 1926.

226. Thompson, R. K., Manganiello, L. O. J., and Nichols, P.: Intraventricular hemorrhage: Some experimental and clinical observations. South. Med. J., *40*:990–996, 1947.

227. Tran-Dinh, H., Williams, L. M., and Jayasinghe, L. S.: Association of intracranial aneurysm and arteriovenous malformation. Med. J. Aust., *1*:521–523, 1983.

228. Tsementzis, S. A.: Surgical management of intracerebral hematomas. Neurosurgery, *16*:562–572, 1985.

229. Ujiie, H., Sato, K., Onda, H., et al.: Clinical analysis of incidentally discovered unruptured aneurysms. Stroke, *24*:1850–1856, 1993.

230. van-Gijn, J., van-Dongen, K. J., Vermeulen, M., et al.: Perimesencephalic hemorrhage: A nonaneurysmal and benign form of subarachnoid hemorrhage. Neurology, *35*:493–497, 1985.

231. VanderArk, G. D., and Kempe, G.: Classification of anterior communicating artery aneurysms as a basis for surgical approach. J. Neurosurg., *32*:300–303, 1970.

232. VanderArk, G. D., Kempe, G., and Smith, D. R.: Anterior communicating artery aneurysms: The gyrus rectus approach. Clin. Neurosurg., *21*:120–133, 1974.

233. Vermeulen, M., Lindsay, K. W., Murray, G. D., et al.: Antifibrinolytic treatment in subarachnoid hemorrhage. N. Engl. J. Med., *311*:432–437, 1984.

234. Verweij, R. D., Wijdicks, E. F., and van-Gijn, J.: Warning headache in aneurysmal subarachnoid hemorrhage: A case-control study [see comments]. Arch. Neurol., *45*:1019–1020, 1988.

235. Viale, G. L., and Pau, A.: Carotid-choroidal aneurysms: Remarks on surgical treatment and outcome. Surg. Neurol., *11*:141–145, 1979.

236. Waga, S., Otsubo, K., and Handa, H.: Warning signs in intracranial aneurysms. Surg. Neurol., *3*:15–20, 1975.

237. Wakai, S., Fukushima, T., Furihata, T., et al.: Association of cerebral aneurysm with pituitary adenoma. Surg. Neurol., *12*:503–507, 1979.

238. Walton, J. N.: The electroencephalographic sequelae of spontaneous subarachnoid hemorrhage. Electroencephalogr. Clin. Neurophysiol., *5*:41–52, 1953.

239. Walton, J. N.: Subarachnoid Hemorrhage. Edinburgh, E & S Livingstone, 1956.

240. Watanabe, K., Wakai, S., Okuhata, S., et al.: Ruptured distal anterior cerebral artery aneurysms presenting as acute subdural hematoma: Report of three cases. Neurol. Med. Chir. Tokyo, *31*:514–517, 1991.

241. Weir, B., Grace, M., Hansen, J., et al.: Time course of vasospasm in man. J. Neurosurg., *48*:173–178, 1978.

242. Weir, B., Myles, T., Kahn, M., et al.: Management of acute subdural hematomas from aneurysmal rupture. Can. J. Neurol. Sci., *11*:371–376, 1984.

243. Weir, B. K.: Aneurysms affecting the nervous system. Baltimore, Williams & Wilkins, 1987.

244. Wiebers, D. O., Whisnant, J. P., and O'Fallon, W. M.: The natural history of unruptured intracranial aneurysms. N. Engl. J. Med., *304*:696–698, 1981.

245. Wiebers, D. O., Whisnant, J. P., Sundt, T., Jr., et al.: The significance of unruptured intracranial saccular aneurysms. J. Neurosurg., *66*:23–29, 1987.

246. Wijdicks, E. F., Ropper, A. H., Hunnicutt, E. J., et al.: Atrial natriuretic factor and salt wasting after aneurysmal subarachnoid hemorrhage. Stroke, *22*:1519–1524, 1991.

247. Williams, R. R., Bahn, R. C., and Sayre, G. P.: Congenital cerebral aneurysms. Proc. Staff Meet. Mayo Clin., *30*:161–168, 1955.

248. Wilson, G., Riggs, H. E., and Rupp, C.: The pathologic anatomy of ruptured cerebral aneurysms. J. Neurosurg., *11*:128–134, 1954.

249. Winn, H. R., Almaani, W. S., Berga, S. L., et al.: The long-term outcome in patients with multiple aneurysms: Incidence of late hemorrhage and implications for treatment of incidental aneurysms. J. Neurosurg., *59*:642–651, 1983.

250. Winn, H. R., Newell, D. W., Mayberg, M. R., et al.: Early surgical management of poor-grade patients with intracranial aneurysms. Clin. Neurosurg., *36*:289–298, 1990.

251. Wirth, F. P., Laws, E., Jr., Piepgras, D., et al.: Surgical treatment of incidental intracranial aneurysms. Neurosurgery, *12*:507–511, 1983.

252. Wise, B. L.: Syndrome of inappropriate antidiuretic hormone secretion after spontaneous subarachnoid hemorrhage: A reversible cause of clinical deterioration. Neurosurgery, *3*:412–414, 1978.

253. Xu, H. Q., and Wang, Y. S.: Insular cistern hematoma: A special type of subarachnoid hemorrhage. Chin. Med. J. (Engl.), *105*:717–720, 1992.

254. Yamamoto, Y., Asari, S., Sunami, N., et al.: Computed angiotomography of unruptured cerebral aneurysms. J. Comput. Assist. Tomogr., *10*:21–27, 1986.

255. Yasargil, M. G.: Microneurosurgery. Vols. I and II. New York, Thieme-Stratton, 1987.

256. Yasargil, M. G., Boehm, W. G., and Ho, R. E.: Microsurgical treatment of cerebral aneurysms at the bifurcation of the internal carotid artery. Acta Neurochir. (Wien), *41*:61–72, 1978.

257. Yasargil, M. G., and Carter, L. P.: Saccular aneurysms of the distal anterior cerebral artery. J. Neurosurg., *40*:218–223, 1974.

258. Yasargil, M. G., and Fox, J. L.: The microsurgical approach to intracranial aneurysms. Surg. Neurol., *3*:7–14, 1975.

259. Yasargil, M. G., Gasser, J. C., Hodosh, R. M., et al.: Carotid-ophthalmic aneurysms: Direct microsurgical approach. Surg. Neurol., *8*:155–165, 1977.

260. Yoshimoto, T., Uchida, K., Kaneko, U., et al.: An analysis of follow-up results of 1000 intracranial saccular aneurysms with definitive surgical treatment. J. Neurosurg., *50*:152–157, 1979.

261. Yoshimoto, T., Uchida, K., and Suzuki, J.: Surgical treatment of distal anterior cerebral artery aneurysms. J. Neurosurg., *50*:40–44, 1979.

262. Zacks, D. J., Russell, D. B., and Miller, J. D.: Fortuitously discovered intracranial aneurysms. Arch. Neurol., *37*:39–41, 1980.

Intracranial Giant Aneurysms†

Intracranial aneurysms 2.5 cm or greater in diameter are classified by convention as giant aneurysms. In spite of advances in techniques in neuroradiology, neuroanesthesiology, and microneurosurgery treatment of these aneurysms remains difficult. Routine clipping of the aneurysm neck is impractical, and combination of multiple clips or occlusion of the parent artery with bypass surgery is often required. The development of the intravascular technique is rapidly changing the treatment strategy for giant aneurysms.

Clinical Presentation

Giant intracranial aneurysms present as either mass signs or subarachnoid hemorrhage. Subarachnoid hemorrhage is seen in 14 to 35 per cent of patients.[10, 21, 36] Intradural saccular aneurysms show a higher incidence of subarachnoid hemorrhage than extradural aneurysms, such as intracavernous internal carotid aneurysms or intradural fusiform aneurysms.[22, 25, 28] However, differentiation between fusiform and saccular aneurysms is not always easy. Many giant aneurysms develop at the trunk of the carotid and vertebrobasilar arteries rather than at bifurcation of branches, and so they have wide necks. Intraluminal thrombosis, found in about 40 per cent of the cases, also contributes to the incidence of subarachnoid hemorrhage.[19] Nonthrombosed aneurysms have a higher incidence of subarachnoid hemorrhage than partially thrombosed aneurysms. Subarachnoid hemorrhage from giant aneurysms causes more severe neurological deficits.[13, 50] It is conceivable that giant aneurysms cause a more severe hemorrhage than small aneurysms because of the higher tension of the wall, as can be calculated by Laplace's law, $T = PR/2e$, where T is the tension of

the aneurysm wall, P is the intramural pressure; R is the radius of the aneurysm, and e is the thickness of the wall.[19]

A higher pressure must be applied to rupture the giant aneurysm wall than to rupture the small aneurysm wall, and a larger amount of hemorrhage occurs once the giant aneurysm ruptures.

Intracranial giant aneurysms are reported to comprise 2 to 5 per cent of all intracranial aneurysms.[58] Localization of intracranial giant aneurysms (Table 54–1) is different from that of small aneurysms.[19, 20, 34, 58] To summarize, about 40 per cent are seen in the carotid artery, 25 per cent in the anterior and middle cerebral arteries, and 30 per cent in the vertebrobasilar arteries. The high percentage of giant aneurysms in the posterior circulation in Peerless's report reflects their referral pattern.[34] The ratio of giant aneurysms to all aneurysms is about six to one in the posterior circulation, much higher than that of anterior circulation. The average age of patients is 50, and a female predominance (60 per cent) is similar to the statistics for all aneurysms.

The location of giant aneurysms determines the characteristic clinical signs demonstrated. Aneurysms of the intracavernous carotid artery manifest by chronic retro-orbital pain, fluctuating diplopia, or ptosis. Massive epistaxis can occur if the aneurysms erode the surrounding bone. Carotid-ophthalmic aneurysms usually cause asymmetrical visual field defects with decreased visual acuity. Carotid bifurcation aneurysms cause visual deficits, epilepsy, and dementia. Subarachnoid hemorrhage is also seen in 50 per cent of these cases. Mental disturbance and visual defects are common in giant aneurysms in the anterior communicating artery. Epilepsy and hemiparesis are common in the middle cerebral aneurysms.

Giant aneurysms in the basilar bifurcation and superior cerebellar artery cause ataxia, dementia, oculomotor palsy, and Weber's syndrome. Features similar to those of pontine tumors, such as abducens palsy, hy-

---

†Dr. Sugita is deceased.

M. Shibuya • K. Sugita

Table 54–1

LOCATIONS OF INTRACRANIAL GIANT ANEURYSMS

	Total No.			
	Weir et al.[58] *573*	*Keravel et al.*[19] *309*	*Kodama et al.*[20] *1023*	*Peerless et al.*[34] *635*
Carotid	39%	42%	51%	34%
Cavernous	6	13		9
Ophthalmic	21	12		15
Pcom	3	7		5
Bifurcation	9	10		5
MCA	16	15	13	8
ACA	12	10	8	3
V-B	25	33	27	56
PCA	3	2		9
BA bifurcation	7	15		21
BA-SCA	8	} 9		8
BA trunk				8
VA junction	3	} 6		5
VA	4			5
Others	8			

ACA, anterior cerebral artery; BA, basilar artery; MCA, middle cerebral artery; PCA, posterior cerebral artery; Pcom, posterior communicating artery; SCA, superior cerebellar artery; VA, vertebral artery; V-B vertebrobasilar artery.

drocephalus, and dementia, are common in basilar trunk aneurysms. Vertebrobasilar junction aneurysms cause signs of cerebellopontine angle tumors such as hearing loss, hemifacial palsy, or hypesthesia. Giant aneurysms of the vertebral artery cause lower cranial nerve palsy, tetraparesis, and respiratory distress.[58] Sleep apnea is often life threatening in patients with giant vertebral aneurysms.

Pathology

Giant aneurysms most probably grow from small aneurysms starting at a site with a congenital or acquired defect in the arterial wall. Walls of giant aneurysms often lack the muscular layer, and very few elastic and muscular fibers can be found. Some giant aneurysms apparently grow with repeated hemorrhages.[12] The laminated clot seen in most giant aneurysms seems to have formed in response to relentless arterial pulsation and progressive accumulation of thrombus on the inner aneurysmal surface from turbulent and slow blood flow in the aneurysms.[36, 58] Sutherland and associates demonstrated platelet deposition within giant aneurysms using a dual radioisotope technique employing indium-111–labeled platelets and technetium-99m–labeled red blood cells.[53] Half of the patients with intraluminal platelet deposition, as calculated by the difference in ratio of the radioisotopes, showed symptoms of ischemia. They concluded that platelet aggregation occurred frequently in giant aneurysms and that platelet metabolites or thrombi could embolize to distal cerebral arteries.

Neuroradiological Examinations

ANGIOGRAPHY

Cerebral angiography is still the most important neuroradiological examination for surgery of giant aneurysms. To clarify the exact anatomy around the neck of the aneurysm, not only straight anteroposterior and lateral views but also various oblique views are important. Manual compression of one carotid artery is important to determine the collateral flow from the other carotid artery through the anterior communicating artery and from the basilar artery through the posterior communicating artery. This maneuver is also useful to visualize the distal aneurysmal neck of a giant carotid ophthalmic aneurysm, which is often obscured on the carotid angiograms because of dilution of the contrast medium in a large aneurysmal sac. Intraoperative angiography is very useful, especially in difficult cases requiring complete examination of the clipping and patency of the parent artery.

COMPUTED TOMOGRAPHY

Computed tomography is useful in diagnosing small aneurysms resulting from subarachnoid hemorrhage to predict the bleeding site. Giant aneurysms can be identified as round masses. Contrast medium–enhanced computed tomography may show a "target sign," a ring enhancement around the aneurysmal wall, the nonenhanced mural thrombus, and the enhanced central region due to residual blood flow.[40] The relationship between the parent artery and the aneurysmal sac, which is often not clearly seen by angiography, can be visualized by high-resolution computed tomography with 0.5- to 1-mm thin slices. Intraluminal thrombi are visualized as iso- or high-density areas, which may clarify the discrepancy between the size of aneurysms as demonstrated by angiography and at surgery. The presence of intraluminal thrombosis also warns of difficulty in clipping without thrombectomy and suggests that great care must be taken not to dislocate the thrombi into the distal artery during manipulation of the aneurysm. Calcification of the wall of the aneurysm, which also causes great difficulty during clipping, is only clearly seen by high-resolution computed tomography. Crushing of the calcification by a hemostat may be needed to close the clip blades.[8]

Thin-sliced bone level computed tomography is helpful to the surgeon who is drilling the bone of the anterior clinoid process, optic canal, or air cells in the case of a giant parasellar aneurysm. It is also important in the transcondylar approach for a high vertebral aneurysm to obtain exact information about the occipital condyle and jugular tubercle. Additionally, it is most useful in following the size and progress of thrombosis in the aneurysms after proximal occlusion of the parent artery. The size of the aneurysm is reduced and density is increased with successful cessation of the blood flow and thrombosis in the sac. Three-dimensional computed tomography seems to facilitate obtaining anatomical detail of a giant aneurysm, parent artery, and adjacent bony structures.[15]

MAGNETIC RESONANCE IMAGING

Magnetic resonance imaging is a noninvasive technique for demonstrating the presence of giant aneurysms and the flow within the aneurysms as well as for differentiating old clots from recent clots. Deoxyhemoglobin, methemoglobin (in red blood cells), and hemosiderin cause low signal intensity on a T2-weighted image. Both free and bound methemoglobin cause high signal intensity on a T1-weighted image. Recent clots remain bright on both T1- and T2-weighted images; and as the water is reabsorbed from the organizing clot, its signal becomes less and less intense. Rapid or turbulent flow gives no signal on a T1-weighted image but may show central phase artifact on a T2-weighted image. Magnetic resonance imaging also gives excellent anatomical detail in and around giant aneurysms.[33, 59]

Surgery of Giant Aneurysms

All information about the aneurysm, angiography, computed tomography, and magnetic resonance imaging must be carefully weighed to select the most appropriate form of treatment: direct clipping and proximal occlusion with or without bypass surgery. Preoperative balloon test occlusion is essential to make such a decision.[24, 27] In addition, one must remember that ischemia due to proximal occlusion during surgery is more severe than by balloon test occlusion due to brain retraction, which limits collateral flow.

EFFECT OF PROXIMAL OCCLUSION

Carotid Artery

Proximal ligation of a parent artery can be expected to prevent rupture of an aneurysm by decreasing the distal blood pressure, since it is known that rupture of an aneurysm correlates well with the blood pressure in the parent artery.[32, 56, 60] Roski and Spetzler collected 348 cases with previous carotid artery ligation, 83 per cent of whom showed either decrease or disappearance of the aneurysms angiographically.[38] The effect was also confirmed by repeated computed tomography.[17, 37] Since giant cavernous aneurysms rarely rupture, with some exceptions carotid occlusion is often the treatment of choice for those who can tolerate the occlusion test, especially in patients older than 70 years of age.[13, 30, 31]

Proximal occlusion of the carotid artery may be complicated by both hemodynamic and embolic ischemia. Nishioka reported ischemic complications after carotid ligation in 30 per cent of patients: 49 per cent of these occurred after ligation of the internal carotid artery and 28 per cent after ligation of the common carotid artery.[31] The ischemic complications were greatly reduced by selection of the patients and by careful preoperative examinations, electroencephalography, and measurement of cerebral blood flow during test occlusion of the carotid artery.[24, 27]

Rupture of aneurysms after carotid ligation still occurs in about 20 per cent of the patients, and improvement in visual deficits takes a long time.[25, 31, 32] Increase of blood flow in the contralateral carotid artery may lead to formation of a new aneurysm in the remaining carotid artery, and development of systemic hypertension is also reported.[19] These facts suggest that carotid artery ligation alone is not recommended for younger patients and that bypass surgery may be needed.

Vertebral Artery

Ligation of one vertebral artery is a relatively safe procedure if the opposite vertebral artery is functioning well.[11] Most deaths reported as resulting from ligation of a vertebral artery for vertebrobasilar aneurysms are related to an atretic opposite vertebral artery, vasospasm, compression of arteries by giant aneurysms, parent vessel thrombosis, or rupture of the aneurysm. Drake reported excellent or good results in 7 of 8 patients who underwent unilateral vertebral occlusion for large vertebrobasilar aneurysms.[7] Shibata and associates, in 1982, gathered from the literature 31 cases of unilateral vertebral artery occlusion for vertebral aneurysms.[41] Eight patients died—7 of 17 (41 per cent) before 1970 and only 1 of 14 (7 per cent) after 1970. Rebleeding from the aneurysm was seen in 8 per cent of the patients with proximal ligation. Shintani and Zervas reported an overall mortality rate of 12 per cent in patients who underwent ligation of a vertebral artery for various reasons.[43] Complications are fewer in patients with good flow in the remaining vertebral artery. Ligation of one vertebral artery is commonly performed in patients with a dissecting aneurysm of the vertebral artery in those patients with good circulation through the contralateral vertebral artery, and the results seem to be satisfactory.[61]

Basilar Artery

Mount and Taveras successfully ligated the basilar artery between the superior cerebellar and posterior cerebral artery in a patient with an aneurysm at the basilar artery bifurcation.[29] They considered that opacification of bilateral posterior cerebral arteries by carotid angiogram was indispensable. Drake clipped the basilar artery in seven patients with unclippable basilar aneurysms; three patients were in good condition, two were in poor condition, and two died.[7] Drake concluded that occlusion of the basilar artery must be done only when the artery filled spontaneously from the carotid circulation. Otherwise, even when reasonable posterior communicating arteries were demonstrated, it was best to perform test occlusion with the use of local anesthesia. Rozario and Stein reported a successful ligation of the basilar artery for a giant basilar apex aneurysm and reviewed five other cases.[39] They stressed the importance of preserving the perforating arteries in addition to collateral flow from the carotid circulation.

In a patient with a ruptured giant aneurysm at the basilar superior cerebellar artery and a large arteriovenous malformation in the cerebellar hemisphere, the authors clipped the basilar artery just proximal to the superior cerebellar artery. The patient's posterior communicating arteries on both sides were of a good size and had partially fed the arteriovenous malformation. Because vital signs did not change and brain stem auditory evoked response was observed for 30 minutes during temporary occlusion, the clip was left permanently. Further operative treatment was not indicated because of the patient's poor cardiac condition. The size of the aneurysm was seen to decrease slightly on the postoperative angiography, and the patient returned home in good condition. Ten months after the clipping, however, the patient died of bleeding from the untreated arteriovenous malformation.[42]

Long-term follow-up of 201 patients with deliberate occlusion of basilar or vertebral artery for aneurysms by Steinberg and co-workers showed that patients with vertebral aneurysms had a higher percentage of excellent or good outcomes (87 per cent) than patients with basilar apex aneurysms (64 per cent).[47]

BYPASS SURGERY

Anterior Circulation

To avoid ischemic complications of carotid ligation, extracranial-intracranial bypass surgery using a superficial temporal artery, a radial artery, or a saphenous vein graft is indispensable.[5, 18, 45, 62] Blood flow supplied by a superficial temporal artery is 20 to 60 mL per minute and is probably not large enough to accommodate normal blood flow of 75 to 120 mL per minute through a middle cerebral artery if there is no collateral flow through the posterior and anterior communicating arteries.[4] Higher flow can be expected by a double superficial temporal–middle cerebral artery anastomosis.[54] Sundt and associates reported bypass flow of 100 to 110 mL per minute in their patients with external carotid–posterior cerebral artery anastomosis by using a saphenous vein graft.[42] Abiko and colleagues obtained a flow of 180 mL per minute through an external carotid–middle cerebral artery anastomosis using a saphenous vein graft.[1] Immediate occlusion of the carotid artery was required, and the aneurysm should be trapped as soon as patency of the bypass was ensured, since rupture of giant aneurysms after anastomoses has been reported.[2, 26] Gradual occlusion of the carotid artery by a Selverstone clamp should be avoided because of the risk of embolic showers when the lumen is narrowed just before final occlusion.

Posterior Circulation

The results of bypass surgery for giant aneurysms in the posterior circulation remain to be improved. Sundt and colleagues reported that only four patients had excellent or good results among nine patients with giant aneurysms in the posterior circulation who received a saphenous vein graft between the carotid and posterior cerebral arteries and underwent occlusion of the vertebrobasilar artery.[52] Those patients who had large fusiform aneurysms of the basilar trunk did not fare well after vertebral artery ligation in spite of the fact that the bypass graft itself remained patent. These patients often suffered from both ischemia and mass effect of the aneurysm itself. Superficial temporal-to-superior cerebellar or temporal-to-posterior cerebral arterial bypass with ligation of the basilar artery was performed in two patients with a giant basilar artery aneurysm by Hopkins and co-workers.[16] One patient recovered from a locked-in state and returned home with minimal neurological deficits. The other patient recovered over several weeks to an awake and communicable state with good movement in all extremities but died of respiratory complications. Wakui and colleagues used a radial arterial graft for external carotid–posterior cerebral artery anastomosis in a patient with a giant aneurysm in the dominant vertebral artery.[57] The patient recovered well except for truncal ataxia.

DIRECT SURGERY: TECHNIQUES AND RESULTS

Giant Carotid Aneurysms

Giant carotid aneurysms are classified by the projection of the domes into the following four types: (1) ventrolateral, (2) ventromedial, (3) dorsomedial, and (4) dorsal. The ventrolateral type is an enlarged aneurysm projecting in the same direction as the internal carotid–posterior communicating aneurysm, which is the most common among the small carotid aneurysms. The ventromedial type is most frequent among the giant carotid aneurysms. Although this type is often designated as giant ophthalmic aneurysm in the literature, the necks are often not well defined, originating from proximal to the origin of the ophthalmic artery to that of the anterior choroidal artery. The dorsomedial type compresses the optic nerve more than the ventromedial type; the dorsomedial type aneurysm elevates the nerve from below, causing visual disturbance. We have operated on 12 giant and 15 large carotid aneurysms and on 5 ventrolateral, 16 ventromedial, and 3 dorsomedial aneurysms (Table 54–2). The ventromedial aneurysm type is the most common type. A detailed explanation of this clipping technique follows.

With the patient in the supine position, the cervical carotid artery is exposed for temporary trapping and a frontotemporal skin flap is made. The frontal branch of the superficial temporal artery is preserved as a possible donor for the extracranial-intracranial bypass surgery. Before approaching the aneurysm, bone in the paraclinoid region should be drilled by both epidural and subdural approaches.[6, 35] The dural sheath of the optic canal and the dural ring are opened widely to loosen the optic nerve and C3 portion of the carotid

Table 54–2
GIANT AND LARGE CAROTID ARTERY ANEURYSMS: PROJECTIONS AND RESULTS

	No.	Size		Outcome			
		Large*	Giant	Good	Fair	Poor	Dead
VL	5	4	1	4	1	0	0
VM	16	7	9	13	0	1	2
DM	3	2	1	3	0	0	0
D	1	1	0	1	0	0	0
Cavern.	2	1	1	2	0	0	0
Total	27	15	12	23	1	1	2

*Aneurysms between 18 and 25 mm in diameter.
VL, aneurysms projecting ventrolaterally; VM, ventromedial; DM, dorsomedial; D, dorsal; Cavern., intracavernous aneurysms.

artery. Brisk bleeding from the cavernous sinus can be controlled by elevating the patient's head 30 degrees and by meticulous packing with oxidized cellulose.

The body of the aneurysm is isolated from its neck. Narrowing of the parent artery by an angled-ring clip is most frequently caused by insufficient dissection of the aneurysmal wall from the surrounding bony or dural structures. Many thick fibrous trabeculae connect the aneurysmal wall to the skull base, and the neurosurgeon must dissect these sharply. More than two thirds of the circumference of the aneurysm must be dissected free for satisfactory clipping (Fig. 54–1). When the intraluminal pressure is too high to isolate the aneurysm, tentative clipping on the neck or temporary trapping of the parent artery is necessary. The patient is heparinized before temporary occlusion. During temporary occlusion, ischemia should be monitored by electroencephalography, somatosensory evoked potentials, or measurement of local cerebral blood flow by a laser Doppler or thermoelectric device. Giant aneurysms usually have a thick base, which makes direct clipping difficult.[51] If it appears that direct clipping is impossible, the aneurysm should not be explored further, since this not only prolongs the procedure but may also damage surrounding nerves, brain,

and blood vessels. In such cases, either proximal ligation or trapping with or without bypass surgery is recommended.

Giant aneurysms often do not collapse by trapping alone. The blood inside the aneurysm must be evacuated by direct tapping from either the internal carotid artery or a branch of the external carotid artery in the neck.[3, 9, 55] We use the direct puncture method. After trapping or tentative clipping, the aneurysm is punctured with a 21-gauge butterfly needle that is connected with an extension tube to a 25- to 50-mL plastic syringe. The plastic flange of the needle is removed except for a small handle that is held by a mosquito clamp. The clamp is held by a self-retaining retractor that is fixed to a multipurpose head frame (Fig. 54–2). The aneurysm should be punctured as far from the neck as possible to leave a space for the blades of multiple clips. Blood is continuously suctioned by an assistant to collapse the aneurysm. Heparinization is indispensable during trapping. In the initial stage of the authors' series, they have encountered an intraoperative thrombosis of the carotid artery in a patient with a giant carotid aneurysm when aneurysmectomy was performed without heparinization.

Holding a puncture needle with a self-retaining re-

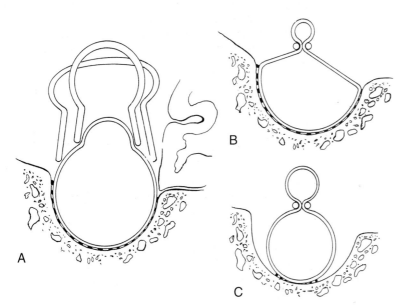

Figure 54–1

Schematic drawing of the clipping of a giant carotid aneurysm. *A and B.* An angled-ring clip cannot close or can slip to hold only a narrow lumen because of insufficient dissection of the dome of the aneurysm from the tight adhesion to the surrounding bony or dural structures. *C.* Correct positioning of the clip blades is possible only after more than two thirds of the aneurysmal circumference has been dissected.

tractor has several advantages; the operating field can be kept clean and the needle can be held in the same position during clip application. Evacuation of the blood by an assistant through the suction device requires that the assistant understands the details of the aneurysm clipping done by a chief surgeon. Usually the amount of blood suctioned is less than 20 mL, but in difficult cases it may be as much as 200 mL. The authors have designed a special puncture needle that occupies less space than the needle held by a mosquito clamp.[23]

Multiple clips are necessary in all cases: usually, two or three clips are applied for a large aneurysm and three or four clips are used for a giant aneurysm, choosing the best combination of clips.[48] To avoid a space between the blades of multiple clips, the clips should be positioned so that the axes of the spring of the clips are parallel when the parent artery is straight or in the same plane when the parent artery is curved. To prevent stenosis of the parent artery, the ring clip should be inserted deep enough so that the near side of the ring almost touches the wall of the parent artery. For a ventromedial giant aneurysm, obliteration by three ring clips with shorter blades is better than by two clips with a longer blade. The residual portion in either the proximal or the distal side of the giant aneurysm should be obliterated with clips without a ring (Fig. 54–3). The position of the clip blade on the blind side can be checked with a mirror.

Giant Aneurysms of the Middle Cerebral Artery

Surgery for giant aneurysms of the middle cerebral artery is generally easier than surgery in other areas

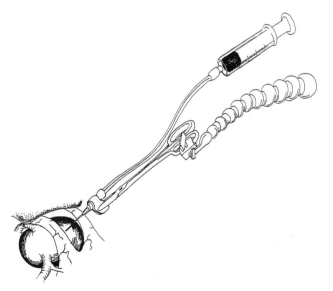

Figure 54–2

"Suction decompression" of a giant carotid aneurysm by direct puncture. The carotid artery is temporarily trapped, and the dome of the aneurysm is punctured with a 21-gauge butterfly needle, which is connected to a plastic syringe. The blood is continuously suctioned by an assistant surgeon. The butterfly needle is steadily held with a mosquito clamp and a self-retaining retractor.

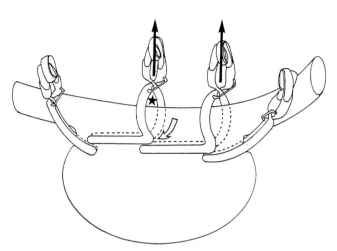

Figure 54–3

Multiple clipping of a giant aneurysm. The axes of the spring portion of the angled-ring clips (*straight arrows*) should be parallel to each other to avoid a gap between the blades of the clips (*open arrow*). The clips should be inserted deep enough, leaving little space between the ring and the parent artery (*star*), to establish a wide lumen in the parent artery. The remaining portions of the aneurysm should be occluded with regular clips without a ring, which are less voluminous and more maneuverable.

because the operating field is wider and shallower. The most important point of the surgery is to avoid stenosis and occlusion of distal parent arteries and lenticulostriate arteries. The best combination of multiple clips with various shapes should be applied, and often wrapping of the remaining portion of the aneurysm must be added to preserve the parent arteries (Fig. 54–4). Occasionally, complete aneurysmectomy, together with parent arteries, followed by anastomosis between branches of the middle cerebral artery or with the superficial temporal artery is required.

Giant Aneurysms of the Anterior Cerebral Artery

To clip giant aneurysms on the anterior cerebral artery, an interhemispheric approach rather than the pterional approach is selected because the first and second segments of the artery are better exposed on both sides. But, when part of the parent arteries is hidden behind the dome of a giant aneurysm, the parent arteries may have to be dissected from the side by including a pterional approach. The lower blood pressure of these aneurysms compared with that of aneurysms in other locations is an advantage. In addition, this area seems to tolerate temporary occlusion better than other areas. However, these aneurysms are more complicated than those of other areas in that the first and second segments of both anterior cerebral arteries and the anterior communicating artery must be preserved. In some cases, side-to-side or side-to-end anastomosis of the second segment of the anterior cerebral artery must be performed.

Giant Aneurysms of the Basilar Bifurcation

The natural course of a giant basilar bifurcation aneurysm is miserable. Most grow by direct pulsation of

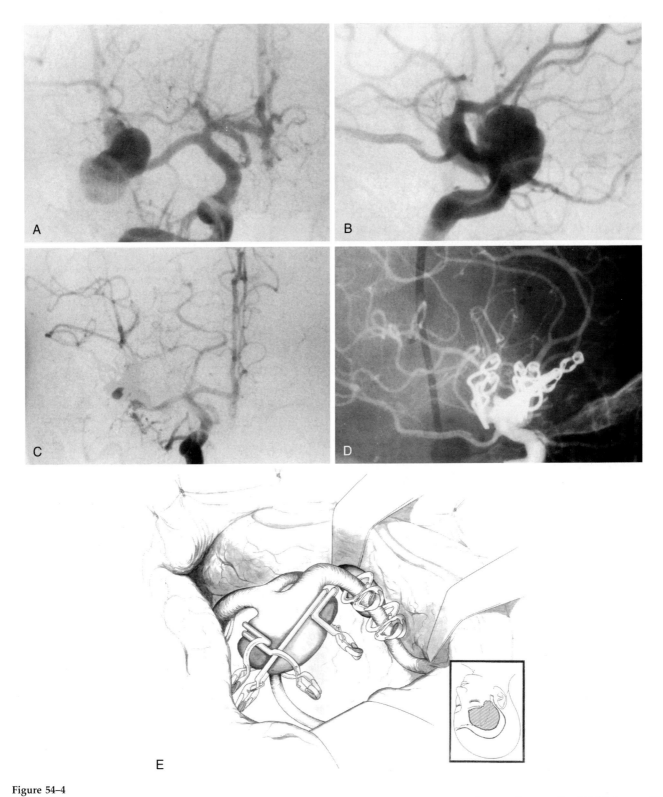

Figure 54–4

A giant middle cerebral aneurysm. *A and B.* Preoperative anteroposterior and lateral views of the right carotid artery. *C and D.* Right carotid angiograms 2 years after the surgery show exclusion of the aneurysm. *E.* Intraoperative schema of clipping. The body of the giant aneurysm was occluded with a 25-mm-long straight clip and a 12-mm straight-ring clip. An L-shaped clip and an angled-ring clip were used to reinforce the aforementioned clips. Two angled-ring clips were used to occlude a fusiform dilatation of the distal portion of the aneurysm. The residual portion of the neck of the aneurysm was wrapped with several pieces of soft cellulose patty.

the blood flow into the dome, resulting in fatal bleeding. The pterional approach with removal of the lateral orbital ridge and zygomatic process is quite useful in widening the operative field.[14] Removal of the anterior clinoid process and excision of the dural ring around the carotid artery may release the tension during direct retraction of the carotid, especially when it is short and sclerotic. In spite of all these tactics, clipping of giant basilar aneurysms is most difficult and surgical results are poor, since perforating arteries behind the huge dome are difficult to preserve. Satisfactory results may only be obtained under cardiac arrest and hypothermia as reported by Silverberg and associates and by Spetzler and colleagues.[44, 46] In our series, direct clipping was successful only when the aneurysms were smaller than 22 mm.

Giant Aneurysms of the Vertebral Artery

Most of the giant vertebral aneurysms are partially thrombosed, presenting as mass lesions. Long tract signs, lower cranial nerve palsy and respiratory distress, and particularly sleep apnea are caused by brain stem compression by the aneurysm. The first treatment choice may be intravascular occlusion of the vertebral artery if the patient can tolerate the occlusion test and has a good vertebral artery on the opposite side. Narrowing in the opposite vertebral artery is sometimes caused by the compression of the giant aneurysm. If the patient can tolerate the balloon occlusion test, direct attack can be carried out. If the patient's condition does not improve after proximal occlusion, trapping with aneurysmectomy may be necessary. Treatment strategy of giant and partially thrombosed aneurysms is shown in Figure 54–5. Surgery must be performed early after the development of these symptoms; otherwise, prolonged neurological deficits do not improve with decompression.[49]

Partially Thrombosed Giant Aneurysms

Partially thrombosed aneurysms make closure of the clip blades impossible by simple application of the clip after puncturing the dome. Clips applied to the neck usually slide to the parent artery and constrict its lumen. Thrombectomy or endaneurysmectomy is indispensable.[50] Great care must be taken not to migrate thrombi into the mainstream. Sectioning of the aneurysm must be done as far from the parent artery as possible so that clips can be applied to the body of the aneurysm.

Results

During the past 12 years, the authors have operated on 29 giant aneurysms measuring 25 mm or larger and on 44 large aneurysms measuring between 18 and 25 mm in diameter. The giant and large aneurysms were only 1.8 per cent and 2.5 per cent of the total operated aneurysm cases. Surgical results of 27 cases with giant and large carotid aneurysms were excellent and good in 23, fair in 1, and poor or dead in 3 cases (Table 54–3; see Table 54–2). Vision improved in six patients and deteriorated in three patients. Two patients died, one of postoperative obliteration of the carotid artery and the other of subarachnoid hemorrhage that occurred during the night after bypass surgery and before direct surgery was performed. After these accidents, systemic heparinization was used for temporary trapping of the aneurysms and direct surgery was performed on the same day as the bypass surgery. Good results were obtained in 16 of 19 (84 per cent) patients with large and giant aneurysms in the anterior and middle cerebral arteries. Among 27 patients with large and giant aneurysms in the posterior circulation, 19 patients (70 per cent) obtained good results, 2 had fair results, 3 had poor results, and 3 patients died.

The treatment goal for giant intracranial aneurysm is prevention of rupture, removal of the mass lesion, and re-establishment of the normal cerebral blood flow without damaging the brain or the cranial nerves. Preoperative studies should include circulation dynamics

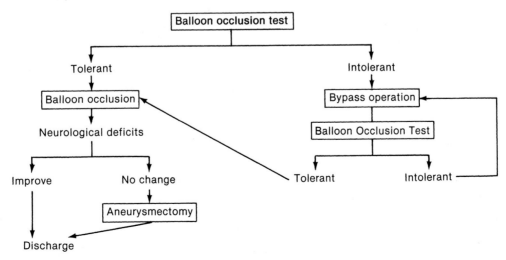

Figure 54–5

Flow chart of treatment plan for partially thrombosed giant aneurysms of the vertebral artery.

Table 54–3
SURGICAL RESULTS OF LARGE AND GIANT ANEURYSMS

	No.	Size		Outcome			
		Large	*Giant*	*Good*	*Fair*	*Poor*	*Dead*
ICA	27	15	12	23	1	1	2
MCA	11	6	5	9	1	0	1
ACA	8	4	4	7	0	1	0
Basilar	15	13	2	10	2	2	1
Vertebral	12	6	6	9	0	1	2
Total	73	44	29	58	4	5	6
	100%	60%	40%	79%	5%	7%	8%

ICA, internal carotid artery; MCA, middle cerebral artery; ACA, anterior cerebral artery.

by four-vessel angiography, balloon test occlusion, and measurement of cerebral blood flow. Then the treatment strategy can be planned, depending on the location of the aneurysm, the collateral flow, and the patient's age. During surgery, ischemic change of the brain should be monitored by electroencephalography, somatosensory evoked potentials, or cerebral blood flow measurement. The brain must be protected from ischemic damage due to temporary trapping by bypass surgery, hypothermia, or "anti-ischemic cocktails." For ideal clipping, the aneurysms must be slackened by suction decompression, thrombectomy, or cardiac standstill. The surgeon should select the best-fitting combination of multiple clips and check the results by intraoperative angiography.

REFERENCES

1. Abiko, S., Yamashita, T., Nakano, S., et al.: Intracranial microvascular anastomosis with ligation and trapping of the internal carotid artery for giant aneurysm at IC-cavernous portion. Surg. Cerebral Stroke (Tokyo), 15:161, 1987.
2. Anson, J. A., Stone, J. L., and Crowell, R. M.: Rupture of a giant carotid aneurysm after extracranial-to-intracranial bypass surgery. Neurosurgery, 28:142, 1991.
3. Batjer, H. H., and Samson, D. S.: Retrograde suction decompression of giant paraclinoid aneurysms. J. Neurosurg., 73:305, 1990.
4. Crowell, R. M.: STA-MCA bypass for acute focal cerebral ischemia. In Schmiedeck, P., ed.: Microsurgery for Stroke. New York, Springer-Verlag, 1977, pp. 244–250.
5. Diaz, F. G., Ausman, J. I., and Pearce, J. E.: Ischemic complications after combined internal carotid artery occlusion and extraintracranial anastomosis. Neurosurgery, 10:563, 1982.
6. Dolenc, V. V.: A combined epi- and subdural approach to carotid–ophthalmic artery aneurysms. J. Neurosurg., 62:667, 1985.
7. Drake, C. G.: Ligation of the vertebral (unilateral or bilateral) or basilar artery in the treatment of large intracranial aneurysms. J. Neurosurg., 43:255, 1975.
8. Drake, C. G.: Giant intracranial aneurysms: Experience with surgical treatment in 174 patients. Clin. Neurosurg., 26:12, 1979.
9. Flamm, E. S.: Suction decompression of aneurysms. J. Neurosurg., 54:275, 1981.
10. Fox, J. L.: Giant aneurysms. In Fox, J. L.: Intracranial Aneurysms. Vol. I. New York, Springer-Verlag, 1983, pp. 149–154.
11. Fox, J. L.: Vertebrobasilar artery ligation. In Fox, J. L., ed.: Intracranial Aneurysms. Vol. II. New York, Springer-Verlag, 1983, p. 814.
12. Fried, L. C., and Yballe, A.: Rapid formation of giant aneurysms. J. Neurol. Neurosurg. Psychiatry, 35:527, 1972.
13. Fujita, K., Yamashita, H., Masumura, M., et al.: Natural history of giant intracranial aneurysms. Neurol. Surg. (Tokyo), 16:225, 1988.
14. Fujitsu, K., and Kuwabara, T.: Zygomatic approach for lesions in the interpeduncular cistern. J. Neurosurg., 62:340, 1985.
15. Harbaugh, R. E., Schlusselberg, D. S., Jeffery, R., et al.: Three-dimensional computerized tomography angiography in the diagnosis of cerebrovascular disease. J. Neurosurg., 76:408, 1992.
16. Hopkins, L. N., Budny, J. L., and Castellani, D.: Extracranial-intracranial arterial bypass and basilar artery ligation in the treatment of giant basilar artery aneurysms. Neurosurgery, 13:189, 1983.
17. Ishii, R., Tanaka, R., Koike, T., et al.: Computed tomographic demonstration of the effect of proximal ligation for giant intracranial aneurysms. Surg. Neurol., 19:532, 1983.
18. Ito, Z.: Long radial artery grafting. In Ito, Z.: Microneurosurgery of Cerebral Aneurysms. Amsterdam/Niigata, Elsevier/Nishimura, 1985, pp. 270–279.
19. Keravel, Y., and Sindou, M.: Giant Intracranial Aneurysms. Berlin, Springer-Verlag, 1988, pp. 1–163.
20. Kodama, N., Sasaki, T., and Goto, K.: Treatment of giant aneurysms. In Saito, I., Hashi, K., eds.: Treatment of Intracranial Aneurysms. Tokyo, Kodama Co., 1987, pp. 41–47 (in Japanese).
21. Koshikawa, N., Kamio, M., Sekino, H., et al.: Giant aneurysm. Neurol. Surg. (Tokyo), 8:79, 1980.
22. Kupersmith, M. J., Hurst, R., Berenstein, A., et al.: The benign course of cavernous carotid artery aneurysms. J. Neurosurg., 77:690, 1992.
23. Kyoshima, K., Kobayashi, S., Wakui, K., et al.: A newly designed puncture needle for suction decompression of giant aneurysms. J. Neurosurg., 76:880, 1992.
24. Linskey, M. E., Sekhar, L. N., Horton, J. A.: Aneurysms of the internal carotid artery: A multidisciplinary approach to treatment. J. Neurosurg., 75:525, 1991.
25. Little, J. R., St. Louis, P., Weinstein, M., et al.: Giant fusiform aneurysm of the cerebral arteries. Stroke, 12:183, 1981.
26. Matsuda, M., Shiino, A., and Handa, J.: Rupture of previously unruptured giant carotid aneurysm after superficial temporal–middle cerebral artery bypass and internal carotid occlusion. Neurosurgery, 16:177, 1985.
27. Miller, J. D., Jawad, K., and Jennett, B.: Safety of carotid ligation and its role in the management of intracranial aneurysms. J. Neurol. Neurosurg. Psychiatry, 40:64, 1977.
28. Morley, T. P., and Barr, H. W. K.: Giant intracranial aneurysms: Diagnosis, course and management. Clin. Neurosurg., 16:73–94, 1969.
29. Mount, L. A., and Taveras, J. M.: Ligation of basilar artery in treatment of an aneurysm at the basilar-artery bifurcation. J. Neurosurg., 19:167, 1962.
30. Nishimaki, K., Koike, T., Takeuchi, S., et al.: Natural history of intracranial giant aneurysms. Surg. Cerebral Stroke (Tokyo), 19:414, 1991.
31. Nishioka, H.: Report on cooperative study on intracranial aneurysms and subarachnoid hemorrhage. J. Neurosurg., 25:660, 1966.
32. Odom, G. L., and Tindall, G.: Carotid ligation in the treatment of certain intracranial aneurysms. Clin. Neurosurg., 15:101, 1968.
33. Olsen, W. L., Brant-Zawadzki, M., Hodges, J., et al.: Giant intracranial aneurysms: MR imaging. Radiology, 163:431, 1987.
34. Peerless, S. J., Wallace, M. C., and Drake, C. G.: Giant intracranial

aneurysms. *In* Youmans, J. R., ed.: Neurological Surgery. 3rd ed. Philadelphia, W. B. Saunders Co., 1990, pp. 1742–1763.

35. Perneczky, A., Knosp, E., Czech, T.: Para- and infraclinoid aneurysms: Anatomy, surgical technique and report of 22 cases. *In* Dolenc, V. V., ed.: The Cavernous Sinus. Vienna, Springer-Verlag, 1987, pp. 253–271.

36. Pia, H. W., Zierski, J.: Giant cerebral aneurysms. Neurosurg. Rev., 5:17, 1982.

37. Pozzati, E., Agioli, L., Servadei, F., et al.: Effect of common carotid ligation on giant aneurysms of the internal carotid artery: Computerized tomography study. J. Neurosurg., 55:527, 1981.

38. Roski, R. A., and Spetzler, R. F.: Carotid ligation. *In* Wilkins, R. H., and Rengachary, S. S., eds.: Neurosurgery. New York, McGraw-Hill, 1985, pp. 1414–1422.

39. Rozario, R. A., and Stein, B. M.: Ligation of the basilar artery as the definitive treatment for a giant aneurysm of the basilar artery apex. Neurosurgery, 6:87, 1980.

40. Schubiger, O., Valavanis, A., and Hayek, J.: Computed tomography in cerebral aneurysms with special emphasis on giant intracranial aneurysms. J. Comput. Assist. Tomogr., 4:24, 1980.

41. Shibata, T., Ito, A., Enomoto, H., et al.: Proximal ligation of the vertebral artery for treatment of vertebral aneurysm. Neurol. Surg. (Tokyo), 10:1327, 1982.

42. Shibuya, M., Takayasu, M., Kanamori, M., et al.: Ligation of the basilar artery in a patient with giant basilar aneurysm and arteriovenous malformation in the cerebellum. Proceedings of the 13th Conference of Surgical Treatment of Stroke, Tokyo, 1984, pp. 67–71.

43. Shintani, A., and Zervas, N. T.: Consequence of ligation of the vertebral artery. J. Neurosurg., 36:447, 1972.

44. Silverberg, G. D., Reitz, B. A., Ream, A. K., et al.: Hypothermia and cardiac arrest in the treatment of giant aneurysms of the cerebral circulation and hemangioblastoma of the medulla. J. Neurosurg., 55:337, 1981.

45. Spetzler, R. F., Schuster, H., and Roski, R. A.: Elective extracranial-intracranial arterial bypass in the treatment of inoperable giant aneurysms of the internal carotid artery. J. Neurosurg., 53:22, 1980.

46. Spetzler, R. F., Hadley, M. N., Rigamonti, D., et al.: Aneurysms of the basilar artery treated with circulatory arrest, hypothermia, and barbiturate cerebral protection. J. Neurosurg., 68:868, 1988.

47. Steinberg, G. K., Drake, C. G., and Peerless, S. J.: Deliberate basilar or vertebral artery occlusion in the treatment of intracranial aneurysms. J. Neurosurg., 79:161, 1993.

48. Sugita, K.: Microneurosurgical Atlas. Berlin, Springer-Verlag, 1985.

49. Sugita, K., Kobayashi, S., Takemae, T., et al.: Giant aneurysms of the vertebral artery. J. Neurosurg., 68:960, 1988.

50. Sundt, T. M., Jr., and Piepgras, D. G.: Surgical approach to giant intracranial aneurysms: Operative experience with 80 cases. J. Neurosurg., 51:731, 1979.

51. Sundt, T. M., Jr., Piepgras, D. G., Houser, O. W., et al.: Interposition saphenous vein grafts for advanced occlusive disease and large aneurysms in the posterior circulation. J. Neurosurg., 56:205, 1982.

52. Sundt, T. M., Jr., Piepgras, D. G., Marsh, W. R., et al.: Saphenous vein bypass grafts for giant aneurysms and intracranial occlusive disease. J. Neurosurg., 65:439, 1986.

53. Sutherland, G. R., King, M. E., Peerless, S. J., et al.: Platelet interaction with giant intracranial aneurysms. J. Neurosurg., 56:53, 1982.

54. Suzuki, J., and Oonuma, T.: A giant intracranial aneurysm which disappeared angiographically following pneumoencephalography. Neurol. Med. Chir. (Tokyo), 16:105, 1976.

55. Tamaki, N., Kim, S., Ehara, K., et al.: Giant carotid-ophthalmic artery aneurysm: Direct clipping utilizing the "trapping-evacuation" technique. J. Neurosurg., 74:565, 1991.

56. Tytus, J. S., and Ward, A. A.: The effect of cervical carotid ligation on giant intracranial aneurysms. J. Neurosurg., 33:184, 1970.

57. Wakui, K., Kobayashi, S., Takemae, T., et al.: Giant thrombosed vertebral aneurysm managed with extracranial-intracranial bypass surgery and aneurysmectomy. J. Neurosurg., 77:624, 1992.

58. Weir, B.: Giant aneurysms. *In* Weir, B., ed.: Aneurysms Affecting the Nervous System. Baltimore, Williams & Wilkins, 1987, pp. 187–206.

59. Worthington, B. S., Kean, D. M., Hawkes, R. C., et al.: NMR imaging in the recognition of giant intracranial aneurysms. A.J.N.R., 4:835, 1983.

60. Wright, R. L., and Sweet, W. H.: Carotid or vertebral occlusion in the treatment of intracranial aneurysms: Value of early and late readings of carotid and retinal pressures. Clin. Neurosurg., 9:163, 1962.

61. Yamaura, A.: Diagnosis and treatment of vertebral aneurysms. J. Neurosurg., 69:345, 1988.

62. Yasargil, M. G.: Microsurgery Applied to Neurosurgery. New York, Academic Press, 1969, pp. 105–117.

Aneurysms of the Cavernous Sinus: Treatment Options and Considerations

The cavernous sinus was long perceived to be the "no man's land" of neurological surgery. However, recent advances in approaches to the skull base, a comprehensive understanding of its microsurgical anatomy, and technical advances in interventional and neuroradiological imaging have revolutionized treatment. Carotid cavernous aneurysms represent a most intriguing and challenging pathological entity within this region. Their management is based on a thorough understanding of the complex anatomy of the cavernous sinus and on cerebral vascular physiological considerations. In this chapter, these considerations are reviewed, management options are discussed, and recommendations for the treatment and study of these challenging vascular lesions are made.

Anatomical Considerations

CAROTID ARTERY ANATOMY

The practical and surgical anatomy of the cavernous carotid artery and its associated soft-tissue, neural, and bony elements have been eloquently described.* The anatomical descriptions within this chapter are based on the modified nomenclature of Dolenc and Fischer and serve as a reference of orientation for future discussion (Fig. 55–1).[22, 28]

The carotid artery enters the petrous portion of the temporal bone at the base of the skull anterior to the jugular foramen. Within the petrous bone, the carotid artery runs vertically for 5.0 to 12.5 mm; it then turns horizontally at its genu (the posterior loop) to travel 14.5 to 24.0 mm in an anteromedial direction (the horizontal segment).[52] Proximal control of the cavernous carotid artery can be obtained within this segment,

*See references 22, 38, 52, 76, 79, 81, 82, 88–90, and 111.

which is anatomically defined as the "posterolateral triangle." Key landmarks for access to the carotid artery within this region include the greater superficial petrosal nerve, the posterior aspect of the mandibular branch of the trigeminal nerve, the foramen ovale, the foramen spinosum, and the arcuate eminence. As the carotid artery passes above the foramen lacerum and under the gasserian ganglion, it pierces the lateral dural ring and turns medially, forming the lateral loop, and enters the cavernous sinus proper. Running in the cavernous sinus, the carotid artery proceeds superomedially toward the posterior clinoid process. Just medial to V_1, the sixth cranial nerve crosses the carotid artery in an intimate fashion. At the level of the posterior clinoid process, the carotid artery makes a forward turn, forming the medial loop. Found at this level are the meningohypophyseal trunk and its branches.[81, 82, 111] Access to the carotid artery in this segment of the cavernous sinus is via Parkinson's triangle or the paramedian triangle. Parkinson's triangle is defined by the medial border of the fourth cranial nerve, the lateral aspect of the fifth cranial nerve, and the posterior dura where the nerves enter. The paramedian triangle is defined by the lateral aspect of the third cranial nerve, the medial aspect of the fourth cranial nerve, and the posterior entry point of these two nerves. Through these two regions, the horizontal segment of the cavernous carotid artery, the medial loop of the internal carotid artery, and the sixth cranial nerve may be identified. The carotid artery then courses forward, giving off the inferior lateral trunk and McConnell's capsular arteries before it turns back on itself to form the carotid siphon (anterior loop) and pierces the proximal dural ring. At this level, the carotid artery is both extracavernous and epidural. Upon piercing the distal dural ring, the carotid artery enters the subarachnoid space. In most patients (85 to 90 per cent), the ophthalmic artery is found originating on its dorsal medial surface. Access to this segment is through the anteromedial

---

T. C. Origitano • O. Al-Mefty

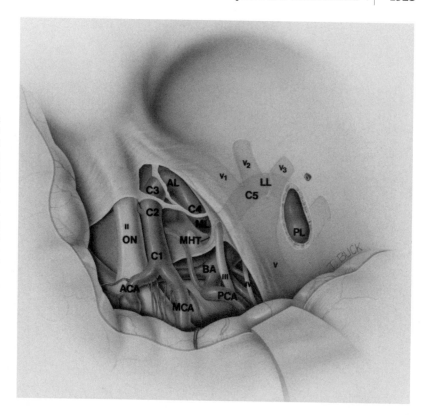

Figure 55–1

Cavernous carotid artery nomenclature taken from Dolenc[22] and Fischer,[28] as proposed by Fukushima (personal communication), with modification by the authors. True cavernous segment is seen from the lateral dural ring (between V_3/V_2) and the proximal dural ring (between C_3/AL). ACA, anterior cerebral artery; AL, anterior loop; BA, basilar artery; C_1, supraclinoid carotid artery from bifurcation to posterior communicating artery; C_2, posterior communicating artery to distal dural ring; C_3, proximal dural ring to distal dural ring, epidural extracavernous segment; C_4, intracavernous horizontal segment, proximal dural ring to MHT; C_5, intracavernous ascending segment, lateral dural ring to MHT; LL, lateral loop; MCA, middle cerebral artery; MHT, meningeal hypophyseal trunk; ML, medial loop; ON, optic nerve; PCA, posterior cerebral artery; PL, posterior loop.

triangle, which lies beneath the base of the anterior clinoid process. Its borders are the lateral aspect of the optic nerve in the optic canal and the medial aspect of the third cranial nerve, as well as their dural entry points. This triangle provides distal epidural control of the cavernous carotid artery and serves as a workhorse for the exposure of aneurysms of the third and fourth segments of the carotid artery.

ANATOMICAL CONSIDERATIONS RELATED TO ANEURYSM LOCATION

A review of the literature reveals that the term "cavernous aneurysm" covers a multitude of anatomically described aneurysms. Included in this group are the true cavernous aneurysms, the paraclinoid aneurysms (originating on the C_2/C_3 segment), the transitional aneurysms (originating intracavernously but extending into the subarachnoid space), and the petrous carotid aneurysms (originating in the temporal bone and extending into the cavernous sinus). True cavernous aneurysms are those that originate between the lateral and proximal dural rings (see Fig. 55–1). In reviewing the literature, it is often difficult to determine the true origin of lesions designated as cavernous aneurysms. However, knowledge of their anatomical origin becomes important when treatment options are considered, as the origin has bearing on the potential risk and natural history of the lesions.

Petrous carotid aneurysms are those that originate proximal to the lateral ring. These relatively rare lesions are generally fusiform in nature and present as

mass lesions within the temporal bone (Fig. 55–2), often affecting cranial nerves VII and VIII.[37]

The variety of aneurysms that originate distal to the proximal dural ring (C_3/C_2) are far more numerous, variable, and problematic. Most traumatic aneurysms of the carotid artery are located on the segment between the proximal and distal dural rings (C_3). They are pseudoaneurysms that generally project medially into the sphenoid sinus (Fig. 55–3). Their presentation is usually associated with the classic triad: head injury with basal skull fracture, unilateral visual loss, and epistaxis.[58, 63, 87] Because they are pseudoaneurysms, treatment generally requires removal of the vascular segment from which they originate.

The largest variety of paracavernous sinus aneurysms originates along the internal carotid artery from the proximal dural ring to the posterior communicating artery. A diverse nomenclature has been used to describe these aneurysms: paraclinoid, infraclinoid, dorsal, carotid cave, transitional, and ophthalmic segment.* These aneurysms may appear to originate from or enter into the cavernous sinus by distention of the dural rings or direct erosion of the cavernous sinus wall (Fig. 55–4). Their presentation or probability of extension into the subarachnoid space endows them with the potential to cause catastrophic subarachnoid hemorrhage with its concurrent morbidity and mortality.

Epidemiological Considerations

Cavernous aneurysms represent 3 per cent of all angiographically identified aneurysms and 11 to 14 per

*See references 4, 11, 12, 13, 20, 30, 33, 39, 45, 46, 72, 75, 85, and 115.

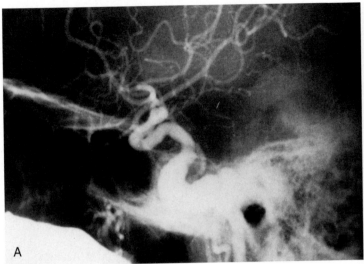

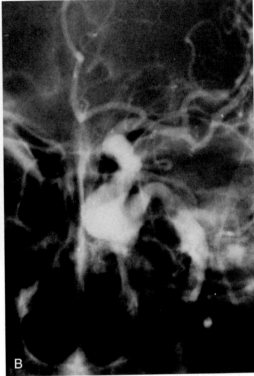

Figure 55–2

Lateral *(A)* and anteroposterior *(B)* angiograms of a petrous carotid aneurysm depicting the fusiform shape and distal extension into the cavernous sinus.

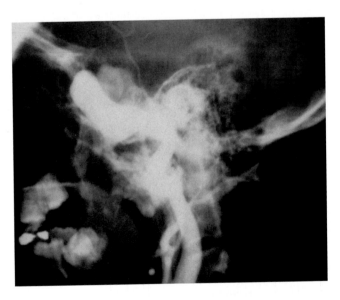

Figure 55–3

Lateral angiogram of a traumatic pseudoaneurysm of the cavernous sinus.

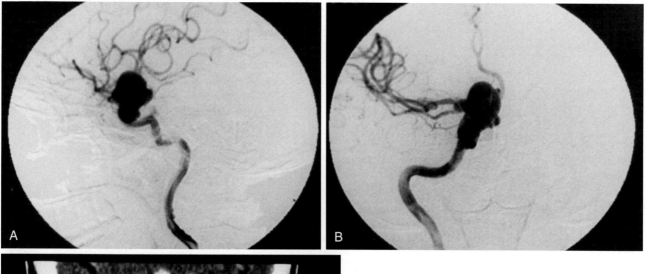

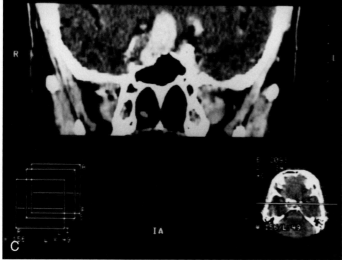

Figure 55–4

Paracavernous sinus aneurysm that involves both the cavernous sinus and the subarachnoid space. *A.* Anteroposterior view. *B.* Lateral view. *C.* Coronal contrast-enhanced computed tomography.

Table 55–1

EPIDEMIOLOGY OF CAVERNOUS ANEURYSMS: SURVEY OF MODERN CASE MATERIAL

Authors	Date	No. of Patients	No. of Aneurysms	Females	Males	Mean Age
Kupersmith et al.[47]	1992	70	79	65	5	62
Linskey and Sekhar et al.[53, 54, 55, 96]	1989	37	44	30	7	61
	1990					
	1990					
	1991					
Inagawa[42]	1991	22	24	18	4	63.3
Lye et al.[61]	1989	23	25	21	2	55.5
Total		152	172	134 (88%)	18 (12%)	60.5 (mean)

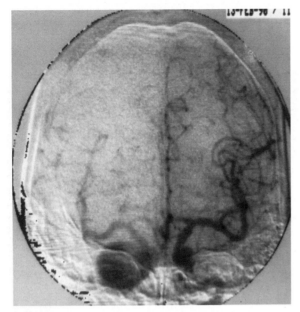

Figure 55–5

Bilateral cavernous aneurysms are encountered in 10 per cent of the cases.

masses, cavernous sinus syndrome, and even pituitary dysfunction and oculomotor paresis.*

The natural history of these lesions is not well known. Series in the literature are heavily oriented toward operative cases. Recent reviews of larger series of case material confirm earlier epidemiological findings (Table 55–1). Mass effect leading to ophthalmoplegia, both painful and painless; headache; and retro-orbital pain predominate among the clinical signs and symptoms.[42, 47, 53, 54, 61] A review of case material consisting of 80 cavernous aneurysms that did not undergo operation revealed a 2.5 per cent occurrence of hemorrhage over a mean follow-up ranging from 2.4 to 6.9 years (Table 55–2).

Treatment Options

A broad spectrum of treatment options has been applied to the management of cavernous aneurysms (Table 55–3). Treatment options can be divided into direct (those that affect only the aneurysms) and indirect (those that are based on parent artery occlusion).

INDIRECT APPROACHES

In the past, common carotid artery and internal carotid artery ligation were the mainstay of treatment.[26, 73, 86] Dissatisfaction with ischemic complication rates ranging from 32 to 59 per cent and the advent of microsurgical techniques led to the development of new and innovative approaches.[91, 92, 103] In the era of microvascular anastomosis, a mainstay of treatment for cavernous or giant aneurysms became the extracranial-to-intracranial bypass in the form of a superficial temporal artery–to–distal middle cerebral artery anastomosis in combination with carotid artery occlusion and/or trapping.† Ischemic complications after bypass with carotid artery occlusion stimulated the development of high-flow conduits of saphenous vein and of methods to gain deeper access to the proximal middle cerebral trunk.[18, 56, 107, 108] Controversy still exists about whether

cent of all aneurysms arising from the internal carotid artery.[42, 59, 93] They are found predominantly in women, usually presenting in the fifth or sixth decade of life. Approximately 10 per cent of cases are bilateral (Fig. 55–5). The causes of cavernous aneurysms can be described as traumatic, mycotic, or spontaneous. Morphologically, they are either saccular or fusiform, and are divided by size as small (less than 1 cm), large (1–2.5 cm), or giant (greater than 2.5 cm) (Fig. 55–6).

Clinical presentation can be compressive, hemorrhagic, or serendipitous (asymptomatic) and has been well documented over a long period.[7, 43, 60, 65] Compressive symptoms include ophthalmoplegia, eye pain, headache, and, if the lesion is sufficiently large, visual loss (Fig. 55–7). Hemorrhage can present as the formation of a carotid-cavernous fistula, subarachnoid hemorrhage, or subdural hematoma, or as epistaxis.[41, 74] Cavernous aneurysms should be included in the differential diagnosis of patients with sellar or parasellar

*See references 24, 34, 48, 62, 69, and 112.
†See references 7, 15, 16, 17, 32, 39, 57, 101, and 106.

Table 55–2
NONOPERATIVE FOLLOW-UP FOR CAVERNOUS ANEURYSMS: SURVEY OF MODERN CASE MATERIAL

Authors	Date	No. of Nonoperated Cavernous Aneurysms	Average Follow-Up Period (yr)	Hemorrhage
Kupersmith et al.[47]	1992	34	2.8	1*
Linskey and Sekhar et al.[53, 54, 55, 96]	1989	20	2.4	0
	1990			
	1990			
	1991			
Inagawa[42]	1991	16	4.7	0
Lye et al.[61]	1989	10	6.9	1
Total		80	4.2 (mean)	2 (2.5%)

*Aneurysm demonstrated a nipple projecting into the subarachnoid space.

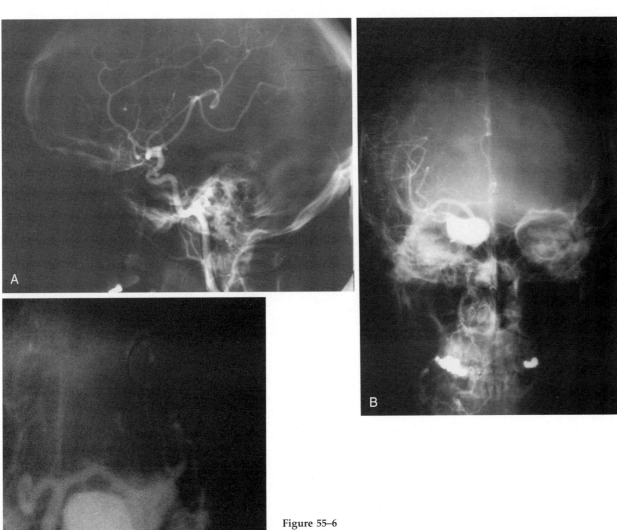

Figure 55–6

Cavernous sinus aneurysms vary greatly in size and morphology and, consequently, in the signs and symptoms they produce. *A.* Small (< 1 cm) asymptomatic aneurysm. *B.* Large (1 to 2.5 cm) aneurysm, with facial pain. *C.* Giant (> 2.5 cm), with ophthalmoplegia.

Figure 55–7

Visual loss in field and acuity from the paracavernous aneurysm presented in Figure 55–4.

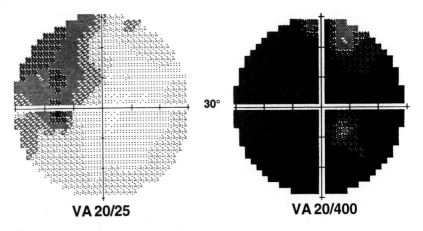

Table 55–3

TREATMENT OPTIONS FOR CAVERNOUS CAROTID ANEURYSMS: LITERATURE REVIEW

Authors	Date	No. of Aneurysms	Treatment
Gelber and Sundt[32]	1980	6 Intracavernous 1 Intrapetrous	ICA ligation plus EC-IC bypass
Sen and Sekhar[95, 98]	1990 1992	2 Cavernous 1 Petrous	Direct vein graft repair
Spetzler et al.[104]	1990	15 Cavernous	Direct vein graft repair
Fukushima[31]	1993 1994†	28 Cavernous* 70	Direct vein graft repair Direct clipping
Matsuoka et al.[64]	1986	4	Direct clipping
Hakuba et al.[35]	1982	3	Direct clipping
Hakuba et al.[36]	1989		
Higashida et al.[40]	1990	87	Endovascular balloon/ICA occlusion 68 (78%) Endovascular balloon/aneurysm occlusion 19 (22%)
Taki et al.[109]	1992	4	Endovascular occlusion/ICA
Berenstein et al.[10]	1984	12 Cavernous and petrous carotid	Endovascular trapping with dual balloon
Fox et al.[29]	1987	37 Cavernous and petrous carotid	Proximal ICA occlusion by endovascular balloon, 11 with EC-IC bypass
Dolenc[19]	1983	3	Direct clipping
Parkinson[83]	1988	3	Diect reconstruction (with hypothermic circulatory arrest)
Al-Rodhan et al.[4]	1993	23	Direct clipping (17) Excision (1) ICA ligation plus STA-MCA (1) Vein graft plus ICA ligation (4)
Kupersmith et al.[47]	1992	36	Embolization (33) Direct surgery (1) Carotid ligation (2)
Linskey and Sekhar[53, 54, 55, 96]	1989 1990 1990 1991	19	Direct clipping (4) Suture repair (2) Saphenous vein bypass and trapping (2) Endovascular occlusion of ICA (5) Endovascular trapping (1) Embolized (5)

Little et al.[57]	1989	15	ICA occlusion:
			  Gradual with Selverstone clamp and
			    anticoagulation (10)
			  Ligation (1)
			  Trapping (4)

Ausman et al.[5]	1990	16	ICA occlusion:
			  EC-IC and gradual occlusion (10)
			  EC-IC and trapping (6)

Diaz et al.[15]	1982	5	ICA occlusion:
Diaz et al.[16]	1988		EC-IC and gradual occlusion (5)

Diaz et al.[17]	1989	32	ICA occlusion:
			  EC-IC and gradual occlusion (10)
			  STA-MCA and trapping (7)
			  Direct clipping (15)

Serbinenko et al.[100]	1990	4	Endovascular ICA occlusion with EC-IC bypass
Silvani et al.[101]	1985	4	EC-IC with Silverstone clamp (1 trapped)
Lye and Jha[61]	1989	23	CCA ligation (11) ICA ligation (2) Observed; no treatment (10)

*Interposed with report of Spetzler et al.
†Personal communication.
ICA, internal carotid artery; EC-IC, external carotid–internal carotid; STA-MCA, superficial temporal to middle cerebral artery; CCA, cavernous carotid artery.

carotid occlusion should be abrupt or gradual, and about the utilization of perioperative anticoagulation.

Technical advances in endovascular neuroradiology have added more options to the therapeutic armamentarium. Endovascular balloon test occlusion has become an important, minimally invasive method for assessing cerebrovascular reserve, especially when it is coupled with cerebral blood flow or cerebral perfusion studies. Proximal endovascular internal carotid artery occlusion, balloon trapping, and direct aneurysm embolization have all been utilized successfully to treat cavernous carotid aneurysms.* Endovascular techniques have the advantage of minimal invasiveness. However, they are limited by aneurysm size, neck configuration, and association with risks of embolization and parent artery occlusion.

DIRECT APPROACHES

The pioneering work of Parkinson on direct operative approaches to vascular lesions of the cavernous sinus demonstrated the feasibility of such approaches.[79-84] Dolenc systematically demonstrated the surgical anatomical principles for operative entry into and management of cavernous sinus lesions.[19, 20-23] Experience with neoplastic lesions has led to the development of management strategies for cavernous vascular lesions.† Two principal approaches for direct treatment have been taken: (1) direct transcavernous clipping or microvascular reconstruction, and (2) direct large vein bypass (petrous carotid artery–to–supraclinoid carotid saphenous vein bypass).‡

Physiological Considerations

Management of cavernous carotid aneurysms depends heavily on cerebrovascular physiological considerations. Demonstration of cerebrovascular reserve, which is the ability to tolerate temporary or permanent carotid artery occlusion, is essential. Cerebrovascular assessment has been refined in recent years as a result of the vast experience with carotid artery sacrifice, endovascular balloon test occlusion, and noninvasive cerebral blood flow analysis.§ Early work by Miller and co-workers and Leech and associates defined parameters for safe carotid artery occlusion that have stood the test of time.[51, 68] Ligation is generally safe if cerebral blood flow is greater than 40 mL per 100 g per minute during test occlusion; it also is safe if cerebral blood flow ranges from 20 to 40 mL per 100 g per minute provided that flow reduction is less than 25 per cent. Ligation is always unsafe if the cerebral blood flow during clamping is less than 20 mL per 100 g per minute.

Endovascular balloon test occlusion with qualitative or quantitative cerebral blood flow/carotid artery pressure measurements have been successfully used to assess the hemodynamic risk of permanent or temporary carotid artery occlusion.* This assessment couples the 20-minute clinical occlusion test with a qualitative or quantitative assessment. A number of caveats regarding this test must be kept in mind. First, the test itself carries a 4 to 7 per cent ischemic complication rate.[77, 110] Second, it cannot predict delayed changes in cerebrovascular reactivity, which may occur in association with carotid artery occlusion. Third, it is a static test and does not evaluate direct effects on cerebrovascular reactivity. Finally, the test does not evaluate the risk of embolic phenomena, the most common complication of carotid artery occlusion.[6, 49] Even with these limitations, this testing is important in guiding decision-making.

Once cerebrovascular reserve has been established, other factors such as the size of the aneurysm, contralateral vascular disease, and the presence of recent subarachnoid hemorrhage must be considered. Patients with contralateral stenosis or aneurysms, or both, are poor candidates for carotid artery sacrifice. Patients with recent subarachnoid hemorrhage are prone to having a decline in cerebral blood flow and reactivity within the perihemorrhage period.[66]

Patients who are found to be without deficits in cerebral blood flow or perfusion on clinical balloon occlusion testing have the full spectrum of treatment options available. At this point, secondary considerations such as the surgeon's skill, the patient's age, and the presence or absence of contralateral disease come into play.

Patients who pass the clinical balloon occlusion test but demonstrate significant cerebral blood flow or cerebral perfusion deficits are at risk for hemodynamic insufficiency. Supplemental extracranial-to-intracranial bypass with subsequent re-evaluation is necessary before indirect treatment can be undertaken. The type of bypass is directly related to the flow deficiency.

Patients who frankly fail the clinical balloon occlusion testing are at the greatest risk and pose the greatest challenge. These patients are generally best treated with direct transcavernous approaches for clipping or with petrous carotid artery–to–supraclinoid carotid artery bypass with the aid of cerebral protective agents, such as barbiturates or etomidate.[9]

Significant drawbacks to large vein petrous to supraclinoid bypass are the 1- to 2-hour carotid artery occlusion time and the technical complexity of the procedure. This procedure is extremely attractive for patients with giant aneurysms that would pose significant technical difficulties if direct clipping were used.

Indications for Treatment

Indications for treatment vary from physician to physician. Generally accepted indications include (1) history of rupture, (2) extension of the aneurysm into the

---

*See references 10, 29, 40, 50, 67, 71, 99, 100, and 109.
†See references 2, 3, 5, 22, 23, 31, 35, 36, 55, 64, 94, 96, 97, and 113.
‡See references 5, 19, 21, 22, 23, 31, 35, 36, 95, 98, and 104.
§See references 14, 25, 27, 44, 70, 105, and 110.

*See references 14, 25, 27, 44, 70, 105, and 110.

subarachnoid space, (3) traumatic etiology, (4) progressive enlargement of the aneurysm, and (5) progressive neurological deficits. The treatment of small, asymptomatic, completely intracavernous (serendipitous) lesions remains a subject of controversy. These aneurysms are most effectively managed with a direct approach that involves their obliteration and preservation of the carotid artery. Unfortunately, postoperative ophthalmoplegia that lasts 3 to 6 months is not uncommon. Arguments for treatment of these lesions emphasize concerns about their potential progression over time.

Management of Cavernous Carotid Aneurysms: Authors' Perspective

The initial evaluation begins with the separation of patients into symptomatic and asymptomatic categories. Patients with small, asymptomatic, wholly intracavernous lesions are followed conservatively (Fig. 55–8). Magnetic resonance imaging is extremely helpful in determining intracavernous locations in three dimensions in correlation with standard four-vessel angiography. Symptomatic patients with lesions who present without hemorrhage (compressive symptoms only) are also evaluated with magnetic resonance imaging and angiography (Fig. 55–9). Again, if no evidence of exposure to the subarachnoid space is observed, a period of conservative management is attempted. Regression has been demonstrated.[47, 54, 61] Unfortunately, it may be impossible to determine clearly which aneurysms have a wholly intracavernous location on the basis of radiographic imaging alone. Surgical exploration may be necessary for establishing definitive anatomical presentation. Aneurysms subject to operative intervention are those that present with any portion within the subarachnoid space, those that have a progressive increase in size or that cause neurological deficit, and those that are located on the C_3 portion.[4]

The work-up consists of four-vessel cerebral angiography with complete cross-compression (side-to-side/back-to-front) for determination of the adequacy of anatomical collateral. Physiological collateral then is assessed with simultaneous balloon occlusion testing and with the injection of a cerebral perfusion agent, or inhalation of stable or radioactive xenon with cerebral blood flow measurements. The relationship to adjacent anatomy can be assessed with magnetic resonance imaging with projection in the sagittal, coronal, and axial planes. Thoughtful consideration of angiographic and magnetic resonance imaging findings with regard to the relationship of the dome and neck to the anterior clinoid process assists in the preoperative planning stage. The work-up is completed with a neuro-ophthalmological assessment for documentation of visual acuity and fields as well as cranial nerve function.

The goal of the authors' surgical intervention is to obliterate the aneurysm and preserve the carotid artery whenever possible. This philosophy has led to the use of direct surgical clipping as the initial treatment for

appropriate aneurysms. Judgment as to whether an aneurysm is clippable remains within the discretion of the surgeon.

APPROACH

After induction of general endotracheal anesthesia, a spinal drain is placed and the head is immobilized with three-point pin fixation, with the head rotated 30 degrees away from the midline and tilted slightly back. This position allows the frontal lobes to fall back and away from the operative area. A cranio-orbital craniotomy is performed with or without zygomatic extension, depending on the size and location of the aneurysm.[1, 102] The carotid artery in the neck is exposed in patients in whom proximal control may be necessary for clipping. With cervical carotid exposure, retrograde aspiration (the Dallas technique) may be utilized if necessary.[8] Intraoperative electrophysiological monitoring of the scalp, electroencephalography, and monitoring of cranial nerves III, IV, and VI via direct intraorbital electrode are performed. The cavernous sinus is unlocked after proximal and distal control has been attained. Proximal control at the level of the petrous carotid artery can be obtained with minimal exposure and with the use of a No. 2 French Fogarty catheter within the petrous carotid canal, as demonstrated by Wascher and colleagues.[114] The anterior clinoid process is then removed in an extradural fashion. In cases in which the dome or neck of the aneurysm appears radiologically to be at risk of injury during extradural drilling, the clinoid process is cored out, with final removal occurring under direct intradural visualization. Dolenc points out that the spinal drain should remain closed throughout the extradural exposure so that a cerebrospinal fluid buffer is present during drilling.* Removal of the clinoid process and opening of the osseous optic canal provide access to ophthalmic segment aneurysms and C_3 segment aneurysms as well as distal control of the cavernous carotid segment.

If additional exposure within the middle cranial fossa is needed, the zygomatic extension of the cranio-orbital craniotomy is performed. This permits total bone removal around the temporal tip. In de novo approaches, the temporal-polar veins may be taken down. This maneuver, along with splitting of the proximal sylvian fissure, allows the temporal lobe to be mobilized up and out of the middle cranial fossa, providing robust exposure of the cavernous sinus.[78]

ENTRY TO CAVERNOUS SINUS

Entry into the cavernous sinus depends on both the location and the size of the aneurysm. Knowledge of the relationships among the anatomical structures of the cavernous sinus gives the surgeon a better understanding of the surgical approaches. Several anatomical triangles have been described and illustrated. The ana-

---

*Personal communication.

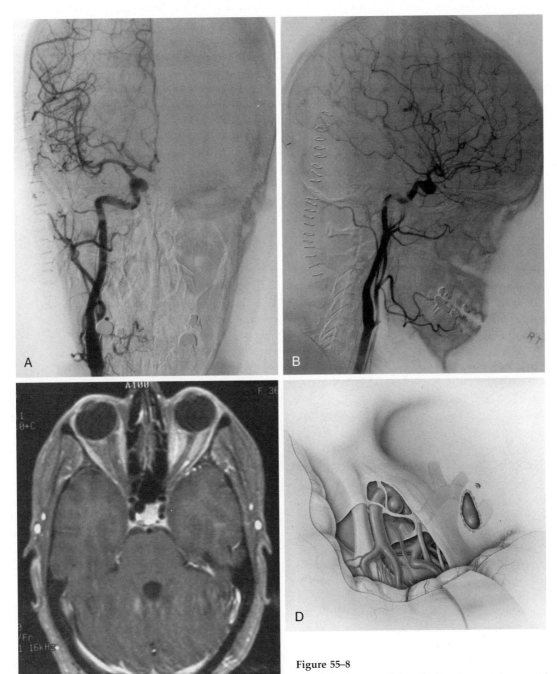

Figure 55–8

Example of a serendipitously found cavernous carotid artery aneurysm. Anteroposterior (A) and lateral (B) angiograms reveal the origin of the neck on the C_4 segment. Magnetic resonance imaging (C) reveals that the aneurysm is totally confined to the cavernous space, without subarachnoid projection. Surgical view of the aneurysm (D) designated (C_4, S, N) by the proposed nomenclature.

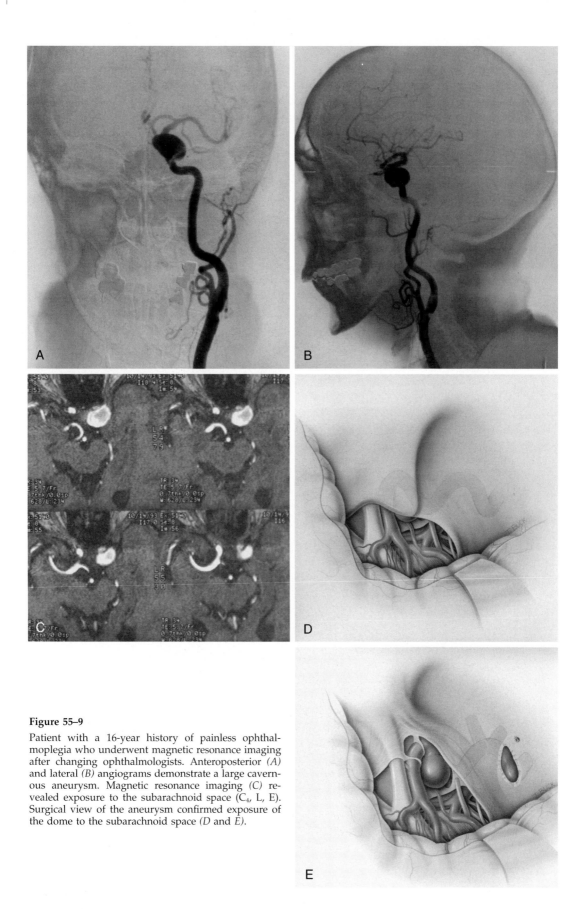

Figure 55–9

Patient with a 16-year history of painless ophthalmoplegia who underwent magnetic resonance imaging after changing ophthalmologists. Anteroposterior (A) and lateral (B) angiograms demonstrate a large cavernous aneurysm. Magnetic resonance imaging (C) revealed exposure to the subarachnoid space (C_4, L, E). Surgical view of the aneurysm confirmed exposure of the dome to the subarachnoid space (D and E).

tomical relationships of dural, osseous, neural, and vascular structures permit the identification of 10 triangles, which can be grouped into three divisions.[22] Four triangles are found in the parasellar region: the anteromedial, the paramedial, the oculomotor, and Parkinson's triangles. The middle cranial fossa area also has four triangles: the anterolateral, the lateral, the posterolateral (Glasscock's), and the posteromedial (Kawase's). Two triangles are in the paraclival region: the inferomedial and the inferolateral (trigeminal).

The cavernous sinus can be entered through any of these windows or triangles, depending on the anatomical variation of the patient and the nature and location of the lesion approached. However, two main avenues of entry into the sinus are used in most surgical procedures that utilize the cranial approach: the lateral and the superior. These routes may be extended or combined.

When the entry is through the superior aspect, the dura is opened in a semicircular fashion and the incision is centered on the pterion. Then, the dura is split along the sylvian fissure toward the anterior clinoid process. Next, the sylvian fissure is opened, the frontal and temporal lobes are separated, and the parasellar area and the roof of the cavernous sinus are exposed. The dural sheath of the optic nerve is incised along the length of the optic canal, starting from the falciform fold through the entire length of the canal. This crucial step mobilizes the optic nerve and fully exposes the origin and course of the ophthalmic artery. The distal dural ring anchoring the carotid artery as it enters the subdural cavity is opened. The opening is extended posteriorly to cranial nerve III; this allows superb entry into the cavernous sinus through its superior wall. This exposure transforms an otherwise high-risk ophthalmic aneurysm into an internal carotid artery aneurysm, with distal and proximal control readily attainable.

To enlarge this exposure, the carotid artery can be freed and mobilized laterally. The posterior clinoid process can be dissected from the dura and removed with a diamond drill along with a portion of the dorsum sella; this allows further exposure of the upper clivus. Use of the zygomatic extension greatly enhances this aspect of the dissection. This maneuver is helpful for exposing aneurysms of the upper basilar artery.

Further medial enlargement of this superior approach can be accomplished with dissection of the dura over the planum sphenoidale, which is then drilled away before the sphenoid sinus is entered. The sphenoid sinus mucosa is pushed downward and medially or is removed. The previously freed optic nerve can then be mobilized laterally while the diaphragma sellae is incised; this permits clear visualization of the pituitary gland and the medial aspect of the carotid artery.

The lateral entry into the cavernous sinus is through Parkinson's triangle, which has the fourth cranial nerve as its medial border and the medial aspect of the first division of the trigeminal nerve as its lateral border. This is the conventional avenue, especially for the approach to a lesion confined to the cavernous sinus. It provides good exposure of the lateral surface of the

horizontal intracavernous carotid artery segment and of the medial loop.

The free margin of the tentorium and the third and fourth cranial nerves are identified. The fourth cranial nerve is more difficult to identify because it courses below the third. The position of both nerves in the superior lateral wall of the cavernous sinus is relatively constant. An incision is made beneath the projected course of the third cranial nerve, centering on the point where the third cranial nerve appears over the horizon of the free margin of the tentorium. The incision extends approximately 8 mm both anteriorly and posteriorly. The outer layer of the lateral wall of the cavernous sinus is then peeled away from the first and second divisions of the trigeminal nerve. The inner layer of the lateral wall remains intact, and venous bleeding is not encountered up to this point. A natural gap exists in the inner layer between the fourth cranial nerve and the first division of the trigeminal nerve. This gap can be enlarged to expose the carotid artery and the sixth cranial nerve on the lateral wall of the carotid artery. This nerve frequently has two divisions, but it is the only cranial nerve coursing inside the cavernous sinus.

The lateral exposure can be further enhanced with the use of one or more maneuvers. The outer layer of the lateral wall can be peeled further posteriorly and inferiorly; this exposes the third division and the trigeminal ganglion and opens Meckel's cavity. For further visualization, the mandibular division can be sectioned to permit retraction of the gasserian ganglion and exposure of the posterior entrance of the carotid artery into the cavernous sinus. This maneuver adds length to the exposed segment of the intrapetrous carotid artery, allowing grafting with a shunt if necessary. Drilling of the petrous tip medial to the carotid artery and anterior to the internal auditory meatus (Kawase's triangle) provides further exposure. This maneuver allows entry into the posterior fossa and reveals the posterior aspect of the cavernous sinus—in particular, the entry of the sixth cranial nerve and Meckel's cavity.

The lateral entry can be combined with the superior entry to achieve complete exposure of the carotid artery from the intracranial entry to the supraclinoid carotid artery.

Clip application can proceed once adequate exposure is obtained, venous bleeding controlled and with proximal and distal arterial control. In patients with small, simple aneurysms, clip application follows the general principles of aneurysm surgery. In those with larger, atherosclerotic aneurysms, a period of temporary occlusion with cerebral protection greatly enhances the clip application. If the neck is atherosclerotic, care should be taken to place the clip sufficiently high to allow for the atheroma. It can be helpful to tailor the neck with initial placement of a clip high on the neck, followed by piggybacking and the placement of a second clip lower than the first.

Retrograde suction from the carotid artery exposure is quite helpful in those cases in which aneurysm size and turgidity limit clip application. Care should be taken to ensure distal occlusion of the parent vessel and feeders and to avoid excessive blood aspiration during decompression.

Intraoperative angiography has proved to be invaluable for direct assessment of clip placement. It can be performed through the carotid artery exposure in the neck or from a preoperatively placed transfemoral angiographic catheter. Immediate confirmation of aneurysm obliteration and carotid artery patency is rewarding for the surgeon and can be life-saving for the patient.

Giant and fusiform aneurysms not amenable to direct clipping or reconstruction are best managed with short vein bypass. This procedure was pioneered by Fukushima and co-workers and popularized by Sekhar and colleagues.[31, 97, 98, 104] It provides high-flow bypass that approximates native carotid artery flow. No manipulation of the aneurysms or cranial nerves is necessary, and thus additional iatrogenic ophthalmoplegia is avoided. However, this procedure is technically demanding and may require 1 to 2 hours of carotid artery occlusion. The prolonged occlusion time raises concern about the versatility of this procedure in patients without cerebrovascular reservoir and about its necessity in those patients without cerebrovascular concerns. Al-Mefty proposed the use of an interpositioned shunt to circumvent the long occlusion time.[3] However, this technique has not found widespread application.

OVERVIEWS

Aneurysms of the cavernous carotid artery are now readily treatable with a broad spectrum of direct and indirect approaches (see Fig. 55–4). Direct approaches are appealing, as they provide obliteration or complete exclusion of the lesion with preservation or reconstruc-

tion of carotid artery flow. Indications for operation, standardized nomenclature for carotid artery and aneurysmal anatomy, and the natural history of these aneurysms remain to be established. The authors support the use of a modification of the Fischer nomenclature, as proposed by Fukushima,* for description of the carotid artery anatomy (Table 55–4).[28] Extrapolation of this nomenclature to describe aneurysm sites is advocated. The increasing availability of magnetic resonance imaging and magnetic resonance angiography will increase the incidence of diagnosis of asymptomatic cavernous aneurysms. Patients with wholly intracavernous lesions should be followed so that natural history data can be collected. Indications for operative intervention can be accurately established only after nomenclature has been standardized and the natural history of these lesions has been studied scientifically.

REFERENCES

1. Al-Mefty, O., and Smith, R. R.: Tailoring the cranioorbital approach. Keio J. Med., 39:217–224, 1990.
2. Al-Mefty, O., Ayoubi, S., and Schenk, M. P.: Unlocking and entering the cavernous sinus. Perspect. Neurol. Surg., 2:49, 1991.
3. Al-Mefty, O., Khalil, N., Elwany, N., et al.: Shunt for bypass graft of the cavernous carotid artery: An anatomical and technical study. Neurosurgery, 27:721, 1990.
4. Al-Rodhan, N. R. F., Piepgras, D. G., and Sundt, T. M.: Transitional cavernous aneurysms of the internal carotid artery. Neurosurgery, 33:993, 1993.
5. Ausman, J. I., Diaz, F. G., Sadasivan, B., et al.: Giant intracranial aneurysm surgery: The role of microvascular reconstruction. Surg. Neurol., 34:8, 1990.
6. Barnett, H. J. M.: Delayed cerebral ischemic episodes distal to occlusion of major cerebral arteries. Neurology, 28:769, 1978.
7. Barr, H. W. K., Blackwood, W., and Meadows, S. P.: Intracavernous carotid aneurysms: A clinical-pathological report. Brain, 94:607, 1971.
8. Batjer, H. H., and Samson, D. S.: Retrograde suction decompression of giant paraclinoidal aneurysms. J. Neurosurg., 73:305, 1990.
9. Batjer, H. H., Frankfurt, A. I., Purdy, P. D., et al.: Use of etomidate, temporary arterial occlusion and intraoperative angiography in surgical treatment of large and giant arachnoid aneurysms. J. Neurosurg., 68:234, 1988.
10. Berenstein, A., Ransohoff, J., Kupersmith, M., et al.: Transvascular treatment of giant aneurysms of the cavernous carotid and vertebral arteries: Functional investigation and embolization. Surg. Neurol., 21:3, 1984.
11. Day, A. L.: Intracavernous carotid artery aneurysms. In Kapp, J. P., and Schmidek, H. H., eds.: The Cerebral Venous System and Its Disorders. Orlando, Grune & Stratton, 1984, pp. 569–580.
12. Day, A. L.: Clinicoanatomic features of supraclinoid aneurysms. Clin. Neurosurg., 36:256, 1988.
13. Day, A. L.: Aneurysms of the ophthalmic segment. J. Neurosurg., 72:677, 1990.
14. DeVries, E. J., Sekhar, L. N., Horton, J. A., et al.: A new method to predict safe resection of the internal carotid artery. Laryngoscope, 100:85, 1990.
15. Diaz, F. G., Ausman, J. I., and Pearce J. E.: Ischemic complications after combined internal carotid artery occlusion and extracranial-intracranial anastomosis. Neurosurgery, 10:563, 1982.
16. Diaz, F. G., Ohaegbulam, S., and Dujovny, M.: Surgical management of aneurysms in the cavernous sinus. Acta Neurochir. (Wien), 91:25, 1988.
17. Diaz, F. G., Ohaegbulam, S, and Dujovny, M., et al.: Surgical alternatives in the treatment of cavernous sinus aneurysms. J. Neurosurg., 71:846, 1989.

Table 55–4

PROPOSED NOMENCLATURE FOR CAVERNOUS CAROTID ANEURYSMS*

Feature	Symbol	Meaning
Location†	C_1	Bifurcation to posterior communicating artery
	C_2	Posterior communicating artery to distal dural ring
	C_3	Proximal dural ring to distal dural ring
	C_4	Intracavernous horizontal segment
	C_5	Intracavernous ascending segment
Size	S (small)	Less than 1.0 cm
	L (large)	1.0–2.5 cm
	G (giant)	Greater than 2.5 cm
Exposure to subarachnoid space	N	Nonexposed
	E	Exposed

*Aneurysms designated on the basis of location, size, exposure. Example: C_3, L, E.

†Cavernous carotid artery nomenclature taken from Dolenc[22] and Fischer,[28] as proposed by Fukushima (personal communication), with modification by the authors.

*Personal communication.

18. Diaz, F. G., Umansky, F., Mehta, B., et al.: Cerebral revascularization to a main limb of the middle cerebral artery in the Sylvian fissure: An alternative approach to conventional anastomosis. J. Neurosurg., 63:21, 1985.

19. Dolenc, V. V.: Direct microsurgical repair of intracavernous vascular lesions. J. Neurosurg., 58:824, 1983.

20. Dolenc, V. V.: A combined epi- and subdural direct approach to carotid ophthalmic artery aneurysms. J. Neurosurg., 62:667, 1985.

21. Dolenc, V. V.: Surgery of vascular lesions of the cavernous sinus. Clin. Neurosurg., 36:240, 1988.

22. Dolenc, V. V.: Anatomy and Surgery of the Cavernous Sinus. New York, Springer-Verlag, 1989, pp. 1–341.

23. Dolenc, V. V., Skrap, M., Sustersic, J., et al.: A transcavernous-transsellar approach to the basilar tip aneurysms. Br. J. Neurosurg., 1:251, 1989.

24. Eguchi, T., Nakagomi, T., and Teraoka, A.: Treatment of bilateral mycotic intracavernous carotid aneurysms. J. Neurosurg., 56:443, 1982.

25. Erba, S. M., Horton, J. A., Latchaw, R. E., et al.: Balloon test occlusion of the internal carotid artery with stable xenon CT cerebral blood flow imaging. A.J.N.R., 9:533, 1988.

26. Faria, M. A., Jr., Fleischer, A. S., and Spector, R. H.: Bilateral giant intracavernous carotid aneurysms treated by bilateral carotid ligation. Surg. Neurol., 14:207, 1980.

27. Feldmann, M., Voth, E., Dressler, D., et al.: ^{99m}Tc-Hexamethylpropylene amine oxime SPECT and x-ray CT in acute cerebral ischemia. J. Neurol., 237:475, 1990.

28. Fischer, E.: Die Lageabweichungen der vorderen Hirnarterie im Gefässbild. Zentralbl. Neurochir., 3:300, 1938.

29. Fox, A. J., Viñuela, F., Pelz, D. M., et al.: Use of detachable balloons for proximal artery occlusion in the treatment of unclippable cerebral aneurysms. J. Neurosurg., 66:40, 1987.

30. Fox, J. L.: Microsurgical treatment of ventral (paraclinoid) internal carotid artery aneurysms. Neurosurgery, 22:32, 1988.

31. Fukushima, T., Day, J., and Tung, H.: Intracavernous carotid aneurysms. In Apuzzo, M. L. J., ed.: Brain Surgery: Complication Avoidance and Management. New York, Churchill Livingstone, 1992, pp. 925–944.

32. Gelber, B. R., and Sundt, T. M., Jr.: Treatment of intracavernous and giant carotid aneurysms by combined carotid ligation and extra- to intracranial bypass. J. Neurosurg., 52:1, 1980.

33. Giannotta, S. L., and Levy, M. L.: Carotid ophthalmic aneurysms. In Apuzzo, M. L. K., ed.: Brain Surgery: Complication Avoidance and Management. New York, Churchill Livingstone, 1992, pp. 944–957.

34. Guy, J. R., and Day, A. L.: Intracranial aneurysms with superior division paresis of the oculomotor nerve. Ophthalmology, 96:1071, 1989.

35. Hakuba, A., Nishimura, S., Shirakata, S., et al.: Surgical approaches to the cavernous sinus: Report of 19 cases. Neurol. Med. Chir. (Tokyo), 22:295, 1982.

36. Hakuba, A., Tanaka, K., Suzuki, T., et al.: A combined orbitozygomatic infratemporal epidural and subdural approach for lesions involving the entire cavernous sinus. J. Neurosurg., 71:699, 1989.

37. Halbach, V. V., Higashida, R. T., Hieshima, G. B., et al.: Aneurysms of the petrous portion of the internal carotid artery: Results of treatment with endovascular or surgical occlusion. A.J.N.R., 11:253, 1990.

38. Harris, F. S., and Rhoton, A. L., Jr.: Anatomy of the cavernous sinus: A microsurgical study. J. Neurosurg., 45:109, 1976.

39. Heros, R. C., Nelson, P. B., Ojemann, R. G., et al.: Large and giant paraclinoid aneurysms: Surgical techniques, complications, and results. Neurosurgery, 12:153, 1983.

40. Higashida, R. T., Halbach, V. V., Dowd, C., et al.: Endovascular detachable balloon embolization therapy of cavernous carotid aneurysms: Results in 87 cases. J. Neurosurg., 72:857, 1990.

41. Hodes, J. E., Fletcher, W. A., Goodman, D. F., et al.: Rupture of cavernous carotid artery aneurysm causing subdural hematoma and death: Case report. J. Neurosurg., 69:617, 1988.

42. Inagawa, T.: Follow-up study of unruptured aneurysms arising from the C3 and C4 segments of the internal carotid artery. Surg. Neurol., 36:99, 1991.

43. Jefferson, G.: On the saccular aneurysms of the internal carotid artery in the cavernous sinus. Br. J. Surg., 26:267, 1932.

44. Jungreis, C. A.: Strategies for embolization of the internal carotid artery for cavernous sinus tumors. Skull Base Surg., 1:191, 1991.

45. Knosp, E., Müller, G., and Perneczky, A.: The paraclinoid carotid artery: Anatomical aspects of a microsurgical approach. Neurosurgery, 22:896, 1988.

46. Kobayashi, S., Kyoshima, K., Gibo, H., et al.: Carotid cave aneurysms of the internal carotid artery. J. Neurosurg., 70:216, 1989.

47. Kupersmith, M. J., Hurst, R., Berenstein, A., et al.: The benign course of cavernous carotid artery aneurysm. J. Neurosurg., 77:690, 1992.

48. Landau, K., Horton, J. C., Hoyt, W. F., et al.: Aneurysm mimicking intracranial growth of optic sheath meningioma. J. Clin. Neuroophthalmol., 10:185, 1990.

49. Landolt, A. M., and Millikan, C. H.: Pathogenesis of cerebral infarctions secondary to mechanical carotid artery occlusion. Stroke, 1:52, 1970.

50. Lapresle, J., Lasjaunias, P., Verret, J. M., et al.: Giant aneurysms of the intracavernous carotid complicated by subarachnoid hemorrhage: Emergency treatment by occlusive balloon and thrombosis in situ. Nouv. Presse Med., 8:3037–3040, 1979.

51. Leech, P. J., Miller, J. D., Fritch, W., et al.: Cerebral blood flow, internal carotid artery pressure and the EEG as a guide to the safety of carotid ligation. J. Neurol. Neurosurg. Psychiatry, 37:854, 1974.

52. Leonetti, J. P., Smith, P. G., and Linthicum, F. H.: The petrous carotid artery: Anatomic relationships in skull base surgery. Otolaryngol. Head Neck Surg., 102:3, 1990.

53. Linskey, M. E., Sekhar, L. N., Hirsch, W. L., Jr., et al.: Aneurysms of the intracavernous carotid artery: Clinical presentation, radiographic features and pathogenesis. Neurosurgery, 26:71, 1990.

54. Linskey, M. E., Sekhar, L. N., Hirsch, W. L., Jr., et al.: Aneurysms of the intracavernous carotid artery: Natural history and indications for treatment. Neurosurgery, 26:933, 1990.

55. Linskey, M. E., Sekhar, L. N., Horton, J. A., et al.: Aneurysms of the intracavernous carotid artery: A multidisciplinary approach to treatment. J. Neurosurg., 75:525, 1991.

56. Little, J. R., Furlan, A. J., and Bryerton, B.: Short vein grafts for cerebral revascularization. J. Neurosurg., 59:384, 1983.

57. Little, J. R., Rosenfeld, J. V., and Awad, I. A.: Internal carotid artery occlusion for cavernous segment aneurysm. Neurosurgery, 25:398, 1989

58. Liu, M. Y., Shih, C. J., Wang, Y. C., et al.: Traumatic intracavernous carotid aneurysm with massive epistaxis. Neurosurgery, 17:569, 1985.

59. Locksley, H. B.: Natural history of subarachnoid haemorrhage, intracranial aneurysms and arteriovenous malformations. J. Neurosurg., 25:219, 1966.

60. Lombardi, G., Passerini, A., and Migliavacca, F.: Intracavernous aneurysms of the internal carotid artery. A.J.R., 89:361, 1963.

61. Lye, R. H., and Jha, A. N.: Unruptured aneurysms of the intracavernous internal carotid artery: Outcome following carotid ligation or conservative treatment. Br. J. Neurosurg., 3:181, 1989.

62. Markwalder, T. M., and Meienberg, O.: Acute painful cavernous sinus syndrome in unruptured intracavernous aneurysms of the internal carotid artery. J. Clin. Neuroophthalmol., 3:31, 1983.

63. Masana, Y., and Taneda, M.: Direct approach to a traumatic giant internal carotid artery aneurysm associated with a carotid-cavernous fistula. J. Neurosurg., 76:524, 1992.

64. Matsuoka, Y., Hakuba, A., Kishi, H., et al.: Direct surgical treatment of intracavernous internal carotid artery aneurysms: Report of four cases. Surg. Neurol., 26:360, 1986.

65. Meadows, S. P.: Intracavernous aneurysms of the internal carotid artery: Their clinical features and natural history. Arch. Ophthalmol., 62:566, 1959.

66. Meyer, C. H. A., Lowe, D., Meyer, M., et al.: Progressive change in cerebral blood flow during the first three weeks after subarachnoid hemorrhage. Neurosurgery, 12:58, 1983.

67. Micheli, F., Schteinschnaider, A., Plaghos, L. L., et al.: Bilateral cavernous sinus aneurysm treated by detachable balloon technique. Stroke, 20:1751, 1979.

68. Miller, J. D., Jawad, K., Jennett, B.: Safety of carotid ligation and its role in the management of intracranial aneurysms. J. Neurol. Neurosurg. Psychiatry, 40:64, 1977.

69. Mindel, J. S., Sachdev, V. P., Kline, L. B., et al.: Bilateral intracavernous carotid aneurysms mimicking a prolactin-secreting pituitary tumor. Surg. Neurol., 19:163, 1983.

70. Morioka, T., Matsushima, T., Fujii, K., et al.: Balloon test occlusion of the internal carotid artery with monitoring of compressed spectral arrays (CSAs) of electroencephalogram. Acta Neurochir. (Wien), 101:29, 1989.

71. Mullan, S.: Carotid cavernous fistulas and intracavernous aneurysms. In Wilkins, R. H., and Rengachary, S. S., eds.: Neurosurgery. New York, McGraw-Hill, 1985, pp. 1483–1494.

72. Nakagawa, F., Kobayshi, S., Takemae, T., et al.: Aneurysms protruding from the dorsal wall of the internal carotid artery. J. Neurosurg., 65:303, 1986.

73. Nishioka, H.: Report on the cooperative study of intracranial aneurysms and subarachnoid hemorrhage: Section VIII, Part I: Results of the treatment of intracranial aneurysms by occlusion of the carotid artery in the neck. J. Neurosurg., 25:660, 1966.

74. Nishioka, T., Kondo, A., Aoyama, I., et al. Subarachnoid hemorrhage possibly caused by a saccular carotid artery aneurysm within the cavernous sinus. J. Neurosurg., 73:301, 1990.

75. Nutik, S.: Carotid paraclinoid aneurysms with intradural origin and intracavernous locations. J. Neurosurg., 48:526, 1978.

76. Ono, M., Ono, M., Rhoton, A. L., Jr., et al.: Microsurgical anatomy of the region of the tentorial incisure. J. Neurosurg., 60:365, 1984.

77. Origitano, T. C., Al-Mefty, O., Leonetti, J. P., et al.: Vascular considerations and complications in base surgery. Cranial Neurosurg., 35:351–363, 1994.

78. Origitano, T. C., Anderson, D. E., Tarassoli, Y., et al.: Skull base approaches to complex cerebral aneurysms. Surg. Neurol., 40:339, 1993.

79. Parkinson, D.: A surgical approach to the cavernous portion of the carotid artery: Anatomical studies and case report. J. Neurosurg., 23:474, 1965.

80. Parkinson, D.: Transcavernous repair of carotid cavernous fistula: Case report. J. Neurosurg., 26:420, 1967.

81. Parkinson, D.: Surgical anatomy of the cavernous sinus. In Wilkins, R. H., and Rengachary, S. S., eds.: Neurosurgery. New York, McGraw-Hill, 1985, pp. 1483–1484.

82. Parkinson, D.: Surgical anatomy of the lateral sellar compartment (cavernous sinus). Clin. Neurosurg., 36:219, 1988.

83. Parkinson, D.: Surgical management of internal carotid artery aneurysms within the cavernous sinus. In Schmidek, H. H., and Sweet, W. H., eds.: Operative Neurosurgical Techniques. 2nd ed. Philadelphia, W. B. Saunders, 1988, pp. 837–844.

84. Parkinson, D., and West, M.: Lesions of the cavernous plexus region in neurological surgery. In Youmans, J. R., ed.: Neurological Surgery. 2nd ed. Philadelphia, W. B. Saunders, 1982, pp. 3004–3023.

85. Perneczky, A., Knosp, E., Vorkapic, P., et al.: Direct surgical approach to infraclinoid aneurysms. Acta Neurochir., 76:36, 1985.

86. Perret, G. E., and Nibbelink, D. W.: Randomized treatment study: Carotid ligation. In Sahs, A. L., Nibbelink, D. W., Torner, J. C., eds.: Aneurysmal Subarachnoid Hemorrhage: Report of the Cooperative Study. Baltimore, Urban & Schwarzenberg, 1981.

87. Ramana Reddy, S. V., and Sundt, T. M., Jr.: Giant traumatic false aneurysm of the internal carotid artery associated with a carotid-cavernous fistula. J. Neurosurg., 55:813–818, 1981.

88. Rhoton, A. L., and Inoue, T.: Microsurgical approaches to the cavernous sinus. Clin. Neurosurg., 37:391, 1989.

89. Rhoton, A. L., Jr., Hardy, D. G., and Chamber, S. M.: Microsurgical anatomy and dissection of the sphenoid bone, cavernous sinus and sellar region. Surg. Neurol., 12:63–104, 1979.

90. Rhoton, A. L., Jr., Harris, F. S., and Fuji, K.: Anatomy of the cavernous sinus. In Kapp, J. P., and Schmidek, H. H., eds.: The Cerebral Venous System and Its Disorders. Orlando, Grune & Stratton, 1984, pp. 61–91.

91. Roski, R. A., and Spetzler, R. F.: Carotid ligation in neurosurgery. In Wilkins, R. H., and Rengachary, S. S., eds.: Neurosurgery. New York, McGraw-Hill, 1985, pp. 1414–1422.

92. Roski, R. A., Spetzler, R. F., and Nilsen, F. S.: Late complications of carotid ligation in the treatment of intracranial aneurysms. J. Neurosurg., 54:584, 1981.

93. Sahs, A. L., Perret, G. E., and Locksley, H. G.: In Nishioka, T., ed.: Aneurysms and Subarachnoid Hemorrhage: A Cooperative Study. Philadelphia, J. B. Lippincott, 1969, p. 296.

94. Sekhar, L. N., Burgess, J., and Akin, O.: Anatomical study of the cavernous sinus emphasizing operative approaches and related vascular and neural reconstruction. Neurosurgery, 21:806, 1987.

95. Sekhar, L., Sen, C., and Jho, H. D.: Saphenous vein graft bypass of the cavernous internal carotid artery. J. Neurosurg., 72:35, 1990.

96. Sekhar, L. N., Linskey, M. E., Sen, C. N., et al.: Surgical management of lesions within the cavernous sinus. Clin. Neurosurg., 37:440, 1989.

97. Sekhar, L. N., Schramm, V. L., Jr., Jones, N. F., et al.: Operative exposure and management of the petrous and upper cervical internal carotid artery. Neurosurgery, 19:967, 1986.

98. Sen, C., and Sekhar, L. N.: Direct vein graft reconstruction of the cavernous petrous and upper cervical internal carotid artery: Lessons learned from 30 cases. Neurosurgery, 30:732, 1992.

99. Serbinenko, F. A.: Balloon catheterization and occlusion of major cerebral vessels. J. Neurosurg., 41:125–145, 1974.

100. Serbinenko, F. A., Filatov, J. M., Spallone, A., et al.: Management of giant ICA aneurysms with combined extracranial-intracranial anastomosis and endovascular occlusion. J. Neurosurg., 73:57, 1990.

101. Silvani, V., Rainoldi, F., Gaetani, P., et al.: Combined STA/MCA arterial bypass and gradual internal carotid artery occlusion for treatment of intracavernous and giant carotid artery aneurysms. Acta Neurochir., 78:142, 1985.

102. Smith, R. R., Al-Mefty, O., and Middleton, T. H.: An orbitocranial approach to complex aneurysms of the anterior circulation. Neurosurgery, 24:385, 1989.

103. Spetzler, R. F., Schuster, H., and Roski, R. A.: Elective extracranial-intracranial arterial bypass in the treatment of inoperable giant aneurysms of the internal carotid artery. J. Neurosurg., 53:22, 1980.

104. Spetzler, R. F., Fukushima, T., Martin, N., et al.: Petrous carotid–to–intradural carotid saphenous vein graft for intracavernous giant aneurysm, tumor and occlusive cerebrovascular disease. J. Neurosurg., 73:496, 1990.

105. Steed, D. L., Webster, M. W., DeVries, E. J., et al.: Clinical observations on the effect of carotid artery occlusion on cerebral blood flow mapped by xenon computed tomography and its correlation with carotid artery blood pressure. J. Vasc. Surg., 11:38, 1990.

106. Sundt, T. M., Jr., and Piepgras, D. G.: Surgical approach to giant intracranial aneurysms: Operative experience in 80 cases. J. Neurosurg., 51:731, 1979.

107. Sundt, T. M., Jr., Piepgras, D. G., Marsh, W. R., et al.: Saphenous vein bypass grafts for giant aneurysms and intracranial occlusive disease. J. Neurosurg., 65:439, 1986.

108. Sundt, T. M., III, and Sundt, T. M., Jr.: Principles of preparation of vein bypass grafts to maximize patency. J. Neurosurg., 66:172, 1987.

109. Taki, W., Nishi, S., Yamashita, K., et al.: Selection and combination of various endovascular techniques in the treatment of giant aneurysms. J. Neurosurg., 77:37, 1992.

110. Tarr, R. W., Jungreis, C. A., Horton, J. A., et al.: Complications of preoperative balloon test occlusion of the internal carotid artery: Experience in 300 cases. Skull Base Surg., 1:240, 1991.

111. Tran-Dinh, H.: Cavernous branches of the internal carotid artery: Anatomy and nomenclature. Neurosurgery, 20:205, 1987.

112. Trobe, J. D., Glaser, J. S., and Post, J. D.: Meningiomas and aneurysms of the cavernous sinus: Neuroophthalmological features. Arch. Ophthalmol., 96:457, 1978.

113. Van Loveren, H. R., Keller, J. R., El-Kalliny, M., et al.: The Dolenc approach for cavernous sinus exploration (cadaveric prosection). J. Neurosurg., 74:837, 1991.

114. Wascher, T. M., Spetzler, R. F., Zabramski, J. M.: Improved transdural exposure and temporary occlusion of the petrous internal carotid artery for cavernous sinus surgery. J. Neurosurg., 78:834, 1993.

115. Yasargil, M. G., Gasser, J. C., Hodosh, R. M., et al.: Carotid-ophthalmic aneurysms: Direct microsurgical approach. Surg. Neurol., 8:155, 1977.

Posterior Circulation Aneurysms

The surgical treatment of aneurysms of the posterior circulation continues to advance. Improvements in microsurgical instrumentation, pharmocological brain protection, neuroradiography, and surgical strategies all have contributed to morbidity and mortality rates approaching those for the surgical treatment of anterior circulation aneurysms. This is certainly the case for most smaller aneurysms in the posterior circulation. For these lesions, the traditional aneurysm approaches to the posterior fossa have been useful (subtemporal, transsylvian, and suboccipital). Difficulties still exist with the therapy for large lesions and those along the basilar trunk. Direct surgical methods have not always proved satisfactory, stimulating intensive work on improving endovascular methodology.[3, 23] The role of endovascular therapy for individual lesions is not clearly defined at this time; however, with continuing advances in technology and analysis of the long-term results, a better understanding of the indications is being gained. In parallel with this trend, innovative approaches to the cranial base, sacrificing bone in lieu of brain retraction, have provided alternative strategies for the direct surgical management of difficult posterior circulation lesions. Current practice is to consider endovascular treatment for those patients harboring giant or complex lesions whose medical condition precludes general anesthesia. Patients who are in otherwise good condition are offered direct surgical therapy for the lesion as the best method of securing the aneurysm. This chapter focuses on the strategies and techniques of direct surgery for posterior circulation aneurysms, including contemporary cranial base strategies.

Incidence

Aneurysms of the posterior circulation account for 10 to 15 per cent of all intracranial aneurysms. The most common of these aneurysms are located at the basilar bifurcation, followed by those at the origins of the superior cerebellar artery and at the posterior inferior cerebellar arteries. Aneurysms arising along the posterior cerebral arteries and at the origins of the anterior inferior cerebellar artery and the vertebrobasilar junction are the least common. The incidences of multiple aneurysms and of aneurysms associated with arteriovenous malformations are the same as those for their anterior circulation counterparts. Giant aneurysms occur in the posterior circulation as frequently as in the anterior circulation, and the predilection for their site of origin follows the pattern for smaller lesions.[12, 32]

Most commonly, these aneurysms are of the saccular type; however, the vertebral artery complex is unusual in its high percentage of dissecting and fusiform lesions, 31 per cent and 9 per cent, respectively.[2, 14, 38, 41] Nontraumatic dissections of the vertebral artery, once thought to be rare, are being discovered more frequently with the advent of modern imaging techniques. The epidemiological pattern of saccular aneurysms of the posterior circulation is similar to the pattern of other cerebral aneurysms. However, the dissecting lesions tend to favor men and to occur at an earlier age.[2, 4, 37, 42] Dolichoectasias of the vertebral and basilar arteries are uncommon lesions that probably represent degenerative fusiform lesions complicated by dissection.[31] Frustrating to manage surgically, these lesions also tend to occur in adult males.

Clinical Presentation

The great majority of aneurysms of the posterior circulation, regardless of morphology, are first manifested by symptoms and signs of subarachnoid hemorrhage. Only occasionally can the clinical picture be

J. Diaz Day • *S. L. Giannotta*

differentiated from that associated with rupture of an anterior circulation aneurysm. Headache, nuchal pain and rigidity, nausea, and vomiting occur with equal frequency. Intraparenchymal hemorrhage and lower cranial nerve deficits are not common presenting problems. A vertebrobasilar catastrophe may be suggested by abrupt loss of consciousness, prolonged coma, middle to lower cranial nerve palsies with associated crossed pareses, pulmonary edema, or cardiac arrest. Fewer than one third of patients, however, present with such a constellation.[13, 32]

Occasionally, a cranial nerve deficit points to a specific posterior circulation lesion. Oculomotor nerve dysfunction may be associated with basilar bifurcation or superior cerebellar or upper basilar trunk aneurysms. Ruptured peripheral anterior inferior cerebellar artery lesions may cause hearing loss or facial nerve palsy. Aneurysms of the vertebrobasilar junction or lower basilar trunk are heralded by abducens dysfunction.

Subarachnoid hemorrhage less often dominates the clinical picture of giant aneurysms of the posterior circulation than it does in those of the anterior circulation.[12] Because of their close anatomical association with the brain stem and the cranial nerves, these larger lesions more frequently present with signs and symptoms referable to mass effect. Obstructive hydrocephalus may also be a presenting feature.

Large or giant dolichoectasias of the basilar artery typically present with symptoms referable to brain stem or cranial nerve compression. Ischemic syndromes may also be expected because of intermittent but progressive obliteration of brain stem–perforating branches.[31, 32] Trigeminal neuralgia and hemifacial spasm, frequently seen in patients with dolichoectasias, can occasionally be treated with transposition of the offending vessel.

Imaging

Angiography remains the gold standard for diagnosis and surgical planning of these lesions. Recent advances in magnetic resonance imaging have produced magnetic resonance angiography that is approaching the resolution necessary to eliminate the need for invasive angiography. At present, both angiography and magnetic resonance imaging are requisite to surgical planning in the posterior fossa. The morphology of the aneurysm influences the surgical treatment of these lesions; therefore, it is important that imaging distinguish between saccular, dissecting, and fusiform aneurysms. Often this requires several views, including oblique and submental vertex projections. The adequacy of filling of both vertebral arteries must be assessed as well as possible collaterals to the basilar circulation, such as the posterior communicating arteries. A venous phase study should also be included in all preoperative studies. This is especially critical if an approach that involves skeletonizing or ligating the sigmoid sinus is being considered.

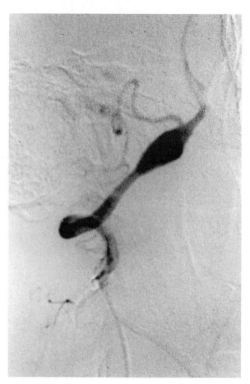

Figure 56–1

Angiography shows a fusiform vertebral aneurysm proximal to the takeoff of the posterior inferior cerebellar artery. Intraoperative findings confirmed a dissection.

Dissecting aneurysms, more common in the vertebral circulation, can have variable angiography signatures (Fig. 56–1). A double lumen, retention of contrast material during the venous phase, a "string sign," and an outpouching of the parent vessel all are features that have been recognized. The double lumen, considered the diagnostic hallmark for these lesions, may be difficult to visualize. Magnetic resonance imaging is a helpful adjunct in this regard. Because treatment may differ for dissecting and fusiform lesions, if the study does not distinguish adequately between the two, it may be advisable to repeat the study.

Surgical Anatomy

VERTEBRAL ARTERY ANATOMY

The vertebral artery enters the subarachnoid space by piercing the atlanto-occipital membrane and dura after giving rise to several muscular branches that supply the deep posterolateral muscles of the neck and, usually, a posterior meningeal artery. Typically, the first branch of the vertebral artery as it enters the subarachnoid space is the posterior spinal artery. The vertebral artery then courses medially and superiorly around the medulla. The twelfth cranial nerve crosses the artery, usually just before the origin of the posterior inferior cerebellar artery. The twelfth cranial nerve rootlets are often split by the posterior inferior cerebellar artery, which usually travels in a posterior and lateral direction, just inferior to the olive. Distal to the origin of the posterior inferior cerebellar artery, the glossopharyngeal, vagus, and spinal accessory nerves cross the lateral surface of the vertebral artery as they traverse the subarachnoid space to the jugular foramen. The spinal portion of the eleventh nerve is located lateral and posterior to the vertebral artery from its dural entrance to the origin of the posterior inferior cerebellar artery. The vertebral artery supplies the medulla through perforating branches along this segment. Aneurysms in this region are typically in close apposition to the lateral medullary surface, displacing and stretching the ninth through twelfth cranial nerves. The hypoglossal nerve is often associated with the aneurysm neck of vertebro–posterior inferior cerebellar artery aneurysms, or the aneurysm may even split the rootlets of the nerve.

The anatomy of the posterior inferior cerebellar artery is best described by dividing this artery into several short segments.[25] Proximal to the crossing of the spinal accessory nerve, the artery is divided into an anterior and a lateral medullary segment. As the artery crosses under the eleventh nerve, it makes an inferior turn around the cerebellar tonsil. This tonsillomedullary segment is the last to possess perforating branches supplying the medulla. Therefore, trapping of aneurysms of the distal posterior inferior cerebellar artery should be done distal to this division. As the artery turns rostral, it becomes the telovelotonsillar division, which branches several times into cortical segments. These cortical branches arise in the interhemispherical fissure of the cerebellum and course over the inferior surface of the cerebellum.

The vertebral artery distal to the origin of the posterior inferior cerebellar artery gives rise to several perforating arteries that also supply the medulla. The vertebral arteries join anterior to the pontomedullary junction to form the basilar artery. Just proximal to the junction, the anterior spinal arteries take their origin from each side and course inferiorly and medially to join into a common anterior spinal trunk, running in the anterior median sulcus of the lower medulla and spinal cord.

BASILAR ARTERY ANATOMY

The basilar artery begins at the vertebrobasilar junction and courses superiorly in the basilar sulcus of the pons toward the interpeduncular fossa. The artery has several major and intermediate branches, all of which may provide a point of origin for an aneurysm. The first major branch of the basilar artery is the anterior inferior cerebellar artery, which arises several millimeters distal to the vertebrobasilar junction and courses laterally and posteriorly to supply the inferior surface of the cerebellum. The superior cerebellar artery originates just proximal to the basilar bifurcation and courses laterally in the pontomesencephalic sulcus to supply the superior cerebellar hemisphere. The basilar artery terminates in the region of the interpedun-

cular fossa as it bifurcates to form the posterior cerebral arteries.

In addition to these major arteries supplying the cerebellum, the basilar artery gives rise to some intermediate-sized vessels.[30] The most proximal is the pontomedullary artery that originates between the vertebrobasilar junction and the takeoff of the anterior inferior cerebellar artery. This vessel travels laterally in the pontomedullary sulcus and terminates in the retro-olivary fossa. The long lateral pontine arteries are the next major branches. Usually consisting of a superolateral and an inferolateral artery, these vessels arise at about the level of the trigeminal nerve and course laterally to supply the paramedian and lateral pontine surface. The posterolateral artery is the most distal intermediate branch, arising just proximal to the takeoff of the superior cerebellar artery. This vessel is responsible for supplying the superolateral pontine surface.

Important in reducing surgical morbidity is the preservation of the critical perforating branches of the basilar artery. Perforators can arise either directly from the basilar artery or from its branches. These vessels may be divided into three groups—the caudal, middle, and rostral.[30] The caudal group originates from the dorsal surface of the initial segment of the basilar artery, between the vertebrobasilar junction and takeoff of the anterior inferior cerebellar artery. This group, comprising from one to four vessels, descends along the basilar sulcus and enters the foramen caecum medullae oblongatae. Occasionally, one or more of these vessels arises from the pontomedullary artery or the anterior inferior cerebellar artery. The middle group of perforators arise from the segment of the basilar artery, between the origins of the anterior inferior cerebellar artery and the posterolateral artery. They also arise from the dorsal surface and course rostrally or caudally for a short distance before penetrating the pons in the basilar sulcus. Some of these vessels may also originate from the anterior inferior cerebellar, long lateral, posterolateral, or pontomedullary arteries. The rostral perforator group usually numbers from one to five vessels and originates from the dorsal surface of the terminal basilar artery. These vessels course rostrally to enter the caudal posterior perforated substance. Importantly, these perforators may, in a small percentage of patients, arise from the superior cerebellar artery or the posterolateral arteries.[30]

POSTERIOR CEREBRAL ARTERY ANATOMY

The posterior cerebral artery is best described according to the nomenclature outlined by Zeal and Rhoton dividing the artery into three major segments.[45] P_1 is defined as that segment from the origin at the basilar bifurcation to the junction with the posterior communicating artery. This segment usually contains the origins of the thalamoperforating arteries and the long and short circumflex vessels. The P_2 segment extends to the region of the pulvinar and courses through the crural and ambient cisterns. This portion may be divided into halves, an anterior and a posterior P_2 segment. The anterior half typically gives rise to the anterior temporal, hippocampal, medial posterior choroidal, and peduncular perforating arteries. The middle and posterior temporal arteries, common temporal artery, and lateral posterior choroidal artery originate from the posterior segment of P_2. According to Zeal and Rhoton's work, the thalamogeniculate perforators arise from the P_2 segment, slightly more commonly from the posterior than from the anterior half.[45] The P_3 segment courses through the lateral part of the quadrigeminal cistern toward the calcarine fissure, where the artery splits into calcarine and parieto-occipital arteries.

Surgical Technique

ANESTHETIC CONSIDERATIONS

Several anesthetic adjuncts are used to minimize brain injury while maximal exposure of the aneurysm is obtained. As a routine, intravenous furosemide (20 to 40 mg) and a 20 per cent mannitol solution (0.5 g per kg) are administered at the time of the skin incision to initiate a diuresis. The P_{CO_2} is maintained in the 25- to 30-mm Hg range to make use of the vasoconstrictive effects of hypocapnia. Hypotension is not used except in the case of uncontrollable rupture. In most patients who undergo a supratentorial approach, a lumbar subarachnoid drain is placed. Aneurysms that are approached through a transmastoid or suboccipital route do not benefit from lumbar cerebrospinal fluid drainage. Rather, cerebrospinal fluid is evacuated through the cisterna magna after dural opening.

The authors routinely employ evoked potential and electroencephalography monitoring in all cases of posterior circulation aneurysms, in the event that temporary arterial occlusion is necessary. Before any temporary occlusion of a parent vessel, electroencephalography burst suppression is induced. The authors' current practice is to administer propofol for this purpose. Alterations in the wave morphology or latencies of the somatosensory evoked potentials are reasonably predictive of ongoing ischemia and reinforce the need for pharmacological agents that provide some protection. In transmastoid approaches, facial nerve electromyography and brain stem auditory evoked response are also monitored. Spinal accessory nerve monitoring during extradural bone removal around the jugular foramen is a helpful adjunct.

Another important consideration is patient positioning. Careful attention must be directed to the maintenance of adequate jugular venous drainage if the head is turned excessively. Increased venous pressure caused by inadequate drainage may inhibit exposure and increase retractor pressure. For most of the posterolateral approaches, the park bench or lateral position is used. For midline suboccipital exposures, the lateral or prone position suffices. Thin patients with supple necks are placed in the supine position if the subtemporal ap-

proach is used. In the authors' opinion, there are few indications for the routine use of the sitting position. The risk of intraoperative air embolism is not compensated by any advantage in exposure, decreased bleeding, or surgeon comfort. The sitting, or Concorde, position is, however, used beneficially in the setting of an anterior or superior cerebellar arteriovenous malformation in association with a distal posterior inferior cerebellar artery or distal superior cerebellar artery aneurysm.[29]

SURGICAL APPROACH

Vertebral Artery Aneurysms

The most common saccular aneurysms involving the vertebral artery complex are aneurysms of the vertebro–posterior inferior cerebellar artery. Most of these lesions can be approached through a simple lateral suboccipital approach. Large or complex saccular aneurysms may require strategies for exposing the posterolateral skull base and posterior fossa.

Lateral Suboccipital Approach

This approach is used for aneurysms located on the proximal vertebral artery up to and including the takeoff of the posterior inferior cerebellar artery. Dissecting aneurysms in which proximal ligation is the goal are readily accessed. True posterior inferior cerebellar artery aneurysms located on the initial segments (anterior medullary, lateral medullary, and tonsillomedullary segments) are also adequately exposed by this method. This approach has several modifications, which have been aptly described by Heros.[22]

The lateral, or park bench, position is used with the head in three-pin fixation. The incision begins at the level of the pinna and extends inferiorly along the posterior body of the mastoid and posterior margin of the sternocleidomastoid to about the C4 level. The muscular attachments to the occiput and the superficial and middle muscular layers in the neck are incised with electrocautery. The vertebral artery as it arches over C1 is avoided by its identification in the suboccipital triangle, delimited by the superior oblique, inferior oblique, and rectus capitis major muscles. The artery's course is quite variable, and it may have a significant extension lateral to the arch of C1, where it is vulnerable.

After dissection of all soft tissues free from the lateral base of the occiput, the craniotomy is made. The opening extends from the transverse sinus to the foramen magnum. The medial limit is usually short of the midline, with the lateral border being the sigmoid sinus. Removal of the rim of the foramen magnum as far lateral as possible is critical in gaining maximal exposure. The dura is then opened to expose the lateral cerebellar hemisphere and the cerebellar tonsil. The tonsil and the caudal hemisphere are gently retracted superiorly and medially to reveal the lateral medulla, the proximal vertebral artery, and the lower cranial nerves.

The arachnoid is opened sharply, liberating spinal fluid, which significantly relaxes structures in the posterior fossa. Under high magnification and with the use of sharp technique, the arachnoid is opened widely along the course of the vertebral artery. The lower cranial nerves easily come into view and must be negotiated gently. Again, sharp dissection is best used. Some of the branches of the ninth and tenth nerves are extremely fragile and occasionally can be mistaken for arachnoid, especially if the cistern is filled with blood from a recent subarachnoid hemorrhage. The aneurysm is identified by following the vertebral artery rostrally, being careful not to injure the twelfth cranial nerve draping over the vessel.

Occasionally, the hypoglossal or jugular tubercle is particularly large, hiding the proximal vertebral artery. In this circumstance, branches of the posterior inferior cerebellar artery may be identified lateral and rostral to the cerebellar tonsil. The trunk can then be followed back to its junction with the vertebral artery, allowing identification of the origin of the aneurysm. Subarachnoid blood is judiciously and carefully suctioned away. The origin of the posterior inferior cerebellar artery must be identified so that a clip occluding the neck of the aneurysm does not inadvertently occlude it. Gentle manipulation of the tenth and eleventh cranial nerves is permissible during placement of the clip; however, excessive traction on these nerves produces hoarseness, with the potential for prolonged vocal cord paralysis and aspiration. The need for aperture clips is uncommon, but they may occasionally accommodate a lower cranial nerve. The benefits of this approach are that it is familiar to most neurosurgeons and does not require complex cranial base dissection. For lesions more distal along the vertebral artery, such a limited approach may be confining, necessitating some element of brain stem retraction. In such circumstances, a more radical approach may be necessary.

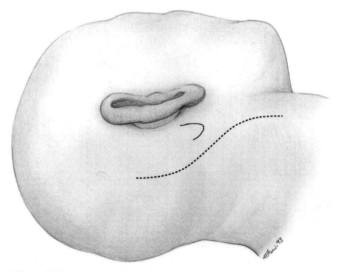

Figure 56–2

Skin incision for the extreme lateral inferior transcondylar exposure approach.

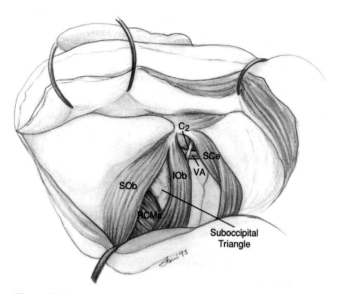

Figure 56–3

Anatomy of the suboccipital triangle shows the C2 nerve root crossing the vertebral artery. SOb, superior oblique muscle; SCe, splenius cervicis muscle; VA, vertebral artery; IOb, inferior oblique muscle; RCMa, rectus capitis major muscle.

Extreme Lateral Inferior Transcondylar Exposure Approach

Clip ligation of distal or complex vertebral artery aneurysms may require visualization from a more anterolateral, caudal-to-rostral trajectory, exposing the anterior surface of the medulla. To accomplish this, a modification of the far lateral approach that includes partial reduction of the posterior occipital condyle and excision of the jugular tubercle removes the bony obstructions to the desired line of sight anterior to the brain stem.

The patient is positioned in the three-quarter lateral position, with the head in three-pin fixation with the vertex oriented slightly downward and the ear as the highest point. The shoulder is moved out of the surgeon's way by pulling it caudally and rotating it anteriorly. The incision is started 2 to 3 cm behind the ear at the level of the external auditory meatus and continued caudad along the posterior body of the mastoid and the posterior aspect of the sternocleidomastoid muscle to the level of C4. The incision is shaped somewhat like a lazy S (Fig. 56–2). The superficial and intermediate muscle layers of the lateral neck are then incised with the monopolar cautery and reflected. The superficial layer is composed of the trapezius and sternocleidomastoid muscles. The intermediate layer includes the splenius capitis, longissimus capitis, and semispinalis capitis muscles. The deep layer of muscles includes the superior and inferior obliques, longissimus cervicis, rectus capitis major, and rectus capitis minor (Fig. 56–3).

Precise localization of the vertebral artery as it arches over C1 to pierce the atlanto-occipital membrane is essential and is accomplished as has been discussed for the far lateral method. The surrounding venous plexus is coagulated with bipolar cautery, and the con-

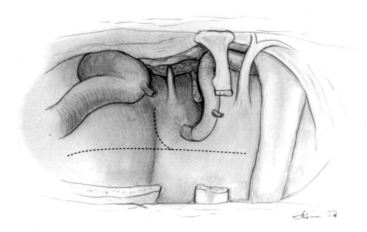

Figure 56–4

Preparation is made for dural opening. The sigmoid sinus and jugular bulb are skeletonized superolaterally. The vertebral artery and extradural branches are exposed above partially resected C1 lamina.

nective tissue is removed. Several muscular branches, which may be coagulated and divided, arise from the artery in this segment. Also, the posterior meningeal artery originating just proximal to the dural entrance of the vertebral artery may be divided. The posterior spinal artery typically arises just distal to the dural entrance of the artery, within the subarachnoid space. The oblique muscles are then detached from the transverse process of C1 and reflected.

The suboccipital craniotomy is next made, the anterolateral margin of which is the sigmoid sinus. By use of a high-speed drill, the sigmoid sinus and jugular bulb are skeletonized and the rim of the foramen magnum removed. The occipital condyle is then partially reduced with the drill. Drilling continues anteromedially and superiorly to expose the undersurface of the jugular bulb. As the bone removal proceeds anteriorly and medially, the jugular tubercle is removed. Depending on the desired degree of exposure, bone removal may proceed until the hypoglossal canal is skeletonized, exposing the extradural portion of the twelfth cranial nerve.

With bone removal complete, the dura is opened, beginning at the transverse–sigmoid sinus junction. The incision proceeds inferiorly to the dura covering the cervicomedullary junction, just posterior to the vertebral artery dural entrance. A second, short incision is made parallel to the vertebral artery dural entrance (Fig. 56–4). A dural ring, which is used for tight dural closure, is preserved around the vertebral artery. The dura is reflected anteriorly. The line of sight provided should allow a view of the anterior surface of the medulla. The hypoglossal nerve is seen crossing over the vertebral artery as the nerve traverses the subarachnoid space. The spinal portion of the eleventh nerve should be clearly seen as it travels rostrally toward the vagus and glossopharyngeal nerves. Here it is joined by its cranial portion, and the nerves exit the pars venosa of the jugular bulb with the vagus nerve. A wide exposure of the vertebral artery as it courses superiorly should be obtained. The line of sight can be adjusted to see along the vertebral artery all the way to the vertebrobasilar junction (Fig. 56–5). Techniques to obliterate the aneurysm are similar to those previously discussed, with the added feature that proximal and distal control of the vertebral vessel is avail-

able. Fusiform aneurysms of the distal vertebral artery can pose a number of strategic problems. The majority of these are dissections and are probably best treated with proximal occlusion or trapping, because brain stem–perforating branches are probably already occluded by the pathological process. Temporary occlusion while the electrophysiology data are observed helps make this tactic safer.

At the completion of the intradural portion of the procedure, the dura is closed in a watertight fashion, and the muscle layers of the neck are reapproximated. Upper cervical spine stability has not been a problem. The degree of condylar removal necessary for maximal exposure does not result in significant disruption of the atlanto-occipital joint.

The far lateral and extreme lateral inferior transcon-

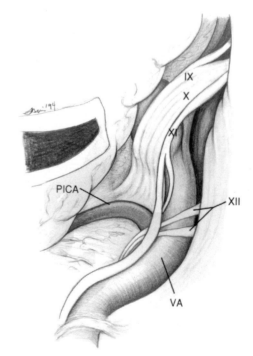

Figure 56–5

Dural opening and cerebellar retraction allow caudal-rostral and lateral-medial trajectory to the vertebrobasilar junction. IX, X, XI, and XII are cranial nerves; PICA, posterior inferior cerebellar artery; VA, vertebral artery.

dylar approaches can be expanded in a number of ways to attack large or complex pathologies. Removal of up to one half of the condyle and all of the jugular tubercle, with skeletonization of the hypoglossal nerve, further enhances visualization anterior to the brain stem. Hemilaminectomy of C1 and C2 provides a more caudal-to-rostral trajectory, and, if necessary, the vertebral artery can be transposed from the C1–C2 transverse foramen.

The benefit of this approach is its anterolateral rostral-caudal trajectory, which allows a sight line parallel with the vertebral artery anterior to the lower brain stem. With judicious handling of the cranial nerves, the vertebral artery can be exposed to its junction with the basilar artery. Lower basilar trunk aneurysms may also be approached with the use of this strategy.

Vertebrobasilar Junction Aneurysms

Retrolabyrinthine-Transsigmoid Approach

The vertebrobasilar junction is typically located at the level of the pontomedullary junction. This anatomical location may be difficult to adequately expose by a routine lateral suboccipital approach without an unacceptable degree of cerebellar or brain stem retraction. Tortuosity of the vertebral artery may additionally place the lesion at a relatively long operative distance through a suboccipital or transcondylar approach. For these situations, the retrolabyrinthine-transsigmoid approach has been developed to provide increased rostral exposure while shortening the operative distance.[18] Preoperative venous phase angiography is important in planning this approach, because the dominance pattern of the venous drainage must be first ascertained. An approach through the side of a dominant drainage pattern may necessitate preservation of the sinus, forcing the surgeon to work on either side of an intact sigmoid sinus.

The patient is positioned on the operating table, either in the lateral position or with the head turned 45 degrees away in the supine position. Both methods use gravity to advantage by allowing the cerebellum to fall away from the petrous bone and clivus, thus decreasing the need for retraction. A slightly curved retroauricular incision is made, from just above the nuchal line to the level of C1. A modified mastoidectomy is then made to expose the presigmoid dura. The mastoidectomy should include exposure from the middle fossa dura above to the jugular bulb below. The anterior limit is the posterior semicircular canal. The sigmoid sinus is then skeletonized, and about 2 cm of retrosigmoid dura is exposed.

The dura posterior to the sinus is then opened. The sigmoid sinus is ligated both at the transverse-sigmoid junction and at the inlet to the jugular bulb. This ligation is performed with either clips or ligatures. The dural opening is then completed across the sigmoid sinus, and the dural flap is reflected anteriorly. The center of the operative field includes the seventh and eighth cranial nerve complex and the flocculus of the cerebellum. The superior portion of the field includes

the fifth cranial nerve, spanning the subarachnoid space to its entrance into Meckel's cave. Inferiorly, the ninth, tenth, and eleventh nerves are in view as they enter the pars nervosa of the jugular foramen. Opening of the arachnoid of the cerebellopontine angle clearly exposes the vertebral artery as it meets its contralateral counterpart to form the vertebrobasilar junction. Aneurysm dissection is accomplished by straddling the relevant cranial nerves; rarely is there enough space for both instruments to fit between the various complexes. This tactic is made easier with the retrolabyrinthine-transsigmoid approach because the line of sight is parallel to the course of cranial nerves V through X. Facial nerve electromyography and brain stem auditory evoked responses are helpful at this juncture. The sixth cranial nerve must be identified and preserved. Proximal and distal control of vertebral and basilar vessels is available. Because of the narrow corridor between cranial nerves, low-profile clip appliers are necessary. In their absence, use of elongated clips may obviate the need to force a large clip applier between two delicate cranial nerves. After clip ligation of the aneurysm, the dura is closed tightly, and the exposed air cells are occluded with bone wax. The bony defect is then packed with a fat graft, harvested from either the thigh or the abdomen, and the fascia and skin are closed (Fig. 56–6).

The key to the use of the retrolabyrinthine-transsigmoid approach is the selection of the side on which the approach is made. Two anatomical factors govern the choice. The first and most important factor is the size and lateralization of the aneurysm. For lesions that are strongly lateralized, meaning that the aneurysm points either to the right or to the left, the side of the approach should usually be on the side of the dome. This is the shortest reach and obviates the need to work across the midline through a nest of basilar artery–perforating vessels. For lesions that are not lateralized, that is, those that point either ventrally or dorsally, an approach on the side of the smaller sigmoid sinus is ideal. Scrutiny of the venous phase results of carotid angiography is necessary to ensure that both lateral sinuses connect with the torcular. Unless one sigmoid sinus is dramatically larger than another, sigmoid ligation should be tolerated nicely. In the circumstance in which the approach is made on what appears to be a dominant sigmoid sinus, temporary occlusion of the sinus with measurement of the venous sinus pressure has been used to predict tolerance. When occlusion of the sinus produced more than a 5-mm Hg rise in venous pressure, the authors have resorted to a variation of the extreme lateral inferior transcondylar approach or the transpetrosal approach (see later) in order to preserve the sigmoid sinus.

Extended Extreme Lateral Inferior Transcondylar Approach

When sacrifice of the sigmoid sinus was not possible, or the complexity or size of the vertebrobasilar junction aneurysm required a wider degree of exposure, the authors have chosen to combine the transmastoid ex-

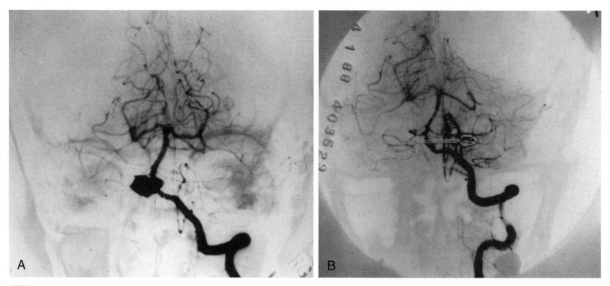

Figure 56–6

Preoperative *(A)* and postoperative *(B)* angiography demonstrates clip ligation of a vertebrobasilar junction aneurysm through a retrolabyrinthine-transsigmoid approach.

posure with the extreme lateral inferior transcondylar approach, which provides several advantages. The first is a wide caudal-to-rostral operative field with minimal cerebellar and brain stem retraction. Similarly, the viewing angle to the anterior surface of the brain stem is relatively flat, providing ready access to the midline. The full vertebral complex is exposed with the use of this strategy, giving ample room for placing temporary clips for proximal control. The rostrocaudal limits of the approach are from the vertebral artery's dural entrance, below, to the point at which the trigeminal nerve enters Meckel's cave, above. The midbasilar artery is also accessible through this strategy. The authors have also used this combination of approaches for processes that involved the jugular foramen.

Essentially, the technique described previously for a limited extreme lateral inferior transcondylar approach is performed, and then a mastoidectomy follows. The extent of mastoid exposure is that of a retrolabyrinthine approach, preserving the labyrinthine structures and stopping short of skeletonization of the fallopian canal. In this approach, the posterior, superior, and inferior surfaces of the jugular bulb are skeletonized, and the jugular tubercle is completely removed.

Basilar Trunk Aneurysms

Aneurysms of the basilar trunk are those arising between the vertebrobasilar junction and the superior cerebellar artery. The majority of these uncommon lesions are located at the takeoff of the anterior inferior cerebellar artery, along the lower and middle thirds of the clivus. These aneurysms in association with the anterior inferior cerebellar artery usually project laterally. True trunk lesions arising at the origin of one of the long lateral pontine arteries or other perforating branches may project posteriorly, into the pons, or anteriorly, pressing against the clivus. They usually have a close relationship to the sixth cranial nerve.

Upper basilar trunk lesions that originate between the origin of the anterior inferior cerebellar artery and the superior cerebellar artery may be approached with one of the aforementioned posterolateral approaches. However, if lesions are located high along the clivus or are large and complex, a trajectory from superolateral to inferomedial may be more beneficial. Peerless and Drake have proposed a subtemporal transtentorial approach.[32] There are a number of drawbacks to this approach, not the least of which is the amount of temporal lobe retraction and the long, narrow corridor through which the lesion is accessed. To obviate some of these drawbacks, the authors have resorted to using two approaches. One is through the petrous apex, which is usually an extradural approach, and one is anterior to the sigmoid through the mastoid.[6, 24, 27, 28] Both allow superior exposure of the upper basilar trunk.

Extended Middle Fossa Approach (Rhomboid Approach)

The patient is placed in the supine position with the head in three-pin fixation and rotated almost 90 degrees away from the side of approach. A small question mark–shaped skin incision is made, and the scalp is reflected anteriorly, held in place by blunt hooks. The fascia overlying the zygoma is incised and elevated circumferentially to reveal the entire length of attachment to the petrous squamosa. The temporalis muscle and fascia are then reflected anteriorly. A 4 cm by 4 cm rectangular bone flap, situated one third behind and two thirds in front of the external auditory canal, is then cut. The bony margin along the middle fossa floor is removed so that the inferior limit of the craniotomy is flush with the floor of the middle fossa.

Dural elevation begins along the petrous ridge, identifying the arcuate eminence as a primary landmark. Elevation is then carried anteromedially to uncover the greater superficial petrosal nerve and tegmen tympani. Any bony irregularities of the middle fossa floor must be drilled flat for better exposure. The middle meningeal artery is coagulated and divided as it joins the dura to allow a greater extent of dural elevation from the middle fossa floor. The medial and posterolateral margins of dural elevation are the third division of the trigeminal nerve and the petrous ridge, respectively. The dura is elevated further from the connective tissue that covers the third division of the fifth cranial nerve, which allows added dural retraction.

The middle fossa landmarks that define the volume of bone to be resected may now be identified. These points are (1) the intersection of the greater superficial petrosal nerve with the trigeminal nerve, (2) the porus trigeminus, (3) the intersection of the arcuate eminence and the petrous ridge, and (4) the intersection of the lines projected along the axes of the greater superficial petrosal nerve and the arcuate eminence. This rhomboid-shaped area, projected through the petrous bone toward the clivus, describes the volume of bone that will be removed to the level just beyond the inferior petrosal sinus.

To begin, the internal auditory canal is unroofed with a high-speed drill. To accomplish this, the angle between lines projected along the axes of the greater superficial petrosal nerve and the arcuate eminence is bisected. Drilling is started along the midpoint of this axis. The dura overlying the internal auditory canal is identified after approximately 3 to 4 mm of bone is removed. With the internal auditory canal dura exposed, the laterally located wedge of bone between it and the superior semicircular canal, termed the "postmeatal triangle," is drilled away to expose posterior fossa dura posterior and superior to the internal auditory canal.[6] By gently unroofing the greater superficial petrosal nerve lateral to the facial hiatus, the geniculate ganglion can be identified as a further landmark defining the lateral extent of the internal auditory canal. The bone anterior to the internal auditory canal is next removed to the level of the inferior petrosal sinus, exposing posterior fossa dura. The cochlea lies within the lateral half of the "premeatal triangle," which is defined by the internal carotid artery genu, the geniculate ganglion, and the medial lip of the internal auditory canal.[6] By skeletonizing the bone of the undersurface of Meckel's cave, toward the foramen lacerum, the entire petrous apex is removed after being sufficiently thinned with the drill. Removal of this bone exposes the lateral margin of Dorello's canal.

After the greater superficial petrosal nerve is sacrificed, the bone overlying Glasscock's triangle is next removed to expose the horizontal intrapetrous carotid artery. The bone medial and inferior to the carotid artery may also be removed without damaging any neural or vascular structures. To maximize exposure, bone under the carotid artery is removed, and the cochlea is "undercut," increasing the amount of posterior fossa dura seen through the exposure.[6] Opening of the dura is preceded by interruption of the superior petrosal sinus medially at the porus trigeminus. An incision is made in the tentorium for increased expo-

sure, and it is retracted with the temporal lobe. The posterior fossa dura in the transpetrosal window is resected at this juncture. The lower to middle basilar artery is seen, as well as the sixth cranial nerve and anterior inferior cerebellar artery (Fig. 56–7).

With the completion of the intradural portion of the procedure, a partial dural closure is made. The periosteal layer that was meticulously preserved at the beginning, with temporalis muscle and fascia, is laid in the defect, along with abdominal fat. This serves to seal off the posterior fossa from the middle fossa and to reduce the chance of a cerebrospinal fluid leak. The bone flap is then secured, and the scalp closed in layers.

Combined Petrosal Approach

The combined petrosal approach provides a true lateral trajectory to the upper basilar trunk, using a corridor through the mastoid and superior petrosal sinus.[1, 21, 35] It may be performed with a number of variations, mostly based on the extent of petrous bone removal. The transmastoid component of the procedure can vary from retrolabyrinthine exposure, preserving hearing, to a transcochlear approach, for maximum access to the midline.[35] For aneurysms of the posterior fossa, it would be unusual to perform more than the retrolabyrinthine drilling in the transmastoid phase of the approach.

The patient is positioned on the operating table in the lateral decubitus position with the head in three-pin fixation. The skin incision is L-shaped around the ear, with a small anterior limb extending downward toward the root of the zygoma, inside the hairline. The height of the incision over the ear should correspond to the squamosal suture, about 45 mm above the external auditory meatus. Posteriorly, the incision extends about 1 cm behind the body of the mastoid, to 1 cm below the mastoid tip. The galeal-cutaneous flap is elevated and reflected inferiorly. The pericranium and temporalis muscle are elevated in a single layer and reflected anteriorly. An L-shaped craniotomy is then made around the mastoid, which exposes the temporal and posterior fossa dura. Burr holes are placed over the temporal squama, on the nuchal line at the level of the asterion, at the posterior body of the mastoid, and 2 cm inferior and posterior to the hole at the posterior body of the mastoid. The latter three burr holes flank the transverse–sigmoid sinus junction. The temporal portion of the craniotomy should be flush with the floor of the middle fossa.

After elevation of the bone flap, the mastoidectomy is performed to completely skeletonize the transverse and sigmoid sinuses to the jugular bulb. Air cells are removed to skeletonize the bony labyrinth, the sinodural angle, and the middle fossa and presigmoid dura. It is not necessary to skeletonize the fallopian canal in this approach for aneurysms.

The dura is opened, beginning over the inferior temporal lobe and continuing to the transverse-sigmoid junction. Here the superior petrosal sinus is ligated as it enters the transverse-sigmoid junction. The incision

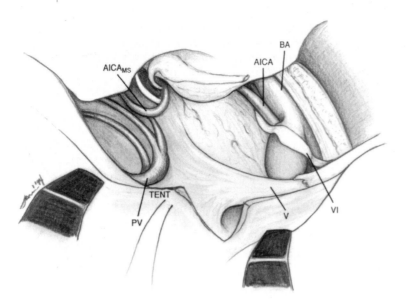

Figure 56–7

Diagram of a left extended extradural middle fossa (rhomboid) approach. The left retractor reflects the tentorium (TENT) and divides the superior petrosal sinus. The right retractor reflects the trigeminal nerve (V), exposing the internal carotid artery in petrous bone. The middle portions of the basilar artery (BA) and anterior inferior cerebellar artery (AICA) are readily exposed.

then continues inferiorly in front of the sigmoid sinus toward the jugular bulb. This dural incision opens both the supratentorial and infratentorial compartments. The tentorium is then incised toward the incisura parallel to the petrous ridge. This allows the sigmoid sinus and underlying cerebellum to be retracted posteriorly and the temporal lobe superiorly, maximizing exposure of the upper basilar trunk, the origin of the anterior inferior cerebellar artery, and cranial nerves V, VII, and VIII. For improved lateral exposure, an incision may also be made in the retrosigmoid dura, effectively skeletonizing the sigmoid sinus. This allows reflection of the sigmoid sinus in both the anterior and the posterior directions and provides enhanced access to the lower cranial nerve structures and upper vertebral artery (Fig. 56–8).

After clip ligation of the aneurysm, the dura is closed in a watertight fashion, with the use of dural grafts as necessary. The mastoid is packed with fat taken from either the lateral thigh or the abdomen. The bone flap is secured, and the scalp is closed in layers.

Basilar Apex Aneurysms

Aneurysms located at the basilar apex include those arising from the basilar bifurcation and from the origin of the superior cerebellar arteries. Important considerations in surgical planning are the size of the aneurysm, the direction or orientation of the dome, the height in relation to the clivus and dorsum sellae, and the presence and location of any associated lesions. The surgical approaches to be considered for these lesions are the subtemporal, pterional-transsylvian, and transcavernous exposures for complex lesions.*

The anatomy surrounding basilar bifurcation aneurysms is some of the most complex with which neurosurgeons must deal. These aneurysms reside among a nest of thalamic and midbrain perforating arteries that originate from the rostral basilar artery, the P_1 portion

of the posterior cerebral artery, and the posterior communicating artery. Straddling the base of the aneurysm are both third nerves, one of which usually must be manipulated to secure the neck of the aneurysm. Working space is limited because of the inability to radically retract the temporal lobe in conjunction with the immobility of surrounding structures, including the tentorial edge. The length and depth of the exposure dramatically complicates even the simplest of surgical maneuvers.

Critical to the decision-making related to selection of the approach and strategies necessary to obliterate the aneurysm are the direction in which the aneurysm

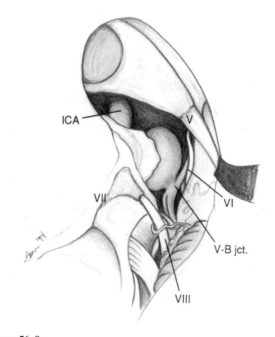

Figure 56–8

Diagram of a left combined petrosal approach. The retractor reflects the sigmoid sinus, which is mobilized by dividing the superior petrosal sinus and the tentorium to the incisura. V-B jct., vertebrobasilar junction.

---

*See references 7, 11, 12, 15, 17, 29, and 43.

points and the height of the aneurysm in relation to the posterior clinoid process. Anteriorly projecting aneurysms are the most favorable. Such a configuration allows easier access to the posterior portion of the dome and neck and, thereby, more facile manipulation of critical perforating vessels. Posterior projecting or globular aneurysms are the most difficult to secure without injuring critical perforators. These aneurysms frequently incorporate the origin of the posterior cerebral artery, thereby causing P_1 perforators also to be intimately related to the base. Inventive clip strategies, including multiple clips and aperture clips to encircle either the posterior cerebral artery or the third nerve, or both, are often necessary.

The height of the aneurysm neck in relation to the dorsum sellae and posterior clinoid can also complicate surgical decision-making. Lesions that lie significantly below the posterior clinoid process may require strategies either to remove the process by drilling or to circumvent it by taking a more lateral or posterior approach. An excessively high-positioned bifurcation potentially provides the most difficult of all situations in that most traditional approaches do not allow adequate superior exposure.

The approaches that follow should provide the surgeon with an array of alternatives to meet most clinical situations. In the final analysis, the surgeon's facility with microsurgical technique and knowledge of regional anatomy are the most critical factors in outcome. For approaches with which the surgeon is not familiar, practice in the Skull Base Anatomy Lab or assistance from an accomplished colleague should lessen operative complications.

Subtemporal Approach

The subtemporal approach is the easiest to master for lesions of the basilar bifurcation. It is highly lateralized and provides access to the anterior and posterior aspects of the lesion without the need for major manipulation of the aneurysm itself. It is useful for solitary basilar bifurcation aneurysms, especially those pointing posteriorly or located below the posterior clinoid process.

The subtemporal approach closely follows the method first popularized by Drake.[9, 10, 11, 12, 32] The patient is placed on the operating table in the lateral decubitus position with the head in three-pin fixation. A linear or small, question mark–shaped incision is made beginning just anterior to the tragus. After reflection of the myocutaneous scalp layer, a temporal craniotomy is made. The bone flap is made anterior to the ear and usually measures about 4 cm by 4 cm. It is important to make the craniotomy flush with the middle fossa floor to help minimize temporal lobe retraction. The dura is then opened, and an inferiorly based dural flap is usually made. A retractor is gently placed over the inferior temporal lobe, and the undersurface of the lobe is inspected for the configuration and location of the basal temporal veins, specifically the vein of Labbé.

Retraction of the temporal lobe during the opening of the cerebrospinal fluid drain exposes the uncus. The retractor is positioned to elevate the uncus, which stretches the arachnoid layer spanning the interval between the mesial temporal lobe and the tentorial edge. Visible through the arachnoid layer, the third cranial nerve crosses the interpeduncular fossa. The arachnoid is sharply divided to increase the retraction of the medial temporal lobe. The fourth cranial nerve is then identified under the edge of the tentorium. Just anterior to the entrance of the nerve into the underside of the tentorial edge, a traction stitch is placed to widen the operative corridor. The suture is passed through the dura of the middle fossa floor and tied tightly.

The arachnoid is widely opened, allowing the third nerve to be retracted upward along with the uncus. Tracing the third nerve back leads to the P_2 portion of the posterior cerebral artery and the superior cerebellar artery passing through the ambient cistern. These vessels can then be followed medially, deep within the cistern, to approach the neck of the aneurysm. The posterior communicating artery can also be used as a landmark and followed posteriorly to its junction with the posterior cerebral artery. After the aneurysm has been sighted, initial dissection should be directed anteriorly. By removing subarachnoid clot, the surgeon should be able to identify the third nerve on the opposite side, which allows ready identification of the P_1 portion of the contralateral posterior cerebral artery. Identification of P_1 perforators on both sides is critical. After this has been accomplished, dissection should be carried to the posterior aspect of the neck. Here, basilar artery perforators are encountered that must be meticulously dissected away from the base. At this point, the size of the neck of the aneurysm and the angle of takeoff of the P_1 portion of the posterior cerebral artery should be analyzed so that appropriate clip selection can be made. Excessive retraction of the P_1 vessel occasionally results in injury to P_1 perforators, so a fenestrated or an aperture-style clip would be best selected. The aperture incorporates the posterior cerebral artery (Fig. 56–9). Unfortunately, the array of clips available may not always provide for the appropriate blade length. In this circumstance, the diamond drill, under the operating microscope, can be used to shorten the blades of an aperture clip so as to avoid injury to structures on the opposite side of the aneurysm. After clip ligation has been accomplished, meticulous inspection should be carried out to ensure that no perforators are included in the clip and that the clip does not injure or distort the third nerve on the opposite side. If there is any doubt as to the adequacy of obliteration, multiple clips should be used in tandem to completely occlude the lesion.

Pterional Transsylvian Approach

The pterional transsylvian approach provides an alternative strategy for lesions of the upper basilar artery complex. Although somewhat more complex because of the need to remove the sphenoid wing, this strategy is commonly used for anterior circulation aneurysms, thus becoming part of most neurosurgeons' surgical

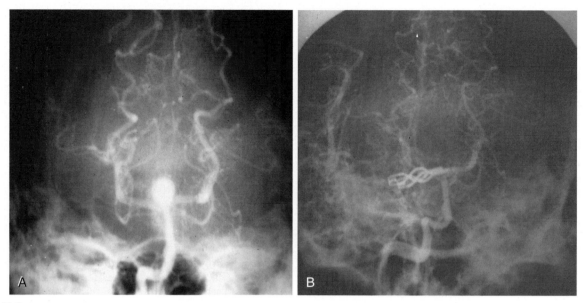

Figure 56–9

Preoperative *(A)* and postoperative *(B)* angiography shows a basilar apex aneurysm approached from the subtemporal trajectory. Tandem fenestrated clips are shown, with the posterior cerebral artery in both apertures.

armamentarium. It is used successfully for the majority of aneurysms of the basilar bifurcation, providing a more anterolateral trajectory than does the traditional subtemporal approach. Manipulation of the aneurysm itself is frequently necessary to identify perforators on the posterior aspect of the aneurysm sac. Manipulation of the third nerve, however, is minimized in comparison with the lateral approach, and lesions excessively above or excessively below the posterior clinoid process may prove difficult to access with this strategy. For basilar bifurcation aneurysms that reside in association with other anterior circulation lesions, the pterional transsylvian approach may provide a strategy for obliteration of multiple pathologies.

In principle, the pterional approach popularized by Yasargil is employed with minor modifications, depending on the aneurysm location and configuration.[43, 44] Compensation for aneurysm location and configuration is effected through differences in the amount of bone removed and the positioning of the head. The pterional bone flap, as described by Yasargil, is used for all routine cases. After the dura has been opened, the sylvian fissure is widely opened. The lumbar drain has remained closed up to this point, and it remains so until the fissure is satisfactorily dissected. The maintenance of cerebrospinal fluid in the fissure provides some buoyancy to the vessels and prevents collapse of the frontal and temporal lobes into the fissure, facilitating microdissection. The surgeon sharply dissects the arachnoid surrounding the optic nerve, taking care to stay close to the nerve while dissecting superiorly, avoiding the perforating arteries entering the anterior perforated substance above. Temporally, the arachnoidal investments of the temporal tip are divided, with care taken to avoid any bridging veins that typically span the temporal pole and the middle fossa dura.

At this point, an assessment is made as to the amount of space existing between the internal carotid artery and the optic nerve medially versus the space between the internal carotid artery and the tentorial incisura laterally. The trajectory to the basilar bifurcation is usually made through the largest space, although intermittent retraction of the carotid artery may provide for working space on either side. The posterior communicating artery is followed through the membrane of Liliequist, which is opened widely. Subarachnoid blood is gently suctioned away, and the many perforators off the posterior communicating artery are dissected free from arachnoidal investments and preserved. The artery is followed to its junction with the posterior cerebral artery, which is then followed medially to the neck of the aneurysm. Rotation of the microscope, deepening of the retractor blade on the uncus of the temporal lobe, and gentle retraction of the internal carotid artery open the necessary space to gain access to the entire neck of the aneurysm. The third nerve may be gently retracted, although, without freeing the nerve from the porus oculomotorius, dramatic movement of the third nerve is limited. Using a combination of blunt and sharp dissection, the surgeon should be able to identify the entire upper basilar artery complex. Both lateral and contralateral origins of posterior cerebral and superior cerebellar arteries should be identifiable, as long as the basilar bifurcation is not significantly below the posterior clinoid process. In that event, the posterior clinoid can be partially removed with careful drilling. This maneuver may open the posterior cavernous sinus. Bleeding is controlled with the use of judicious packing with a hemostatic agent.

For small basilar bifurcation aneurysms, the perforator dissection is relatively straightforward, and by moving the microscope, the surgeon can observe and dissect most of the neck. For larger aneurysms, deflection of the aneurysm sac is necessary to identify posteriorly directed perforators.

The trajectory afforded by the transsylvian approach frequently allows simple clip application without the need for aperture or fenestrated configurations. As always, care must be taken to completely occlude the entire neck without injuring or including P_1 perforators on the contralateral side.

Proximal control of the basilar artery can be accomplished in certain circumstances, especially if the basilar bifurcation is particularly high-riding. In general, however, most approaches for upper basilar aneurysms provide little room for the placement of temporary clips. If necessary, the posterior clinoid can be radically removed to further increase the ability to gain more proximal exposure of the basilar artery.

Occasionally, the need to divide the posterior communicating artery arises. Although it is best avoided, this procedure can allow more maneuverability. It is best to use small clips to preserve working space and avoid touching the clips with the bipolar, which could cause cautery to spread and inadvertently to injure adjacent perforators.

Extradural Anterior Temporopolar Approach

Complex basilar aneurysms and those that are high-riding above the dorsum sellae may not be adequately exposed through the more traditional approaches to this area. The temporopolar approach is based on a transsylvian pterional trajectory and borrows heavily from the principles of Dolenc and colleagues' transcavernous approach and Sano's temporopolar strategy to expand the classic exposure.[8, 34] The principal advantages of the approach are the preservation of anterior temporal venous drainage, decreased brain retraction, and a wider operative field that allows the surgeon to move the microscope through almost a 90-degree arc.[7]

The preparation, positioning, and skin incision are the same as those used for a routine pterional approach. The incision extends over the root of the zygoma. For exposure of aneurysms that extend above the dorsum sellae, a more basal-to-vertex trajectory may be needed. In that situation, removal of the zygoma, alone or in combination with removal of the orbital rim, can add significantly to the exposure. Zygoma removal is begun with a cut made parallel to the long axis of the zygoma at its junction with the temporal bone. The second cut, perpendicular to the first, is made along the orbital zygomatic process near the lateral orbital rim. This manuever increases inferior retraction of the temporalis muscle, enabling the operating microscope to be radically deviated to gain a more lateral-to-medial and inferior-to-superior trajectory.[16] The zygoma is resecured using one of the titanium miniplate systems. If anterior orbital retraction is desired to enhance an inferior-to-superior viewing angle from a more frontal direction, the orbital rim is removed with the bone flap as a single unit.[20, 26]

Dural elevation begins from the anterolateral middle fossa to expose the foramen rotundum and superior orbital fissure and continues medially to expose the floor of the anterior cranial fossa. The limits of dural elevation are the foramen ovale laterally and the anterior superior ethmoidal artery medially. Using a high-speed drill with cutting and diamond burrs, the sphenoid ridge is shaved entirely flat, along with all irregularities of the orbital roof and anterior middle fossa floor. To provide some mobility of the superior orbital fissure contents, meticulous drilling is performed to skeletonize the lateral wall of the superior orbital fissure. The foramen rotundum is also unroofed, exposing the second trigeminal branch. The optic canal is additionally unroofed to achieve modest mobility of the optic nerve.

The anterior clinoid process is removed by drilling the center of the process, as if debulking a mass, leaving a thin shell of bone that is either extracted or chipped away. When removal of the extradural bone is completed, the dura propria of the temporal tip is elevated from the outer cavernous membrane. Beginning at the apex of the superior orbital fissure, the meningo-orbital vessels are divided. The surgeon develops a cleavage plane beginning at the junction of the temporal dura and the periorbital fascia, elevating the dura from the outer cavernous membrane. This plane is sharply developed from the superior orbital fissure along the second trigeminal branch, continuing posteriorly to the foramen ovale. The outer cavernous membrane is composed of thin connective tissue contiguous with the nerve sheaths of the third, fourth, and fifth cranial nerves and surrounds the venous plexus of the cavernous sinus. The limits of dural reflection are the third trigeminal branch posteriorly and the tentorial edge medially. It is necessary to incise the medial tentorial incisura, separating it from the inner cavernous membrane near the third cranial outer. By intermittently positioning a self-retaining retractor blade over the temporal fossa dura during exposure of the cavernous sinus membrane, the temporal lobe is automatically retracted posteriorly.

The dura over the sylvian fissure is incised, extending the incision to the optic nerve sheath dura. An L-shaped incision is made by medially extending the incision along the frontal base for 2 or 3 cm. Perneczky's fibrous ring is opened laterally to free the carotid artery from its dural attachment. The temporal lobe is retracted posterolaterally with dural protection, and the frontal lobe posteromedially in like fashion. In this manner, the temporal tip veins are preserved with the anterior temporal dura.

Opening of the anterior 2 cm of the sylvian fissure adds to the exposure of the superior clival area. The internal carotid and proximal A_1 and M_1 segments are well exposed at this point. Opening of the superior triangle of the cavernous sinus (between the oculomotor and the trochlear nerves) and the porus oculomotorius permits the mobilization of the oculomotor and trochlear nerves. The oculomotor nerve is exposed from its origin at the midbrain to its dural entrance into the superior orbital fissure. The third cranial nerve can be gently retracted laterally after first covering it

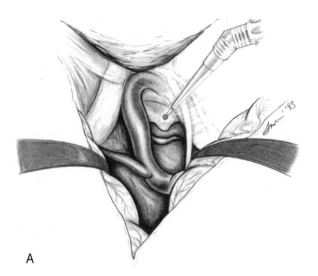

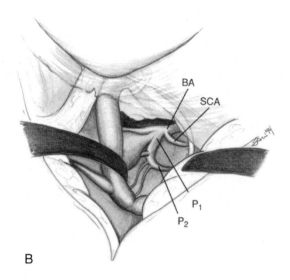

Figure 56–10

A and *B*. Diagram of the exposure gained with the right extradural temporopolar approach prior to removal of the posterior clinoid process. The oculomotor and trochlear nerves are skeletonized and retracted. The carotid siphon is exposed by removing the anterior clinoid process. The temporal lobe is retracted posterior to the porus oculomotorius, and the medial edge of the tentorium is reflected. Removal of the posterior clinoid process allows exposure of the basilar artery (BA) to its midportion as well as the superior cerebellar (SCA) and posterior cerebral artery (P_1 and P_2) branches.

with a soft Cottonoid. The internal carotid artery may be mobilized medially or laterally, because it has been freed from its dural attachment anteriorly. This gentle retraction widens the corridor to the sella, posterior clinoid, and membrane of Liliequist. To visualize the basilar artery, the arachnoid membrane is sharply opened, lateral to the internal carotid artery. To complete the exposure, the posterior clinoid is removed with a high-speed drill, increasing exposure of the basilar artery below the sella and allowing for proximal temporary occlusion (Fig. 56–10). Cavernous sinus bleeding is controlled with Surgicel packing and bipolar cautery. With the temporal lobe retracted and the zygoma removed, the microscope can be swung through a widened arc, allowing large or superiorly positioned lesions to be better visualized.

At the conclusion of the procedure, the surgeon closes the dura in a watertight fashion, using a fascial patch graft if necessary. The pericranium is preserved during opening for this purpose (Fig. 56–11).

Basilar-Superior Cerebellar Artery Aneurysms

Strategies for treatment of aneurysms of the superior cerebellar artery vary little from those used to deal with basilar bifurcation lesions. Because most superior cerebellar lesions are relatively small and strongly lateralized, they are for the most part technically less difficult than basilar bifurcation aneurysms: the reach is usually shorter and the number of adherent perforating vessels is almost always less than for basilar apex lesions.

From the standpoint of approach, either the subtemporal or the transsylvian technique can be used, according to surgeon preference and the location of the

aneurysm with respect to the dorsum sellae. With the transsylvian approach, the surgeon may elect a contralateral approach because the trajectory allows both sides of the basilar artery to be visualized. Such a contralateral tactic may be desirable if a coexisting anterior circulation aneurysm is present. Short, straight fenestrated clips may be appropriate in some circumstances, allowing the posterior cerebral artery to exit through the aperture of the clip. Frequently, the entire lesion can be collapsed with one or two clips placed on the dome parallel to the path of the superior cerebellar artery and the posterior cerebral artery (Fig. 56–12). For low-lying aneurysms, either selection of the subtemporal approach on the ipsilateral side or removal of the posterior clinoid using a high-speed drill may be employed.

The third cranial nerve always has an intimate relation to these aneurysms. The nerve is located either above or below the lesion, rarely being stretched over the dome laterally. Also in close apposition is the ipsilateral P_1 segment. The perforators of the P_1 segment (thalamoperforators) are often involved over the backside of these lesions and must be freed either by elevating the P_1 and dissecting them free or by looking over the top of the basilar caput and P_1 segment to expose and free them superiorly. The rostral group of basilar artery perforators are less often involved because of their predominantly midline and superior projection.

Posterior Cerebral Artery Aneurysms

These uncommon lesions usually arise from the P_1 and P_2 segments of the artery, usually in conjunction with thalamoperforating or short circumflex arteries. The traditional strategies for basilar apex aneurysms suffice for these lesions.

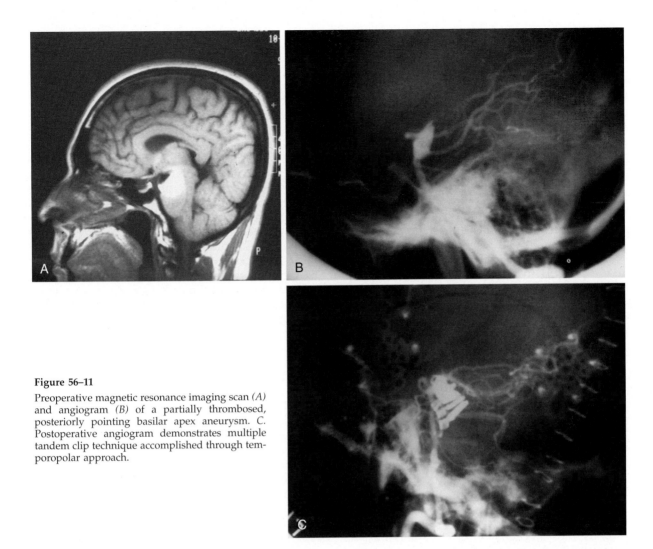

Figure 56–11

Preoperative magnetic resonance imaging scan (A) and angiogram (B) of a partially thrombosed, posteriorly pointing basilar apex aneurysm. C. Postoperative angiogram demonstrates multiple tandem clip technique accomplished through temporopolar approach.

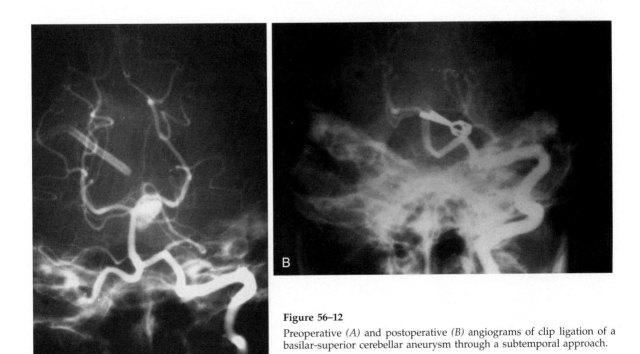

Figure 56–12

Preoperative (A) and postoperative (B) angiograms of clip ligation of a basilar-superior cerebellar aneurysm through a subtemporal approach.

Aneurysms located on the anterior and posterior P_2 segments (roughly half of all posterior cerebral artery aneurysms) may be best approached subtemporally. These lesions are located in the crural and ambient cisterns, regions that are well exposed through this route. Because the artery courses at the level of the choroidal fissure, it is typically covered by the mesial temporal lobe, which requires a degree of temporal lobe retraction. A disadvantage to this approach in exposure of larger lesions is the probability of increasing the retraction of the temporal lobe to the point of a high risk of occlusion of the basal temporal veins. Any protracted period of sluggish flow through these major veins may result in postoperative temporal lobe edema and possibly infarction. Aggressive maneuvers to relax the brain help reduce the risk. In some cases, it may be necessary to perform a limited subpial resection of the parahippocampal gyrus; however, this maneuver is reserved for extreme circumstances (Fig. 56–13).

The P_3 segment begins at the pulvinar in the lateral quadrigeminal cistern and harbors only a small percentage of posterior cerebral artery aneurysms. Proximal aneurysms along this segment can be treated with a subtemporal approach; however, as the need for more distal access increases, exposure may not be satisfactory. Distal P_3 aneurysms most commonly require exposure through an occipital interhemispherical approach. Through this approach, the occipital lobe is retracted superiorly and laterally to reveal the junction between the falx cerebri and the tentorium. This junction is followed anteriorly to expose the calcarine fissure on the mesial occipital lobe. The anterior aspect of this fissure typically harbors the calcarine artery branch of P_3, located in the posterior quadrigeminal cistern. The aneurysm is thus exposed in this region.

A rich collateral supply to this artery has been documented through both anatomical studies and clinical experience with trapping segments of the artery to treat complex aneurysms.[33] Peerless and Drake observed occipital lobe infarctions after occlusion of ei-

ther the P_1 or the proximal P_2 segments in only 2 of 27 patients, most likely because of the rich collateral supply of the distal posterior cerebral artery through the anterior choroidal, middle and anterior cerebral, and contralateral posterior cerebral arteries.[32] The anterior choroidal artery anastomoses with the medial and lateral posterior choroidal arteries. The choroidal branches of the contralateral posterior cerebral artery also communicate across the midline to help reconstitute the vessels. The middle cerebral artery and anterior cerebral artery contribute to the cortical branches, and the splenial arteries receive collateral supply from the pericallosal branches of the anterior cerebral artery. The collateral network dominates distal to the anterior P_2 segment; therefore, trapping for fusiform or other complex lesions of the posterior cerebral artery should be reserved for those arising on the P_1 or anterior P_2 segments.

Complications

INTRAOPERATIVE ISCHEMIA

The major source of complications in the direct surgical treatment of aneurysms of the posterior circulation is ischemia. Because of the critical nature of the neural structures supplied by the perforating branches of the basilar and vertebral artery complexes, perforator occlusion is typically dramatically symptomatic. For this reason, the anatomy of these vessels and the techniques necessary for their meticulous preservation must be mastered. Maneuvers that ensure the identification and liberation of all perforating branches from the aneurysm sac before clip placement are of paramount importance. Inspection after clip positioning is also crucial to be sure that any proximate vessels are continuing to fill. Major arterial branch occlusions, although much less common, have dramatic consequences as well. These problems are most often secondary to poor

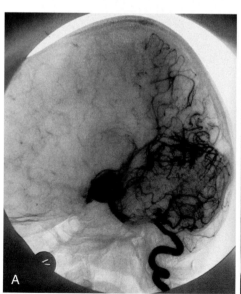
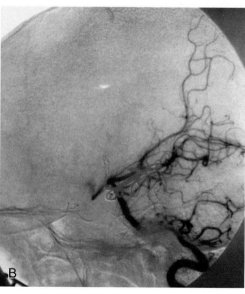

Figure 56–13

Preoperative (A) and postoperative (B) angiograms demonstrate a poorly filling P_2 aneurysm and obliteration through a subtemporal approach.

clip placement. Intraoperative angiography should be routinely incorporated to ensure proper clip placement. There is no substitute for perfect clip placement.

Ischemic complications from intraoperative events can be ameliorated in part with the use of pharmacological brain protection, the maintenance of euvolemia and normal blood pressure, and the use of strategies to decrease retractor pressure. For all complex posterior circulation lesions, burst suppression is induced with the use of the appropriate pharmacological agents at the beginning of the dissection of the lesion. In many circumstances, temporary occlusion of important vessels does not occur, but ischemia is better tolerated if the protective agent is infused before it is needed.

INTRAOPERATIVE RUPTURE

Perhaps the most devastating complication of posterior circulation aneurysms is intraoperative rupture. The morbidity and mortality rates of such events, especially with basilar bifurcation aneurysms, are exceedingly high. It is critical for the operating surgeon to have a practiced set of steps, not only to avoid this complication but also to treat it as quickly and efficiently as possible.

Batjer and Samson have reviewed the surgical techniques designed to reduce the incidence of intraoperative aneurysm rupture. Heavy reliance on sharp dissection is of paramount importance. Complete dissection of the lesion before any attempt at clip ligation reduces the incidence of premature rupture. Should intraoperative rupture occur, tamponade is usually the quickest and most effective method for initial management. Should tamponade fail to significantly reduce the hemorrhage, temporary arterial occlusion should be considered. Only in the most dire circumstances should hypotension be induced, and for only the brief period that it takes to gain control of the situation. The experience of the authors has suggested that induced hypotension is rarely necessary to gain control, and, when utilized, it may be associated with poorer outcome.[19]

CRANIAL NERVE INJURY

Cranial nerve deficits are a well-recognized concomitant of the treatment of posterior circulation aneurysms. Most common in the treatment of basilar bifurcation aneurysms is a temporary third cranial nerve palsy that results in ptosis and ophthalmoplegia. The likely cause is operative manipulation. Deficits are usually short-lived, with most patients recovering within 3 months. Other causes include injury from poor clip placement or occlusion of midbrain tectum perforators. The fourth nerve is vulnerable in the subtemporal approach, especially during retraction of the incisural edge and placement of a tacking suture. The nerve is typically no more than 2 to 3 mm from the edge of the tentorium until it turns anteriorly to lie in the roof of the cavernous sinus; therefore, the stitch must stay very close to the dural edge to avoid the nerve. Sixth nerve involvement is most often encountered in midbasilar trunk lesions and some vertebrobasilar junction aneurysms. Anatomically, the sixth nerve is located close to the vertebrobasilar junction and can be injured at the time of aneurysm rupture. Patients with sixth nerve pareses have recovered even after 6 months.

Compromise of function of the seventh or the eighth cranial nerve is usually related to approaches for vertebrobasilar junction, anterior inferior cerebellar artery, or upper trunk lesions. The most common cause of hearing loss is retraction injury to the cochlear nerve. However, hearing loss can result from injury to the labyrinth or cochlea during the bony exposure. Peculiar to the middle fossa rhomboid approach and the extradural temporopolar approach has been the occurrence of postoperative trigeminal distribution dysesthetic pain. This has always been self-limiting and is no doubt secondary to extradural trigeminal manipulation.

Approaches to vertebral artery aneurysms expose the lower cranial nerves, placing them at risk. Sharp dissection and gentle retraction are critical in avoiding injury. Approaches that allow trajectories parallel to the course of the lower cranial nerves as opposed to tangential approaches, such as the retrolabyrinthine-transsigmoid approach, may also reduce injury. The tenth cranial nerve supplies the motor innervation to the pharyngeal muscles and the arytenoids through the superior laryngeal nerve. The recurrent laryngeal branch of the vagus innervates the muscles and mucosa below the vocal folds. Swallowing dysfunction and airway protection may necessitate gastrostomy tube placement to ensure adequate nutrition until function recovers.

VENOUS INJURIES

Ischemic or hemorrhagic complications are reduced by employing strategies that reduce the need for excessive or prolonged retraction of nervous tissue. The obstruction of venous drainage is another consequence of excessive retraction or the use of methods that interrupt major venous drainage outlets. Procedures that use retraction on the inferior temporal lobe place the temporal basal veins, most importantly the anastomotic vein of Labbé, at risk. Employing strategies of extradural bone removal, such as making the subtemporal craniotomy flush with the middle fossa floor or using a posterior transpetrosal approach, reduces the stress placed on this critical venous structure. Interruption of the temporal tip bridging veins to the sphenoparietal sinus may be tolerated by some individuals; however, in the absence of an accurate method of predicting this resilience preoperatively, the authors do not recommend this as a routine practice.

Conclusion

Expertise implies continual improvement. Improvement requires recognition of true advances, mastery of

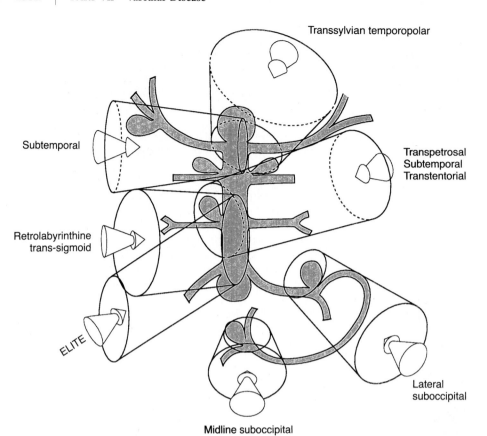

Transsylvian temporopolar

Subtemporal

Transpetrosal
Subtemporal
Transtentorial

Retrolabyrinthine
trans-sigmoid

ELITE

Lateral
suboccipital

Midline suboccipital

Figure 56–14

Paradigm for decision-making regarding approaches and trajectories for posterior circulation aneurysms. Note the overlap between the various approaches. ELITE, extreme lateral inferior transcondylar exposure.

the salient features of those advances, and addition of one's own innovations. The advances of Drake, Sundt, Sano, Chou, Yasargil, Sugita, Peerless, and others form the framework within which current innovations are evaluated and adopted.* Currently, the influence of cranial base techniques on the management of posterior circulation aneurysms is being evaluated as to whether or not true advances will be realized. The foregoing discussion and Figure 56–14 present a framework for clinical decision-making incorporating the basic approaches to the vertebrobasilar circulation and contemporary posterior cranial base strategies. The challenge remains to analyze, practice, select, and develop true expertise.

REFERENCES

1. Al-Mefty, O., Ayoubi, S., and Smith, R. R.: The petrosal approach: Indications, technique, and results. Acta Neurochir. Suppl. (Wien), *53:*166–170, 1991.
2. Andoh, T., Shirakami, S., Nakashima T, et al.: Clinical analysis of a series of vertebral aneurysm cases. Neurosurgery, *31:*987–993, 1992.
3. Aymard, A., Gobin, Y. P., Hodes, J. E., et al.: Endovascular occlusion of vertebral arteries in the treatment of unclippable vertebrobasilar aneurysms. J. Neurosurg., *74:*393–398, 1991.
4. Berger, M. S., and Wilson, C. B.: Intracranial dissecting aneurysms of the posterior circulation. J. Neurosurg., *61:*882–894, 1984.
5. Chou, S. H., and Ortiz-Suarez, H. J.: Surgical treatment of arterial aneurysms of the vertebrobasilar circulation. J. Neurosurg., *41:*671–680, 1974.
6. Day, J. D., Fukushima, T., and Giannotta, S. L.: Microanatomical study of the extradural middle fossa approach to the petroclival and posterior cavernous sinus region: Description of the rhomboid construct. Neurosurgery, *34:*1009–1016, 1994.
7. Day, J. D., Giannotta, S. L., and Fukushima, T.: Extradural temporopolar approach to lesions of the upper basilar artery and infrachiasmatic region. J. Neurosurg, *81:*230–235, 1994.
8. Dolenc, V., Skrap, M., Sustersic, J., et al.: A transcavernoustranssellar approach to the basilar tip aneurysms. Br. J. Neurosurg., *1:*251–259, 1987.
9. Drake, C.: Bleeding aneurysms of the basilar artery: Direct surgical management in four cases. J. Neurosurg., *18:*230–238, 1961.
10. Drake, C. G.: Surgical treatment of ruptured aneurysms of the basilar artery. J. Neurosurg., *23:*457–473, 1965.
11. Drake, C. G.: The surgical treatment of aneurysms of the basilar artery. J. Neurosurg., *29:*436–446, 1968.
12. Drake, C. G.: The treatment of aneurysms of the posterior circulation. Clin. Neurosurg., *26:*12–95, 1979.
13. Duvoisin R. C., and Yahr, M. D.: Posterior fossa aneurysms. Neurology, *15:*231–241, 1965.
14. Friedman, A. H., and Drake, C. G.: Subarachnoid hemorrhage from intracranial dissecting aneurysm. J. Neurosurg., *60:*325–334, 1984.
15. Fujimoto, Y., Ikeda, H., and Yamamoto, S.: Pterional transcavernous approach for large basilar tip aneurysm: Significance of the exposure of Dolenc's triangle. Surg. Cereb. Stroke (Jpn.), *20:*191–195, 1992.
16. Fujitsu, K., and Kuwabara, T.: Zygomatic approach for lesions in the interpeduncular cistern. J. Neurosurg., *62:*340–343, 1987.
17. Fukushima, T., Day, J. D., and Tung, H.: Intracavernous carotid artery aneurysms. *In* Apuzzo, M. L. J., ed.: Brain Surgery: Complication Avoidance and Management. New York, Churchill Livingstone, 1992, pp. 925–944.
18. Giannotta, S. L., and Maceri, D.: Retrolabyrinthine transsigmoid approach to basilar trunk and vertebrobasilar artery junction aneurysms. J. Neurosurg., *69:*461–466, 1988.

*See references 5, 12, 32, 36, 39, 40, and 43.

19. Giannotta, S. L., Oppenheimer, J. H., Levy, M. L., et al.: Management of intraoperative rupture of aneurysm without hypotension. Neurosurgery, 28:531–536, 1991.
20. Hakuba, A., Tanaka, K., Suzuki, T., et al.: A combined orbitozygomatic infratemporal epidural and subdural approach for lesions involving the entire cavernous sinus. J. Neurosurg., 71:699–704, 1991.
21. Hashi, K., Nin, K., and Shimotake, K.: Transpetrosal combined supratentorial and infratentorial approach for midline vertebrobasilar aneurysms. In Brock, M., ed.: Modern Neurosurgery I. Berlin-Heidelberg, Springer-Verlag, 1982, pp. 442–448.
22. Heros, R. C.: Lateral suboccipital approach for vertebral and vertebrobasilar artery lesions. J. Neurosurg., 64:559–562, 1986.
23. Higeshida, R. T., Halback, V. V., Cahan, L. D., et al.: Detachable balloon embolization therapy of posterior circulation intracranial aneurysms. J. Neurosurg., 71:512–519, 1989.
24. House, W. F., Hitselberger, W. E., and Horn, K. L.: The middle fossa transpetrous approach to the anterior-superior cerebellopontine angle. Am. J. Otol., 7:1–4, 1986.
25. Hudgins, R. J., Day, A. L., Quisling, R. G., et al.: Aneurysms of the posterior inferior cerebellar artery: A clinical and anatomical analysis. J. Neurosurg., 58:381–387, 1983.
26. Ikeda, K., Yamashita, J., Hashimoto, M., et al.: Orbitozygomatic temporopolar approach for a high basilar tip aneurysm associated with a short intracranial internal carotid aretery: A new surgical approach. Neurosurgery, 28:105–110, 1991.
27. Kawase, T., Shiobara, R., and Toya, S.: Anterior transpetrosal-transtentorial approach for sphenopetroclival meningiomas: Surgical method and results in 10 patients. Neurosurgery, 28:869–876, 1991.
28. Kawase, T., Toya, S., Shiobara, R., et al.: Transpetrosal approach for aneurysms of the lower basilar artery. J. Neurosurg., 63:857–861, 1985.
29. Kobayashi, S., Sugita, K., Tanaka, Y., et al.: Infratentorial approach to the pineal region in the prone position: Concorde position: Technical note. J. Neurosurg., 58:141–143, 1983.
30. Marinkovic, S., and Gibo, H.: The surgical anatomy of the perforating branches of the basilar artery. Neurosurgery, 33:80–87, 1993.
31. Mizutani, T., and Aruga, T.: "Dolichoectatic" intracranial vertebrobasilar dissecting aneurysms. Neurosurgery, 31:765–773, 1992.
32. Peerless, S. J., and Drake, C. G.: Posterior circulation aneurysms. In Wilkins, R. H., and Rengachary, S. S., eds.: Neurosurgery. New York, McGraw-Hill, 1985, pp. 1422–1436.
33. Sakata, S., Fujii, K., Matsushima, T., et al.: Aneurysm of the posterior cerebral artery: Report of eleven cases. Surgical approaches and procedures. Neurosurgery, 32:163–168, 1993.
34. Sano, K.: Temporo-polar approach to aneurysms of the basilar artery at and around the distal bifurcation: Technical note. Neurol. Res., 2:361–367, 1980.
35. Spetzler, R. F., Daspit, C. P., and Pappas, C. T. E.: The combined supra- and infratentorial approach for lesions of the petrous and clival regions: Experience with 46 cases. J. Neurosurg., 76:588–599, 1992.
36. Sugita, K., Kobayashi, S., Shintani, A., et al.: Microneurosurgery for aneurysms of the basilar artery. J. Neurosurg., 51:615–620, 1979.
37. Tanaka, K., Waga, S., Kojima, T., et al.: Non-traumatic dissecting aneurysms of the intracranial vertebral artery: Report of six cases. Acta Neurochir. (Wein), 100:62–66, 1989.
38. Tiyaworabun, S., Wanis, A., Schirmer, M., et al.: Aneurysms of the vertebro-basilar system: Clinical analysis and follow-up result. Acta Neurochir. (Wein), 63:221–229, 1982.
39. Wilson, C. B., and U, H. S.: Surgical treatment for aneurysms of the upper basilar artery. J. Neurosurg., 44:537–543, 1976.
40. Wright, D. C., and Wilson, C. B.: Surgical treatment of basilar aneurysms. Neurosurgery, 5:325–333, 1979.
41. Yamaura, A.: Diagnosis and treatment of vertebral aneurysms. J. Neurosurg., 69:345–349, 1988.
42. Yamaura, A., Watanabe, Y., and Saeki, N.: Dissecting aneurysms of the intracranial vertebral artery. J. Neurosurg., 72:183–188, 1990.
43. Yasargil, G., Antic, J., Laciga, R., et al.: Microsurgical pterional approach to aneurysms of the basal bifurcation. Surg. Neurol., 6:83–91, 1976.
44. Yasargil, M. G., and Fox, J. L.: The microsurgical approach to intracranial aneurysms. Surg. Neurol., 3:7–14, 1975.
45. Zeal A., and Rhoton, A.: Microsurgical anatomy of the posterior cerebral artery. J. Neurosurg., 48:534–559, 1978.

Endovascular Management of Intracranial Aneurysms

During the past decade, endovascular techniques for the treatment of intracranial aneurysms have been extensively developed. The original indication, giant unclippable intracranial aneurysms, has been extended to include small aneurysms and those that have recently ruptured. The introduction of coils and hardening materials in addition to balloons has allowed extension of the technique to virtually any aneurysm of the intracranial circulation.

The initial efforts in endovascular surgery involved a variety of novel techniques, such as the injection of hair into an aneurysm, the use of magnetically focused thrombogenic particles, and electric current delivered through stereotactically placed electrodes. Early attempts centered on arterial occlusion for otherwise untreatable aneurysms, such as giant or fusiform aneurysms, and for aneurysms located within the cavernous sinus.[1, 2, 10] Later, the application spread to smaller aneurysms, with the goal of parent artery patency.

In 1978, DeBrun and co-authors presented their experience with balloon catheter systems, including their use in the treatment of aneurysms.[7] This clinical series and careful approach helped establish the indications for endovascular treatment of aneurysms. DeBrun described two types of balloon catheters: one was similar to that described by Serbinenko and required the use of a hardening agent.[28] The other type, a self-sealing balloon catheter, did not require hardening agents but mandated the use of a coaxial detachment system. Serbinenko treated 14 aneurysms, 10 of which were in the cavernous sinus. DeBrun concluded that the indications for use of detachable balloons for intradural aneurysms were limited.[7]

Also in 1978, Laitinen and Servo described a model for a self-sealing, noncoaxial detachable balloon, which would eliminate the need for hardening agents.[19] Taki and colleagues also described a model for a balloon catheter system, later adding a solidifying agent to prevent deflation.[32]

Large series began appearing from various centers in the 1980's.[9, 11, 15, 17] In 1984, Berenstein and associates published their experience with balloon trapping of giant aneurysms.[5] Higashida and co-workers reported the results of the endovascular treatment of cavernous carotid artery aneurysms in 87 patients. Later, a series of 26 aneurysms involving the posterior circulation was described.[16] The results were acceptable, considering that these were largely unclippable aneurysms.

Many factors influence results after acute aneurysmal subarachnoid hemorrhage. The configuration, size, and location of the aneurysm and its relation to intracranial structures are important. The clinicoanatomical form of the hemorrhage and the presence of vasospasm, hydrocephalus, intracranial hypertension, and rebleeding affect outcome. The age of the patient, the associated systemic pathology, hypertension, heart disease, and other conditions associated with the ictal event (e.g., heart failure) all are significant. Neurological condition is a significant variable but yet an integral of all other factors.[31] Decisions made by the surgeon also affect survival. The timing of the operation, the choice of operative approach, complications related to and accompanying any surgical treatment, and the tactics of the surgeon all can be modified to improve outcome.

Toward the end of the decade, the focus of endovascular therapy began to broaden. The potential for endovascular techniques to become the primary and definitive treatment for cerebral aneurysms was explored.[6, 9, 16, 17] In 1991, Moret and associates reported a series from Paris, wherein he treated 124 patients with detachable balloon therapy. Twenty-two of these patients had suffered an acute subarachnoid hemorrhage; many of those were "berry" aneurysms classically referred for direct surgical therapy.[24] Shcheglov detailed 867 patients treated only by detachable balloon techniques, reporting a greater than 90 per cent rate of parent artery patency.[30]

Y. N. Zubkov • L. Alexander • R. R. Smith

Gianturco and co-workers were among the first to report the use of intravascular coils to abet vessel thrombosis of the renal artery.[10] Hilal and colleagues extended this idea with the use of platinum microcoils to thrombose intracranial lesions.[17] A variety of coils, with various thrombogenic attachments, have been introduced.[6, 8, 11] However, these techniques suffered from a lack of control of the coil after it was expelled from the catheter and also from the physical characteristics of the coil itself.

The use of electrolytic coils has been pioneered by Guglielmi. These supple platinum coils can be delivered through superselective catheter systems and thus can be placed with a high degree of accuracy. The coils remained attached to the guide wire and can be repositioned or removed if necessary. After optimal positioning has been achieved, a small direct current passed through the catheter and coil effects detachment and abets thrombosis.[12–14]

Braun and co-workers used intravascular metal coils to treat two patients with internal carotid artery aneurysms.[6] The aneurysm was located in the cavernous sinus in one patient and in the extracranial carotid artery in the other. In each case, the internal carotid artery was occluded successfully without production of any deficits.[6] Hilal and co-authors used synthetic fiber–coated platinum coils to treat patients with aneurysms in the distal lenticulostriate arteries.[17]

Graves and associates studied the makeup of coils and their effects.[11] Simple coils consisted of a single coil; complex coils were fabricated with and without silk fibers. They introduced these coils into artificial aneurysms formed by suturing venous pouches onto the carotid arteries of dogs. Complex coils with silk fibers formed into complex configurations, such as a flower-petal design, produced the most stable patterns, which lessened the chance of migration from the pouch. Dowd and colleagues described three cases of posterior inferior cerebellar artery aneurysms treated with coils to preserve the parent arteries.[8] They used .018-in. platinum coils interwoven with Dacron fibers.* Since 1990, the number of reports describing the use of coils and the number of patients treated with this method have increased tremendously. There is clear inference in recent reports that coils produce better results than microballoons; fewer complications and wider applications of the technique are now reported. Guglielmi described the results of treating 37 patients with intracranial aneurysms by this method.[12, 13] Intra-aneurysmal thrombus developed in 70 to 100 per cent, but complete thrombosis of the aneurysm occurred in only 7 patients. In 16 patients, the aneurysm was 90 to 95 per cent occluded. One patient developed temporary neurological deficits, and another permanent ones. Four patients died: three in Hunt-Hess grade 5, and one in grade 4.

Berenstein and co-workers described the treatment of 31 patients using the Guglielmi detachable coil system.[5] Complete obliteration of the aneurysm was achieved in only 53 per cent. In 12 patients, 95 per

cent occlusion was accomplished. In one patient, the aneurysm was 90 per cent obliterated, and in two, 80 per cent occlusion occurred. The total morbidity was 9.7 per cent, and there were no deaths. These authors concluded that this technique showed promise for aneurysm treatment. Lylyk and co-workers described the use of this technique in 66 patients.[21] There were 41 complete occlusions (66 per cent), 19 subtotal occlusions (28 per cent), and 6 partial (9 per cent). The mortality rate was 9 per cent. Tortuous vessels and vasospasm were described as remaining challenges to the technique.

The early results with this technique seem promising, as several users have indicated. However, major shortcomings include less than satisfactory occlusion of the aneurysm, the primary aim of therapy. The method often leaves significant rests from which growth and rupture may later occur. Electrothrombosis is not a simple process, and regulation of the amount of clot that forms is difficult. Clot lysis is also greatly determined by the patient's fibrinolytic system. The procedure is currently under trial and may not be widely applicable because of its inherent complexity. The final chapter in this encouraging development must be written later.

Each aneurysm requires a special technique, but commonalities apply. Equipment in the operating room, monitoring of the procedure, preoperative and postoperative care, and preparation of catheters are essential to all procedures.[20, 22]

Endovascular Ergonomics

High-resolution imaging equipment is the number one priority for endovascular neurosurgery. Digital methods, subtraction angiography, and road mapping are required for best results. The radiation source must be mobile in relation to the head. Good lateral, anterioposterior, oblique, and submentovertex views are important. The power of the system is perhaps of less importance than the software used to display the image. The energy source must be checked periodically to ensure a consistent and safe dose. Annually, the endovascular team should review the hazards of radiation and methods for protecting themselves and the patient. The procedure may be carried out in the radiology suite or in the operating room, depending on the patient's condition and needs. In the operating room, either fixed-beam or mobile sources may be used. These instruments emit 10 to 20 rad per minute in the boost mode and perhaps more in some instances. Careful attention must be paid to safe usage. Doses exceeding 1,500 rad may cause superficial skin reactions.

Equipment for monitoring is also required. Transcranial Doppler ultrasound and intra-arterial lines for continuous arterial pressure monitoring should be available, and intracranial pressure lines and monitors should be used if needed.

*Hilal microcoils, manufactured by Cook Inc., Chicago.

BALLOON CATHETERS

Serbinenko's latex balloon catheter was first developed in 1971.[28] Two types of balloons were used, detachable and nondetachable. Polyethylene was used for the catheter and latex for the balloon itself. For nondetachable balloons, the balloon was annelled to the catheter with a fine monofilament suture. The first detachable balloon prepared by Serbinenko was affixed to a catheter that was slightly flared at the tip. The orifice of the balloon contained a thickened area of latex that functioned as a valve. After placement, the balloon was inflated with hardening material. After hardening, it was possible to detach the balloon from the flared catheter while inflation of the balloon was maintained. However, this balloon did not lend itself well to liquid materials because the liquid escaped from the orifice, and deflation occurred. Later, Serbinenko and Filatov developed a valve system designed to prevent deflation.[29]

INFLATING MATERIALS

Both liquid and polymerizing materials may be used to inflate the balloon. Contrast materials used for angiography, such as Venografin, Omnipaque, or Conray, are acceptable. Nonionic contrast materials are less toxic and are therefore preferred. Sometimes, inflation with isotonic saline is preferred. If, for instance, the balloon has been placed in a position that will produce stenosis of the parent vessel, this would not be seen on angiography if the balloon were inflated with contrast material. Therefore, the lumen of the parent vessel may be more adequately evaluated if the balloon is inflated with saline. The ideal properties of a polymerizing material are as follows[36]:

1. Polymerization must be accurately controlled and measured.
2. The polymerizing material must be inert in relation to the balloon material so that erosion and rupture do not occur.
3. The material must be of low viscosity so that it can be injected through fine catheters within a reasonable period of time.
4. The material must be biocompatible and approved for medical use.
5. The volume of the material must not expand or contract during polymerization from the liquid phase. The liquid and solid states must not vary in volume more than 1 to 2 per cent. If the aneurysm shrinks, it may fill angiographically; if the aneurysm expands, it may rupture.
6. The material should be visible radiologically.

Popular polymerizing agents include silicone, 5-hydroxyethyl methacrylate, and isobutyl 2-cyanoacrylate. Each of these materials must be combined with its own catalyst in order to polymerize. The polymerization time is determined by the amount of catalyst in proportion to polymer. Currently, no radiologically opaque polymer is available.

The aneurysm is first filled with liquid contrast material, and it is determined angiographically that the aneurysm is completely occluded. The contrast material is then withdrawn, and the amount that was used to produce the desired effect is carefully measured. Only this amount of polymerizing agent is then injected back into the balloon. During the polymerization process, angiography is used to make certain that the balloon occludes the aneurysm. If insufficient polymer is present, more may be added with its catalyst to achieve the desired effect.

COILS

During recent years, many endovascular surgeons have turned to platinum microcoils to induce thrombosis in intracranial aneurysms. Various materials (e.g., wool, silk, cotton, Dacron) have also been incorporated into the microcoils to form a fibrous network or mesh to entrap the blood particles and enhance clot formation. Gianturco and co-workers were the first to use coils to occlude the vasculature to a hypernephroma.[10] The diameter of these coils was large, and the delivery system was not suitable for neurosurgical use. Originally, the coils consisted of fragments of the guide wire used for angiography catheters. At first, 5-cm lengths of 0.89-mm wire were used in the renal system. In 1979, Anderson and co-workers introduced "mini" Gianturco stainless steel coils for transcatheter vascular occlusion. The mini coils are made from segments of guide wires 5 cm long by 0.46 mm in diameter.[10] Dacron threads were included in these original stainless steel coils, which were introduced through a 5-French catheter, but these were still not appropriate for neurosurgical use.

Yang and co-authors reported on the use of platinum wire in patients with arteriovenous fistulas.[33, 34] They used distal tips with .014- and .013-in. steerable guide wires. The length of the coils produced was 0.5 to 1.5 cm. Hilal and co-workers used coils of platinum coated with synthetic fibers.*[5] Guglielmi and colleagues developed a new type of coil, the so-called detachable coil, that could be used for electrothrombosis before separation.[12, 13]

Endovascular Treatment Techniques

The two widely practiced methods for producing occlusion of aneurysms by endovascular techniques are balloon catheters and thrombogenic coils. In Russia, many neurosurgeons employ detachable balloons, which are introduced through direct puncture of either the carotid or the vertebral artery and applied to a large number of aneurysms. In the United States and some European countries, femoral approaches are used to deliver some detachable balloons, but chiefly coils, to a much more narrow number of lesions. A thorough

---

*Hilal microcoils, Cook Inc., Chicago.

discussion of the subject must include both methodologies.

In making the balloon, the size of the form needed depends on the size of the aneurysm to be occluded. The larger the diameter of the aneurysm, the larger the form required. Forms measuring 0.4 to 1.0 mm create balloons in the range of 0.5 to 1.0 cm after they are fully inflated. The length of the balloon is determined by the length of exposed latex on the end of the catheter. The balloon and catheter may be sterilized by several methods. Air must be removed, and the balloon must be trained to inflate properly to accommodate the space it will occupy when inflated.

The balloon is connected to the catheter by the use of magnification and manipulation. The balloon should be inserted over the catheter until it comes in contact with the apex. A radiological marker is usually placed in its apex. The balloon is then fixed to the catheter, using 8-0 nylon or Prolene suture material. The ends of the suture are then trimmed closely with microscissors, and the nondetachable balloon is thus secured. Finally, the affixed balloon is dipped into the latex mixture once more. The latex is allowed to cover the balloon entirely, extending over about 0.1 mm of the catheter to further affix the balloon to the catheter. This produces a smooth, nonthrombogenic surface connecting the catheter to the balloon. The diameter of the finished balloon is critical. In no case should the inflated diameter of the balloon exceed 115 per cent of the normal vessel diameter.[31] However, the latex balloon is so flexible that it assumes a sausage shape in the vessel. Balloons made from silicone assume a globular shape and may cause vessel rupture.[31]

For detachable balloons, both the catheter tip and the balloon must be prepared differently. Again, the catheter tip should be stretched and lengthened in its terminal 8 to 10 cm. No flare is placed on the end of the catheter. Detachable balloons are fixed and hardened by a method similar to that used for nondetachable balloons. The diameter of the noninflated balloon must be small enough to pass through any stenotic area in the vessel leading to the aneurysm and into the orifice of the aneurysm itself.

INTRODUCTION OF THE CATHETER

Russian neurosurgeons use a styletted needle for direct arterial puncture. For puncture of the cervical common carotid artery, a needle 5 cm long with an internal diameter of at least 2 mm is needed. The stylet is sharp and abets the initial puncture. The needle has a terminal, atraumatic bevel. Two ports are available on the proximal end of the needle: one in line with the axis of the needle, and another 45 degrees from the primary axis. The in-line port is used for the introduction of balloons and guide wires; the 45-degree port is for introduction of contrast or flush material. A special diaphragm mechanism is attached to the in-line port to allow introduction of balloons and prevent the backflow of blood.[27]

The Seldinger method may be used to introduce the catheter into the carotid, brachial, or femoral system. The skin should be punctured with a no. 11 blade in order to pass the dilator over the guide wire. In this technique, the artery is punctured and the stylet withdrawn. A short guide wire is introduced into the Seldinger needle, and the vessel dilator is then placed over the guide wire. After the opening of the carotid artery is dilated, finger pressure is continued to prevent bleeding from the dilated opening. A plastic sheath is then passed over the guide wire, and attempts are made to direct it into the internal carotid artery. If the sheath is not absolutely straight and in the center of the arterial stream as the balloon is withdrawn, it may be detached prematurely by kinks in the tip of the plastic sheath. This method has the advantage, however, of having a closable diaphragm. This diaphragm covers the side port and prevents backbleeding at the time of introduction of the balloon catheter.

The final balloons are directed toward the aneurysm by the endovascular surgeon. The balloon is not inflated until the radiological marker can be seen near the orifice of the aneurysm in question. Periodically, injections are made, and road-mapping techniques are employed. In this way, the orifice of the aneurysm is identified before the balloon reaches the target site.

In some cases, the aneurysms may be occluded by use of only a single balloon, but two balloons are preferred for most aneurysms. The helper balloon is used, first, to alter the flow of blood in the arterial tree. By inflation or deflation of this balloon, the primary balloon may be directed into whatever flow channel results from the occlusion by the helper balloon.[7] Second, the helper balloon may be used as a deflector of the primary balloon. The helper balloon is advanced beyond the orifice of the aneurysm. The primary balloon is then advanced until it deflects into the orifice of the aneurysm. The helper balloon is then deflated and retracted slightly. Thirdly, the helper balloon is used to safely detach the primary balloon. After inflation of the primary balloon in the aneurysm, the helper balloon is advance into a position in which it occludes the orifice of the aneurysm. The catheter from the primary balloon passes it in contact with the side wall of the parent artery. This provides safety because the very flexible latex balloon tends to deform and pull into the arterial lumen as the catheter is retracted. Last, the helper balloon is deflated after the catheter is detached from the primary balloon, and both catheters and the helper balloon are removed from the artery. The helper balloon may be held in a waiting position near the orifice of the aneurysm while the primary balloon is being inflated. Should the artery or the aneurysm rupture, the helper balloon is rapidly advanced and inflated, reducing blood flow and causing tamponade. Then, the patient is taken immediately to the operating room for direct surgical repair of the bleeding site by craniotomy.

ENDOVASCULAR MANIPULATION

As the balloon catheter or catheters are advanced slowly, direct and continuous imaging is essential. Inflation of the balloon is normally not required. Inflation is contraindicated as long as the radiological marker proceeds along the vascular channel of interest. If the balloon catheter stops its distal migration because tortuosity or a bifurcation of a vessel is encountered, minimal inflation may be needed to create a bolus for flow-directed movement. Maximal inflation, on the other hand, produces tamponade and retards forward migration.

The balloon is directed slowly toward the orifice of the aneurysm. Special maneuvers may be needed to force the balloon into the aneurysm, where flow is slow. Occasionally, minimal inflation of the balloon causes turbulent flow, directing the balloon into the orifice of the aneurysm. The direction of blood flow may be altered by compression of the opposite cervical carotid artery, directing the balloon toward the aneurysm or collateral artery. This is a useful maneuver if the balloon must be directed into the A_1 branch. Occlusion of the opposite carotid artery augments flow in the ipsilateral A_1 segment, reversing flow in the opposite A_1 segment. It may also create enough flow aberration to direct the balloon into an anterior communicating artery aneurysm. The contrast material that is used to inflate the balloon may be somewhat heavier than the blood in which it passes. Therefore, when the balloon is inflated, gravity can be used to direct the movement of the balloon. The patient's head may be turned so that the aneurysm lies in the most dependent portion, thus facilitating passage of the heavier balloon into the aneurysm.

After the balloon is introduced into the aneurysm cavity, temporary inflation is carried out in order to assess its position. At this time, the balloon is inflated from the fundus proximally toward the orifice. This prevents the entrapment of blood within the aneurysm and the creation of abnormal stresses on the aneurysm wall.

Temporary occlusion allows testing of the effect of the balloon on local circulation. Occasionally, an inflated balloon may protrude into the lumen, blocking distal flow. The volume necessary to produce the desired balloon size must be calculated carefully. The usual temporary occlusion time is 20 to 30 minutes, and this provides ample opportunity to study intracranial flow patterns that will result after detachment. The clinical status of the patient is evaluated, keeping in mind that inflation of the balloon may precipitate vasospasm or produce ischemic signs. In addition, the transcranial Doppler ultrasound may be used to monitor cerebral blood flow velocity. During test occlusion, a significant (50 per cent) fall in velocity alerts the surgeon that balloon occlusion probably will not be tolerated.

In the next stage, permanent occlusion is carried out. The balloon is deflated by gentle suction applied to the catheter by a small syringe. The decision must be made as to what the permanent inflating or hardening agent will be. In each case, the decision is based on the individual characteristics of the patient and the aneurysm to be treated. Aneurysms that have a large internal diameter (greater than 10 mm) should be treated with soft balloons filled with contrast material. For smaller aneurysms, a hardening agent is usually preferred. Silicone may be used as a hardening agent before detachment of the catheter. With large and giant aneurysms, some shrinkage is desirable. If the hardening agent is firm, this will not occur. Soft balloons filled with contrast material permit thrombosis and fibrosis, eventually leading to shrinkage of the aneurysm. Invariably, there is some leakage through the latex membrane. Smaller aneurysms (less than 10 mm) rarely produce mass effect even locally, and therefore shrinkage is not required.

After permanent occlusion of the aneurysm, detachment is the final stage. If the balloon is filled with contrast material, it may be detached at any time. If it is filled with a hardening agent, it must be left in place until solid. This can often be determined by examination of the residual material that remains after mixture of the compounds; similar hardening has usually taken place within the aneurysm, and the balloon may be detached at the appropriate time. The amount of agent placed in the balloon for temporary occlusion is determined by measuring the amount removed after temporary inflation. Only that amount can be reintroduced into the balloon for permanent detachment. Before the balloon is detached, aneurysm occlusion is evaluated angiographically, and the status of the parent artery is examined. Occasionally, a small amount of additional hardening agent is needed to produce total occlusion. A helper balloon is always preferred in detachment, whether the aneurysm has been preliminarily filled with soft or hard materials. If the balloon seems well seated and unlikely to migrate back into the artery, detachment proceeds.

After detachment of the balloon, the operation may be terminated. This requires gentle retraction of the catheter to which the balloon was attached, and, subsequently, removal of the catheter and the helper balloon. The patient should be observed at this time for the development of ischemic and hemorrhagic complications. Anticoagulation should not be reversed, but control of blood pressure is essential. Preoperative coagulography allows identification of potential bleeding complications. The evaluation of neurological signs of ischemia and hemorrhage is carried out at regular intervals. Postoperatively, the patient should be observed closely.

OCCLUSION OF THE PARENT VESSEL

Occasionally, the vessel on which an aneurysm arises must be sacrificed for definitive treatment. If the balloon can be passed directly into an aneurysm, thus preserving the parent artery from which it arises, the term *reconstruction* is applied. This operation is not always feasible, however, and depends on the relation of the parent artery to the aneurysm, the size of the aneurysm, its orifice, and its location in the arterial tree. In some cases, the parent artery on which the aneurysm arises may be occluded along with the aneurysm. This is referred to as a *deconstructive operation*, and it is sometimes acceptable, even when minor deficits are anticipated, if overall risks are weighed against a possible subarachnoid hemorrhage. Deconstructive operations are feasible if the vessel on which the aneurysm arises can be sacrificed without profound neurological impairment. The determination of collateral patterns and the safety of a deconstructive operation can be made only by temporary balloon occlusion of the artery in question combined with careful monitoring and neurological testing.

Deconstructive operations are applicable under certain circumstances, for example, if there is a fusiform aneurysm or if the aneurysm involves the cavernous portion or surgically inaccessible arteries. These lesions are prone to form intravascular thrombi and embolize. Therefore, in certain instances, proximal balloon placement is preferable to placement of balloons directly into the thrombus-filled sac. Additionally, these lesions may become symptomatic because of compression, embolization, or hemorrhage.

OCCLUSION TESTS

Preoperative evaluation gives information on how aggressive the surgical procedure can be with regard to carotid artery sacrifice, and it also identifies patients who are potential candidates for revascularization procedures, such as superficial temporal artery anastomosis to the middle cerebral artery or a direct saphenous vein bypass of the cavernous internal carotid artery.

Clinical Balloon Occlusion Test. The balloon is passed into the artery from which the aneurysm arises. Inflation excludes both the parent artery and the aneurysm from cerebral flow. For approximately 30 minutes thereafter, vital signs, the electroencephalogram, and appropriate neurological signs are monitored. If an aneurysm of the vertebrobasilar circulation is being excluded, visual fields and eye findings are of interest. If anterior circulation vessels are to be occluded, motor, speech, and consciousness are important. If vital signs remain normal, the neurological status does not change, and the electroencephalogram is not altered in amplitude or frequency, it may be concluded that this procedure carries low risk. After 30 minutes, if the patient is stable and the electroencephalogram is unchanged, the balloon may be detached from the catheter.

Temporary Occlusion with Distal Back Pressure. In this test, a special balloon is prepared in which a catheter passes through the balloon and projects into the lumen distal to it.[2] A smaller catheter attaches to the balloon for inflation and deflation. Thus, a double-lumen catheter is passed. The balloon is slowly inflated with contrast material in the parent artery as angiography is carried out. After the vessel is occluded, the syringe is left attached and the balloon is maintained at a constant volume and pressure. The catheter passing through the balloon into the distal lumen is connected to a transducer, and intra-arterial pressure is measured before and after balloon occlusion. If back pressure does not fall more than 30 per cent below baseline, balloon occlusion should be tolerated. A decrease of 30

to 50 per cent in back pressure defines the intermediate zone, in which there is greater risk of ischemic deficits. If pressure falls more than 50 per cent, ischemic complications are virtually ensured.

Balloon Occlusion with Transcranial Doppler Testing. In the authors' center, patients have been studied with the use of the Matas compression test and transcranial Doppler ultrasound. They were placed in either the high-risk or the low-risk group based on the results. Patients whose middle cerebral artery velocity was reduced by less than 50 per cent during external compression of the carotid artery and whose anterior communicating artery flow reversed were placed in the low-risk group. None developed neurological deficits after permanent occlusion. High-risk patients were those who had a reduction of greater than 50 per cent in the middle cerebral artery velocity or whose anterior communicating artery flow failed to reverse on compression. Fifteen per cent of those in our small series of patients who underwent permanent occlusion developed ischemic deficits.[31]

Endovascular Surgery Techniques for Specific Aneurysms

CAVERNOUS ANEURYSMS

Because of the complexity of a direct operative approach, cavernous aneurysms have come more and more frequently to the attention of endovascular therapists.[5, 18, 26] Reconstructive operations, in which the internal carotid artery is spared, should be pursued in any endovascular procedure involving its cavernous portion. However, because of the special configuration of aneurysms in this region, achievement of this goal is not always feasible. Accordingly, the functional significance of the internal carotid artery to the hemispherical circulation must be known. After test occlusion, the tactics of the endovascular approach may need modification. If the aneurysm is fusiform and the artery is not essential to neurological function, a deconstructive procedure may be performed, in which the aneurysm and the parent vessel (or the parent vessel alone) can be occluded with a detachable balloon. Symptomatic lesions of the cavernous sinus are usually encountered after they attain a size of about 1 cm or more in greatest dimension. Much depends on the location of the aneurysm within the sinus as to the symptoms produced and the indications for treatment. There are anatomical spaces in the cavernous sinus, especially underneath the first forward curve of the carotid artery, that would accommodate an aneurysm of 1 cm or larger without causing any signs of compression.

Based on age at onset, clinical signs, and the few anatomical studies from the pathology literature, a degenerative origin, at least in part, must be considered for cavernous aneurysms. Arteriosclerosis is probably the underlying disorder causing derangement of the arterial wall in most cases. Fusiform dilatations of the cavernous portion of the internal carotid artery occur commonly in the fifth decade and beyond. Direct surgical management of fusiform cavernous aneurysms by craniotomy requires special operative skills. Only neurosurgeons thoroughly familiar with the anatomy and surgical approaches to this region should consider direct operation, and all the alternatives should be exercised beforehand.

The configuration of the usual aneurysms that arise from the internal carotid artery in the cavernous sinus are appropriate for treatment using endovascular methods. These procedures usually allow preservation of the carotid artery. In those cases in which the carotid artery must be sacrificed, the endovascular approach, with test occlusion, indicates to the surgeon which vessel can be sacrificed safely. Test occlusion is indicated not only in all endovascular procedures involving the cavernous portion but also as a preliminary to any direct surgical approach or carotid occlusion procedure or trapping (Fig. 57–1). All these reasons combine to emphasize the need for experience in endovascular therapy and testing by the neurosurgeon.

Before the definitive therapy is begun, test occlusion should be carried out for a period of not less than 30 minutes, evaluating all aspects of carotid artery circulation and neurological function during occlusion. If test occlusion is not tolerated or if blood flow data, measured by either velocity or volume flow determinations, indicate that ischemic problems are likely to arise, modification in therapy is required. The final decision must be predicated on the overall experience of the surgeon or clinic involved. If only an endovascular approach is to be considered, then this should be attempted without sacrifice of the parent artery. Likewise, direct surgical treatment must be structured in order to preserve the artery. Overall, the endovascular approach is preferred because the risk of cranial nerve injury is greatly reduced. Also, the endovascular operation may be abandoned without deficit if the balloon has not been detached in the primary artery or parent artery.

If an occlusion test indicates that the deficits associated with arterial occlusion may be mild or absent and it is not possible to introduce the balloon into the aneurysm directly, occlusion of the parent artery or a trapping procedure may be acceptable. Conversely, if occlusion testing indicates that the deficit anticipated with a deconstructive operation would be severe and the balloon cannot be introduced directly into the aneurysm, the endovascular approach should be discontinued. A bypass procedure may be performed before the definitive interventional procedure is carried out. Further test occlusions are required after maturation of the bypass, however, to confirm its adequacy for protection of the arterial territory in question.

Only cavernous sinus aneurysms that are symptomatic should be considered for either endovascular or direct surgical treatment. Many patients harbor aneurysms in this location for years before they become symptomatic, and many aneurysms reach a stable size and never cause problems. Perhaps some lesions in this location even undergo spontaneous resolution. Since most postmortem examinations do not include this area, the incidence of asymptomatic lesions is not known.

The endovascular approach may be carried out through a common carotid artery puncture. Either of two deconstructive procedures may be employed for fusiform aneurysms. In one of these, the internal carotid artery is occluded proximal to the aneurysm. In the other, the aneurysm is occluded along with the internal carotid artery. In this procedure, a long balloon is used to occlude the aneurysm at its origin and along all or a greater part of the fusiform segment. This lessens the risk of bleeding or growth of the lesion from back pressure.

Acute occlusion may be carried out. In this case, the balloon is immediately detached after inflation and left in place. The effects of blood flow and pressure tend to force the balloon upstream distally. This may lead to subtotal occlusion with distal embolization into the middle cerebral artery and its terminal branches, either by the balloon or by clot in the aneurysm.

Delayed occlusion may be preferred; in this case, the balloon and catheter are left in place in the carotid

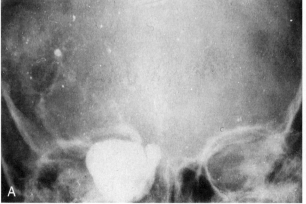 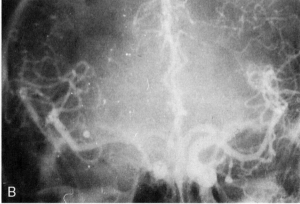

Figure 57–1

A. Giant aneurysm of the cavernous segment of the internal carotid artery. *B.* The aneurysm has been treated with a latex balloon, using the deconstructive method. After test occlusion, the balloon was detached within the carotid artery. There is good postocclusion perfusion by means of the anterior communicating artery.

artery. The balloon is later deflated sequentially over an interval of 7 to 10 days as thrombus replaces the balloon and catheter. The delayed occlusion procedure, with the proximal end of the catheter fixed in the neck by a suture, prevents proximal migration of the balloon until after the thrombus has become well fixed. With delayed occlusion, a few drops of contrast material are allowed to leak from the balloon each day for several days until the balloon is completely deflated. Then, angiography is carried out to ensure that occlusion is complete. At this point, the catheter and balloon may be safely withdrawn.

In deconstructive procedures, the balloon extends along the longest axis of the aneurysm, beyond the orifice, and back into the main channel of the internal carotid artery, blocking it permanently. In this way, the balloon cannot become displaced by pressure or flow. If more than one balloon is required to completely block an aneurysm from the circulation, these balloons must be impacted tightly so that no movement is possible. Blood volume and pressure must be maintained, and clinical parameters must be assessed at frequent intervals after deconstructive procedures to recognize ischemia early. Even if the balloon test occlusion indicates low risk for the development of these complications, postoperative monitoring should be used to indicate embolic complications. The two major hemodynamic problems are reduction in flow in the distal branches of the internal carotid artery and thromboembolic complications related to distal embolization. The blood pressure must be maintained in a normal to slightly hypertensive state, and coagulation must be controlled by the administration of aspirin or heparin.

Reconstructive operations are done in patients who harbor an aneurysm that has a good aneurysmal neck and can be entered easily and safely from the internal carotid artery. The goal for reconstructive operations, in which the carotid artery is spared, is to place the balloon along the longest axis of the aneurysm, permitting simultaneous occlusion of the orifice and fundus. Otherwise, the balloon may be displaced and become free in the aneurysm cavity. Technically, occlusion with balloons or coils is usually not difficult for aneurysms in this location. Absence of tortuosity of the artery facilitates the maneuver, especially if the aneurysm occurs proximal to the siphon. Manipulations and test occlusions may be carried out relatively safely proximal to the major communicating arteries. If the diameter of the aneurysm orifice is half that of the internal carotid artery or more, there is usually no difficulty in introducing the balloon into this orifice. If the orifice is smaller than half the diameter of the parent artery, a helper balloon may be placed above the aneurysm to direct the primary balloon into the smaller orifice. In the case of large or giant aneurysms, one balloon may not be sufficient to produce satisfactory occlusion.

Liquid contrast material is preferred for inflation of the balloons, allowing some leakage through the latex and later shrinkage of the aneurysm after thrombosis has occurred. It is almost always possible to produce occlusion of a giant aneurysm with balloons placed sequentially into the fundus. Preferably, three or more balloons of varying size should be introduced into the cavity without inflation. All balloons are then inflated to slowly obliterate the cavity from the most distal site proximally. The last balloon to be totally inflated projects into the orifice and occludes it, hopefully without compromise of the parent artery. Then, all balloons are detached sequentially. Total occlusion of some aneurysms may not be required or possible; even partial occlusion may result in shrinkage, freeing cranial nerves from compression.

SUPRACLINOID ANEURYSMS

The supraclinoid aneurysm is perhaps the best suited of all aneurysms for management with the innovative techniques recently developed. Aneurysms of the supraclinoid portion of the internal carotid artery arise preferentially at certain sites (i.e., at the takeoff of the ophthalmic, posterior communicating, or anterior choroidal artery branches or at the bifurcation). Aneurysms at each site must be evaluated individually for endovascular therapy. Before the surgeon elects an endovascular procedure over a direct approach or decides on a specific endovascular operation, the functional significance of the parent artery from which the aneurysm arises must be estimated. The terminal distribution of the artery and any neurological deficit that would result from its closure must be anticipated. All possible complications must be kept in clear focus. Of importance to outcome are the results of occlusion of an ophthalmic artery or the short branches of any major artery that may supply the internal capsule, midbrain, or thalamus. During the endovascular procedure, termination of the operation may be necessary to avert complications, and test occlusions are therefore an important part of the endovascular procedure.

Before any operation is contemplated, the endovascular surgeon, like the direct surgeon, must have a clear understanding of the hemodynamics of the arterial tree. He or she must know whether vasospasm is present, whether good collateral circulation is present, and whether there are distal infarcts or abnormalities in cerebral blood flow. Before definitive occlusion of the aneurysm, all complications of the acute period must be dealt with individually. Hydrocephalus, syndrome of inappropriate antidiuretic hormone, brain edema, intracerebral hemorrhage, and all the other complications of subarachnoid hemorrhage must be managed in order to prepare the patient for the endovascular procedure. Otherwise, worsening of complications may be expected in a patient in poor neurological grade, as in the direct surgery. Before a procedure for definitive occlusion is chosen, the structure of the aneurysm, its size, its relation to the parent vessel, its relation to other brain structures nearby, and the size of its neck are important parameters to be considered.[35, 36]

For approaches to the supraclinoid aneurysm, a cervical carotid artery puncture is the preferred route. The introduction of a catheter (onto which is fixed a detachable balloon) into the supraclinoid portion of the carotid artery is usually not difficult. However, catheters may be directed more easily into aneurysms that project medially from the internal carotid artery than into those projecting laterally or inferiorly. In this location, the use of helper balloons or methods whereby the direction of blood flow is altered are not usually necessary. Those aneurysms arising from the artery bifurcation are in a direct line of flow, and balloon catheters naturally progress along the arterial wall toward this lesion. If the orifice of the aneurysm projects toward the origin of the A_1 or M_1, the position and direction of travel of the balloon catheter must be altered.

More difficult still are arterial aneurysms that arise along the posterior surface of the internal carotid artery, such as those that arise near the ostium of the posterior communicating artery. The balloon tends to migrate anteriorly and medially along the surface of the carotid artery because it is filled with contrast material that is lighter than blood. To introduce the balloon into an aneurysm with a posterior location, adjunctive measures, such as occlusion of the contralateral artery with the finger, turning of the head to either side, and a helper balloon, are needed.

Aneurysms of the internal carotid artery often consist of two or more lobules. They may also be elongated or otherwise irregular. With aneurysms that are multilobulated, it is imperative that the balloon be interposed along the longest trajectory to the distal fundus, simultaneously blocking the orifice. Aneurysms originating with long, thin necks must be handled in a different manner. In this case, a balloon may be introduced and partially inflated, leaving the uninflated portion remaining in the neck. The balloon must be specially trained to inflate distally and retain some

uninflated portion proximally. The distal portion of the balloon must be inflated first and the proximal portion left uninflated in the neck, causing thrombosis within the aneurysm later.

Giant aneurysms that produce their symptoms by virtue of their mass should preferably be filled with a soft material so as not to increase the mass effect. Contrast material is effective in this regard because it leaks from the balloon gradually over time as the aneurysm shrinks in volume. On the other hand, small aneurysms may also be filled with a hardening material such as silicone or hema. With aneurysms with a wide neck or orifice, the use of helper balloons makes detachment safer. Otherwise, as the catheter is extracted, the balloon may be pulled into the orifice of the parent artery, obstructing it. The helper balloon holds gently against the primary balloon, keeping it well placed within the orifice during attachment.[10] Examples of endovascular occlusion of aneurysms using endovascular methods are shown in Figure 57–2.

There are many options for managing aneurysms of the supraclinoid segment. The choice depends on the size and configuration of the lesion, its location, its relation to the hemorrhage, and, most important, the expertise and experience of the aneurysm team. Quality preoperative studies with test occlusion render decision-making easier and more accurate.

MIDDLE CEREBRAL ARTERY ANEURYSMS

In deconstructive procedures, those in which the main arterial trunk is sacrificed, the distal territory

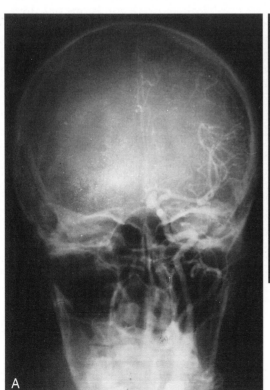
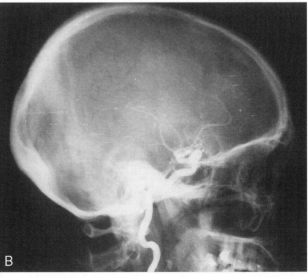

Figure 57–2

A and B. The aneurysm involves the carotid artery within the cavernous segment. In this case, the balloon occludes the carotid artery at the takeoff of the aneurysm neck. The deconstructive operation should be preceded by physiological monitoring of awake neurological signs.

must be nourished by collateral channels. These procedures are rarely applicable to the middle cerebral artery. The main trunk of the artery must be preserved if neurological deficits are to be avoided. Overall, however, endovascular approaches to these aneurysms are gaining in utility and feasibility. Because of the importance of the middle cerebral artery to perfusion of the hemisphere, temporary test occlusion with the balloon in the aneurysm is essential for a safe endovascular approach. Procedures for test occlusion are similar to those used with other aneurysms. The detachable balloon is placed in the aneurysm and inflated to its permanent size and configuration. Afterward, the patient is evaluated neurologically and with physiological methods to assess flow in the artery. In addition, angiography is carried out after the balloon has been inflated to its maximum permanent size. After 30 minutes, if the patient's neurological condition remains stable and if there is no retardation of flow, consideration is given to permanent detachment. If signs (e.g., hemiparesis, hemisensory function, speech disturbances, or visual impairment) appear during this 30-minute interval, the balloon must be deflated and the procedure terminated.

Test occlusion also serves a useful purpose by demonstrating to the surgeon who is planning direct clipping which vessels are important. Those arising from the fundus of the aneurysm can be critically assessed, and then the surgical planning can be finalized. If the patient develops ischemic symptoms during the 30-minute occlusion testing period, if velocity falls 50 per cent or more in the middle cerebral artery, or if there is an inadequate flow pattern on angiography, further deterioration is likely after permanent occlusion. In the patient who fails the first balloon occlusion test, a second balloon occlusion test may be carried out with a more successful result. This usually requires modification of systemic arterial pressure and anticoagulation. Thus, a single failure of temporary test occlusion may not always negate the endovascular option for permanent occlusion.

Complex aneurysms of the middle cerebral bifurcation may bear a complex relation to the M_1 or M_2 branches, with preservation unlikely if clipping is used. An extracranial-to-intracranial bypass may be considered as a preliminary procedure. Thereafter, a second test occlusion may be carried out, recognizing that sacrifice of major vessels may still be needed but may perhaps be better tolerated. Permitting the bypass to mature for 3 to 4 months is advisable. During this time, blood flow through it may increase significantly. Occasionally, however, the bypass does not remain open because of high flow and pressure within the median cerebral artery. The function of the extracranial bypass should be evaluated both with Doppler ultrasound and with angiography before a second endovascular testing procedure.[31, 35, 36]

Two possibilities for endovascular treatment arise after a successful bypass. In one of these, the endovascular surgeon may perform a deconstructive procedure in which the M_1 or M_2 branch is sacrificed. In the other, the balloon is again detached in the main body of the aneurysm, sparing these vessels. Sacrifice of the M_1 should always be carried out with trepidation, realizing the importance of this artery to the circulation of the hemisphere and the likelihood that deficits will follow, even with a successful extracranial-to-intracranial bypass. For permanent balloon occlusion of the median carotid artery, the short branches must be spared and the balloon must be placed as close to the orifice of the aneurysm as feasible. On the M_2 side, the balloon must also be as close to the aneurysm as possible to spare the short branches that exit the M_2 branches and penetrate the operculum to supply deep structures.

Reconstructive operations are those in which the M_1 and M_2 branches are spared by placing the balloon or coil directly in the aneurysmal sac (Fig. 57–3). This, of course, is the preferred treatment, and it is often feasible with median cerebral artery aneurysms. If neurological deficits do not appear within 30 minutes of test occlusion, velocity is not significantly reduced, and the angiography shows good filling of the distal branches, then permanent occlusion may be carried out safely. Both liquid and hard material are useful for producing the final permanent balloon inflation. For large and giant aneurysms, liquid contrast material is preferred because, as weeks go by, leakage from the balloon allows thrombosis and shrinkage of the aneurysmal mass. For smaller aneurysms, those of 1 cm or less, the use of hard material is preferred because immediate protection is provided, and late thrombosis in this aneurysm is less likely to occur because of its flow characteristics.

In detaching the balloon, after it has been permanently inflated with either hard material or liquid, the use of a helper balloon is preferred. The helper balloon is placed in the parent artery adjacent to the orifice to occlude the aneurysm. The catheter onto which the balloon is attached inside the aneurysm is held against the wall of the aneurysm by the inflated helper balloon. On detachment, the helper balloon places tension against the orifice of the aneurysm, keeping the detachable balloon in place and preserving the parent artery. The balloon also allows some protection against bleeding should it occur during detachment.

The introduction of the balloon into the aneurysm is perhaps easiest with middle cerebral bifurcation aneurysms, because the aneurysm often arises in a direct line with the M_1 segment through which the balloon passes. Aneurysms that arise from the M_1 segment usually exit at an acute angle from the M_1, pointing anteriorly and inferiorly. Placing a detachable balloon in this particular aneurysm may require all of the techniques available. Changing the patient's head position in relation to the balloon may be necessary, but, always, a helper balloon is placed near the orifice to reduce flow in the artery and to serve as a deflector for the primary balloon.[31]

Postoperatively, maintenance of homeostasis in the circulatory system is important. The blood pressure should not be allowed to fall greatly, and coagulation should be reduced with aspirin or heparin. After 24 hours of observation, it is unlikely that deficits will

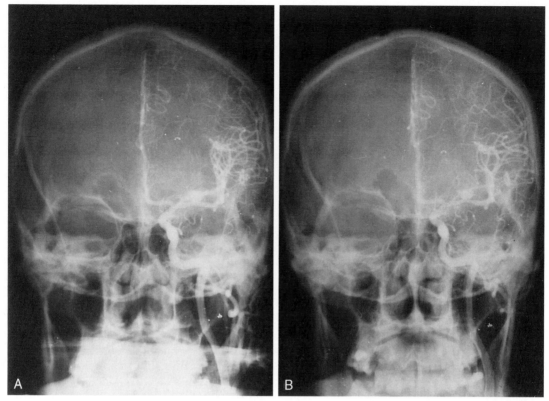

Figure 57–3

A. Aneurysm shown on the M_1 segment of the middle cerebral artery. *B.* The aneurysm has been occluded with a single balloon placed within the cavity.

appear if they have not already done so, and the patient may be discharged to home.

ANTERIOR CEREBRAL ANEURYSMS

The endovascular operation, like the direct operation, is best applied to patients in good neurological condition. The size and configuration of the aneurysm is also most important with aneurysms of the anterior communicating artery and A_1 segments. With direct clipping, surgical results are best for aneurysms that are less than 2 cm in size. Endovascular operations may be better for larger aneurysms and less suitable for smaller lesions, those measuring less than 1 cm. The endovascular approach is useful not only for aneurysmal occlusion but also for diagnosis. Balloon occlusion of parent arteries indicates to the surgeon whether a vessel can be safely occluded temporarily or permanently.

Historically, aneurysms of the anterior communicating artery complex have been the most difficult ones for endovascular methods. The first reports of successful management by endovascular techniques appeared in 1973.[35] In this case, an arteriovenous malformation fed by both anterior cerebral arteries was associated with an aneurysm involving the anterior communicating artery. An arteriovenous malformation occupied the posterior frontal lobes bilaterally in the interhemispherical fissure. The patient had had two previous

hemorrhages, from either the aneurysm or the malformation. A small latex balloon, introduced into the carotid artery, passed rapidly into the A_1 segments intracranially, aided by the abnormal flow patterns. Then, the balloon was manipulated into the anterior communicating artery and into the aneurysm, where it was inflated and detached. The aneurysm was thus occluded, sparing feeders to the malformation, which were subsequently embolized with polysterol. Since 1973, endovascular techniques have flourished. Perhaps Shcheglov in Kiev has now accumulated the largest series of patients with lesions of the anterior communicating artery, numbering in the hundreds.[28, 30]

Several problems had to be overcome in order to pass a catheter into the A_1 segment consistently.[29] Many types of arterial balloons and catheters were developed and tested in order to negotiate the sharp turns encountered at the takeoff of the A_1 from the internal carotid artery. The microballoons that can be passed through these small vessels may still be of insufficient size to occlude large aneurysms of the anterior communicating artery complex, the lesion regarded as most applicable for this technique. Before deciding on any endovascular approach, complete studies of both carotid arterial circulations, including oblique views of the anterior cerebral–anterior communicating artery complex, are necessary. Oblique projections through the orbit provide good visualization of the artery and allow the surgeon to make decisions concerning the neck of the aneurysm in relation to the parent artery.

The internal carotid artery from which the aneurysm fills best is preferred for initial catheterization. If the aneurysm is not fed equally from the right or the left arteries, the nondominant carotid artery should almost always be chosen for the entry site. Configuration of the takeoff of the A_1 from the internal carotid artery is important. An A_1 that leaves with an obtuse angle of more than 90 degrees is more easily entered than one that take an inferior course or leaves the artery at an angle of 90 degrees or less. Contralateral occlusion of the carotid artery in the neck with simple compressive techniques may be helpful in changing the flow pattern so that the catheter can be introduced into the A_1 segment. Otherwise, a balloon may be placed into the ipsilateral median carotid artery and inflated to direct flow into the ipsilateral A_1 for manipulation of the balloon catheter. The aim of endovascular surgery for this aneurysm is to maintain flow in the anterior communicating artery as well as in both A_1 and A_2 segments. It is perhaps easier to introduce balloons into those aneurysms that point anteriorly, because the contrast material that fills the balloon is somewhat lighter than blood and tends to migrate upward when the patient is placed in the supine position on the operating table. Deconstructive operations (wherein the parent artery is sacrificed) must sometimes be carried out in those cases in which the aneurysm occupies all of the anterior communicating artery. In these cases, occlusion of the anterior communicating artery is almost universal with balloon inflation. This effectively separates the two anterior circulations but is usually well tolerated. Test occlusions are employed with the patient awake to identify those patients who are dependent on cross-flow through the anterior communicating artery branch.

The second endovascular procedure found useful is occlusion of the dominant A_1 that feeds the aneurysm. The size of the balloon to be used and its position within the A_1 segment are important for this procedure. Because the perforating arteries from A_1 feed the medial basal forebrain, internal capsule, and caudate nucleus, the balloon must be short and well placed distally in the segment, as close to the aneurysm as possible. After A_1 occlusion, angiography should be repeated to see if the aneurysm fills from the opposite side. If it does, other procedures may be needed to effectively exclude this lesion from the arterial circulation. Test occlusions must be carried out before the balloon is detached to make certain that the balloon does not occlude important perforators such as Heubner's artery. A large aneurysm associated with an arteriovenous malformation is shown in Figure 57–4.

POSTERIOR CIRCULATION ANEURYSMS

Both transaxillary and transfemoral approaches have been used to gain access to the posterior cranial circulation. The transaxillary approach places the surgeon at a shorter distance from the lesion and therefore makes manipulation much easier in the vertebrobasilar circulation. Full four-vessel angiography is necessary for adequate decision-making about whether a balloon, clip, or coil is the most appropriate method of treating the lesion (Fig. 57–5). The collateral circulation to the aneurysm, its location and takeoff position, and any perforating or short branches that surround the aneurysm must be identified. The approach depends on the location of an aneurysm in relation to the vertebral artery. Aneurysms arising from the left vertebral artery must be approached from the left axillary artery. Conversely, those arising on the right should be approached from the right side. To pass a balloon catheter retrograde down a vertebral artery from the opposite one is a difficult task. If the aneurysm arises at the vertebrobasilar junction or at the basilar artery per se, the nondominant artery that has the fewest curves and serpentine movements throughout its course should be selected.

Preocclusion testing is important in making a decision about whether deconstructive or reconstructive procedures are to be carried out. If the parent artery is to be sacrificed, the functional significance of this vessel must be determined by use of preliminary balloon occlusion for a 30-minute test interval before its final detachment. Even if the balloon is to be placed into the aneurysmal sac, a preliminary test period of 30 minutes should be carried out to ensure that any small perforating branches that may reside near the fundus of the aneurysm will not be compromised by the balloon. If the patient's condition does not change during the test interval, permanent occlusion with the detachable balloon is possible. Again, with small aneurysms, a hardening material is preferred to fill the aneurysm before deflation. However, for large and giant aneurysms, a liquid inflating material is preferred because it allows shrinkage of the aneurysm over time.

In patients with large and giant aneurysms, the decision must be made as to whether to place multiple balloons within the aneurysmal sac to achieve complete obliteration. In these cases, it is preferable to place two, three, or more balloons within the aneurysm, adjust their volume and position under radiological and clinical control, and then detach them together if occlusion seems favorable. Deconstructive operations, in which the parent artery is occluded, are not always possible, especially with aneurysms along the basilar trunk. Here, many short arteries penetrate the paramedian areas of the pons and midbrain to supply vital reticular and nuclear areas. In these cases, symptoms may appear on inflation, and then the balloon must be deflated and the operation aborted. Fox and colleagues emphasized the complications that may arise during temporary occlusion testing in this group of patients, in whom short arteries must be compromised if a balloon is to be detached permanently in the basilar artery.[9] Postoperatively, maintenance of vascular homeostasis is essential. Blood pressure, viscosity, and coagulation must be monitored and controlled effectively.

Large and giant aneurysms require special considerations:

1. The carotid artery approach is preferred because

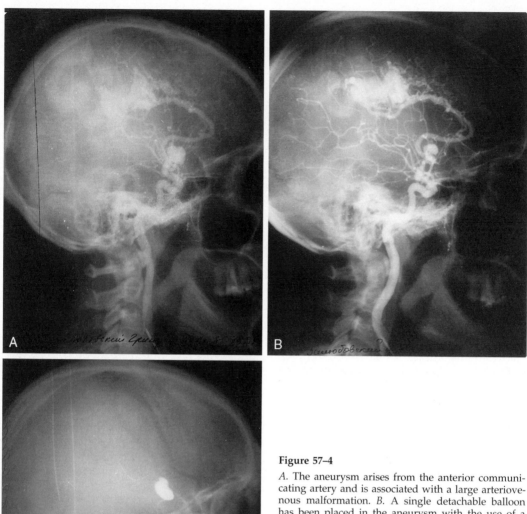

Figure 57–4

A. The aneurysm arises from the anterior communicating artery and is associated with a large arteriovenous malformation. *B.* A single detachable balloon has been placed in the aneurysm with the use of a helper balloon. *C.* Plain radiography of the skull shows the balloon in place.

access is shorter and manipulation is easier from this route. Multiple catheters and balloons must usually be manipulated within a small channel.

2. Large-diameter catheters and needles should be employed because large balloons and coils may be needed for occluding these lesions.

3. Patients harboring giant aneurysms often have stenosis proximal to the lesion in question. Sometimes dilatation must be performed before an endovascular approach can be used effectively.

4. The endovascular treatment of giant aneurysms usually requires a helper balloon. This assists in directing the primary balloon into the aneurysmal orifice.

5. Multiple balloons are usually a better solution than a single large balloon. Necessary materials should be prepared before this approach is elected.

6. Liquid material, rather than hardening material,

should be used to fill the cavity of the aneurysm. This allows for shrinkage and reduction in size of the lesion.

7. Coils, fibers, and other coagulants may be required.

8. After the endovascular procedure, an observation period follows. Occasionally, the giant aneurysm requires later excision; it shrinks more often than not.

9. In the deconstructive procedure, in which the parent vessel must be occluded, the balloon should be placed proximal to the neck of the aneurysm. If the balloon is placed adjacent to the neck, shrinkage of the aneurysm is delayed.

10. During the postoperative period, systemic anticoagulation is helpful in preventing distal thrombosis and embolization in patients in whom deconstructive procedures are used. Blood pressure and volume should be maintained.

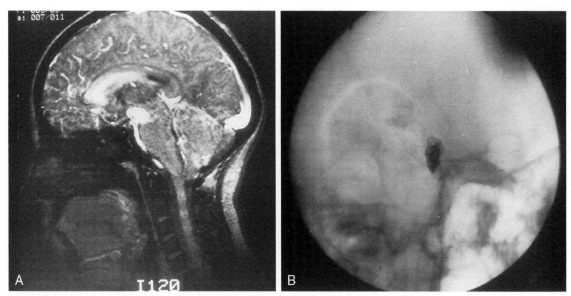

Figure 57–5
A. Giant unclippable aneurysm of the basilar artery apex. *B.* After treatment with detachable coils, thrombosis of the aneurysm is achieved.

Fusiform aneurysms are usually large if they produce symptoms. They have no neck and almost always contain thrombi. Fusiform aneurysms recanalize, and a central channel forms through the thrombus. These anatomical features mandate special requirements for surgical treatment. Preliminary diagnostic tests are essential to evaluate the fusiform aneurysm. The relation of the fusiform segment to the normal parent artery and the relation of the short branches to the fusiform segment must be determined individually. The careful use of distal occlusion during low-volume pressure injection allows the surgeon to evaluate perforating channels that may arise from the fusiform segment. This method must be used with caution because pressure can lead to progression or rupture.

Endovascular techniques do not permit reconstruction of fusiform aneurysms. The endovascular approach is always deconstructive, because the parent artery must be sacrificed. As with giant aneurysms, the placement of the balloon is a critical feature of the deconstructive procedure. The balloon should be placed proximally in the fusiform aneurysm. This permits shrinkage of the lesion and preserves penetrating arteries that are required for vital perfusion. Preliminary angioplasty may be needed. Thrombosed aneurysms are often in evolution. Part of the aneurysm may be well thrombosed with firm thrombus and other portions with soft thrombus. A balloon placed in an aneurysm in this configuration may shift or move. Postoperative angiography is needed to evaluate the status of the balloon in the aneurysm. Migration or movement of the balloon requires further treatment.

Because of structural peculiarities, the choice of a procedure, either direct or endovascular, is a complex problem. The best endovascular surgical candidate is one in whom the aneurysm is greater than 5 mm in diameter at its greatest dimension; the aneurysm should have a generous orifice for introduction of the balloon, and there must be no major branches exiting from the fundus. Before placement of a temporary balloon, test occlusion should be carried out to ensure that blood flow to the hemisphere and to the deep structures has not been compromised. In this test, the vessel or aneurysm is occluded with the test balloon for a period of 30 minutes. Monitoring of neurological and physiological parameters is carried out continuously during test occlusion.

Endovascular therapy can be applied more appropriately to patients with large or giant aneurysms than to those with small aneurysms. During the hemorrhagic period (the first 6 weeks after onset), the endovascular procedure should be performed only in patients who are compensated (Hunt-Hess grade 1). It should be applied only after vasospasm, if it is present, has been treated with angioplasty or has abated as determined by angiography or transcranial Doppler ultrasound. In this time period, the coagulogram should be normal or there should be a tendency toward hypocoagulability.

Special Difficulties of Balloon Occlusion of Aneurysms

Unusual anatomy and patterns of blood flow create special challenges for the endovascular surgeon. Inadequate equipment for imaging and for performing balloon occlusion testing leads to poor results. Inadequate training or poor technical skills can also lead to complications.

The endovascular treatment of a patient with recent subarachnoid hemorrhage carries special risks and complications not usually associated with the unruptured aneurysm. The surgeon must be aware of these special problems when planning early treatment. In addition to hemorrhagic complications, the patient's general cerebrovascular reserve may be compromised because of ischemia or local coagulopathic defects. The arterial wall after acute subarachnoid hemorrhage is covered with a platelet fibrin deposit, and there is a widespread degeneration in the endothelial layer. These events promote a coagulopathic reaction that may lead to thrombus formation in the vessel to be treated or around the balloon and distally.

Angioplasty, like surgery, can precipitate a cascade of events leading to severe neurological deficit if the surgeon does not exercise due care. If endovascular surgery is to be undertaken in the acute phase (e.g., 1 week after a major hemorrhage), the patient must be in good neurological condition and compensated (Hunt-Hess grade 1 or 2). There should be no evidence of cerebral vasospasm based on clinical examination, transcranial Doppler ultrasound, cerebral blood flow study, or the angiography done immediately before balloon therapy. The exception, of course, is the angioplastic treatment for vasospasm in which the aneurysm is to be managed concurrently.[31]

Aneurysms develop peculiar shapes (L-shaped configurations or multiple lobulations), and these create special problems for the endovascular surgeon. Peculiarly shaped balloons may be designed to facilitate closure of the orifice of the unusually shaped aneurysm. The size of the balloon must be configured carefully in order to occlude the neck and rest on the dome of the aneurysm distally. When inflated, it extends across the longest length of the aneurysm, with the proximal end projecting almost to the parent artery orifice. The remainder of the aneurysm need not be filled with a balloon. If the orifice is sufficiently blocked or occluded, thrombus will form in the aneurysm, and it will gradually shrink as balloon volume decreases.

The next major challenge that the endovascular surgeon faces relates to the size of the blood vessel and the orifice of the aneurysm to be treated. If the parent artery presents a stenotic channel, flow may be accelerated. Guidance of the catheter in the channel distal to the stenosis may be impossible. Sometimes, stenosis is so great that the balloon catheter itself cannot pass. Tortuous and serpentine arteries also sometimes present difficulties to the endovascular surgeon because catheters and balloons tend to hang up at sharp angles. If the communicating arteries are inadequate, the balloon catheter may not pass through these small channels in which blood flow is reduced. Aberrations in the circle of Willis must also be considered. If the A_1 is hypoplastic or absent, the endovascular surgeon may be unable to modify blood flow adequately by carotid compression. These obstacles may be overcome by modification of technique.

As with surgery elsewhere, knowledge of the angiographic anatomy, of the physiology of the cerebral circulation, and of the particular vessel in question is also required. Familiarity with acceptable occlusion times for the various vessels is also needed. Balloon occlusion of large arterial trunks along the base may be well accepted in a patient who has good collateral and cross-filling. Skills and training are required to prepare a small balloon, attach it to a catheter, and

pass it into the intracranial circulation, just as they are for microdissection of an aneurysm away from the middle cerebral artery.

PREVENTION OF ENDOVASCULAR COMPLICATIONS

In patients harboring recently ruptured cerebral aneurysms, in contrast to those with arteriovenous malformations and fistulae, reduced blood flow may be expected. Recognition of the threat of ischemia prepares the surgeon for managing ischemic complications associated with passage of a balloon through vessels that are already compromised. Patients who have the poorest collateral circulation and the poorest reserve are the ones most likely to develop complications. The situation is similar for patients with vasospasm and subarachnoid hemorrhage: the patient who is becoming lethargic or febrile in the early stages of vasospasm is at greatest risk for balloon occlusion of the aneurysm.

Clinical testing is an essential feature of balloon occlusion of aneurysms. Test occlusion must be carried out to assess the patient's tolerance for manipulation. During test occlusion, the balloon is advanced into the intracranial internal carotid artery and inflated with contrast material. If the patient tolerates 3 to 5 minutes of occlusion, planned treatment proceeds. If the patient does not tolerate brief balloon occlusion, then modifications in technique must be made. Volume augmentation, hypertension, or balloon angioplasty of the stenotic vessels is needed before balloon occlusion of the aneurysm is carried out. Intolerance or even brief periods of ischemia also require modification of the helper balloon technique because the balloon partially occludes the parent artery.

The endovascular surgeon should have some knowledge concerning the wall of the cerebral vessel to be treated and the unique rheology of the circulating blood. Blood clotting may be a factor. In addition to heparinization and blood volume expansion, the use of dextran is helpful in preventing catheter complications; 500 mL of dextran 40 may be administered initially.

Patients who harbor intracranial aneurysms often have vascular disease proximally in the arterial tree. The endovascular surgeon must be familiar with the status of the vessels preoperatively so as not to dislodge plaque material by the introduction of the catheter and balloons. Collateral blood supply and the peculiarities of the circle of Willis should be known. If a balloon projects from the aneurysm and blocks the parent artery to a minor degree, the surgeon should know whether collateralization from the opposite hemisphere or from nearby vessels would be sufficient to maintain the distal tissue. Monitoring of blood flow and functional physiology is therefore essential in the endovascular operating area and may be accomplished by electroencephalography or by volume or velocity flow measurements, all supplemented by the clinical examination. In the event that ischemic events, as measured by these methods, do not clear in minutes, the operation should be terminated immediately. If the patient develops a deficit with temporary balloon occlusion of a parent artery, the operation should be terminated and started again on another day when the patient is hemodynamically stable. Sometimes, other treatment methods must be chosen.[31]

Angioplasty for Vasospasm Treatment

Angiography is carried out to verify the position of the needle and the status of the intracranial vessels, allowing confirmation of vasospasm and the status of the aneurysm and ensuring correct positioning. The balloon must be modified for entering the cerebral circulation. The ideal balloon is sausage-shaped and soft, and, when fully inflated, it does not exceed by more than 10 to 15 per cent the normal diameter of the vessel to be dilated. A specially prepared latex balloon fulfills these demands best. To date, silicone balloons are harder and globular in shape, tending to rupture the thin intracranial arteries. They are fixed to fine catheters, secured with fine suture, and dipped in latex to cover the connection.[36]

The balloon catheter is then fed through an adapter that prevents backbleeding around it. The catheter is advanced in the needle and moved into the artery by flushing. As the catheter and balloon are advanced, saline may be injected into the side port to assist carriage into the internal carotid artery. The catheter is gently fed into the vessel until it reaches the intracranial circulation. The balloon usually stops spontaneously as it reaches the vasospastic portion of the median cerebral artery or carotid artery.

At this point, the proximal part of the balloon is gradually inflated. As this takes place, the proximal inflated balloon comes in contact with a wall of the artery, securing it. Subsequently, as the distal portions are inflated, the balloon assumes a sausage shape and expands into the constricted portion of the vessel. This inflation requires only a few seconds to be carried out, and then the balloon is quickly deflated. The balloon and catheter are then advanced along the vessel, dilating 1.0 to 1.5 cm of the vessel on each successive turn. The limits of angioplasty for the middle cerebral artery usually are reached at the bifurcation. The balloon and catheter may be advanced into the M_2 branches, but these arteries, being smaller, may rupture when the balloon is fully inflated. Usually vasospasm terminates at the distal end of the M_1 branch. This procedure, however, allows augmentation of blood flow to the important short branches that enter the basal nuclei, usually proximal to the M_2 branches.

The same balloon catheter may be used to perform angioplasty on the supraclinoid portion of the internal carotid artery and the M_1 branches. Anatomical peculiarities of the A_1 and the anterior cerebral artery make them somewhat more difficult. The A_1 segment may originate from the internal carotid artery at an acute, an obtuse, or a straight angle. The maneuvers employing two balloon catheters help introduce the dilating balloon into the A_1 portion. One is advanced into the M_1 segment and inflated briefly while the other is pushed into the A_1 from the internal carotid artery. Inflation of the M_1 balloon deflects flow, and the balloon, into the A_1 branch. Then, the M_1 balloon is deflated and removed.

Angioplasty in the vertebrobasilar system is best performed with a catheter having an internal diameter of 2.0 to 2.5 mm. An axillary artery puncture allows quick entry, but longer catheters must be employed for a femoral route. The short length through the axillary approach allows easy manipulation of the catheters after they enter the intracranial vasculature, with less dead space. The patient should be monitored neurologically throughout the angioplasty, and transcranial Doppler ultrasound is also helpful. The Doppler measures cerebral blood flow and ensures that compromise by catheter or balloon has not occurred. After angioplasty, the catheter is removed from the vessel, and the needle is removed under direct imaging. Bleeding from the vessel is controlled by 10 to 15 minutes of compression.

The following general observations apply to balloon angioplasty for vasospasm:

1. Local anesthesia is preferred because it allows constant neurological evaluation during the procedure.

2. Angioplasty should be performed on the most severely affected hemisphere first. This choice is based on both radiological and clinical criteria.

3. A single dilatation provides permanent relief from vasoconstriction. Dilatation for more than a few seconds causes deterioration from worsening ischemia.

4. Control of intracranial pressure is essential to successful angioplasty.

5. The coagulation system must be normal.

6. Heparinization with 3,000 to 5,000 U is required during manipulation of the balloon and catheter.

COMPLICATIONS OF VASODILATATION

Three primary complications are associated with vasodilatation: ischemic complication, hemorrhagic complication, and general complications of the endovascular approach.

Ischemic complications occur as a result of excessive occlusion times during the procedure. Stenosis can also occur because the diameter of the noninflated balloon is equivalent to the vessel's diameter. In this situation, the balloon adds to ischemia of the vasospasm even before dilatation. Occasionally, the procedure is carried out in patients whose blood flow has been critically reduced even before dilatation. Only short periods of vasodilatation are tolerated.

The most feared complication of angioplasty is separation of the balloon from the catheter and distal migration into the intracranial arterial tree. This occurs most often when a detachable balloon has been used for occlusion of an aneurysm. To prevent ischemic complications, the balloon and catheter should be as small as possible and firmly attached to the catheter, and the dilatations should be carried out rapidly. The balloon should then be rapidly deflated to augment flow. Acute local vasospasm may be precipitated by manipulation of the artery. The injection of a small amount of papaverine may relieve this kind of vasospasm. The segment of vasospastic artery to be dilated should be a short one. The segment to be dilated should include, if possible, the primary collateral channels and penetrating branches. If further dilatation is needed, a second session should be scheduled. If the balloon separates and migrates into the arterial tree, prompt craniotomy is required. In this case, the artery containing the balloon must be exposed surgically and opened, and the embolus extracted. The artery is then closed with a few interrupted 10-0 nylon sutures.[31]

Hemorrhagic complications occur because of rupture of the primary vessel or the aneurysm. Fortunately, among more than 100 patients, this complication has occurred in only one. The complication probably arises when dilatation exceeds normal diameter of the artery. In no case should the balloon diameter exceed 115 per cent of the normal vessel diameter. Also, if there is any clear evidence of arteriosclerotic vessels, these should be spared, because the hard artery tends to fracture more easily. Older patients with aneurysms have arteriosclerotic plaques that may be confused with vasospasm.

Aneurysms rupture coincidental to angioplasty because of loss of coagulation, as a result of traction or maneuvering during the angioplasty near the aneurysmal neck, or because of a misplaced balloon in the neck of an aneurysm that causes increased arterial pressure or dynamic pressures within the aneurysm. During test occlusion, only a short segment of the vessel should be closed, the balloon size should be correct, and test occlusion should not be carried out near the aneurysm. The surgeon should always be prepared for an open prompt craniotomy and should try to preserve flow in the affected arterial branches if they become obstructed by catheter, balloon, or thrombus.

Certain complications are common to all endovascular procedures. These arise because of difficulties during puncture. Subintimal threading of the catheter or needle may give rise to dissection syndromes and subsequent ischemic complications. Neck hematomas may develop, requiring termination of the procedure. Occasionally, a punctured artery develops thrombus and becomes a surgical emergency. Neurological deficits may appear even during primary vessel puncture.

Endovascular operations, much like direct operations, are invasive and carry with them inherent risks. Because the endovascular procedure is done remotely, from the end of a fine catheter, control and manipulation are also issues. Unusual complications arise because of these variables, and the endovascular surgeon should always have these possibilities in mind. The loss of a balloon into the distal arterial tree or rupture of a parent artery aneurysm may lead to serious morbidity or mortality. Preparation and prompt action by craniotomy may lessen the ultimate risk of these serious complications.

Endovascular Approach Versus Craniotomy

The decision regarding whether to use a direct intracranial operation or an endovascular approach must take into account many factors. They include the experience of the surgeon, the facilities available, the patient's condition, the peculiarities in configuration and location of the aneurysm, and the patient's desires and wishes. The decision is influenced by how recently the aneurysm has ruptured, its size, its location in relation to the parent vessel, and its orifice size. In patients with a recent rupture, the risk of rupture and rebleeding is substantially greater than in those with a "cold aneurysm." If the decision is made that an aneurysm should be treated with an endovascular method, preliminary plans should have been made to perform an emergency craniotomy, with all of the advance planning requisite for that procedure. If the aneurysm ruptures during the endovascular procedure, bleeding may be arrested with a balloon placed in the parent artery at the aneurysm orifice. Only a short period of time (depending on many factors, including the reserve energy state of the arterial territory in question) is available in which to make necessary decisions and to carry out a craniotomy and direct clipping of the aneurysm.

REFERENCES

1. Anderson, J. H., Wallace, S., Gianturco, C., et al.: "Mini" Gianturco stainless steel coils for transcatheter vascular occlusion. Radiology, 132:301–303, 1979.
2. Benashvili, G. M.: Treatment of giant intracranial aneurysms [Thesis]. St. Petersburg, Polenov Neurosurgical Institute, 1990 [Russian].
3. Benedetti, A., Curri, D., Volpin, L., et al.: Our experience in early aneurysm operation: A preliminary report. Neurochirurgia (Stuttg.) 29:25–27, 1986.
4. Berenstein, A., Choi, I. S., Setton, A., et al.: Endovascular treatment of cerebral aneurysms using the Guglielmi detachable coil: The NYU experience. Annual Meeting of the American Association of Neurological Surgeons, Boston, April 24–29, 1993. Abstract #750, 1993, pp. 182–183.
5. Berenstein, A., Ransohoff, J., Kupersmith, M., et al.: Transvascular treatment of giant aneurysms of the cavernous carotid and vertebral arteries. Surg. Neurol., 21:3–12, 1984.
6. Braun, I. F., Hoffman, J. C., Jr., Casarella, W. J., et al.: Use of coils for transcatheter carotid occlusion. A.J.N.R., 6:953–956, 1985.
7. DeBrun, G., Lacour, P., Caron, J. P., et al.: Treatment of certain vascular lesions by released balloon. Ann. Radiol. (Paris), 21:497–514, 1978.
8. Dowd, C. F., Halbach, V. V., Higashida, R. T., et al.: Endovascular coil embolization of unusual posterior inferior cerebellar artery aneurysms. Neurosurgery, 27:954–961, 1990.
9. Fox, A. J., Viñuela, F., Pelz, D. M., et al.: Use of detachable balloons for proximal artery occlusion in the treatment of unclippable cerebral aneurysms. Neurosurgery, 66:40–46, 1987.
10. Gianturco, C., Anderson, J. H., and Wallace, S.: Mechanical devices for arterial occlusion. A.J.R., 129:428–435, 1975.
11. Graves, V. B., Partington, C. R., Rufenacht, D. A., et al.: Treatment of carotid artery aneurysms with platinum coils: An experimental study in dogs. A.J.N.R., 11:249–252, 1990.
12. Guglielmi, G: Embolization of intracranial aneurysms with detachable coils and electrothrombosis. In Viñuela, F., Halbach, V. V., and Dion, J. E., eds.: Interventional Neuroradiology: Central Nervous System. New York, Raven Press, 1992, pp. 63–65.

13. Guglielmi, G., Viñuela, F., Dion J., et al.: Electrothrombosis of saccular aneurysms via endovascular approach: Part 2. Preliminary clinical experience. J. Neurosurg., *75*:8–14, 1991.
14. Guglielmi, G., and Viñuela, F: Endovascular electrothrombosis of aneurysms: Experimental research and initial clinical applications. First Congress of the World Federation of Interventional and Therapeutic Neuroradiology. Neuroradiology, *33*(Suppl):137, 1991.
15. Hieshima, G. B., Higashida, R. T., Wapenski, J., et al.: Balloon embolization of a large distal basilar artery aneurysm. J. Neurosurg., *65*:413–416, 1986.
16. Higashida, R. T., Halbach, V. V., Cahan, L. D., et al.: Detachable balloon embolization therapy of posterior circulation intracranial aneurysms. J. Neurosurg., *71*:512–519, 1989.
17. Hilal, S. K., Khandji, A., Solomon, R. W., et al.: Obliteration of intracranial aneurysms with preshaped thrombogenic coils [Presentation]. Annual Meeting of the Radiological Society of North America, Chicago, November 26–December 1, 1989.
18. Khilko, V. A., and Zubkov, Y. N.: Intravascular surgery of intracranial aneurysms. *In* Endovascular Neurosurgery. Leningrad, Medicina, 1982.
19. Laitinen, L., and Servo, A.: Embolization of cerebral vessels with inflatable and detachable balloons: Technical note. J. Neurosurg., *48*:307–308, 1978.
20. Lasarev, V. A.: Endovascular surgery of arterial aneurysms of the internal carotid artery [Thesis]. Moscow, 1983 [Russian].
21. Lylyk, P., Guglielmi, G., Viñuela, J., et al.: Endovascular neurosurgery in intracranial aneurysms with G.D.C. coils: Buenos Aires experience [Presentation]. Annual Meeting of the American Association of Neurological Surgeons, Boston, April 24–29, 1993.
22. Montero, K. I.: Diagnostic and endovascular treatment of giant aneurysms of the brain vessels [Thesis]. Kiev, Kiev Neurosurgical Institute, 1986 [Russian].
23. Moret, J., Boulin, A., Mawad, M., et al.: Endovascular treatment of berry aneurysms by endovascular balloon occlusion. Neuroradiology, *33*(Suppl):S135, 1991.
24. Moret, J., Boulin, A., Mawad, M., et al.: Endovascular treatment of berry aneurysms by endosaccular balloon occlusion. First Congress of the World Federation of Interventional and Therapeutic Neuroradiology. Neuroradiology, *33*(Suppl):135–136, 1991.
25. Moret, J.: Endovascular treatment of berry aneurysms by endosaccular occlusion. International Symposium, Vienna, Austria, May 21–25, 1990. Acta Neurochir. Suppl. (Wien), *53*:48–49, 1991.
26. Ohmoto, T., Nagao, S., Mino, S., et al.: Exposure of the intracavernous carotid artery in aneurysm surgery. Neurosurgery, *28*:317–324, 1991.
27. Romodanov, A. P., and Shcheglov, V. I.: Intravascular occlusion of saccular aneurysms of the cerebral arteries by means of a detachable balloon catheter: Kiev Research Institute of Neurosurgery, Kiev (USSR). Adv. Tech. Stand. Neurosurg., *9*:25–49, 1982.
28. Serbinenko, F. A.: Catheterization and occlusion of magistral brain vessels. *In* The Abstract Book of the First Congress of Neurosurgeons of USSR. Vol. 1. Moscow. 1971, pp. 121–123.
29. Serbinenko, F. A., and Filatov, Y. M.: Method of catheterization of anterior cerebral artery. *In* The Proceedings of the Third Congress of Neurosurgeons. Baltic Republic, Riga, 1972, pp. 160–762.
30. Shcheglov, V. I.: Endovascular interventions in neurosurgical pathology. *In* Sjezd Neirokhirurgov USSR. Moscow, 1979, pp. 558–559 [Russian].
31. Smith, R. R., Zubkov, Y. N., and Tarassoli, Y.: Cerebral Aneurysm. New York, Springer-Verlag, 1994.
32. Taki, W., Handa, H., Yamagata, S., et al.: Balloon embolization of a giant aneurysm using a newly developed catheter. Surg. Neurol., *12*:363–365, 1979.
33. Yang, P. J., Halbach, V. V., Higashida, R. T., et al.: Platinum wire: A new transvascular embolic agent. A.J.N.R., *9*:547–550, 1988.
34. Yang, P. J., Halbach, V. V., Higashida, R. T., et al.: Platinum wire: A new transvascular embolic agent [Abstract]. A.J.N.R., *9*:1030, 1988.
35. Zubkov, Y. N.: Catheterization of brain vessels [Russian]. Neurosurgery: Ann. Polenov Neurosurg. Inst. (Leningrad), *5*:218–227, 1973.
36. Zubkov, Y. N.: Intravascular surgery of intracranial aneurysms. *In* Endovascular Neurosurgery. Leningrad, Medicina, 1982, pp. 150–153.

Arteriovenous Malformations of the Brain

It would be nothing less than foolhardy to attack one of the deep-seated racemose lesions. . . . The surgical history of most of the reported cases shows not only the futility of an operative attack upon one of these angiomas but the extreme risk of serious cortical damage which it entails. . . . How many less successful attempts, made by surgeons less familiar with intracranial procedures, have gone unrecorded may be left to the imagination.

HARVEY CUSHING[22]

Despite technical breakthroughs in microneurosurgery and despite the development of radiological diagnosis in the more than 100 years since the first reported surgical procedures for treatment of arteriovenous malformations of the brain, the therapy for these lesions, perhaps more than that for any other neurosurgical disease, demands the synthesis of all of the neurosurgeon's clinical skills. Astute judgment, microsurgical proficiency, and clinical expertise are required of any surgeon contemplating excision of a given arteriovenous malformation. The modern neurosurgical literature is rife with reports of surgical misadventures and poor outcomes in the treatment of arteriovenous malformations. Describing one such case with intraoperative hyperemia and hemorrhage during resection, Cushing related the following incident:

Finally bleeding began to occur from around the sides of the varix and a rupture seemed imminent. There was evidently only one thing to do—to catch the base of the protruding lesion with a large curved clip and to throw a ligature around the whole mass. This desperate step was taken and the cavity, which continued to bleed after the ligature was placed, was finally filled with a slab of muscle taken from the patient's leg, before the excessive venous hemorrhage could be controlled. . . . One could hardly have chosen a worse place than over the lower motor area of the leading hemisphere in which to attempt the surgical removal of a racemose varix.[22]

Any surgeon who has resected a number of these lesions has probably encountered similar predicaments and futile attempts to stem tenacious bleeding.

The treatment of these lesions has challenged a number of exemplary neurosurgeons throughout the years, including Cushing, Dandy, Olivecrona, Yasargil, and many others. The treatment results have progressively improved with the evolution of improved microsurgical techniques, culminating in the superior results of Yasargil in a series of 414 arteriovenous malformations: 2.4 per cent operative mortality and 2.9 per cent major morbidity.[116] More recently, adjunctive and primary therapies in the form of embolization and radiosurgery have been introduced in an attempt to lessen the morbidity attendant in open surgical resection of some lesions. This chapter describes the diagnosis and surgical treatment of arteriovenous malformations of the brain with respect to their natural history and with particular emphasis on the rationale behind the decision for surgical as opposed to conservative therapy. The treatment of malformations in specific anatomical locations is discussed.

Definitions

Arteriovenous malformations are but one of a heterogeneous group of vascular developmental anomalies of the brain. McCormick's widely accepted pathological classification includes arteriovenous malformations, cavernous malformations, venous malformations, and telangiectasias.[60] This classification scheme is based strictly on pathology, and several authors have described mixed or transitional types of malformations that include characteristics of more than one type of malformation within the same lesion.[6]

ARTERIOVENOUS MALFORMATIONS

Arteriovenous malformation may not be the most common type of vascular anomaly in the brain, but it

P. J. Camarata • R. C. Heros

is the one most familiar to clinicians. Grossly, these lesions are composed of a mass of abnormal arteries (with walls containing elastin and smooth muscle) and veins of different sizes. Functionally, they represent direct artery-to-vein shunting with no intervening capillaries, and they are seen angiographically as early filling of veins. Occasionally, some of these lesions, although pathologically identical to standard arteriovenous malformations, are "angiographically occult" or "cryptic" and resemble the cavernous lesions at surgery.

Although there are no normal capillary beds in an arteriovenous malformation, an abnormal proliferation of capillaries adjacent to the malformation is frequently seen. Histologically, there may be small amounts of intervening neural tissue, which is often gliotic and is generally believed to be nonfunctional.[62] However, a subtype of "diffuse arteriovenous malformation," reported primarily in younger patients, has been shown to have pathologically normal-appearing neurons with varying amounts of gliosis.[17] Gross and microscopic evidence of remote hemorrhage and thrombosis, including hemosiderin-laden macrophages, thickened arachnoid, and hyalinized, calcified vascular walls, is almost always found. Some degree of microscopic inflammation is invariably seen. Most of this chapter is devoted to the diagnosis and treatment of this particular type of vascular malformation.

CAVERNOUS MALFORMATIONS

Cavernous malformations (angiomas) are found throughout the central nervous system. Pathologically, they consist of compact masses of cavernous or sinusoidal channels of varying sizes with thin walls and no intervening neural tissue.[62] Grossly, they appear as purplish, berry-like clusters containing hemorrhage in various stages of organization. The vessels in these lesions contain no elastin or smooth muscle but may be hyalinized and thickened. The presence of large amounts of hemosiderin around the malformation, seen both pathologically and radiologically with magnetic resonance imaging, provides evidence of multiple previous episodes of microscopic hemorrhage (Fig. 58–1). Computed tomography often reveals a hyperdense lesion that enhances little or not at all with contrast administration. These lesions are not visible on angiography and represent the largest percentage of angiographically occult vascular malformations.[71, 86] As many as 10 per cent of individuals present with multiple cavernous angiomas.[85] Most commonly, these lesions cause seizure, focal neurological deficit (usually secondary to hemorrhage), or headache, although they are frequently found incidentally with the routine use of magnetic resonance imaging. Robinson and associates found 76 lesions with typical magnetic resonance imaging characteristics in a review of more than 14,000 head magnetic resonance images performed at the Cleveland Clinic in a 6-year period. They demonstrated an annualized bleeding rate of 0.7 per cent.[85]

Surgical extirpation of such a lesion is relatively straightforward because there is usually a gliotic plane with evidence of hemosiderin from old hemorrhage around it. The surgical procedure can be likened more to removal of a metastatic tumor than to removal of a true arteriovenous malformation. Bleeding is much less of a problem with cavernous malformations than with arteriovenous malformations, because there are never large feeding vessels or draining veins. Except for lesions deep in the brain or brain stem, most can be resected with minimal morbidity. The most difficult aspect of the management is to decide when surgery is indicated, because the natural history of these lesions is relatively poorly understood. In very general terms, the authors recommend excision of newly diagnosed asymptomatic or questionably symptomatic lesions—that is, those discovered on magnetic resonance study ordered because of headaches or because of a single seizure—only if they are single, the patient has no family history of cavernous angioma, and the lesion is in a location for which the probability of surgical morbidity is minimal. The authors generally recommend excision of clearly symptomatic lesions—those in patients with appropriate neurological deficit or difficult-to-control epilepsy—unless they are located deep in the brain stem or in the internal capsule, where surgical excision would be expected to worsen the neurological deficit.

VENOUS MALFORMATIONS

Venous malformations (angiomas) have been called the most common type of malformation.[62] They consist of collections of small, histologically normal veins that usually drain into one or more large central veins, creating a "caput medusae" appearance on angiography or magnetic resonance imaging (Fig. 58–2). Normal brain tissue is present between the venous channels. Microscopic hemorrhage and calcification are usually not observed in pathological specimens. These lesions are found most often in the white matter and may represent a developmental anomaly that occurs when the normal pattern of venous drainage fails to develop in the maturing embryo.[6] They contain only venous blood and have been proved to hemorrhage only very rarely. Several authors have pointed out that these lesions frequently occur in combination with cavernous malformations; older reports of hemorrhage from venous malformations may actually have resulted from undetected associated cavernous malformations.* Venous malformations are most often asymptomatic and are detected incidentally with computed tomography scanning, angiography, or, increasingly, magnetic resonance imaging. Because the veins of the "angioma" drain normal brain tissue, surgical obliteration could produce venous congestion and infarction; therefore, most neurosurgeons agree that venous angiomas should not be resected. In cases of mixed lesions containing cavernous and venous malformations, the venous lesion should be preserved if possible.

---

*See references 21, 56, 70, 74, 84, 85, and 90.

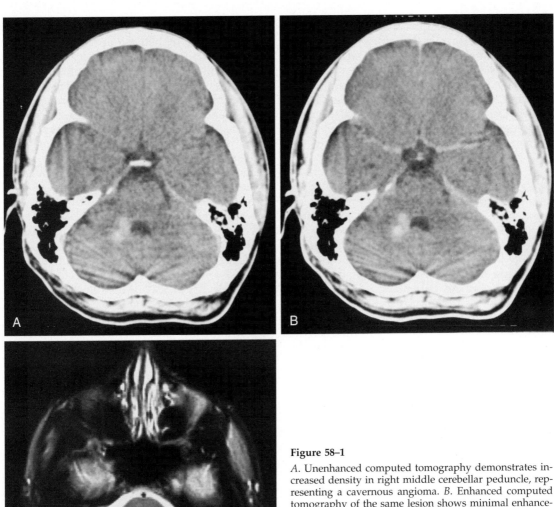

Figure 58–1

A. Unenhanced computed tomography demonstrates increased density in right middle cerebellar peduncle, representing a cavernous angioma. *B*. Enhanced computed tomography of the same lesion shows minimal enhancement. *C*. T2-weighted magnetic resonance imaging shows characteristic dark signal of hemosiderin around the lesion.

CAPILLARY MALFORMATIONS

Capillary malformations (telangiectasias) are small clusters of capillary-sized vessels with normal intervening neural parenchyma.[62] They are commonly found in the pons and the roof of the fourth ventricle but can occur anywhere in the brain. Histologically, the vessels are identical to normal capillaries. The telangiectasias do not usually appear on angiography and rarely show any histological evidence of hemorrhage and gliosis. They are seen most commonly in the Rendu-Osler-Weber syndrome and only rarely come to clinical attention.

Mixed or transitional forms of vascular malformations have also been identified and may be more common than originally thought. Stressing the frequent simultaneous presentation of two or more of these lesions, Awad and co-workers reported a series that included four main types: mixed cavernous and venous malformations, mixed cavernous and arteriovenous malformations, mixed cavernous and capillary malformations, and mixed venous and arteriovenous malformations.[6]

Embryology

Arteriovenous malformations, like most cerebral vascular malformations, are believed to arise congenitally. The most popular theory holds that the problem develops between the 45th and the 60th days of embryogen-

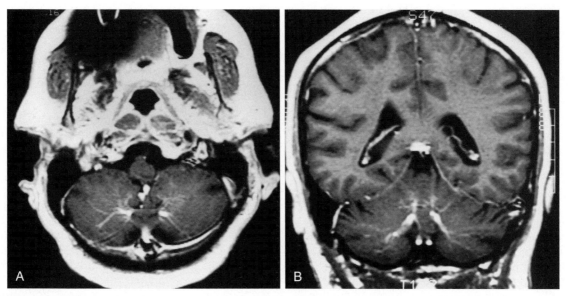

Figure 58–2

Axial *(A)* and coronal *(B)* magnetic resonance imaging enhanced with gadolinium shows bilateral cerebellar venous angiomas draining into large peritonsillar tributaries.

esis. The primitive circulation to the brain begins at about the fourth week of embryogenesis, by which time a capillary meshwork exists over the entire brain. Some of the capillaries coalesce into larger luminal structures as this primitive plexus differentiates into afferent, efferent, and capillary components.[57] Another theory holds that arteriovenous malformations result from persistent direct connections between the future arterial and venous sides of the plexus.

The etiology is less clear for cavernous and capillary malformations. Venous malformations have been postulated to occur as the result of a defect somewhat later in embryological life in which a more mature cortical and deep drainage pattern fails to replace a primitive venous drainage system.[6]

Mullan has put forward yet another interesting postulate for development of arteriovenous malformations.[66] Dural arteriovenous fistulae have been shown to arise from traumatic or spontaneous occlusion of major venous sinuses. Mullan reasons that the malformations of the brain might also arise, in an analogous manner, from a "fistulization" of a thrombosed major vein, perhaps early in embryogenesis. This fistula could mature throughout life into a typical arteriovenous malformation. Several cases and anatomical studies have shown this to be a convincing argument, at least for some malformations.

Pathophysiology

Neurosurgeons and neuropathologists have studied the complex pathophysiology of arteriovenous malformations since the first surgical excision. Because of the complex nature of the vascular physiology and the difficulty in studying the lesions in vivo, knowledge of

the flow patterns in and around the malformations remains limited. The experimental study of these malformations has been limited to mathematical modeling and the study of extracerebral shunts because there is no satisfactory animal model.

The majority of symptoms from arteriovenous malformations are in some way referable to the abnormal hemodynamic situation. The direct anastomosis of arteries and veins creates a high-flow, low-resistance shunt. Structurally, the thin, dilated feeding arteries are abnormal because of decreased amounts of smooth muscle and elastin; hyalinization and calcification of the vessels are common. The dilated, thin-walled, venous side of the malformation is also abnormal from long-standing high arterial pressure undampened by the presence of a capillary bed. Segmental dilatations and sacculations are commonly found on the venous side. Pathologically, areas of thrombosis are also often seen, accompanied sometimes by marked inflammation.

It is thought that initially, in the absence of any capillary resistance in the arteriovenous malformation, pressure in the feeding vessels is reduced. This creates a sumping effect, which concomitantly increases blood flow and causes dilatation of the arteries feeding the malformation. In turn, this reduced intravascular pressure causes further recruitment of flow into the arteriovenous malformation. It is possible the malformation itself could promote the ingrowth of further vasculature, perhaps as a result of intermittent thrombosis or through some as yet unrecognized angiogenesis factor released by adjacent brain tissue.

The increased flow through arteriovenous malformations and the pathological changes in feeding arteries are believed to account for the relatively increased incidence of saccular aneurysms in patients with these lesions.[7, 13, 20, 30] Ten to fifteen per cent of patients with these lesions are found to have aneurysms, most on vessels hemodynamically related to the arteriovenous malformation. This is a higher incidence than that suggested by the results of major autopsy series in unselected populations. Cunha e Sa and co-workers have recently categorized the aneurysms into those occurring proximally on major arteries feeding the arteriovenous malformation, those occurring distally on feeders, those occurring on deep feeders, and those unrelated to the malformation.[20] These aneurysms have been known to decrease in size or even disappear after resection of the lesion.[36, 47, 50]

Because most arteriovenous malformations do not become symptomatic until the third decade of life, it is reasonable to assume that physiological and anatomical changes occur that eventually cause these symptoms. An increase in size is caused not only by enlargement of feeding vessels and draining veins but presumably by additional recruitment of adjacent vessels initially uninvolved in the malformation. This is demonstrated by the growth that is seen over time in partially embolized malformations or in those not completely obliterated by surgery. This growth can manifest as increased symptoms owing to increased mass, increased flow recruitment and subsequent "steal" from adjacent brain, and venous hypertension.

Many of arteriovenous malformations show at least microscopic evidence of old hemorrhage, even if there has not been a clinically significant hemorrhage.[62] Varying degrees of thrombosis are also seen frequently in these lesions. Thrombosis can occasionally be quite dramatic, resulting in almost complete obliteration of the malformation with disappearance on angiography. At times, these lesions present with hemorrhage after what appears to be a major thrombosis, and all that remains angiographically are large, blunted feeding vessels or perhaps a late-filling, large, draining vein. Although angiographic steal from adjacent brain is commonly seen with these lesions, the presence of a neurological deficit attributable to steal is much less frequent. Progressive neurological deficit in some patients in the absence of true volume growth of the malformation has been attributed to steal. Pathologically, the areas around the malformation undergoing vascular steal demonstrate gliosis, necrosis, and calcification.[62] Venous hypertension from arterialization, occlusion, or stenosis of the drainage system has also been implicated in the pathophysiology of progressive neurological deficits.[3, 111]

One theory, "normal perfusion pressure breakthrough," holds that the vascular bed in brain adjacent to the malformation is chronically exposed to decreased pressure and, as a result of hypoxia, loses its normal autoregulatory response and becomes maximally vasodilated. Swelling from edema and hemorrhage can occur after removal of the shunt if this dysautoregulated vascular bed is exposed to normal perfusion pressure.[100] Vessels chronically hypoperfused are known to undergo structural changes, with reduction of the medial layer and increased luminal diameter.[28] However, cerebrovascular responsiveness to carbon dioxide and blood pressure changes has been shown to be preserved in some studies.[11, 119, 120] This is discussed in more detail in a later section.

Natural History

After an arteriovenous malformation has become manifest by hemorrhage, seizures, progressive neurological deficit, or headache, the history often progresses with further episodes of bleeding and deterioration. This seems to be true regardless of whether the malformation has hemorrhaged in the past. The study by Ondra and associates is perhaps the most comprehensive in terms of numbers and length of follow-up of patients followed conservatively, with a mean follow-up of 24 years.[73] They estimated a 4 per cent yearly hemorrhage rate for both ruptured and previously unruptured arteriovenous malformations. The annual mortality rate in both the ruptured and unruptured malformations was 1 per cent, and the major morbidity and mortality rate, when both groups were considered together, was 2.7 per cent per year. Twenty-three per cent of their patients died as a direct result of hemorrhage from an arteriovenous malformation, and the mean age at death in those dying from hemorrhage was significantly lower (15 years) than for patients dying from other causes. Both the annual rehemorrhage rate and the annual mortality rate did not vary over the entire length of the study.

Others have followed patients with arteriovenous malformations who were treated conservatively for a number of years and have come to similar conclusions. Graf and co-workers estimated the risk of rebleeding after hemorrhage from such a lesion to be 6 per cent during the first year and 2 to 4 per cent per year after that.[33] In a study of 168 patients with unruptured arteriovenous malformations at the Mayo Clinic, 18 per cent bled during a mean follow-up period of 8.2 years. Of these, 29 per cent died of the hemorrhage, and 23 per cent had significant long-term morbidity.[14] After following 217 patients with arteriovenous malformations treated conservatively for a mean of 10.4 years, Crawford and associates estimated that the risk of a neurological deficit from hemorrhage was 27 per cent during the 20 years of follow-up. The yearly hemorrhage rate was 2.6 per cent for ruptured lesions and 1.7 per cent for unruptured ones.[19] In a 1985 review of previous clinical studies encompassing over 1,500 patients, Wilkins concluded that unruptured arteriovenous malformations carry an annual risk of hemorrhage of 2 to 3 per cent and an annual mortality rate of about 1 per cent.[113] The rate of hemorrhage after an initial bleed was 6 per cent in the first year and the same as for unruptured lesions in subsequent years.

Several conclusions can be drawn from a comprehensive review of these studies. First, unruptured arteriovenous malformations appear to be much less benign than had previously been thought, and they appear to follow a very similar course to those that present with hemorrhage. Second, although in the year after hemorrhage the risk may be slightly greater, after that the annual rate of hemorrhage is identical in ruptured and unruptured lesions: 3 to 4 per cent per year. Third, the risk of death associated with each hemorrhage appears to be about 10 to 15 per cent, with an annual rate of death secondary to hemorrhage of 1 per cent in both ruptured and unruptured malformations. Fourth, there is a significant permanent neurological morbidity associated with these malformations that approaches 2 to 3 per cent per year, or 20 to 30 per cent from each episode of hemorrhage.

Current diagnostic imaging modalities, such as magnetic resonance imaging, have increased the number of asymptomatic arteriovenous malformations diagnosed. Insufficient data are available to make any assessment as to the natural history of these lesions, but there is little reason to assume that their risk of yearly hemorrhage is significantly different from that of previously unruptured arteriovenous malformations that present with seizures or with other neurological symptoms unrelated to hemorrhage.

Clinical Presentation

Spontaneous hemorrhage is the most common presentation of an arteriovenous malformation, accounting for 41 to 79 per cent in selected series.* The hemorrhage is most commonly intraparenchymal, but occasionally it is subdural or subarachnoid. In 5 to 10 per cent of cases, intraventricular hemorrhage is present.[72] The hemorrhage presumably occurs from rupture of abnormally arterialized venous channels in the malformation nidus.

There has been some speculation that smaller arteriovenous malformations bleed more frequently or have an increased propensity for both initial and recurrent hemorrhage.[36, 49, 61] Spetzler and co-workers speculate and provide some evidence to the effect that there is an inverse relation between the size of the malformation and both the risk of hemorrhage and the size of the resulting hematoma.[98] They believe that this is explained by the fact that the pressure in the feeding arteries tends to be higher in the smaller lesions. Others have speculated that venous obstruction may increase the risk of hemorrhage or that certain angioarchitectural factors such as intranidal or pedicular aneurysms may render the malformation more likely to hemorrhage.[3, 111, 114] Pre-existing hypertension or activities that elevate arterial blood pressure or venous pressure (e.g., Valsalva maneuver) have not been shown to be associated with higher rates of hemorrhage.[104]

Hemorrhage from an arteriovenous malformation is frequently less catastrophic than that from an aneurysm. One reason is that the hemorrhage is more likely to arise from the venous end of the arteriovenous shunt and therefore to occur under lower pressure. Furthermore, vasospasm, which occurs frequently with ruptured aneurysms, rarely occurs with arteriovenous malformations because of the smaller volume of blood entering the basal subarachnoid space. In addition, Mohr has noted that because the hemorrhage arises within the substance of the malformation, which generally is thought to include only nonfunctional brain tissue, it often has less disruptive impact on cerebral function than a hypertensive hemorrhage, which occurs in normally functioning and usually critical brain tissue.[65] Eighty to 90 per cent of patients who hemorrhage from an arteriovenous malformation survive the initial rupture, but only 50 to 60 per cent survive the initial impact of an aneurysmal hemorrhage.[33]

The second most common presentation of an arteriovenous malformation is seizures, which occur in 11 to 33 per cent of cases.* Other common presenting symptoms include headache, progressive neurological deficit, and cardiac failure.[51, 115, 117] All types of seizures have been reported with these lesions.[40] Apart from the absence of seizures from lesions in the posterior fossa, the specific location of an arteriovenous malformation correlates poorly with the frequency of seizures.[65] However, focal seizures with visual aurae have often been associated with lesions in the occipital lobe.

Both classic and common migraine have been reported with arteriovenous malformations. The incidence in these patients may be no greater than in the normal population.[78] However, it is believed that when patients with arteriovenous malformations have migraines, the lesion is most frequently in the occipital lobe and, furthermore, that the headache and the visual symptomatology are usually unilateral and consistently referable to the side of the lesion.[108] Other headaches, not involving hemorrhage, may be associated with these malformations. The cause is thought to be stretching of dura and venous sinuses and dilation of feeding arterial vessels. Progressive neurological deficit over time may be related to additional recruitment of adjacent vessels and resulting cerebrovascular steal.

Diagnosis

Most patients who come to clinical attention because of hemorrhage, seizure, or neurological deficit undergo a computed tomography or magnetic resonance study as the initial diagnostic test. In addition to hemorrhage, the unenhanced computed tomography study frequently shows speckled calcifications within and surrounding a malformation. With the addition of contrast, large tortuous feeders or dilated veins are often visualized. These same features in greater anatomical detail are seen on magnetic resonance imaging.

Angiography remains the definitive study both for diagnosis of an arteriovenous malformation and for the operative planning and decision-making. Angiography of ipsilateral and contralateral vessels is necessary, and it is also important that the study be done in close temporal proximity to the definitive surgical therapy. Arteriovenous malformations are known to change in size and patterns of drainage with time. In

---

*See references 2, 19, 37, 43, 73, 80, 87, and 117.

*See references 2, 19, 37, 73, 87, and 117.

addition, vessels that were not seen because of compression from a hemorrhage on initial angiography may be visible on follow-up studies several weeks later. Multiple views, magnifications, and high-speed filming techniques are helpful. In particular, digital subtraction equipment enables rapid sequence imaging throughout the arterial and venous stages, allowing for precise delineation of feeding vessels and arteriovenous shunting. Magnetic resonance angiography is still unable to give this temporal detail, so critical in operative planning and decision-making.

The authors rarely operate on a malformation without having obtained a recent magnetic resonance imaging study for precise anatomical localization. On several occasions, the operative plan and approach have been changed by subtle anatomical nuances regarding location that could not be precisely defined on angiography. The angiography and magnetic resonance imaging results provide complementary information to help the surgeon formulate a three-dimensional view of the location of the malformation, its feeders, and its drainage system.

The precise role of other diagnostic modalities, such as xenon computed tomography blood flow imaging and functional magnetic resonance imaging, in the diagnosis of arteriovenous malformations has yet to be defined. The xenon computed tomography technique can be useful in following patterns of blood flow surrounding the lesion before and after operation. Some have advocated its use to determine the likelihood of perioperative perfusion-related complications.[9, 58, 106] Functional magnetic resonance imaging has been able to detect the proximity of a malformation to eloquent areas of brain such as primary motor cortex or Broca's area (Fig. 58–3; see color section in this volume). Such information can be used to guide operative planning, although one would be unlikely to leave residual arteriovenous malformation simply because of its proximity to eloquent cortex. More likely, these studies can be helpful in determining whether a given malformation is operable or not.

Treatment

In few instances in neurosurgery is the decision about whether and how to treat as difficult as it is in the case of a patient with an arteriovenous malformation. In such a case, the Hippocratic dictum, "primum non nocere," rings particularly true. The decision not to treat becomes obvious if the neurosurgeon is faced with a very large hemispheric lesion involving primary motor or speech cortex and extending into the deep gray matter. At the other end of the spectrum, it is generally recognized that small lesions in "noneloquent" areas of the brain should be surgically excised, although even this assumption has been called into question.[102] Between these extremes, there is a large gray area that calls for the surgeon's highest decision-making skills. The decision can be arrived at only after a careful assessment of the natural history of the dis-

ease as it is known, the location and type of malformation, the condition of the patient, and—not to be forgotten—the surgeon's experience with the particular form of therapy. The natural history has already been described, and the other factors are briefly discussed here.

PATIENT FACTORS

Age. Some believe the patient's age to be the most critical factor in making a decision to operate on a given malformation. There is evidence to suggest that the likelihood of hemorrhage from a malformation decreases in later life, although some studies indicate otherwise.[19, 29, 33, 53, 80] The age of the patient determines the number of years during which the patient will be at risk for hemorrhage if the lesion is left untreated. This can be important, given the apparent 4 per cent annual cumulative risk of hemorrhage. One may therefore take a more conservative approach with an elderly patient, even with a malformation that has hemorrhaged previously. Conversely, a young person with a malformation has a substantial cumulative risk of hemorrhage and attendant morbidity throughout the rest of his or her life. A younger patient also is better able to tolerate the extended surgical procedure and the prolonged postoperative course that is often necessary. In addition, a younger patient is more capable of recovering from the potential morbidity associated with surgery.

General Health and Clinical Condition. The general medical condition of a patient with an arteriovenous malformation must be taken into consideration when deciding on a given form of therapy. An elderly patient with a cardiac condition that prohibits prolonged general anesthesia would be better advised to undergo radiosurgical treatment or no therapy for the malformation. A patient with a life-limiting condition has fewer years at risk for hemorrhage than a healthier patient of the same age.

There is general agreement among experienced surgeons that unless a life-threatening hemorrhage has occurred, arteriovenous malformation surgery should be an elective procedure. Most surgeons prefer to wait several weeks after a clinically significant hemorrhage has occurred to allow the patient to improve neurologically and reach optimal neurological condition. It is difficult to ascertain surgical morbidity in those series in which patients were operated on before given such a chance for improvement. The surgeon must resist the temptation to operate early after a hemorrhage that results in a major neurological deficit under the assumption that the patient "cannot be made worse." Such ill-advised operations can turn what may have been a reversible deficit into a permanent one.

Although the common indications for surgical treatment of these lesions include hemorrhage, seizures, progressive neurological deterioration, and severe headaches, the neurosurgeon is increasingly faced with the diagnosis of an asymptomatic malformation. It is in these patients, who are in optimal clinical condition

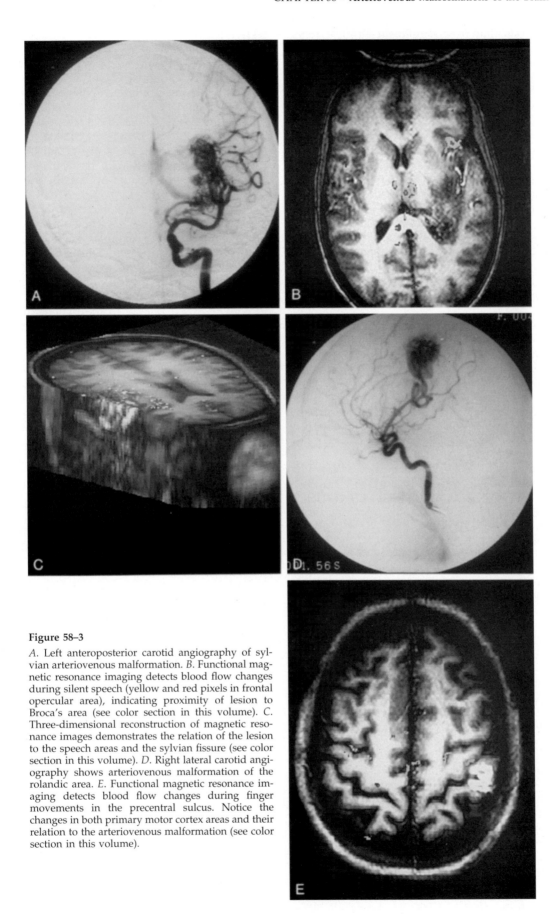

Figure 58–3

A. Left anteroposterior carotid angiography of sylvian arteriovenous malformation. *B.* Functional magnetic resonance imaging detects blood flow changes during silent speech (yellow and red pixels in frontal opercular area), indicating proximity of lesion to Broca's area (see color section in this volume). *C.* Three-dimensional reconstruction of magnetic resonance images demonstrates the relation of the lesion to the speech areas and the sylvian fissure (see color section in this volume). *D.* Right lateral carotid angiography shows arteriovenous malformation of the rolandic area. *E.* Functional magnetic resonance imaging detects blood flow changes during finger movements in the precentral sulcus. Notice the changes in both primary motor cortex areas and their relation to the arteriovenous malformation (see color section in this volume).

but have lesions that pose significant surgical risks, that the surgeon's decision-making expertise is most severely tested.

Occupation and Lifestyle. These are more subjective factors that, nevertheless, must be considered in arriving at a decision to treat. The patient must consider the risks as described by the surgeon and be aware of how any deficit would affect the ability to function and carry on his or her previous occupation and lifestyle. Young, physically active athletes may consider a hemiparesis an unacceptable complication and may be willing to live with the risk of future hemorrhage. On the other hand, a patient may be unable to deal with the fact that he or she has an arteriovenous malformation and may desire to have it surgically excised no matter what the cost. Whereas a hemianopsia may be an unacceptable complication for a truck driver and an apraxia of the hand may likewise be unacceptable to a sculptor, neither deficit may be inconvenient to a teacher or a lawyer.

It is of utmost importance that the treating surgeon take into consideration the psychological makeup of the individual with the malformation. Many patients with inoperable lesions are devastated after having been told that they have a "time bomb" or a "cocked pistol" in their heads. Others are well able to live with the knowledge that they will have a risk of hemorrhage year after year but would not want to live with a "handicap" or be "crippled."

FACTORS RELATED TO ARTERIOVENOUS MALFORMATION

Location and Type of Lesion. There have been many attempts to grade malformations or to identify those important characteristics of the lesion that correlate with outcome.* From these classifications, it can be gleaned that the larger malformations present the greater technical challenge to the treating surgeon, and their removal is fraught with increased morbidity. Deep lesions, those adjacent to or involving eloquent cortex, and those in the posterior fossa, are generally associated with increased surgical morbidity and difficulty.[4, 54, 96, 97] In addition, excision of a lesion at some sites (e.g., the deep substance of the brain stem or the posterior limb of the internal capsule) predictably leads to an unacceptable deficit, and the malformation is therefore "inoperable." Most proposed grading systems have included an assessment of the size, location, and number of the arterial feeding vessels as important determinants of operative difficulty.[42] The system described by Shi and Chen also includes an assessment of the pattern of venous drainage.[91] The authors have found the system of Spetzler and Martin, with its emphasis on size, eloquence, and whether there is deep venous drainage (indicative of deep location or extension), to be simple, easy to use, and reproducible.[97]

---

*See references 12, 31, 45, 52, 76, 91, 97, and 105.

SURGEON'S EXPERIENCE

Although not included in any of the grading systems and difficult to quantify, the experience that a surgeon has with lesions similar to that being considered for surgery should be honestly assessed by the surgeon when entertaining the prospect of operating on a given malformation. The treating surgeon has a responsibility to do what is best for the patient, and that may entail referral to a physician with more experience or to a radiosurgeon. It is unjust and perhaps unethical for a neurosurgeon who sees one to two arteriovenous malformations a year to attempt surgical excision of a large, complex malformation in eloquent brain. On the other hand, many less complex malformations are well within the scope of competence of any well-trained neurosurgeon.

If the surgeon has a clear opinion as to the correct course for an individual patient, he or she has a duty to convey this explicitly to the patient during discussion of the options. It is unacceptable to simply present all of the options in an equal manner and leave all the burden of the decision up to the patient—unless, of course, the surgeon truly believes that the available options are equal in their merit. More than likely, the patient will ask what the surgeon advises. Occasionally, the patient decides against what the surgeon has recommended. In this case, the surgeon must be supportive, perhaps referring the patient for other opinions if he or she believes the patient has chosen a less desirable course of action. Under no circumstance should a surgeon perform open surgery or radiosurgery if the surgeon believes it is not the optimal form of therapy for that patient. The excuse that the surgery is "what the patient wanted" does not justify doing other than what the surgeon believes is best for the patient.

General Surgical Techniques

TIMING OF SURGERY AND PREPARATION

Surgery for arteriovenous malformation should ideally be performed in an elective fashion. Occasionally, an intraparenchymal hemorrhage must be removed on an emergency basis because of life-threatening mass effect. In this situation, the authors prefer to do the most conservative operation possible, removing most of the hemorrhage but steering clear of the malformation vessels. After the brain edema has subsided, one can return for definitive therapy. In most cases, the hemorrhage can be treated conservatively for 3 to 4 weeks after a moderate hemorrhage before approaching the malformation for definitive surgical excision. This allows the patient's clinical condition to improve and usually to reach a plateau. In addition, the hematoma begins to liquefy, which can facilitate surgery. During this waiting period, it is important to evaluate the forms of therapy that can be offered, and arteriography must be repeated before any definitive therapy is undertaken.[88] As the clot is reabsorbed, the configuration of the arteriovenous malformation often changes.[68] In addition, there may be some new changes on angiography, such as thrombosis of existing feeders or the appearance of vessels not initially visualized.

As with most intracranial operations requiring significant brain retraction, the authors routinely use steroids preoperatively and in the immediate perioperative period. Prophylactic antibiotics are also administered preoperatively, as are anticonvulsants in the case of supratentorial lesions. Lumbar drainage or mannitol may be required for brain relaxation. A standard anesthetic induction for intracranial cases is employed, with the use of fentanyl and pentobarbital along with an agent for neuromuscular blockade. After anesthesia has been accomplished, the PCO_2 is steadily decreased with hyperventilation to a level of approximately 25 to 30 mm Hg. Maintenance of anesthesia is continued, usually with 30 per cent nitrous oxide and an inhalation agent such as isoflurane combined with intermittent doses of fentanyl. The authors have usually preferred not to use hypotensive agents to control bleeding except in very rare circumstances. Most often, patients have a slightly lower than normal blood pressure during anesthesia.

POSITIONING AND CRANIOTOMY

Positioning is critical to the planning of an arteriovenous malformation operation. The position is different for lesions in different locations, but in general the head should be positioned so as not to cause compression of the neck veins, which could significantly impede venous drainage. The positioning should be such that brain retraction during resection is minimal and is aided by gravity whenever possible. Ideally, the least amount of cerebral tissue should be transgressed, and the cisternal and sulcal anatomy should be used to the fullest. In most cases, the head is rigidly fastened in a fixation device; with a cortical representation, the surface of the lesion is placed parallel to the floor so that the approach to the arterial feeders is as perpendicular as possible.

A generous craniotomy and dural opening is the rule with this surgery, particularly if the malformation is of moderate or large size. The authors routinely expose a large portion of brain tissue around what is believed to be the nidus of the malformation, for easier orientation to the positions of the arterial feeders, draining veins, and other cortical landmarks. Frequently, the malformation is not visible on the cortical surface and is only located by recognition of one or more arterial feeders dipping into a distal sulcus or a large draining vein remote from the exact nidus. In addition, a generous craniotomy allows the surgeon to adjust the angle of the microscope over a wide field and to deal with any unforeseen hemorrhage remote from the operative site. In spite of the best preoperative planning, there is always the possibility of an intraoperative discovery that may call for a slightly different approach and a wider craniotomy.

SURGICAL ADJUNCTS

The operating microscope is the *sine qua non* of modern arteriovenous malformation surgery. The authors prefer to bring in the operating microscope early in dissection of the arachnoid, just after opening of the dura. The magnification and illumination provided by the operating microscope are invaluable in defining the precise margins of the malformation. Although one could argue that the microscope limits the field of vision, there is no substitute for a precise, magnified view. Modern microscopes are equipped with controls to allow free and wide access at the touch of a button to the entire operative field.

Coagulation of vessels with the bipolar cautery is now routine. The forceps are also useful for dissection along the planes of the malformation or along individual vessels. If standard bipolar forceps are used, they must frequently be returned to the scrub nurse for cleaning of the tips. This helps avoid sticking of the tips during coagulation of smaller vessels, which can cause tearing and meddlesome bleeding. The senior author has begun to use the newer irrigating tips, which, if properly employed, can significantly reduce the amount of charring and, concomitantly, the time the scrub nurse spends cleaning the tips. Microsurgical suction tips that are most narrow at their distal end and have a graduated, thumb-regulated suction power have also proved invaluable. The tip of the suction is small enough to be used adjacent to the bipolar tips in microdissection.

Microclips of various sizes are used, and temporary clipping is employed at times to confirm dampening of pulsations of feeding arteries or to determine whether a particular vessel in the vicinity of a malformation is a vessel "en passage." Permanent small hemoclips are useful to occlude the larger feeding vessels (>1 mm). These are now magnetic resonance–compatible and are made of titanium. In addition, the small removable microclips introduced by Sundt are extremely useful to occlude the tiny vessels often found at the depths of arteriovenous malformation dissections.[103] These vessels, despite exposure and identification, are all too often extremely resistant to bipolar cauterization, necessitating further suctioning of brain tissue and identification of longer segments of vessels to coagulate, which frequently only aggravates the problem.

Ultrasound studies have occasionally been useful in determining the most direct approach to the nidus. Although the authors have no experience with stereotactic guidance in the approach to deep arteriovenous malformations, others have found this to be helpful.[27, 93]

SURGICAL TECHNIQUES

The process of excision of the lesion can be thought of in five stages: identification of the malformation and elimination of superficial feeding vessels, circumferential dissection, dissection of the apex of the lesion, division of the final vascular pedicle with complete removal, and absolute hemostasis. These are each discussed in detail in chronological order.

Identification and Elimination of Feeding Vessels

If the malformation is not visible on the surface after the surgeon has turned a large bone flap and made a generous dural opening, a decision must be made as to the site of entry. Any visible superficial feeders should be identified under the microscope by opening the arachnoid over them with an arachnoid hook. The feeder should be dissected, identified, and followed until it enters the malformation, at which point it can be divided, but only after confirmation that the vessel does not supply any adjacent brain tissue. The latter occurs with vessels "en passage," which are found particularly in perisylvian lesions and those of the corpus callosum. Should the malformation nidus not be visible on the surface, ultrasound may be useful to identify it. Frequently, an enlarged cortical artery can be identified and followed into a sulcus to the malformation nidus; alternatively, a red arterialized vein may be visible and can be traced to the lesion.

In identifying and taking the superficial feeders, it is of utmost importance not to confuse them with "red" draining veins, which should almost always be preserved until the end of the procedure. The exception may be a malformation that drains largely by one or more deep veins, with only minor superficial drainage. Premature obliteration of the main venous drainage can lead to disastrous intraoperative swelling and hemorrhage. With experience, it is often easy to differentiate these veins from arteries under high-power magnification, because their walls are thinner and they are less turgid than arteries of the same size; also, the veins tend to be larger in diameter than most of the feeding arteries. If the identification is doubtful, the application of a temporary clip will clearly indicate whether the pulsations are dampened toward or away from the malformation. In addition, the veins and arteries can often be identified by tactile sensation by gently compressing the vessel between the tips of the bipolar forceps. The difference between the thin, easily compressible venous wall and the firmer arterial feeders can often be ascertained. Finally, during coagulation of these vessels, the application of a small, short current from a bipolar forceps can readily differentiate artery from vein: the vein more quickly shrinks toward occlusion. During division of the feeders, the authors use microhemoclips in addition to bipolar coagulation for vessels greater than 1 mm in diameter.

Circumferential Dissection

After the surgeon has used the angiography results to ascertain that all the large superficial feeding vessels have been identified and divided, circumferential dissection around the malformation can begin. It is imperative that the dissection be carried as close to the margin of the lesion as possible to avoid any injury to adjacent brain. Only in those malformations situated far from neurologically critical areas (e.g., at the extreme frontal or temporal tips) can the plane of dissection be slightly more peripheral. Contrary to reports in the older literature regarding an avascular plane surrounding a malformation, there is rarely such a plane around an entire lesion; indeed, if the plane becomes too avascular, it may be that the surgeon has strayed too far from the malformation itself.

In general, the oozing encountered at the margin can be controlled with Cottonoids compressed under a retractor onto the lesion. It is often fruitless and potentially disastrous to pack bleeding from the brain side. Doing so could lead to intraparenchymal or intraventricular hemorrhage that may not be recognized until catastrophic swelling occurs. In lesions on the cerebral convexity, the initial circumferential cortisectomy should proceed to a depth of about 2.5 cm, which is the maximum depth of the sulci, before the dissection is deepened. The reason is that the superficial arterial supply may be entering the malformation at the depth of a sulcus and not be visible at the surface. Usually, after elimination of the feeders at this depth, no larger feeding vessels are encountered until the apex of the malformation is reached.

Dissection of the Apex

The circumferential dissection is continued in a conical fashion until this, the most difficult step in resection, is reached. It is at this stage that the final feeding vessels are encountered. The most vexing of these are the small, friable, subependymal vessels that resist any attempts at coagulation. This stage of the resection is also frustrating and often lengthy because the vessels stubbornly resist identification and coagulation, and hemorrhage persists. The authors have found hemoclips and small aneurysm clips difficult to use at this depth, and, at times, the vessels continue to bleed through the clips. The Sundt microclips are most useful in this situation, although they are expensive. With persistence and patience, the surgeon can eventually secure hemostasis. Again, one must avoid packing into the white matter, which simply allows the vessels to retract and continue bleeding farther away. Some surgeons have found hypotension valuable to control bleeding at this stage; however, if hypotension is used, it is advisable to keep the patient sedated and hypotensive for 2 or 3 days after surgery.[107]

Final Vascular Pedicle and Removal

After circumferential dissection and control of the apex, the malformation should literally "dangle" from its venous pedicle. Frequently, the veins are still somewhat arterialized at this stage, owing to small feeders that lie directly underneath or adjacent to draining veins. Careful attention should be paid to this possibility as the veins are clipped and divided.

Absolute Hemostasis

At this point, the resection cavity should be carefully inspected for the presence of any bleeding or residual malformation. Frequently, a number of Cottonoids have been placed in the resection cavity to mark the planes. These must be carefully removed one by one under constant irrigation so as not to cause additional bleeding. The entire wall of the resection cavity is inspected under magnification. Careful attention must be paid to this portion of the procedure because it could mean the difference between a smooth postoperative course and a catastrophic hemorrhage. If bleeding or clotted blood is identified, the walls of the resection are gently rubbed with a Cottonoid to discover any residual malformation or microscopic bleeding sites. If residual malformation is encountered, a careful removal at this stage is usually straightforward. After the surgeon is sure that all malformation has been removed and all hemorrhage controlled, the entire cavity is lined with a single layer of Surgicel. The anesthesiologist is then asked to gently raise the blood pressure to 15 to 20 mm Hg above the resting pressure to check for any bleeding from the cavity walls. If any bleeding sites are recognized, these should be dealt with, relined with Surgicel, and then reinspected with increased blood pressure. Only after 10 to 15 minutes of inspection of the cavity under the microscope should the surgeon allow the blood pressure to return to its spontaneous anesthetic level. The anesthesiologist is then instructed not to allow the blood pressure to rise above this point of artificial elevation.

POSTOPERATIVE CARE

The introduction of the anesthetic agent propofol has allowed prompt awakening of patients after even the most prolonged period under anesthesia. The infusion of propofol is begun approximately 1 to 2 hours before the end of a particularly lengthy procedure. This allows a quick wake-up so that the patient's neurological condition can be assessed in an expeditious fashion. Careful attention, however, must be paid to the type of emergence from anesthesia. Of all neurosurgical procedures, the resection of an arteriovenous malformation demands the smoothest awakening, without blood pressure elevation, Valsalva maneuvers, or untoward coughing or straining that could raise intracranial pressure. Instantaneous control of blood pressure must be possible. The blood pressure is artificially kept below the value that was tested after the resection for 24 to 48 hours. No patient is discharged without first undergoing cerebral angiography to demonstrate complete obliteration of the arteriovenous malformation. The authors also use intraoperative angiography before the wound is closed in complicated arteriovenous malformations or if there is any uncertainty about the completeness of the resection.

SPECIAL TECHNIQUES

Staged Resection

During the final stages of resection or during the first day or two after resection of large, high-volume arteriovenous malformations, some patients develop swelling or hemorrhage in the operative bed and surrounding brain tissue that cannot be explained by residual lesion or by early obstruction or obliteration of draining veins. Although it occurs infrequently, the syndrome has been recognized by other neurosurgeons.* It was first described by Spetzler and associates, who attributed it to the restoration of normal perfusion pressure, after removal of the shunt, into the surrounding vascular bed, which is thought to be dysautoregulated because of chronic hypoperfusion from the steal into the shunt, as previously described.[100] Since the original description, several theories have been proposed to explain this problem, and some experienced surgeons have expressed doubt about its importance.[3, 11, 117]

The angiography characteristics that predispose to this complication include large size of the nidus, the presence of large-caliber and long feeding vessels, and preferential shunting into the malformation with relative paucity of filling of vessels in adjacent brain. In addition, other clinical and physiological characteristics are thought to be associated with the occurrence of this syndrome: progressive neurological deficit of the kind associated with cerebral hypoperfusion (steal), increased carotid flow as measured by Doppler ultrasound, impaired autoregulation as measured by decreased responsiveness to carbon dioxide (although others have reported paradoxical increased responsiveness to carbon dioxide in these patients), and significant increase in proximal feeder pressure and surrounding cerebral blood flow after distal occlusion of a feeding vessel.[9]

To prevent this complication, whatever its cause, staged obliteration has been proposed.† Staged obliteration is gradual reduction of flow into the malformation by embolization or feeder occlusion before definitive resection. With the advent of modern neurointerventional embolization procedures, the authors prefer the use of embolization by closed endovascular navigational techniques almost exclusively for this purpose.

Embolization

The particular techniques, indications, and complications involved in intraoperative or endovascular embolization are detailed in Chapter 59. There is no doubt that arteriovenous malformation surgery has been made safer and technically less demanding with the availability of preoperative embolization. Nevertheless, embolization carries an intrinsic risk, which is substantial even in the best hands. Therefore, careful judgment is in order and, in the authors' opinion, embolization should never be used routinely simply to make surgery "easier" or "faster." It should be used only if, in the judgment of the surgeon after discussion with the interventionalist, the combined risk of embolization and surgery is lower than the risk of surgery alone.

---

*See references 5, 11, 23, 26, 48, 67, 69, 82, and 99.
†See references 5, 25, 26, 53, 67, 69, 72, 77, 81, 82, 88, 89, 99–101, 109, and 110.

Blood Flow Measurements

Though the authors have limited experience with the use of these techniques in arteriovenous malformation surgery, others have reported on the use preoperative and intraoperative measurements of cerebral blood flow. Stable xenon with single photon emission computed tomography (SPECT) and with standard computed tomography has been used preoperatively combined with acetazolamide to assess the carbon dioxide autoregulatory capacity.[9, 106] In the SPECT studies, patients who later developed hyperemic complications actually had a hyper-responsiveness to acetazolamide in ipsilateral steal regions, indicating increased carbon dioxide reactivity. In the more sensitive xenon computed tomography studies, decreased vascular reserve (decreased carbon dioxide reactivity) was found in 27 per cent of the sites adjacent to malformation. However, no correlation was made to the later development of any hyperemic complications. It is possible that, with further refinement and research, these techniques will allow for a reliable preoperative identification of those individuals likely to encounter problems with perfusion breakthrough. Blood flow velocity measurements obtained by insonating feeding vessels with transcranial Doppler ultrasound have been touted as a means of identifying those patients at risk for hyperemic complications or of deciding when to proceed or halt embolization.[18, 46]

Several techniques are available to quantify intraoperative blood flow during resection of the malformation. Laser Doppler flowmetry and thermal diffusion methods have been used during resection to detect changes in cortical blood flow.[16] Intravenous xenon-133 has been used to detect changes in regional cerebrospinal fluid that occur during surgical resection.[119, 120] All studies suggest an increase in perfusion of areas surrounding the malformation after resection. Whether these changes can be used to guide intraoperative decision-making remains to be seen.

Additional intraoperative monitoring techniques that others have found useful during resection include electrophysiological monitoring of somatosensory evoked potentials and electrocorticography.[15, 34]

Intraoperative Angiography

Newer, high-quality digital subtraction angiography equipment that is essentially portable and can be used with a minimum of disruption during surgery has facilitated the use of intraoperative arteriography. Radiolucent carbon head frames are available that provide minimal distortion of the images. Most arteriovenous malformation surgeons agree that one of the most common causes of postoperative hemorrhage is retained malformation, so it is important to confirm that the malformation has been completely excised. The senior author has, on at least two occasions, removed residual malformation on the basis of intraoperative angiography, and others have reported similar experiences.[8, 59]

Approaches to Arteriovenous Malformations in Specific Anatomical Locations

Classification schemes have been developed based on (1) anatomical divisions, with terms such as "lobar," "convexity," or "paraventricular"; (2) vascular patterns, with descriptions such as "anterior choroidal artery" or "pericallosal"; and (3) functional units, with designations such as "medial hemispherical-limbic" or "thalamocaudate." Although any given malformation may defy classification under one heading, the authors have chosen to consider here the supratentorial lesions in the somewhat arbitrary anatomical categories of "superficial" and "deep" (similar to Yasargil's "convexial" and "central" divisions), and to consider infratentorial lesions in a separate section (Fig. 58–4). In each case, the authors describe their approach to lesions occupying predominantly one anatomical location and describe potential pitfalls and concerns characteristic of lesions in that given area. Patient positioning and general desired approach to each lesion are summarized in Table 58–1.

SUPERFICIAL SUPRATENTORIAL ARTERIOVENOUS MALFORMATIONS

Convexity Lesions

The positioning of patients for surgery of lesions of the cerebral convexities is dictated by the location of the lesion and the location of its primary arterial supply. Lesions primarily involving the parasagittal convexity areas are discussed separately below. Frontal arteriovenous malformations usually are supplied by the anterior and middle cerebral arteries and their branches. Except for small lesions, parietal malformations are most often supplied by all three major vascular territories. Temporal convexity lesions usually derive their supply from distal branches of the middle and posterior cerebral arteries. Uncal and temporal branches of the anterior choroidal arteries may also supply these lesions. Convexity lesions of the occipital lobe are usually supplied by distal branches of the posterior and, in some cases, the middle cerebral arteries. If they are medially situated, there may be some supply from distal anterior cerebral feeders as well.

For the smaller convexity lesion, the techniques described in the section on general surgical techniques apply. The head is elevated, and the plane of the lesion is kept parallel to the floor as much as possible, to allow a perpendicular approach. Large lesions present special problems. By virtue of their size, these lesions are usually supplied by vessels from two or three major vascular divisions. They often reach the ventricular surface and have both superficial and deep venous drainage; at times, extracranial supply can be a problem. Their margins are often poorly defined, and it can be difficult to tell whether large, dilated vessels near the periphery belong to the malformation proper or to

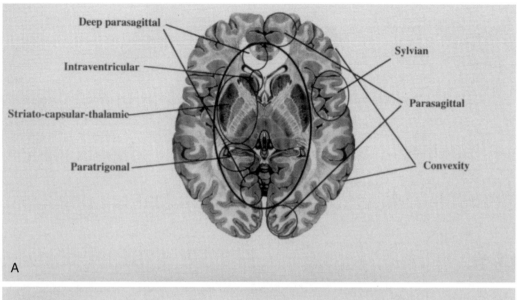

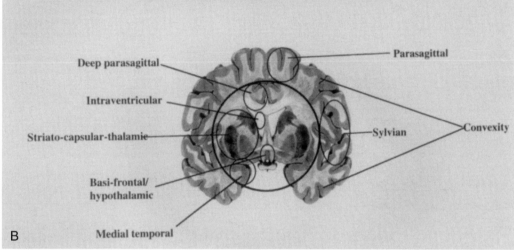

Figure 58–4

Anatomical classification of arteriovenous malformations: axial *(A)* and coronal *(B)*. (Adapted from Nieuwenhuys, R., Voogd, J., and vanHuijzen, C.: The Human Central Nervous System: A Synopsis and Atlas. 3rd rev. ed. Berlin, Springer-Verlag, 1988, pp. 70 and 91. Reprinted by permission.)

surrounding brain. These lesions are often those that are at risk for hyperemic complications. Presurgical embolization can be particularly helpful in decreasing the flow through the lesion and in cutting down the external carotid supply.

Whenever there is significant meningeal supply, extreme caution must be used in turning the craniotomy flap; the authors use multiple burr holes and a careful stripping of the dura, sometimes coagulating enlarged meningeal feeders through the burr holes before removing the bone flap. The dural opening should begin far away from the surface presentation of the arteriovenous malformation to avoid bleeding from tearing of involved vessels or meningeal vascular pedicles. At times, it is most prudent to leave malformation attached to a circle of free dura, as one does with a dural-based meningioma, and graft the dural defect at the conclusion of the case.

Because of the size and multiplicity of the arterial

supply, the surgeon may need to use several different positions to obliterate the feeding vessels early in the procedure. For example, with large parieto-occipital malformations, the procedure may begin with the head turned 90 degrees and parallel to the floor, in a subtemporal approach designed to take the posterior feeders, and be followed by a second stage with the head straight up, to eliminate pericallosal feeders. Alternatively, large feeding vessels from one or more of the arterial distributions may be eliminated preoperatively by embolization to facilitate operative removal (see the section on parasagittal lesions).

Sylvian (Insular) Lesions

In spite of their appearance on angiography, which may seem to show these lesions to be located in the angular gyrus or opercular cortex, surgically they are most frequently located on the cortical surface of the

Table 58–1

OPERATIVE APPROACHES TO ARTERIOVENOUS MALFORMATIONS

Lesion Location	Position	Operative Approaches
Supratentorial		
Superficial		
Convexity	Surface of malformation parallel to floor	Wide craniotomy centered over nidus of lesion
Sylvian		
Anterior	Supine, head turned 45 degrees	Pterional, anterior temporal craniotomy
Posterior	Supine, head turned 90 degrees, or lateral	Posterior parietotemporal craniotomy
Parasagittal		
Anterior	1st stage, supine, head straight up	Broad-based craniotomy to midline
	2nd stage, lateral or head turned 90 degrees ipsilateral side up	
Posterior frontal/parietal	Same as above	—
Occipital	Prone or semisitting	Large craniotomy extending to sagittal and transverse sinuses
Deep		
Medial hemispheric		
Medial temporal		
Anterior	Supine, head turned 45 degrees	Pterional, anterior temporal craniotomy, exposure of zygoma, wide splitting of fissure
Midtemporal	Supine, head turned 90 degrees, or lateral	Temporal craniotomy with subtemporal approach or through inferior temporal gyrus
Paratrigonal	If medial and superior to trigone, semisitting	Posterior parietal-occipital craniotomy extending to midline, approach through posterior parietal cortisectomy
	If lateral and inferior to trigone, lateral	Temporoparietal craniotomy with subtemporal/transtemporal approach
Splenial/posterior third ventricle	Semisitting or lateral with side with greatest lateral extension down	Parasagittal craniotomy on side of greatest lateral extension
Deep parasagittal		
Anterior	Semisitting, head neutral	Parasagittal craniotomy
Posterior frontal, parietal, occipital	Lateral ipsilateral side down	—
Anterior callosal	Small lesions—semisitting, head neutral	Parasagittal craniotomy
	Large lesions—reclining, head neutral	Large bifrontal craniotomy, subfrontal followed by interhemispheric approach
Hypothalamic/inferior frontal	Supine, head turned 45 degrees	Unilateral pterional/subfrontal approach
Intraventricular	Supine	Approach is through corpus callosum, through middle frontal gyrus, transtemporal, or through posterior parietal cortisectomy depending on location and presence or absence of ventriculomegaly
Striato-capsular-thalamic	Approach discussed with other lesions above	—
Infratentorial		
Mesencephalic	Tectal lesions—sitting	Supracerebellar infratentorial approach
	Lateral lesions—lateral	Temporal craniotomy, subtemporal-transtentorial or presigmoid approach
Cerebellar		
Hemispheric	Prone or lateral	Unilateral suboccipital craniectomy
Vermian	Sitting	Bilateral suboccipital craniectomy
Brain stem		
Floor or fourth ventricle	Prone or lateral	Midline suboccipital craniectomy with approach through inferior vermis
Lateral pons	Lateral	Temporal, suboccipital craniotomies, subtemporal-presigmoid transtentorial approach

insula, with venous drainage into the sylvian fissure.[117] These arteriovenous malformations are particularly important because of their arterial supply "en passage" from normal middle cerebral artery branches. This anatomical fact often renders these lesions difficult if not impossible to embolize because of the risk to normal surrounding eloquent tissue.

These malformations can be subdivided into anterior and posterior lesions. For anteriorly located malforma-

tions, a pterional or combined pterional–anterior temporal craniotomy is used to facilitate access to the anterior sylvian fissure.[41] The carotid artery is exposed, and the medial sylvian fissure is carefully opened. Care is taken to preserve any anteriorly draining arterialized veins initially, but any small veins draining across the sylvian fissure may be coagulated, clipped, and divided, provided there is adequate drainage posteriorly. Dissection then proceeds along the second and third division branches of the middle cerebral artery (M_2 and M_3), making certain that only those vessels entering the malformation are divided. The senior author has often found it helpful to apply temporary clips to these vessels while continuing distal dissection until he is assured that the vessel enters only the malformation. Not infrequently, a vessel that appears to enter the arteriovenous malformation actually passes by or through the lesion to supply normal brain beyond. An additional problem with these lesions is bleeding from deep lenticulostriate feeders. These vessels are fragile and often difficult to coagulate, and the temptation to "pack them away" must be resisted in every case.

For more posteriorly situated malformations (Fig. 58–5), the authors prefer a straight lateral head position with a standard horseshoe-shaped incision extending over the ear. One must avoid placement of the incision too far anterior to the tragus, because injury to the frontalis branch of the facial nerve could occur. It is not necessary to extend the craniotomy to the pterional area or to open the medial sylvian fissure for these lesions. The vein of Labbé can be used as a landmark, with arterialized veins traced in a retrograde fashion back to the malformation. Most of these malformations are small to moderately sized, although some may extend 5 to 6 cm deep with medial drainage. A small

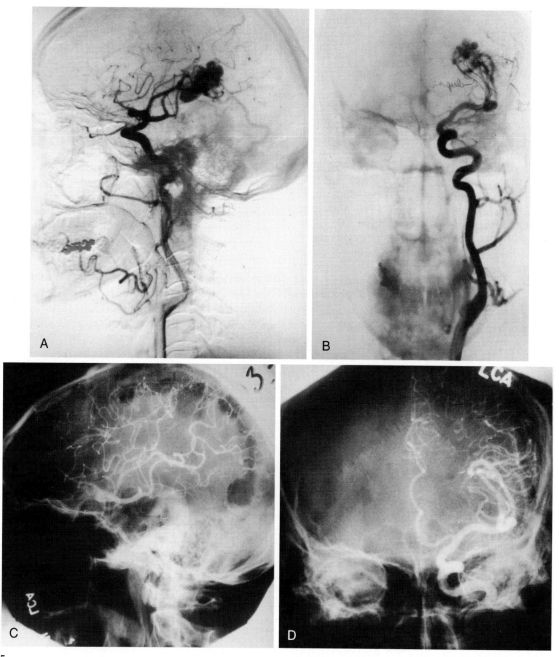

Figure 58–5

Left posterior sylvian anteriovenous malformations. *A and B.* Preoperative angiography. *C and D.* Postoperative angiography demonstrates no residual malformation.

amount of subpial dissection may be necessary, but eventually the sylvian fissure can be identified. Feeding vessels are then skeletonized, taking only the side branches as they enter the lesion, with liberal use of temporary clipping to aid in their identification. As the malformation shrinks, it can often be pulled from the surrounding neurologically critical areas with minimal deficit.

Parasagittal Lesions

Anterior frontal malformations are best approached through a frontal craniotomy extending to the midline, with the head straight up and the patient in the supine position initially to control the interhemispheric feeders. Alternatively, these anterior cerebral feeding vessels can be dealt with by endovascular occlusion and embolization before the procedure; then the lesion is removed with the head turned 90 degrees and the ipsilateral side up. In this manner, the arteriovenous malformation can be retracted against the falx as the middle cerebral artery feeders are taken laterally around the lesion (Fig. 58–6).

Posterior frontal and parietal lesions are more of a problem because (1) they often have blood supply from more than one arterial distribution, (2) they have large arterialized draining veins traversing the field into the sagittal sinus that limit entry into the interhemispheric fissure, and (3) they are intimately involved with critical primary motor and sensory areas. Again, preoperative embolization is frequently helpful, with the aim of occluding the interhemispheric anterior cerebral artery feeders. If embolization is not feasible, a first surgical stage with the patient in the semisitting position and the head straight up is frequently advisable to occlude the anterior cerebral feeders. Injury to arterialized draining veins is a potentially disastrous complication in the larger lesions. It is therefore prudent to use a broad-based bone flap so that the surgeon can tailor

the approach to the interhemispheric fissure between these vessels. The second stage is carried out with the patient in the supine position (or full lateral) with the head turned 90 degrees, elevated, and the ipsilateral side up; this facilitates occlusion of the convexity middle cerebral feeders. This method can be used only if the pericallosal feeding vessels have first been dealt with, because they are the last vessels encountered laterally during the progression around the lesion to the falx.

Occipital parasagittal lesions that reach the convexity are best approached through a generous craniotomy extending to the sagittal and transverse sinuses with the patient in either prone or semisitting position. Again, embolization is a tremendous help in obliterating medial feeders from the anterior and posterior cerebral arteries in the interhemispheric fissure.

DEEP SUPRATENTORIAL ARTERIOVENOUS MALFORMATIONS

Medial Hemispheric Lesions

Medial Temporal Lesions

Basomedial temporal lobe arteriovenous malformations frequently present a question as to whether resection can be undertaken with low morbidity because they often extend upward to involve parts of the basal ganglia, the internal capsule, or the thalamus. The following angiographic features favor operability of these lesions:[72]

1. Primary blood supply by the anterior choroidal artery and laterally directed posterior cerebral branches, as opposed to medially directed vessels

2. Venous drainage into the basal vein of Rosenthal and the medial sylvian vein, as opposed to the internal cerebral or galenic veins

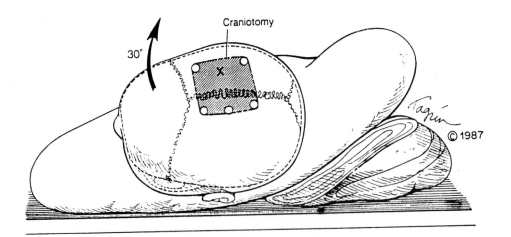

Figure 58–6

Single-operation approach to a parasagittal lesion. The initial stage of the resection should be parasagittal to gain control of interhemispheric anterior cerebral feeders unless these have been eliminated by preoperative embolization; for the interhemispheric approach, the head should be in the neutral position and flexed 30 to 45 degrees relative to the floor. The second stage would be to come around the malformation laterally, with the ipsilateral side up and the head turned parallel to the floor. (From Ojemann, R. G., Heros, R. C., and Crowell, R. M.: Surgical Management of Cerebrovascular Disease. 2nd ed. Baltimore, Williams & Wilkins, 1988, p. 376. Reprinted by permission.)

3. Projection beneath the plane of the middle cerebral artery on lateral angiography, not above as in thalamocapsular lesions

4. Projection lateral to the sweep of the posterior cerebral artery on anteroposterior angiography

These lesions can be subdivided into those involving the uncus, amygdala, and anterior hippocampal and parahippocampal areas (anterior); those involving primarily the midhippocampus, temporal horn, and parahippocampal region (middle); and those in the posterior paratrigonal area.

Anterior Temporal Lesions. The anterior lesions are primarily supplied by anterior choroidal branches, the anterior temporal branches of the middle cerebral artery, and branches of the posterior communicating and posterior cerebral arteries. Venous drainage is primarily into the basal vein but occasionally into the sphenoparietal sinus or vein of Labbé, especially if there is underlying central venous occlusive disease.[117] Although they may be approached transtemporally through the inferior temporal gyrus, the anterior-most group is best approached through a combined pterional–anterior temporal approach, as described by the senior author.[38, 41] Initially, the sylvian fissure is widely opened to sequentially control, first, the middle cerebral feeders, then the anterior choroidal feeders, and finally, the posterior communicating and posterior cerebral branches.

Midtemporal Lesions. For midtemporal lesions, which often involve the choroid plexus of the temporal horn, a horseshoe-shaped incision extending over the ear is used with a low temporal craniotomy. The head is positioned parallel to the floor with the vertex slightly down to allow the temporal lobe to fall away by gravity. The authors prefer to approach the smaller lesions subtemporally to get early control of the posterior cerebral feeders if the vein of Labbé does not present a problem. The larger lesions can be approached through the inferior temporal gyrus with a cortisectomy anterior or posterior to the vein of Labbé, at times combined with a subtemporal approach. After the temporal horn has been entered, the anterior choroidal feeders are controlled through the choroidal fissure, and the lesion is gradually removed in an anterior-posterior fashion, until, ultimately, the draining venous pedicle at the basal vein is reached. This resection usually produces a superior quandrantanopia from damage to the inferior optic radiations. An approach to these lesions through the superior or middle temporal gyri may seem more direct, but it is also more apt to leave the patient with a severe visual field deficit or dysphasia in the dominant temporal lobe.

Paratrigonal or Posterior Temporal-Occipital Lesions. The paratrigonal malformations are those that involve the superior, medial, and inferior walls of the trigone and, occasionally, the adjacent pulvinar of the thalamus. The supply is primarily from posterior cerebral and posterolateral choroidal artery branches, with medial venous drainage into the basal vein of Rosenthal.

The surgical approach to these lesions depends on whether the lesion is located superior and medial or inferior and lateral to the trigone. In the first of these groups, which Yasargil called "parasplenial" lesions, the authors prefer a transcortical approach through the posterior parietal area with the patient in the semisitting position (Fig. 58–7). The cortical incision is made at a point 2 cm lateral to the falx and 9 cm above the inion (7 cm above the occipital pole) (Fig. 58–8). The transcortical dissection proceeds through a relatively noneloquent area between visual and somatosensory association fibers until the trigonal area is reached. The approach is directed from the cortical incision toward the ipsilateral pupil. Ultrasound imaging can also be helpful in localizing the atrium of the ventricle. If the bone flap is extended to the midline, the splenium can be visualized through the interhemispheric fissure and used as a guide to the location of the atrium (approximately 3 cm lateral in the same axial plane). The inferior dural cut must be diagonal so as not to allow the occipital lobe to herniate over the edge. In this approach, the malformation is encountered before the blood supply has been interrupted; preoperative embolization can be helpful in this respect. Additionally, if the lesion is located mainly posterior to the atrium, the feeding vessels coming from the anteroinferior direction can be interrupted by working in a plane anterior to the malformation. The senior author has found this approach preferable to the interhemispheric approach through the precuneus that is advocated by others because there is essentially no retraction on the occipital lobe, minimizing the likelihood of postoperative visual field deficits.[10, 94, 117]

For those lesions largely situated lateral or inferior to the trigone, the authors prefer a subtemporal-transtemporal approach.[38] With the patient in the lateral position, a lumbar drain in place for brain relaxation, and the head parallel to the floor or tilted with the vertex slightly down, a horseshoe-shaped skin incision is made, and a generous temporo-occipital craniotomy is performed. The initial approach is subtemporal to locate and divide the posterior cerebral feeders, being careful to preserve the vein of Labbé by working anterior and posterior to it if necessary. A transtemporal approach through the inferior temporal gyrus (or perhaps through the middle temporal gyrus on the nondominant side) is used to arrive at the malformation (Fig. 58–9). Dissection proceeds circumferentially, leaving the medial draining vein intact until the end. The difficult aspect of the lesion in this approach is the posterolateral choroidal artery feeding vessels, which are encountered late and deep in the dissection. Operation through the inferior temporal gyrus is likely to leave the patient with a superior quadrantal visual field deficit, but this deficit is pre-existing in many patients and is not very disabling.

Splenial and Posterior Third Ventricle Lesions

Arteriovenous malformations of the splenium are primarily fed by pericallosal branches of the posterior cerebral and distal anterior cerebral arteries as well as

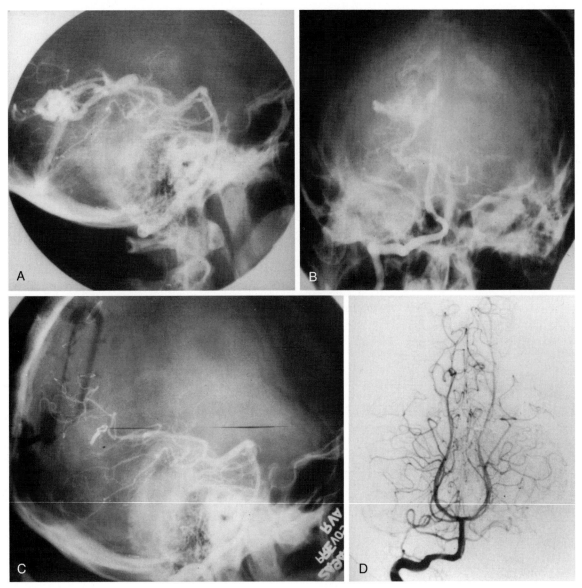

Figure 58–7

Paratrigonal arteriovenous malformation approached through the posterior parietal lobule. Preoperative *(A and B)* and postoperative *(C and D)* vertebral angiography.

by posteromedial choroidal vessels. Additionally, with significant lateral extension, these lesions often recruit posterolateral choroidal feeders (Fig. 58–10). Drainage is usually into the internal cerebral veins and galenic system. Although they appear to be deeply situated on angiography, these lesions are actually seated on the surface of the brain at the base of the interhemispheric fissure. The approach, therefore, is parasagittal on the side with the greatest lateral extension of the lesion.

The authors have used the semisitting position with a generous parieto-occipital craniotomy that extends both 7 to 8 cm in an anteroposterior direction (to allow for different angles of approach between medially draining veins) and across the midline. In addition, the authors have successfully resected several of these lesions using the lateral position with the head parallel to the floor and the ipsilateral side down to allow the occipital lobe to "fall away" with gravity. In these

cases, it is imperative that the medially based dural flap be thin so that the brain falls under the dura and not against the cut edge.

The pericallosal blood supply is approached anteriorly along the posterior part of the corpus callosum. The posterior pericallosal supply is also identified as it originates in the quadrigeminal cistern. Next, the anterior and superior limits of the malformation are identified by an incision through the posterior cingulate gyrus. Delineation of the medial extent of the malformation is aided by dividing the falx, because it often lies across the midline. With gentle retraction on the malformation to the side of its greater bulk, the feeding vessels from the posterior medial choroidal artery can be put on gentle stretch and divided. Lastly, the lateral extent of the lesion is defined by splitting the splenium in the direction of its fibers. If the lesion extends beyond the confines of the splenium, this plane of dissec-

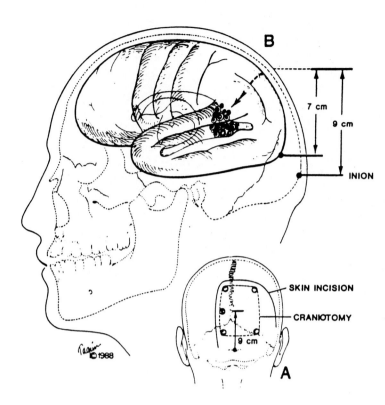

Figure 58–8

Diagram of approach to paratrigonal lesions that are primarily superior and medial to the trigone. The approach is through the posterior parietal lobule (*B*). The craniotomy is centered at a point approximately 9 cm above the inion, and the point of cortical entry is located 7 cm above the occipital pole and about 3 cm off midline (*A*). (From Heros, R. C.: Brain resection for exposure of deep extracerebral and paraventricular lesions. Surg. Neurol., *34*:188–195, 1990. Copyright 1990 by Elsevier Science Inc. Reprinted by permission.)

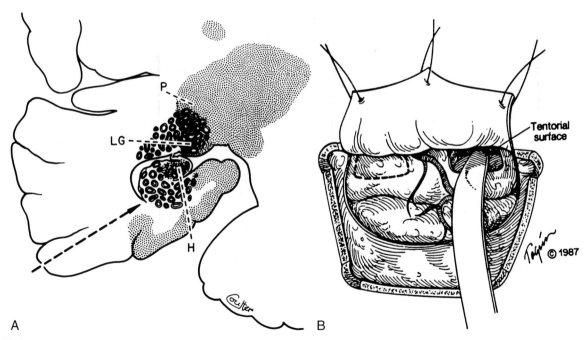

Figure 58–9

A. Diagram of approach through the inferior temporal gyrus to paratrigonal lesions located primarily lateral or inferior to the trigone. H, hippocampus; LG, lateral geniculate body; P, pulvinar. *B.* To minimize retraction of the temporal lobe, brain resection in the inferior temporal gyrus anterior and posterior to the vein of Labbé can be used to resect lesions of the paratrigonal area. (*B* From Heros, R. C.: Brain resection for exposure of deep extracerebral and paraventricular lesions. Surg. Neurol., *34*:188–195, 1990. Copyright 1990 by Elsevier Science Inc. Reprinted by permission.)

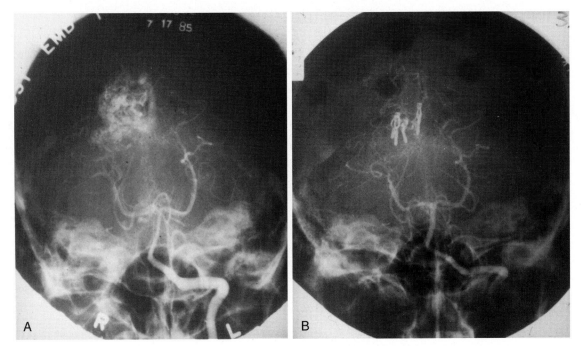

Figure 58–10
Preoperative *(A)* and postoperative *(B)* vertebral angiography of a right parasplenial arteriovenous malformation.

tion can begin through the precuneus anterior to the calcarine fissure. With significant lateral extension, it may be difficult to secure posterolateral choroidal feeders without significant brain retraction. As is always the case, the important medial drainage must be preserved until the end of the resection.

The contralateral parafalcial approach has been advocated by some for resection of these lesions.[24]

Deep Parasagittal and Callosal Lesions

Branches of the pericallosal and callosal marginal arteries supply arteriovenous malformations in this area (the corpus callosum and deep medial hemispheres), and they are drained into the superior and inferior sagittal sinuses. The frontal lesions can be approached through a unilateral frontal craniotomy extending to the midline with the patient in the semireclining position and the head in the neutral position; for more posterior frontal, parietal, and occipital lesions, the patient can be placed in the lateral position with the ipsilateral side down. This latter position should be used only for those lesions that do not reach the cerebral convexities. Lesions that reach the convexity invariably obtain supply from the middle cerebral artery that must be controlled over the convexity with a wider dural flap, which can result in cortical injury against the dural edge in this position. One must always preserve any large, posterior draining veins because, if taken, they can produce disabling venous infarction and hemiplegia.

Anterior Callosal Lesions

The smaller of these malformations involve only the corpus callosum, the cingulate gyrus, and the immedi-

ate subcallosal area, with blood supply from the pericallosal and callosal marginal arteries and drainage superiorly into the sagittal sinus and intraventricularly into the septal vein. The approach is through a unilateral frontal craniotomy extending to the midline. These arteriovenous malformations can be resected by skeletonizing the pericallosal arteries as they pass through the lesion, being careful to preserve the main trunks and taking only the side branches to the malformation.

Resection of larger lesions can be a formidable surgical challenge because they begin to involve the medial aspect of the striatum and anterior hypothalamus (Fig. 58–11). With lateral extension, these malformations recruit feeders from the recurrent artery (Heubner's) and from medial lenticulostriate arteries. With larger lateral extension, they obtain lateral lenticulostriate supply. If this occurs, the lesion is usually inoperable because it involves the internal capsule. These lesions also have blood supply from perforators of the anterior cerebral and anterior communicating arteries, requiring a subfrontal approach. In these large lesions, the approach is through a large bifrontal craniotomy extending from the low frontal area to the coronal suture. Initially, the subfrontal approach allows identification and division of the feeding vessels from the anterior communicating complex and the anterior cerebral arteries. This can be followed by an anterior interhemispheric approach to follow the A_2 vessels distally and then through the callosum to complete the dissection of the medial and intraventricular planes of the lesion.

Hypothalamic and Inferior Frontal Lesions

These lesions are usually small and involve the septal, anterior hypothalamic, and medial subfrontal re-

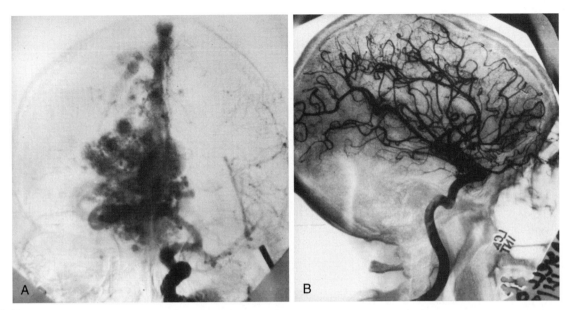

Figure 58–11

Large anterior callosal arteriovenous malformation extending into the basal ganglia. Preoperative *(A)* and postoperative *(B)* carotid angiography.

gions, with feeding vessels from the anterior communicating complex. They are best dealt with through a unilateral pterional subfrontal approach, which provides a direct approach to the feeding vessels.[72] As in the operative approach to anterior communicating aneurysms, a small gyrus rectus cortisectomy may be useful to secure feeders.

Intraventricular Lesions

Although many arteriovenous malformations have some ependymal representation, purely intraventricular ones are relatively rare, comprising only 4 to 13 per cent of large series.[112] In the senior author's opinion, the operability of these lesions is determined by the relative contributions of feeding vessels from perforator as opposed to choroidal arteries. Those lesions fed mostly by deep perforating vessels involve the deep substance of the basal ganglia and thalamus. During dissection around the lesion and within the ganglionic substance, the small friable perforators shrink away, and deep hemorrhage can cause major neurologic morbidity. Conversely, choroidal supply can be controlled at the ependymal surfaces of the lesion and usually indicates that the bulk of the lesion is superficial within the ventricle and therefore operable.

These lesions have, in part, been discussed under other categories. Arteriovenous malformations of the head of the caudate are supplied by choroidal branches, Heubner's artery, and medial lenticulostriate vessels. They are approached through the anterior corpus callosum or, if ventriculomegaly is present, through the lateral frontal horn. The anterior callosal approach can also be used for malformations of the anterior forniceal-septal region.

Arteriovenous malformations in the area of the atrium of the lateral ventricle were discussed under medial temporal lesions. Dorsal thalamic lesions medial to the fornix can be supplied by medial posterior choroidal branches if they are situated medially, or by the posterior lateral choroidal arteries if they are more laterally located. The approach depends on the primary arterial supply. An interhemispheric approach through the splenium is used in the case of lesions in the area of the posterior third ventricle and the velum interpositum, and a transcortical posterior parietal approach is used for the more lateral lesions.

Some lesions located mainly in the region of the lateral ventricle are essentially arteriovenous malformations of the choroid plexus. These can be resected through a variety of approaches: through the corpus callosum or transcortically through the middle frontal gyrus if hydrocephalus is present, through the inferior temporal gyrus if the lesion is situated primarily in the anterior temporal horn, or though the posterior parietal approach if it is located in the atrium. The larger lesions can be so extensive as to involve the entire distribution of the choroid plexus from the temporal tip to the trigone; in these cases, a wide exposure is used to work through the sylvian fissure to control the middle cerebral branches and then across the isthmus of the insula and into the ambient cistern, where posterior cerebral and choroidal branches can be controlled (Fig. 58–12). Subcallosal lesions can be resected by an interhemispheric approach (Fig. 58–13).

Lesions located primarily in the third ventricle can be resected through an anterior transcallosal approach by use of either a transforaminal, interforniceal, or subchoroidal approach, depending on the situation.

Striato-Capsular-Thalamic Lesions

These are lesions of the caudate and putamen, the thalamus, and the internal capsule located lateral to

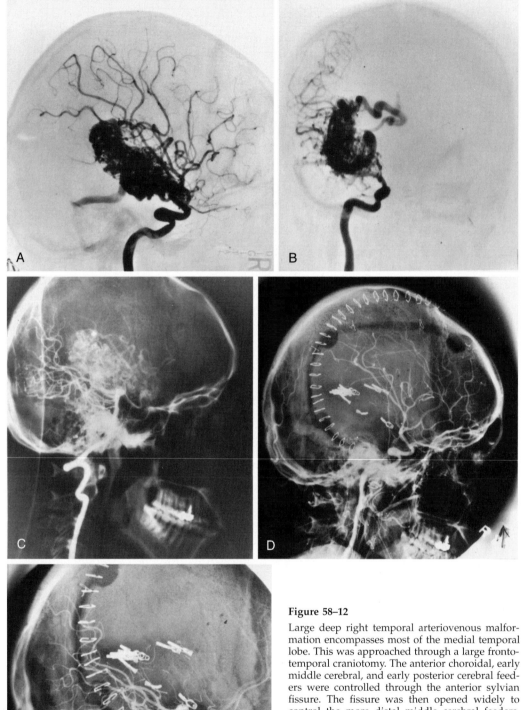

Figure 58–12

Large deep right temporal arteriovenous malformation encompasses most of the medial temporal lobe. This was approached through a large frontotemporal craniotomy. The anterior choroidal, early middle cerebral, and early posterior cerebral feeders were controlled through the anterior sylvian fissure. The fissure was then opened widely to control the more distal middle cerebral feeders, and an incision was made through the isthmus of the insula to gain access to the cisterna ambiens and the distal posterior cerebral and posterolateral choroidal feeders. Preoperative carotid (A and B) and vertebral (C) angiography. Postoperative carotid (D) and vertebral (E) angiography demonstrates complete resection.

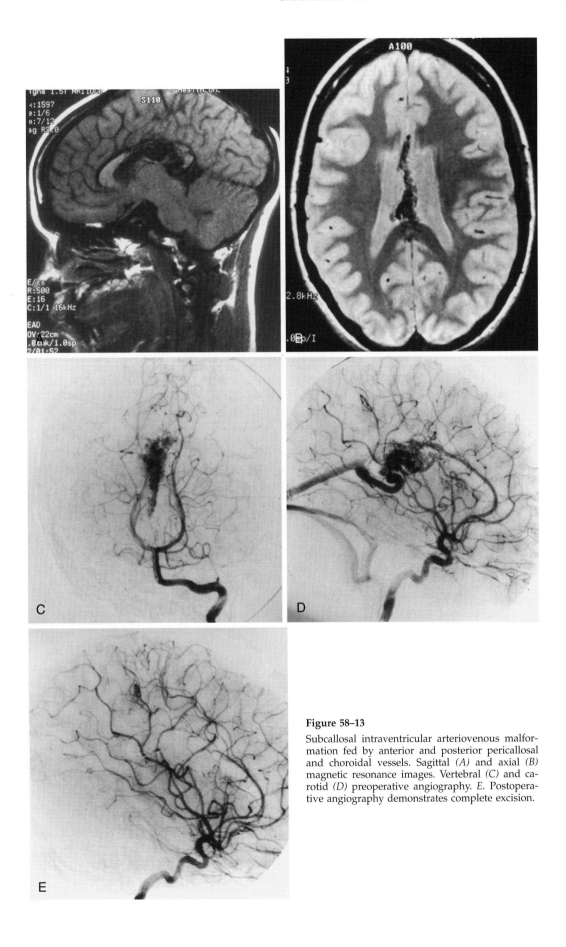

Figure 58–13

Subcallosal intraventricular arteriovenous malformation fed by anterior and posterior pericallosal and choroidal vessels. Sagittal *(A)* and axial *(B)* magnetic resonance images. Vertebral *(C)* and carotid *(D)* preoperative angiography. *E.* Postoperative angiography demonstrates complete excision.

the ventricle and medial to the insula. If they are large and have supply primarily from deep perforators, the authors consider these lesions to be inoperable. However, some can be resected with low morbidity, and they fall into the following categories:

1. Smaller lesions with primarily choroidal vascular supply

2. Small arteriovenous malformations of the head of the caudate nucleus

3. Lesions located lateral to the internal capsule (lateral basal ganglia and insular)

4. Lesions of the dorsal aspect of the pulvinar, as described above

5. Lesions of the inferolateral thalamus fed primarily by circumferential and thalamogeniculate branches of the posterior cerebral artery. Surgical removal of these lesions leaves the patient with a complete homonymous hemianopsia because they involve the lateral geniculate body; however, if hemorrhage has occurred, the patient usually has this deficit already.

Other surgeons have taken a more aggressive approach to these difficult lesions, with good results in selected patients.[55, 92, 95, 109]

INFRATENTORIAL ARTERIOVENOUS MALFORMATIONS

Mesencephalic Lesions

Only the smallest and most superficial of these lesions are readily operable. The small tectal lesions supplied by the posteromedial choroidal and circumferential branches can be approached by a supracerebellar, infratentorial approach. This approach has the advantage of being below most of the important venous structures (i.e., basal, internal cerebral, and galenic veins). Alternatively, a paraoccipital transtentorial approach can be used. As Yasargil has noted, these malformations, which usually present with hemorrhage, may be barely detectable on angiography and are discovered only by the presence of an early filling vein (Fig. 58–14).

Those lesions involving the lateral surface of the mesencephalon can be approached by the subtemporal-transtentorial route with good results (Fig. 58–15).[94] The authors have also used a combined subtemporal-presigmoid approach to these lesions.

Cerebellar Hemispheric Lesions

If the lesion is small and restricted to one hemisphere, a unilateral suboccipital craniotomy is sufficient. If large, these lesions can have blood supply from all three of the major long circumferential arteries that supply the cerebellum. In large lesions, it is necessary to carry the craniectomy from the transverse sinus superiorly, to give access to superior cerebellar artery feeders; to the sigmoid sinus laterally, to allow control of anterior inferior cerebellar artery feeders at the cerebellopontine angle; and past the midline into the foramen magnum inferiorly, to control intertonsillar feeders from the posterior inferior cerebellar artery. The craniectomy can be carried far laterally to the occipital condyle for early control of the posterior inferior cerebellar artery as well.[39] With the larger lesions, feeding vessels can be taken at some distance from the nidus, a technique generally to be avoided in arteriovenous malformation surgery.

Vermian Cerebellar Lesions

The deeper lesions, involving the vermis and deep nuclei or the cerebellar peduncles and lateral brain stem, are more difficult (Fig. 58–16). The vermian lesions are almost always supplied by branches of the superior cerebellar artery, with prominent drainage into the precentral cerebellar vein and the galenic system. They also usually have significant supply from the posterior inferior cerebellar artery, and occasionally they have feeders from the anterior inferior cerebellar artery.

The patient is placed in the sitting position with the head flexed, and a generous bilateral suboccipital exposure is performed with the transverse sinuses and torcula as the superior limit. Initially, a relatively small, superiorly based dural flap is used to control the superior cerebellar artery feeders; in this manner, the cerebellum does not fall against the cut dural edge. After sacrifice of some superficial, superiorly draining veins, the cerebellum falls away by its own weight. These veins can usually be taken because there is prominent drainage anteriorly into the vein of Galen. If there is prominent supply from the posterior inferior cerebellar artery, the dura can later be opened in the midline and the cerebellar tonsils exposed. Dissection between the tonsils reveals the posterior inferior cerebellar artery, which can be traced upward to the choroidal point, after which any significant branches going toward the arteriovenous malformation can be taken with impunity. Significant supply from the anterior inferior cerebellar artery can be controlled laterally in the cerebellopontine angle. The malformation can then be resected by dissecting medially to the floor of the fourth ventricle, laterally, then finally anteriorly.

Resection of unilateral lesions is usually well tolerated. Removal of deep vermian lesions can be expected to produce significant postoperative ataxia that improves with time. This can be particularly disabling in an elderly patient, however, and it must be considered during the discussion of treatment alternatives.

Brain Stem Lesions

Few intrinsic brain stem arteriovenous malformations should be considered operable. In addition to the mesencephalic lesions that have been discussed, small lesions on the floor of the fourth ventricle with circumferential (as opposed to transpontine) arterial supply can be approached suboccipitally. Superficial, laterally situated lesions on the pons or lesions that are partially on the surface of the pons and partially in the cerebellopontine angle can be resected with the use of the

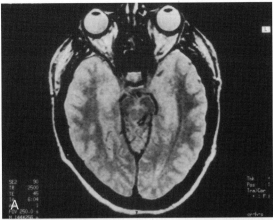

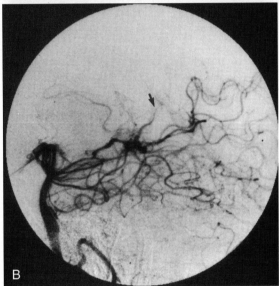

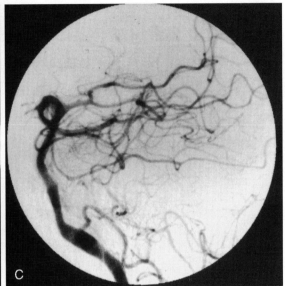

Figure 58–14

A. This magnetic resonance image was performed 2 months after a small hemorrhage into the left tectal area. *B.* Vertebral angiography showed only the hint of an early filling vein draining into the straight sinus *(arrow).* At surgery, a small arteriovenous malformation on the surface of the tectum was found, with an arterialized precentral cerebellar vein. *C.* Postoperative vertebral angiography shows no early filling vein.

combined subtemporal-presigmoid transtentorial approach.

Complications

The types of complications that occur in the surgical treatment of arteriovenous malformations involve all aspects of the patient's preoperative evaluation, intraoperative time, and postoperative course. Each of these is discussed in temporal order.

PREOPERATIVE

In the authors' estimation, faulty surgical judgment is the most frequent cause of complications in arteriovenous malformation surgery. The most common error in this category is misjudgment of the exact topography of a lesion that encroaches on primary motor-sensory, speech, or capsular areas or the brain stem. Spatial misconception is a much less frequent occurrence now that high-resolution magnetic resonance imaging can delineate the exact extent of a given lesion

and its proximity to the motor strip, internal capsule, or brain stem. In the authors' experience, there have been several cases in which surgery would have been recommended based on angiography alone, but definite involvement of the motor strip or brain stem was discovered on magnetic resonance imaging.

If the lesion is found by imaging studies to involve a critical area, a deficit must be expected. Some patients are willing to accept this type of morbidity, depending on their age, occupation, and willingness to live with the uncertain threat of future hemorrhage. Cortical mapping has proved helpful to some.[31, 32] However, this does not alter the technique of arteriovenous malformation resection, which dictates resection exactly at the margin between the lesion and adjacent brain—unless one were to retreat and leave malformation behind, which is clearly dangerous. In the senior author's opinion, intraoperative mapping is useful only if the surgeon is willing to abandon the attempt to resect the arteriovenous malformation before it begins, should the mapping show that the lesion indeed involves critical brain. Most recently, the authors have preferred to use preoperative functional magnetic resonance mapping for that purpose.[44]

Another error in surgical judgment involves surgery

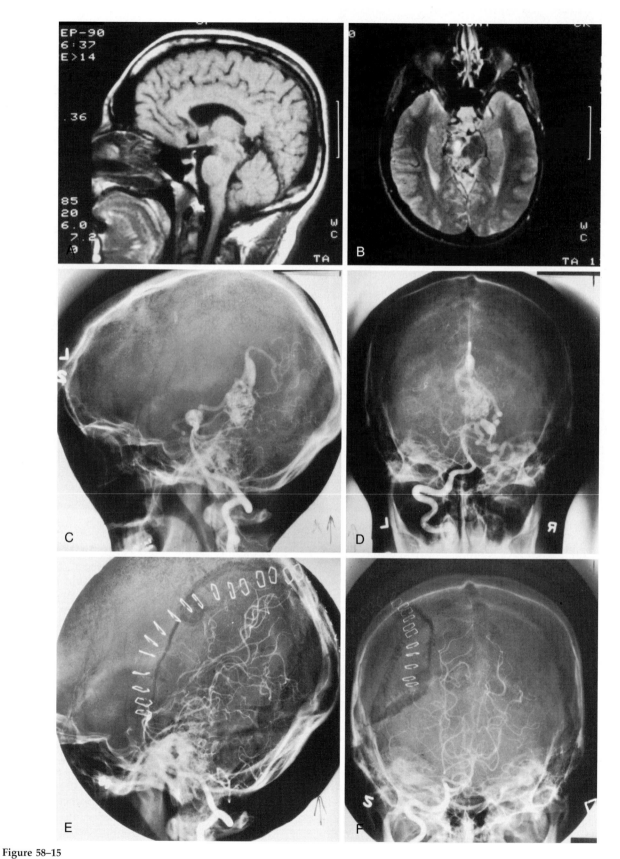

Figure 58–15

Sagittal (A) and axial (B) magnetic resonance imaging of an arteriovenous malformation of the lateral mesencephalon and superior cerebellar peduncle. The lesion was resected through a subtemporal-transtentorial approach. C and D. Preoperative angiography. E. and F. Postoperative vertebral angiography.

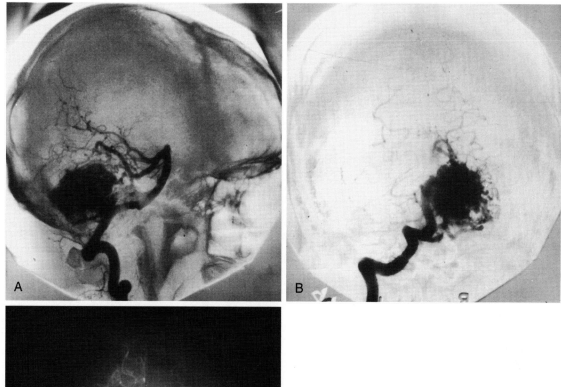

Figure 58–16

Preoperative *(A and B)* and postoperative *(C)* angiography of deep cerebellar arteriovenous malformation fed by branches of superior, anterior inferior, and posterior inferior cerebellar arteries.

on a patient with significant medical risk. The patient must be able to withstand a prolonged time under anesthesia, with significant hemodynamic alterations and, often, major blood loss. A thorough clinical evaluation of pulmonary and cardiovascular systems is warranted in every patient.

At times, a surgeon may underestimate the capacity of a patient to recover from the initial hemorrhage. In a patient with a significant deficit, early operation may be considered, with the thought that the deficit will not be made any worse by surgery. Although this may be true, a potentially reversible deficit can be converted into a permanent one by proceeding with operation in the acute phase, with the difficulties attendant in operating through hemorrhage and increased intracranial pressure. Waiting several weeks often allows patients to recover significantly, and this wait poses minimal additional risk because the chance of early rebleeding is low with arteriovenous malformations. In addition, waiting and repeating the angiography stud-

ies several weeks later often reveals changes in the arteriovenous malformation or even complete thrombosis.

INTRAOPERATIVE

Parenchymal Injury

The next most common cause of complications in our series is parenchymal injury, although at times it can be difficult to separate this result from errors caused by preoperative spatial misconceptions and resection of lesions too close to eloquent brain. Parenchymal injury can be caused by taking too extensive a margin of resection around the malformation while searching for a more "bloodless" plane. The plane of resection must always be kept exactly on the loops of the malformation, regardless of how bloody the field becomes. Indeed, working in a "bloodless" field often means that one has strayed too far from the edge of the malformation into adjacent white matter. As has been mentioned, a relatively avascular gliotic plane surrounding arteriovenous malformations is often incomplete and even nonexistent in most unruptured malformations. The only instance in which a more distant plane can be developed is with polar lesions situated in the frontal or temporal poles, and even then the plane of resection need not be far from the nidus.

Ischemia and infarction of normal tissue, caused by taking feeders at a distance from the malformation, is another cause of parenchymal injury. This can be a problem with arteriovenous malformations supplied by vessels "en passage" that ultimately go on to supply normal brain or by "transitional" vessels, those that supply both the malformation and adjacent brain. All feeding vessels must carefully be followed to the nidus of the lesion before sacrifice. In superficial feeding vessels, the arachnoid must be opened and the vessel must often be followed deep into a sulcus before finally being identified as going to the nidus. Sylvian and anterior callosal arteriovenous malformations, in particular, are often supplied by middle cerebral and anterior cerebral vessels that must carefully be skeletonized as they pass through the lesion so as not to occlude the main trunks, which ultimately supply normal brain.

Retraction injury in the periarteriovenous malformation tissue and its consequent edema are believed by many to be the cause of most transient postoperative deficits. Certainly, major frontal, temporal, or occipital lobe retraction can result in significant edema and often in venous infarction from occlusion of major draining veins. This is why the authors prefer certain approaches that involve some resection of noneloquent brain to prevent vigorous retraction.[40] For instance, retraction on the temporal lobe and potential injury to the vein of Labbé for the subtemporal approach to midtemporal and posterior medial temporal lobe lesions can be obviated by operating through the inferior temporal gyrus. Excessive frontal retraction (with potential injury to major draining veins) for the interhemispheric, transcallosal approach to a lesion in the head of the caudate could be avoided by operating transcortically in the presence of ventriculomegaly. Injury to the occipital lobe from retraction in an interhemispheric approach to a lesion in the medial paratrigonal area can be minimized by a transcortical posterior parietal approach.

By virtue of their long course through the temporal and occipital lobes, the visual radiation fibers must be given special consideration in arteriovenous malformation resections. They are intimately related to the location of many deep temporal, paratrigonal, and occipital arteriovenous malformations, and therefore are often damaged. The senior author has analyzed the effect of surgery on the visual field in 174 patients.[48] Eighteen of these patients experienced a new deficit or worsening of a pre-existing field cut. A careful consideration of the approach to these lesions can often minimize injury to the geniculocalcarine fibers. For instance, in the above-mentioned series, approach to anteriomedial temporal lobe lesions through the sylvian fissure re-

sulted in no visual field deficits in 8 cases. Approach to the larger medial midposterior temporal lesions through the inferior temporal gyrus resulted in hemianopsia in only 3 of 14 cases.

Hemorrhage

Intraoperative hemorrhage can result from premature venous occlusion that causes hyperemia and engorgement of the brain and the remaining malformation. As has been stressed, only if more than one substantial vein drains the malformation can a vein be ligated and divided to help mobilize the nidus. It is good practice, therefore, to leave any arterialized vein intact until the lesion is circumferentially dissected. After excision of the nidus, bleeding from the walls of the cavity most likely represents retained malformation. The authors' approach to identification and resection of these areas has been detailed in the sections on surgical technique.

As discussed, hemorrhage from deep perforating branches can be troublesome. In addition, substantial parenchymal injury can occur during attempts to stop the bleeding from these fragile vessels in the white matter, either from suctioning to identify the vessels or from packing away from the field. As discussed, packing bleeding from these vessels must be avoided at all costs because it can lead to unrecognized parenchymal or intraventricular bleeding.

POSTOPERATIVE

Hemorrhage

The most common cause of hemorrhage in the postoperative period is retained arteriovenous malformation. There are often small rests of this tissue left on the walls of the resection cavity as a natural consequence of carrying the plane of resection as close as possible to the malformation. Under high magnification, it is possible to cut through a small peripheral portion of the lesion. For this reason, careful inspection of the resection wall is absolutely necessary. The authors advise even raising the blood pressure and inspecting the resection bed for at least 15 minutes to provoke bleeding from unrecognized residual arteriovenous malformation fragments. Intraoperative angiography can be extremely helpful in disclosing arteriovenous malformation remnants.

Normal perfusion pressure breakthrough bleeding is probably a rare occurrence, but it can be a cause of postoperative hemorrhage. In our series of almost 300 patients, there were only 4 patients who were thought to have suffered a hemorrhage secondary to perfusion breakthrough. These patients all had large, high-flow malformations in which this complication might have been expected. Two of these patients, who were operated on early in the series, were not embolized, and the other two underwent what proved to be inadequate embolization. This complication could theoretically occur intraoperatively as well, as reported by Day and associates.[23] Treatment includes evacuation of hematoma, careful blood pressure control, institution of barbiturate coma, and antiedemic therapy. With similar treatment, three of the four patients have made good long-term recoveries. This complication may have been seen much more often had preoperative embolization not been used for many of these lesions.

Vascular Thrombosis

After excision of high-flow lesions with the sudden interruption of long draining veins, there exists a theoretical risk of retrograde venous thrombosis with its attendant possibilities of venous infarction and hemorrhage. There is at least one well-documented case of this occurring postoperatively.[63] Retrograde arterial thrombosis is also a theoretical possibility after resection, particularly if long, tortuous feeding arteries are interrupted just as they enter the nidus of the lesion. Miyakasa has demonstrated this occurrence in 5 of 76 patients, only 3 of whom developed neurological deficit.[64]

Although vasospasm may be seen on postoperative angiography in or around a bed, ischemic deficits attributed to cerebral vasospasm of the type seen after aneurysmal subarachnoid hemorrhage are exceedingly rare after arteriovenous malformation surgery. Although the authors have not seen vasospasm in any of the patients in their series, Yasargil reports two postoperative deficits he believes were attributable to vasospasm.[116] The authors do not routinely give prophylaxis with calcium channel blockers to their patients who have bled previously, although in those rare cases with extensive cisternal blood clot this may be a good idea.

Epilepsy

The onset of seizures in patients who were without seizures preoperatively occurs in 6 to 22 per cent of cases, depending on the site of the lesion and the length and thoroughness of follow-up.* In the senior author's series, 15 per cent of the patients had new-onset seizures, but half of them had only one or two seizures in the immediate postoperative period. If patients with an arteriovenous malformation present with intractable epilepsy, intraoperative electrocorticography can be helpful in guiding resection of epileptogenic tissue around the lesion.[118]

Surgical Results

Table 58–2 gives the updated early results of surgical excision of arteriovenous malformations by the senior author. The lesions are categorized by the classification scheme of Spetzler and Martin. The numbers shown represent the status of the patients at the time of discharge from the hospital. It is clear from long-term

---

*See references 1, 29, 35, 43, 75, 79, 83, and 116.

Table 58–2

EARLY SURGICAL RESULTS IN ARTERIOVENOUS MALFORMATION SURGERY* (RCH, 1981–1993)

Grade†	Number of Patients	Good	Fair	Poor	Dead
I	38	38	0	0	0
II	70	67	3	0	0
III	76	60	11	4	1
IV	72	53	13	5	1
V	37	2	8	17	0
TOTALS	293	220	35	26	2

*Results at time of discharge from hospital.
†Grade according to the classification of Spetzler and Martin.

longitudinal studies that there is significant improvement in patients' neurological status after discharge home or to a rehabilitation facility, and many patients are able eventually to move up one or more grades.[43] The overall long-term rate of major morbidity (poor result) in the series of Heros, Korosue, and Diebold was 1.9 per cent, and the mortality rate was also 1.9 per cent (1 of 153 patients); however, for grade V arteriovenous malformations, the combined major morbidity and mortality rate was 19.1 per cent, and another 19.1 per cent of these patients had serious although not disabling morbidity (fair result).

In Table 58–2, "good" refers to a patient with minimal or no neurological deficit who is completely independent, "fair" refers to someone with a mild to moderate neurological deficit who is less than completely independent, and "poor" denotes a patient who is severely incapacitated by a neurological deficit.

With modern microsurgical techniques, all but the most difficult arteriovenous malformations (Spetzler-Martin grades IV or V) can be resected with a minimum of morbidity and mortality, usually less than 5 per cent. However, serious morbidity is attendant in resection of the most difficult lesions, even with the best of care.

Conclusions

The surgical treatment of arteriovenous malformations of the brain can be challenging for the surgeon and perilous for the patient. However, with experience and meticulous attention to detail, the neurosurgeon can resect many of these lesions with a minimum of risk to the patient. Perhaps the most important skill to acquire in dealing with arteriovenous malformations is not a proficiency with microsurgery but rather the ability to wisely determine for which lesions and in what patients an operation is indicated. Although hemorrhage from an arteriovenous malformation can be disabling or deadly, the course in many untreated patients can be quite benign. This may justify conservative treatment or treatment with radiosurgery in some lesions. To leave a young patient with a serious, permanent neurological deficit as a result of an ill-advised surgical resection of a difficult arteriovenous malformation in a neurologically critical area is unjustified. Ultimately, the rational approach to surgery of these lesions must always involve careful assessment of the characteristics of the lesion, the patient and his or her occupation and capacity to cope with a potentially severe deficit, and the surgeon's experience.

REFERENCES

1. Abad, J. M., Alvarez, F., and Manrique, M.: Cerebral arteriovenous malformations: Comparative results of surgical vs. conservative treatment in 112 cases. J. Neurosurg. Sci., 27:203, 1983.
2. Albert, P.: Personal experience in the treatment of 178 cases of arteriovenous malformations of the brain. Acta Neurochir., 61:297, 1982.
3. Al-Rodhan, N. R. F., Sundt, T. M., Jr., Piepgras, D. G., et al.: Occlusive hyperemia: A theory for the hemodynamic complications following resection of intracerebral arteriovenous malformations. J. Neurosurg., 78:167, 1993.
4. Amacher, A. L., Allock, J. M., and Drake, C. G.: Cerebral angiomas: The sequelae of surgical treatment. J. Neurosurg., 37:571, 1972.
5. Andrews, B. T., and Wilson, C. B.: Staged treatment of arteriovenous malformations of the brain. Neurosurgery, 21:314, 1987.
6. Awad, I. A., Robinson, J. R., Jr., Mohanty, S., et al.: Mixed vascular malformations of the brain: Clinical and pathogenetic considerations. Neurosurgery, 33:179, 1993.
7. Azzam, C. J.: Growth of multiple peripheral high flow aneurysms of the posterior inferior cerebellar artery associated with a cerebellar arteriovenous malformation. Neurosurgery, 21:934, 1987.
8. Barrow, D. L., Boyer, K. L., and Joseph, G. J.: Intraoperative angiography in the management of neurovascular disorders. Neurosurgery, 30:153, 1992.
9. Batjer, H. H., and Devous, M. D., Sr.: The use of acetazolamide-enhanced regional cerebral blood flow measurement to predict risk to arteriovenous malformation patients. Neurosurgery, 31:213, 1992.
10. Batjer, H. H., and Samson, D.: Surgical approaches to trigonal arteriovenous malformations. J. Neurosurg., 67:511, 1987.
11. Batjer, H. H., Devous, M. D., Sr., Meyer, Y. J., et al.: Cerebrovascular hemodynamics in arteriovenous malformation complicated by normal perfusion pressure breakthrough. Neurosurgery, 22:503, 1988.
12. Batjer, H. H., Devous, M. D., Seibert, G. B., et al.: Intracranial arteriovenous malformation: Relationship between clinical factors and surgical complications. Neurosurgery, 24:75, 1989.
13. Batjer, H., Suss, R. A., and Samson, D.: Intracranial arteriovenous malformations associated with aneurysms. Neurosurgery, 18:29, 1976.
14. Brown, R. D., Jr., Wiebers, D. O., Forbes, G., et al.: The natural history of unruptured intracranial arteriovenous malformations. J. Neurosurg., 68:352, 1988.
15. Burchiel, K. J., Clarke, H., and Ojemann, G. A.: Use of stimulation mapping and corticography in the excision of arteriovenous malformations in the sensorimotor and language-related neocortex. Neurosurgery, 16:154, 1985.
16. Carter, L. P.: Surface monitoring of cerebral cortical blood flow. Cerebrovasc. Brain Metab. Rev., 3:246, 1991.
17. Chin, L. S., Raffel, C., Gonzalez-Gomez, I., et al.: Diffuse arteriovenous malformations: A clinical, radiological, and pathological description. Neurosurgery, 31:863, 1992.
18. Chioffi, F., Pasqualin, A., Beltramello, A., et al.: Hemodynamic effects of preoperative embolization in cerebral arteriovenous malformations: Evaluation with transcranial Doppler sonography. Neurosurgery, 31:877, 1992.
19. Crawford, P. M., West, C. R., Chadwick, D. W., et al.: Arteriovenous malformations of the brain: Natural history in unoperated patients. J. Neurol. Neurosurg. Psychiatry, 49:1, 1986.
20. Cunha e Sa, M. J., Stein, B. M., Solomon, R. A., et al.: The

21. Curling, O. D., Jr., and Kelly, D. L., Jr.: The natural history of intracranial cavernous and venous malformations. Perspect. Neurol. Surg., 1:19, 1990.
22. Cushing, H., and Bailey, P.: Tumours Arising from the Blood Vessels of the Brain: Angiomatous Malformations and Hemangioblastomas. Vol. 3. Springfield, Charles C. Thomas, 1928, pp. 19–34.
23. Day, A. L., Friedman, W. A., and Sypert, G. W.: Successful treatment of the normal perfusion pressure breakthrough syndrome. Neurosurgery, 11:625, 1982.
24. DeAlmeida, G. M., Shibata, M. K., and Nakagawa, E. J.: Contralateral parafalcine approach for parasagittal and callosal arteriovenous malformations. Neurosurgery, 14:744, 1984.
25. Debrun, G., Vinuela, F., Fox, A., et al.: Embolization of cerebral arteriovenous malformations with bucrylate: Experience in 46 cases. J. Neurosurg., 56:615, 1982.
26. Drake, C. G.: Cerebral arteriovenous malformations: Considerations for an experience with surgical treatment in 166 cases. Clin. Neurosurg., 26:145, 1979.
27. Ehricke H. H., Schad, L. R., Gademann, G., et al.: Use of MR angiography for stereotactic planning. J. Comput. Assist. Tomog., 16:35, 1992.
28. Folkow, B., and Sivertsson, R.: Adaptive changes in "reactivity" and wall/lumen ratio in cat blood vessels exposed to prolonged transmural pressure difference. Life Sci., 7:1283, 1968.
29. Forster, D. M. C., Steiner, L., and Håkanson, S.: Arteriovenous malformations of the brain: A long-term clinical study. J. Neurosurg., 37:562, 1972.
30. Fox, J. L.: Concurrent intracranial aneurysm and arteriovenous malformation. In Wilkins, R. H., and Rengachary, S. S., eds.: Neurosurgery Update. II.: Vascular, Spinal, Pediatric, and Functional Neurosurgery. New York, McGraw-Hill, 1991, pp. 126–128.
31. Garretson, H. D.: Intracranial arteriovenous malformations. In Wilkins, R. H., and Rengachary, S. S., eds.: Neurosurgery. New York, McGraw-Hill, 1985, pp. 1448–1458.
32. Girvin, J. P., Fox, A. J., Vinuela, F., et al.: Intraoperative embolization of cerebral arteriovenous malformations in the awake patient. Clin. Neurosurg., 31:188, 1983.
33. Graf, C. J., Perret, G. E., and Torner, J. C.: Bleeding from cerebral arteriovenous malformations as part of their natural history. J. Neurosurg., 58:331, 1983.
34. Grundy, B. L., Nelson, P. B., Lina, A., et al.: Monitoring of cortical somatosensory evoked potentials to determine the safety of sacrificing the anterior cerebral artery. Neurosurgery, 11:64, 1982.
35. Guidetti, B., and Delitala, A.: Intracranial arteriovenous malformations: Conservative and surgical treatment. J. Neurosurg., 53:149, 1980.
36. Hayashi, S., Arimoto, T., Itakura, T., et al.: The association of intracranial aneurysms and arteriovenous malformation of the brain: Case report. J. Neurosurg., 55:971, 1981.
37. Hernesniemi, J., and Keranen, T.: Microsurgical treatment of arteriovenous malformations of the brain in a defined population. Surg. Neurol., 33:384, 1990.
38. Heros, R. C.: Arteriovenous malformations of the medial temporal lobe: Surgical approach and neuroradiological characterization. J. Neurosurg., 56:44, 1982.
39. Heros, R. C.: Lateral suboccipital approach for vertebral and vertebrobasilar artery lesions. J. Neurosurg., 64:559, 1986.
40. Heros, R. C.: Brain resection for exposure of deep extracerebral and paraventricular lesions. Surg. Neurol., 34:188, 1990.
41. Heros, R. C., and Lee, S. H.: The combined pterional/anterior temporal approach for aneurysms of the upper basilar complex: Technical report. Neurosurgery, 33:244, 1993.
42. Heros, R. C., and Tu, Y. K.: Unruptured arteriovenous malformation: A dilemma in surgical decision making. Clin. Neurosurg., 33:187, 1986.
43. Heros, R. C., Korosue, K., and Diebold, P. M.: Surgical excision of cerebral arteriovenous malformations: Late results. Neurosurgery, 26:570, 1990.
44. Hinke, R. M., Hu, X., Stillman, A. E., et al.: Functional magnetic resonance imaging of Broca's area during internal speech. Neuroreport, 4:675, 1993.

45. Höllerhage, H. G., Dewenter, K. M., and Dietz, H.: Grading of supratentorial arteriovenous malformations on the basis of multivariate analysis of prognostic factors. Acta Neurochir. (Wien), *117*:129, 1992.

46. Kader, A., Young, W. L., Massaro, A. R., et al.: Transcranial Doppler changes during staged surgical resection of cerebral arteriovenous malformations: A report of three cases. Surg. Neurol., *39*:392, 1993.

47. Kondziolka, D., Nixon, B. J., and Lasjaunias, P.: Cerebral arteriovenous malformations with associated arterial aneurysms: Hemodynamic and therapeutic considerations. Can. J. Neurol. Sci., *150*:130, 1988.

48. Korosue, K., and Heros, R. C.: Complications of complete surgical resection of arteriovenous malformations of the brain. *In* Barrow, D. L., ed.: Intracranial Vascular Malformations: Neurosurgical Topics. Park Ridge, IL, American Association of Neurological Surgeons, 1990, pp. 157–168.

49. Krayenbuhl, H., and Wiebenmann, R.: Small vascular malformations as a cause of primary intracerebral hemorrhage. J. Neurosurg., *22*:7, 1965.

50. Lasjaunias, P., Piske, R., and Terbrugge, K.: Cerebral arteriovenous malformations (C. AVM malformation) and associated arterial aneurysms (AA): Analysis of 101 C. AVM cases, with 37 AA in 23 patients. Acta Neurochir., *91*:29, 1988.

51. Luessenhop, A. J.: Cerebral arteriovenous malformations: Parts I and II. Contemp. Neurosurg., *11*:1, 1989.

52. Luessenhop, A. J., and Gennarelli, T. A.: Anatomical grading of supratentorial arteriovenous malformations for determining operability. Neurosurgery, *1*:30, 1977.

53. Luessenhop, A. J., and Rosa, L.: Cerebral arteriovenous malformation: Indications for and results of surgery, and the role of intravascular techniques. J. Neurosurg., *60*:14, 1984.

54. Malik, G. M., and McCormick, P. W.: Surgical resection of thalamocaudate arteriovenous malformations. *In* Wilkins, R. H., and Rengachary, S. S., eds.: Neurosurgery Update: II. Vascular, Spinal, Pediatric, and Functional Neurosurgery. New York, McGraw-Hill, 1991, pp. 149–156.

55. Malik, G. M., Umansky, F., and Patel, S.: Microsurgical removal of arteriovenous malformations of the basal ganglia. Neurosurgery, *23*:209, 1988.

56. Malik, G. M., Morgan, J. K., Boulos, R. S., et al.: Venous angiomas: An underestimated cause of intracranial hemorrhage. Surg. Neurol., *30*:350, 1988.

57. Marin-Padilla, M.: Embryology. *In* Yasargil, M. G.: AVM of the Brain: History, Embryology, Pathological Considerations, Hemodynamics, Diagnostic Studies, Microsurgical Anatomy. *In* Microneurosurgery: IIIA. Stuttgart, Georg Thieme Verlag, 1987, pp. 23–47.

58. Marks, M. P., O'Donahue, J., Fabricant, J. I., et al.: Cerebral blood flow evaluation of arteriovenous malformations with stable xenon CT. A.J.N.R., *9*:1169, 1988.

59. Martin, N., Doberstein, C., and Bentson, J.: Intraoperative angiography in cerebrovascular surgery. Clin. Neurosurg., *37*:312, 1991.

60. McCormick, W. F.: The pathology of vascular ("arteriovenous") malformations. J. Neurosurg., *24*:807, 1966.

61. McCormick, W. F.: Classification, pathology and natural history of angiomas of the central nervous system. Neurol. Neurosurg. Weekly Update, *1*:3, 1978.

62. McCormick, W. F.: Pathology of vascular malformations of the brain. *In* Wilson, C. B., and Stein, B. M., eds.: Intracranial arteriovenous malformations. Baltimore, Williams & Wilkins, 1984, pp. 44–65.

63. Miyakasa, Y., Yada, K., and Ohwada, T.: Retrograde thrombosis of feeding arteries after removal of arteriovenous malformations. J. Neurosurg., *72*:540, 1990.

64. Miyakasa, Y., Yada, K., and Ohwada, T.: Hemorrhagic venous infarction after excision of an arteriovenous malformation: Case report. Neurosurgery, *29*:265, 1991.

65. Mohr, J. P.: Neurological manifestations and factors related to therapeutic decisions. *In* Wilson, C. B., and Stein, B. M., eds.: Intracranial Arteriovenous Malformations. Baltimore, Williams & Wilkins, 1984, pp. 1–11.

66. Mullan, S.: Personal communication, 1993.

67. Mullan, S., Brown, F. D., and Patronas, N. J.: Hyperemic and ischemic problems of surgical treatment of arteriovenous malformations. J. Neurosurg., *51*:757, 1979.

68. Newton, T. H., Troost, B. T., and Moseley, I.: Angiography of arteriovenous malformations and fistulas. *In* Wilson, C. B., and Stein, B. M., eds.: Intracranial Arteriovenous Malformations. Baltimore, Williams & Wilkins, 1984, pp. 64–104.

69. Nornes, H., and Grip, A.: Hemodynamic aspects of cerebral arteriovenous malformation. J. Neurosurg., *53*:456, 1980.

70. Numaguchi, Y., Kitamura, K., Fukui, M., et al.: Intracranial venous angiomas. Surg. Neurol., *18*:193, 1982.

71. Ogilvy, C. S., Heros, R. C., Ojemann, R. G., et al.: Angiographically occult arteriovenous malformations. J. Neurosurg., *69*:350, 1988.

72. Ojemann, R. G., Heros, R. C., and Crowell, R. M.: Arteriovenous malformations of the brain. *In* Ojemann, R. G., ed.: Surgical Management of Cerebrovascular Diseases. 2nd ed. Baltimore, Williams & Wilkins, 1988, p. 347.

73. Ondra, S. L., Troupp, H., and George, E. D.: The natural history of symptomatic arteriovenous malformations of the brain: A 24 year follow-up assessment. J. Neurosurg., *73*:387, 1990.

74. Pak, H., Patel, S. C., Malik, G. M., et al.: Successful evacuation of a pontine hematoma secondary to rupture of a venous angioma. Surg. Neurol., *15*:164, 1981.

75. Parkinson, D., and Bachers, G.: Arteriovenous malformations: Summary of 100 consecutive supratentorial cases. J. Neurosurg., *53*:285, 1980.

76. Pasqualin, A., Barone, G., Cioffi, F., et al.: The relevance of anatomic and hemodynamic factors to a classification of cerebral arteriovenous malformations. Neurosurgery, *28*:370, 1991.

77. Pasqualin, A., Scienze, R., Cioffi, F., et al.: Treatment of cerebral arteriovenous malformations with a combination of preoperative embolization and surgery. Neurosurgery, *29*:358, 1991.

78. Paterson, J. H., and McKissock, W.: A clinical survey of intracranial angiomas with special reference to their mode of progression and surgical treatment: A report of 110 cases. Brain, *79*:233, 1956.

79. Pelletieri, L., Carlsson, C. A., Grevsten, S., et al.: Surgical versus conservative treatment of intracranial arteriovenous malformations. Acta Neurochir. (Wien), *29*(Suppl.):1, 1980.

80. Perret, G., and Nishioka, H.: Arteriovenous malformations: An analysis of 545 cases of cranio-cerebral arteriovenous malformations and fistulae reported to the cooperative study. J. Neurosurg., *25*:467, 1966.

81. Pertuiset, B., Ancri, D., Kinuta, Y. P., et al.: Clipping of the anterior communicating artery to eliminate the contralateral blood supply in supratentorial large AVM of the carotid system: A report of 22 cases. Acta Neurochir. (Wien), *109*:87, 1991.

82. Pertuiset, B., Ancri, D., Sichez, J. P., et al.: Radical surgery in CVM: Tactical procedures based upon hemodynamic factors. *In* Krayenbuhl, H., ed.: Advances and Technical Standards in Neurosurgery, New York, Springer-Verlag, 1983, pp. 81–144.

83. Piepgras, D. G., Sundt, T. M., Jr., Raggowanksi, A. T., et al.: Seizure outcome in patients with surgically treated cerebral arteriovenous malformations. J. Neurosurg., *78*:5, 1993.

84. Rigamonti, D., and Spetzler, R. F.: The association of venous and cavernous malformations: Report of four cases and discussion of the pathophysiological, diagnostic, and therapeutic implications. Acta Neurochir. (Wien), *92*:100, 1988.

85. Robinson, J. R., Awad, I. A., and Little, J. R.: Natural history of the cavernous angioma. J. Neurosurg., *75*:709, 1991.

86. Robinson, J. R., Jr., Awad, I. A., Masaryk, T. J., et al.: Pathological heterogeneity of angiographically occult vascular malformations of the brain. Neurosurgery, *33*:547, 1993.

87. Samson, D.: Surgical treatment of intracranial arteriovenous malformations. Tex. Med., *79*:52, 1983.

88. Samson, D. S., and Batjer, H. H.: Surface lesions: Lobar arteriovenous malformations. *In* Apuzzo, M. L. J., ed.: Brain Surgery: Complication Avoidance and Management. New York, Churchill Livingstone, 1993, pp. 1142–1176.

89. Samson, D., Ditmore, Q. M., and Beyer, C. W., Jr.: Intravascular use of isobutyl 2-cyanoacrylate: Part I. Treatment of intracranial arteriovenous malformations. Neurosurgery, *8*:43, 1981.

90. Sasaki, O., Tanaka, R., Koike, T., et al.: Excision of cavernous angioma with preservation of coexisting venous angioma: Case report. J. Neurosurg., *75*:461, 1991.

91. Shi, Y., and Chen, X.: A proposed scheme for grading intracranial arteriovenous malformations. J. Neurosurg., 65:484, 1986.

92. Shi, Y-Q., and Chen, X-C.: Surgical treatment of arteriovenous malformations of the striatothalamocapsular region. J. Neurosurg., 66:352, 1987.

93. Sisti, M. B., Kader, A., and Stein, B. M.: Microsurgery for 67 intracranial arteriovenous malformations less than 3 cm in diameter. J. Neurosurg., 79:653, 1993.

94. Solomon, R. A., and Stein, B. M.: Surgical management of arteriovenous malformations that follow the tentorial ring. Neurosurgery, 18:708, 1986.

95. Solomon, R. A., and Stein, B. M.: Interhemispheric approach for the surgical removal of thalamocaudate arteriovenous malformations. J. Neurosurg., 66:345, 1987.

96. Solomon, R. A., and Stein, B. M.: Surgical resection of medial hemispheric arteriovenous malformations of the brain. In Wilkins, R. H., and Rengachary, S. S., eds.: Neurosurgery Update: II. Vascular, Spinal, Pediatric, and Functional Neurosurgery. New York, McGraw-Hill, 1991, pp. 140–148.

97. Spetzler, R. F., and Martin, N. A.: A proposed grading system for arteriovenous malformations. J. Neurosurg., 65:476, 1986.

98. Spetzler, R. F., Hargraves, R. W., McCormick, P. W., et al.: Relationship of perfusion pressure and size to risk of hemorrhage from arteriovenous malformations. J. Neurosurg., 76:918, 1992.

99. Spetzler, R. F., Martin, N. A., Carter, L. P., et al.: Surgical management of large AVM's by staged embolization and operative excision. J. Neurosurg., 67:17, 1987.

100. Spetzler, R. F., Wilson, C. B., Weinstein, P., et al.: Normal perfusion pressure breakthrough theory. Clin. Neurosurg., 25:651, 1978.

101. Stein, B. M., and Wolpert, S. M.: Surgical and embolic treatment of cerebral arteriovenous malformations. Surg. Neurol., 7:359, 1977.

102. Steiner, L., Lindquist, C., Cail, W., et al.: Microsurgery and radiosurgery in brain arteriovenous malformations. J. Neurosurg., 79:647, 1993.

103. Sundt, T. M., Jr.: Operative techniques for arteriovenous malformations of the brain. In Barrow, D. L., ed.: Intracranial Vascular Malformations: Neurosurgical Topics. Park Ridge, IL, American Association of Neurological Surgeons, 1990, pp. 111–123.

104. Szabo, M. D., Crosby, G., and Sundaram, P.: Hypertension does not cause spontaneous hemorrhage of intracranial arteriovenous malformations. Anesthesiology, 70:761, 1989.

105. Tamaki, N., Ehara, K., Lin, T. K., et al.: Cerebral arteriovenous malformations: Factors influencing the surgical difficulty and outcome. Neurosurgery, 29:856, 1991.

106. Tarr, R. W., Johnson, D. W., Rutigliano, M., et al.: Use of acetazolamide-challenge xenon CT in the assessment of cerebral blood flow dynamics in patients with arteriovenous malformations. A.J.N.R., 11:441, 1990.

107. Tew, J.: Personal communication.

108. Troost, B. T., and Newton, T. H.: Occipital lobe arteriovenous malformations: Clinical and radiologic features in 26 cases with comments on differentiation from migraine. Arch. Ophthalmol., 93:250, 1975.

109. U, H. S.: Microsurgical excision of the paraventricular arteriovenous malformations. Neurosurgery, 16:293, 1985.

110. Vinuela, F., Dion, J. E., Duckwiler, G., et al.: Combined endovascular embolization and surgery in the management of cerebral arteriovenous malformations: Experience with 101 cases. J. Neurosurg., 75:856, 1991.

111. Vinuela, F., Nombela, L., Roach, M. R., et al.: Stenotic and occlusive disease of the venous drainage system of deep brain AVM's. J. Neurosurg., 63:180, 1985.

112. Waga, S., Shimosaka, S., and Kojima, T.: Arteriovenous malformations of the lateral ventricle. J. Neurosurg., 63:185, 1985.

113. Wilkins, R. H.: Natural history of intracranial vascular malformations: A review. Neurosurgery, 16:421–430, 1985.

114. Willinsky, R., Lasjaunias, P., and Terbrugge, K.: Brain arteriovenous malformations: Analysis of angio-architecture in relationship to hemorrhage (based on 152 patients explored and/or treated at the Hôpital de Bicetre between 1981 and 1986). J. Neuroradiol., 15:225, 1988.

115. Woodard, E. J., and Barrow, D. L.: Clinical presentation of intracranial arteriovenous malformations. In Barrow, D. L., ed.: Intracranial Vascular Malformations: Neurosurgical Topics. Park Ridge, IL, American Association of Neurological Surgeons, 1990, pp. 53.

116. Yasargil, M. G., ed.: AVM of the brain: Clinical considerations, general and special operative techniques, surgical results, nonoperated cases, cavernous and venous angiomas. In Microneurosurgery: IIIB. Stuttgart, Georg Thieme Verlag, 1988.

117. Yasargil, M. G., ed.: AVM of the brain: History, embryology, pathological considerations, hemodynamics, diagnostic studies, microsurgical anatomy. In Microneurosurgery: IIIA. Stuttgart, Georg Thieme Verlag, 1988.

118. Yeh, H. S., Tew, J. M., Jr., and Gartner, M.: Seizure control after surgery on cerebral arteriovenous malformations. J. Neurosurg., 78:12, 1993.

119. Young, W. L., Kader, A., Prohovnik, I., et al.: Pressure autoregulation is intact after arteriovenous malformation resection. Neurosurgery, 32:491, 1993.

120. Young, W. L., Prohovnik, I., Ornstein, E., et al.: The effect of arteriovenous malformation resection on cerebrovascular reactivity to carbon dioxide. Neurosurgery, 27:257, 1990.

Endovascular Treatment of Arteriovenous Malformations

The treatment of neurovascular disorders has undergone great change in the past 25 years with the development of a variety of novel and technically sophisticated therapeutic strategies. The development of the operating microscope and the subsequent advent of the microsurgical era spawned renewed interest in difficult and complex neurovascular disorders, especially in the treatment of arteriovenous malformations. Endovascular therapy, in particular, was developed to enhance the neurosurgeon's margin of safety in treating these lesions and has evolved to be an essential component of multimodal management of neurovascular disorders. Endovascular therapy for these lesions may be employed in combination with microsurgical or radiosurgical therapy or, in rare circumstances, as the sole treatment. The goals of embolization are to enhance the safety of surgical resection, to reduce nidus size to that of a lesion treatable with radiosurgery, or, in rare circumstances, to reduce symptoms of cerebral steal in inoperable lesions. The ultimate goal is elimination of the lesion, although permanent obliteration may not be possible with embolization alone.

HISTORY OF ENDOVASCULAR TREATMENT

Embolization of an intracerebral arteriovenous malformation was first performed in 1960 by Luessenhop and Spence via a direct surgical exposure of the internal carotid artery, through which Silastic spheres were flow-directed into the nidus.[58] In 1970, Boulos and colleagues reported a similar technique with the use of Teflon-coated spheres.[12] The era of endovascular therapy was begun by Serbinenko, who treated a variety of neurovascular lesions, including arteriovenous malformations, with a detachable balloon technique, although few details of the procedure were reported.[91]

In 1975 Debrun and associates followed with a description of the detachable balloon technique and their results.[22] Kerber's development of the calibrated-leak balloon for the first time allowed the direct embolization of the nidus of an arteriovenous malformation through the introduction of a rapidly solidifying polymer.[49]

The development of a microcatheter that could reach the high-order bifurcations of the cerebrovascular system was pioneered in the United States by Target Therapeutics. Their microcatheter, the Tracker microcatheter*, was manipulated by means of a steerable guide wire. The larger lumen of this catheter allowed the use of particulate emboli, such as polyvinyl alcohol particles. Therapeutic embolization with the use of a compressed polyvinyl alcohol sponge was introduced by Tadavarthy and co-workers.[100] Other solid and particulate endovascular agents were developed, including metallic coils, balloon catheters, and polymer threads.[8, 37, 109, 112] In Europe, flow-directed microcatheters, such as the Magic microcatheter,† allowed catheterization of high-order vessels, although only for use with liquid embolic agents.

The development of digital subtraction angiography and other software and technological advances in radiography allowed the refinement of routine and safe catheterization of high-order vessels. The introduction of low-osmolarity, nonionic contrast media lessened the risk of contrast reaction considerably, enhancing the safety of angiography procedures.[92, 93] Real-time fluoroscopy was added to digital subtraction angiography, in the so-called roadmapping technique, to further limit the contrast burden.[89]

OBJECTIVE OF ENDOVASCULAR THERAPY

As the sophistication of endovascular therapy has developed, the role of this modality has become better

*Manufactured by Target Therapeutics, Fremont, California.
†Manufactured by Balt, Montmorency, France.

S. C. Standard • *L. R. Guterman* • *A. K. Wakhloo* • *L. N. Hopkins*

defined. Endovascular therapy aims to change the fundamental hemodynamics of the arteriovenous malformation to enhance the success of additional treatment and ameliorate the malignant natural history of the lesion. As more knowledge is gained in predicting the biological and pathological response to intervention, the precise risks can be more accurately predicted and the procedures more specifically tailored to each lesion. Although modification of the hemodynamics of a malformation in an acute manner with staged embolization may enhance the ease of surgical excision, this benefit must carefully be weighed against the cumulative risks of the additional intervention and compared with the probable natural history of the lesion. Adjunctive therapy is of benefit only if the overall treatment morbidity and mortality are less than those anticipated in the absence of treatment.

ROLE OF THE NEUROVASCULAR MANAGEMENT TEAM

The contemporary management of complex cerebrovascular disorders is best accomplished by a neurovascular team composed of a neurosurgeon, an endovascular therapist, a radiosurgeon, an anesthesiologist with a special interest in neurovascular physiology, and a critical care specialist. The neurosurgeon must direct the overall management of the patient, ensuring that the cumulative risk to the patient is minimized and the natural history of the patient's malformation is considered.

Theoretical Considerations in Endovascular Treatment

HEMODYNAMICS AND CONSEQUENCES OF THERAPY

The nidus of the arteriovenous malformation is defined as the central compartment of the lesion, as distinct from the surrounding normal parenchyma and gliosis. The nidus is composed of a series of compartments, each fed by a discrete arterial supply of pedicles. These compartments have a complex interrelationship and may communicate (Fig. 59–1). The fact that individual compartments are usually fed by individual feeding pedicles means that the appearance on angiography is able to reflect the dissection of these compartments as successive feeding pedicles are embolized.

Despite a limited understanding of the pathogenesis of arteriovenous malformations, their hemodynamic effects have been the subject of a number of reports. The placement of a low-resistance circuit in the cerebrovascular tree increases flow and blood velocity within the regional major arterial conduits.[16] Angiography assessment of flow is qualitative at best, and it is affected by the injection pressure and the concentration of contrast material within the vessel. It is difficult to compare

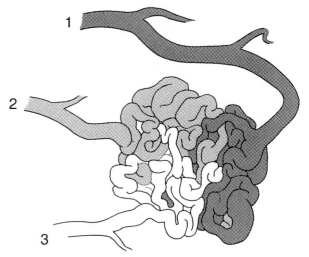

Figure 59–1

Arteriovenous malformations are composed of one or more compartments within a single nidus. Individual compartments are supplied by one or more arterial pedicles (1, 2, 3) and have venous drainage by one or more veins. Compartments may have differing geometric configurations that interdigitate and communicate.

progressive angiograms, especially during the course of embolization.[38] However, rapid flow is commonly identified in the transit time between contrast injection and appearance of the earliest draining vein on angiography. Especially rapid flow may indicate the presence of significant intranidal fistulae.

Flow within an arteriovenous malformation is between 150 and 900 mL per minute, with an average value of 490 mL per minute.[73] The flow (Q) within a feeding pedicle is approximated by the Hagen-Poiseuille equation:

$$Q = \Delta P \pi r^4 / 8\eta L$$

where ΔP is the drop in intraluminal pressure along the vessel, r is the radius of the vessel, η is the viscosity of the fluid, and L is the length of the vessel. The flow is directly related to the difference in pressure between the feeding artery and the draining vein and also to the fourth power of the radius of the vessel. It is inversely related to the length of the feeding artery and the blood viscosity. Thus, arteriovenous malformations with long feeding pedicles and low pressure differentials tend to have slower flow.[57]

A great deal of attention has been focused on the disordered autoregulation of the brain adjacent to the nidus of an arteriovenous malformation. According to the classic theory of Spetzler and colleagues, the parenchymal vessels adjacent to the lesion are exposed to a prolonged condition of low perfusion pressure and have disordered autoregulation.[98] When exposed to high pressure after surgical excision or embolization, these vessels may produce striking cerebral edema or hemorrhage. This disordered autoregulation has been confirmed by studies of stable xenon–enhanced computed tomography with and without acetazolamide challenge and by direct measurement of local cerebral blood flow during craniotomy with thermistor–Peltier stack arrays.* [4, 103] These experiments demonstrated a marked increase in postexcision local cerebral blood flow and disordered carbon dioxide reactivity in two patients who displayed evidence of normal perfusion pressure breakthrough. The staged embolization of malformations through endovascular means or direct cannulation at craniotomy may allow the gradual normalization of autoregulation and prevent this complication.

The hemodynamic profile of an arteriovenous malformation is a function of the number, position, and caliber of its feeding pedicles and their length as well as the resistance of the nidus, venous drainage, and associated fistulae. Several authors have proposed the measurement of the intraluminal pressure of the feeding pedicle as an important index of these parameters. Spetzler and colleagues correlated the pedicle pressure as measured at craniotomy with lesion size and risk of hemorrhage.[96] They reported that small lesions presented more often with hemorrhage and that the difference between the mean arterial pressure and the mean pedicle pressure in lesions that presented with hemorrhage was small (i.e., the lesions that bled had a high mean pedicle pressure). The malformations that presented with other neurological symptoms, such as seizure or steal, tended to have a large difference between mean arterial pressure and mean pedicle pressure; that is, they had a low mean pedicle pressure (Fig. 59–2).

Miyasaka and co-workers have extended these observations to note that high pressure within the draining vein of a malformation has a high correlation with history of hemorrhage.[69] This finding was also significantly correlated with the number of draining veins from the nidus, in that lesions with few draining veins had a higher incidence of hemorrhage. This information should be considered in light of the possibility that small, asymptomatic arteriovenous malformations are less likely to cause seizures or steal and may not come to the attention of the neurosurgeon unless there is hemorrhage.

The relation between pressure and hemorrhage has important implications for embolization in that the pressure in the feeding arterial pedicles tends to rise as the embolization progresses. Jungreis and Horton studied the changes in feeding pedicle pressures in pedicles undergoing embolization and reported an abrupt rise just before angiographic stasis was achieved.[46] Duckwiler and colleagues reported that an accurate measurement of intraluminal pressure may be obtained through a microcatheter and that an abrupt rise may signal a dangerous change in the risk of developing normal perfusion pressure breakthrough in the surrounding parenchyma, as well as an increase in the pressure experienced by untreated compartments of the nidus.[24] Measurement of draining vein pressure has not been performed during therapeutic embolization, but Nornes and Grip noted a significant drop in draining vein pressure during craniotomy for the surgical removal of arteriovenous malformations.[73]

Rapid flow within major vessels is associated with

*Manufactured by Flowtronics, Phoenix, Arizona.

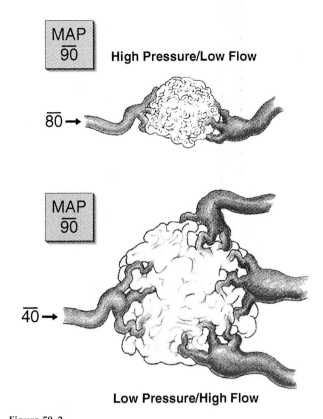

Figure 59–2

Schematic drawing of two types of arteriovenous malformations characterized by flow, size, and mode of presentation. Small lesions *(top)* tend to present with hemorrhage and have high mean pedicle pressures. Notice also the low flow and compact nidus with a single draining vein. Large lesions *(bottom)* tend to have low mean pedicle pressures and high flow rates. Notice the multiplicity of draining veins.

changes of the vessel walls. Histological evaluation of experimental chronic arteriovenous fistulae has revealed a high-flow angiopathy affecting all three layers of the vessel wall.[78] Endothelial cells are plump and irregular, with denuded areas to which platelet aggregates may adhere. Changes in the media consist of an irregular, duplicated, and thinned elastic lamina with invasion of mesenchymal cells; in addition, the adventitia may exhibit neovascularity. Vessels that feed the malformations as well as the nidal and arterialized veins may be abnormal and potentially more subject to the trauma of catheterization. Therefore, meticulous angiography technique is essential in catheterization of these lesions.

An adequate model of an intracranial arteriovenous malformation has not been developed for analysis of hemodynamics or for evaluation of endovascular therapy. Hecht and colleagues developed a computer model for the analysis of the progress of particulate embolization; it assumes no fistulous component and a series of parallel channels that are occluded at a constant rate by uniformly and randomly distributed emboli.[38] Flow was observed to diminish rapidly as the terminal phase of embolization was reached, with a precipitous change in percentage of flow within the last bolus of particulate emboli. These results explain the observation that no apparent change in flow is seen on angiography during the first phase of embolization but that just before stasis is achieved, the flow changes precipitously.

Massoud and colleagues presented a novel swine model for the simulation of intracranial arteriovenous malformations.[65] Pigs have a well-defined rete mirabile, composed of fine vessels (75 to 150 microns in diameter), which is supplied by the ascending pharyngeal arteries. By creating a low-resistance circuit in one carotid artery through anastomosis with the internal jugular vein and ligation of the proximal carotid artery, the blood flow is preferentially directed through the "nidus" of the pig rete and into a low-resistance outflow. Although this model does not accurately reproduce the hemodynamics of an arteriovenous malformation and the surrounding neural elements, it may be appropriate for the implementation of some endovascular techniques.

Indications for Treatment and Timing of Procedure

CLINICAL PRESENTATION

Patients who present with intracerebral or subarachnoid hemorrhage are stabilized and treated by a coordinated neurovascular team. Diagnostic angiography is performed, and a treatment strategy is devised. Optimal timing of initiation of therapy after hemorrhage is controversial. Most authorities recommend waiting at least 4 to 8 weeks before embolization.[106] Embolization should proceed after the acute effects of the hemorrhage are over and the patient's neurological condition has stabilized. The deferment of treatment for a few weeks does not add an appreciable risk to the patient, unless an aneurysm is found on diagnostic angiography. In such a case, the authors prefer to treat the aneurysm acutely and the arteriovenous malformation as the clinical condition of the patient permits.

RADIOLOGICAL GRADING CRITERIA

Spetzler and Martin have devised a grading system for arteriovenous malformations that correlates with the risk of neurological complications after surgical resection.[95] Lesions are given a score based on size, pattern of venous drainage, and location, from 1 (small, superficial, and easily resected) to 5 (deep, large, and complex in eloquent cortex). This grading system has become widely accepted and is helpful in describing the complexities of these malformations, but it has not yet been shown to correlate with the risk of postembolic complications. Other factors, such as feeding pedicle pressure, number and tortuosity of feeding pedicles, presence of intranidal fistulae, and angioarchitecture, play a role in the difficulty and thus the risk of embolization.

Magnetic resonance imaging and magnetic resonance angiography can add significantly to the understanding of pre-embolization and postembolization flow dynamics. Magnetic resonance imaging allows some characterization of the size of the nidus and may eventually provide a quantitative volumetric measurement of the progress of staged embolization. Phase-contrast magnetic resonance angiography allows quantification of flow velocity and provides significant information regarding nidus and feeding pedicle morphology.[44] However, significant artifacts, caused by metallic clips and hemosiderin, are present in the imaging, especially in time-of-flight magnetic resonance angiography. Phase-contrast magnetic resonance angiography is susceptible to flow-aliasing artifacts.

Chappell and colleagues demonstrated the usefulness of magnetic resonance angiography in the delineation of single-pedicle malformations but showed that the detection of intranidal aneurysms and angiomatous changes was unreliable, especially in large lesions.[15] The ability to precisely delineate vessels en passage and venous outflow obstructions will be necessary if magnetic resonance angiography is to replace digital subtraction angiography. Further progress in this area may allow more precise noninvasive quantification of the hemodynamics of these lesions throughout the treatment period.

STAGING OF PROCEDURE

Preoperative embolization of arteriovenous malformations may be performed at a single session, but more commonly a staged approach to the lesion is adopted to allow a gradual adjustment of the regional hemodynamics. Serial examination of arteriovenous malformation hemodynamics has demonstrated that vasoreactivity in adjacent parenchyma is normalized within 10 days to 2 weeks after embolization.[103] However, a delay in definitive treatment allows the recruitment of alternative pial and dural collateral feeding vessels, and recanalization of previously embolized pedicles may occur with both particulate and liquid polymer embolization.[27, 75, 107]

Typically, one to four pedicles of a malformation are embolized per session, and then the patient is allowed to recover. The optimum schedule for staged embolization is controversial, ranging from 48 hours to 2 weeks to 1 month.[56, 98a, 107] In a patient with several arterial feeding pedicles, the number of sessions required varies from one to five.[28] Specifically, deep, surgically inaccessible feeders are selected for embolization first, and staged embolization proceeds to obliteration of accessible feeding pedicles immediately before surgery. This decision must be tempered by the relative number of pedicles encountered in a given major vascular territory. Usually, only one major vascular territory is addressed per session. The authors recommend staged embolization in sessions 3 to 6 weeks apart in patients in whom surgical intervention is planned.

General Endovascular Techniques

PREOPERATIVE EVALUATION

Patients are evaluated by the neurovascular team and selected for endovascular therapy. An extensive neurological examination and a screening medical evaluation are carried out. Particular emphasis is placed on focal neurological deficits and examination of cerebral functions at risk during the embolization of specific vascular territories. Also of importance is the attention span and cooperativeness of the patient, because of the often long duration of the embolization procedure and the necessity of cooperation with serial neurological examinations.

Medical history of cardiopulmonary or, more importantly, renal disease is carefully assessed; complete blood count, coagulation profile, bleeding time, and metabolic profile screenings are performed. Evidence of peripheral vascular disease, especially of the common femoral artery, is important because it may alter the percutaneous access route of the procedure. Alternative access may be provided through brachial or axillary arterial approaches.

History of contrast allergy is not an absolute contraindication to the performance of endovascular procedures, given the low incidence of severe hypersensitivity reactions to nonionic contrast media, reported to be 0.04 per cent.[48] Life-threatening reactions to nonionic contrast media occur in 0.004 per cent of patients, although mild symptoms may occur in as many as 3 per cent of patients. A history of contrast reaction increases the rate of severe reactions to 0.1 per cent. Premedication of patients with suspected contrast allergy or allergy to shellfish is performed with intravenous steroids and histamine antagonists.

Radiological evaluation of the patient includes high-quality three-vessel or, occasionally, four-vessel cerebral angiography. If a notable period has passed since the diagnostic angiography, thorough diagnostic angiography of the internal and external carotid system must be repeated before embolization. Evaluation of the number and caliber of the feeding pedicles and their surgical accessibility is performed, and the nidus volume is calculated by multiplying $0.52 \times$ length $\times$ width $\times$ height.[74] The pattern of venous drainage is identified. The clinician should be alert to the presence of arteriovenous fistulae and any aneurysms or venous stenoses that may be present. An assessment of the eventual microsurgical strategy is made in collaboration with the neurosurgical staff, and a therapeutic plan is devised.

PREOPERATIVE COUNSELING

Consultation with the patient and the family is extremely important, especially in light of the lengthy and complex course of the treatment of these lesions. The natural history of arteriovenous malformations and the relative risk of the patient's individual lesion are reviewed. Therapeutic options, including the option of nontreatment, are reviewed. The procedure of embolization is explained, as is the importance of perseverance until definitive treatment is achieved, and the patient is informed that except in rare cases embolization is not a substitute for eventual treatment by surgical excision. Female patients must be advised of the risk of radiation exposure to the unborn fetus should they become pregnant during the treatment interval. The possible complications of contrast reaction and stroke in the distribution of the vessel and the risks of hemorrhage and death are also explained.

PREOPERATIVE TREATMENT

Patients are routinely admitted the night before the procedure. Completion of the preoperative assessment is ensured, and the patient is given nothing to eat or drink after midnight. Intravenous corticosteroids help to prevent any postembolization intracerebral edema, but they must be instituted 8 to 12 hours before the procedure for maximal effect.[13] Corticosteroids have an additional benefit in ameliorating the effects of contrast reaction, should it occur. However, complications of corticosteroid therapy, particularly hyperglycemia and inhibition of fibrinolysis, may develop and must be carefully avoided.[64]

Twelve to 24 hours of intravenous crystalloid hydration therapy is instituted, and two large-bore intravenous infusion lines are placed. Hydration minimizes the nephrotoxicity caused by the considerable contrast load that these patients receive and enhances perfusion of jeopardized neural tissues should embolic complications occur.

Cerebroselective calcium channel blockers, such as nimodipine, are usually favored; administration is begun 12 to 24 hours before the procedure for the prevention of cerebral vasospasm and for cerebral protection. Experimental data have implicated the influx of calcium through voltage-dependent channels as a final common pathway in irreversible cell injury.[17] Nimodipine has been shown to be cytoprotective in clinical and experimental models of ischemia.[31] Therefore, the authors attempt to provide an environment that is conducive to limiting neuronal loss should vessel occlusion or hemorrhage occur.

Patients also receive a low dose of benzodiazepine and, sometimes, narcotic analgesic to lessen preoperative apprehension and provide smooth induction of neuroleptic analgesia during the procedure. Intramuscular atropine inhibits reflex bradycardia when the carotid bifurcation is manipulated during placement of the guiding catheter. A Foley catheter is placed to avoid reflex hypertension during bladder expansion and to provide for patient comfort during lengthy embolization sessions.

EMBOLIZATION TECHNIQUE

Monitoring and Anesthesia

Patients are monitored throughout the procedure by electrocardiography and measurements of blood pressure, pulse rate, and oxygen saturation. Electroencephalography is rarely indicated, except if the patient requires general anesthesia and is undergoing embolization near eloquent neural structures. Neuroleptic analgesia is obtained by administration of short-acting benzodiazepines (midazolam, 1 to 2 mg, or diazepam, 2 to 5 mg) in combination with narcotic analgesics. Especially in the elderly patient, the oxygen saturation must be carefully monitored because of the synergistic respiratory depressive effects of these drugs.[68]

Arterial Access

Arterial access is usually obtained by cannulation of the common femoral artery through the Seldinger technique.[90] A large-bore (7- to 9-French) introducer catheter is inserted, sutured in place, and connected to heparinized saline irrigation. Sometimes, if significant arteriosclerosis of the femoral artery or aorta exists, alternative arterial access points can be used. Transaxillary brachial or direct carotid access is possible but is associated with a significant incidence of local complications, including brachial plexopathy, hematoma, and arterial dissection.

Anticoagulation

The use of anticoagulation during embolization of arteriovenous malformations is controversial, although it is widely employed. The risk of cerebral embolism is low if meticulous angiography technique is maintained and the duration of the procedure is short. Emboli may form around or within a catheter owing to irregularities in the catheter or trauma from passage of the guide wire. Thrombus can be identified in almost all catheters on microscopy, and emboli may derive from improperly handled flushing solutions or contrast solutions.[52] The purpose of heparinization is to limit the propagation of thrombus on catheters, guide wires, and adjacent portions of arteries undergoing therapeutic manipulation. Anticoagulation may also be of benefit if iatrogenic arterial dissection occurs.

The disadvantage of anticoagulation is that devastating hemorrhagic complications may ensue from intranidal hemorrhage or inadvertent vascular perforation. Hemorrhagic complications may prove overwhelming before physiological inactivation of heparinization can be achieved by administration of protamine sulfate (20 to 30 minutes), or before operative management can be undertaken.[79] Vascular perforations are most commonly caused by guide wires and can usually be controlled by endovascular means.

In most institutions, heparinization is routinely applied during endovascular procedures, especially if the procedure is expected to be lengthy. Maintenance of the activated clotting time at 300 seconds or longer (two to three times control) provides an adequate and easily reversible level of anticoagulation. Protamine sulfate (1 mg per 100 U of heparin) may be used to reverse the effects of heparinization at the termination of the procedure.

Catheters

Diagnostic angiography is performed through a guiding catheter inserted coaxially through the introducer sheath (Fig. 59–3) and then navigated into final position. In the anterior circulation, the guide catheter is positioned in the petrous portion of the internal carotid artery; in the posterior circulation, the catheter is positioned adjacent to the C2 arch. The guide catheter is positioned as close as possible to the malformation to minimize the distance traversed by the microcatheter. Positioning of the catheter beyond the carotid siphon is associated with an increased risk of carotid dissection. If significant tortuosity of the carotid artery exists, the catheter may be positioned proximal to the curve and steered with the microcatheter, or the artery may be straightened by navigating the catheter beyond the coiled segment, although this risks dissection or occlusion of the vessel. If extreme tortuosity exists, surgical correction of the course of the artery by end-to-end anastomosis may be performed before embolization, or a microcatheter may be inserted by direct percutaneous puncture of the internal carotid artery.[54] Alternatively, the patient may be treated by selective cannulation of selected feeding pedicles during craniotomy.[97]

Microcatheters are available in flow-directed* and steerable guide wire† versions. They are available with external terminal dimensions as low as 2.2 French (Fig. 59–4). Guide wires of various configurations are available with easily shaped tips of variable stiffnesses. Commonly available sizes are 0.016 inch and 0.010 inch. The microcatheter is inserted coaxially through

---

*Magic, manufactured by Balt, Montmorency, France; Zephyr, manufactured by Target Therapeutics, Fremont, California.

†Tracker, manufactured by Target Therapeutics, Fremont, California.

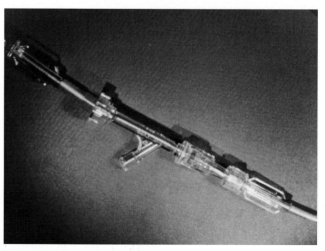

Figure 59–3

Guiding catheter with coaxial microcatheter and guide wire in position. Typically, the guiding catheter is placed at the level of the petrous internal carotid artery or in the vertebral artery at the C2 level. Notice the rotating hemostatic valve connector, which allows attachment of a heparinized saline flush pack along with microcatheter.

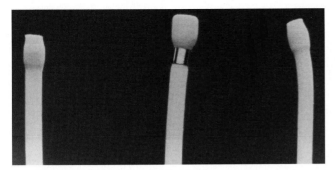

Figure 59–4

Typical flow-directed microcatheters are available in sizes as small as 2.2 French. Tips may be shaped by gentle steam heating. Notice the dilatation at the end to allow flow-direction of the catheter.

the guide catheter by use of a Y-shaped rotating hemostatic adapter that allows movement of the microcatheter through an O-ring type of hemostatic valve and simultaneous infusion of heparinized saline through the side port (Fig. 59–5). The steerable guide wire is moved into the feeding pedicle, and the microcatheter is advanced over the wire. Considerable technical skill is required to perform catheterizations of the higher-order (sixth- to seventh-order) vessels that often comprise the feeding pedicles to the malformation. As the tip of the microcatheter is advanced further distally, considerable mechanical energy may be stored in the catheter, so that the correlation of the manipulation of the proximal catheter with the movement of the distal catheter is not congruent.

Flow-directed catheters are placed through a guiding catheter in a fashion similar to that used with the steerable guide wire microcatheter. The end of the catheter has a small dilatation that allows the catheter to be carried by the blood column. The surgeon selects the vessel by trial and error, using blood flow and small pulses of saline given through the catheter with a syringe. The small size of the flow-directed microcatheter makes it best suited for liquid adhesive agents.

Angioarchitecture

The pedicle for embolization is selected preoperatively, based on the overall treatment strategy for the malformation. If the lesion has several arterial feeding pedicles, deep and inaccessible vessels are embolized first to facilitate surgical resection. Consideration of the difficulty of catheterization of vessels and the relative contribution of each vessel to the overall nidus is also important. Embolization of feeding pedicles in eloquent cortex is possible and gives the surgeon the advantage of performing a functional challenge test in an awake patient rather than dealing with these vessels at surgical resection in an anesthetized patient. The patient's neurological status is evaluated, and then a small bolus of sodium amobarbital (Amytal) or sodium methohexital (Brevital) is slowly injected into the vessel to be embolized. If no subsequent neurological dysfunction is observed on repeat examination, embolization can usually be performed safely. Any vessel can be embolized if the catheter can be positioned distal to all branches supplying normal neural tissue. Anatomical localization alone is an inadequate method of determining safety of embolization.

The development of collateral blood supply after embolization is complex; theoretically, an advantage exists in embolizing these pedicles in close temporal proximity to the surgical resection. Fournier and colleagues suggest that the occipital cortex is especially prone to recanalization through collateral supply and deserves special consideration.[28] Arteriovenous malformations are known to acquire both leptomeningeal and dural supply, and therefore careful angiography of the possible dural collaterals should be performed before operative excision (Fig. 59–6).

Aneurysms are found on feeding pedicles in 2.7 to 9.3 per cent of patients harboring arteriovenous malformations.[5, 40, 76] The significance of these aneurysms has been debated, but they have been reported to be associated with a high incidence of hemorrhage. In one series, of the patients harboring arteriovenous malforma-

Figure 59–5

Rotating hemostatic adapter allows constant irrigation of the dead space of the coaxial catheter system while it maintains torque control of the catheter. Notice the guide wire being rotated by a torque vise.

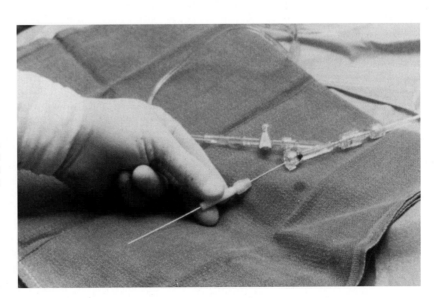

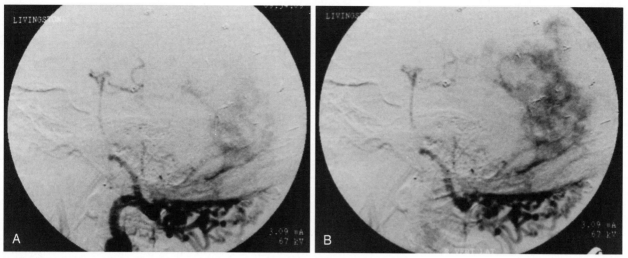

Figure 59–6

A and B. Lateral left vertebral angiography of a 43-year-old patient with a large left temporoparietal arteriovenous malformation after staged embolization of anterior circulation pedicles, showing revascularization through transcranial collateral vessels from muscular branches of the vertebral artery. Notice the intense recruitment of the blood supply at a site remote from the arteriovenous malformation. Preoperative embolization of these vessels lessens blood loss during craniotomy.

tions that presented with intracerebral hemorrhage, 78 per cent were thought to have bled from the aneurysm.[5] Marks and colleagues distinguished between proximal aneurysms on the circulus arteriosus and aneurysms occurring on the feeding pedicles.[62] In this report, aneurysms occurring on the feeding pedicles were not associated with an increased frequency of hemorrhage.[63] More recently, Cunha and associates have classified five types of aneurysms that occur in association with arteriovenous malformations.[19] In this series, the aneurysms on feeding pedicles were often symptomatic, and all symptomatic aneurysms were treated by direct surgical clipping before embolization. No cases of aneurysmal rupture followed therapeutic embolization in this series.

Although aneurysms on feeding pedicles may regress after treatment, pedicles that harbor aneurysms should be embolized first to minimize the risk of hemorrhage.[28] The risk of aneurysmal rupture increases secondary to rises in intraluminal pressure and flow that occur after embolization of feeding pedicles. Guide wire perforation of pedicle aneurysms has also been reported.[36] Garcia-Monaco and associates reported that pseudoaneurysms within arteriovenous malformations are associated with a relatively high incidence of rebleeding.[29] Their report suggests that liquid adhesive embolization should be employed to definitively obliterate the pedicle aneurysm and the nidus of the malformation simultaneously. Aneurysms of the circulus arteriosus should be managed in accordance with their size and clinical history.

The presence of significant arteriovenous fistulae is a major consideration in planning embolization of a feeding pedicle because they represent the least resistant pathway for blood flow through the malformation. Although fistulae may be difficult to accurately visualize even with rapid-sequence angiography, their presence may be inferred by extremely rapid flow within the lesion. Fistulae are thought to occur in a majority of arteriovenous malformations. Typical diameters of intranidal vessels are thought to be 70 to 275 microns.[55] The size of a fistula is difficult to measure but may be as large as 1,200 microns. Particulate embolization of arteriovenous malformations relies on the embolization of nidus vessels, but particles have been documented by radiolabeled monitoring to pass through the arteriovenous fistulae of the nidus to the pulmonary circuit.[26] Clinically, the presence of fistulae may prevent successful particulate embolization of the nidus, necessitating the use of solid embolic materials (i.e., coils or silk) to occlude the fistulae before definitive embolization of the nidal vessels may be performed.

Measurement and Significance of Pedicle Pressure

Pressure within the feeding arterial pedicle of an arteriovenous malformation has been correlated with the risk of hemorrhage from the nidus.[96] Measurement of the pedicle pressure through a microcatheter was confirmed by Duckwiler and co-workers to be an accurate reflection of the intraluminal pressure in most cases, although elevation of 10 mm Hg was observed with the use of a Tracker 18 microcatheter.[24] Pedicle pressures tend to rise during embolization and to approach the mean arterial pressure.[47] Takemae and associates measured systolic pedicle pressures in embolization and reported that in well-embolized pedicles the final pressure tended to be higher.[101]

More recent investigations have revealed that a rise of more than 75 per cent in the mean pedicle pressure is associated with an increased incidence of hyperemic and hemorrhagic complications.[1] Sudden rises in perfusion pressure to surrounding cerebral cortex are thought to underlie the development of normal perfusion pressure breakthrough and therefore should be avoided during therapeutic embolization. More importantly, significant rises in pedicle pressures may be transmitted to untreated compartments of the lesion and result in an increased possibility of hemorrhage.

Provocative Testing

One of the significant advantages of endovascular techniques is the ability to assess neurological function during the procedure. Wada and Rasmussen first employed intra-arterial sodium amobarbital (Amytal) within the internal carotid artery to evaluate cerebral dominance before epilepsy surgery.[108] Rauch and colleagues adapted this technique for the superselective injection of cerebral arteries.[83] Reversible neurological changes in the distribution of the cerebrovascular tree may be assessed by this method before definitive embolization of the vessel. The rate of positive Amytal tests is approximately 20 per cent, depending on the adjunctive assessment with electroencephalography.

The predictive value of the Amytal test is high. Forty per cent of patients develop neurological deficit if embolization is performed in the face of a positive test. The rate of neurological deficit with a negative Amytal test (false-negative result) is reported to be 5 to 8 per cent, although in one case the test changed from negative to positive as the embolization progressed. This phenomenon may be caused either by the changing hemodynamics of the malformation during the course of embolization or by reflux of embolic materials into the normal vasculature. Rising intraluminal pressure diminishes the sump effect of the malformation and allows greater perfusion of collateral vascular pedicles and normal cortical vessels as the nidus is occluded. Therefore, the Amytal test should be repeated whenever there is a change in the lesion on angiography.

Because multiple injections of amobarbital may result in significant sedation, some authors have advocated a shorter-acting barbiturate, sodium methohexital. Evidence indicates that there is a low incidence of arterial vasospasm and seizure with this agent in a 1 per cent concentration, and no false-negative results have been reported; no embolizations were performed in the face of a positive Brevital test.[77]

The evaluation of cranial nerve function during therapeutic embolization is performed with the use of intra-arterial injection of lidocaine in the external carotid system.[42] Thirty to 70 mg of lidocaine in 2 per cent solution are injected. Evaluation of dural supply of the lesions should always include both barbiturate and lidocaine injection to rule out the risk of cerebral or cranial nerve dysfunction after embolization.

Embolic Agents and Technical Considerations

The ideal material for endovascular embolization of arteriovenous malformations does not exist. Ideally, an embolic agent should be nonbiodegradable, nontoxic, and nonmutagenic. It should be easily delivered through a microcatheter, should be easily seen at fluoroscopy, and should bond to the walls of the vessels without extravasation or recanalization. Finally, ideal embolic materials should be soft enough to allow retraction of the lesion from surrounding normal tissues during surgical excision.[56, 80]

Liquid Adhesive Polymers

The development of the earliest microcatheter with a calibrated-leak balloon allowed the delivery of rapidly solidifying liquid adhesive polymers for the treatment of arteriovenous malformations. The alkylcyanoacrylates have been most widely used, especially isobutyl 2-cyanoacrylate.[23, 50] The exposure of the monomer solution to an ionic environment, such as blood, results in polymerization, the essential step being the addition of a negative ion to open the carbon-carbon double bond.[14] The resultant polymer forms extremely strong bonds with tissue and has been used as a tissue adhesive in various settings.[11, 66] Histopathological studies indicate that there is some resorption of the material at follow-up angiography with recanalization of the nidus of the malformation, especially if the nidus is large and complex.[82] Complete disappearance of the glue cast has been documented on follow-up of 12 to 20 months. Therefore, although liquid adhesive embolizate is the longest-lasting agent used in neuroendovascular procedures, it is by no means permanent.

The technique of embolization with liquid adhesives is to maneuver the microcatheter into definitive position for embolization. The catheter is irrigated with a nonionic solution, such as dextrose solution. Any contact with ionic solution will initiate the polymerization process, and significant precautions must be taken to prevent the premature occurrence of polymerization. In order to determine the appropriate polymerization time, the transit time of the malformation is calculated; this is done by measuring the time between injection and the appearance of the earliest draining vein on angiography.

The polymerization time must be precisely adjusted by the addition of iophendylate or acetic acid. If the polymerization time is too long, the material traverses the malformation and polymerizes within its venous drainage, resulting in venous occlusion and resultant venous infarction or intranidal hemorrhage[23] (Fig. 59–7). If the polymerization is too fast, the arterial feeding pedicle is occluded before the nidus, allowing revascularization of the nidus and the development of collateral supply.[27, 37] As an alternative, the flow may be diminished by the inflation of a proximal calibrated-leak balloon in order to keep to the standard polymerization time, but this may risk gluing the balloon in place.[3] If the transit time of the malformation is too fast, embolization during craniotomy may be considered.[86]

Because of concerns over the carcinogenicity and brittleness of isobutyl 2-cyanoacrylate, N-butyl cyanoacrylate has been employed as an alternative embolic agent.[45] This polymer has a slightly shorter polymerization time; it is also softer and, therefore, more easily retracted and cut at surgery. The carcinogenicity of the cyanoacrylates remains uncertain but is thought to be inversely proportional to the length of the alkyl side chain.[14] Consequently, N-butyl cyanoacrylate offers a

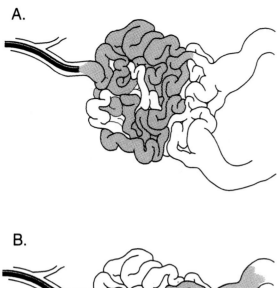

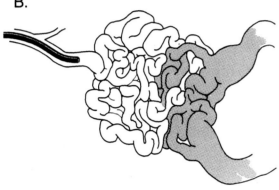

Figure 59–7

Schematic drawing of liquid adhesive polymer embolization of an arteriovenous malformation compartment. *A.* Accurate calculation of the polymerization time results in filling of the nidus of the malformation and occlusion of the feeding pedicle. *B.* Prolonged polymerization time allows migration of the polymer into the draining veins, resulting in the possibility of venous occlusion and hemorrhage.

theoretical benefit in this regard as well. No instance of intracranial carcinogenicity of implanted polymeric adhesive has been documented, despite their use in interventional procedures throughout the last 15 years.

Liquid adhesive polymers tend to provoke a moderately intense foreign body reaction over the first 4 weeks, followed by a lymphocytic infiltration.[14, 105] At 4 weeks after embolization, focal necrosis of the vessels has been documented, with occasional extravascular migration of the polymer. No difference in the histological reaction to the two polymers could be discerned.

Taki and co-workers proposed an ethylene vinyl alcohol copolymer as an embolic agent and have used it in the embolization of arteriovenous malformations.[102] Concerns over the solvent, dimethyl sulfoxide, have limited its widespread use. Another promising technique uses a combination of estrogen alcohol and polyvinyl acetate.[99] Alcohols tend to promote thrombosis in vessels with diameters of 20 to 40 microns and to progress to thrombose the larger vessels. Long-term data on the use of these materials have not yet been reported.

Particulate Materials

To diminish the hazard of liquid polymer adhesives, a technique for gradual occlusion of arteriovenous mal-

formations with finely graded particles was developed.[88] The most common agent is polyvinyl alcohol particles, which are commercially available in sizes ranging from 150 to 2,000 microns in diameter.[51] The particles are suspended in isosmotic contrast medium, placed in an infusion chamber, and injected in small aliquots of 0.1 to 1.0 mL. The particles are sized according to the component of the lesion: the smaller particles are used earlier, for deep penetration of the nidus, and the pedicle is brought to stasis with increasingly larger particles. Polyvinyl alcohol was initially developed as a pulmonary prosthesis for use after pneumonectomy; it was applied to transarterial embolization because of its extreme compressibility.[100] Histopathological examination of malformations embolized with polyvinyl alcohol revealed a mild foreign body reaction with areas of focal angionecrosis.[32] The pathophysiology of occlusion was by intra-arterial thrombosis and flow obstruction. Recanalization was identified in 18 per cent of vessels.

The advantage of polyvinyl alcohol is that it is easily compressed and retracted at surgery.[81] An additional advantage is that the embolization may proceed in a more controlled fashion, and there is no risk of catheter gluing. There is, however, the risk of inadvertent reflux of particulate material into adjacent blood vessels as the embolization progresses; this was thought to account for a significant number of the complications reported by Schumacher and Horton.[87] Particulate embolization is time-consuming, and the particles must be sized to penetrate the nidus without traversing the fistulae within the nidus. Alternatively, a solid embolic agent (i.e., silk or coils) may be used to occlude any significant fistulae.[72] At the conclusion of the procedure, the feeding pedicle may be occluded with a coil (Fig. 59–8).

Mixtures of thrombogenic agents may be added to polyvinyl alcohol to enhance retrograde thrombosis of intranidal vessels after embolization has occurred. Microfibrillary collagen (Avitene) is commonly employed and does not appear to increase the risk of complications significantly. A mixture of Avitene and dilute alcohol has been reported to be very effective in promoting intravascular thrombosis in an animal model.[55]

Horton and colleagues reported the use of an absorbable gelatin powder as a temporary embolic agent.[43]* Gelfoam embolization results in predictable recanalization within 2 to 4 weeks and may be used if temporary occlusion of a vessel is desired. Tissue reaction to Gelfoam is mild. The experimental studies of Razack and co-workers demonstrated that recanalization occurs within 4 weeks without residual angiopathic inflammation.[84] Particulate Gelfoam is particularly useful because of its small size (average, 150 microns) for the occlusion of vessels 125 to 175 microns in diameter.

Solid Materials

Occlusion of high-flow fistulae within arteriovenous malformations and occlusion of feeding pedicles after

---

*Gelfoam, manufactured by The Upjohn Co., Kalamazoo, Michigan.

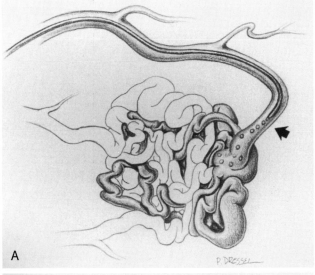

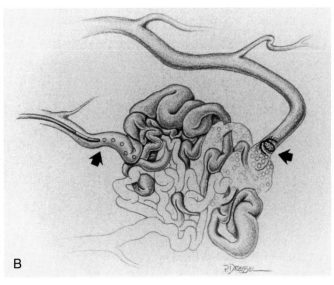

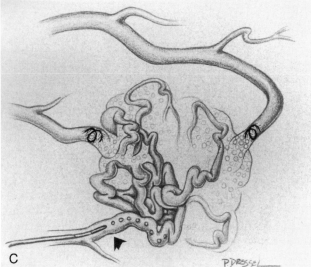

Figure 59–8

Staged particulate embolization of an arteriovenous malformation. *A.* First stage: catheterization of a feeding pedicle and introduction of particles of polyvinyl alcohol. *B.* Second stage: superselective catheterization of a separate pedicle and subsequent embolization. Notice the coil in the previously embolized pedicle. *C.* Third stage: notice anatomical dissection of the separate compartments as the embolization progresses.

embolization may require solid embolic materials, such as minicoils and silk, to evenly distribute the embolic material throughout the lesion. Several varieties of coils made of platinum have been developed for this purpose.[41, 94, 112] Hilal and Solomon have introduced coils into which Dacron fibers have been interwoven to enhance thrombogenicity and prevent coil migration.[41] Coils are available in a variety of straight and helical shapes and sizes (Fig. 59–9).

After it has been introduced into the microcatheter, the coil is advanced through the catheter with saline injection or by a special introducer wire designed for this purpose. The coil is flow-directed to the fistula of the nidus or deposited in the vessel as stasis through the feeding pedicle is achieved. These solid materials should not be employed for proximal vessel occlusion because of the risk of revascularization of the nidus.

Surgical silk sutures and polylene threads may also be used to occlude high-flow fistulae within the lesion.[8] These materials are not radiopaque, so precise localization of their deposition is not possible. The catheter may be seen to recoil as the strands exit so that embolization is confirmed.

Inflatable, detachable balloons (Fig. 59–10) have also been used to occlude the feeding pedicles before surgical resection.[37] This technique does not treat the nidus, but it has been shown to decrease the need for postoperative blood transfusion and shorten the duration of surgical resection. Unless immediate postembolization resection is planned, this method is not currently favored because of the risk of development of collateral revascularization.

Pediatric Arteriovenous Malformations

Embolization of malformations in the pediatric population follows guidelines similar to those described, although certain special considerations should be observed. Most endovascular procedures done on children should be performed under general anesthesia, sometimes necessitating continuous electroencephalography monitoring during the procedure. Fluid balance is also a primary consideration in terms of flush solutions and infusion of anesthetic agents. Similarly, blood loss from repeated aspiration through catheters and withdrawal for diagnostic purposes should be carefully

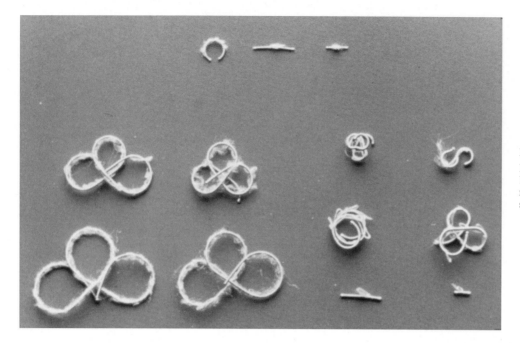

Figure 59–9

Platinum coils with interwoven Dacron fibers are available in a number of configurations and sizes.

monitored. Finally, contrast load should be kept to a minimum (5 mL per kg) to avoid contrast toxicity. The authors routinely employ the assistance of a pediatric anesthesiologist in the treatment of these lesions.

End Point of Embolization

The end point of embolization depends on the treatment goal. Embolization should proceed to reduce as much of the accessible blood supply as possible. Staged

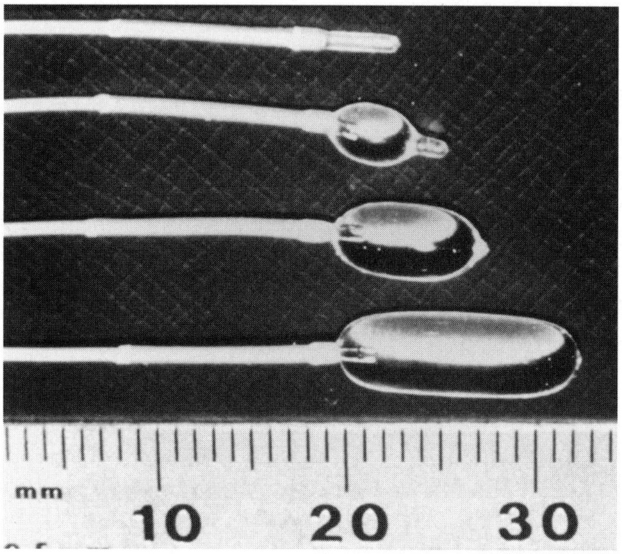

Figure 59–10

Silicone balloons on delivery catheters. As the balloon is inflated, it assumes an elliptical shape. (From Hopkins, L. N., Guterman, L. R., Livingston, K., Gibbons, K. J., et al.: Endovascular treatment of aneurysms and cerebral vasospasm. *In* Awad, I. A., ed.: Current Management of Cerebral Aneurysms. Vol. 15, Neurosurgical Topics Series. Park Ridge, IL, American Association of Neurological Surgeons, 1993, pp. 219–242. Reprinted by permission.)

embolization allows the surrounding parenchyma to regain autoregulatory capacity. The number of feeding pedicles embolized at each session varies and is dependent on patient compliance and contrast burden. Typically, one to four pedicles are embolized at any one session, although some clinicians attempt a more aggressive embolization. The endovascular therapist must maintain a perspective on the overall management strategy to achieve a timely reduction in the blood flow within the nidus without allowing an inordinate time between embolizations, during which recanalization may occur. Surgically inaccessible feeders should be embolized first, and accessible high-flow feeders should be embolized last, just before surgery.

Complications of Endovascular Procedures

Endovascular therapy can result in local, systemic, and cerebral complications, which should be carefully explained to the patient before the procedure. Actual complication rates for embolization procedures are difficult to assess because of rapidly evolving technology, differences in technique, and the varying grades of lesions treated. The risk of selective angiography without embolization is considered to be 0.45 per cent or lower.[34] Viñuela and colleagues, reporting on a series of 101 cases, noted the following long-term rates of embolization morbidity: 3.9 per cent mild, 6.9 per cent moderate, and 1.9 per cent severe.[107] Mortality in this series was 0.9 per cent. Berenstein and co-workers reported a similar mortality rate in their early experience but noted that the mortality rate later improved, from 4.4 to less than 1 per cent, and severe morbidity improved from 3.4 to 2.3 per cent.[9] In a more recent review by the same group, the rate of immediate and delayed hemorrhage was 15 per cent.[45] Viñuela later reported similar results, with a mortality of 1.3 per cent, a long-term morbidity with severe neurological deficit in 2.5 per cent, and a moderately severe deficit in 3.1 per cent.[106] Most centers report a short-term complication rate of between 8 and 10 per cent.[87]

LOCAL COMPLICATIONS

Local complications are uncommon but include femoral hematoma, infection, arterial dissection or occlusion, and arterial laceration. Groin hematomas occur in approximately 2 to 5 per cent of patients undergoing diagnostic angiography, and this rate may be increased by heparinization without adequate reversal or by leaving the introducer sheath in place for more than 2 days. Infection of the puncture site is unusual, occurring in less than 0.1 per cent of cases. Meticulous angiography technique is necessary to minimize these local complications.

Dosages of radiation received by patients and personnel are small during the procedure, but the cumulative dose effect may be substantial.[10] Annual dosages to personnel are well below established limits, but strict radiation safety must be practiced. Focal alopecia has been reported in relation to multiple prolonged interventional procedures.

SYSTEMIC COMPLICATIONS

Systemic complications of embolization are usually related to contrast allergy or adverse reaction to neuroleptic analgesia. Severe adverse contrast reactions are rare, less than 0.04 per cent, and may be ameliorated by pretreatment with steroids and H_2-blockers. Nonionic contrast material may also lower serum calcium levels and promote a significant osmotic diuresis; careful postoperative monitoring is warranted.

Hemingway and Allison have described a postembolization syndrome, consisting of malaise, low-grade fever, and slight leukocytosis, that was reported to be present in as many as 40 per cent of patients undergoing therapeutic embolization for peripheral indications.[39] This syndrome has occurred rarely in neurological embolization cases. Management of these systemic reactions is centered on the removal of the offending agent and supportive care.

The authors encountered significant pulmonary embolism during a case of therapeutic embolization of a facial arteriovenous malformation that was documented by ventilation-perfusion scanning (Fig. 59–11). During therapeutic embolization, particles may pass through the nidus and may be visualized by radiation scintigraphy in the pulmonary vasculature.[26] A significant amount of embolic material may reach the pulmonary circulation, resulting in ventilation-perfusion mismatch. Care must be taken to reduce the risk of particulate embolization of the lung by closing large fistulae before particulate embolization. The clinician should be aware of this possibility and be prepared to treat the patient with respiratory support. Anticoagulation should not be necessary if the embolization procedure is terminated.

CEREBRAL COMPLICATIONS

Hemorrhage

The rate of hemorrhage from arteriovenous malformations treated by therapeutic embolization ranges from 3 to 11 per cent.[79] Hemorrhage may be caused by deranged hemodynamics and resultant hemorrhage from the nidus, in either an acute or a delayed fashion. Alternatively, the catheter may perforate the wall of the vessel, resulting in extravasation of contrast material and blood.

The risk of vessel wall perforation is reduced by the use of soft-tipped guide wires and flexible microcatheters. Flow-directed microcatheters are somewhat less prone to perforate than steerable guide wire catheters. Perforation is reported to occur in 1.1 per cent of patients undergoing interventional procedures.[36] It occurs most commonly when the microcatheter is wedged against the side of a vessel, usually at a sharp bend, and the guide wire is advanced through the microcatheter or fluid is forcefully injected (Fig. 59–12). Perforation may be more prone to occur in the anterior choroidal artery. Evidence of perforation is the extravasation of contrast material on careful injection and the appearance of a gyral pattern (Fig. 59–13). Often the patient has a severe headache, and the neurological status may change.

This complication is managed by, first, reversing the anticoagulation as quickly as possible. The temptation to remove the catheter should be resisted.[79] Removal of the catheter may result in worsening of the hemorrhage because the catheter may be tamponading the bleeding. In many cases, a coil or other embolic agent may be placed at the perforation site after reversal of heparinization to prevent catastrophic hemorrhage and avoid neurological injury.[36] If a flow-directed catheter is being used, this technique may not be possible because of the small internal diameter of the catheter; after reversal of the anticoagulation, the catheter may be removed without placement of an occlusive coil.

Hemorrhage from the nidus may occur on either an acute or a delayed basis. Acute hemorrhage from the malformation after embolization is probably related to the rise in pressure within the feeding pedicles, which may be transmitted to untreated compartments of the malformation. Alternatively, occlusion of the venous outflow may occur, especially if liquid adhesive polymers are used, resulting in dramatic increases in intranidal pressure. These hemorrhages occur within the first hours after embolization and necessitate prompt intervention. The institution of prompt measures to control blood pressure and correct coagulation factors, along with standard management of increased intracranial pressure, is vital to successful management of these problems. Purdy and colleagues also strongly argue for the prompt surgical evacuation of any sig-

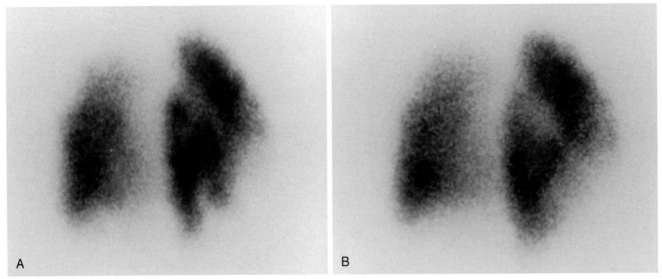

Figure 59–11

Ventilation-perfusion scan of a 30-year-old patient after embolization of a facial arteriovenous malformation. A perfusion defect evident in the left basal pulmonary segment *(A)* resolved after 48 hours *(B)*. Clinically, the patient developed symptomatic respiratory distress immediately after embolization of a fistulous compartment of the arteriovenous malformation.

nificant hematoma, along with the excision of the lesion, to achieve the maximum rate of neurological salvage.[79]

Delayed hemorrhage after embolization of arteriovenous malformations may occur but is uncommon. Hemorrhage may result from further hemodynamic changes or from delayed thrombosis of enlarged draining veins. Duckwiler and co-workers reported delayed venous occlusion 2 weeks after treatment.[25] Venous structure of draining veins from malformations is known to be abnormal and may contribute to the development of this syndrome.[67] Prompt treatment is predicated on cautious hydration therapy and the control of increased intracranial pressure.

Hyperperfusion Syndrome

The development of the hyperperfusion syndrome after treatment of arteriovenous malformations has been controversial because of the difficulty of documenting deranged hemodynamics in the parenchyma surrounding the nidus. Batjer and colleagues documented the development of normal perfusion pressure breakthrough after surgical resection by analysis with stable xenon-133 computed tomography and suggested a rate as high as 21 per cent in postoperative patients, although this rate has recently been challenged by the demonstration of normal autoregulation in cortex surrounding the lesion after surgical excision.[6, 7, 113] The phenomenon of normal perfusion pressure breakthrough has not occurred within the author's experience with staged embolization of these lesions, possibly because of the gradual normalization of autoregulation in surrounding cortex.

The idea of "occlusive hyperemia," as proposed by Al-Rodhan and colleagues, is a unifying concept.[2] They propose that post-therapeutic cerebral edema in the presence or absence of hemorrhage is caused by a

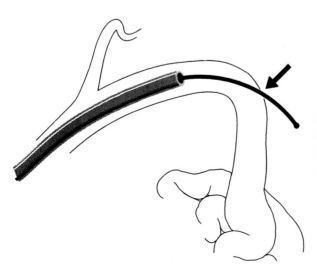

Figure 59–12

Most perforations occur at a sharp angulation of a vessel, especially in a region containing a large number of perforators. The guide wire may be inadvertently advanced through the wall of the artery *(arrow)*, and the catheter may follow.

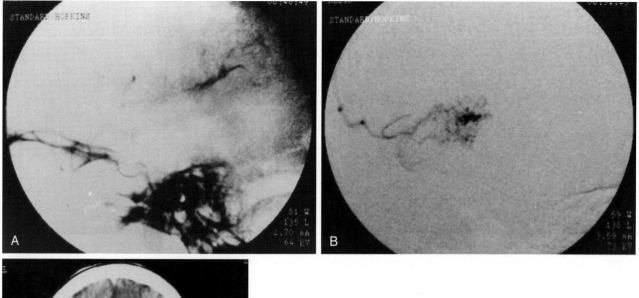

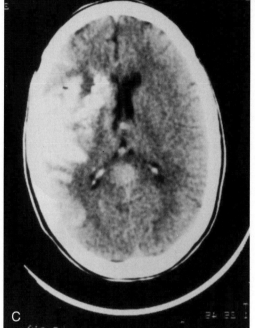

Figure 59–13

A 25-year-old female who developed a sudden headache during embolization of a thalamic arteriovenous malformation. *A.* Lateral fluoroscopic image demonstrates the gyral pattern of extravasated contrast material. A coil was placed, and the catheter was withdrawn into the feeding pedicle. *B.* Embolization of the remaining pedicle was performed. *C.* Postoperative computed tomography demonstrates contrast material within the left sylvian fissure and subarachnoid space. The region of the embolized portion of the malformation is seen adjacent to the ventricle. The right side of the patient is on the right side of the image. The patient suffered no ill effects.

combination of venous outflow restriction, with subsequent passive hyperemia and stagnant flow in the malformation arterial feeders, and worsening of existing hypoperfusion and ischemia. Miyasaka and associates have characterized these stagnating arteries as having high pressure and slow flow owing to persistent vessel dilatation after treatment.[70] Delayed restoration of vessel diameter may be caused by decrease of elasticity as a result of long-standing hemodynamic stresses. Neuroeffector mechanisms have also been postulated.[61]

Hyperemic complications can be prevented by careful avoidance of venous outflow occlusion during therapeutic embolization of large malformations. Furthermore, embolization should be performed as close to the nidus as possible to protect nutrient transient vessels and the precarious cortex surrounding the nidus. Significant hypotension should be avoided because of the resulting exacerbation of venous outflow restriction and arterial stagnation.

Hyperemic complications are managed by ensuring adequate blood volume and perfusion pressure. Volume contraction as a standard method for treating increased intracranial pressure should be avoided. In addition, hemoconcentration should be avoided; an optimum hematocrit below 35 per cent should be maintained.[110] Intravenous steroids should be used, and hyperventilation therapy may be instituted as warranted by the patient's clinical condition. Prompt administration of barbiturate coma has also been reported to be successful in the management of hyperperfusion syndrome by globally reducing cerebral blood flow and allowing the normal brain to develop normal autoregulation.[20, 104]

Embolization and Reflux

The technique of embolization of arterial feeding pedicles aims to prevent the inadvertent embolization of normal cortical vessels and the reflux of particulate or liquid adhesive embolic materials into normal vasculature. Constant fluoroscopy monitoring during embolization and placement of the microcatheter as close to the nidus as possible are the two most important means of preventing this complication. The use of functional challenge testing with Amytal also limits inadvertent embolization of functional cortex.

The embolization of small amounts of small particulate materials is unlikely to result in neurological compromise, whereas liquid polymers tend to be less forgiving. Management of this complication is by aggressive fluid resuscitation and by preoperative use of corticosteroids and calcium channel blockers. Collateral circulation to an ischemic zone allows salvage of a significant portion of neural tissue within the "ischemic penumbra"; therefore, any deficit manifested by the patient is assumed to be ischemic rather than infarcted tissue and is treated accordingly. The judicious use of hypervolemic hemodilution is also employed.[111]

Retrograde Thrombosis

Retrograde thrombosis of feeding pedicles is thought to occur after therapeutic embolization and to account for some cases of delayed neurological deficit. Retrograde thrombosis is thought to occur in cases in which high-flow fistulae are converted to slow-flow vessels in the setting of long-standing arterial injury. Sudden neurological decline should prompt emergent computed tomography scanning to rule out intracerebral hemorrhage. Repeat angiography should be considered if computed tomography results are negative. Stagnating arteries may be observed, and vessel occlusion may be identified owing to retrograde thrombosis (Fig. 59–14). If the occlusion is less than 6 to 8 hours old, the use of intra-arterial thrombolysis may be considered. The use of volume expansion and hemodilution in addition to heparinization is encouraged to limit further propagation of thrombus.

Cerebral Steal

The development of an altered hemodynamic profile after therapeutic embolization may result in worsening of perfusion to adjacent brain by a shift in the pattern of steal. Although this phenomenon has not been well studied, Livingston and colleagues (unpublished data) report the occurrence of worsening steal in the middle cerebral artery distribution in a patient with a large parietal malformation who underwent an anterior cerebral artery embolization. This exacerbation of steal responded to treatment with volume expansion and hypertension and gradually resolved over several days.

Development of Collateral Supply

The development of collateral supply after embolization procedures may be observed, especially in large and complex malformations. Again, deep and surgically inaccessible pedicles may develop if the superficial arterial supply is embolized early in the course of therapy. Pial collateral vessels of 150 to 200 microns in diameter, which are not angiographically visible, may enlarge to provide significant blood supply to the nidus. Revascularization is thought to occur as early as 3 weeks after embolization and may involve the dural vascular supply.[28] Patients who develop recurrent headaches after embolization are likely to have developed dural collaterals. Thorough diagnostic angiography examinations should be performed at regular intervals after therapeutic embolization, and the total length of staged embolization sessions should be relatively short.

Infection

Mourier and colleagues reported a case of staphylococcal abscess after cerebral embolization of an arteriovenous malformation.[71] Potential sources of contamination include the embolic agent and embolization of thrombus contaminated by unsterile catheters or guide wires. Strict aseptic technique is essential in the performance of therapeutic angiography procedures.

Postoperative Care

The goal of postoperative management is to prevent and rapidly treat complications, should they occur. All patients are admitted to the intensive care unit for neurological and hemodynamic monitoring. Intravenous hydration therapy is continued, and hypotension is carefully avoided. Serum electrolytes, complete blood count, platelet count, and coagulation studies are monitored. Intravenous steroids and nimodipine are continued for the first 48 hours, and then the patient is placed on a tapering steroid dose. Neurovascular observation of the extremity and arterial circulation distal to the puncture site is performed. The extremity is placed flat for at least the first 4 to 6 hours. Any undue swelling or compromise of the distal pulses should prompt evaluation by a vascular surgeon. Complaints of abdominal or back pain may signify the development of a retroperitoneal hematoma or aortic dissection and should be evaluated by abdominal computed tomography.

Neurological changes are evaluated by emergent cranial computed tomography. If the results are negative, emergent angiography should be performed to evaluate the arterial and venous supply to the lesion as well as the proportion of steal. Carotid dissection is also a diagnostic possibility. Superselective delivery of thrombolytic agents for intra-arterial thrombus can be strongly considered if vessel occlusion is confirmed on angiography. In the author's institution, intra-arterial thrombolysis is performed with a special microcatheter that has side holes in the distal portion to deliver thrombolytic agents directly into the thrombus.* The catheter may be manipulated into and beyond the

---

*Softstream, manufactured by Target Therapeutics, Fremont, California.

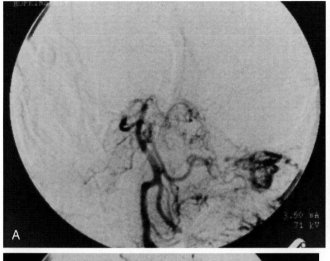

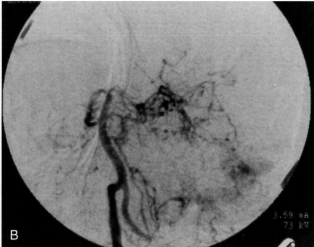

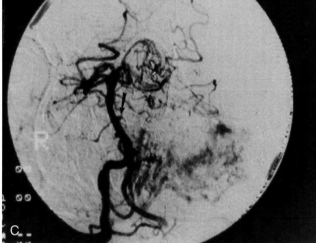

Figure 59–14

Oblique vertebral angiography of a 63-year-old male with a left cerebellar arteriovenous malformation. *A.* Initial embolization was performed on major feeders from the superior cerebellar artery, but supply remained from the left anterior inferior cerebellar artery (AICA). *B.* Postembolization angiography demonstrates patency of the anterior inferior cerebellar artery. *C.* Two weeks after the procedure, the patient developed sudden hearing loss and cerebellar dysfunction. Cerebral angiography demonstrates retrograde thrombosis of the left anterior inferior cerebellar artery *(arrow).*

thrombus. Surveillance angiography is performed to assess the resolution of thrombus every 10 to 15 minutes.

Conclusion

Considering the natural history of arteriovenous malformations, with a cumulative hemorrhage rate of 3 to 4 per cent per year, the goal of management of these lesions should be complete obliteration. The end point for endovascular therapy is changing as technology and techniques are improved and as a more complete understanding of the pathophysiology of these lesions is obtained. Currently, endovascular therapy is employed as a preoperative or intraoperative adjunct to definitive surgical excision, as an adjunct to radiosurgery, as a palliative treatment for inoperable lesions, and as definitive therapy in selected cases.

As an adjunct to surgical resection of these lesions, embolization has the potential to reduce mortality and morbidity and make surgery easier. Flow-related aneurysms and venous ectasias may be obliterated by preoperative embolization.[28] Embolization has been shown to reduce intraoperative blood loss and to reduce trans-

fusion requirements during resection of the malformations.[18, 75] The incidence of new major deficits and death after surgical resection and the rate of postoperative seizure disorder have also been reduced by preoperative embolization.[35, 75] This is thought to be a result of the reduction in size and flow within the nidus, which reduces the number of deep and inaccessible feeders and eliminates intranidal aneurysms.

Although staged occlusion of feeding pedicles of a lesion carries a significant theoretical advantage in reduction of the incidence of hyperemic complications after resection, there is no conclusive evidence to support this hypothesis.

Embolization may also be used as adjunctive therapy for radiosurgical obliteration of an arteriovenous malformation. The endovascular strategy is to obliterate as much of the lesion as possible and to tailor the shape of the lesion to make it more amenable to radiosurgery.[21] Rodesch and Lasjaunias suggest that liquid embolic agents should be used for preoperative embolization because of a lower degree of post-treatment recanalization, but the basis for this statement remains to be confirmed.[85] In the series of Dawson and colleagues, seven lesions were treated by preoperative embolization followed by stereotactic radiosurgery with a cobalt-60 Gamma unit.[21] At 2-year follow-up, two of seven malformations were cured, and two had 98 per cent reduction in volume. Lesions that were larger than 3 cm in diameter after embolization were less likely to be cured. The optimum diameter for stereotactic radiosurgery is thought to be less than 4 cm.[59]

Angiographically confirmed cure rates for stereotactic radiosurgery alone are reported to be 84 per cent if the nidus size is less than 28 mm. Reports of a large series of patients undergoing radiosurgery with a cobalt-60 Gamma radiosurgery unit demonstrated similar obliteration rates for small malformations (4 cm[3] or smaller) and 58 per cent obliteration rates for large ones (diameter greater than 4 cm).[60] Two (0.88 per cent) of 227 patients died of intracerebral hemorrhage within 2 years of treatment. Ten per cent of patients had symptomatic postirradiation changes on magnetic resonance imaging at a mean of 10 months after treatment. Endovascular therapy may therefore serve as an adjunct to radiosurgery in selected patients, although the delay in effecting "cure" of the lesion, as evidenced by negative angiography results, is a disadvantage to this technique.

Endovascular embolization may be used as palliative therapy if the lesion is inoperable or if the patient refuses traditional therapy. By halting the process of dural recruitment, embolization may produce dramatic relief in headache or make migrainous attacks more amenable to traditional medications.[30] Judicious embolization can also reduce or halt steal phenomena by altering the hemodynamics of the malformation.[53, 97] Protection from rebleeding in these cases has not been documented.

Fewer than 15 per cent of arteriovenous malformations can be angiographically obliterated through an endovascular approach.[28, 33] As definitive therapy, endovascular therapy must eliminate the nidus entirely and demonstrate its persistent and unequivocal obliteration on long-term follow-up.[56] Usually, those malformations that are capable of angiographic obliteration are small, low-grade lesions supplied by a single feeding pedicle and having a very low surgical morbidity. The authors experienced recanalization of a small, single-feeder lesion 2 years after embolization with polyvinyl alcohol particles. This lesion had demonstrated obliteration on 1-year follow-up angiography. Long-term follow-up is necessary to verify the permanence of angiographic "cure" in these patients, depending on the technique and substance used for occlusion.

Preoperative embolization is clearly beneficial in reducing perioperative morbidity, particularly in the treatment of Spetzler-Martin grade III to V lesions.[95] In inoperable lesions, embolization reduces symptoms of seizure or steal and reduces the size of the nidus for radiosurgical therapy.

REFERENCES

1. Ahuja, A., Gibbons, K. J., Guterman, L. R., et al.: Pedicle pressure changes in cerebral arteriovenous malformations during therapeutic embolization: Relationship to delayed hemorrhage [Abstract]. Stroke, 24:185, 1993.
2. Al-Rodhan, N. R. F., Sundt, T. M., Jr., Piepgras, D. G., et al.: Occlusive hyperemia: A theory for the hemodynamic complications following resection of intracerebral arteriovenous malformations. J. Neurosurg., 78:167, 1993.
3. Bank, W. O., Kerber, C. W., and Cromwell, L. D.: Treatment of intracerebral arteriovenous malformations with isobutyl 2-cyanoacrylate: Initial clinical experience. Radiology, 139:609, 1981.
4. Barnett, G. H., Little, J. R., Ebrahim, Z. Y., et al.: Cerebral circulation during arteriovenous malformation operation. Neurosurgery, 20:836, 1987.
5. Batjer, H., Suss, R. A., and Samson, D.: Intracranial arteriovenous malformations associated with aneurysms. Neurosurgery, 18:29, 1986.
6. Batjer, H. H., Devous, M. D., Sr., Seibert, G. B., et al.: Intracranial arteriovenous malformation: Relationship between clinical factors and surgical complications. Neurosurgery, 24:75, 1989.
7. Batjer, H. H., Purdy, P. D., Giller, C. A., et al.: Evidence of redistribution of cerebral blood flow during treatment for an intracranial arteriovenous malformation. Neurosurgery, 25:599, 1989.
8. Benati, A., Beltramello, A., Colombari, R., et al.: Preoperative embolization of arteriovenous malformations with polylene threads: Techniques with wing microcatheter and pathologic results. A.J.N.R., 10:579, 1989.
9. Berenstein, A. B., Choi, I. S., Kupersmith, M. J., et al.: Complications of endovascular embolization in 202 patients with cerebral AVMs [Abstract]. A.J.N.R., 10:876, 1989.
10. Berthelsen, B., and Cederblad, Å.: Radiation doses to patients and personnel involved in embolization of intracerebral arteriovenous malformations. Acta Radiol., 32:492, 1991.
11. Bonutti, P. M., Weiker, G. G., and Andrish, J. T.: Isobutyl cyanoacrylate as a soft tissue adhesive: An in vitro study in the rabbit Achilles tendon. Clin. Orthop., 229:241, 1988.
12. Boulos, R., Kricheff, I. I., and Chase, N. E.: Value of cerebral angiography in the embolization of treatment of cerebral arteriovenous malformation. Radiology, 97:65, 1970.
13. Braughler, J. M., and Hall, E. D.: Current application of "high-dose" steroid therapy for CNS injury: A pharmacological perspective. J. Neurosurg., 62:806, 1985.
14. Brothers, M. F., Kaufmann, J. C. E., Fox, A. J., et al.: N-butyl 2-cyanoacrylate: Substitute for IBCA in interventional neuroradiology. Histopathologic and polymerization time studies. A.J.N.R., 10:777, 1989.
15. Chappell, P. M., Steinberg, G. K., and Marks, M. P.: Clinically documented hemorrhage in cerebral arteriovenous malformations: MR characteristics. Radiology, 183:719, 1992.
16. Chioffi, F., Pasqualin, A., Beltramello, A., et al.: Hemodynamic effects of preoperative embolization in cerebral arteriovenous malformations: Evaluation with transcranial Doppler sonography. Neurosurgery, 31:877, 1992.
17. Choi, D. W.: Glutamate neurotoxicity in cortical cell culture is calcium dependent. Neurosci. Lett., 58:293, 1985.
18. Cromwell, L. D., and Harris, A. B.: Treatment of cerebral arteriovenous malformations: A combined neurosurgical and neuroradiological approach. J. Neurosurg., 52:705, 1980.
19. Cunha, M. J., Stein, B. M., Solomon, R. A., et al.: The treatment of associated intracranial aneurysms and arteriovenous malformations. J. Neurosurg., 77:853, 1992.
20. Day, A. L., Friedman, W. A., Sypert, G. W., et al.: Successful treatment of the normal perfusion pressure breakthrough syndrome. Neurosurgery, 11:625–630, 1982.
21. Dawson, R. C., Tarr, R. W., Hecht, S. T., et al.: Treatment of arteriovenous malformations of the brain with combined embolization and stereotactic radiosurgery: Results after 1 and 2 years. A.J.N.R., 11:857, 1990.
22. Debrun, G. M., Lacour, P., and Caron, J.-P., et al.: Traitement des fistules arterioveineuses et d'anéurysmes par ballon gonflable et largable. Nouv. Presse Med., 4:2315, 1975.
23. Debrun, G., Viñuela, F., Fox, A., et al.: Embolization of cerebral arteriovenous malformations with bucrylate: Experience in 46 cases. J. Neurosurg., 56:615, 1982.
24. Duckwiler, G., Dion, J., Viñuela, F., et al.: Intravascular microcatheter pressure monitoring: Experimental results and early clinical evaluation. A.J.N.R., 11:169, 1990.
25. Duckwiler, G. R., Dion, J. E., Viñuela, F., et al.: Delayed venous

occlusion following embolotherapy of vascular malformations in the brain. A.J.N.R., 13:1571, 1992.

26. DuCret, R. P., Adkins, M. C., Hunter, D. W., et al.: Therapeutic embolization: Enhanced radiolabeled monitoring. Radiology, 177:571, 1990.

27. Fournier, D., TerBrugge, K., Rodesch, G., et al.: Revascularization of brain arteriovenous malformations after embolization with brucrylate [bucrylate]. Neuroradiology, 32:497, 1990.

28. Fournier, D., TerBrugge, K. G., Willinsky, R., et al.: Endovascular treatment of intracerebral arteriovenous malformations: Experience in 49 cases. J. Neurosurg., 75:228, 1991.

29. Garcia-Monaco, R., Rodesch, G., Alvarez, H., et al.: Pseudoaneurysms within ruptured intracranial arteriovenous malformations: Diagnosis and early endovascular management. A.J.N.R., 14:315, 1993.

30. Gawel, M. J., Willinsky, R. A., and Krajewski, A.: Reversal of cluster headache side following treatment of arteriovenous malformation. Headache, 29:453, 1989.

31. Gelmers, H. J., Gorter, K., deWeerdt, C. J., et al.: A controlled trial of nimodipine in acute ischemic stroke. N. Engl. J. Med., 318:203, 1988.

32. Germano, I. M., Davis, R. L., Wilson, C. B., et al.: Histopathological follow-up study of 66 cerebral arteriovenous malformations after therapeutic embolization with polyvinyl alcohol. J. Neurosurg., 76:607, 1992.

33. Gibbons, K. J., Guterman, L. R., Ahuja, A., et al.: Angiographic obliteration of arteriovenous malformations following embolization. Neuroradiology, 33(Suppl.):S175, 1991.

34. Grzyska, U., Freitag, J., and Zeumer, H.: Selective cerebral intraarterial DSA: Complication rate and control of risk factors. Neuroradiology, 32:296, 1990.

35. Halbach, V. V., Higashida, R. T., and Hieshima, G. B.: Interventional neuroradiology. A.J.R., 153:467, 1989.

36. Halbach, V. V., Higashida, R. T., Dowd, C. F., et al.: Management of vascular perforations that occur during neurointerventional procedures. A.J.N.R., 12:319–327, 1991.

37. Halbach, V. V., Higashida, R. T., Yang, P., et al.: Preoperative balloon occlusion of arteriovenous malformations. Neurosurgery, 22:301, 1988.

38. Hecht, S. T., Horton, J. A., and Kerber, C. W.: Hemodynamics of the central nervous system arteriovenous malformation nidus during particulate embolization: A computer model. Neuroradiology, 33:62, 1991.

39. Hemingway, A. P., and Allison, D. J.: Complications of embolization: Analysis of 410 procedures. Radiology, 166:669, 1988.

40. Higashi, K., Hatano, M., Yamashita, T., et al.: Coexistence of posterior inferior cerebellar artery aneurysm and arteriovenous malformation fed by the same artery. Surg. Neurol., 12:405, 1979.

41. Hilal, S. K., and Solomon, R. A.: Endovascular treatment of aneurysms with coils [Letter]. J. Neurosurg., 76:337, 1992.

42. Horton, J. A., and Kerber, C. W.: Lidocaine injection into external carotid branches: Provocative test to preserve cranial nerve function in therapeutic embolization. A.J.N.R., 7:105, 1986.

43. Horton, J. A., Marano, G. D., Kerber, C. W., et al.: Polyvinyl alcohol foam: Gelfoam for therapeutic embolization. A synergistic mixture. A.J.N.R., 4:143, 1983.

44. Huston, J., III, Rufenacht, D. A., Ehman, R. L., et al.: Intracranial aneurysms and vascular malformations: Comparison of time-of-flight and phase-contrast MR angiography. Radiology, 181:721, 1991.

45. Jafar, J. J., Davis, A. J., Berenstein, A., et al.: The effect of embolization with N-butyl cyanoacrylate prior to surgical resection of cerebral arteriovenous malformations. J. Neurosurg., 78:60, 1993.

46. Jungreis, C. A., and Horton, J. A.: Pressure changes in the arterial feeder to a cerebral AVM as a guide to monitoring therapeutic embolization. A.J.N.R., 10:1057, 1989.

47. Jungreis, C. A., Horton, J. A., and Hecht, S. T.: Blood pressure changes in feeders to cerebral arteriovenous malformations during therapeutic embolization. A.J.N.R., 10:575, 1989.

48. Katayama, H., Yamaguchi, K., Kozuka, T., et al.: Adverse reactions to ionic and nonionic contrast media: A report from the Japanese committee on the safety of contrast media. Radiology, 175:621, 1990.

49. Kerber, C.: Balloon catheter with a calibrated leak: A new system for superselective angiotherapy and occlusive catheter therapy. Radiology, 120:547, 1976.

50. Kerber, C.: Use of balloon catheters in the treatment of cranial arterial abnormalities. Stroke, 11:210, 1980.

51. Kerber, C. W., Bank, W. O., and Horton, J. A.: Polyvinyl alcohol foam: Prepackaged emboli for therapeutic embolization. A.J.R., 130:1193, 1978.

52. Kido, D. K., King, P. D., Manzione, J. V., et al.: The role of catheters and guidewires in the production of angiographic thromboembolic complications. Invest. Radiol. 23(Suppl. 2):S359, 1988.

53. Kusske, J. A., and Kelly, W. A.: Embolization and reduction of the "steal" syndrome in cerebral arteriovenous malformations. J. Neurosurg., 40:313, 1974.

54. Lasjaunias, P., and Berenstein, A.: Surgical Neuroangiography. Vol 2. Endovascular treatment of craniofacial lesions. New York, Springer-Verlag, 1987, p. 12.

55. Lee, D. H., Wriedt, C. H., Kaufmann, J. C. E., et al.: Evaluation of three embolic agents in pig rete. A.J.N.R., 10:773, 1989.

56. Livingston, K. L., and Hopkins, L. N.: Endovascular treatment of intracerebral arteriovenous malformations. Clin. Neurosurg., 39:331, 1992.

57. Lo, E. H.: Perfusion pressure and risk of AVM hemorrhage [Letter]. J. Neurosurg., 78:156, 1993.

58. Luessenhop, A. J., and Spence, W. T.: Artificial embolization of cerebral arteries: Report of use in a case of arteriovenous malformation. J.A.M.A., 172:1153, 1960.

59. Lunsford, L. D., Flickinger, J., Lindner, G., et al.: Stereotactic radiosurgery of the brain using the first United States 201 cobalt-60 source Gamma knife. Neurosurgery, 24:151, 1989.

60. Lunsford, L. D., Kondziolka, D., Flickinger, J. C., et al.: Stereotactic radiosurgery for arteriovenous malformations of the brain. J. Neurosurg., 75:51, 1991.

61. MacFarlane, R., Moskowitz, M. A., Sakas, D. E., et al.: The role of neuroeffector mechanisms in cerebral hyperperfusion syndromes. J. Neurosurg., 75:845, 1991.

62. Marks, M. P., Lane, B., Steinberg, G. K., et al.: Hemorrhage in intracerebral arteriovenous malformations: Angiographic determinants. Radiology, 176:807, 1990.

63. Marks, M. P., Lane, B., Steinberg, G. K., et al.: Intranidal aneurysms in cerebral arteriovenous malformations: Evaluation and endovascular treatment. Radiology, 183:355, 1992.

64. Marshall, L. F., King, J., and Langfitt, T. W.: The complications of high-dose corticosteroid therapy in neurosurgical patients: A prospective study. Ann. Neurol., 1:201, 1977.

65. Massoud, T. F., Ji, C., Viñuela, F., et al: A new in vivo model following experimental carotid-jugular fistula in swine: A preliminary angiographic study [Abstract]. Thirty-first Annual Meeting of the American Society of Neuroradiology, Vancouver, Canada, 1993.

66. Matsumoto, T., and Heisterkamp, C. A., III: Long-term study of aerosol cyanoacrylate tissue adhesive spray: Carcinogenicity and other untoward effects. Am. Surg., 35:825, 1969.

67. Mawad, M. E., Hilal, S. K., Michelsen, W. J., et al.: Occlusive vascular disease associated with cerebral arteriovenous malformations. Radiology, 153:401, 1984.

68. Midazolam. Med. Lett. Drugs Ther., 28:73, 1986.

69. Miyasaka, Y., Yada, K., Kurata, A., et al.: Correlation between intravascular pressure and risk of hemorrhage due to arteriovenous malformations. Surg. Neurol., 39:370, 1993.

70. Miyasaka, Y., Yada, K., Ohwada, T., et al.: Pathophysiologic assessment of stagnating arteries after removal of arteriovenous malformations. A.J.N.R., 14:15, 1993.

71. Mourier, K. L., Bellec, C., Lot, G., et al.: Pyogenic parenchymatous and nidus infection after embolization of an arteriovenous malformation: An unusual complication [Case report]. Acta Neurochir. (Wien), 122:130, 1993.

72. Nakstad, P. H., Bakke, S. J., and Haid, J. K.: Embolization of intracranial arteriovenous malformations and fistulas with polyvinyl alcohol particles and platinum fiber coils. Neuroradiology, 34:348, 1992.

73. Nornes, H., and Grip, A.: Hemodynamic aspects of cerebral arteriovenous malformations. J. Neurosurg., 53:456, 1980.

74. Pasqualin, A., Barone, G., Cioffi, F., et al.: The relevance of anatomic and hemodynamic factors to a classification of cerebral arteriovenous malformations. Neurosurgery, 28:370, 1991.

75. Pasqualin, A., Scienza, R., Cioffi, F., et al.: Treatment of cerebral arteriovenous malformations with a combination of preoperative embolization and surgery. Neurosurgery, 29:358, 1991.

76. Patterson, J. H., and McKissock, W.: A clinical survey of intracranial angiomas with special reference to their mode of progression and surgical treatment: A report of 110 cases. Brain, 79:233, 1956.

77. Peters, K. R., Quisling, R. G., Gilmore, R., et al.: Intraarterial use of sodium methohexital for provocative testing during brain embolotherapy. A.J.N.R., 14:171, 1993.

78. Pile-Spellman, J. M. D., Baker, K. F., Liszczak, T. M., et al.: High-flow angiopathy: Cerebral blood vessel changes in experimental chronic arteriovenous fistula. A.J.N.R., 7:811, 1986.

79. Purdy, P. D., Batjer, H. H., and Samson, D.: Management of hemorrhagic complications from preoperative embolization of arteriovenous malformations. J. Neurosurg., 74:205, 1991.

80. Purdy, P. D., Batjer, H. H., Risser, R. C., et al.: Arteriovenous malformations of the brain: Choosing embolic materials to enhance safety and ease of excision. J. Neurosurg., 77:217, 1992.

81. Purdy, P. D., Samson, D., Batjer, H. H., et al.: Preoperative embolization of cerebral arteriovenous malformations with polyvinyl alcohol particles: Experience in 51 adults. A.J.N.R., 11:501, 1990.

82. Rao, V. R. K., Mandalam, K. R., Gupta, A. K., et al.: Dissolution of isobutyl 2-cyanoacrylate on long-term follow-up. A.J.N.R., 10:135, 1989.

83. Rauch, R. A., Viñuela, F., Dion, J., et al.: Preembolization functional evaluation in brain arteriovenous malformations: The ability of superselective Amytal test to predict neurologic dysfunction before embolization. A.J.N.R., 13:309–314, 1992.

84. Razack, N., Soloniuk, D. S., Perkins, E., et al.: Cerebrovascular histopathology after intracarotid infusion of Gelfoam in the rat. Neurosurgery, 33:116, 1993.

85. Rodesch, G., and Lasjaunias, P.: Treatment of arteriovenous malformations [Letter]. A.J.N.R., 12:1023, 1991.

86. Samson, D., Ditmore, Q. M., and Beyer, C. W., Jr.: Intravascular use of isobutyl 2-cyanoacrylate: Part 1. Treatment of intracranial arteriovenous malformations. Neurosurgery, 8:43, 1981.

87. Schumacher, M., and Horton, J. A.: Treatment of cerebral arteriovenous malformations with PVA: Results and analysis of complications. Neuroradiology, 33:101, 1991.

88. Scialfa, G., and Scotti, G.: Superselective injection of polyvinyl alcohol microemboli for the treatment of cerebral arteriovenous malformations. A.J.N.R., 6:957, 1985.

89. Seeger, J., Weinstein, P. R., Carmody, R. F., et al.: Digital video subtraction angiography of the cervical and cerebral vasculature. J. Neurosurg., 56:173, 1982.

90. Seldinger, S. I.: Catheter replacement of the needle in percutaneous arteriography. Acta Radiol., 39:368, 1952.

91. Serbinenko, F. A.: Balloon catheterization and occlusion of major cerebral vessels. J. Neurosurg., 41:125, 1974.

92. Skalpe, I. O.: The toxicity of non-ionic water-soluble monomeric and dimeric contrast media in selective vertebral angiography: An experimental study in rabbits. Neuroradiology, 24:219, 1983..

93. Skalpe, I. O., and Aulie, Å.: The toxicity of non-ionic water-soluble contrast media in selective vertebral angiography: An experimental study in rabbits with special reference to the difference between monomeric and dimeric compounds. Neuroradiology, 27:77, 1985.

94. Smith, M. D., Russell, E. J., Levy, R., et al.: Transcatheter obliteration of a cerebellar arteriovenous fistula with platinum coils. A.J.N.R., 11:1199, 1990.

95. Spetzler, R. F., and Martin, N. A.: A proposed grading system for arteriovenous malformations. J. Neurosurg., 65:476, 1986.

96. Spetzler, R. F., Hargraves, R. W., McCormick, P. W., et al.: Relationship of perfusion pressure and size to risk of hemorrhage from arteriovenous malformations. J. Neurosurg., 76:918, 1992.

97. Spetzler, R. F., Martin, N. A., Carter, L. P., et al.: Surgical management of large AVMs by staged embolization and operative excision. J. Neurosurg., 67:17, 1987.

98. Spetzler, R. F., Wilson, C. B., Weinstein, P., et al.: Normal perfusion pressure breakthrough theory. Clin. Neurosurg., 25:651, 1978.

98a. Stein, B. M., and Kader, A.: Intracranial arteriovenous malformations. Clin. Neurosurg., 39:77, 1992.

99. Su, C. C., Takahashi, A., Yoshimoto, T., et al.: Histopathology studies of a new liquid embolization method using estrogen alcohol and polyvinyl acetate: Experimental evaluations with a model of cortical arterial cannulation in the canine brain. Surg. Neurol., 36:4, 1991.

100. Tadavarthy, S. M., Moller, J. H., and Amplatz, K.: Polyvinyl alcohol (Ivalon)—a new embolic material. A.J.R., 125:609, 1975.

101. Takemae, T., Kobayashi, S., and Sugita, K.: Perinidal hypervascular network on immediate postoperative angiogram after removal of large arteriovenous malformations located distant from the arterial circle of Willis. Neurosurgery, 33:400–406, 1993.

102. Taki, W., Yonekawa, Y., Iwata, H., et al.: A new liquid material for embolization of arteriovenous malformations. A.J.N.R., 11:163, 1990.

103. Tarr, R. W., Johnson, D. W., Horton, J. A., et al.: Impaired cerebral vasoreactivity after embolization of arteriovenous malformations: Assessment with serial acetazolamide challenge xenon CT. A.J.N.R., 12:417, 1991.

104. U, H. S.: Microsurgical excision of paraventricular arteriovenous malformations. Neurosurgery, 16:293, 1985.

105. Vinters, H. V., Debrun, G., Kaufmann, J. C. E., et al.: Pathology of arteriovenous malformations embolized with isobutyl-2-cyanoacrylate (bucrylate): Report of 2 cases. J. Neurosurg., 55:819, 1981.

106. Viñuela, F.: Functional evaluation and embolization of intracranial arteriovenous malformations. In Viñuela, F., Halbach, V. V., and Dion, J. E., eds.: Interventional Neuroradiology: Endovascular Therapy of the Central Nervous System. New York, Raven Press, 1992, pp. 77–86.

107. Viñuela, F., Dion, J. E., Duckwiler, G., et al.: Combined endovascular embolization and surgery in the management of cerebral arteriovenous malformations: Experience with 101 cases. J. Neurosurg., 75:856, 1991.

108. Wada, J., and Rasmussen, T.: Intracarotid injection of Sodium Amytal for the lateralization of cerebral speech dominance: Experimental and clinical observations. J. Neurosurg., 17:266–282, 1960.

109. Wallace, S., Gianturco, C., Anderson, J. H., et al.: Therapeutic vascular occlusion utilizing steel coil technique: Clinical applications. A.J.R., 127:381, 1976.

110. Wilson, C. B., and Hieshima, G. B.: Occlusive hyperemia: A new way to think about an old problem [Editorial]. J. Neurosurg., 78:165, 1993.

111. Wood, J. H., Simeone, F. A., Fink, E. A., et al.: Hypervolemic hemodilution in experimental focal cerebral ischemia. J. Neurosurg., 59:500, 1983.

112. Yang, P., Halbach, V. V., Higashida, R. T., et al.: Platinum wire: A new transvascular embolic agent. A.J.N.R., 9:547, 1988.

113. Young, W. L., Kader, A., Prohovnik, I., et al.: Pressure autoregulation is intact after arteriovenous malformation resection. Neurosurgery, 32:491, 1993.

CHAPTER 60

Radiosurgery for Arteriovenous Malformations

radiosurgery was first espoused more than 40 years ago by Leksell.[2, 24] Recent developments in computer technology for dose planning, as well as refinements in radiation delivery systems, have led to an increase in interest in radiosurgery as a treatment methodology. Perhaps of equal importance is the increasing evidence that it is a useful treatment option for a variety of challenging neurosurgical disorders.

The History of Radiosurgery

GAMMA KNIFE SYSTEMS

In 1951, Leksell described the concept of focusing many beams of external radiation on a stereotactically defined intracranial target.[24] He coined the term "radiosurgery" to describe this process. He and his colleagues experimented with a variety of radiation sources, including orthovoltage x-ray machines, particle beams,[25] and early linear accelerators, before designing a completely new device, called the "Gamma knife."

The first Gamma knife was installed in Stockholm in 1968. It contained 179 ^{60}Co sources, all collimated and focused on one point (Fig. 60–1). The unit was designed to produce an elliptically shaped lesion, similar to that produced by a radiofrequency lesion electrode. It was to be used primarily as a functional neurosurgery tool, for example, to treat pain, movement disorders, or psychiatric disease. It subsequently became clear that the inability to stimulate or record before lesion-making, as well as the long latency period before the lesion developed, limited the use of radiosurgery in functional neurosurgery.

PARTICLE ACCELERATOR SYSTEMS

Wilson, a physicist, has been credited with first suggesting the medical usage of particle beams, in the 1940's.[26] Early radiosurgical groups utilized the proton beam produced by synchrocyclotrons. Workers in Sweden employed high-energy intersecting proton beams, in a fashion analogous to the intersecting cobalt beams of the gamma knife. Groups in Boston and Berkeley, however, used the Bragg peak effect (see next section) to maximize the radiosurgical effectiveness of the proton beam. Single-dose and fractionated treatments have been devised (Fig. 60–2).[39]

A 160-MeV proton beam with a 10-mm-wide Bragg peak is used in Boston.[21] The radiation is delivered through 12 portals in one fraction. Since 1980, 130-MeV helium ion beams have been used at the Berkeley installation.[32] The limiting factor on the use of particle beam radiosurgery appears to be the requirement for a synchrocyclotron to generate the radiation source. These facilities are available only at a small number of high-energy physics research institutes.

LINEAR ACCELERATOR SYSTEMS

Linear accelerators were simultaneously developed in the United States and Great Britain in the 1950's.[11] They are devices that accelerate electrons to nearly the speed of light. The electron beam is aimed at a heavy metal alloy target. The resulting interactions produce x-rays, which can be collimated and focused on a patient. Linear accelerators have, over the ensuing decades, become the favored treatment device for conventional radiation therapy.

In 1984, Betti and Derechinsky described a radiosurgical system using the linear accelerator as the source of radiation.[3] Colombo and colleagues described their system in 1985.[7] Subsequently, many investigators have modified these systems in a variety of ways to achieve the requirements of radiosurgical systems.[16, 35, 40] Winston and Lutz first developed methods for quantifying the accuracy of linear accelerator radiosurgery

W. A. Friedman • F. J. Bova

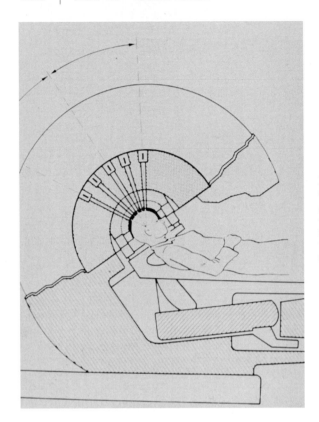

Figure 60–1

The Gamma knife is a hemispherical device that contains 201 cobalt sources, all collimated and focused on one point. The patient is stereotactically positioned within one of four collimator helmets (producing 4-mm, 8-mm, 14-mm, or 18-mm radiation beams), such that the intracranial target coincides with the focal point of the machine. This results in a high target dose with relatively little radiation to surrounding structures.

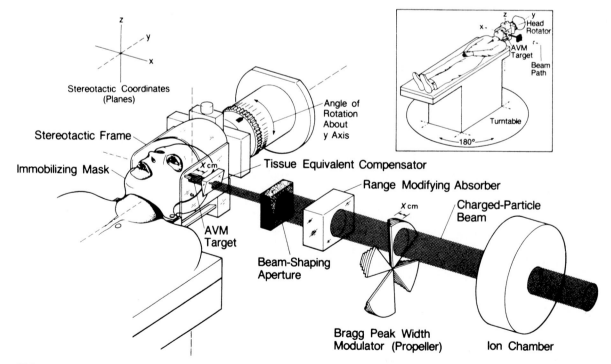

Figure 60–2

Diagram of charged-particle beam delivery system at the University of California at Berkeley-Lawrence Laboratory 184-in. synchrocyclotron. The stereotactic positioning system allows translation along three orthogonal axes and rotation around the y and z axes. The width of the Bragg ionization peak can be spread to the prescribed size by interposing a modulating filter (here a propeller with variable-thickness blades) in the beam path. The depth in tissue is determined by a range-modifying absorber. Individually designed apertures shape the beam cross section to conform to the shape of the lesion. Multiple beams at different angles are used to produce the lowest possible dose to sensitive adjacent brain structures.

systems.[31, 54] In 1988, workers on the University of Florida radiosurgery system improved the work of Winston and Lutz by eliminating the inherent inaccuracy of the linear accelerator bearings and by incorporating ultra-high-speed computer dose planning[13] (Fig. 60–3).

All linear accelerator radiosurgical systems rely on a single basic paradigm: A collimated x-ray beam is focused on a stereotactically identified intracranial target. The gantry of the linear accelerator rotates over the patient, producing an arc of radiation focused on the target. The patient's couch is then rotated in the horizontal plane, and another arc is performed. In this manner, multiple, non-coplanar intersecting arcs of radiation are produced. In a fashion exactly analogous to the multiple intersecting cobalt beams in the gamma knife, the intersecting arcs produce a high target dose, with minimal radiation to the surrounding brain.

The Physics of Radiosurgery

Radiosurgery delivers high doses of energy to treatment volumes while delivering smaller, less effective doses to nontarget tissues. One basic radiosurgery technique used by all teletherapy units, whether isotope units (the Gamma knife) or electronically produced photon units (linear accelerators), relies on averaging the effects of multiple photon beams focused at a single point. Both x-rays and gamma rays are photons; the only difference between these two types of radiation is the source. Gamma rays, such as those produced by cobalt-60, originate in the nuclei of that isotope. Each time a cobalt-60 atom decays, it produces two photons. These photons have an average energy of 1.25 MeV.

Linear accelerators do not use stored isotopes but produce their photons through the slowing down of high-energy electrons. Through the use of microwave power, they accelerate electrons to high energies. For stereotactic radiosurgery, energies between 4 and 15 MeV have been used. These electrons are focused onto a target, usually a heavy metal alloy. As electrons interact with the target, they are slowed down. As they slow down, they give off their energy through two mechanisms: collisional losses and radiative losses. The collisional losses result in heat and produce no therapeutic radiation. The radiation losses, however, produce photons. These photons, which are produced outside the nucleus, are called x-rays. Although these x-rays are produced over a spectrum of energies up to the maximum energy of the linear accelerator, their effective energy is approximately equal to one third of the maximum energy. Hence, a 6-MeV accelerator produces an x-ray beam with an average energy of approximately 2 MeV.

Because the energies of the Gamma knife and the linear accelerator are similar, their photon absorption characteristics in tissue are also similar. In "average" body tissue, the cobalt-60 beam loses approximately 5 per cent of its intensity per centimeter, and the 6-MeV accelerator beam loses approximately 4 per cent of its intensity per centimeter. Because this loss is constant, after a small initial build-up depth, the photon beam possesses no special properties that allow any significant concentration of its energy over a target volume. The technique used for concentration of the energy at the target site is a simple averaging process. For example, if six beams are aimed at a target at the center of a 15-cm sphere, each beam is attenuated, by tissue absorption of energy, to approximately 70 per cent of its surface value. The intersection of the six beams, however, has a value of 6 × 70%, or 420 per cent of the

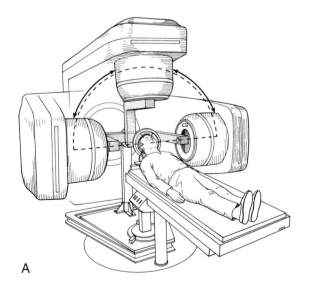
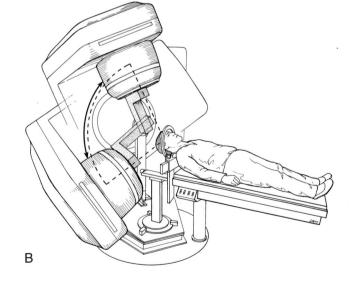

A   B

Figure 60–3

A linear accelerator is a device that accelerates electrons almost to the speed of light. The electrons collide with a heavy metal alloy, producing a beam of photon energy, called x-rays. *A.* The target is stereotactically positioned to coincide with the isocentric rotation point of the gantry of the linear accelerator. *B.* After one arc of radiation is delivered, the patient is horizontally repositioned at a new "table angle," and another arc is performed. Typically, 5 to 9 arcs of radiation are used per isocenter.

surface dose. This averaging process is accomplished in the gamma knife by using 201 separate cobalt-60 sources, all focused at the same point. For linear accelerators, multiple non-coplanar arcs of radiation are used to achieve the same effect.

The second physics approach to radiosurgery involves the use of heavy charged-particle beams. Particle beams lose energy uniformly until the particle nears the end of its range. At this point, the particle sharply increases its energy loss, depositing a well-defined maximum dose. This region of increased dose is termed the "Bragg peak." The depth at which the Bragg peak occurs can be varied by changing the entrance energy of the particle beam. In practice, this depth adjustment is achieved through the use of absorbing materials. Absorbers are also used to spread out the width of the Bragg peak to match the target width. Although the Bragg peak effect has an advantage over the exponentially decreasing dose profile of photon beams, it alone does not produce a satisfactorily steep dose gradient at the target site. As with photon beams, an averaging technique is employed. Because of the Bragg peak, fewer cross-fired beams are necessary to produce a steep gradient.

General Radiosurgical Paradigm

Although the details of radiosurgical treatment techniques differ somewhat from system to system, the basic paradigm is similar everywhere. The following is a detailed description of a typical radiosurgical treatment at the University of Florida.

Almost all radiosurgical procedures in adults are performed on an outpatient basis. A stereotactic head ring is applied under local anesthesia. No skin shaving or preparation is required. If the treatment is for an arteriovenous malformation, the patient is transported to the angiography suite, where a stereotactic angiogram is performed. Subsequently, stereotactic computed tomography or stereotactic magnetic resonance imaging is performed. To maximize resolution, a bolus of intravenous contrast material is given just before imaging through the lesion. Because the stereotactic angiogram provides a relatively poor three-dimensional database,[5, 6, 46] the authors also rely on the appearance of the nidus on contrast-enhanced computed tomography for treatment planning. After computed tomography scanning, the patient is transported to the outpatient radiology area for postangiography observation.

The angiogram, computed tomogram, or magnetic resonance image are transferred by Ethernet to the radiation physics suite for dosimetry. The nidus of the lesion is outlined on the angiogram, which is then mounted on a digitizer board. A mouse-like device is used to identify the stereotactic frame markers and to trace the nidus; they simultaneously appear on the computer screen. The computer then generates anteroposterior, lateral, and vertical coordinates of the center of the lesion as well as its demagnified diameter. Next,

the computer determines the position of all of the computed tomography images or magnetic resonance images within the stereotactic coordinate system. The angiography target center point is displayed on the scan image. Dosimetry then begins and continues until an optimal dose plan has been developed (Fig. 60–4). A final computer printout shows all of the treatment parameters in a checklist format.

Patients rest comfortably until the end of the normal radiation therapy treatment day. The radiosurgical device is attached to the linear accelerator. The patient then is attached to the device and treated. The radiation treatment time averages approximately 20 minutes. Afterward, the head ring is removed and, after a short observation period, the patient is discharged.

Radiosurgery for Arteriovenous Malformations

Many studies have demonstrated a substantial risk of hemorrhage (3 to 4 per cent per year), often associated with morbidity or mortality, in patients harboring arteriovenous malformations.[38] Refinements in microsurgical technique and the development of increasing effective endovascular treatments have rendered many of the lesions amenable to successful, safe, surgical cure.[15, 18, 42, 45] Those lesions that are not suitable for surgical removal are often considered for radiosurgical management.

ANGIOGRAPHIC THROMBOSIS RATES

Radiosurgery appears to produce thrombosis of the malformations by inducing a pathological process in the nidus, leading to gradual thickening of the vessels until thrombosis occurs.[37, 56] Several radiosurgical series have systematically evaluated this process by obtaining 1-year and 2-year follow-up angiograms. Steiner has published reports on Gamma knife radiosurgery for arteriovenous malformations.[36, 50–52] He has reported 1-year occlusion rates ranging from 33.7 to 39.5 per cent and 2-year occlusion rates ranging from 79 to 86.5 per cent. However, these results were "optimized" by retrospectively selecting patients who received a minimum treatment dose. For example, in one report, Linquist and Steiner stated, "a large majority of patients received at least 2,000 to 2,500 rad of radiation . . . . Of the 248 patients treated before 1984, the treatment specification placed 188 in this group."[27] The reported thrombosis rates in this paper applied only to these 188 patients (76 per cent of his total series).[27] Yamamoto and colleagues reported on 25 Japanese patients who were treated on the gamma unit in Stockholm but followed in Japan.[56] The 2-year thrombosis rate in the lesions that were completely covered by the radiosurgical field was 64 per cent. One additional patient had complete thrombosis at 3-year angiography and one more at 5-year angiography, for a total cure rate of

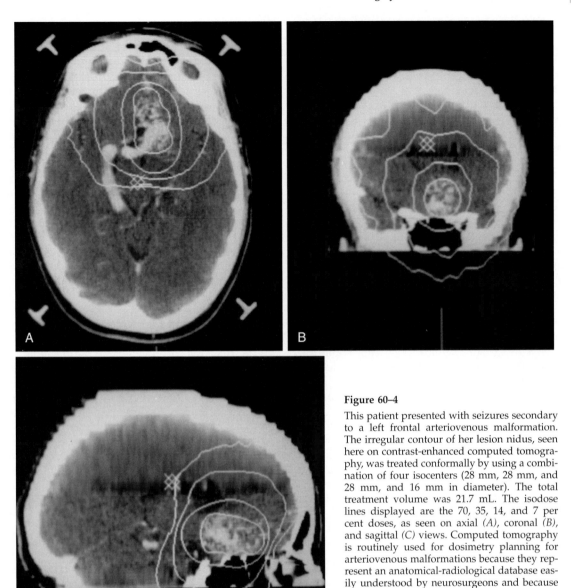

Figure 60–4

This patient presented with seizures secondary to a left frontal arteriovenous malformation. The irregular contour of her lesion nidus, seen here on contrast-enhanced computed tomography, was treated conformally by using a combination of four isocenters (28 mm, 28 mm, and 28 mm, and 16 mm in diameter). The total treatment volume was 21.7 mL. The isodose lines displayed are the 70, 35, 14, and 7 per cent doses, as seen on axial (A), coronal (B), and sagittal (C) views. Computed tomography is routinely used for dosimetry planning for arteriovenous malformations because they represent an anatomical-radiological database easily understood by neurosurgeons and because of inherent limitations of stereotactic angiography.

73 per cent. In another paper, these authors reported angiographic cures in 6 (67 per cent) of 9 children treated in Stockholm or Buenos Aires and followed in Japan.[55]

Kemeny, Dias, and Forster reported on 52 patients with arteriovenous malformations who were treated with Gamma knife radiosurgery.[20] They all received 2,500 rad to the 50 per cent isodose line. At 1 year, 16 patients (31 per cent) had complete thrombosis, and 10 patients (19 per cent) had "almost complete" thrombosis. He found that the results were better in younger patients and in patients with a relatively lateral location of malformations. There was no difference in outcome between small (less than 2 mL), medium (2 to 3 mL), and large (more than 3 mL) lesions.

Lunsford and colleagues reported on 227 patients treated with Gamma knife radiosurgery.[30] The mean dose delivered to the nidus margin was 2,120 rad.

Multiple isocenters were used in 48 per cent of the patients. Seventeen patients underwent 1-year angiography, which confirmed complete thrombosis in 76.5 per cent. As indicated in the paper, "this rate may be spurious since many of these patients were selected for angiography because their [magnetic resonance] image had suggested obliteration." Of the 75 patients who were followed for at least 2 years, 2-year angiography was performed in only 46 (61 per cent). Complete obliteration was confirmed in 37 (80 per cent) of 46. This thrombosis rate strongly correlated with malformation size: 100 per cent for lesions of less than 1 mL, 85 per cent if between 1 and 4 mL, and 58 per cent if between 4 and 10 mL.

Steinberg and associates reported 86 patients who were treated with a particle-beam radiosurgical system, reporting a 29 per cent rate of thrombosis at 1 year, 70 per cent at 2 years, and 92 per cent at 3 years.[48] The best results were obtained with smaller lesions and higher doses. Initially, a treatment dose of 3,460 rad was used, but a higher than expected neurological complication rate (20 per cent for the entire series) led to the currently used dose range of 770 to 1,920 rad. No patients treated with the lower dose range had complications.

Betti and colleagues reported on 66 patients treated with a linear accelerator radiosurgical system.[4, 21] Doses of no more than 4,000 rad were used in 80 per cent of patients. He found a 66 per cent thrombosis rate at 2 years. The percentage of cured patients was highest if the entire malformation was included in the 75 per cent isodose line (96 per cent cured) or if the maximum diameter of the lesion was less than 12 mm (81 per cent cured).

Colombo reported on 97 patients treated with a linear accelerator system.[7, 8] Doses from 1,870 to 4,000 rad were delivered in one or two sessions. Of 56 patients who were followed longer than 1 year, 50 underwent 12-month follow-up angiography. In 26 patients (52 per cent) complete thrombosis was demonstrated. Fifteen (75 per cent) of 20 patients undergoing 2-year angiography had complete thrombosis. He reported a definite relationship between malformation size and thrombosis rate, as follows. Lesions less than 15 mm in diameter had a 1-year obliteration rate of 76 per cent and a 2-year rate of 90 per cent. Lesions 15 to 25 mm in diameter had a 1-year thrombosis rate of 37.5 per cent and a 2-year rate of 80 per cent. Lesions greater than 25 mm in diameter had a 1-year thrombosis rate of 11 per cent and a 2-year rate of 40 per cent. In a more recent study, Colombo and colleagues reported follow-up on 180 radiosurgically treated malformations.[8] The 1-year thrombosis rate was 46 per cent, and the 2-year rate was 80 per cent.

Souhami and associates reported on 33 patients who were treated with a linear accelerator system. The prescribed dose at isocenter varied from 5,000 to 5,500 rad.[43] A complete obliteration rate of 38 per cent was seen on 1-year angiography. For patients whose arteriovenous malformation nidus was covered by a minimum dose of 2,500 rad, the total obliteration rate was 61.5 per cent, whereas none of the patients who received less than 2,500 rad at the edge of the nidus obtained a total obliteration.

Loeffler and colleagues reported on 16 arteriovenous malformations treated with a linear accelerator system.[29] The prescribed dose was 1,500 to 2,500 rad, typically to the 80 to 90 per cent line. The total obliteration rate was 5 (45 per cent) of 11 at 1 year and 8 (73 per cent) of 11 at 2 years after treatment.

Between May 18, 1988, and August 31, 1993, 158 of these lesions were treated on the University of Florida radiosurgical system.[14] There were 80 men and 78 women in the series. The mean age was 39 (range: 13 to 70). Presenting symptoms included hemorrhage (61), seizure (63), headache/incidental (30), and progressive neurological deficit (4). Twenty-two patients had undergone prior surgical attempts at excision of the malformations. Fourteen patients had undergone at least one embolization procedure. All patients were screened

by a vascular neurosurgeon before consideration of radiosurgery. The mean radiation dose to the periphery of the lesion was 1,560 rad (range: 1,000 to 2,500 rad). This treatment dose was almost always delivered to the 80 per cent isodose line (range: 70 to 90 per cent). One hundred thirty-nine patients were treated with one isocenter, 12 patients with two isocenters, 6 patients with three isocenters, and 1 patient with four isocenters. The mean lesion volume was 9 mL (range: 0.5 to 45.3 mL). Median lesion volume was 7.1 mL. In an effort to provide data comparable to that in other publications in the radiosurgical literature, the following size categories were used in this analysis: A (less than 1 mL), B (1 to 4 mL), C (4 to 10 mL), and D (more than 10 mL). The treatment volume was determined in all cases by performing a computed dose-volume histogram of the treatment isodose shell (which was constructed so as to be conformal to the lesion's nidus).

Mean follow-up duration for the entire group was 33 months (range: 6 to 70 months). Follow-up consisted of clinical examination and magnetic resonance imaging every 6 months after treatment.[41] If possible, follow-up was performed in Gainesville; otherwise scan and examination results were forwarded by the patient's local physician. Clinical information is available on 153 of 158 patients. Initially, all patients were asked to undergo angiography at yearly intervals, regardless of the magnetic resonance imaging findings. After the first 50 patients had been treated, it was decided to defer angiography until magnetic resonance imaging strongly suggested complete thrombosis. Furthermore, if complete thrombosis was not identified 3 years after radiosurgery, repeat radiosurgery was undertaken in an effort to obliterate any remaining nidus. By angiography, a cure required that no nidus or shunting remain on the study, as interpreted by a radiologist and the treating neurosurgeon (Figs. 60–5 and 60–6). A total of 48 patients had such cures, of 60 angiograms performed (80 per cent). These patients are considered to have achieved a definitive successful end point for radiosurgery. The following cure rates were seen in the various size categories: A, no angiograms; B, 81 per cent; and C, 89 per cent, D—69 per cent. Two patients with 2-year angiograms showing small amounts of remaining nidus had complete occlusion on 3-year follow-up angiograms.

COMPLICATIONS

Hemorrhage

Many series report that the hemorrhage rate for arteriovenous malformations treated but not yet obliterated with radiosurgery is the same as if they had not been treated.[37] Most recently, Steiner and colleagues analyzed clinical outcomes in 247 consecutive patients treated with the Gamma knife.[53] No patient with angiographically proven thrombosis had a hemorrhage. The protective effect of radiosurgery against hemorrhage in incompletely obliterated lesions was evaluated, using both the person-year and Kaplan-Meier life table meth-

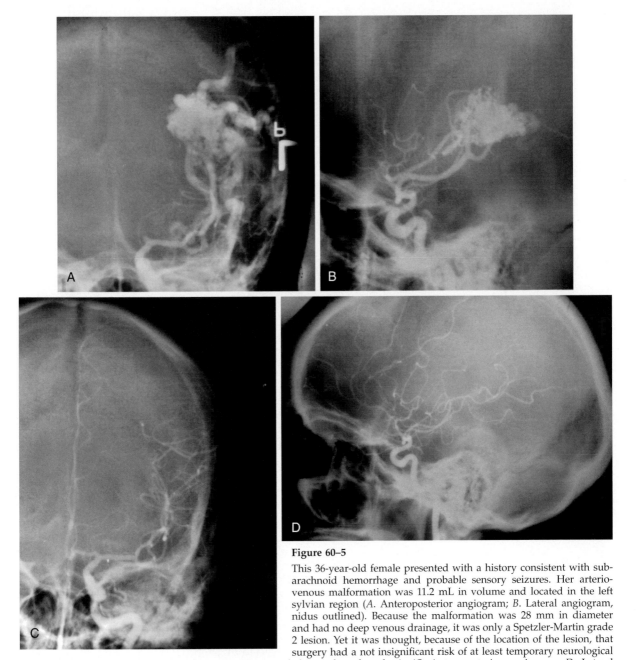

Figure 60–5

This 36-year-old female presented with a history consistent with subarachnoid hemorrhage and probable sensory seizures. Her arteriovenous malformation was 11.2 mL in volume and located in the left sylvian region (*A.* Anteroposterior angiogram; *B.* Lateral angiogram, nidus outlined). Because the malformation was 28 mm in diameter and had no deep venous drainage, it was only a Spetzler-Martin grade 2 lesion. Yet it was thought, because of the location of the lesion, that surgery had a not insignificant risk of at least temporary neurological deficits. Angiography 24 months after treatment revealed complete thrombosis (*C.* Anteroposterior angiogram; *D.* Lateral angiogram).

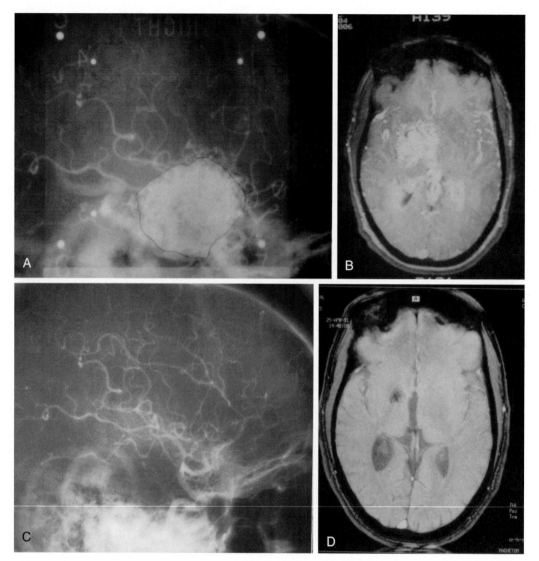

Figure 60–6

This 39-year-old male presented with a history of headaches, seizures, and a progressive visual field cut. He was referred for radiosurgery. He received 1,000 rad to the 70 per cent isodose line, through a 35-mm collimator (*A.* Lateral view, pretreatment angiogram; *B.* Pretreatment magnetic resonance image). One-year angiography revealed substantial but incomplete thrombosis of the lesion. Two-year angiography revealed complete nidus thrombosis (*C.* Lateral view, post-treatment angiogram; *D.* Post-treatment magnetic resonance image).

ods of analysis. The person-year method showed a rebleed rate of 2 to 3 per cent per year—very similar to the known natural history of the disease. The Kaplan-Meier analysis showed a risk of 3.7 per cent per year until 5 years after radiosurgery. At that point, the risk seemed to plateau. Steiner and his associates believe this plateau, which has long been a source of controversy in the radiosurgery literature, to be an artifact of this statistical method when it is applied to a relatively small group of patients. In general, most authors believe that radiosurgery has no protective effect against hemorrhage until the malformation has thrombosed. This lack of protection is, in fact, the major known drawback of radiosurgery compared with microsurgery.

Colombo and colleagues studied the risk of hemorrhage after radiosurgery in 180 patients.[8] In totally irradiated lesions (163), the bleeding rate decreased from 4.8 per cent in the first 6 months to 0 per cent after 12 months. In subtotally irradiated lesions, the bleeding risk increased from 4 per cent in the first 6 months, to 10 per cent from 12 to 18 months, and then decreased to 5.5 per cent from 18 to 24 months. There were no hemorrhages observed in this group after 24 months had elapsed.

Radiation-Induced Complications

Several authors have reported that radiosurgery can acutely exacerbate seizure activity.[17, 44] Others have reported nausea, vomiting, and headache occasionally occurring after radiosurgical treatment.[1] Delayed radiation-induced complications have been reported by all groups performing radiosurgery. Steiner found symptomatic radiation necrosis in approximately 3 per cent of his patients.[50] Statham and colleagues described one patient who developed radiation necrosis 13 months after Gamma knife radiosurgery of a 5.3-mL arteriovenous malformation with 2,500 rad to the margin.[47] Lunsford and colleagues reported that 10 patients in their series (4.4 per cent) developed new neurological deficits thought to be secondary to radiation injury.[30] Symptoms were dependent on location and developed between 4 and 18 months after treatment. All patients were treated with steroids, and all improved. Only two patients were reported to have residual deficits that appeared permanent. The radiation dose and isodose line treated did not correlate with this complication. As he noted, the failure of correlation of dose and complications may relate to the fact that the dose was selected to fall below Flickinger's computed 3 per cent risk line. This is a mathematically derived line that prescribes lower doses for larger lesions.[10, 12]

Steinberg and colleagues reported a definite correlation between lesion dose and complications.[48] As has been indicated, the initial treatment dose of 3,460 rad led to a relatively high complication rate. No patients treated with the subsequently used lower dose range had complications. In an earlier report on 75 patients treated with helium particles at a dose of 4,500 rad, 7 (11 per cent) of 75 patients experienced radiation-induced complications.[19] Kjellberg and associates, using a compilation of animal and clinical data, constructed a series of log-log lines relating prescribed dose and lesion diameter.[21, 22] Kjellberg's 1 per cent isorisk line is similar to Flickinger's mathematically derived 3 per cent risk line.

In the series reported by Colombo and colleagues, 9 (5 per cent) of 180 patients experienced symptomatic radiation-induced complications.[8] Four (2.2 per cent) were permanent. Loeffler and associates reported 1 of 21 patients developed a similar problem, which responded well to steroids.[29] Souhami and colleagues reported severe side effects in 2 (6 per cent) of 33 patients.[43] Marks recently reviewed six radiosurgical series and found a 9 per cent incidence of clinically significant radiation reactions.[34] Seven of 23 cases received doses below Kjellberg's 1 per cent risk line.

In the University of Florida series, three patients (2 per cent) have experienced transient delayed complications directly attributable to radiosurgery. One of these patients experienced headache, and two had mild dysphasia. The onset of symptoms occurred at 14, 14, and 15 months after radiosurgery, respectively. All had documented areas of edema around their malformations, which resolved after several months of steroid therapy. All now have no deficit, and their magnetic resonance images are normal (Fig. 60–7). It has been subsequently documented by angiography that two of these patients have been cured, and one has refused further radiological follow-up. Two patients (1 per cent) have experienced permanent radiation-induced complications. One patient has mild lower extremity weakness. The other has Parinaud's syndrome and hemibody analgesia. The onset of symptoms was 11 and 14 months after radiosurgery, respectively. Both patients had documented areas of edema, which resolved after months of steroid therapy. Subsequently, it

has been documented by angiography that both patients have been cured. Figure 60–8 shows the treatment dose and lesion size of all patients treated. The two patients with permanent complications received doses higher than those the authors subsequently used in other lesions of similar volume. Conversely, the three patients with transient complications received doses that have been safely used in other patients with malformations of similar size.

Others have reported that asymptomatic radiation-induced changes appear frequently (24 per cent in Lunsford's series) on magnetic resonance images.[33] The authors have also observed this phenomenon. These changes tend to be asymptomatic if the lesion is located in a relatively "silent" brain area and symptomatic if the lesion is located in an "eloquent" brain area. Therefore, lesion location may be another important consideration in radiosurgical treatment planning and dose selection.

Most radiosurgical series report their radiation-induced complications as a percentage of the total patient population treated. The fact that most radiation-induced complications do not appear until 12 to 18 months after treatment results in a systematic underestimate of the true complication rate.

MULTIMODALITY TREATMENT

Radiosurgery may be used alone in the treatment of malformations smaller than 3.5 cm in diameter. Occasionally, larger lesions are treated with a combination of endovascular therapy, surgery, and radiosurgery.[9] Embolization and radiosurgery have been applied with increasing frequency (Fig. 60–9). Many questions remain to be answered regarding this combination of therapies, such as what type of embolic material is best. The authors treat the nidus that remains after embolization. Because radiosurgery frequently takes 2 years to produce nidus thrombosis, the possibility exists that the embolic material will "wash out" during this latent period.

It does seem clear that radiosurgery combined with embolization exposes the patient to the risks of both procedures. Because embolization alone rarely produces a cure, it should be used only if the malformation is too large to be safely treated with radiosurgery alone.

CAVERNOUS MALFORMATIONS

The advent of magnetic resonance imaging as a neurological screening test has resulted in the identification of substantial numbers of cavernous malformations. This vascular malformation differs pathologically from true arteriovenous malformations. The role of radiosurgery in the treatment of these lesions is not well defined. Kondziolka and colleagues reported on 24 patients treated with the Gamma knife at the University of Pittsburgh.[23] Radiosurgery was used conservatively; each patient had sustained two or more hemorrhages and had a lesion defined by magnetic resonance im-

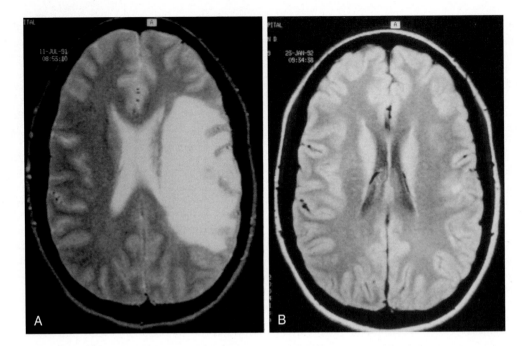

Figure 60–7

This 30-year-old female developed a grand mal seizure disorder and was discovered to have a left frontoparietal arteriovenous malformation. She was treated with 1,500 rad to the 80 per cent isodose line, through a 26-mm collimator. One-year angiogram showed more than 90 per cent thrombosis. One month later she presented with complaints of headache. *A.* T2-weighted magnetic resonance image revealed an area of probable radiation necrosis, in the exact area treated with radiosurgery, surrounded by considerable edema. She was treated with steroids, which produced a prompt and dramatic clinical improvement. *B.* After months of therapy, her magnetic resonance image became normal. Two-year angiography revealed complete thrombosis of the malformation.

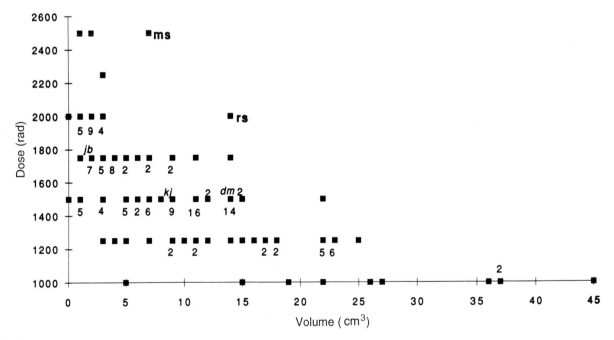

Figure 60–8

This figure displays the dose prescribed to the periphery of every arteriovenous malformation versus that malformation's volume. Numbers displayed adjacent to data points indicate the number of patients treated at that particular volume and dose. In general, the larger the volume, the lower the dose that can be safely prescribed. The two patients with minor, permanent neurological complications are indicated with bold initials. They were treated early in the series and received doses that were higher than those now employed for lesions of similar volume. The three patients with transient radiation-induced complications are indicated with nonbold initials. They received doses that have been safely employed in other patients.

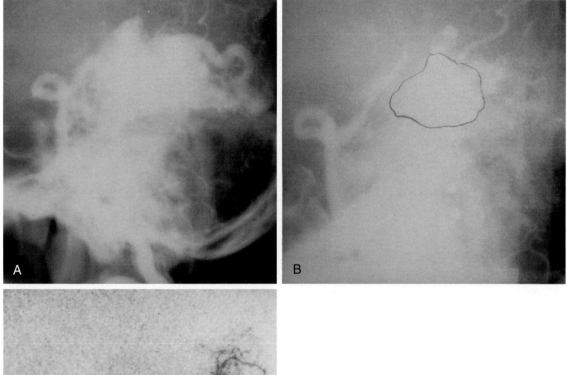

Figure 60–9

This 40-year-old male presented with a history of headaches and seizures. *A.* Pre-embolization lateral angiography. *B.* Post-embolization lateral angiography, with nidus outlined. He underwent multiple endovascular treatments for a large left occipitoparietal arteriovenous malformation. The residual nidus was treated with radiosurgery (1,500 rad, 80 per cent isodose line, 28-mm collimator). *C.* Lateral digital angiogram 1 year after treatment shows complete thrombosis.

aging that was located in a region of the brain in which microsurgical removal was judged to pose an excessive risk. Fifteen malformations were in the medulla, pons, or mesencephalon, and five were located in the thalamus or basal ganglia. Follow-up ranged from 4 to 24 months. Nineteen patients either improved or remained clinically stable and did not hemorrhage again during the follow-up interval. One patient suffered another hemorrhage 7 months after radiosurgery. Five patients experienced temporary worsening of pre-existing neurological deficits that suggested delayed radiation injury. Magnetic resonance imaging demonstrated signal changes and edema surrounding the radiosurgical target.

Steinberg and colleagues reported 35 patients treated for angiographically occult vascular malformations.[49] The clinical outcome was excellent or good in 80 per cent and poor in 14 per cent. Six per cent of the patients died. Six patients experienced recurrent hemorrhage. Four patients worsened from probable radiation injury.

These reports indicate a significantly higher complication rate for radiosurgical treatment of cavernous malformations than for similar treatment of true arteriovenous malformations. In addition, the fact that they are angiographically occult means that no objective criteria for successful treatment exist. Only by following patients with a proven propensity for hemorrhage and demonstrating a significant decrease in hemorrhage rate can benefit be shown. Proof of such benefit does not currently exist. At the University of Florida, aggressive surgical therapy is used on the majority of patients with symptomatic cavernous malformation. Radiosurgery is regarded as a last resort.

Conclusions

In summary, many reports indicate that approximately 80 per cent of arteriovenous malformations in the radiosurgery size range are angiographically obliterated 2 years after radiosurgical treatment. Permanent neurological complications are rare (2 to 3 per cent). The major drawback of this treatment method is that the patients are unprotected against hemorrhage during the 2-year latent period. Although radiosurgery was used primarily as a single modality of treatment in previous studies, it has been increasingly employed as part of a multimodality treatment approach incorporating surgical and endovascular methods. Radiosurgery is of unproven value in the treatment of cavernous malformations.

REFERENCES

1. Alexander, E., III, Siddon, R. L., and Loeffler, J. S.: The acute onset of nausea and vomiting following stereotactic radiosurgery: Correlation with total dose to area postrema. Surg. Neurol., 32:40–44, 1989.
2. Backlund, E. O., Johansson, L., and Sarby, B.: Studies on craniopharyngiomas: II. Treatment by stereotaxis and radiosurgery. Acta Chir. Scand., 138:749–759, 1972.
3. Betti, O. O., and Derechinsky, V. E.: Hyperselective encephalic irradiation with a linear accelerator. Acta Neurochir. Suppl. (Wien), 33:385–390, 1984.
4. Betti, O. O., Munari, C., and Rosler, R.: Stereotactic radiosurgery with the linear accelerator: Treatment of arteriovenous malformations. Neurosurgery, 24:311–321, 1989.
5. Blatt, D. L., Friedman, W. A., and Bova, F. J.: Modifications in radiosurgical treatment planning of arteriovenous malformations based on CT imaging. Neurosurgery, 33:588–596, 1993.
6. Bova, F. J., and Friedman, W. A.: Stereotactic angiography: An inadequate database for radiosurgery? Int. J. Radiat. Oncol. Biol. Phys., 20:891–895, 1991.
7. Colombo, F., Benedetti, A., Pozza, F., et al.: External stereotactic irradiation by linear accelerator. Neurosurgery, 16:154–160, 1985.
8. Colombo, F., Pozza, F., Chierego, G., et al.: Linear accelerator radiosurgery of cerebral arteriovenous malformations: An update. Neurosurgery, 34:14–21, 1994.
9. Dawson, R. C., III, Tarr, R. W., Hecht, S. T., et al.: Treatment of arteriovenous malformations of the brain with combined embolization and stereotactic radiosurgery: Results after 1 and 2 years. Am. J. Neuroradiol., 11:857–864, 1990.
10. Flickinger, J. C.: An integrated logistic formula for prediction of complications from radiosurgery. Int. J. Radiat. Oncol. Biol. Phys., 17:879–885, 1989.
11. Flickinger, J. C., Lunsford, L. D., Coffey, R. J., et al.: Radiosurgery of acoustic neurinomas. Cancer, 67:345–353, 1991.
12. Flickinger, J. C., Schell, M. C., and Larson, D. A.: Estimation of complications for linear accelerator radiosurgery with the integrated logistic formula. Int. J. Radiat. Oncol. Biol. Phys., 19:143–148, 1990.
13. Friedman, W. A., and Bova, F. J.: The University of Florida radiosurgery system. Surg. Neurol., 32:334–342, 1989.
14. Friedman, W. A., and Bova, F. J.: LINAC radiosurgery for arteriovenous malformations. J. Neurosurg., 77:832–841, 1992.
15. Hamilton, M. G., and Spetzler, R. F.: The prospective application of a grading system for arteriovenous malformations. Neurosurgery, 34:2–7, 1994.
16. Hartmann, G. H., Schlegel, W., Sturm, V., et al.: Cerebral radiation surgery using moving field irradiation at a linear accelerator facility. Int. J. Radiat. Oncol. Biol. Phys., 11:1185–1192, 1985.
17. Heifetz, M. D., Whiting, J., Bernstein, H., et al.: Stereotactic radiosurgery for fractionated radiation: A proposal applicable to linear accelerator and proton beam programs. Stereotact. Funct. Neurosurg., 53:167–177, 1989.
18. Heros, R. C., Korosue, K., and Diebold, P. M.: Surgical excision of cerebral arteriovenous malformations: Late results. Neurosurgery, 26:570–578, 1990.
19. Hosobuchi, Y., Fabrikant, J. I., and Lyman, J. T.: Stereotactic heavy-particle irradiation of intracranial arteriovenous malformations. Appl. Neurophysiol., 50:248–252, 1987.
20. Kemeny, A. A., Dias, P. S., and Forster, D. M.: Results of stereotactic radiosurgery of arteriovenous malformations: An analysis of 52 cases. J. Neurol. Neurosurg. Psychiatry, 52:554–558, 1989.
21. Kjellberg, R. N., and Abbe, M.: Stereotactic Bragg peak proton beam therapy. In Lunsford, L. D., ed.: Modern Stereotactic Neurosurgery. Boston, Martinus Nijhoff, 1988, pp. 463–470.
22. Kjellberg, R. N., Hanamura, T., Davis, K. R., et al.: Bragg-peak proton-beam therapy for arteriovenous malformations of the brain. N. Engl. J. Med., 309:269–274, 1983.
23. Kondziolka, D., Lunsford, L. D., Coffey, R. J., et al.: Stereotactic radiosurgery of angiographically occult vascular malformations: Indications and preliminary experience. Neurosurgery, 27:892–900, 1990.
24. Leksell, L.: The stereotaxic method and radiosurgery of the brain. Acta Chir. Scand., 102:316–319, 1951.
25. Leksell, L., Larsson, B., Andersson, B., et al.: Lesions in the depth of the brain produced by a beam of high energy protons. Acta Radiol., 54:251–264, 1960.
26. Levy, R. P., Fabrikant, J. I., Frankel, K. A., et al.: Charged-particle radiosurgery of the brain. Neurosurg. Clin. North Am., 1(4):955–990, 1990.
27. Lindquist, C., and Steiner, L.: Stereotactic radiosurgical treatment of malformations of the brain. In Lunsford, L. D., ed.: Modern Stereotactic Neurosurgery. Boston, Martinus Nijhoff, 1988, pp. 491–506.
28. Linskey, M. E., Lunsford, L. D., and Flickinger, J. C.: Radiosurgery for acoustic neurinomas: Early experience. Neurosurgery, 26:736–744, 1990.
29. Loeffler, J. S., Alexander, E., III, Siddon, R. L., et al.: Stereotactic radiosurgery for intracranial arteriovenous malformations using a standard linear accelerator. Int. J. Radiat. Oncol. Biol. Phys., 17:673–677, 1989.
30. Lunsford, L. D., Kondziolka, D., Flickinger, J. C., et al.: Stereotactic radiosurgery for arteriovenous malformations of the brain. J. Neurosurg., 75:512–524, 1991.
31. Lutz, W., Winston, K. R., and Maleki, N.: A system for stereotactic radiosurgery with a linear accelerator. Int. J. Radiat. Oncol. Biol. Phys., 14:373–381, 1988.
32. Lyman, J. T., Phillips, M. H., Frankel, K. A., et al.: Stereotactic frame for neuroradiology and charged particle Bragg peak radiosurgery of intracranial disorders. Int. J. Radiat. Oncol. Biol. Phys., 16:1615–1621, 1989.
33. Marks, M. P., Delapaz, R. L., Fabrikant, J. I., et al.: Intracranial vascular malformations: Imaging of charged-particle radiosurgery: Part II. Complications. Radiology, 168:457–462, 1988.
34. Marks, L. B., and Spencer, D. P.: The influence of volume on the tolerance of the brain to radiosurgery. J. Neurosurg., 75:177–180, 1991.
35. McGinley, P. H., Butker, E. K., Crocker, I. R., et al.: A patient rotator for stereotactic radiosurgery. Phys. Med. Biol., 35:649–657, 1990.
36. Nedzi, L. A., Kooy, H., Alexander, E., et al.: Variables associated with the development of complications from radiosurgery of intracranial tumors. Int. J. Radiat. Oncol. Biol. Phys., 21:591–599, 1991.
37. Ogilvy, C. S.: Radiation therapy for arteriovenous malformations: A review. Neurosurgery, 26:725–735, 1990.
38. Ondra, S. L., Troupp, H., George, E. D., et al.: The natural history of symptomatic arteriovenous malformations of the brain: A 24-year follow-up assessment. J. Neurosurg., 73:387–391, 1991.
39. Phillips, M. H., Kessler, M., Chuang, F. Y., et al.: Image correlation of MRI and CT in treatment planning for radiosurgery of intracranial vascular malformations. Int. J. Radiat. Oncol. Biol. Phys., 20:881–889, 1991.
40. Podgorsak, E. B., Olivier, A., Pla, M., et al.: Dynamic stereotactic radiosurgery. Int. J. Radiat. Oncol. Biol. Phys., 14:115–126, 1988.
41. Quisling, R. G., Peters, K. R., Friedman, W. A., et al.: Persistent nidus blood flow in cerebral arteriovenous malformation after stereotactic radiosurgery: MR imaging assessment. Radiology, 180:785–791, 1991.
42. Sisti, M. B., Kader, A., and Stein, B. M.: Microsurgery for 67 intracranial arteriovenous malformations less than 3 cm in diameter. J. Neurosurg., 79:653–660, 1993.

43. Souhami, L., Olivier, A., Podgorsak, E. B., et al.: Radiosurgery of cerebral arteriovenous malformations with the dynamic stereotactic irradiation. Int. J. Radiat. Oncol. Biol. Phys., 19:775–782, 1990.

44. Souhami, L., Olivier, A., Podgorsak, E. B., et al.: Dynamic stereotactic radiosurgery in arteriovenous malformation: Preliminary treatment results. Cancer, 66:15–20, 1990.

45. Spetzler, R. F., and Martin, N. A.: A proposed grading system of arteriovenous malformations. J. Neurosurg., 65:476–483, 1985.

46. Spiegelmann, R., Friedman, W. A., and Bova, F. J.: Limitations of angiographic target localization in radiosurgical treatment planning. Neurosurgery, 30:619–624, 1992.

47. Statham, P., Macpherson, P., Johnston, R., et al.: Cerebral radiation necrosis complicating stereotactic radiosurgery for arteriovenous malformation. J. Neurol. Neurosurg. Psychiatry, 53:476–479, 1990.

48. Steinberg, G. K., Fabrikant, J. I., Marks, M. P., et al.: Stereotactic heavy-charged particle Bragg peak radiation for intracranial arteriovenous malformations. N. Engl. J. Med., 323:96–101, 1990.

49. Steinberg, G. K., Levy, R. P., Fabrikant, J. I., et al.: Stereotactic helium ion Bragg peak radiosurgery for angiographically occult intracranial vascular malformations. Stereotact. Funct. Neurosurg., 57:64–71, 1991.

50. Steiner, L.: Treatment of arteriovenous malformations by radiosurgery. In Wilson, C. B., and Stein, B. M., eds.: Intracranial Arteriovenous Malformations. Baltimore, Williams & Wilkins, 1984, pp. 295–313.

51. Steiner, L.: Radiosurgery in cerebral arteriovenous malformations. In Fein, J. M., and Flamm, E. S., eds.: Cerebrovascular Surgery. Vol. 4. New York, Springer-Verlag, 1985, pp. 1161–1215.

52. Steiner, L., Leksell, L., Greitz, T., et al.: Stereotaxic radiosurgery for cerebral arteriovenous malformations: Report of a case. Acta Chir. Scand., 138:459–464, 1972.

53. Steiner, L., Lindquist, C., Adler, J. R., et al.: Clinical outcome of radiosurgery for cerebral arteriovenous malformations. J. Neurosurg., 77:1–8, 1992.

54. Winston, K. R., and Lutz, W.: Linear accelerator as a neurosurgical tool for stereotactic radiosurgery. Neurosurgery, 22:454–464, 1988.

55. Yamamoto, M., Jimbo, M., Ide, M., et al.: Long-term follow-up of radiosurgically treated arteriovenous malformations in children: Report of nine cases. Surg. Neurol., 38:95–100, 1992.

56. Yamamoto, M., Jimbo, M., Kobayashi, M., et al.: Long-term results of radiosurgery for arteriovenous malformation: Neurodiagnostic imaging and histological studies of angiographically confirmed nidus obliteration. Surg. Neurol., 37:219–230, 1992.

Special Problems Associated with Subarachnoid Hemorrhage

Debate continues on whether environment, stress factors, or congenital defects are the most important contributors to the pathogenesis of the cerebral aneurysm. Forbus found medial degeneration and fragmentation of the internal elastic membrane caused by continued overstretching.[17] On the other hand, Stehbens questioned the role of medial defects. He found medial defects in all animal species that he studied, but in only one animal, an 8-year-old chimpanzee, was he able to identify an intracranial aneurysm that had been responsible for subarachnoid hemorrhage.[54, 55] Wilson and co-workers concluded that anomalous formations of the circle of Willis can contribute to the development of aneurysms.[69] Hyperplasia of one or more segments or persistence of channels is significant. Vessels that perform the most work, such as those that supply an arteriovenous malformation, are often those from which cerebral aneurysms arise. Likewise, if hypoplasia occurs in one segment (e.g., the A_1 segment), the opposite vessel supplies both anterior cerebral arteries and usually harbors the aneurysm when one is present.[18] Alpers and Berry and also Riggs and Rupp noted that the configuration of the cerebral circulation is important.[1, 46] Among patients with aneurysms, the basal circulation was "normal" in 21 per cent, and some type of deformity occurred in 79 per cent. Many investigators have recognized that onset between 50 and 60 years of age favors some degenerative condition.[27]

Aneurysmal rupture has been associated with pregnancy and the puerperium.[72] According to Pedowitz and Perell, subarachnoid hemorrhage is the most common cerebral vascular complication encountered during pregnancy.[41] They reviewed 79 cases and reported 2 others. The risk of rupture of cerebral aneurysm appears to parallel the hemodynamic changes, reaching an apex in the third trimester, in concert with blood volume changes. One per cent of the reported cases occurred near or at term. However, hemorrhage was recorded in 25 per cent of those who bled either during labor or in the first 24 postpartum hours. Pedowitz and Perell concluded that the hemodynamic changes of pregnancy were a much greater precipitating factor for hemorrhage than the stress of labor and vaginal delivery. The location of aneurysms on the arterial tree in pregnancy is not unique, and they occur in approximately the proportion seen in nonpregnant patients. Treatment must be individualized, however, to take into consideration labor and delivery. Aneurysms seem prone to rupture during the seventh and eighth months of pregnancy and at delivery. There are a number of reasons why the pregnant patient is more susceptible to subarachnoid hemorrhage. Increased blood volume, increased generalized edema, and increased arterial pressure occur during pregnancy, labor, and delivery.[9]

In the series of Cannell and Botterell, some patients underwent cesarean section and others delivered vaginally.[6] The series was small, but there was no clear advantage for cesarean section, according to these authors. Diaz and Sekhar reviewed the records of 154 pregnant patients with verified intracranial hemorrhage.[9] One hundred eighteen (77 per cent) of these lesions were caused by intracranial aneurysm. The 30th to 34th weeks seemed to be a particularly risky period for intracranial hemorrhage, but the method of delivery was not significantly important. Eleven patients died before delivery. The fetal mortality was 11 per cent with cesarean section and 20 per cent with vaginal delivery. Currently, with safer surgical and anesthetic methods, it seems appropriate to perform cesarean section if a survivable infant is to be expected, and then to immediately clip the aneurysm.

Aneurysms are rare in both infants and children.[22] Patients younger than 20 years of age make up only 1.5 to 4.6 per cent of cases. The sites of origin are somewhat different from those in adults, and the configuration may be unusual. Heiskanen reviewed the children's cases encountered among 1,346 patients with aneurysm in Helsinki.[26] Sixteen (1.2 per cent) were younger than 20 years of age. In this series, the most common sites were the anterior communicating artery and the internal carotid artery at the posterior communicating junction. Multiple aneurysms were rare. One case was associated with coarctation of the aorta. Heiskanen believed that the results of microsurgery on aneurysms in children are better than those in adults, provided that good clinical grade patients are seen. Overall management mortality, however, is still high, 39 to 46 per cent.

A familial relation in the development of intracranial aneurysms has been established. Ayer mentioned cases among cousins aged 6 and 10.[3] Chambers and associates were the first to emphasize intracranial aneurysm development in a father and a son.[7] Hemorrhage occurred in these two patients within a few months of each other. Phillips reported aneurysms in sisters, both of whom presented with subarachnoid hemorrhage caused by aneurysms at the internal carotid artery.[42] The reasons for familial clustering are not clear and are probably multifactorial.

Arterial aneurysms also are found in patients with moyamoya disease. Aneurysms occur in 10 to 15 per cent of patients in whom a diagnosis of moyamoya disease is established angiographically. Aneurysms occur on both the diseased segment and the counterpart normal vessels. Because the hemorrhagic form of moyamoya disease is characterized by spontaneous hemorrhage, the differential diagnosis becomes especially complex in the patient harboring an aneurysm.[58] There are two forms of moyamoya disease. In the childhood type, the ischemic symptoms prevail. In the adult type, and in those who survive childhood and carry their disease into the adult situation, intracranial hemorrhage becomes a factor to be considered. The prognosis in patients with cerebral aneurysm and moyamoya disease is quite unfavorable. Further discussion of moyamoya disease is given in Chapter 49.

Cerebral aneurysms develop in patients with sickle cell disease or occur coincidentally with it. Multiple aneurysms have been described in some patients with this disease. Also, widespread arterial lesions have been observed in patients with sickle cell anemia. The vessels of the conjunctiva are similarly affected, showing more profound changes in those afflicted with the homozygous entity.[52] The arterial lesions, at least in children, may be demonstrated with magnetic resonance angiography, which shows an intraluminal defect in the vascular distribution of the affected territory and correlates well with the arterial lesions observed on conventional angiography.[70] Because patients with sickle cell anemia undergo arteriography with great risk, they should be subjected first to studies that do not require the injection of contrast materials.

Intracranial arterial aneurysms arise commonly in patients with anomalies of the basal cranial vessels and in those with diseases or structural abnormalities of these vessels. It is now possible to detect many of these anomalies and variations in anatomical structure with the use of ultrasound, magnetic resonance imaging, and selective angiography.

Abnormal embryogenesis results in the retention of primitive vessels and peculiarities in collateralization and anastomotic patterns.[40] George and co-workers reported that 14 per cent of patients who had persistence of the primitive trigeminal artery also had intracranial aneurysms.[21]

From dissection studies, it is known that the ideal circle of Willis, in which each vessel is made up of its average size, occurs rarely in any individual. More often, hypoplasia and asymmetry occur, especially in patients with intracranial arterial aneurysms. In 1966, Kirgis and co-authors studied 1,000 circles of Willis, 7 per cent of which harbored aneurysms.[31] Of the 26 patients with aneurysms of the anterior communicating artery, 58 per cent also had hypoplasia of one A1 segment. Rhoton and colleagues found a normal circle of Willis in 54 per cent of their cases.[45] The most common variation was hypoplasia of one posterior communicating artery, and this occurred in 32 per cent of the cases examined. Kayembe and co-authors studied 44 patients with intracranial arterial aneurysms and found only 11 per cent with the "normal" circle of Willis.[29]

Arteriosclerosis, infection, other inflammatory diseases, disorders of connective tissue, and tumors all have been implicated in the formation of aneurysms. The role that arteriosclerosis plays is unclear. Some aneurysms originate within an area of atheroma that involves the parent artery and the neck of the aneurysm. Courville described pyramidal, fusiform, spherical, and multiple small outpouchings on arteries containing atheroma.[8] Arteriosclerotic aneurysms may develop after the atheroma has destroyed the medial layer, allowing herniation of the intima. They commonly originate at the bifurcation of an intracranial artery, which is also the most common site of atheroma formation. They also occur at the bifurcations of arteries in patients older than 50 years of age who have arterial hypertension. Classification is made more complex by the fact that atheroma forms in the walls of some aneurysms secondarily, much as it forms in the artery walls.

The association of intracranial aneurysm with bacterial endocarditis was made early. In the series reported by Roach and Drake, 2.6 per cent had bacterial aneurysms.[47] Bacterial endocarditis fosters aneurysms infrequently, in fewer than 5 per cent of affected patients. Roach and Drake postulated that a microscopic infected embolus lodges in the vasa vasorum. However, vasa vasorum have been found only on the first segment of the internal carotid artery, and this is not the usual site of the development of bacterial aneurysms. The middle cerebral arteries and their branches are frequently involved, but the site is usually that at which an embolus impacts with the orifice of a small central perforating branch.

Intracranial arterial aneurysms develop in as many as 10 per cent of patients with subacute bacterial endocarditis.[74] Most of these aneurysms subsequently lead to intracranial hemorrhage. Summarizing the available data, Fox found 175 arterial aneurysms in 140 patients with subacute bacterial endocarditis.[19] Eleven per cent were on the internal carotid artery, 64 per cent were on the middle cerebral artery, 11 per cent were on the anterior communicating artery, 8 per cent were on the posterior communicating artery, and 6 to 7 per cent were on the vertebrobasilar system. Usually, the bacterial aneurysm is peripherally placed, and it may be either saccular or fusiform in type. In 25 cases, Fox found more than one bacterial aneurysm. Typical subarachnoid hemorrhage occurred in 18 per cent of patients. Ischemic disorders occurred in 11 per cent, and tumor and epilepsy were encountered rarely. In 12 per cent, the aneurysm was discovered incidentally. Seventy-one per cent of the cases were associated with endocarditis. Eleven per cent of patients had meningitis; 10 per cent had septicemia; rarely, thrombophlebitis of the cavernous sinus, osteomyelitis, and skin abscess were also encountered. The bacteria involved in most cases were beta-hemolytic streptococci and *Staphylococcus aureus; Pneumococcus* and *Corynebacterium* also were encountered. Fungal, syphilitic, spirochetal, and amebic aneurysms also occur, but rarely.

Bacterial aneurysms seem to localize on peripheral branches intraparenchymally. The predilection for these sites apparently is determined by the course of the infected embolus. After embolization, the organisms flourish, causing injury to the internal elastic membrane and endothelial layers. Later, the muscular layers and medial collagen network are broken through, allowing herniation of the newly formed endothelial layer through the defect produced. The microembolus apparently lyses and passes on, preserving blood flow in the vessel.[33, 34, 56]

Bacterial aneurysms have unpredictable bleeding rates, and rebleedings have occurred while patients were waiting for antibiotic treatment to be effective. In the cases in which the aneurysm is embedded in eloquent brain and significant resection would be required to obliterate the aneurysm, a course of antibiotic therapy is still warranted. If the lesion can be excised or clipped at low risk, this treatment should prevail.[53]

Connective tissue disorders cause aneurysms by contributing to early degeneration of connective tissue layers. Among the causes are fibromuscular dysplasia, Ehlers-Danlos syndrome, Marfan's syndrome, pseudoxanthoma elasticum, lupus erythematosus, and the Rendu-Osler-Weber syndrome. Rubinstein and Cohen reported the first association of an intracranial aneurysm with Ehlers-Danlos syndrome.[48] The patient had defective collagen tissue and skin, hyperelastic skin, and elastic joints. An aneurysm developed on the internal carotid artery and caused a subarachnoid hemorrhage. At operation, the surgeon described the intracranial carotid artery as flimsy, virtually falling to pieces when touched. Other vessels seemed to be defective in collagen content. Neil-Dwyer and colleagues studied the ratio of type III to type I collagen in 17 patients undergoing surgery for ruptured cerebral aneurysm.[37] Among this group, 11 of the 17 were deficient in type III collagen. All control subjects had normal collagen ratios. Type IV Ehlers-Danlos syndrome is caused by a type III collagen deficiency, and these

patients are known to harbor intracranial aneurysms with increased frequency.[42, 43]

Weir listed the aneurysms associated with systemic tumors.[65] Metastatic carcinoma of the arterial wall leads in frequency. Cardiac myxoma, choriocarcinoma, and carcinoma are the most likely offending neoplasms. Aneurysms also develop from invasions by contiguous neoplasms, such as carcinoma, glioma, and lymphoma; some aneurysms are associated with primary central nervous system tumors, such as meningiomas (29 per cent), adenomas (26 per cent), and gliomas (22 per cent). In some cases, these aneurysms grow to giant size and present clinical features similar to those of intracranial tumors.

Neoplastic aneurysms develop where implantation of a malignant tumor occurs in a penetrating vessel. This most often occurs from tumors arising in the heart that embolize to the peripheral intracranial circulation. Other neoplastic aneurysms evolve from the invasion of adjacent vessels by nearby malignant tumors. In each case, the neoplastic cells penetrate the vessel wall and cause destruction of the internal elastic membrane.

In addition to the known etiological agents responsible for intracranial aneurysms, there are a number of conditions that have been weakly linked to the development of arterial aneurysms and yet, by association, must be included. The coexistence of an intracranial aneurysm and an arteriovenous malformation is widely appreciated. The exact relation between the aneurysm and the malformation has never been established, however. In general, the aneurysm occurs on vessels supplying the angioma. Whether both lesions represent an underlying defect in vascular development is unclear. More likely, arteries that supply angiomas are subject to more flow and stress, which somehow weakens the vessel wall.[30, 53, 61]

Arteriovenous malformations often harbor intracranial arterial aneurysms, both on their feeding arteries and on adjacent normal arteries. Arterial aneurysms are found in about 5 per cent of patients who harbor arteriovenous malformations, and, likewise, about 5 per cent of patients with aneurysms harbor such malformations. Identification of the source of an intracranial hemorrhage in a patient who has both an aneurysm and an arteriovenous malformation may present a diagnostic dilemma. In addition to hemorrhage, patients who harbor both aneurysm and arteriovenous malformation may have only seizures as a first manifestation.

Over time, the development of aneurysms seems to be logarithmic. Stehbens identified two other anomalies in which intracranial arterial aneurysms have been found.[57] Both coarctation of the aorta and polycystic kidney disease are congenital disorders associated with intracranial arterial hypertension that may place additional stress on the cerebral vessels. Stehbens found that although many patients with coarctation also have bacterial endocarditis, the intracranial aneurysms almost invariably arise from mechanical factors.

Other conditions seem to predispose to aneurysm or at least to make the presence of an aneurysm more difficult to manage. Bigelow reported 42 cases and reviewed the literature relating to cystic renal disease and intracranial aneurysms.[5] By 1953, many patients with polycystic renal disease had suffered intracranial hemorrhage. At least 20 of these, and perhaps more, demonstrated aneurysms that had ruptured. The underlying problem leading to the development of both lesions is not clear. Hypertension commonly accompanies polycystic renal disease and could be the underlying factor. Also, defects in connective tissue deposition may be present in both disorders. The link to hypertension, however, has been made in other instances. Coarctation of the aorta is a well-known progenitor of intracranial aneurysm. Wright collected 304 cases of coarctation of the aorta and found 16 intracranial aneurysms, which caused death in 11 instances.[71]

Traumatic aneurysms may be divided according to spontaneous or iatrogenic arterial wall injury. These groups may be further classified into true aneurysms, in which part of the arterial wall is present, and false aneurysms, in which a remnant of the blood clot forms the outer wall. Traumatic aneurysms occur on virtually any artery but more often on those susceptible to external trauma. The anterior cerebral artery in its relation to the falx is a favorable site. Other susceptible sites include the carotid artery in relation to the clinoid processes and the middle cerebral artery as it becomes peripheral. Aneurysms may also arise from surgical manipulation along the tract of needle puncture sites or at the site of arterial anastomosis.[71]

Traumatic aneurysms have been reported almost since the cause of subarachnoid hemorrhage became known.[3] There are several types. Pseudoaneurysms form when a major artery is torn and hematoma forms about it. If only the elastic lamina is torn, the intima bulges through the defect, producing true traumatic aneurysm. These are found on susceptible vessels, such as the anterior cerebral artery in juxtaposition to the falx, the carotid artery adjacent to the tentorium, and the middle cerebral artery near a bone flap or depressed fracture.

Additional discussion of subarachnoid hemorrhage and aneurysms is given in Chapter 50.

Ischemic Deficits

The complex structural alterations that occur in cerebral arterial walls after subarachnoid hemorrhage have been extensively reviewed by Mayberg and colleagues.[36] Regardless of whether vasospasm is caused primarily by vascular smooth muscle contraction, structural changes, or a combination, perhaps with different mechanisms predominating at different times, there is no doubt that it is common after subarachnoid hemorrhage. The likelihood of its occurrence is related to the amount of blood present in the basal cisterns on an early computed tomography study.[16] The occasional development of vasospasm in other situations is probably also related to the presence of subarachnoid blood (e.g., in trauma or hemorrhage from an arteriovenous malformation) or inflammatory exudate (e.g., in meningitis). Vasospasm is a leading cause of death or morbidity after subarachnoid hemorrhage and, if it goes untreated, leads to death or permanent disability in about 20 per cent of cases.

INCIDENCE AND DIAGNOSIS OF VASOSPASM

Vasospasm, defined as a reduction in the caliber of basal arteries seen on a second cerebral angiogram compared with an earlier study, is very common. If it were possible to do daily angiography on patients with subarachnoid hemorrhage and to visualize very small vessels, spasm would possibly be seen in all cases.[66] If transcranial Doppler ultrasound studies are done daily, it is common to see an increase in velocity of flow with time in most patients.[50]

Delayed ischemia caused by vasospasm is less common, because arterial narrowing needs to be very severe before blood flow is reduced enough to cause symptomatic ischemia. The increase in velocity (measured by Doppler ultrasound), in itself, helps maintain flow through a narrowed segment, and a good collateral circulation is also useful in maintaining tissue perfusion.[51] In normal situations, the brain has a reserve of blood flow and, by increasing oxygen extraction, can tolerate a considerable reduction in flow before there is loss of function. Furthermore, flow can be reduced below even this level before ionic fluxes develop that warn of impending permanent membrane dysfunction.[24] Finally, even after ischemia is clinically apparent, the risk of permanent infarction depends on both its severity and its duration; there is often a window of time during which restoration of flow can prevent permanent damage.

In the clinical situation of a patient with subarachnoid hemorrhage, there are often other, treatable factors involved in delayed deterioration, apart from pure vasospasm.[38] Examples include raised intracranial pressure as a result of hydrocephalus or brain edema, hyponatremia, hypoxia, and hypotension. Deterioration associated with less severe vasospasm can often be improved by attention to these factors.

Incidence of Vasospasm Diagnosed by Angiography

In a review of the literature on cerebral vasospasm, angiographic narrowing was reported, in 223 studies involving 31,168 patients, to occur in 13,490, or 43.28 per cent.[13] A wide range of reported incidence, from 19 to 97 per cent, was found. This probably depends partly on the timing of angiography and partly on looseness in the definition of vasospasm: some papers defined a specified reduction in lumen diameter as significant, and others accepted any narrowing. In some papers, absolute sizes were defined; in others, a second angiogram was compared with an initial study. In 38 studies in which angiography was specified as being performed some days after subarachnoid hemorrhage, the reported incidence was 67.3 per cent in 2,738 cases, with a range from 40 to 97 per cent. This much higher figure is probably closer to the true incidence.

Incidence and Timing of Delayed Ischemia

Symptomatic vasospasm, or delayed ischemic deficit, has been widely reported, occurring in about 30 to 35 per cent of cases. There is a wide range of incidence, between 5 and 90 per cent, probably owing to differences in definition, strictness of exclusion of other causes of hemorrhage or of deterioration, or reporting bias. It is known that the significant, delayed spasm that follows subarachnoid hemorrhage develops over a period of several days, in contrast with the common, transient spasm that occurs immediately after the hemorrhage. Indeed, the blood and its breakdown products probably need to be present for at least 2 or 3 days for spasm to develop.[14] Classically, the onset of angiographic spasm occurs late in the first week after hemorrhage.[49] This equates with the onset of increased velocities seen on Doppler ultrasound.[50, 51] Spasm usually begins and is most severe in vessels near the ruptured aneurysm, although it can be much more widespread (Fig. 61–1). It reaches a peak of severity at about 8 to 10 days, and in most cases it has resolved by 3 weeks.

Symptomatic vasospasm is delayed in onset by 1 to 3 days after angiographic changes. The most common time of onset is around the end of the first week, and peak severity 1 to 4 days later.

CLINICAL ASPECTS OF VASOSPASM

Clinical Picture. The onset of delayed ischemic deficit is usually insidious, starting with a subtle deterioration in higher functions rather than focal symptoms. An increase in headache is commonly the first symptom, and there may be a mild fever. Focal signs such as hemiparesis or dysphasia may follow hours or even days later. More rarely, the onset is rapid, with full development of the entire clinical picture over one to several hours, or even catastrophic, with deterioration over a few minutes. In such cases, the delayed ischemia may be mistaken for a recurrent hemorrhage.[35] This is probably the reason for the erroneous view, once widely held, that there was a secondary peak of recurrent bleeding early in the second week.

Specific syndromes depend on the location of the most severe vasospasm and thus of the ruptured aneurysm itself. In the case of internal carotid or middle cerebral artery aneurysms, the syndrome most commonly includes hemiparesis or hemiplegia, with or without sensory loss or hemianopia. For the anterior cerebral territory, there is more severe disturbance of cognitive function, occasionally with paraparesis, or varying degrees of coma or akinetic mutism in severe

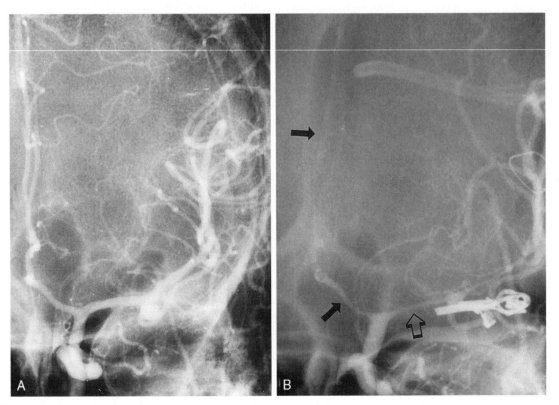

Figure 61–1

A. Left carotid anteroposterior angiography taken 10 days after subarachnoid hemorrhage shows a middle cerebral artery aneurysm. *B.* Repeat study 4 days later, 2 days after the operation, shows widespread spasm involving both the middle cerebral artery *(open arrow)* and the proximal and distal anterior cerebral arteries *(closed arrows)*. (Dorsch, N. W. C.: Picking the haemorrhage: Diagnosis and management of cerebral aneurysm. Modern Medicine of Australia, June 1988, p. 42. Reprinted by permission.)

cases. The posterior circulation may produce long tract, cranial nerve, cerebellar, or vegetative disturbance, hemianopia, or even cortical blindness.

Investigation. The definitive test for confirming vasospasm as a cause of deterioration is cerebral angiography. It shows arterial narrowing in the appropriate distribution in most cases. Occasionally it fails to do so, possibly because of spasm in small perforating vessels that are not easily visible on angiography or because there is only mild spasm in conjunction with another problem. The importance of confirming the diagnosis needs to be balanced against the risks of angiography (including the possibility that it may worsen the spasm or cause other ischemic complications) and the possible delays in starting definitive treatment that may result.

Transcranial Doppler ultrasound is a useful tool in diagnosis, particularly if the patient is being monitored with daily or second-daily studies and an increase in flow velocity has already been shown. In general, a mean flow velocity of 100 cm per second is accepted as suspicious, a velocity greater than 120 cm per second is considered diagnostic of vasospasm, and values of 200 cm per second or more are almost always associated with clinical deterioration. Doppler ultrasound has the advantage of being a quick, bedside, repeatable diagnostic test with no known harmful effects. However, it can insonate only large vessels, and the results depend considerably on the skill of the operator. In many cases, signals can be obtained only from the middle cerebral arteries, and the test is not possible at all in 5 to 10 per cent of subjects.

Direct measurement of cerebral blood flow has been widely used, more in a clinical research setting than for diagnosis in individual cases. Radioactive xenon clearance, single photon emission computed tomography, and stable xenon computed tomography techniques have been used, both for prediction of delayed ischemia and to monitor progress or response to treatment in individuals.[73]

Other investigations are essential to exclude other causes of deterioration that may be the real problem or that may coexist with vasospasm. Computed tomography is used particularly to look for hydrocephalus but also to exclude recurrent subarachnoid hemorrhage, intracerebral hematoma, or postoperative hemorrhage, and to check whether brain edema or infarction caused by vasospasm is already present, because these conditions may alter the rigor with which the spasm is to be treated. Hemoglobin, serum electrolytes and glucose, and arterial gases must also be measured, with particular attention to hyponatremia or hypoxia, and liver function should be checked if treatment with a calcium antagonist is planned. Chest examination and radiography are necessary to exclude pneumonia.

Effects of Vasospasm. The influence of vasospasm on the overall outcome of patients with subarachnoid hemorrhage was assessed by Dorsch and King.[13] Highly significant effects were found, both on the death rate (30.6 per cent in those with vasospasm versus 16.6 per cent in its absence) and on the proportion of patients recovering (44.4 and 70.0 per cent, respec-

tively). Of 3,327 reported patients, 30.3 per cent died, another 34.0 per cent were left with a permanent neurological deficit, and 35.7 per cent made a good recovery. In summary, the natural history of vasospasm after aneurysmal subarachnoid hemorrhage is for clinical deterioration to affect about 30 per cent, leading to death in about 10 per cent and permanent disability in about 11 per cent. In other words, outcome is adversely affected by vasospasm in about 21 per cent of patients.

PREVENTION OF VASOSPASM

Principles of Management

An important landmark in the history of vasospasm, after early reports on the use of induced hypervolemia, was the realization that most patients with subarachnoid hemorrhage were subject to a number of changes as a result of their severe intracranial disturbance, immobilization in bed, and, often, active dehydration in a bid to prevent brain swelling.[34] Both plasma and erythrocyte volumes are reduced, and all these changes contribute, if not to vasospasm itself, to worsening of its adverse effects.

The importance of fluid management in subarachnoid hemorrhage cannot be overemphasized. In contrast to many other conditions in neurosurgery, dehydration must be strenuously avoided. Even if doing so does not prevent the development of vasospasm, maintenance of a normal or high circulating blood volume may well prevent the resultant ischemia. Fluid loading alone has often been used for both prevention and treatment of delayed ischemic deficit.

Other complications of subarachnoid hemorrhage or of a depressed state of consciousness must also be monitored and corrected, lest they convert an asymptomatic vasospasm into a dangerous ischemic state. These include hydrocephalus, electrolyte imbalance, and infections.

Hypervolemia, Hypertension, and Hemodilution

Induced hypertension was used first in the treatment of delayed ischemic deficit rather than for prophylaxis.[32] The application of this therapy for both prevention and treatment has been variable. In many reported studies, hypervolemia was used, often with fluid loading of several liters daily. Some used fluid loading plus pressor drug–induced hypertension, and others used a combination of hypervolemia, induced hypertension, and active hemodilution to a hematocrit of about 30 per cent, with blood withdrawal if necessary (triple H therapy).[39] A considerable reduction in the incidence of delayed ischemic deficit was seen when variations of this therapy were used; in 2,516 reported patients, it occurred in only 17.6 per cent.[11] Although no controlled trial of this type of management has been reported, this result compares favorably with the incidence of 32.7 per cent seen with no specific preventive treatment.

Calcium Antagonists

Several calcium antagonist drugs have been used in the prevention or treatment of vasospasm. By far the largest reported experience has been with the dihydropyridine analogue, nimodipine. This drug has undergone a number of trials, summarized by Tettenborn and Dycka.[60] Further analysis of these and other studies showed an odds ratio for bad outcome after subarachnoid hemorrhage (death or permanent deficit in all patients, regardless of cause) of 1.68 for nimodipine prophylaxis compared with control patients (95% confidence interval, 1.40 to 2.01).[11] The incidence of delayed ischemic deficit in 5,826 reported patients treated with nimodipine was 15.9 per cent. It is possible that the intravenous preparation of the drug, with which deficits occurred in 14.3 per cent of 4,555 cases, is more effective than oral treatment, with which deficits occurred in 21.7 per cent.[11]

Other studies have involved prophylaxis with nicardipine, including two large trials by the Cooperative Aneurysm Study group. Although the first of these showed significantly less delayed ischemic deficit with nicardipine, outcome was not improved, possibly because of the greater use of fluid-hypertensive therapy in the control group.[23] Overall, with nicardipine prophylaxis in 1,643 patients (16 studies), ischemic deficits occurred in 24.6 per cent. Flunarizine, diltiazem, and verapamil have been used in smaller numbers, flunarizine giving the most impressive results.[11]

Calcium antagonists are used with the intention of preventing or reversing arterial spasm, but there are other possible mechanisms of action. If they have a role, it may include the opening of collateral vessels, direct protection of ischemic neurons, intracellular actions, rheological changes in the blood, reduced mitogenesis in vessel walls, or an influence on fluid management.[12]

21-Aminosteroids

These drugs act as potent inhibitors of iron-dependent lipid peroxidation, which is involved both in the development of vasospasm and in membrane breakdown in ischemic neurons. Clinical experience has been gained with tirilazad mesylate, which in a phase II study showed some reduction in delayed ischemic deficit and improvement in outcome.[28] Two large controlled studies of this drug have shown encouraging results in males only (Kassell, N. F., et al., in preparation).

Recombinant Tissue Plasminogen Activator

In less than a decade, a reversal in one aspect of the management of subarachnoid hemorrhage has occurred, from the regular use of antifibrinolytic agents to decrease aneurysmal rebleeding to the use of fibrinolytic drugs, such as urokinase and tissue plasminogen activator. The rationale is the dissolution of cisternal blood (after early operation to secure at least the ruptured aneurysm) by local application or infusion. Animal studies on the use of tissue plasminogen activator have shown significantly less vasospasm if treatment is started within 48 hours.[14] Encouraging results have come from a number of clinical trials. In 11 studies of a total of 268 patients, the incidence of the deficit was less than 10 per cent (26 cases). Controlled studies are also underway with this drug. A potential hazard is postoperative bleeding, and special care with wound hemostasis is essential. Severe bruising and subgaleal collections are common, and a number of significant hemorrhages have been reported, four of them fatal.[11]

Transluminal Angioplasty

Transluminal angioplasty is another technique that was developed initially for treatment. In some centers, it is now being used more for prophylaxis, that is, if spasm is seen angiographically but is not symptomatic.[75] There have been a few reported cases of aneurysm or vessel rupture with this technique, which requires sophisticated radiological equipment and a highly skilled staff. A refinement that may allow more general use is that of chemical angioplasty (see the section on transluminal angioplasty treatment).

Other Methods

A number of other drugs have been used in efforts to prevent vasospasm since the extensive reviews of Wilkins.[68] They include the "intracellular" calcium antagonist AT877, methylprednisolone acetate, and heparin. Impressive results have occasionally been recorded.[11]

TREATMENT OF DELAYED ISCHEMIC DEFICIT

A large number of drugs and other techniques were used in the 1970s and 1980s for the treatment of vasospasm. Many seemed to produce favorable results in initial reports, but this did not continue with wider use.[68] More recent studies have involved hydrocortisone, the oxygen-carrying blood substitute Fluosol, and barbiturates.[11] Three types of treatment have been used more widely, with apparent success: induced hypertension, calcium antagonists, and transluminal angioplasty.

Induced Hypertension

As with prophylaxis of vasospasm, variations on the use of fluid loading, induced hypertension, and hemodilution have been described. They are applied more vigorously when used for treatment; in many centers, this includes measures such as detailed monitoring in an intensive care setting, Swan-Ganz catheterization, and drug-induced systolic blood pressures of 200 mm Hg or more. In a summation of studies involving variations of this type of treatment, with a total of more than 2,000 patients, death occurred in 17.5 per cent; 28.5 per cent were left with permanent deficits;

Table 61–1
SUMMARY OF VASOSPASM MANAGEMENT

Subarachnoid Hemorrhage Admission Computed tomography Angiography with or without surgery	Central line fluids: 3–4 L/day; crystalloids, colloids; central venous pressure 8–12 mm Hg with or without variations of triple H therapy Daily transcranial Doppler measurement	EITHER OR	Oral nimodipine, 60 mg every 4 hr, for 2–3 wk Intravenous nimodipine, beginning at 2.5 mL/hr, with up to 10 mL over 2 hr; duration 2 wk, then 1 wk oral
Development of Delayed Ischemic Deficit	Angiogram for confirmation Increase fluid intake Intravenous nimodipine to 15 mL/hr With or without pressor drug, Swan-Ganz, etc. Angioplasty		

and the outcome was good in 54.0 per cent.[11] These figures are considerably better than would be expected without treatment.

Calcium Antagonists

The largest experience has been with nimodipine. When used for treatment only (i.e., not started until ischemic deficits have already developed), it has given good results, with a death rate of 13 per cent and good outcome in 67 per cent.[11] In other studies, which analyzed outcome in patients who developed delayed ischemic deficit while already receiving nimodipine for prophylaxis, the outcome figures were not as good; the death rate was 18 per cent, and good outcomes were achieved in only 50 per cent. These patients, having shown that they were "resistant" to the use of nimodipine for prevention of delayed ischemic deficit, would not be expected to respond well to its continued use as treatment.

Other calcium antagonists have been less frequently used for treatment of delayed ischemic deficit. Among 191 patients receiving nicardipine (seven studies), death occurred in 12 per cent and good outcomes in 71 per cent.

Transluminal Angioplasty

This treatment was first reported for vasospasm in 1984.[76] It has since been used mainly for treatment of established delayed ischemic deficit. Mechanical dilatation by balloon in spastic segments of artery, often at multiple points, is effective and long-lasting. If one considers that until recently it has mainly been reserved until other forms of treatment, including induced hypertension and a calcium antagonist, have failed, the results have often been surprisingly good. In only 10 reports with 199 patients, 23 per cent died, and 54 per cent made a good recovery. The complication rate was acceptably low.

It may be difficult to pass a catheter into smaller branches, especially if they are in spasm, and balloon transluminal angioplasty is in general not feasible past the first bifurcation of the middle cerebral artery. Because of the curves involved, the anterior cerebrals often also cannot be cannulated. For this reason, and to reduce the risk from mechanical dilatation, chemical angioplasty has been used, usually by injection of ei-

ther papaverine or a calcium antagonist. Results in 43 cases (three studies) have again been good, with 3 patients dying and 20 recovering.

DISCUSSION

The principles of vasospasm management are presented in Table 61–1. With the large numbers of reported cases, there is little doubt, even in the absence of controlled studies, that fluid loading–hypertensive therapy is useful both in lowering the incidence of delayed ischemic deficit and in improving its outcome. Nimodipine has also been shown to be effective in improving the overall outcome of patients with subarachnoid hemorrhage.

Cost-effectiveness is increasingly a consideration in assessing the usefulness of a form of treatment. The high cost of calcium antagonists may be offset by their safety and ease of use, especially compared with the intensive care and monitoring needed for the most rigorous application of hypertensive treatment. Similar considerations may apply to the use of tissue plasminogen activator and aminosteroids if they prove effective.

The problem of cerebral vasospasm is perhaps less than in the past, but it certainly is not solved yet. Apart from techniques under trial or already shown to be effective, future possibilities include the N-methyl-D-aspartate antagonists, endothelin antagonists, and other antioxidant treatments such as glycolated superoxide dismutase. The process of development of vasospasm and consequent ischemia is undoubtedly a long cascade of events, starting with the presence and then the breakdown of subarachnoid blood. In the absence of a single, totally effective drug, it is most likely that successful management of this process will require treatment at different points along the cascade, such as early operation and tissue plasminogen activator to remove cisternal blood, a calcium antagonist and a free radical scavenger to decrease the chance of spasm and to minimize ischemic damage if spasm does occur, and chemical or balloon angioplasty if vasospasm develops in spite of other measures or for patients who present late after hemorrhage with spasm already present.

Fluid and Electrolyte Disturbances

Transient minor disturbances, particularly in sodium balance and serum sodium levels, are common after subarachnoid hemorrhage, especially in the postoperative period when surgery has followed within hours or days of hemorrhage. In one series of 134 patients, hyponatremia developed in 33 per cent.[67] Disturbances of balance may be compounded by overenthusiastic administration of saline or fluids in the perioperative period or during prophylaxis or treatment of vasospasm. The resultant diuresis and natriuresis may also cause diagnostic confusion.

DIABETES INSIPIDUS

Diabetes insipidus is a complication caused by a deficiency of antidiuretic hormone (vasopressin) that is occasionally seen after subarachnoid hemorrhage, usually from an anterior circulation aneurysm, particularly those around the anterior communicating area. Involvement of small perforating vessels around the hypothalamus, either with the initial hemorrhage or later as a result of vasospasm, is possibly a factor. The onset is often delayed for several days and can be quite abrupt.

Polyuria is the most prominent feature, and in severe cases the loss of fluid may exceed 10 L daily. The diagnosis is confirmed by the finding of high volumes (>400 mL per 2 hours) of dilute (specific gravity 1.000) urine of very low osmolality, at the same time as high serum osmolality (often over 300 mOsm per kg), with hypernatremia in severe cases. A water deprivation test may be necessary in mild episodes, but extreme care must be taken to avoid further dehydration.

The prime purpose of management of diabetes insipidus is the maintenance of normovolemia. The importance of avoiding significant dehydration cannot be overemphasized, especially at about the end of the first week after hemorrhage, when the risk of ischemia caused by vasospasm is at its peak. Intravenous fluid maintenance, often with dextrose rather than saline solutions, is usually necessary. In more severe cases, treatment with an antidiuretic hormone analogue, such as desmopressin acetate, may be needed. Although this is less dangerous than earlier preparations of Pitressin (particularly the oily form), care is still needed not to administer too much, which would risk precipitating the opposite situation with overhydration and the danger of brain swelling.

Diabetes insipidus usually is temporary and resolves after a few days or weeks. Occasionally, it becomes chronic, and long-term treatment with nasal desmopressin acetate is needed.

SYNDROME OF INAPPROPRIATE ANTIDIURETIC HORMONE

The syndrome of inappropriate antidiuretic hormone secretion is more common than diabetes insipidus and is often more difficult to manage. Its onset is usually several days after hemorrhage, and occasionally a period of syndrome of inappropriate antidiuretic hormone precedes the onset of diabetes insipidus, possibly because of the release of antidiuretic hormone from damaged pituitary cells.

This condition is the opposite of diabetes insipidus, with oliguria and fluid retention, high urine osmolality, low serum sodium, and, if severe, cerebral swelling. Management is primarily with fluid restriction, which may need to be stringently applied; occasionally, small amounts of hypertonic saline are helpful. This may seem difficult if the patient is at the same time being treated with fluids for vasospasm, but careful monitoring with central line or pulmonary wedge pressure measurement is needed.

A number of other factors can lead to apparent syndrome of inappropriate antidiuretic hormone, such as hypotension or hypovolemia. Differentiation of fluid balance problems is discussed at length by Walker and in several other articles in a useful supplement to *Acta Neurochirurgica*.[63]

CEREBRAL SALT-WASTING SYNDROME

Cerebral salt-wasting syndrome is another condition that can cause hyponatremia, but one that is accompanied by dehydration and a low plasma volume. It is possibly related to overproduction by the hypothalamus of the atrial natriuretic peptide or factor. Serum levels of atrial natriuretic factor were raised in a high proportion of patients with subarachnoid hemorrhage in one study, although the correlation with hyponatremia was poor.[10]

In theory, it could be of vital importance to differentiate this complication from syndrome of inappropriate antidiuretic hormone, because loss of sodium (and water) rather than retention of fluid is the primary problem, and management must be directed toward replenishing sodium (or limiting its loss) rather than simple fluid restriction. Measurement of plasma volume and total sodium balance is needed to be certain of what is happening in many cases. Treatment with fludrocortisone has been shown in one study to minimize natriuresis after subarachnoid hemorrhage.[25]

SUMMARY

Problems of water and sodium balance can have devastating effects in some patients, and minor degrees of disturbance are common. The specific cause is not always clear, and other factors, such as surgery, infection, diuretics, and renal disease, may worsen the situation. Attention to fluid balance is important both in reducing the risk of delayed ischemia and in preventing overload and cerebral edema.

Occasionally, hypothalamic dysfunction can lead to dangerous combinations of disturbances of fluid homeostasis, particularly in the medium to long term, if these include derangement of the thirst mechanism. The combination of diabetes insipidus with loss of the thirst drive is especially dangerous, as is polydipsia combined with treated diabetes insipidus.

Retinal and Preretinal Hemorrhage

Subarachnoid hemorrhage is commonly associated with subdural or subarachnoid bleeding in the optic nerve sheaths, and in 20 per cent or more of patients intraocular hemorrhage occurs. In the past, the latter was often attributed to the tracking of subarachnoid blood directly from the cranial subarachnoid space along the nerve sheath and through the lamina cribrosa at the back of the optic disc. However, no communication that would allow this has been found, and it would not explain the occasional development of intraocular hemorrhage in other conditions such as head injury, or after a sudden severe rise in intracranial pressure. A more likely explanation is that the increased intracranial pressure, known to occur after subarachnoid hemorrhage, is transmitted along the sheath and obstructs venous drainage from the globe, via both the central retinal vein and the retinochoroidal anastomotic veins.[27, 28] Hemorrhage may occur in one or more of several layers, including occasionally behind the retina.[20, 64] More common is bleeding in the layers of the retina itself. A typical flame-shaped hemorrhage results from bleeding into the nerve fiber layer. Hemorrhage between this layer and the internal limiting membrane of the retina can cause larger, round collections of blood. If the internal limiting membrane is ruptured, collection of the blood between it and the cortical vitreous layer enclosing the vitreous is known as a preretinal or subhyaloid hemorrhage, the most common variety of intraocular hemorrhage. Finally, if the cortical vitreous layer is breached, vitreous hemorrhage or Terson's syndrome occurs, with loss of the red reflex and of ophthalmoscopic detail of the retina.[62] Different types and severity of hemorrhage may be seen in each eye.

Retinal and vitreous hemorrhages are generally held to be more common in cases involving aneurysms on the internal carotid or anterior communicating arteries, perhaps because of their proximity to the optic nerves and the more immediate and direct transmission of pressure. The outlook for the patient is also thought to be worse if such hemorrhages are present, although this was not the case in one small, prospective study.[20] The ocular bleeding is usually seen immediately after the hemorrhage and may then be a useful aid in the diagnosis, but occasionally it is not seen until several days later, especially in the case of the breakthrough into the vitreous that occurs with Terson's syndrome.

In a conscious patient, symptoms caused by retinal or vitreous hemorrhage range from complete blindness to moderate reduction in visual acuity or scotomata. The usual clinical course is for the blood to be absorbed over weeks or months, with gradual recovery of vision. Treatment consisting of a pars plana vitrectomy with evacuation of blood and pigment may be needed, and the result is good in most cases. It should usually be delayed until the patient has gone at least 6 months with no further improvement, although it may be needed earlier on one side in those with bilateral hemorrhages and severe effects on vision in both eyes.

REFERENCES

1. Alpers, B. J., and Berry, R. G.: Circle of Willis in cerebral vascular disorders: The anatomical structure. Arch. Neurol., 8:398–402, 1963.
2. Auld, A. W., and Shafey, S.: Transient ischemic attacks not produced by extracranial vascular disease: A plea for complete and early angiographic investigation. South Med. J., 69:722–724, 1978.
3. Ayer, W. D.: So-called spontaneous subarachnoid hemorrhage: A resume with its medicolegal consideration. Am. J. Surg., 26:143–151, 1934.
4. Ball, M. J.: Pathogenesis of the "sentinel headache" preceding berry aneurysm rupture. Can. Med. Assoc. J., 112:78–79, 1975.
5. Bigelow, N. M.: The association of polycystic kidneys with intracranial aneurysms and other related disorders. Am. J. Med. Sci., 255:485–494, 1953.
6. Cannell, D. C., and Botterell, E. H.: Subarachnoid hemorrhage and pregnancy. Am. J. Obstet. Gynecol., 2:844–855, 1956.
7. Chambers, W. R., Harper, B. F., Jr., and Simpson, J. R.: Familial incidence of congenital aneurysms of cerebral arteries: Report of cases of ruptured aneurysms in father and son. J.A.M.A., 155:358–359, 1954.
8. Courville, C. B.: Arteriosclerotic aneurysms of the circle of Willis: Some notes on their morphology and pathogenesis. Bull. Los Angeles Neurol. Soc., 27:1–13, 1962.
9. Diaz, M. S., and Sekhar, L. N.: Intracranial hemorrhage from aneurysms and arteriovenous malformations during pregnancy and the puerperium. Neurosurgery, 27:855–866, 1990.
10. Diringer, M. N., Lim, J. S., Kirsch, J. R., et al.: Suprasellar and intraventricular blood predict elevated plasma atrial natriuretic factor in subarachnoid hemorrhage. Stroke, 22:577, 1991.
11. Dorsch, N. W. C.: A review of cerebral vasospasm in aneurysmal subarachnoid haemorrhage: II. Management. J. Clin. Neurosci., 1:78–92, 1994.
12. Dorsch, N. W. C.: A review of cerebral vasospasm in aneurysmal subarachnoid haemorrhage: III. Mechanisms of action of calcium antagonists. J. Clin. Neurosci., 1:151–160, 1994.
13. Dorsch, N. W. C., and King, M. T.: A review of cerebral vasospasm in aneurysmal subarachnoid haemorrhage: I. Incidence and effects. J. Clin. Neurosci., 1:19–26, 1994.
14. Findlay, J. M., Weir, B. K. A., Kanamaru, K., et al.: The effect of timing of intrathecal fibrinolytic therapy on cerebral vasospasm in a primate model of subarachnoid hemorrhage. Neurosurgery, 26:206, 1990.
15. Fisher, C. M.: Clinical syndromes in cerebral thrombosis, hypertensive hemorrhage and ruptured saccular aneurysms. Clin. Neurosurg., 22:117–147, 1975.
16. Fisher, C. M., Kistler, J. P., and Davis, T. M.: Relation of cerebral vasospasm to subarachnoid hemorrhage visualized by computerized tomographic scanning. Neurosurgery, 6:1, 1980.
17. Forbus, W. D.: On the origin of miliary aneurysms of the superficial cerebral arteries. Bull. Johns Hopkins Hosp., 47:239–284, 1930.
18. Forster, F. M., and Alpers, B. J.: Anatomical defects and pathological changes in congenital cerebral aneurysms. J. Neuropathol. Exp. Neurol., 4:146–154, 1945.
19. Fox, J. L.: Intracranial Aneurysms. Vol. 1. New York, Springer-Verlag, 1983, pp. 418–431.
20. Garfinkle, A. M., Danys, I. R., Nicolle, D. A., et al.: Terson's syndrome: A reversible cause of blindness following subarachnoid hemorrhage. J. Neurosurg., 76:766, 1992.
21. George, A. E., Lin, J. P., and Morantz, R. A.: Intracranial aneurysm on a persistent primitive trigeminal artery: Case report. J. Neurosurg., 35:601–604, 1971.
22. Graf, C. J., and Nibbelink, D. W.: Cooperative study of intracranial aneurysms and subarachnoid hemorrhage: III. Intracranial surgery. Stroke, 5:559–601, 1974.
23. Haley, E. C., Jr., Kassell, N. F., Torner, J. C., et al.: A randomized controlled trial of high-dose intravenous nicardipine in aneurysmal subarachnoid hemorrhage: A report of the cooperative aneurysm study. J. Neurosurg., 78:537, 1993.
24. Harris, R. J., Symon, L., Branston, N. M., et al.: Changes in extracellular calcium activity in cerebral ischaemia. J. Cereb. Blood Flow Metab., 1:203, 1981.
25. Hasan, D., Lindsay, K. W., Wijdicks, E. F. M., et al.: Effect of

fludrocortisone acetate in patients with subarachnoid hemorrhage. Stroke, 20:1156, 1989.

26. Heiskanen, O.: Ruptured intracranial arterial aneurysms of children and adolescents: Surgical and total management results. Child's Nerv. Syst., 5:66–70, 1989.

27. Housepian, E. M., and Pool, J. L.: A systematic analysis of intracranial aneurysms from the autopsy file of the Presbyterian Hospital, 1914 to 1956. J. Neuropathol. Exp. Neurol., 17:409–423, 1958.

28. Kassell, N. F., Haley, E. C., Alves, W. M., et al.: Phase two trial of tirilazad in aneurysmal subarachnoid hemorrhage: A preliminary report of the cooperative aneurysm study. In Findlay, J. M., ed.: Cerebral Vasospasm: Developments in Neurology 8. Amsterdam, Elsevier, 1993, pp. 411–415.

29. Kayembe, K. N., Sasahara, M., and Hazama, F.: Cerebral aneurysms and variations in the circle of Willis. Stroke, 15:846–850, 1984.

30. Khilko, V. A.: About aneurysms of cerebral vessels [Thesis]. Leningrad, 1964.

31. Kirgis, H. D., Fisher, W. L., Llewellyn, R. C., et al.: Aneurysms of the anterior communicating artery and gross anomalies of the circle of Willis. J. Neurosurg., 25:73–78, 1966.

32. Kosnik, E. J., and Hunt, W. E.: Postoperative hypertension in the management of patients with intracranial arterial aneurysms. J. Neurosurg., 45:148, 1976.

33. Kudrjashov, B. A.: Modern condition knowledge about the antihemostatic system of blood. Probl. Hematol. Blood Transfusion, 12:3–13, 1962.

34. Maroon, J. C., and Nelson, P. B.: Hypovolemia in patients with subarachnoid hemorrhage: Therapeutic implications. Neurosurgery, 4:223, 1979.

35. Maurice-Williams, R. S.: Ruptured intracranial aneurysms: Has the incidence of early rebleeding been over-estimated? J. Neurol. Neurosurg. Psychiatry, 45:774, 1982.

36. Mayberg, M. R., Okada, T., and Bark, D. H.: Morphologic changes in cerebral arteries after subarachnoid hemorrhage. Neurosurg. Clin. North Am., 1:417, 1990.

37. Neil-Dwyer, G., Bartlett, J. R., Nicholls, A. C., et al.: Collagen deficiency and ruptured cerebral aneurysms: A clinical and biochemical study. J. Neurosurg., 59:16–20, 1983.

38. Okawara, A.: Warning signs prior to rupture of an intracranial aneurysm. J. Neurosurg., 38:575–580, 1973.

39. Origitano, T. C., Wascher, T. M., Reichman, O. H., et al.: Sustained increased cerebral blood flow with prophylactic hypertensive hypervolemic hemodilution ("Triple-H" therapy) after subarachnoid hemorrhage. Neurosurgery, 27:729, 1990.

40. Ozaki, T., Handa, H., Tomimoto, K., et al.: Anatomical variations of the arterial system of the base of the brain. Arch. Jpn. Chir., 46:3–17, 1977.

41. Pedowitz, P., and Perell, A.: Aneurysms complicated by pregnancy: Part II. Aneurysms of the cerebral vessels. Am. J. Obstet. Gynecol., 73:736–749, 1957.

42. Phillips, R. L.: Case reports and technical notes: Familial cerebral aneurysms case reports. J. Neurosurg., 20:701–703, 1963.

43. Pope, F. M., Kendall, B. E., Slapak, G. I., et al.: Type III collagen mutations cause fragile cerebral arteries. Br. J. Neurosurg., 5:551–574, 1991.

44. Pope, F. M., Limburg, M., and Schievink, W. I.: Familial cerebral aneurysms and type III collagen deficiency. J. Neurosurg., 72:156–158, 1990.

45. Rhoton, A. L., Jr., Saeki, N., and Perlmutter, D.: Microsurgical anatomy of the circle of Willis. In Rand, R. W., ed.: Microneurosurgery. 2nd ed. St. Louis, C. V. Mosby, 1978, pp. 278–310.

46. Riggs, H. E., and Rupp, C.: Variation in form of circle of Willis. Arch. Neurol., 8:8–14, 1963.

47. Roach, M. R., and Drake, C. G.: Ruptured cerebral aneurysms caused by micro-organisms. N. Engl. J. Med., 273:240–244, 1965.

48. Rubinstein, M. K., and Cohen, N. H.: Ehlers-Danlos syndrome associated with multiple intracranial aneurysms. Neurology, 14:125–132, 1964.

49. Saito, I., and Sano, K.: Vasospasm after aneurysm rupture: Incidence, onset, and course. In Wilkins, R. H., ed.: Cerebral Arterial Spasm. Baltimore, Williams & Wilkins, 1980, pp. 294–301.

50. Seiler, R. W., Grolimund, P., Aaslid, R., et al.: Cerebral vasospasm evaluated by transcranial ultrasound correlated with clinical grade and CT-visualized subarachnoid hemorrhage. J. Neurosurg., 64:594, 1986.

51. Seiler, R. W., and Newell, D. W.: Subarachnoid hemorrhage and vasospasm. In Newell, D. W., and Aaslid, R., eds.: Transcranial Doppler. New York, Raven Press, 1992, pp. 101–107.

52. Sigueira, W. C., Figueiredo, and Cruz, A. A., et al.: Conjunctival vessel abnormalities in sickle cell disease: The influence of age and genotype. Acta Ophthalmol. (Copenh.), 68:515, 1990.

53. Smith, R. R., Zubkov, Y. N., and Tarassoli, Y.: Cerebral Aneurysms. New York, Springer-Verlag, 1994.

54. Stehbens, W. E.: Histopathology of cerebral aneurysms. Arch. Neurol., 8:272–281, 1963.

55. Stehbens, W. E.: Cerebral aneurysms of animals other than man. J. Pathol. Bacteriol., 86:161–168, 1963.

56. Stehbens, W. E.: Pathology of the Cerebral Blood Vessels. St. Louis, C. V. Mosby, 1972, p. 559.

57. Stehbens, W. E.: The pathology of intracranial arterial aneurysms and their complications. In Fox, J. L., ed.: Intracranial Aneurysms. Vol. 1. New York, Springer-Verlag, 1983, pp. 272–357.

58. Suzuki, J.: Cerebral Aneurysms. Tokyo, Neuron, 1979.

59. Suzuki, J., Onuma, T., and Ioshimoto, T.: Results of early operations on cerebral aneurysms. Surg. Neurol., 11:407–412, 1979.

60. Tettenborn, D., and Dycka, T.: Prevention and treatment of delayed ischemic dysfunction in patients with aneurysmal subarachnoid hemorrhage. Stroke, 21(Suppl. 4):85, 1990.

61. Turnbull, F., and Dolman, C. L.: Simultaneous hemorrhage from multiple intracerebral aneurysms: A case report. Can. J. Surg., 5:87–92, 1962.

62. Vanderlinden, R. G., and Chisholm, L. D.: Vitreous hemorrhages and sudden increased intracranial pressure. J. Neurosurg., 41:167, 1974.

63. Walker, V.: Fluid balance disturbances in neurosurgical patients: Physiological basis and definition. Acta Neurochir. Suppl. (Wien), 47:95, 1990.

64. Weingeist, T. A., Goldman, E. J., Folk, J. C., et al.: Terson's syndrome: Clinicopathologic correlations. Ophthalmology, 93:1435, 1986.

65. Weir, B.: Aneurysms Affecting the Nervous System. Baltimore, Williams & Wilkins, 1987.

66. White, R. P.: Vasospasm: II. Clinical considerations. In Fox, J. L., ed.: Intracranial Aneurysms. New York, Springer-Verlag, 1983, pp. 250–271.

67. Wijdicks, E. F. M., Vermeulen, M., and van Gijn, J.: Hyponatraemia and volume status in aneurysmal subarachnoid haemorrhage. Acta Neurochir. Suppl. (Wien), 47:111, 1990.

68. Wilkins, R. H.: Attempts at prevention or treatment of intracranial arterial spasm: An update. Neurosurgery, 18:808, 1986.

69. Wilson, G., Riggs, H. E., and Rupp, C.: The pathologic anatomy of ruptured cerebral aneurysms. J. Neurosurg., 11:128–134, 1954.

70. Wizniter, M., Ruggier, P. M., Masaryk, T. J., et al.: Diagnosis of cerebrovascular disease in sickle cell anemia by magnetic resonance angiography. J. Pediatr., 117:551–555, 1990.

71. Wright, C. J. E.: Coarctation of the aorta with death from rupture of cerebral aneurysms. Arch. Pathol., 48:382–386, 1949.

72. Yasargil, M. G.: Subarachnoid hemorrhage: Diagnosis and therapy. Praxis, 64:439–444, 1975.

73. Yonas, H.: Cerebral blood flow measurements in vasospasm. Neurosurg. Clin. North Am., 1:307, 1990.

74. Ziment, I.: Nervous system complications in bacterial endocarditis. Am. J. Med., 47:593–607, 1969.

75. Zubkov, Y. N., Alexander, L. F., Benashvili, G. M., et al.: Cerebral angioplasty for vasospasm. In Findlay, J. M., ed.: Cerebral Vasospasm: Developments in Neurology 8. Amsterdam, Elsevier, 1993, pp. 321–324.

76. Zubkov, Y. N., Nikiforov, B. M., and Shustin, V. A.: Balloon catheter technique for dilatation of constricted arteries after aneurysmal SAH. Acta Neurochir. (Wien), 70:65, 1984.

Spontaneous Intracerebral and Intracerebellar Hemorrhage

Sudden hemorrhage into the cerebral parenchyma is a devastating form of hemorrhagic stroke affecting all ages. The peak incidence of hemorrhage from this group of disorders occurs earlier in life than does that for ischemic stroke. Hemorrhagic stroke therefore produces not only an unacceptable risk of death and disability but also a major loss of productive years during which individuals could have contributed to the work force and their family environment.

The causes of spontaneous cerebral hemorrhage are diverse and often multifactorial. Various forms of congenital and acquired cerebrovascular disease are the most commonly invoked etiological mechanisms, but similar structural hematomas can also occur as complications of primary and secondary cerebral neoplasms, inflammatory and autoimmune brain diseases, or traumatic brain injury, or as manifestations of systemic illnesses producing hypertension or coagulopathy. Iatrogenic causes of cerebral hemorrhage are also becoming more common with the availability of thrombolytic therapy for myocardial and cerebral infarction. Endovascular therapy and its complications are also commonly seen on most neurosurgical units and can result in arterial or venous hemorrhage into the brain.

Because of this heterogeneity of etiological factors, specific therapeutic recommendations and interventions must be carefully tailored to the individual circumstances. Often, simple correction of systemic hemodynamic or coagulation defects suffices for management of the cerebral complication, but not infrequently life-threatening brain distortion or herniation syndromes require emergency surgical consideration. In this chapter, the diagnostic and therapeutic approaches applicable to patients with sudden neurological changes caused by brain hemorrhage are discussed. Consideration is given to the major pathophysiological mechanisms encountered in modern neurological and neurosurgical practice. Emphasis is placed on the multidisciplinary approach to diagnosis and management, which, in the authors' opinion, is critical to optimizing outcome.

Diagnostic Evaluation

The initial diagnostic work-up of a patient with sudden neurological deficit seen by a physician must be a detailed history, usually from a family member or witness to the ictus, followed by a general physical and neurological examination. Although the age of the patient can be helpful in alerting the physician that a cerebral hemorrhage may have occurred, the touchstone of the clinical diagnosis is the presence of severe headache, usually sudden in onset, with or without vomiting, concurrent with neurological deficit. Most types of cerebral hemorrhage, regardless of cause, are heralded by headache. The unconscious patient may have been seen to clutch his or her head before losing consciousness. Although headache points strongly toward hemorrhagic stroke as opposed to ischemic stroke, a number of additional historical details help refine the differential diagnosis.

A history of chronic hypertension should alert the clinician that some form of hypertensive parenchymal event has occurred but not blind the evaluation to other possibilities. The presence of arterial hypertension may predispose the patient to rupture of other congenital or acquired cerebrovascular lesions. A history of valvular heart disease is also important to elicit, because vegetations may have produced infectious cerebral aneurysms. The recent onset of a headache disorder preceding the ictus may also be helpful and suggest primary or secondary brain tumor as a possible cause of hemorrhage. Particularly in young patients, a history of drug abuse is critical to obtain. Cocaine or crack use can produce cerebral hemorrhage by several mechanisms. Associated episodic hypertension can be severe

H. H. Batjer • *T. A. Kopitnik, Jr.* • *L. Friberg*

enough to result in bleeding of its own accord or to predispose to rupture of an unrelated aneurysm or vascular malformation. In addition, a vasculitis can result, which can also lead to hemorrhagic stroke. Cocaine may also complicate the early management of these patients because of persisting hemodynamic effects of the drug, which may last several days. Evidence of intravenous drug use should immediately alert the clinician to the possibility of endocarditis and infectious intracranial aneurysm. A history of prior neurological events, either ischemic or hemorrhagic, is important in the initial evaluation, because degenerative brain disease, hemorrhagic transformation of ischemic lesions, or vascular malformation may be implicated.

The initial neurological examination should be expeditious and focused and should follow a general physical examination. The key neurological elements are the level of consciousness, the presence of lateralizing motor signs, and, critically, the presence or absence of brain stem signs, particularly third cranial nerve dysfunction. The unconscious patient with appropriate history must be presumed to harbor a potentially life-threatening cerebral mass lesion and must undergo emergency resuscitative measures regarding airway and hemodynamic stabilization. The prognosis depends, at least in part, on the avoidance of secondary brain insults, including hypoxia, hypercarbia, and hypotension. Emergency referral of all patients suspected of having brain hemorrhage to appropriate hospital facilities with neurological and neurosurgical coverage should be initiated immediately on diagnosis. Certain types of hemorrhagic lesions can prove fatal within minutes if they are not decompressed. Clearly, the radiological evaluation should be pursued in a hospital setting with efficient access to computed tomography, magnetic resonance imaging, and cerebral angiography.

The initial radiological study to be requested in the work-up of a patient suspected of having cerebral hemorrhage is unenhanced computed tomography.[24, 80] This study identifies the size and location of a parenchymal hematoma in almost all patients if it is obtained within 48 to 72 hours of hemorrhage. It may also provide additional valuable anatomical information, such as associated subarachnoid hemorrhage, calcification of vascular lesions or tumors, and the presence of brain edema unlikely to be caused by the acute hemorrhage alone. The impact of the hematoma may be inferred from evidence of uncal or subfalcial herniation or loss of basal cisterns. The precise location of the hematoma has great significance and often clarifies the etiological diagnosis. This point is expanded in the next section.

Magnetic resonance imaging is a powerful diagnostic tool that is especially important in the clarification of the diagnosis if hypertension alone is unlikely to have caused the hemorrhage. This modality is particularly useful in the identification of vascular malformations (Fig. 62–1), tumors, and giant intracranial aneurysms. Certain drawbacks persist in the application of magnetic resonance imaging to the acutely ill and unstable patient because of the problems in monitoring and

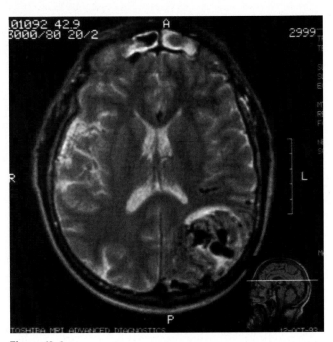

Figure 62–1

Magnetic resonance imaging is an extremely helpful diagnostic adjunct, particularly in the patient with subcortical hemorrhage. This case clearly illustrates the identification of an arteriovenous malformation as the cause of a parieto-occipital hematoma in a 60-year-old man.

ventilating the patient imposed by the magnetic field. In most instances, these studies are performed after the initial work-up and stabilization of the patient have been completed.

Cerebral angiography provides key definitive diagnostic information in patients with aneurysms, vascular malformations, and some neoplasms. It also provides reassuring data, if negative, in cases of lobar or subcortical hematomas. A negative arteriogram in the setting of large cerebral hemorrhage must be interpreted with some caution, however. Occasionally a ruptured aneurysm may become transiently occluded by thrombus and thus rendered invisible angiographically. The mass effect produced by the clot itself may compress and apparently obliterate an associated vascular malformation, particularly if it is small. Therefore, indirect evidence of arterial pathology, such as focal vasospasm or an abnormally large artery that could represent the afferent side of an arteriovenous shunt, should be carefully sought.

The use of infusion computed tomography has been reported to be of great value in the acutely ill aneurysm patient with a large hematoma.[60, 72, 102] This technique emerged in an attempt to gain definitive diagnostic information on the presumed aneurysm patient in whom the delay imposed by cerebral angiography could prove fatal. LeRoux and colleagues have detected the offending aneurysm in each of 25 such patients.[60] Infusion studies can be performed within a 10- to 15-minute interval.

Because of the ready availability of computed tomography in most modern medical centers and the rapid acquisition times that are now commonplace, empirical surgical exploration of patients with presumed cerebral or cerebellar hematomas is almost never indicated. The imprecision of the neurological examination in identifying the cause or even the exact anatomical location of a hematoma is now clear. Empirical exploration has a reasonable chance of missing the hematoma and of producing neurological damage in searching for it.

Differential Diagnosis

Many of the known causes of brain hemorrhage have been mentioned, and the specific therapeutic implications of these conditions are discussed in subsequent sections. The purpose of including a separate discussion of differential diagnosis is to point out that the radiological finding of cerebral hematoma does not represent a diagnosis at all; rather, hemorrhage should always be presumed to be the result of a primary disease or degenerative condition whose correct identification usually has important implications in developing a treatment plan.

Perhaps the most important information relevant to clarifying the underlying diagnosis is the history. The age of the patient may suggest drug abuse or vascular lesion in the young and neoplasm or amyloid angiopathy in the elderly. The use of anticoagulant or antiplatelet medications is becoming more prevalent and is associated with spontaneous cerebral hemorrhage or bleeding after minor trauma. Because intracranial hemorrhage often causes reflex hypertension, a history of chronic hypertension is very important and carries more significance than elevated blood pressure during the acute evaluation.

The location of the hemorrhage is also significant. The classic putaminal or the thalamic hematoma in an untreated hypertensive patient probably does not warrant further diagnostic evaluation, and hypertension may be relied on as the causal factor. Lobar or subcortical hematomas, on the other hand, should be considered diagnostic problems worthy of further evaluation, such as magnetic resonance imaging or angiography. The computed tomography scan should be carefully scrutinized to determine whether the hematoma contacts the basal subarachnoid space or is associated with even a small amount of subarachnoid blood. These circumstances should alert the clinician that intracranial aneurysm could be the cause of hemorrhage. This diagnostic possibility is of paramount importance because early rebleeding is common; if operative decompression is unwittingly performed without the achievement of proximal control, catastrophic intraoperative hemorrhage may be encountered.[7]

The presence of a ruptured arteriovenous malformation may also be suggested (but not proved) by computed tomography. Further diagnostic evaluation with angiography in suspicious cases is helpful in those unusual situations in which a patient presents with life-threatening hematoma, even if direct violation of the malformation can be avoided. The detailed anatomical features of afferent and efferent vasculature allow precise placement of the craniotomy flap and corticotomy to achieve decompression, minimal trauma to the vascular malformation, and full exposure of the offending lesion for delayed treatment or for acute resection if difficult bleeding develops.

Hypertensive Cerebral Hemorrhage

The past three decades have witnessed major advances in the identification of individuals afflicted with hypertension. Because of pharmacological advances, treatment now exists for most compliant patients. A general impression exists that these developments have been instrumental in decreasing stroke, cerebral hemorrhage, and other systemic complications of hypertension.[34] Data from the Framingham Study suggest that aneurysmal subarachnoid hemorrhage is almost three times more prevalent than intracerebral hemorrhage.[81] Similar data from other population groups support the general impression that cerebral hemorrhage is not the critical contributor to early death and disability that it was previously.[15] These impressions and population surveys, coupled with technological and pharmacological advances in the care of the aneurysm patient, have de-emphasized the importance of the problem of spontaneous cerebral hemorrhage in the minds of many neurosurgeons and neurologists. A study by Broderick and colleagues, however, appears to refute this impression.[14] These investigators studied the prevalence of causes of hemorrhagic stroke in the Cincinnati, Ohio, area during 1988. This study is important in that all stroke patients were screened by computed tomography, providing an ideal means of identifying the presence of hemorrhage. These investigators found that the annual incidence of intracerebral hemorrhage was 15 cases per 100,000 population, which was more than twice the incidence of subarachnoid hemorrhage (6 cases per 100,000 population). The mortality rates were almost identical for the intracerebral and subarachnoid groups (44 per cent versus 46 per cent, respectively). Hypertension was the presumed cause in more than two thirds of the intracerebral hemorrhage patients studied.[14] It is therefore clear that hypertensive cerebral hemorrhage is still a major cause of stroke whose management remains controversial and largely unsuccessful. In general, intracerebral hemorrhage accounts for approximately 10 per cent of all strokes, and the median age of victims is 56 years, as opposed to 65 years for patients with ischemic stroke.[10, 32, 55, 70, 103]

PATHOPHYSIOLOGY OF HYPERTENSIVE DISEASE

Chronic arterial hypertension induces a variety of physiological aberrations that lead to destructive and often permanent gross and microscopic cerebrovascular structural changes. A brief review of some of these effects that are relevant to the causation and treatment of hypertensive cerebral hemorrhage is given here.

Cerebral blood flow is extremely responsive to systemic and local environmental changes. Increases in neuronal activity have been shown to increase regional blood flow; this linkage has led most investigators to conclude that tissue metabolism and cerebral blood flow are coupled.[56, 101] A number of other factors, however, affect the cerebral vasculature, including hemodynamic changes, biochemical influences, and hormonal changes, which also determine delivery of substrate to brain tissue.[101]

Chronic elevation of blood pressure (even to very high levels) has remarkably little impact on cerebral blood flow, and tissue perfusion can be maintained at normal levels over wide ranges in systolic blood pressure.* Hypertension leads to an increase in cerebrovascular resistance as a result of adaptive morphological changes in healthy cerebral vessels.[101] Chronic hypertension ultimately leads to medial hypertrophy in cerebral arteries, which increases wall thickness.[101] This change allows cerebral arterioles to withstand higher pressures and minimizes adverse effects on the fragile downstream capillaries.[40, 77] Unfortunately, these protective changes limit the capacity of cerebral vessels to dilate in the face of acute hypotension,[101] thus shifting the autoregulatory capability of the cerebral vessels toward higher pressures.

Autoregulation of the cerebral vasculature maintains cerebral blood flow at approximately 50 mL per 100 g per minute despite variations in mean systemic blood pressure from 60 to 150 mm Hg.[77] After a brief delay, cerebral vessels constrict in response to hypertension and dilate if hypotension develops. The mechanisms responsible for these changes are beyond the scope of this discussion, but both metabolic and myogenic hypotheses have been put forward.[56, 77] The autoregulatory mechanisms appear to vary among different brain regions. The upper limit of autoregulation is lower in the cortex than in the thalamus or brain stem.[9, 94] Such anatomical heterogeneity does not apply to P_{CO_2} reactivity, however.[9]

Long-standing hypertension accelerates atherosclerosis in both large and small cerebral vessels.[35] Although the chronic changes in the large conducting vessels have been well described, more pertinent degenerative changes occur in the penetrating vessels of the brain. Perforating vessels such as the lenticulostriates and thalamoperforates are in general end-arteries and arise from large conducting vessels, often at 90-degree angles. This anatomical characteristic may subject these fragile vessels to intraluminal pressures much higher than those found in arterioles of similar size elsewhere in the brain.[35, 36] Histological changes ultimately result from chronic hypertension. In the deep penetrating vessels, numerous effects may be seen, including microatheroma, lipohyalinosis,[28] fibrinoid necrosis, and microaneurysm.[35] Originally described by Charcot and Bouchard, microaneurysms have been studied intensively over the past 100 years.[17] Fisher demonstrated

---

*See references 8, 12, 20, 33, 39, 98, and 99.

clear points of arteriolar rupture in patients with hypertensive brain hemorrhage and noted microaneurysms in the near vicinity.[29] Although their role in the causation of hemorrhage has not been clarified, it is likely that the morphological changes induced by hypertension lead to small-vessel occlusive phenomena as well as microaneurysm formation and may explain the frequent concurrence of lacunes and hemorrhage in the same patient. The distribution of these histological changes correlates with the common sites of cerebral hemorrhage.

DISTRIBUTION OF HEMORRHAGE

It is difficult to determine the precise anatomical distribution of hypertensive brain hemorrhage because many stroke registries include cerebral hemorrhage from all causes. Considering all spontaneous brain hematomas, about 40 to 50 per cent occur in a lobar pattern, 40 per cent occur in the putaminal and capsular regions, 5 per cent in the thalamus, 5 to 10 per cent in the cerebellum, and 5 per cent in the pons.[10, 32, 70, 103] Wityk and Caplan surveyed the prevalence of hypertension in patients with hematomas in varying sites and reported that 20 to 50 per cent of patients with lobar hemorrhage were hypertensive; in lenticular-capsular hematomas, 40 to 70 per cent of patients were hypertensive; 60 to 100 per cent of thalamic hematomas were hypertensive in origin; and 50 to 70 per cent of cerebellar and brain stem hemorrhages were caused by hypertension.[103] The most common site of hypertensive cerebral hemorrhage is the putamen; these classic hematomas account for approximately 50 per cent of all hypertensive bleeds.[25, 37, 74]

TREATMENT OF HYPERTENSIVE CEREBRAL HEMORRHAGE

The initial management of a patient with spontaneous hypertensive cerebral hemorrhage involves primary medical stabilization and reversal of any coagulation defects. Standard airway and hemodynamic stabilization should be initiated immediately. For patients who are obtunded or comatose, immediate intubation and hyperventilation is appropriate, with a target P_{CO_2} of approximately 25 to 30 mm Hg. Severe hypertension should also be treated gently, and the authors prefer a reduction in mean systemic pressure by about 25 per cent over the first 24 hours. Because of the upward shift in the autoregulatory curve in chronically hypertensive patients, drastic reduction in blood pressure to normal ranges can result in serious brain hypoperfusion. This problem can be further compounded by the frequently associated intracranial hypertension, which can synergistically reduce cerebral perfusion pressure. After the initial medical stabilization has been accomplished, the radiological diagnosis should be pursued expeditiously. Specific medical and surgical strategies and controversies are discussed here as they apply to each anatomical location of the hema-

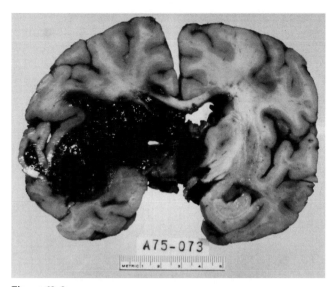

Figure 62–2

This autopsy specimen demonstrates a large medially located putaminal hemorrhage with rupture into the lateral ventricle. This patient died shortly after hemorrhage.

toma. Throughout the discussion, key significance is ascribed to the patient's neurological status, particularly the level of consciousness. The authors empirically treat most patients with high-dose corticosteroids for several days despite their unproven role.

Putaminal Hemorrhage

Substantial variability exists within the subgroup of patients with putaminal hematoma regarding the exact location and extension of the hematoma and the neurological impact of the ictus. Medially located putaminal hematomas usually involve the internal capsule and globus pallidus and often rupture into the ventricular system (Fig. 62–2). Laterally located lesions expand into the insula (Fig. 62–3) and, if large, may present to the insular cortex. Despite the fact that putaminal hematomas are the most common of hypertensive hemorrhages, general and surgical management issues remain highly controversial.

The majority of patients with such lesions, who present with acute onset of hemiplegia but who remain alert or lethargic, can be well managed medically with blood pressure control and diuresis to control intracranial pressure. The decision-making problems center on the obtunded or comatose patient. Most natural history data suggest at least 50 per cent mortality for conservatively treated patients with putaminal hemorrhage, and this number is much higher for the patients who are severely affected neurologically.[43, 57, 84]

Because of the lateral displacement of the insular cortex, surgical evacuation appears to be a logical approach, particularly with microsurgical techniques. In 1959, McKissock and colleagues reported a surgical series in which the mortality of ganglial hemorrhage patients was 93 per cent.[68] Although the microsurgical era may be expected to offer substantially better re-

sults, interpretation of the literature must be done cautiously. Nonrandomized comparisons are often flawed in that patients who undergo surgery are usually deteriorating or severely impaired and would be expected to fare poorly, whereas less severely ill patients often are treated medically. Historical control groups are difficult to interpret because critical care techniques, anesthetic management, and surgical techniques evolve rapidly. Paradoxically, some purely surgical series may report overly optimistic results if all patients are offered surgery; patients whose hematoma is small and who are in good condition would probably do well regardless of therapy.

In 1983, Waga and Yamamoto reported a historically controlled series in which the surgical group had a mortality rate of 28 per cent and the medical cohort had a 14 per cent mortality.[96] In 1984, Kanno and colleagues reported 265 putaminal hemorrhages in which medical and surgical patients had similar outcomes.[48] A subsequent nonrandomized experience published in 1986, involving 182 patients, reported no evidence of surgical advantage.[95] A highly optimistic report appeared in 1983 in which patients operated on within 7 hours of the onset of symptoms did extremely well, with only 9 per cent of patients dead or bedridden at follow-up.[47]

The authors are aware of only four randomized trials of medical versus surgical management for putaminal hemorrhage. In 1961, before the advent of microsurgery, McKissock and colleagues found a mortality rate of 62 per cent in medically treated patients and 75 per cent in those treated surgically.[67] In 1989, Auer and colleagues reported a subgroup of putaminal hemorrhages in which no benefit from surgery was seen.[4] A concurrent randomized study reported by Juvela and associates included 52 patients with hypertensive hemorrhage; the basal ganglia was involved in 39 of the 52 cases.[46] The conservatively treated group was found to have a 38 per cent mortality rate, with 31 per cent of survivors living independently; 46 per cent of the surgical patients died, and only 7 per cent of survivors were independent. Therefore, no surgical benefit was

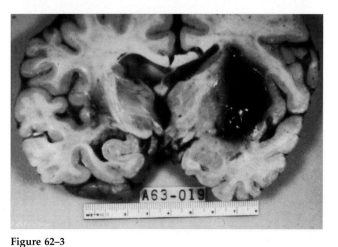

Figure 62–3

Laterally situated putaminal hematomas expand into the insula into the sylvian fissure, as shown in this pathological specimen.

established. Batjer and colleagues reported a randomized study involving best medical management, best medical management plus intracranial pressure monitoring, and microsurgical transsylvian hematoma evacuation.[6] This study was terminated prematurely because of unexpectedly high mortality in each of the three treatment groups. In light of the randomized trials available as evidence, it appears that surgical evacuation as it is currently practiced has no clear benefit over empirical medical management.[91]

These disappointing medical and surgical results clearly suggest the need for further development and strategies. It is possible that stereotactic evacuation or the use of thrombolytic substances can have some impact in the future.[54, 86] At the present time, the authors continue to offer surgical treatment to selected patients with large putaminal hemorrhage. Case selection is done on an individualized basis. In general, surgery is considered for the otherwise healthy patient younger than 70 years of age who has a 3- to 5-cm hematoma, who either deteriorates under optimal medical management or has a nondominant hematoma with radiological evidence of herniation, and who is not posturing on initial evaluation. These management decisions are reached after close consultation among the attending neurosurgeon, neurologist, and neuroanesthesiologist and, often, a critical care specialist.

The surgical procedure offered by the authors is a variant of the standard pterional craniotomy. The head is positioned with an approximately 45-degree rotation and stabilized with three-point fixation. A curvilinear scalp incision is made, extending behind the hairline (if possible) from the zygoma across the superior temporal line and, gently curving medially and anteriorly, ending at the midline. A generous frontotemporal craniotomy is performed, and the sphenoid ridge is removed with the anterior temporal squama. During craniotomy, mannitol, 1 g per kg, is rapidly administered

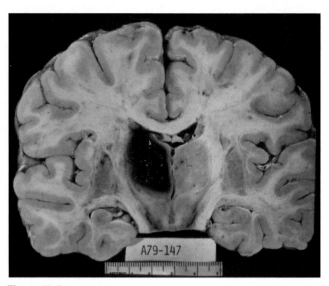

Figure 62–5

Moderate-sized thalamic hematomas like this case may produce minimal mass effect and only moderately severe contralateral motor and sensory signs. The patient survived this hemorrhage for 2 weeks before suffering fatal pulmonary embolism.

intravenously. The P_{CO_2} is maintained at about 25 mm Hg. After dural opening, the microscope is used to perform a microsurgical opening of the opercular-insular portion of the sylvian fissure. The fissure is usually confining because of the mass effect, but the insula is displaced laterally and is therefore encountered superficially. The insular cortex is incised over a distance of approximately 2 cm, and the hematoma is entered. Using the microscope, the major portion of the hematoma is evacuated with care to avoid removing the last adherent portions of the medial aspect of the clot. Operative trauma to the internal capsule and thalamus is not warranted, and simple decompression of the mass is the therapeutic goal, not complete elimination of all components of the hematoma. The blood pressure is then pharmacologically lowered to approximately 150 mm Hg systolic while hemostasis is achieved with bipolar coagulation and gentle tamponade. Closure is routine, and the bone flap is replaced. Postoperative care must respect the fact that the distorted autoregulatory curve requires time for recovery. Therefore, hypotension is avoided at all costs.

Thalamic Hemorrhage

The clinical presentation and ultimate prognosis of patients with primary thalamic hemorrhage is largely dependent on the exact anatomical site and the size of the hematoma. Large, medially located hemorrhages, as shown in Figure 62–4, often produce unconsciousness and frequently rupture into the ventricular system. Smaller hematomas, as shown in Figure 62–5, may produce only mild distortion of the posterior limb of the internal capsule.

In general, the recommended treatment for patients with this condition is nonsurgical. Duff and colleagues and Ropper and King have reported favorable out-

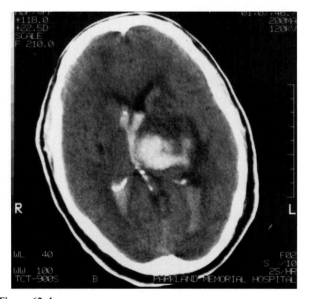

Figure 62–4

Computed tomography scan of a comatose patient with a large medial thalamic hematoma with extension into the third ventricle.

comes with aggressive medical control of intracranial pressure.[26, 79] The surgical options in thalamic hemorrhage are less favorable than those in the putaminal location because of the depth of the lesion and the amount of cerebral tissue that must be dissected to reach it. In the patients of Auer and colleagues who had thalamic hematomas, no surgical benefit was demonstrated.[4] Large thalamic hematomas carry a dismal prognosis, but patients with small or moderate-sized hematomas seem to recover quite well even in terms of memory function if good medical support is provided.[103]

Not infrequently, patients deteriorate 24 to 72 hours after thalamic hemorrhage and are found to have third ventricular compression and obstructive hydrocephalus. These patients respond well to temporary ventricular drainage and only rarely require permanent ventricular shunting. Surgical approaches through the parietal cortex have been attempted as life-saving maneuvers in the deteriorating patient, but considerable normal brain tissue must be violated. An interhemispheric, transcallosal approach through the foramen of Monro is perhaps a more physiological procedure, but, in the patient with major mass effect, excessive retraction is often required. The authors recommend aggressive medical treatment with adjunctive ventricular drainage, if necessary, for the overwhelming majority of patients.

Pontine Hemorrhage

Pontine hemorrhage caused by hypertension is an unmistakable clinical catastrophe, often producing immediate coma with pinpoint pupils and quadriplegia.[103] If these hemorrhages are large (Figs. 62–6 and

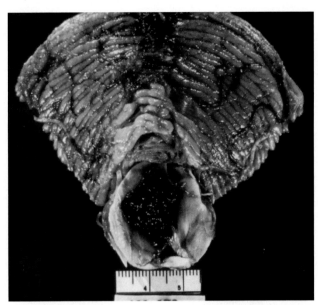

Figure 62–7
Autopsy specimen delineates central pontine hematoma.

62–7), they have a dismal prognosis, and aggressive medical or surgical therapy probably is unethical. The widespread use of computed tomography and, more recently, of magnetic resonance imaging has permitted diagnosis of many smaller hematomas that may have, in general, a much more favorable prognosis. Da Pian and colleagues compared patients treated with direct surgery to those treated medically and were unable to demonstrate a surgical benefit.[23] Although large hematomas (greater than 1.8 cm in diameter) were uniformly devastating in their series, smaller lesions were associated with good outcome in 90 per cent of patients regardless of therapy.

Pontine hemorrhage occurs most commonly in the midpons at the junction of the tegmentum and basis pontis. This region is supplied by paramedian perforating arteries arising from the basilar artery.[103] With expansion, the hematomas may extend into the midbrain or rupture into the fourth ventricle rostrally.

The exquisite resolution of magnetic resonance imaging has allowed identification of pial representation in a small number of pontine hematomas. This anatomical information allows the consideration of a microsurgical procedure chosen to optimally access the hematoma through the subarachnoid space or the floor of the fourth ventricle. This type of procedure may have some merit for selected patients who deteriorate during optimal medical treatment.

Cerebellar Hemorrhage

Although the clinical onset of pontine hemorrhage may be marked by sudden coma, the patient with cerebellar hemorrhage usually complains of a sudden headache, vomiting, dizziness, and inability to stand.[103] Clinical deterioration to the comatose state usually results from hematoma enlargement with direct brain stem compression or fourth ventricular compression

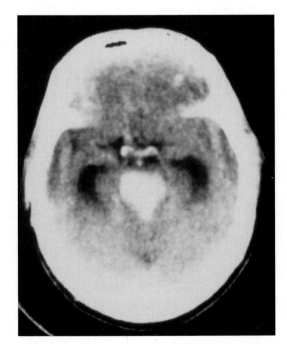

Figure 62–6
Computed tomography of a massive pontine hemorrhage producing coma and aqueductal obstruction.

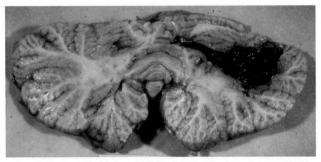

Figure 62–8

A small hypertensive cerebellar hemorrhage arising in the region of the dentate nucleus. This hematoma is in the healing phases of evolution and was not the cause of death.

with acute hydrocephalus. The majority of cerebellar hypertensive hematomas develop in the area of the dentate nuclei (Fig. 62–8), but occasionally the vermis is the probable site (Fig. 62–9). It is the authors' impression that vermian hematomas may carry a more severe prognosis because of earlier brain stem compression or, on occasion, direct brain stem extension.

Clinical management decisions are complex because of the frequent concurrence of obstructive hydrocephalus as a potential explanation for altered level of consciousness or neurological deterioration. Some practitioners were taught that evacuation of cerebellar hematomas could result in awakening and salvage of the brain-dead patient; however, this teaching has not proved true in the authors' experience. Clinical decisions must consider several factors: the neurological status, the neurological course over time, the size of the hematoma, and the presence of acute hydrocephalus. A final, local consideration concerns the surgeon's operating room facility and the length of time required between notification to the operating room and achievement of the craniotomy. Understanding the surgical environment is an especially critical issue if the surgeon is considering an initial course of conservative therapy. The time required for operative positioning and craniotomy or craniectomy in the patient with posterior fossa hematoma is somewhat longer than if the lesion is supratentorial. In the neurologically deteriorating patient with cerebellar hemorrhage, fatal brain stem compression can easily occur if time is wasted before craniotomy.

Evidence is accumulating that the deeply comatose patient with cerebellar hemorrhage is only rarely salvaged. Da Pian and colleagues reported 100 per cent mortality in these patients with surgical decompression.[23] Similar results have been confirmed by other centers.[3, 13, 69] The authors' experience has been somewhat better in patients who were initially alert after the ictus but who subsequently deteriorated during medical evaluation. Some patients who became decerebrate preoperatively nevertheless responded to emergency ventriculostomy and surgical evacuation of the hematoma. Patients who arrived at the hospital in similar condition did not respond as well, which probably implies a significant delay in discovery of the patient by the family.

Patients presenting in excellent condition, with small hematomas, with no clinical evidence of brain stem compression, and without hydrocephalus are well managed medically and usually recover. Patients who are stuporous or develop coma during evaluation should undergo immediate ventriculostomy and craniotomy for decompression. In these critically ill patients, brain stem compression should be assumed to be the cause of the altered state of consciousness. Ventricular drainage alone in this setting is dangerous because excessive time is lost if the patient does not clinically respond.

Decisions become difficult, however, for the lethargic patient. The authors' philosophy has been biased toward aggressive intervention in this group of patients, partially because of the somewhat longer time required between a decision for surgery and achievement of decompression. In the absence of confirmation of hydrocephalus by computed tomography, it seems reasonable to assume that the altered state of consciousness relates to direct brain stem compression; therefore craniotomy would seem appropriate. The lethargic patient *with hydrocephalus* represents an even more difficult decision for the clinician. In an excellent neurosurgical critical care unit with high-quality nursing surveillance, treatment with ventriculostomy alone probably is indicated. Excessive drainage should be avoided in this setting, because upward herniation may occur.[3] The authors' practice has used a system of constant drainage at about 15 cm H_2O. If the patient deteriorates in this setting, emergency computed tomography is repeated to determine whether rebleeding has occurred or whether the ventricular drain has failed or resulted in pneumocephalus. If no immediately correctable cerebrospinal fluid problems are identified, a craniotomy is performed immediately.

After the decision for craniotomy has been made, several points should be kept in mind. If hydrocepha-

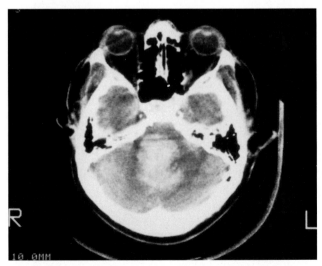

Figure 62–9

Computed tomography of a primary vermian hemorrhage that ruptured into the fourth ventricle. The patient was comatose on arrival at hospital and did not respond to surgical decompression.

lus is present, the authors recommend that ventriculostomy be performed in the operating room, where conditions of lighting and aseptic technique are better than in an emergency facility. The anesthesiologist can therefore be carefully involved in the details of the drainage tubing so as to be of more effective help should problems develop later. The authors prefer to avoid the sitting position for craniotomy in this setting for several reasons. In many cases, the neurological state is explained by impaction of the cerebellar tonsils into the foramen magnum with medullary compression. Hemodynamic and cardiac irregularities may develop over time, which could prove disastrous in the sitting patient if serious hypotension were a component. The risk of air embolization is also well known and could delay the procedure significantly. The authors prefer to use the lateral position for cerebellar hemispheric hemorrhage and the Concorde position for vermian hemorrhage because of these concerns.

These procedures are often performed in an emergency setting with only computed tomography for diagnostic work-up. The possibility of encountering an underlying vascular anomaly or tumor should be kept in mind. If a cerebellar arteriovenous malformation is identified, every attempt should be made to decompress the hematoma and not disturb the malformation. Distal aneurysms of the posterior inferior cerebellar artery have occasionally produced typical hematomas. If such a lesion is encountered, microsurgical dissection should be used through the hematoma to clip the lesion. If abnormal surrounding brain tissue is encountered, frozen and permanent histological sections should be obtained to identify an underlying tumor.

Lobar (Subcortical) Hemorrhage

Lobar cerebral hemorrhage, even in the hypertensive patient, should be further investigated because of the many possible diagnostic explanations for the hematoma. Considerations such as arteriovenous malforma-

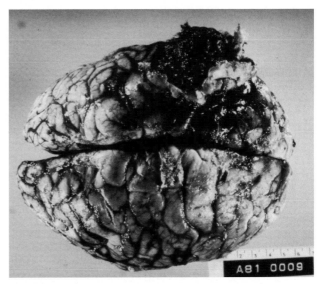

Figure 62–11

This autopsy specimen depicts a massive subcortical hemorrhage that ruptured externally through the cortical pia-arachnoid, producing subdural hematoma and death.

tion, tumor, amyloid angiopathy, sagittal sinus thrombosis, and mycotic (infectious) aneurysm should always be kept in mind. If these hematomas are caused by hypertensive disease, they typically develop beneath the gray matter–white matter junction and dissect among white matter tracts (Fig. 62–10). If they become large, they may rupture into the ventricular system. Figure 62–11 illustrates an unusual case in which the hematoma ruptured through the cortical pia-arachnoid and decompressed into the subdural space.

The specific management issues are dependent on the neurological condition of the patient, the probable diagnostic possibilities, and the need for the histological diagnosis. The location of the lesion determines its neurological consequences, with one exception. Temporal lobe hematomas may produce uncal hematoma and death quickly and without associated elevations in intracranial pressure. For that reason, the authors recommend aggressive surgical decompression of large temporal hematomas. If the hematoma contacts the sylvian fissure or is associated with any subarachnoid hemorrhage, angiography should be performed to exclude an underlying vascular cause.

In the patient presenting with subcortical hemorrhage, even if the patient is hypertensive, many diagnostic possibilities exist, and appropriate work-up with magnetic resonance imaging or angiography should be pursued in most cases.

Cerebral Hemorrhage from Vascular Malformations

Intraparenchymal "congenital" vascular malformations may be considered to be of several types: telangiectasias, venous angiomas, cavernous angiomas, and

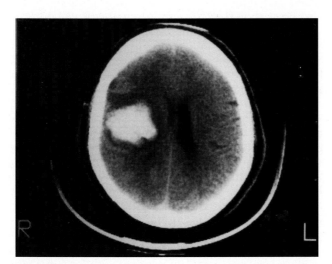

Figure 62–10

Computed tomography of a typical subcortical hematoma arising at the gray matter–white matter junction.

arteriovenous malformations.[66] Of these four major categories of vascular lesions, only two play a major role in intracerebral hemorrhage: arteriovenous malformations and cavernous angiomas. In addition, certain dural vascular malformations, many of which are acquired, can produce cerebral hemorrhage.

Spontaneous hemorrhage is the most common clinical presentation of patients harboring arteriovenous malformations; it occurs in 40 to 50 per cent of these patients in most large series.[85, 90, 104] If hemorrhage occurs, it is most commonly intraparenchymal, although subarachnoid extensions are present occasionally. The identification of a subarachnoid component on computed tomography should strongly suggest an underlying vascular cause. Rarely, the hematoma may extend into the subdural compartment. The age of the patient should also help identify those who have an underlying arteriovenous malformation, because the initial hemorrhage typically occurs in the third decade of life.[63, 85] The heightened suspicion that such a lesion underlies the hemorrhage should lead the clinician to obtain cerebral angiography to delineate the lesion. Although magnetic resonance imaging identifies evidence of the malformation itself, associated aneurysms, which may be present in approximately 5 to 10 per cent of patients, are likely to be missed.

Management of the patient with intracerebral hemorrhage from an arteriovenous malformation should initially involve medical stabilization and nonsurgical control of the intracranial pressure, except for the rare patient in extremis from life-threatening mass effect. For this latter situation, an emergency craniotomy should be performed with the goal of removing the majority of the hematoma and avoiding the malformation. A similar strategy is appropriate for the patient initially treated medically who fails this therapy and worsens clinically. Two factors are important in making this recommendation. First, the incidence of rebleeding from vascular malformations is not increased in the early weeks, as it is after aneurysmal rupture. The risk of rebleeding during the first 6 months is only 4 to 6 per cent.[38, 75, 85] Second, the chances of performing an elegant microsurgical resection with sparing of all brain tissue is extremely unlikely during an operation with a severely swollen brain soon after hemorrhage. Almost always, the patient can be managed medically, and surprising recovery occurs over the few weeks and months after hemorrhage. Figure 62–12 illustrates a patient who had a major frontal opercular and ganglial hemorrhage and was initially hemiplegic. With nonoperative management, he became ambulatory within 2 weeks and recovered to his baseline within 6 weeks. For this reason and for the technical reasons that have been mentioned, there is little support for the argument that the patient with a large hematoma and a dense neurological deficit should undergo early resection of the malformation. The authors prefer to wait about 4 weeks after a hemorrhage of this severity before making a decision about operability, with due consideration given to the characteristics of the malformation and the patient's current neurological status. After the 4-week delay, the brain should be reasonably relaxed.

Even if it is tense early in the procedure, it should become relaxed after the liquefied hematoma is decompressed.

Certain dural malformations and fistulae appear predisposed to intracerebral hemorrhage. Both location and angiography pattern seem to be predictive. Most series suggest that dural malformations involving the anterior cranial fossa or tentorial incisura carry a high risk of cerebral hemorrhage as part of their natural history.[52] In addition, the identification of cortical or pial venous drainage or venous aneurysms by angiography appears to be predictive of hemorrhage.[52] The authors have seen a few cases of dural sinus malformations with pial arterial supply; these lesions have presented with hemorrhage also.

Angiographically occult vascular malformations and cavernous angiomas will generally tend to produce low-pressure, small-volume hemorrhages, which allow their clinical diagnosis but do not place the patient in immediate danger (except in brain stem lesions). Their management is straightforward, and the timing of optimal surgical resection does not differ from that for true arteriovenous malformations.

Cerebral Hemorrhage from Intracranial Aneurysm

Approximately 20 per cent of all large intracerebral hematomas are caused by ruptured aneurysms.[65, 71] Although some degree of intraparenchymal bleeding is often seen during aneurysmal hemorrhage, large and potentially life-threatening hematomas are seen in only 4 to 17 per cent of patients.[11, 61, 82, 87] Significant intraparenchymal hemorrhage is a catastrophe for the aneurysm patient and has been shown to sharply increase mortality to 43.6 per cent.[1] Although the comatose patient after rupture of any aneurysm is well known to have extremely high mortality,[44] the presence of intracerebral hematoma, even in the good-grade patient, has also been shown to be a strong predictor of poor outcome. A series reported by Auer and colleagues noted that 90 per cent of patients in good neurological condition after subarachnoid hemorrhage (grades I and II) had a favorable outcome, but of those with significant intracerebral hemorrhage, 50 per cent recovered well.[2, 5]

Remarkable controversy persists about the optimal timing of surgical intervention for the uncomplicated patient with subarachnoid hemorrhage.* Nevertheless, many cerebrovascular centers, in consideration of the known risk of early rebleeding in the first 2 days[51] and the frequent need for hypertensive or endovascular therapy for vasospasm, now recommend early craniotomy for the awake patient. Unfortunately, the currently utilized grading scales,[44] which play a very helpful role in the determination of timing of intervention for diffuse subarachnoid hemorrhage patients, have little value in the assessment of patients with large hemato-

---

*See references 45, 49, 50, 51, 61, and 62.

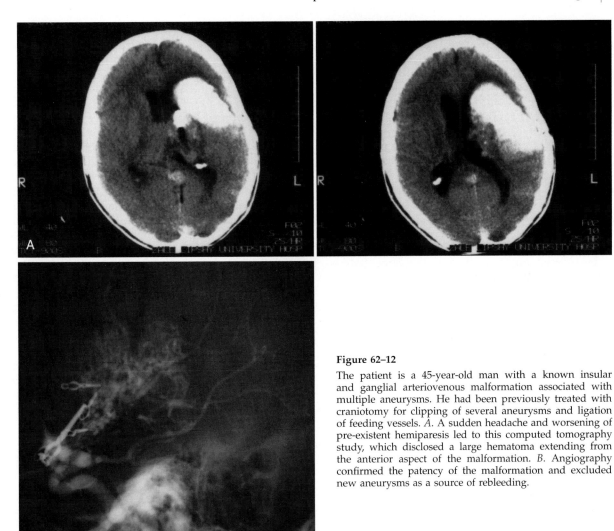

Figure 62–12

The patient is a 45-year-old man with a known insular and ganglial arteriovenous malformation associated with multiple aneurysms. He had been previously treated with craniotomy for clipping of several aneurysms and ligation of feeding vessels. *A.* A sudden headache and worsening of pre-existent hemiparesis led to this computed tomography study, which disclosed a large hematoma extending from the anterior aspect of the malformation. *B.* Angiography confirmed the patency of the malformation and excluded new aneurysms as a source of rebleeding.

mas and unconsciousness or coma related to mechanical brain stem compression.

In 1981, Ljunggren and colleagues reported urgent surgery for hematoma in 30 patients and noted that 50 per cent died.[61] Pasqualin and associates reviewed more than 300 cases of parenchymal hemorrhage from aneurysm and found that delayed surgery was associated with 79 per cent mortality and that early surgery provided some improvement, with a 44 per cent mortality.[76] In 1983, Wheelock and colleagues reviewed data from 11 centers and identified 132 patients with intracerebral aneurysmal hemorrhage.[100] Forty-one per cent of these patients had evidence of herniation. Of the subgroup of moribund patients, early surgery resulted in discharge of 21 per cent to home or rehabilitation centers. All nonoperated patients died. If craniotomy was performed only for hematoma evacuation and the aneurysm was left intact, 75 per cent of patients died. Mortality was decreased to 29 per cent if the aneurysm was secured during the same operation.[100] A prospective randomized trial of alternative treatment strategies was reported by Heiskanen and

colleagues.[42] Thirty patients with hematomas were treated, 15 of whom underwent emergency craniotomy. The interval between hemorrhage and craniotomy varied from 5 to 48 hours (mean: 12 hours). Overall, 80 per cent of the nonoperated patients died, whereas the surgical patients had a 27 per cent mortality.[42]

Based on the evidence that is available, it appears that the patient with a large hematoma caused by aneurysmal rupture who is unconscious or comatose has a poor prognosis regardless of therapy. It is likely that early decompressive craniotomy with hematoma evacuation and aneurysm clipping can salvage some critically ill patients. In an attempt to minimize the time from hemorrhage to decompression in patients with brain stem compression and decerebration, Batjer and Samson have advocated exploration without angiography, because computed tomography suggests the probable source of hemorrhage in almost all cases.[7] LeRoux and colleagues have reported that infusion computed tomography documented the offending aneurysm in each of 25 similar patients so studied, with an additional time delay of only 10 to 15 minutes.[60]

Regardless of the diagnostic strategy employed, the authors have noted that patients of this type operated in extremis frequently have severe primary brain injury that is manifested within 24 to 72 hours. For that reason, several specific technical points are recommended. First, the craniotomy should be large and associated with generous temporal craniectomy, particularly for a middle cerebral aneurysm. The hematoma should be entered and partially decompressed initially under microsurgical guidance. The appropriate subarachnoid space should then be entered with standard clipping of the offending aneurysm using temporary arterial occlusion if necessary. At that point, the authors recommend resection of the remaining hematoma and usually subtotal frontal or temporal lobectomy, depending on the actual site of hemorrhage. The dura is closed with a pericranial patch graft, and the bone flap is left out for decompressive purposes. Any unruptured aneurysms diagnosed angiographically should not be treated in these acutely ill patients. These procedures are fraught with complications and frequent intraoperative premature aneurysm rupture. Yet it is the belief of the authors that some patients will be saved by these aggressive maneuvers.

Infectious and post-traumatic aneurysms often come to clinical attention because of intracerebral bleeding. Their management, in the authors' opinion, does not differ significantly from the aforementioned strategy in terms of timing of intervention. Technically, however, the surgeon must presume that a large portion of the parent vessel's circumference has been damaged by the infectious or traumatic process and that surgical correction will probably require sacrifice of the involved vessel. Therefore, provisions for distal revascularization should be kept in mind for these aneurysms affecting the proximal conducting vessels.[19]

Cerebral Hemorrhage from Vasculitis

Cerebral vasculitis is a general category of disorders that result in inflammation of the blood vessel wall. This inflammation can lead to wall necrosis, vessel occlusion, or aneurysm formation. The vascular insult can involve the major conducting vessels or any of the branches, including arterioles and venules of microscopic size. The precipitating causes comprise many systemic inflammatory disorders, including autoimmune conditions and infections. In addition, some vasculitides appear to be confined to the intracranial circulation. The vascular injuries are of a variety of types, including the deposition of immune complexes into the vessel wall with complement activation and granulomatous processes with lymphocytic infiltration.[21] A detailed description of each type of vasculitis that may result in intracranial hemorrhage is beyond the scope of this chapter, but potential offending conditions have been summarized by Cohen and Biller.[21]

The diagnosis of vasculitis may be suggested by dysfunction of other organ systems, including the kidneys, lungs, and gastrointestinal tract. Other systemic evidence of an inflammatory process may include a skin rash, fever, arthritis, or a history of myalgia. In the absence of systemic symptoms and signs, the diagnosis can be difficult. Computed tomography and magnetic resonance imaging accurately delineate the cerebral hemorrhage, but other signs may be nonspecific or absent. The classic signs of segmental narrowing and dilation on angiography are helpful if present but may also be seen with other conditions, including migraine.[27, 59] Angiography may be negative in 20 to 30 per cent of pathologically verified cases because involved vessels are smaller than can be identified angiographically.[16, 105] The hallmark of definitive diagnosis rests on histopathological verification, a point that should be kept in mind for patients requiring craniotomy for hematoma decompression.

The patient presenting with intracranial hemorrhage of unknown cause, in whom no obvious external site for biopsy (e.g., skin, muscle, temporal artery) is apparent, may well be a candidate for leptomeningeal biopsy or biopsy of the hematoma wall. Although the neurological management of patients with these conditions does not differ from that previously discussed, corticosteroids and immunosuppressive agents have been shown to be effective in the long-term course of these patients.[21]

Cerebral Hemorrhage from Amyloid Angiopathy

Cerebral amyloid angiopathy is primarily a disease of the elderly and is becoming an increasingly prevalent cause of intracerebral hemorrhage. Several features of this condition are relevant to the neurosurgeon because they impact not only treatment of individuals with intracranial hemorrhage but also prognostic recommendations. Amyloid angiopathy is characterized by the finding of amyloid beta-protein within the media and adventitia of cerebral arteries and arterioles.[22, 58, 92] After the arterial wall is weakened and rendered brittle by this protein deposition, the patient is predisposed to spontaneous cerebral hemorrhage or to bleeding into the brain after minor trauma or unrelated intracranial surgery.[58] The hallmark of the clinical diagnosis is multifocal cerebral hemorrhage occurring at different times.[58]

Amyloid in affected patients can be demonstrated in cortical vessels and arterioles and also in senile plaques and neurofibrillary tangles, if present.[58] This material is strongly eosinophilic and has a strong affinity for Congo red stain. Some degree of anatomical specificity may be present, and various series have noted predilection for parieto-occipital,[93] temporo-parietal, or frontal lobe involvement.[22, 58] It is estimated that cerebral hemorrhage will eventually occur in 40 to 67 per cent of affected individuals.[22]

Although familial cases are well known,[92] the sporadic form is clearly age-related. Various investigators have demonstrated histological evidence of amyloid angiopathy in 5 to 8 per cent of autopsies in the seventh decade of life, 23 to 43 per cent in the eighth decade, 37 to 46 per cent in the ninth decade, and 58 per cent of autopsies after age 90.[88, 93] The most severe forms usually have ample histological evidence to support the diagnosis of Alzheimer's disease.

The implications of this condition for the treating physicians are significant. Hematomas from amyloid angiopathy are usually lobar and cortical and, if massive, have a tendency to rupture into the ventricle or subdural space. Management of small hematomas is usually conservative unless histological diagnosis is thought to be critical for the family. If pushed to surgery by major mass effect or clinical deterioration, the surgeon must be prepared for difficulty in achieving hemostasis. The brittle and fragile walls that characterize this disease do not respond well to bipolar cautery and often rupture during manipulation. Leblanc has demonstrated that the methodical use of tamponade and topical hemostatic agents is usually successful.[58] If the diagnosis is in doubt at the time of surgery, biopsies of the hematoma wall should be taken. The postoperative course is often complicated by recurrent bleeding into the hematoma cavity; therefore, blood pressure should be carefully controlled. The patient's family should also be counseled that long-term follow-up may be marked by recurrent cerebral hemorrhage and progressive dementia.

Hemorrhagic Transformation of Cerebral Infarction

Hemorrhage into areas of cerebral infarction, although well known in the past, has assumed new neurosurgical importance. The incidence of some degree of hemorrhage into embolic cerebral infarction is high, and reports following Fisher and Adams' autopsy series[31] have suggested that 51 to 71 per cent of embolic infarctions develop some degree of hemorrhagic transformation.[89] Differentiating between spontaneous cerebral hemorrhage and hemorrhagic cardioembolic infarction is extremely important, because failure to treat the primary embolic source results in recurrent infarction in as many as 21 per cent of patients within the first 3 weeks.[30, 41] Careful scrutiny of the patient's computed tomography scan usually allows accurate differentiation between primary and secondary hemorrhage. The brain slices in hemorrhagic infarction usually demonstrate mixed low and high density and usually conform to a specific vascular territory. If cortical structures are involved, the hemorrhage is usually gyriform in pattern.[89]

In addition to the importance of establishing an accurate diagnosis, neurosurgeons must be aware of the increasing frequency of therapeutic interventions that can risk converting a minor hemorrhagic infarction into a massive intracranial hematoma. Antiplatelet agents, anticoagulants, thrombolytic agents, and intracranial angioplasty are being investigated to improve the prognosis for stroke patients in general. Yet, even as the

most effective reperfusion interval is being established, cases are encountered in which this "window" is exceeded and hemorrhage develops. If surgical decompression is required, a careful consultation with the attending neurologist and, occasionally, a hematologist should be performed to balance the often conflicting objectives of ensuring hemostasis and minimizing the risk of recurrent embolic or occlusive events.

Cerebral Hemorrhage from Tumors

Hemorrhage into the brain related to an underlying neoplasm is a relatively uncommon but not rare occurrence with obvious relevance to the neurosurgeon. In general, about 5 to 10 per cent of all brain tumors develop hemorrhage of some type. Hemorrhage is more common in metastatic tumors and has been estimated to occur in approximately 10 per cent of cases.[73] Primary brain tumors bleed in approximately 5 per cent of cases.[73] Wakai and colleagues found that in 24 per cent of patients developing tumor-related hemorrhage the hemorrhage was the initial presentation of the tumor.[97]

The tissue type of the tumor itself clearly relates to its propensity to bleed. Metastatic lesions, including bronchogenic carcinoma, melanoma, choriocarcinoma, and hypernephroma, are known to carry a high risk of hemorrhage, and, in some series, as many as 40 per cent of metastatic melanoma brain lesions were found to bleed.[53, 64, 83] Of the primary brain tumors, glioblastoma appears to be the most common source of intracerebral hemorrhage; slightly more than 5 per cent of cases are complicated by bleeding.[73] Oligodendrogliomas also have a predilection for hemorrhage and do so more frequently than astrocytomas. Ependymomas and medulloblastomas also have been associated with intracranial hemorrhage.[18, 78] Benign tumors have been known to hemorrhage, although rarely, and pituitary adenomas and meningiomas are the lesions most likely to develop this complication.

Nutt and Patchell have discussed the pathophysiology of hemorrhage into tumors and believe that four factors are contributory: (1) structural abnormalities in tumor vessels, (2) tumor invasion of blood vessel walls, (3) tumor or brain necrosis, and (4) coagulation defects, either related to systemic cancer or iatrogenically induced.[73] The diagnosis should be suspected in patients with known primary malignancy and in new cases in which the hemorrhage is in an unusual location or associated with excessive edema. Computed tomography with or without enhancement can help identify an enhancing mass, although the presence of tumor calcification often makes this distinction difficult. Magnetic resonance imaging is the most sensitive diagnostic aid and should correctly identify tumor tissue in most cases.

The surgical treatment of hemorrhagic lesions in this context should be guided by the severity of the hemorrhage and the offending tumor type. Some attempt at debulking the tumor in cases of massive hemorrhage is highly recommended if serious edema develops postoperatively.

REFERENCES

1. Adams, H. P., Kassell, N. F., and Torner, J. C.: Usefulness of computed tomography in predicting outcome after aneurysmal subarachnoid hemorrhage: A preliminary report of the Cooperative Aneurysm Study. Neurology, 35:1263, 1985.
2. Auer, L. M.: Unfavorable outcome following early surgical repair of ruptured cerebral aneurysms: A critical review of 238 patients. Surg. Neurol., 35:152, 1991.
3. Auer, L. M., Auer, T., and Sayama, I.: Indications for surgical treatment of cerebellar haemorrhage and infarction. Acta Neurochir. (Wien)., 79:74, 1986.
4. Auer, L. M., Deinsberger, W., Niederkorn, K., et al.: Endoscopic surgery versus medical treatment for spontaneous intracerebral hematoma: A randomized study. J. Neurosurg., 70:530, 1989.
5. Auer, L. M., Schneider, G., and Auer, T.: Computed tomography and prognosis in early aneurysm surgery. J. Neurosurg., 65:217, 1986.
6. Batjer, H. H., Reisch, J. S., Allen, B. C., et al.: Failure of surgery to improve outcome in hypertensive putaminal hemorrhage: A prospective randomized trial. Arch. Neurol., 47:1103, 1990.
7. Batjer, H. H., and Samson, D. S.: Emergent aneurysm surgery without angiography for the comatose patient. Neurosurgery, 28:283, 1991.
8. Baumbach, G. L., and Heistad, D. D.: Effects of sympathetic stimulation and changes in arterial pressure on segmental resistance of cerebral vessels in rabbits and cats. Circ. Res., 52:527, 1983.
9. Baumbach, G. L., and Heistad, D. D.: Heterogeneity of brain blood flow and permeability during acute hypertension. Am. J. Physiol., 249:H629, 1985.
10. Bogousslavsky, J., Van Melle, G., and Regli, F.: The Lausanne Stroke Registry. Stroke, 19:1083, 1988.
11. Bohm, E., and Hugosson, R.: Experiences of surgical treatment of 400 consecutive ruptured cerebral arterial aneurysms. Acta Neurochir. (Wein), 40:33, 1978.
12. Bray, L., Lartaud, I., Muller, F., et al.: Effects of the angiotensin I converting enzyme inhibitor perindopril on cerebral blood flow in awake hypertensive rats. Am. J. Hypertens., 4:246, 1991.
13. Brennan, R., and Bergland, R.: Acute cerebellar hemorrhage: Analysis of clinical findings and outcome in 12 cases. Neurology, 27:527, 1977.
14. Broderick, J. P., Brott, T., Tomsick, T., et al.: Intracerebral hemorrhage more than twice as common as subarachnoid hemorrhage. J. Neurosurg., 78:188, 1993.
15. Broderick, J. P., Phillips, S. J., Whisnant, J. P., et al.: Incidence rates of stroke in the eighties: The end of the decline in stroke? Stroke, 20:577, 1989.
16. Calabrese, L. H., and Malleck, J. A.: Primary angiitis of the central nervous system: Report of 8 new cases, review of the literature and proposal for diagnostic criteria. Medicine (Balt.), 67:20, 1987.
17. Charcot, J. M., and Bouchard, C.: Nouvelles recherches sur la pathogenie de l'hemorrhagie cérébrale. Arch. Physiol. Norm. Pathol., 1:110, 1868.
18. Chugani, H. T., Rosenblat, A. M., Lavenstein, B. L., et al.: Childhood medulloblastoma presenting with hemorrhage. Child's Brain, 11:135, 1984.
19. Clare, C. E., and Barrow, D. L.: Infectious intracranial aneurysms. Neurosurg. Clin. North Am., 3:551, 1992.
20. Clozel, J.-P., Kuhn, H., and Hefti, F.: Effects of cilazapril on the cerebral circulation in spontaneously hypertensive rats. Hypertension, 14:645, 1989.
21. Cohen, B. A., and Biller, J.: Hemorrhagic stroke due to cerebral vasculitis and the role of immunosuppressive therapy. Neurosurg. Clin. North Am., 3:611, 1992.
22. Cosgrove, G. R., Leblanc, R., Meagher-Villemure, K., et al.: Cerebral amyloid angiopathy. Neurology, 35:625, 1985.
23. Da Pian, R., Bazzan, A., and Pasqualin, A.: Surgical versus medical treatment of spontaneous posterior fossa hematomas: A cooperative study on 205 cases. Neurol. Res., 6:145, 1984.
24. Drury, I., Whisnant, J. P., and Garraway, W. M.: Primary intracerebral hemorrhage: Impact of CT on incidence. Neurology, 34:653, 1984.
25. Ducker, T. B.: Spontaneous intracerebral hemorrhage. In Wilkins, R. H., and Rengachary, S. S., eds.: Neurosurgery. New York, McGraw-Hill, 1985, pp. 1510–1517.
26. Duff, T. A., Ayeni, S., Levin, A. B., et al.: Nonsurgical management of spontaneous intracerebral hematomas. Neurosurgery, 9:387, 1981.
27. Ferris, E. J., and Levine, H. L.: Cerebral arteritis: Classification. Radiology, 109:327, 1973.
28. Fisher, C. M.: Lacunes, small deep cerebral infarcts. Neurology, 15:774, 1965.
29. Fisher, C. M.: Pathological observations in hypertensive cerebral hemorrhage. J. Neuropathol. Exp. Neurol., 30:536, 1971.
30. Fisher, C. M.: Reducing risks of cerebral embolism. Geriatrics, 34:59, 1979.
31. Fisher, C. M., and Adams, R. D.: Observations on brain embolism with special references to the mechanism of hemorrhagic transformation. J. Neuropathol. Exp. Neurol., 10:92, 1951.
32. Foulkes, M. A., Wolf, P. A., Price, T. R., et al.: The Stroke Data Bank. Stroke, 19:547, 1988.
33. Fredrikson, K., Ingvar, M., and Johansson, B. B.: Regional cerebral blood flow in conscious stroke-prone spontaneously hypertensive rats. J. Cereb. Blood Flow Metab., 4:103, 1984.
34. Furlan, A. J., Whisnant, J. P., and Elveback, L. R.: The decreasing incidence of primary intracerebral hemorrhage: A population study. Ann. Neurol., 5:367, 1979.
35. Garcia, J. H., and Ho, K.-L.: Pathology of hypotensive arteriopathy. Neurosurg. Clin. North Am., 3:497, 1992.
36. Gautier, J. C.: Cerebral ischemia in hypertension. In Russell, R., ed.: Cerebral Arterial Disease. London, Churchill Livingstone, 1978, p. 181.
37. Goldstein, R. J., Bleich, H. L., Caplan, L. R., et al.: Computer stroke registry and diagnosis program. Neurology, 25:356, 1975.
38. Graf, C. J., Perret, G. E., and Torner, J. C.: Bleeding from cerebral malformations as part of their natural history. J. Neurosurg., 58:331, 1983.
39. Harper, S. L.: Effects of antihypertensive treatment on the cerebral microvasculature of spontaneously hypertensive rats. Stroke, 18:450, 1987.
40. Harper, S. L., and Bohlen, H. G.: Microvascular adaptation in the cerebral cortex of adult spontaneously hypertensive rats. Hypertension, 6:408, 1984.
41. Hart, R. G., Coull, B. M., and Hart, D.: Early recurrent embolism associated with nonvalvular atrial fibrillation: A retrospective study. Stroke, 14:688, 1983.
42. Heiskanen, O., Poranen, A., Kuurne, T., et al.: Acute surgery for intracerebral hematomas caused by rupture of an intracranial arterial aneurysm: A prospective randomized study. Acta Neurochir. (Wien), 90:81, 1988.
43. Helweg-Larsen, S., Sommer, W., Strange, P., et al.: Prognosis for patients treated conservatively for spontaneous intracerebral hematomas. Stroke, 15:1045, 1984.
44. Hunt, W. E., and Hess, R. M.: Surgical risk as related to time of intervention in the repair of intracranial aneurysms. J. Neurosurg., 28:14, 1968.
45. Jane, J. A., Kassell, N. F., Torner, J. C., et al.: The natural history of aneurysms and arteriovenous malformations. J. Neurosurg., 62:321, 1985.
46. Juvela, S., Heiskanen, O., Poranen, A., et al.: The treatment of spontaneous intracerebral hemorrhage: A prospective randomized trial of surgical and conservative treatment. J. Neurosurg., 70:755, 1989.
47. Kaneko, M., Tanaka, K., Shimada, T., et al.: Long-term evaluation of ultra-early operation for hypertensive intracerebral hemorrhage in 100 cases. J. Neurosurg., 58:838, 1983.
48. Kanno, T., Sano, H., Shinomiya, Y., et al.: Role of surgery in hypertensive intracerebral hematoma: A comparative study of 305 non-surgical and 154 surgical cases. J. Neurosurg., 61:1091, 1984.
49. Kassell, N. F., and Drake, C. G.: Timing of aneurysm surgery. Neurosurgery, 10:514, 1982.
50. Kassell, N. F., and Torner, J. C.: The International Cooperative Study on Timing of Aneurysm Surgery. Acta Neurochir. (Wien), 63:119, 1982.

51. Kassell, N. F., and Torner, J. C.: Aneurysmal rebleeding: A preliminary report from the Cooperative Aneurysm Study. Neurosurgery, 13:479, 1983.

52. King, W. A., and Martin, N. M.: Intracerebral hemorrhage due to dural arteriovenous malformations and fistulae. Neurosurg. Clin. North Am., 3:577, 1992.

53. Kondziolka, D., Bernstein, M., Resch, L., et al.: Significance of hemorrhage into brain tumors: Clinico-pathological study. J. Neurosurg., 67:852, 1987.

54. Kopitnik, T. A., and Kaufman, H. H.: The future: Prospects of innovative treatment of intracerebral hemorrhage. Neurosurg. Clin. North Am., 3:703, 1992.

55. Kunitz, S. C., Gross, C. R., Heyman, A., et al.: The Pilot Stroke Data Bank. Stroke, 15:740, 1984.

56. Kuschinsky, W.: Physiology and general pathophysiology of the cerebral circulation. In Olesen, J., and Edvinsson, L., eds.: Basic Mechanisms of Headache. New York, Elsevier, 1988, p. 69.

57. Kutsuzawa, T., Itoh, K., and Kawakami, H.: Conservative treatment of hypertensive cerebral hemorrhage: Results of 104 patients in acute stage. Neurol. Med. Chir. (Tokyo), 16:29, 1976.

58. Leblanc, R.: Cerebral amyloid angiopathy and moyamoya disease. Neurosurg. Clin. North Am., 3:625, 1992.

59. Leeds, N. E., and Goldberg, H. I.: Angiographic manifestations in cerebral inflammatory disease. Radiology, 98:595, 1971.

60. LeRoux, P. D., Dailey, A. T., Newell, D. W., et al.: Emergent aneurysm clipping without angiography in the moribund patient with intracerebral hemorrhage: The use of infusion computed tomographic scans. Neurosurgery, 33:189, 1993.

61. Ljunggren, B., Brandt, L., Kagstrom, E., et al.: Results of early operations for ruptured aneurysms. J. Neurosurg., 54:473, 1981.

62. Ljunggren, B., Saveland, H., and Brandt, L.: Early operation and overall outcome in aneurysmal subarachnoid hemorrhage. J. Neurosurg., 62:547, 1985.

63. Luessenhop, A. J., and Rosa, L.: Cerebral arteriovenous malformations: Indications for and results of surgery, and the role of intravascular techniques. J. Neurosurg., 60:14, 1984.

64. Mandybur, T. I.: Intracranial hemorrhage in metastatic tumors. Neurology, 27:650, 1977.

65. Masson, R. L., and Day, A. L.: Aneurysmal intracerebral hemorrhage. Neurosurg. Clin. North Am., 3:539, 1992.

66. McCormick, W. F.: Classification, pathology and natural history of angiomas of the central nervous system. Neurol. Neurosurg. Weekly Update, 1:3, 1978.

67. McKissock, W., Richardson, A., and Taylor, J.: Primary intracerebral haemorrhage: A controlled trial of surgical and conservative treatment in 180 unselected cases. Lancet, 2:221, 1961.

68. McKissock, W., Richardson, A., and Walsh, L.: Primary intracerebral haemorrhage: Results of surgical treatment in 244 consecutive cases. Lancet, 1:683, 1959.

69. Mohadjer, M., Eggert, R., May, J., et al.: CT-guided stereotactic fibrinolysis of spontaneous and hypertensive cerebellar hemorrhage: Long-term results. J. Neurosurg., 73:217, 1990.

70. Mohr, J. P., Caplan, L. R., Melski, J. W., et al.: The Harvard Cooperative Stroke Registry. Neurology, 28:754, 1978.

71. Mutlu, N., Berry, R. G., and Alpers, B. J.: Massive cerebral hemorrhage: Clinical and pathological characteristics. Arch. Neurol., 8:644, 1963.

72. Newell, D. W., Leroux, P. D., Dacey, R. G., et al.: CT infusion scanning for the detection of cerebral aneurysms. J. Neurosurg., 71:175, 1989.

73. Nutt, S. H., and Patchell, R. A.: Intracranial hemorrhage associated with primary and secondary tumors. Neurosurg. Clin. North Am., 3:591, 1992.

74. Ojemann, R. G., and Mohr, J. P.: Hypertensive brain hemorrhage. Clin. Neurosurg., 23:220, 1976.

75. Ondra, S. L., Troupp, H., George, E. D., et al.: The natural history of symptomatic arteriovenous malformations of the brain: A 24-year follow-up assessment. J. Neurosurg., 73:387, 1990.

76. Pasqualin, A., Bazzan, A., Cavazzani, P., et al.: Intracranial hematomas following aneurysmal rupture: Experience with 309 cases. Surg. Neurol., 25:6, 1986.

77. Paulson, O. B., Strandgaard, S., and Edvinsson, L.: Cerebral autoregulation. Cerebrovasc. Brain Metab. Rev., 2:161, 1990.

78. Poon, T. P., and Solis, O. G.: Sudden death due to massive intraventricular hemorrhage into unsuspected ependymoma. Surg. Neurol., 24:63, 1985.

79. Ropper, A. H., and King, R. B.: Intracranial pressure monitoring in comatose patients with cerebral hemorrhage. Arch. Neurol., 41:725, 1984.

80. Rowe, C. C., Donnan, G. A., and Bladin, P. F.: Intracerebral haemorrhage: Incidence and use of computed tomography. B. M. J., 297:1177, 1988.

81. Sacco, R. L., Wolf, P. A., Bharucha, N. E., et al.: Subarachnoid and intracerebral hemorrhage: Natural history, prognosis and precursive factors in the Framingham Study. Neurology, 34:847, 1984.

82. Sano, K.: Intracerebral hematomas. In Pia, H. W., Langmaid, C., and Zierski, J. eds.: Cerebral Aneurysms. Advances in Diagnosis and Therapy. Berlin, Springer-Verlag, 1979, pp. 402–407.

83. Scott, M.: Spontaneous intracerebral hematoma caused by cerebral neoplasms. J. Neurosurg., 42:338, 1975.

84. Scott, M., and Werthan, M.: The fate of hypertensive patients with clinically proven spontaneous intracerebral hematomas treated without surgery. Stroke, 1:286, 1970.

85. Shah, M. V., and Heros, R. C.: Intracerebral hemorrhage due to cerebral arteriovenous malformations. Neurosurg. Clin. North Am. 3:567, 1992.

86. Shields, C. B., and Friedman, W. A.: The role of stereotactic technology in the management of intracerebral hemorrhage. Neurosurg. Clin. North Am., 3:703, 1992.

87. Tapaninaho, A., Hernesniemi, J., and Vapalahti, M.: Emergency treatment of cerebral aneurysms with large hematomas. Acta Neurochir. (Wien), 91:21, 1988.

88. Taveras, J. M.: Multiple progressive intracranial arterial occlusion: A syndrome of children and young adults. A. J. R., 106:235, 1969.

89. Teal, P. A., and Pessin, M. S.: Hemorrhagic transformation: The spectrum of ischemia-related brain hemorrhage. Neurosurg. Clin. North Am., 3:601, 1992.

90. Tonnis, W., Schieffer, W., and Walter, W.: Signs and symptoms of supratentorial arteriovenous malformations. J. Neurosurg., 15:471, 1958.

91. Unwin, D. H., Batjer, H. H., and Greenlee, R. G.: Management controversy: Medical versus surgical therapy for spontaneous intracerebral hemorrhage. Neurosurg. Clin. North Am., 3:533, 1992.

92. Vinters, H. V.: Cerebral amyloid angiopathy: A critical review. Stroke, 18:311, 1987.

93. Vinters, H. V., and Gilbert, J. J.: Amyloid angiopathy: Its incidence and complications in the aging brain. Stroke, 14:915, 1983.

94. Vlahov, V., and Bacracheva, J.: Autoregulation of the regional cortical and thalamic cerebral blood flow in cats. Arch. Int. Pharmacodyn. Ther., 289:93, 1987.

95. Waga, S., Miyazaki, M., Okada, M., et al.: Hypertensive putaminal hemorrhage: Analysis of 182 patients. Surg. Neurol., 26:159, 1986.

96. Waga, S., and Yamamoto, Y.: Hypertensive putaminal hemorrhage: Treatment and results: Is surgical treatment superior to conservative one? Stroke, 14:480, 1983.

97. Wakai, S., Yamakawa, K., Manaka, S., et al.: Spontaneous intracranial hemorrhage caused by brain tumor: Its incidence and clinical significance. Neurosurgery, 10:437, 1982.

98. Waldemar, G., Paulson, O., Barry, D., et al.: Angiotensin converting enzyme inhibition and the upper limit of cerebral blood flow autoregulation: Effect of sympathetic stimulation. Circ. Res., 64:1197, 1989.

99. Waldemar, G., Schmidt, J. F., Andersen, A. R., et al.: Angiotensin converting enzyme inhibition and cerebral blood flow autoregulation in normotensive and hypertensive man. J. Hypertens., 7:229, 1989.

100. Wheelock, B., Weir, B., Watts, R., et al.: Timing of surgery for intracerebral hematomas due to aneurysm rupture. J. Neurosurg., 58:476, 1983.

101. Williams, J. L., and Furlan, A. J.: Cerebral vascular physiology in hypertensive disease. Neurosurg. Clin. North Am., 3:509, 1992.

102. Winn, H. R., Newell, D. W., Mayberg, M. R., et al.: Early surgical management of poor-grade patients with intracranial aneurysms. Clin. Neurosurg., 36:289, 1990.

103. Wityk, R. J., and Caplan, L. R.: Hypertensive intracerebral hem-

orrhage: Epidemiology and clinical pathology. Neurosurg. Clin. North Am., *3*:521, 1992.

104. Woodard, E. J., and Barrow, D. L.: Clinical presentation of intracranial arteriovenous malformations. *In* Barrow, D. L., ed.: Intracranial Vascular Malformations: Neurosurgical Topics. Park Ridge, IL, American Association of Neurological Surgeons, 1990, p. 53.

105. Younger, D. S., Hays, A. P., Brust, J. C. M., et al.: Granulomatous angiitis of the brain: An inflammatory reaction of diverse etiology. Arch. Neurol., *45*:514, 1988.

Lesions of Cerebral Veins and Dural Sinuses

Advances in microneurosurgical equipment and techniques, coupled with the evolution of neurointerventional treatment modalities, have facilitated the surgical treatment of lesions of the cerebral veins and dural venous sinuses. Combined endovascular and surgical intervention should now be considered the standard of care in the treatment of venous sinus pathology. Endovascular therapy may reduce the blood loss and morbidity associated with surgical procedures. This chapter focuses on the most prevalent venous lesions, including dural arteriovenous fistulae, carotid cavernous fistulae, and sagittal sinus thromboses, and their treatment. In particular, the authors elaborate the endovascular therapy for intracranial dural lesions.

Venous Anatomy

The intracranial venous drainage can best be considered in a centrifugal fashion and divided into deep, cortical, and dural venous systems. Embryological variation in any of these systems may result in anomalies, including fenestrations, duplications, and alterations in regions of venous drainage.[78] Usually, these are of little clinical relevance, but they may be associated with dural arteriovenous malformations. Also, unrelated cerebral or dural anatomical anomalies may be evident in up to 30 per cent of patients with cerebral arteriovenous malformations.[78]

The deep venous system is composed primarily of large, deep, named vessels (e.g., Galen, Rosenthal, and internal cerebral veins) and the more occult transcerebral system. This system is the partial exception to the general rule of centrifugal venous drainage because the medullary veins drain into the subependymal veins of the ventricle before the formation of the larger veins that drain to the periphery. The superficial veins, radiating in spokelike fashion from the root of the sylvian fissure, are variable in number and position. Three named and relatively constant veins are those of Trolard and Labbé and the superficial middle cerebral (sylvian) vein. Although they are relatively inconspicuous under normal circumstances, anastomoses exist between superficial and deep systems. The dural venous sinuses, the main conduit for venous drainage from the cranial cavity and its contents, communicate directly with the superficial system and, through emissary veins, with the extracranial venous system.

The true and potential anastomotic channels between these venous strata may be particularly relevant in relation to venous disease processes. Hemodynamic changes in one area may be associated with compensation and collateral drainage in other areas. For example, hemodynamic alteration in venous drainage pathways may occur with venous obstruction or arteriovenous shunting in arteriovenous malformations or fistulae.

Dural Arteriovenous Fistulae and Carotid Cavernous Fistulae

Dural arteriovenous fistulae represent 10 to 15 per cent of all intracranial arteriovenous malformations.[88] Arteriovenous fistulae occur most frequently in the region of the transverse and sigmoid sinuses. They may, however, occur at other dural locations, including the superior sagittal sinus, inferior petrosal sinus, anterior cranial fossa, and around the deep cerebral venous system or vein of Galen.[2, 4, 44, 48, 84] Arteriovenous fistulae are thought to be acquired lesions that, in adults, develop from small vessels that form in a thrombosed sinus or vein.[62] The majority of dural sinus fistulae develop spontaneously. However, trauma and hypercoagulable states have been suggested as predisposing factors in the development of some fistulae.[62]

S. L. Barnwell • O. R. O'Neill

Carotid cavernous fistulae are classified into two major categories, direct and indirect.[8] The direct, or type A, carotid cavernous fistula usually results from traumatic fracture of the sphenoid bone that produces a hole in the cavernous segment of the internal carotid artery (Fig. 63–1). Occasionally, iatrogenic injury to the carotid artery, as a complication of sphenoid sinus biopsy, retrogasserian rhizotomy, or use of Fogarty catheters during carotid endarterectomy, may predispose to fistula formation.[38, 53, 80, 122] Congenital weakness of the cavernous carotid artery, as is seen with collagen vascular diseases or fibromuscular dysplasia, may be associated with tears in the vessel wall and direct fistula formation.* Rupture of cavernous internal carotid artery aneurysms may also produce a direct carotid cavernous fistula.[21, 38] Direct carotid cavernous fistulae are more common in males than females, as is the craniocerebral trauma that predisposes to their formation.

_____

*See references 18, 31, 38, 40, 76, and 105.

The indirect carotid cavernous fistula, a dural arteriovenous fistula involving the cavernous sinus, is subdivided into three types based on the nature of the arterial supply (Fig. 63–2). Type C fistulae receive arterial supply from dural branches of the external carotid artery. Type D fistulae are supplied by branches of both the internal and external carotid arteries. Fistulae receiving arterial supply entirely from small branches of the cavernous segment of the internal carotid artery, type B, are considered to be exceedingly rare.[21] There is a marked female prevalence for indirect carotid cavernous fistulae, and the lesions are most commonly spontaneous in onset. An association with pregnancy has been suggested by Walker and Allegre, although the overwhelming majority of cases occur in postmenopausal women in the fifth and sixth decades of life.[8, 41, 46, 118, 121] Trauma may occasionally result in the indirect type of carotid cavernous fistula. This occurs if there is injury to the intracavernous branches of the internal carotid artery.[95]

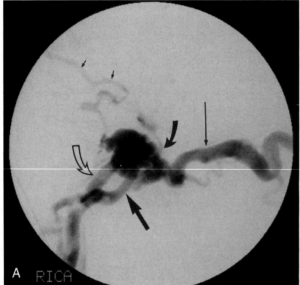

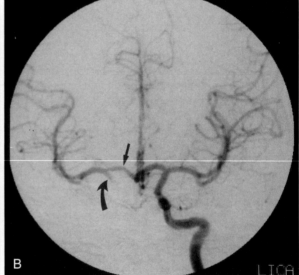

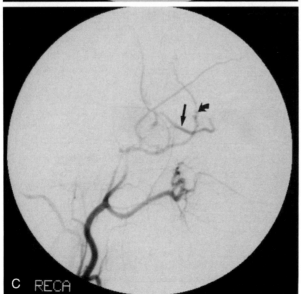

Figure 63–1

Direct, post-traumatic, carotid cavernous fistula in a 12-year-old boy involved in a motor vehicle accident. _A._ Right internal carotid artery angiogram, lateral projection, demonstrates typical features of a direct carotid cavernous fistula. The laceration is in the cavernous portion of the internal carotid artery (_large straight arrow_). There is a small amount of blood flowing distal to the tear in the artery and to the supraclinoid internal carotid artery (_solid curved arrow_). The venous drainage from the fistula is to the superior ophthalmic vein (_long thin arrow_), to the inferior petrosal sinus (_open curved arrow_), and to a subarachnoid cortical vein (_short arrows_). The drainage to the subarachnoid vein gives this fistula a higher risk of hemorrhage. _B._ Left internal carotid artery angiogram, anteroposterior projection, demonstrates steal of this carotid cavernous fistula from the left internal carotid artery. Flow is from the right anterior cerebral artery (_straight arrow_) retrograde into the supraclinoid internal carotid artery (_curved arrow_) to the fistula. The fistula is not well opacified because of additional steal of unopacified blood from the posterior communicating artery. _C._ Right external carotid artery angiogram, lateral projection, demonstrates that the external carotid artery, as in most cases, is not directly involved with the direct carotid cavernous fistula. There is retrograde filling of the ophthalmic artery (_straight arrow_) from the anterior division of the middle meningeal artery (_curved arrow_).

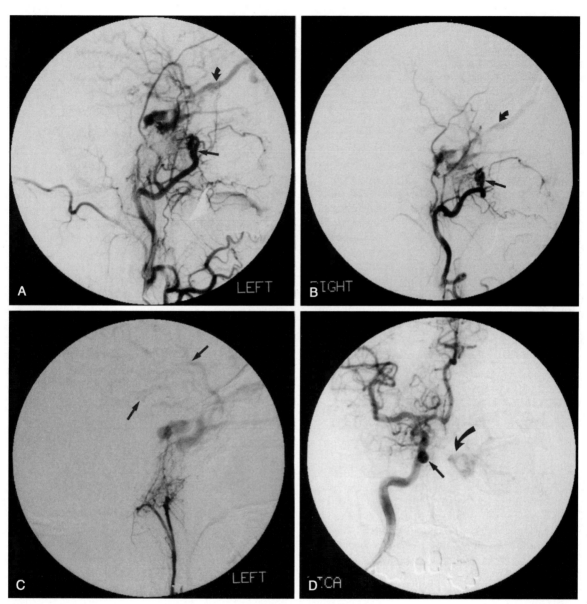

Figure 63–2

A 67-year-old woman with left-sided, type D, indirect, spontaneous dural carotid cavernous fistula. In type D dural carotid cavernous fistulae, the supply is often bilateral and from both the internal and the external carotid arteries. *A.* Left external carotid artery angiogram, lateral projection, demonstrates supply to the left-sided fistula from multiple branches of the distal internal maxillary artery (*straight arrow*). Venous drainage is primarily to the left superior ophthalmic vein (*curved arrow*). *B.* Right external carotid artery angiogram, lateral projection, demonstrates supply to the fistula from branches of the distal right internal maxillary artery (*straight arrow*) that cross the midline to the left-sided dural fistula. The opacified vein (*curved arrow*) is the left superior ophthalmic vein. *C.* Left ascending pharyngeal artery angiogram, lateral projection, shows multiple small vessels supplying this dural fistula. Venous drainage to cortical subarachnoid veins (*arrows*) is well demonstrated on this selective injection. The cortical venous drainage puts this fistula at higher risk for hemorrhage. The multitude of small arterial feeders makes transarterial embolization difficult in terms of curing these lesions. *D.* Right internal carotid artery angiogram, anteroposterior projection, demonstrates supply to the left-sided dural carotid cavernous fistula (*curved arrow*). The arterial supply is from small cavernous branches of the carotid artery (*straight arrow*).

Clinical Manifestations of Dural-Based Arteriovenous Fistulae

The clinical manifestations of dural arteriovenous fistulae may range from asymptomatic lesions to life-threatening hemorrhage.[36, 79, 82, 103, 119] The majority of dural arteriovenous fistulae are asymptomatic or present with a bruit. Symptom complexes associated with fistulae are often vague but may also be site-specific. Mild headaches or ocular symptoms are often the only clinical features, and evaluation may not be performed if these symptoms are not particularly bothersome. Some fistulae, however, may present with a major hemorrhage before any evaluation can be performed. General features of dural fistulae, which may be apparent with any lesion, include bruit, headache, loss of vision, altered mental status, and neurological deficits.[119] Headache is very common and may be related to distention of the dura or compression of the trigeminal nerve. Carotid cavernous fistulae may present with any of the features of dural fistulae, but they frequently present with a constellation of symptoms specific to the location and pathway of venous drainage. Direct and indirect carotid cavernous fistulae present with similar findings, although the direct fistulae may be associated with more severe clinical features.

Angioarchitecture of Dural Arteriovenous Malformations and Clinical Manifestations

The relationship between the angioarchitecture of dural arteriovenous fistulae and their clinical manifestations has been elucidated by Lasjaunias and colleagues.[79] In a review of 195 cases of dural fistulae, the arterial inflow, the location of the nidus, and the venous drainage pattern were related to a variety of syndromes.[79] Regardless of the size or location of the dural arteriovenous fistula, it is the abnormal venous drainage pattern that is associated with the more serious clinical manifestations.*

The arterial contribution from meningeal arteries to a dural fistula may be significant enough that cranial nerves suffer from a steal phenomenon.[79] Lasjaunias and colleagues described this in a patient with Bell's palsy and a cavernous sinus fistula. Neurological deficits as the result of a possible steal mechanism have also been described by Vinuela and co-workers.[119] In one patient, a large ethmoidal groove fistula was associated with amaurosis fugax, presumably from diversion of flow from the ophthalmic artery. In this case, there were no other atheromatous or cardiac diseases to explain the problem. A second patient had a lesion in the region of the foramen magnum and cerebellar dysfunction, possibly related to steal from the vertebral basilar circulation.

---

*See references 1, 36, 58, 79, 82, 97, 103, and 119.

The nidus of a fistula may also be responsible for the clinical findings with arteriovenous fistulae. Shunts within the nidus may be the cause of the pulsatile tinnitus or bruit that is evident in many patients. A bruit is present in virtually all direct carotid cavernous fistulae and in about one half of the indirect types.[66] High-flow fistulae that drain into large sinuses usually have a bruit. Lesions that involve any part of the petrous pyramid frequently cause tinnitus.[79] The source of headaches in patients is not clear, although it may be related to the increased pressure in the dura around the nidus.

High-flow lesions may be associated with hydrocephalus, intracranial hypertension, and macrocephaly. Hydrocephalus and intracranial hypertension may be caused by high pressures in the dural sinuses and the resultant imbalance in cerebrospinal fluid absorption dynamics. Macrocephaly, in the appropriate age group, and papilledema and visual loss are secondary responses to the hydrocephalus and intracranial hypertension.

Venous hypertension, as a result of high flow rates from fistulae into the dural sinuses, may be further exacerbated by associated dural sinus thrombosis, which may be complete or partial. Alternative, usually smaller, venous outflow pathways become responsible for drainage of the arterial supply from the lesions as well as that from their normal cerebral drainage region. This restricted outflow results in venous hypertension, which may affect other areas of the brain by way of passive congestion of veins. The flow in veins may be either anterograde or retrograde.

Venous hypertension can result in seizures, focal neurological deficits, cerebellar abnormalities, dementia, and transient ischemic attacks.[63, 79, 119] Cases of brain stem edema related to post-traumatic direct carotid cavernous fistulae have been described.[115] As expected, this problem results from abnormal venous drainage from the carotid cavernous fistulae to veins in the posterior fossa. Successful treatment of the fistula results in resolution of these problems.

The large dilated veins draining a fistula may produce neurological effects by way of a mass effect. Lasjaunias and colleagues described the case of a patient with an anterior fossa fistula and visual field deficit associated with a large dilated basal vein of Rosenthal.[79] Dural fistulae within the cavernous sinus present with signs that presumably result from compression of nerves by the arterialized veins. The abducens nerve, which is free within the sinus, is usually affected, although a total ophthalmoplegia may result if pressure is sufficiently high to damage the other cavernous cranial nerves. In addition, the proptosis and chemosis result from interference with the venous drainage from the orbit, usually through the superior ophthalmic vein. The greatest risk to vision is ischemia; if untreated, it may result in irreversible blindness and optic atrophy.[104] That the venous drainage is the cause of these problems rather than the site of the fistula itself is supported by the clinical findings with dural arteriovenous fistulae of the inferior petrosal sinus (Fig. 63–3). These lesions, although located distant from the

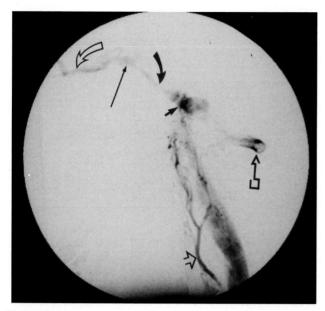

Figure 63–3

A 60-year-old woman with dural arteriovenous fistula of the left inferior petrosal sinus. The patient presented with typical findings of a carotid cavernous fistula, including chemosis, proptosis, and scleral injection of the left eye. Left ascending pharyngeal artery (*open straight arrow*) injection, lateral projection, demonstrates supply to the fistula located in the inferior petrosal sinus (*short straight arrow*). Venous drainage is up the inferior petrosal sinus (*solid curved arrow*) to the cavernous sinus (*long thin arrow*) and out the superior ophthalmic vein (*open curved arrow*). The venous drainage accounts for the clinical syndrome of almost all dural arteriovenous fistulae. Notice the collateral vessel that fills the vertebral artery (*open block arrow*). Such collaterals can make transarterial embolization dangerous.

cavernous sinus, usually drain to the cavernous sinus and produce a syndrome indistinguishable from that of fistulae located within the cavernous sinus.[2] Any dural fistulae that drain to the cavernous sinus may also present with the cavernous sinus syndrome, even if the fistula is located distant from the cavernous sinus.[50]

The occlusive lesions that occur in dural sinuses produce partial thrombosis and stenosis of the sinus and may manifest with neurological deficits distant from the lesion. These deficits may include increased intracranial pressure, mental deterioration, hemorrhage, and focal deficits remote from the site of the fistula. However, in cases in which there is direct shunting to cortical veins without changes in the sinuses, the deficits or hemorrhages tend to be spatially located near the fistula.[63]

Drainage into parenchymal or cortical veins may result in headache, neurological deficits from venous hypertension, or hemorrhage from rupture of thin-walled veins. Houser and co-workers first described the relationship between cortical venous drainage and intracranial hemorrhage.[62] Obrador and colleagues noted that hemorrhage occurred in about 20 per cent of patients with dural fistulae, although no correlation was made with the pattern of venous drainage among these patients.[92] Castaigne, as described by Lasjaunias

and co-workers, was the first to note that 42 per cent of patients with cortical venous drainage presented with bleeding.[14, 92] A review of 213 patients with dural fistulae revealed that 33 patients, all of whom demonstrated cortical venous drainage, presented with hemorrhage.[82] This association has been reported in numerous other series.[36, 79, 92, 103, 119] It may be postulated that dural arteriovenous fistulae do not cause intracranial hemorrhage unless they are associated with cortical venous drainage.[14, 79]

Magnetic Resonance Imaging of Dural Sinuses

Magnetic resonance imaging has proved to be a valuable asset in the evaluation of dural sinuses and is used primarily to evaluate thrombosis.* Several studies have shown the advantage of magnetic resonance imaging compared with computed tomography in the evaluation of dural sinuses.[93, 102, 113] Spin-echo and gradient echo imaging can usually differentiate the slow flow through dural sinuses from thrombosis. Retrograde sinus flow is a sensitive indicator of distal sinus occlusion or high-grade stenosis. Magnetic resonance imaging may also be useful in identifying cortical venous drainage patterns related to dural arteriovenous fistulae by demonstrating dilated vascular structures on the cortical surface adjacent to dural fistulae.[4]

Angiographic Evaluation of Dural Arteriovenous Fistulae

The vascular supply to the intracranial dura is extensive, with the main supply comprising internal and external carotid arteries, vertebral arteries, and dural branches of the posterior cerebral arteries.[62] Occasionally, the dural supply may in part originate from the middle or anterior cerebral arteries. This variation is associated with fistulae that have been present for a prolonged period or cases in which prior surgery has resulted in the interruption of the normal dural supply. Extensive and complete evaluation of all of these vessels is required to fully investigate a dural arteriovenous fistula. In addition, there are cases of multiple dural fistulae that may not be recognized unless all vessels are studied (Fig. 63–4).[3, 70, 103]

The angiographic evaluation of carotid cavernous fistulae is also complex and requires extensive imaging.[22, 89] High-flow direct carotid cavernous fistulae may pose particular problems, because flow through the fistula may be so rapid that all of the contrast injected goes into the cavernous sinus and does not opacify the internal carotid artery distal to the rent. Visualization of the internal carotid artery may also be obscured by the rapid filling of veins in the cavernous

*See references 24, 93, 102, 108, 113, and 116.

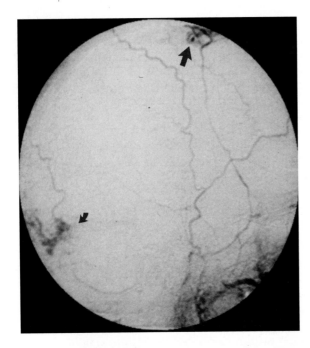

Figure 63–4

A 35-year-old woman with multiple dural arteriovenous fistulae. Right external carotid artery angiogram, lateral projection, demonstrates two dural arteriovenous fistulae involving the superior sagittal sinus (*straight arrow*) and transverse sigmoid sinus (*curved arrow*). Multiple dural arteriovenous fistulae may be unilateral or bilateral.

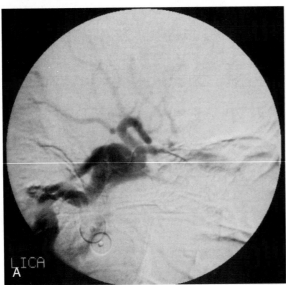

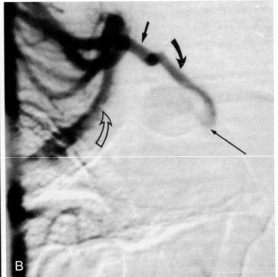

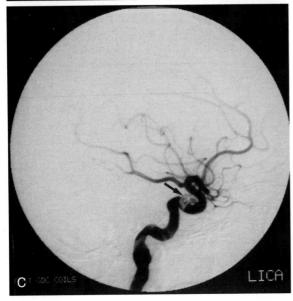

Figure 63–5

A 42-year-old man with Ehlers-Danlos syndrome and spontaneous development of direct carotid cavernous fistula. *A.* Left internal carotid artery angiogram, lateral projection, shows direct carotid cavernous fistula. The site of the hole in the internal carotid artery cannot be well visualized because of rapid opacification of the cavernous sinus by contrast. *B.* Left vertebral artery angiogram, lateral projection, while compressing the left common carotid artery, shows contrast filling the basilar artery (*open curved arrow*) and the posterior communicating artery (*short straight arrow*), down the supraclinoid internal carotid artery (*solid curved arrow*), and out into the fistula at the distal portion of the hole in the internal carotid artery (*long thin arrow*). Understanding the exact site of the hole in the carotid artery allows the proper navigation of catheters through the hole in the internal carotid artery to the cavernous sinus for embolization. *C.* Left internal carotid artery angiogram, lateral projection, after transarterial embolization of the fistula with detachable platinum coils (*arrow*). The coils have been placed at the hole in the internal carotid artery, which corresponds to the site detected by the vertebral artery injection. No coils are actually within the internal carotid artery, although on the lateral projection they overlie this artery.

sinus. Rapid image acquisition, with up to 30 images per second, may help overcome these problems by demonstrating the carotid artery before venous obscuration. Another technique is to perform a vertebral artery injection in the lateral projection, which fills the internal carotid artery distal to the hole through the posterior communicating artery, allowing the site of the rent to be determined (Fig. 63–5). It is vital to define the size of the hole in the carotid artery. Complete transsections often cannot be treated with preservation of the internal carotid artery, whereas a smaller fistula may be successfully closed with preservation of flow in the internal carotid artery.

Dural arteriovenous fistulae are acquired lesions, with dural sinus thrombosis or venous thrombosis as major etiological factors.[15, 62] Cases have been described in which the initial angiogram showed dural sinus occlusion and subsequent angiography demonstrated fistulae in the previously occluded sinus.[62] Post-traumatic venous sinus pathology with an abnormal or thrombosed sinus and subsequent angiographic evidence of the development of a dural arteriovenous fistula has also been described.[15] Graeb and Dolman reported 11 cases of dural fistulae, among which 9 had some degree of sinus thrombosis.[35] These facts highlight the importance of complete evaluation of the venous drainage in the assessment of dural arteriovenous fistulae.

The angiographic evaluation of the venous drainage of a dural fistula should demonstrate the anatomy and flow dynamics of the sinuses. Determination of whether the sinus is normal, partly thrombosed, or completely occluded is important. The distinction between partial and complete occlusion may be a difficult one. Also of importance is the demonstration of the direction of venous drainage. With transverse and sigmoid sinus fistulae, flow may be anterograde down the sigmoid sinus to the jugular bulb, or retrograde from the involved transverse sinus toward the torcula (Fig. 63–6). This pattern may be present if the transverse-sigmoid sinus junction is occluded or if the flow is so high from the fistula that there is reversal of flow in the involved transverse sinus. Distinguishing between these two possibilities is particularly relevant for fistulae involving the transverse-sigmoid sinus junction because surgical resection or induced thrombosis of this segment may be necessary to treat the lesion.

As well as determining venous sinus pathology, the angiogram must completely assess the veins draining to the involved sinus. Again, this factor is most critical in understanding lesions involving the transverse-sigmoid sinus junction. In particular, the vein of Labbé must be analyzed carefully. Retrograde flow in the vein of Labbé may be identified in cases in which a high-flow fistula exists in the region where the vein of Labbé normally empties into the transverse sinus. In this situation, the vein of Labbé is carrying only arterialized blood and, because of this, it may be safely occluded (Fig. 63–7). Vein of Labbé occlusion under these circumstances may be beneficial by diminishing the cerebral venous hypertension associated with retrograde flow.

However, anterograde flow of the vein of Labbé with venous drainage into the transverse sinus, mandates preservation of the vein. Occlusion of the vein of Labbé in this situation carries a high risk of causing a venous infarct (Fig. 63–8).

There are a number of veins from the posterior fossa and supratentorial regions that empty into the transverse and sigmoid sinuses. These small veins, although draining into the sinus in a normal anterograde fashion, may generally be occluded without complication. If treatment of the fistula requires therapeutic thrombosis of the transverse and sigmoid sinuses, it is important to disconnect or occlude these veins because they may become a conduit for venous outflow as the dural sinus is occluded. Diversion of venous drainage from a fistula to these cortical veins may result in disastrous hemorrhage or neurological deterioration.

Measurement of Pressure in Dural Sinuses

Intravascular pressure measurements are being used more frequently in the assessment of cerebrovascular lesions. Pressure measurements may be performed during embolization of the arterial supply to arteriovenous malformations and are used as guidelines to monitor the embolization.[23, 67, 68] As distal outflow in an arterial feeding pedicle is occluded, pressure in the proximal vessel rises. This rise in pressure is used to indicate successful occlusion of the vessel and may be more sensitive to the occlusion of the distal outflow than is fluoroscopic examination.[67] In order to prevent rupture of the artery, embolization is halted when the pressure rises.

Dural sinus pressures, also easily measured, may be valuable in certain clinical settings. In cases of meningioma invasion of a dural sinus, pressures taken on both sides of the tumor can show whether a pressure gradient exists. A significant pressure gradient can be used as an indication of whether the sinus can be sacrificed or must be left open.[49] A test occlusion may be performed to define the patient's tolerance to permanent occlusion of the sinus.

Pressures have been monitored on the arterial and venous sides of dural arteriovenous malformations during treatment.[23] Transarterial embolization was associated with elevation of arterial pedicle pressures and a fall in pressure draining in the draining vein. Transvenous embolization resulted in a significant elevation in the venous pressure until it equilibrated with the arterial pressure, and there was no change in the arterial pedicle pressure. This rise in the venous pressure indicated there was no flow through the fistula, and the fistula went on to thrombose.

Embolic Agents

Vascular occlusion for the treatment of dural arteriovenous fistulae can be accomplished with a wide vari-

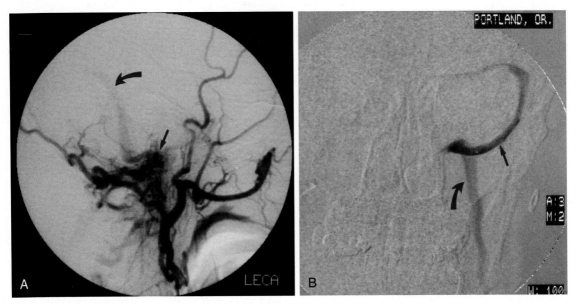

Figure 63–6

A 75-year-old woman with left base-of-skull dural arteriovenous fistula located around jugular bulb. *A.* Left external carotid artery angiogram, lateral projection, demonstrates dural arteriovenous fistula (*straight arrow*) that appears to drain retrograde to the transverse sinus (*curved arrow*) and toward the torcula. The jugular vein appears to be occluded. *B.* Left sigmoid sinus venogram, anteroposterior projection, demonstrates, however, that there is a connection between the sigmoid sinus (*straight arrow*) and the jugular vein (*curved arrow*). Selective venous injections are often helpful in completely elucidating the flow and patency of dural sinuses.

ety of agents. These agents can be grouped into those that result in proximal occlusion of vessels supplying the lesion and those that penetrate into the nidus of the lesion.

Proximal vessel occlusion is of value in the treatment of lesions before surgical resection. Surgical resection is facilitated by a reduction in the size of, and pressure within, the nidus as well as by a reduction in the number of patent feeding arteries. The disadvantage of proximal occlusion is that it cannot be used as the sole form of therapy because of enlargement and hypertrophy of collateral feeders and the ultimate reconstitution of the nidus and return of high flow. Proximal occlusion also precludes later use of this pedicle if more selective catheterization and embolization is planned for the future. Large embolic agents, such as platinum coils or silk suture, are most often used for proximal vessel occlusion.

Agents that penetrate into the small vessels composing the nidus of a fistula include cyanoacrylates, polyvinyl alcohol particles, ethanol, and microfibrillar collagen. Cyanoacrylates and polyvinyl alcohol are the most frequently used agents. Any of these materials has the potential for causing proximal vessel occlusion if delivered proximally.

Isobutyl 2-cyanoacrylate is the cyanoacrylate that has been used for most embolization procedures performed since the initial description by Cromwell and Kerber in 1979.[17] Because of concerns about the carcinogenicity of this agent, *N*-butyl 2-cyanoacrylate has been substituted.[13] However, there are no data that show the risk with this agent is less than with isobutyl 2-cyanoacrylate, and they perform similarly in vivo. Adjustment of the polymerization time for these agents may be achieved by altering the amount of soluble contrast agent or adding glacial acetic acid.[109] Variables used to define the appropriate polymerization time include the speed of the flow through the malformation and the distance between the catheter tip and the nidus. The glue is not radiopaque, so an oil-based contrast agent with tantalum powder is added to make it visible on fluoroscopy. The long-term effects of the cyanoacrylates are not well known, although, acutely, they produce pathological changes, including angionecrosis, within the walls of the vessels.[117] Although the occlusion is generally thought to be permanent, there can be dissolution of the glue over a period of months.[100, 117] One advantage of the liquid glues is the ability to deliver the agents through flow-directed catheters. These catheters are very soft and are less likely to cause vascular perforations than the stiffer catheters through which particles are delivered.

Polyvinyl alcohol is the most frequently used particulate agent.[61, 65, 103] Particle embolization has several advantages over glue, including a reduction in the risk of proximal vessel occlusion and a diminishment in the potential for the delivery catheter to become "glued" to the wall of the blood vessel.[106] The particles are sized from 150 to 1,000 microns in diameter or may be hand cut from larger pieces. Particle size is determined from an estimation of the size of the arteriovenous shunts within the malformation. Occlusion is best obtained if the particles lodge in the nidus rather than proximally. There is a well-demonstrated need for the appropriate choice of particle size. Particles that are too small can pass through the malformation and lodge in the lung, causing fatal pulmonary insufficiency.[101] Small particles may also pass into tiny vessels that cannot be seen on angiography because they are beyond the resolution of the imaging equipment. Occlusion of these vessels, if

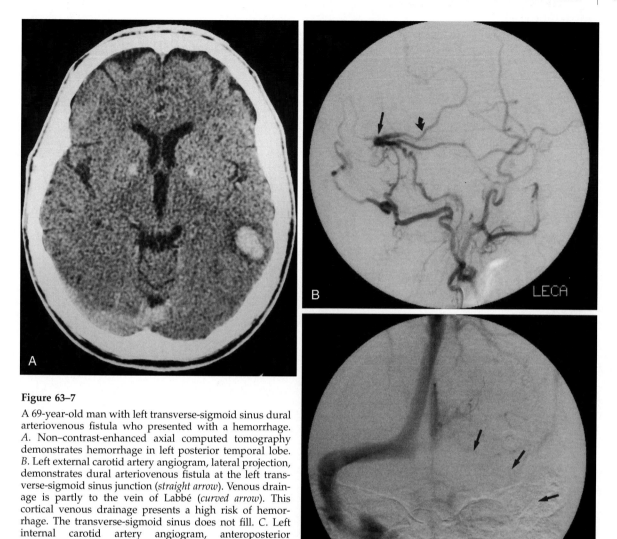

Figure 63–7

A 69-year-old man with left transverse-sigmoid sinus dural arteriovenous fistula who presented with a hemorrhage. *A.* Non–contrast-enhanced axial computed tomography demonstrates hemorrhage in left posterior temporal lobe. *B.* Left external carotid artery angiogram, lateral projection, demonstrates dural arteriovenous fistula at the left transverse-sigmoid sinus junction (*straight arrow*). Venous drainage is partly to the vein of Labbé (*curved arrow*). This cortical venous drainage presents a high risk of hemorrhage. The transverse-sigmoid sinus does not fill. *C.* Left internal carotid artery angiogram, anteroposterior projection, venous phase, demonstrates occlusion of the left transverse and sigmoid sinuses (*arrows*). The venous drainage from the left hemisphere is to the superior sagittal sinus and to the right transverse sinus. The vein of Labbé does not fill from the internal carotid artery circulation; rather, it fills only from the fistula that is supplied by the external carotid artery. In this case, treatment of this fistula would involve, in part, occlusion of the vein of Labbé to prevent the flow of blood from the fistula to the cortical subarachnoid veins. The fistula could also be treated by resection or coagulation of the involved dura.

they supply cranial nerves or parenchyma, may result in damage to those structures.[65] Because the particles are radiolucent, their effectiveness in vascular occlusion is evaluated by the flow patterns of the contrast medium in which the particles are suspended. The occlusive mechanism of action of polyvinyl alcohol appears to be adherence to the walls of vessels. Small particles, therefore, may not necessarily pass through a malformation even if the vessel diameter is larger than the particle.[99] Vessels that have been occluded by polyvinyl alcohol show an angionecrosis similar to that seen in vessels occluded with isobutyl 2-cyanoacrylate.[77]

Fistulous connections within the nidus of a dural arteriovenous malformation may complicate the endovascular treatment. These larger fistulae may allow a high proportion of the embolic material to pass

through the nidus and into the venous side of the lesion, where they may occlude the venous outflow or go to the lung. The use of silk suture has been shown to be effective in closing large fistulous connections within arteriovenous malformations.[27] Larger, hand-cut pieces of polyvinyl alcohol may also be useful in closing fistulous connections. Both are disadvantageous because they are radiolucent, although, if used with contrast medium in selected instances, they are safe. As the fistulous connections are closed, smaller agents may be used.

A variety of embolic agents are currently under investigation.[96, 110, 114] An ethylene vinyl alcohol copolymer sponge (ethylene vinyl alcohol copolymer and metrizamide dissolved in dimethylsulfoxide) has been designed that obstructs both the feeding artery and the nidus.[114] This agent may be advantageous compared

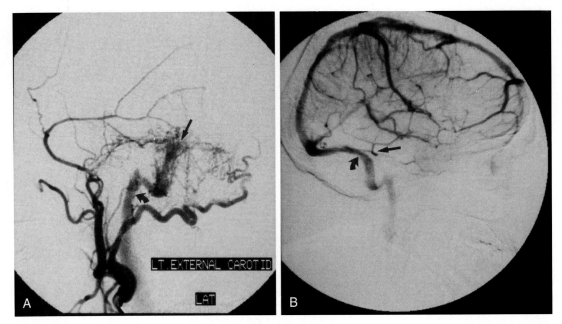

Figure 63–8

A 53-year-old woman with left transverse-sigmoid sinus dural arteriovenous fistula. *A.* Left external carotid angiogram, lateral projection, demonstrates dural arteriovenous fistula of the left transverse-sigmoid sinus junction (*straight arrow*) supplied by multiple branches of the external carotid artery. Venous drainage is entirely down the ipsilateral sigmoid sinus to the jugular vein (*curved arrow*). *B.* Left internal carotid angiogram, lateral projection, demonstrates anterograde flow in the vein of Labbé (*straight arrow*) to the transverse and sigmoid sinuses (*curved arrow*). This anterograde flow of the vein of Labbé means that during treatment of the fistula the transverse-sigmoid sinus junction cannot be safely occluded because the vein of Labbé would be blocked. A venous infarct may occur in the posterior temporal lobe if this vein is occluded. Complete evaluation of drainage of normal veins, primarily the vein of Labbé, is necessary to evaluate these dural fistulae.

with glue in that it stays liquid and does not hold the catheter in the blood vessel. Ethyl alcohol results in vessel occlusion if it is administered in sufficient concentration.[96] It may be useful in obliterating the nidus of a lesion and is relatively easy to deliver. Its disadvantages are the potential to destroy any normal tissue, including vessels or nerves, that it contacts and its propensity to be very painful in the awake patient.

Use of Provocative Testing Before Embolization

Before occlusion of the arterial supply to a dural arteriovenous fistula or carotid cavernous fistula, provocative testing of the vessel is performed. This procedure enables prediction of any potential functional loss associated with blockage of that vessel. Superselective injection of amobarbital (Amytal) into intracranial arteries before embolization has been performed for more than 10 years.[29, 30, 59] This test, a variation of the Wada and Rasmussen test of intracarotid amobarbital injection for language function, is generally considered to be reliable, although there may be false-positive or false-negative results.[120] The pressure and speed of the drug injection should replicate that which will be used with injection of the embolic agents. Overinjection of amobarbital may result in a false-positive test as a result of reflux of the drug into normal vessels.[60] Underinjection may lead to false-negative tests by

sumping of the drug into the fistula, thus bypassing normal branches that might have filled with higher pressure injections. As the embolization of a pedicle proceeds and flow is altered, it is necessary to retest the vessel because normal vessels that did not previously fill may begin to do so. A negative amobarbital test does not necessarily indicate that it will be safe to embolize that pedicle.

Amobarbital has been used extensively for testing the intracranial circulation but may not affect cranial nerve function, although it may affect optic nerve function.[59, 60] Therefore, lidocaine has been used—and is more effective—for testing of cranial nerve function and sight. Lidocaine is toxic to the central nervous system, and precautions should be taken to ensure that it does not enter the cerebral circulation through reflux or collateral flow between the external carotid artery and intracranial circulation.[60]

Indications for Treatment of Dural Arteriovenous Fistulae

The indications for treatment of dural arteriovenous fistulae are changing as our understanding of the natural history of these lesions is elucidated. The factors that predispose to an aggressive clinical course have been clearly described in numerous studies.* Cortical

---

*See references 1, 38, 63, 79, 82, 119, and 124.

and dilated venous structures are significantly associated with an aggressive course leading to hemorrhage or neurological impairment. Awad and colleagues stressed that the first clinical manifestation of aggressive behavior in dural arteriovenous malformations is often associated with major morbidity. Therefore, it is suggested treatment should be initiated as soon as these risk factors have been identified.[1] Dural fistulae that do not demonstrate these risk factors are rarely associated with neurological deficits or bleeds. Bilateral arterial inflow, high-flow shunting, bruit, and location of the fistula are not of particular prognostic significance.[1] However, fistulae involving the tentorial ring or anterior cranial region usually have cortical venous drainage and thereby present with hemorrhage or neurological dysfunction.

Indications for Treatment of Carotid Cavernous Fistulae

The indications for treatment of carotid cavernous fistulae must also be considered in relation to their natural history. Spontaneous closure is more common for indirect than for direct carotid cavernous fistulae, but an accurate estimate of the frequency of such closures is not known.[107] Newton and Hoyt reported spontaneous closure of dural carotid cavernous fistulae in 5 of 11 patients followed without treatment.[89] In another report, 18 of 20 consecutive patients with indirect carotid cavernous fistulae who were followed for 9 months to 9 years demonstrated complete regression of symptoms.[91] Given the natural history of these lesions in cases with mild symptoms, a conservative approach is indicated.[118, 124]

Noninterventional treatment may facilitate closure. Higashida and colleagues reported closure of carotid cavernous fistulae by external compression of the carotid artery and jugular vein.[57] This technique was used on both direct and indirect fistulae. Of the 71 patients in whom compression therapy was used, closure of the fistula was obtained in 7 of 23 patients with indirect carotid cavernous fistulae and 8 of 48 patients with direct carotid cavernous fistulae. The time for fistula closure varied from a matter of minutes to 6 months and, at follow-up after 1 year, none of the fistulae had reopened. This technique should not be used if indications for urgent treatment of the fistula are evident.[20, 38]

The indications for the urgent treatment of either direct or indirect carotid cavernous fistulae have been clearly defined by Halbach and colleagues.[38] In a review of 155 patients with direct and indirect carotid cavernous fistulae, a poor clinical outcome was related primarily to epistaxis and cortical venous drainage (Fig. 63–9).[38] Risk features identified on angiography of carotid cavernous fistulae include the presence of a large varix in the cavernous sinus, venous drainage to cortical veins, and thrombosis of venous drainage pathways distant to the cavernous sinus.[38] Clinical factors indicating a poor prognosis include increased in-

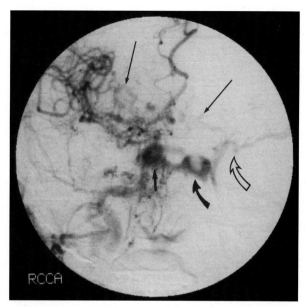

Figure 63–9

A 76-year-old woman with a high-risk bilateral dural carotid cavernous fistula. Right common carotid artery injection, anteroposterior projection, demonstrates dural arteriovenous fistula involving both the right (*short straight arrow*) and the left (*solid curved arrow*) cavernous sinuses. Of particular interest is filling of multiple small subarachnoid cortical veins (*long thin arrows*). This cortical venous drainage makes this fistula a high-risk lesion. The drainage out the left superior ophthalmic vein (*open curved arrow*) accounts for most of the patient's clinical symptoms, although this does not, in itself, present a high risk.

tracranial pressure, progressive proptosis, diminishing vision, and transient ischemic attacks. Progressive diminishment in visual acuity is a particularly important symptom. Based on the results of treatment of 132 patients with carotid cavernous fistulae, Debrun and colleagues recommended treatment of fistulae that are producing worsening vision.[21] Vinuela and colleagues also recommended therapy for patients losing vision or with progressing exophthalmos or ophthalmoplegias.[118] Additional discussion of this subject is given in Chapter 55.

Treatment of Dural and Carotid Cavernous Arteriovenous Fistulae

The treatment of dural arteriovenous fistulae is a potentially complex affair. Compression therapy and embolization through feeding arteries can ameliorate symptoms related to these fistulae, particularly those in anatomical locations such as the cavernous sinus. If transarterial embolization is incomplete, and it usually is, collateral supply will develop and symptoms may recur. Surgical therapy is difficult because of the tremendous blood flow into many of these lesions. There is a 15 per cent incidence of major morbidity and mortality for surgical therapy of nonembolized dural fistulae in the transverse and sigmoid sinuses, mostly related to massive blood loss.[111] However, in certain locations, such as the anterior cranial fossa, surgical treatment is preferred and is usually associated with little morbidity.[4, 84]

A contemporary concept in the treatment of dural arteriovenous fistulae and carotid cavernous fistulae includes a combination of transarterial embolization, transvenous embolization, and, if necessary, surgery.[4, 5, 47] This approach has resulted in improved outcomes in lesions that previously would have been very difficult to treat. In a series of 16 patients treated by combined therapy, all patients were either cured or improved, and there was no serious permanent morbidity.[47] This technique has also led to improved results in lesions previously considered untreatable, such as those in the deep cerebral venous system around the vein of Galen.[48]

Treatment of direct carotid cavernous fistulae may involve intentional or inadvertent occlusion of the parent carotid artery. This possibility must be considered before delivering embolic agents into the artery. Evaluation of collateral circulation, including the demonstration of patent anterior and posterior communicating arteries, allows the neurointerventionalist to make some prediction about the patient's tolerance of carotid occlusion. Traumatic injuries may affect more than one vessel, and these other lesions must be recognized before proceeding with treatment. If the patient lacks sufficient collateral circulation, the physician must be very cautious not to occlude the artery during treatment. The appropriate evaluation of patients before permanent carotid occlusion is complex and controversial. A variety of tests, including temporary balloon occlusion with pressure measurements and quantitative or qualitative cerebral blood flow measurements, may be used to predict a patient's tolerance to permanent occlusion.[26, 34, 54, 85, 86] These tests are probably of little value in the evaluation of direct carotid cavernous fistulae before treatment because the fistula, as a result of steal, acts as a test occlusion itself. Typically, preservation of the carotid artery is expected when one is treating direct carotid cavernous fistulae.

Dural Fistulae Involving the Transverse and Sigmoid Sinuses

The surgical treatment of dural fistulae involving the transverse and sigmoid sinuses has been well described. Sundt and Piepgras, in a series of 27 patients who had progressed during nonoperative management, performed surgery without embolization. They had an excellent outcome in 23 cases, poor outcome in 2 cases, and death in 2 cases.[111] An important observation concerning the surgical treatment of these lesions is the potential for tremendous hemorrhage. Rates of blood loss of up to 1 unit per minute have been documented.[111]

Ligation of feeding arteries to dural arteriovenous fistulae of the transverse and sigmoid sinuses, or elsewhere, has been abandoned.[74, 75] Development of collateral supply and recurrence of the fistula is a predictable consequence, and the subsequent therapeutic approach is, as a result, even more complicated.

Transarterial embolization of dural fistulae was the first major technical advance in the treatment of these lesions. The embolization technique involved superselective catheterization of feeding vessels, evaluation for collaterals to the intracerebral circulation, and functional testing with lidocaine. Embolic agents included mostly polyvinyl alcohol particles and isobutyl 2-cyanoacrylate. Among a series of 23 patients treated with transarterial embolization, 10 were cured and 6 improved by that percutaneous procedure alone.[42] A total of six patients went on to have surgical exposure of feeding vessels for embolization because of restricted percutaneous access. This therapy resulted in cure for four patients and improvement in two patients.

Complications documented with transarterial embolization of these fistulae include reflux of isobutyl 2-cyanoacrylate from a muscular branch into the vertebral artery with subsequent posterior cerebral artery stroke.[42] In another patient, glue went through the fistula and lodged in a vein draining the occipital lobe, leading to a venous infarct.

The transarterial embolization of these fistulae, regardless of the embolic agent used, usually results in a subtotal eradication of the fistula. In a series of four patients treated with transarterial embolization using liquid adhesives, all had subtotal closure of the fistula.[119] There were no complications from this therapy in this small series. Use of conjugated estrogens as an embolic agent resulted in little or no change in three of three patients so treated.[112] Polyvinyl alcohol particles, used to treat five patients with dural fistulae, resulted in complete obliteration in only one patient.[99]

The apparent inability of transarterial embolization to achieve a cure for dural fistulae led to other innovative techniques involving transvenous embolization (Fig. 63–10). The ultimate goal, to lodge embolic material into the fistula itself, can rarely be completed by the transarterial route because of complex and extensive collateral arterial supply to the nidus. The occlusion of dural fistulae by thrombosis from the venous side was developed as an alternative approach. The transvenous route often provides direct access to the fistula and may be used to deliver embolic materials.

Halbach and colleagues were the first to describe the percutaneous transvenous approach to lesions involving the transverse and sigmoid sinuses.[47] Transvenous embolization was performed using coils or glue in a series of 11 patients. Seven patients, treated initially by transarterial embolization to reduce flow, had surgical exposure of the sinus to facilitate the injection of coils or glue into the venous side of the fistula. Four patients were cured, and three had greater than 95 per cent closure of the fistula. The transfemoral approach for both arterial and venous embolization was used in four patients. One of these patients had a cure, there was a 95 per cent reduction in another, and two patients had a 50 per cent decrease in flow. There were only two complications, both temporary, in this series.

There are complications unique to the transvenous therapy.[47] Incomplete closure of the fistula with occlu-

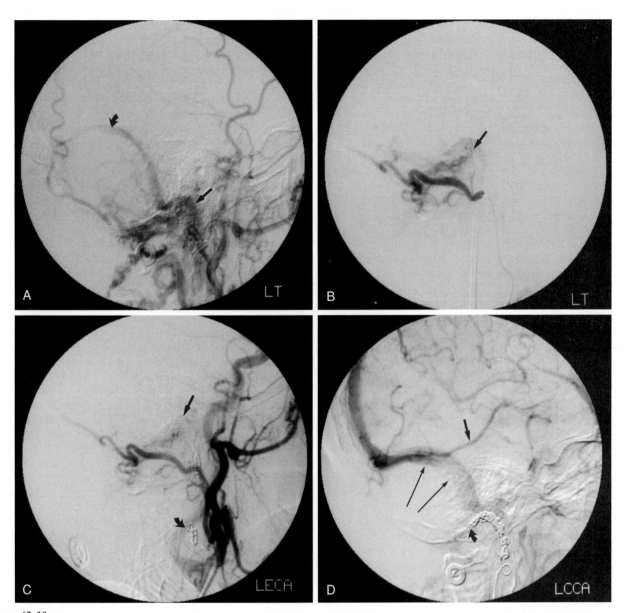

Figure 63–10

A 75-year-old woman with left base-of-skull dural arteriovenous fistula. The patient was treated with a combination of transarterial and transvenous embolization. *A.* Left external carotid artery angiogram, lateral projection, demonstrates dural arteriovenous fistula at the base of the skull (*straight arrow*) with supply from multiple external carotid artery branches. Venous drainage is retrograde in the transverse sinus (*curved arrow*) toward the torcula. *B.* Selective left occipital artery injection, lateral projection, demonstrates multiple small branches supplying the fistula (*arrow*). Eight separate arterial feeders supplying the fistula were embolized with a combination of polyvinyl alcohol particles and small platinum coils. *C.* Left external carotid artery angiogram, lateral projection, after transvenous and transarterial embolization. Coils (*straight arrow*) can be seen within the occluded segment of the sigmoid sinus and jugular bulb. There is no shunting of blood through the fistula. One coil (*curved arrow*) migrated into the jugular vein. *D.* Left common carotid artery angiogram, lateral projection, venous phase, demonstrates preservation of the left vein of Labbé (*short straight arrow*). Flow in the vein of Labbé was anterograde and therefore had to be preserved during the transvenous embolization of this fistula. The coils are placed in the low sigmoid sinus and jugular bulb region (*curved arrow*). Flow in the vein of Labbé is retrograde in the transverse sinus toward the torcula and then down the contralateral right transverse and sigmoid sinuses (*long thin arrows*).

sion of the venous outflow can result in diversion of flow into cortical veins, causing venous hypertension with bleeding or infarction. The placement of an adequate amount of the embolic agent into the fistula to promote thrombosis should prevent this problem. Migration of coils out of the vein may result in a pulmonary or cardiac embolus. The use of appropriately sized coils can prevent this complication. Finally, normal veins draining near the fistula must be preserved. Although this problem is not unique to the transvenous approach, if liquid adhesive agents enter normal veins, the occlusion can lead to a venous infarct.

Complex dural arteriovenous fistulae involving the transverse and sigmoid sinuses are probably most effectively treated with a combined approach using transarterial embolization, transvenous embolization, and surgery.[5] In one series of 11 patients with this type of lesion, 9 were cured, with complete fistula occlusion, and 2 had subtotal occlusion of the fistula.[5] Complications in two patients were related to occlusion of normal veins, and hydrocephalus occurred in a third patient. None of these complications led to a poor outcome.

Dural Arteriovenous Fistulae

SUPERIOR SAGITTAL SINUS

Superior sagittal sinus dural arteriovenous fistulae have been described but are rare. In a series of 65 patients with dural fistulae, the superior sagittal sinus was the site in 7 patients (11 per cent).[44] The cause of the fistula was unknown in four patients and was possibly related to traumatic skull fractures in three patients. Two patients presented with intracranial hemorrhage, one with a fixed neurological deficit, and four with headache. Bruit is an uncommon feature with these fistulae, perhaps because of their distance from the auditory apparatus, and was the presenting symptom in only one patient. The fistulae are most often located in the midportion of the sinus. The arterial supply to these lesions always includes the middle meningeal artery and occasionally involves the superficial temporal, occipital, or meningeal branches of the vertebral artery. The venous drainage is usually to the superior sagittal sinus, but if this sinus is thrombosed, either over a long segment or at the site of the fistula, drainage may be to cortical veins (Fig. 63–11).

Endovascular therapy for dural fistulae of the superior sagittal sinus has been described in eight patients.[44, 119] A transarterial approach using polyvinyl alcohol particles or isobutyl 2-cyanoacrylate was successful in closing the fistula completely in five of six patients. An operative exposure of the middle meningeal artery was necessary in one case.[44] Cases in which endovascular therapy alone was successful exhibited supply from dural vessels only, usually the middle meningeal artery. Arterial supply to the fistula from dural branches of the intracranial vessels makes the endovascular approach less likely to provide a cure.

The combination of transarterial embolization and surgical resection was curative in two of two cases.[44] The involved segment of sinus contains only arterialized, high-pressure blood. For this reason, it can be removed without fear of producing the venous hypertension that is often associated with the surgical resection of this sinus for other indications.[11]

TENTORIAL AND TORCULAR REGIONS

Dural arteriovenous fistulae occurring in the posterior fossa are most frequently in the straight sinus or torcula.* These lesions all drain into subarachnoid veins and have a high risk of hemorrhage, which is the usual presentation. The external carotid artery and the vertebral artery are the usual sources of the arterial branches that supply these generally small fistulae. Transarterial embolization alone is rarely curative but has been reported using particles.[118] A combination of preoperative transarterial embolization followed by surgical resection is the optimal approach and has been shown to be curative in a high percentage of cases (Fig. 63–12).[4, 5, 69, 97, 119]

BASE OF THE SKULL

A distinction must be made between dural arteriovenous fistulae of the base of the skull and foramen magnum and those of the inferior petrosal sinus.[32, 97] Lesions of the skull base and foramen frequently drain to subarachnoid veins and appear to have a risk of hemorrhage and poor prognosis. In the only reported case of a lesion treated by transarterial embolization alone, the patient died from a later hemorrhage.[97] Presumably, the embolization did not result in complete occlusion of the fistula, although complete details are not available. In the authors' experience with unpublished cases, these lesions are often benign or spontaneously thrombose (Fig. 63–13).

INFERIOR PETROSAL SINUS

Dural arteriovenous fistulae of the inferior petrosal sinus are uncommon. Among a series of 105 patients, there were 6 patients with lesions involving the inferior petrosal sinus, all of which were on the left side.[2] The typical presentation is similar to that seen in cavernous carotid fistulae, with bruit, proptosis, diplopia, and headache. The arterial supply is usually from the middle meningeal artery, ascending pharyngeal arteries, dural branches of cavernous internal carotid artery, or, occasionally, dural branches of the vertebral artery. The clinical features are a result of the venous drainage pattern, which most often runs superiorly into the cavernous sinus and superior ophthalmic vein.

There are six reported cases of inferior petrosal sinus fistulae treated by endovascular therapy.[2, 125] The

---

*See references 4, 5, 28, 69, 97, and 119.

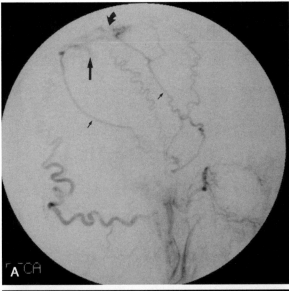

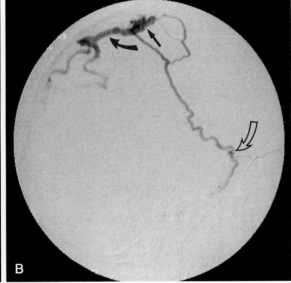

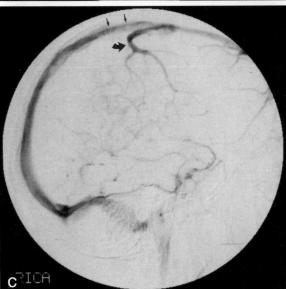

Figure 63–11

A 53-year-old man presenting with subarachnoid hemorrhage from a superior sagittal sinus dural arteriovenous fistula. *A.* Right external artery angiogram, lateral projection, demonstrates multiple hypertrophied middle meningeal artery branches (*small straight arrows*) that supply the dural fistula along the superior sagittal sinus (*curved arrow*). Venous drainage is through cortical subarachnoid veins (*large straight arrow*). *B.* Right middle meningeal artery (*open curved arrow*) angiogram, lateral projection, shows that this dural arteriovenous fistula is located within the wall of the superior sagittal sinus. There is a small collection of vessels, composing the nidus of the fistula (*straight arrow*), that drain to the cortical subarachnoid veins (*solid curved arrow*). *C.* Right internal carotid artery angiogram, lateral projection, venous phase, demonstrates that the superior sagittal sinus is patent at the site (*short arrows*) of the fistula. During treatment of this fistula, flow through the superior sagittal sinus and vein of Trolard (*curved arrow*) must be preserved. The approach to this fistula was preoperative transarterial embolization with polyvinyl alcohol particles and platinum coils, followed by surgical coagulation of the nidus and vessels in the wall of the superior sagittal sinus. The vein that drained the fistula was then ligated.

Figure 63–12

An 81-year-old man with tentorial dural arteriovenous fistula. Left external carotid artery angiogram, lateral projection, demonstrates hypertrophied occipital artery branches (*large straight arrows*) that supply the dural fistula located on the tentorium in the region of the straight sinus and torcula (*curved arrow*). The large dilated varices in the draining vein present a high risk of hemorrhage, which this patient had. This fistula is located in the wall of the straight sinus because there is anterograde flow in the straight sinus (*small straight arrows*). Flow through the involved sinus must be preserved because it is carrying blood in anterograde fashion.

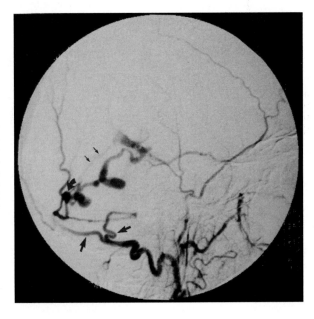

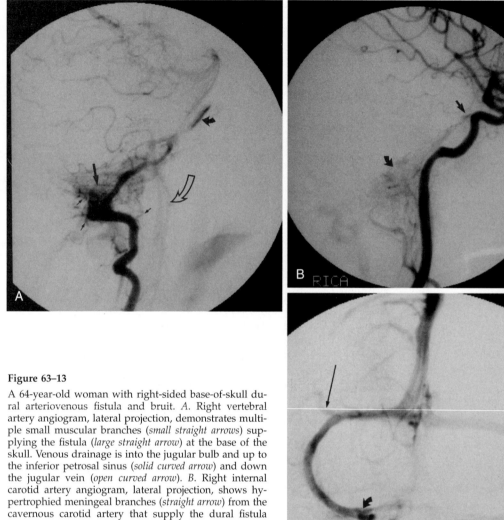

Figure 63–13

A 64-year-old woman with right-sided base-of-skull dural arteriovenous fistula and bruit. *A.* Right vertebral artery angiogram, lateral projection, demonstrates multiple small muscular branches (*small straight arrows*) supplying the fistula (*large straight arrow*) at the base of the skull. Venous drainage is into the jugular bulb and up to the inferior petrosal sinus (*solid curved arrow*) and down the jugular vein (*open curved arrow*). *B.* Right internal carotid artery angiogram, lateral projection, shows hypertrophied meningeal branches (*straight arrow*) from the cavernous carotid artery that supply the dural fistula (*curved arrow*). There is usually supply from the external carotid artery also. *C.* Right internal artery angiogram, anteroposterior projection, venous phase, shows that the sigmoid sinus and jugular bulb (*curved arrow*) are open and normal. The vein of Labbé (*straight arrow*) flows in an anterograde fashion. Such base-of-skull dural arteriovenous fistulae are usually benign lesions unless there is cortical venous drainage. This fistula thrombosed spontaneously.

transvenous approach is most valuable in achieving complete closure of the lesion. The fistulae may also drain into the ipsilateral jugular bulb, and this area can ordinarily be catheterized. Platinum coils have been shown to be successful in promoting thrombosis of fistulae if they are placed in the venous drainage pathway.[125] It is critical that flow not be diverted into the orbit during embolization of these lesions from the venous side. The embolic agents most widely used are silk suture and platinum coils. Although the pathway between the jugular bulb and the inferior petrosal sinus may not be evident angiographically, the small microcatheters and guide wires can often identify and traverse this connection. Even sinuses filled with clot may be entered with these catheter systems.

As previously indicated, numerous arterial feeders make complete closure of the fistula by the transarterial approach difficult. There are always numerous small arterial feeders, and occasionally the supply is bilateral. In addition, anastomoses between the ascending pharyngeal artery and the internal carotid or vertebral arteries may make transarterial embolization with liquid adhesives dangerous. Particulate embolic agents may not give a permanent result. However, transarterial embolization is helpful in slowing flow through the fistula and may ultimately result in complete thrombosis even if the fistula is not completely closed at the time of treatment.

The six patients treated by endovascular therapy all had clinical cure of the fistula with complete resolution of signs and symptoms after follow-up of 3 months to 5 years.[2, 125] Complete angiographic closure of the fistula at the time of treatment was seen in only one patient. The remaining five patients went on to develop clinical and angiographic cures within 8 weeks of undergoing the procedure.

Complications related to treatment included sinus thrombosis in two patients. One of these cases developed palsies of cranial nerves IX, X, and XII; the other case was asymptomatic.[2]

SUPERIOR PETROSAL SINUS

Of 150 patients with dural arteriovenous fistulae, 4 had lesions located in the region of the superior petrosal sinus[7] (Fig. 63–14). These patients included three men and one woman between the ages of 42 and 63 years. Two patients presented with disturbances of vision, one with headaches, and one with trigeminal neuralgia. All of these fistulae were located on the right side and were supplied by cavernous branches of the internal carotid artery, by the middle meningeal artery, and, occasionally, by dural branches of the vertebral artery. The venous drainage exhibited anomalies associated with a higher incidence of hemorrhage, including venous restrictive disease, varices, and sinus thrombosis. Lesions draining to the cavernous sinus presented with disturbances of vision.

The endovascular therapy for fistulae involving the superior petrosal sinus has been limited to preoperative transarterial embolization with polyvinyl alcohol particles. The supply from the middle meningeal artery may be safely treated, but embolizing the small branches off of the internal carotid and vertebral arteries is probably associated with a high risk. If combined with preoperative embolization, surgical treatment of

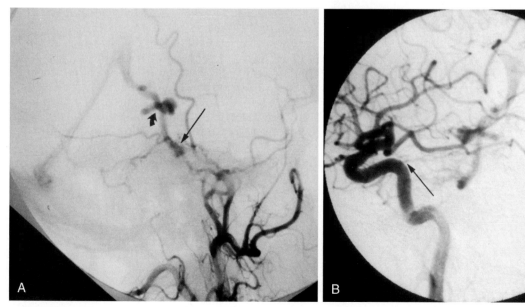

Figure 63–14

A 58-year-old man with dural arteriovenous fistula of the superior petrosal sinus who presented with a subarachnoid hemorrhage. *A.* Left external carotid artery angiogram, lateral projection, shows dural arteriovenous fistula in the region of the superior petrosal sinus (*straight arrow*). Venous drainage from such a fistula is almost always to veins in the posterior fossa (*curved arrow*). Surgical therapy must include occlusion of these veins. *B.* Left internal carotid artery angiogram, lateral projection, shows the same fistula and venous drainage supplied by meningeal branches (*arrow*) of the cavernous internal carotid artery.

the fistula by coagulation of the nidus and occlusion of the draining veins has been completely successful.

ANTERIOR CRANIAL FOSSA

Dural arteriovenous fistulae of the anterior cranial fossa or ethmoidal groove have usually been the subject of case reports, although two series of patients have been presented, and the subject has been reviewed.[50, 84] The presenting symptoms in more than 90 per cent of cases are related to hemorrhage. The second most common presentation is similar to that of cavernous carotid fistulae, with either diplopia or disturbances of vision. The arterial supply is almost always by way of ethmoidal branches of the ophthalmic artery (Fig. 63–15). Venous drainage is usually through cortical veins. These draining veins may be associated with pseudoaneurysms if the lesion has caused a hemorrhage. The lesions that present with findings of diplopia or decreased vision drain to the cavernous sinus.

The arterial supply to fistulae in this location is generally from ethmoidal branches of the ophthalmic artery.[50, 84] Branches of the anterior cerebral artery and the external carotid artery, particularly the internal maxillary, middle meningeal, and superficial temporal arteries, may also supply these fistulae. Attempts at obliteration of these fistulae with embolic materials, including the liquid adhesive isobutyl 2-cyanoacrylate, have been described but have not been successful.[119] Direct surgical approach and resection of fistulae in

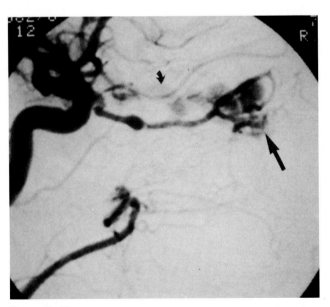

Figure 63–15

A 64-year-old man with dural arteriovenous fistula of the anterior cranial floor ethmoid groove. This patient presented with a subarachnoid hemorrhage. Right common carotid artery angiogram, lateral projection, demonstrates a dural arteriovenous fistula in the region of the ethmoidal groove (*straight arrow*). These fistulae virtually always drain to subarachnoid veins (*curved arrow*) and present with hemorrhage. The treatment involved coagulation of this draining vein.

this location is very successful and is the treatment of choice. Endovascular therapy, with a potentially high risk of occluding the central retinal artery, probably has no role in the treatment of these fistulae.

WALLS OF MAJOR DURAL SINUSES

A variant of dural arteriovenous fistulae has been described within the walls of major dural sinuses, including the superior sagittal, transverse, and straight sinuses (see Figs. 63–11 and 63–12). An unusual feature of these lesions is that the adjacent sinus is open and drains normal venous blood. From one series of 105 patients, this type of fistula was identified in 7 cases.[4] Fistulae in the walls of patent dural sinuses are associated with a higher frequency of hemorrhage or neurological dysfunction than most other dural fistulae. Arterial supply, although usually from the middle meningeal artery, may also be derived from the dural branches of the internal carotid and vertebral arteries. This type of fistula drains most commonly to cortical veins rather than to the adjacent sinus. This alternative drainage pattern may be a consequence of an acquired occlusion of the connection between the fistula and the sinus.

The endovascular approach to these lesions is limited by complexities in their arterial supply and venous drainage and is seldom curative.[4] Transarterial embolization would only be curative if the embolic agent could be lodged in the fistula itself, and the multitude of small arterial feeders makes this possibility remote. However, the treatment may be helpful in reducing blood supply to the fistula before surgical resection. Liquid adhesives have the major risk of penetrating through fistulae and occluding normal veins. The percutaneous transvenous approach is not possible because of cortical venous drainage, which is too circuitous for catheterization. Transarterial embolization, followed by direct surgical approach, is probably the safest and most efficacious treatment of these lesions. Exposure of the involved segment of the dural sinus allows the arterial inflow to be coagulated and the venous drainage to be occluded. This therapy decompresses veins draining onto the brain and prevents hemorrhage. The sinus should always be left intact.

MIDDLE FOSSA

A single report describes the endovascular therapy of a dural arteriovenous fistula of the middle fossa by the transarterial approach with subsequent surgical resection and cure.[119] Although this lesion was not fully described, it was apparently located outside the cavernous sinus. The embolic agent used was isobutyl 2-cyanoacrylate. Dural fistulae of the middle cranial fossa, outside of the cavernous sinus, are very rare (Fig. 63–16).

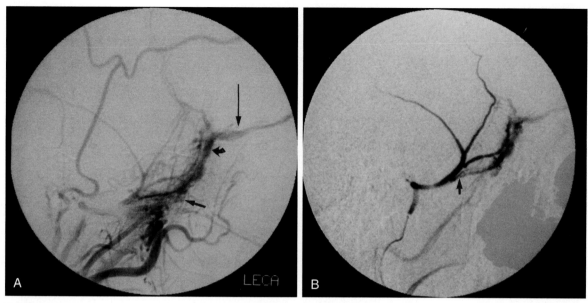

Figure 63–16

A 60-year-old man with middle fossa dural arteriovenous fistula. The patient presented with cavernous sinus syndrome. *A.* Left external carotid artery angiogram, lateral projection, demonstrates a dural arteriovenous fistula (*short straight arrow*) supplied by branches from the external carotid artery. The venous drainage is to the cavernous sinus (*curved arrow*) and up the superior ophthalmic vein (*long thin arrow*). The drainage out the superior ophthalmic vein accounts for the clinical symptoms. *B.* Selective left middle meningeal artery angiogram, lateral projection, shows that arterial supply to the fistula is from a small branch (*arrow*) of the middle meningeal artery. Selective injections are often useful for better defining the angioarchitecture of these lesions.

Multiple Dural Arteriovenous Fistulae of the Cranium

Bilateral cavernous sinus fistulae are a relatively common occurrence, but fistulae that occur at two separate sites are rare. Ten cases have been reported.[3, 70, 103] Among a series of 105 patients, multiple fistulae, other than bilateral cavernous sinus lesions, were found in 7 cases.[3] The clinical presentation and angiography findings in these cases suggest a higher risk of hemorrhage for multiple lesions than for single lesions because all of the patients presented with catastrophic hemorrhage or neurological deficits. The reasons for this worsened prognosis is not known. The angiography findings usually show cortical venous drainage, venous ectasias, and stenotic veins. Arterial supply is typically dependent on location. The therapeutic approach to multiple lesions involves directing treatment initially toward the symptomatic lesion. Treatment techniques are determined by the site of the fistula, the arterial supply, and venous drainage, as if the lesion were an isolated one.[3]

There is some concern that low-risk fistulae may progress to develop high-risk features. This possibility raises the question as to the indications for treatment of a second, incidentally discovered dural fistula. The indications for treatment of these fistulae are not well defined. The authors are not aware of any data supporting progression of low-risk to high-risk fistulae. It is known that some fistulae may spontaneously disappear, whereas others may progress to involve other sites.[9, 25, 52, 70] If there are risk factors for hemorrhage, such as collateral cortical venous drainage, disabling bruits or headaches, or neurological deficits related to

the fistula, the lesions should probably be treated as soon as possible. In the series in which multiple fistulae were found, only symptomatic lesions were treated.[3] If none of these risk factors is present, treatment is elective and may be determined by ease of therapy.

Direct Carotid Cavernous Fistulae

TRANSARTERIAL EMBOLIZATION

The transarterial route is the preferred approach for embolization of most direct carotid cavernous fistulae. A microcatheter, introduced through a guiding catheter in the internal carotid artery, is navigated to the level of the fistula. The most commonly used embolic agents are platinum coils and detachable balloons.* The agent is mechanically firm (wire coils, balloons, glue) or adheres to the wall of the cavernous sinus (silk suture) so that it does not flow out the cavernous sinus away from the fistula. The agent is introduced through the internal carotid artery fistula into the cavernous sinus and deposited in an attempt to occlude the fistula while maintaining the patency of the carotid artery.

There are three large series describing the treatment of direct carotid cavernous fistulae, primarily by transarterial embolization.[20] The goal of closure of the fistula with preservation of flow through the carotid artery was obtained in 59 to 88 per cent of the patients. In the remaining patients, the fistula was usually closed with occlusion of the internal carotid artery. The majority

---

*See references 20, 39, 72, 90, 123, and 125.

of complications were not serious and required no treatment. Pseudoaneurysm formation, from residual filling of the enlarged cavernous sinus, may occur in up to 44 per cent of cases, but often the aneurysm becomes smaller with time.[21] Oculomotor palsies also occur and probably relate to stretching of the cavernous sinus by the embolic agent, particularly if a balloon was used. Usually, these palsies resolve over a period of weeks to months. Stroke from the embolization procedure appears to be very uncommon. The patient is to a large degree protected because errant embolic agents or clots tend to enter the fistula and go to the vein rather than migrating into the cerebral vasculature. The incidence of stroke is approximately 2 to 4 per cent.[20, 55, 72]

There are several reports of endovascular therapy of direct carotid cavernous fistulae associated with persistent trigeminal artery.[19, 20, 37, 107] This arterial anomaly persists in fewer than 1 per cent of the adult population and has been associated with a variety of cerebrovascular abnormalities. Proper recognition of this entity may allow closure of the fistula with preservation of flow in both the basilar and carotid arteries.[19, 73]

TRANSVENOUS EMBOLIZATION

The femoral transvenous approach to direct carotid cavernous fistulae has been described.[43] This route is used if the transarterial approach has failed or is not possible. Such cases include traumatic occlusion of the proximal internal carotid artery or prior trapping procedures that did not cure the fistula. These techniques are further refinements of procedures that were described by Mullan, Manelfe and Berenstein, and Debrun and colleagues.[20, 83, 87, 95] The technique has largely depended on the development of steerable microcatheters. The introduction of balloons through the veins draining carotid cavernous fistulae is very difficult because of the multiple septations in these vascular structures. The embolic agents used in the transvenous approach typically are platinum coils. A variety of other agents have been used, including liquid adhesives, balloons, and silk suture, all of which led to thrombosis of the cavernous sinus and closure of the fistula.[20, 43, 55, 83, 87] In a report of 165 cases of direct carotid cavernous fistulae, 14 (8.5 per cent) were treated using the transvenous route.[43] In this series, 11 patients were cured and 1 patient was improved. There were two complications related to perforation of the inferior petrosal sinus or diversion of blood flow from the cavernous sinus to cortical veins, and in one of these cases, in a patient with Ehlers-Danlos syndrome, a fatal hemorrhage occurred. For selected cases, this approach is effective (Fig. 63–17).

Indirect Carotid Cavernous Fistulae

TRANSARTERIAL EMBOLIZATION

The treatment of indirect carotid cavernous fistulae by transarterial embolization was developed as an al-

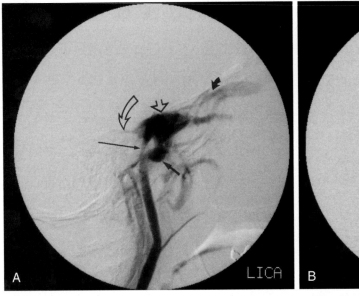
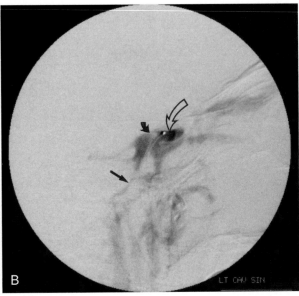

Figure 63–17

A 76-year-old woman with post-traumatic direct carotid cavernous fistula. *A.* Left internal carotid artery angiogram, lateral projection, demonstrates large, high-flow, direct carotid cavernous fistula with flow from the internal carotid artery (*short straight arrow*) to the cavernous sinus (*open straight arrow*) and then into the superior ophthalmic vein (*solid curved arrow*) and down the inferior petrosal sinus (*long thin arrow*) and superior petrosal sinus (*open curved arrow*). Typically, the transarterial route is efficacious at closing the hole in the artery while preserving flow through the artery. However, if the fistula cannot be entered through a transarterial route, the transvenous route may be used. *B.* Left internal carotid artery angiogram, lateral projection, by way of a catheter that has been introduced through the inferior petrosal sinus (*straight arrow*), through the cavernous sinus (*solid curved arrow*), and into the internal carotid artery (*open curved arrow*). The tip of the catheter is visible in the internal carotid artery. The transvenous route allows delivery of embolic agents to the outside of the artery with less risk of parent vessel occlusion in some cases. This same approach can be used for indirect dural carotid cavernous fistulae.

ternative to surgery.[10, 64, 81, 98] Early techniques involved unselective catheterization of the external carotid artery for embolization, but they have advanced to superselective catheterization of multiple vessels close to the fistula. The procedure involves superselective angiography to evaluate the vessels that supply the fistula, to identify the dangerous anastamoses between the external carotid artery and the internal carotid artery or vertebral artery, and to delineate the regional normal vessels not contributing to the lesion.[41] Embolization is performed with a variety of embolic agents, similar to those described for treatment of dural fistulae, with the principal objective of depositing these agents close to, or preferably within, the fistula. Proximal vessel occlusion commonly results in recurrence of the fistula and often makes subsequent treatment difficult because access is more troublesome.

The results of transarterial embolization for the treatment of indirect carotid cavernous fistulae have been good. In a series of 22 patients treated by transarterial embolization, a complete cure was obtained in 77 per cent, and clinical improvement was observed in 18 per cent.[41] Only one patient required surgical therapy. Nine of 10 patients in another series were cured by transarterial embolization.[118] In five of these patients, the clinical cure was not immediate but occurred within 6 months of the treatment. Debrun and co-workers described the results of transarterial embolization of carotid cavernous fistulae on the basis of arterial supply to the lesion.[8, 21] If the arterial supply was only from the external carotid artery (type C), the transarterial route was almost always successful in curing the problem. However, with type D fistulae, which have supply from the internal and external carotid arteries, the technical challenge was greater and fewer than 50 per cent of patients were cured by transarterial embolization. These poorer results were in part caused by the inability to catheterize the small branches arising from the cavernous internal carotid artery. The development of microcatheters that enable selective catheterization of these small cavernous internal carotid artery branches has improved the results of treatment of type D carotid cavernous fistulae.[45]

Cerebral ischemic complications are principally related to errant movement of the embolic agents into the cerebral circulation or clot formation on the catheter. A major source of this potential complication is lack of recognition of collaterals between the external carotid artery and the intracranial circulation. These anastomoses may occur at many sites. For example, the artery of the foramen rotundum may directly communicate between the distal internal maxillary artery and the internal carotid artery. Fortunately, these complications appear to be infrequent, although both of the large series mentioned had such complications.[41, 118] Angle-closure glaucoma caused by embolization of an indirect carotid cavernous fistula has been reported, probably as a result of thrombosis of the superior ophthalmic vein when the fistula was acutely closed.[33] Prompt recognition and management may prevent any permanent sequelae. Cranial nerve deficits may also occur

and are related to damage of the vascular supply to cranial nerves.[71]

TRANSVENOUS EMBOLIZATION

The treatment of choice for indirect, or dural, carotid cavernous fistulae is through a transvenous route. The many arterial feeders supplying these lesions make transarterial embolization less likely to succeed. Any residual arterial supply tends to enlarge, and the fistula reopens to the same degree as before treatment. The transvenous approach was proposed by Mullan in 1974 for direct carotid cavernous fistulae, based on his own work and that of Parkinson.[87, 94] The first report of a percutaneous approach to indirect carotid cavernous fistulae through the superior ophthalmic vein was by Courtheoux and colleagues in 1987.[16] They surgically exposed the superior ophthalmic vein and inserted a catheter into the vein to deliver wire coils and the sclerosing agent tetrasulfate. A complete closure of the fistula was obtained. Teng and associates described five patients with indirect carotid cavernous fistulae who were treated by direct percutaneous puncture of the superior ophthalmic vein and embolization with Gelfoam, liquid adhesives, or wire coils; all five were cured.[115] Monsein and colleagues described this technique in otherwise difficult cases of indirect carotid cavernous fistula, using balloon embolization of the cavernous sinus.[85] The superior ophthalmic vein approach may be complicated by a narrowing of the vein as it exits the superior orbital fissure.[51] If the vein is damaged, there can be retro-orbital hemorrhage. Occlusion of the superior ophthalmic vein can result in diversion of flow to cortical veins, with risk of intracranial hemorrhage.[38, 118]

The largest and most comprehensive series reporting on the transvenous approach comes from the group at the University of California, San Francisco.[46] They described the transvenous embolization of 13 patients with indirect carotid cavernous fistulae. The report is notable for describing femoral vein access to the inferior petrosal sinus as the preferred route of embolization of indirect carotid cavernous fistulae. Even in cases in which the inferior petrosal sinus could not be visualized, the route was successful. Twelve of the 13 patients were cured, and 1 patient improved. This approach is easier and has fewer risks than using the superior ophthalmic vein. There is a risk of rupturing the inferior petrosal sinus and causing a subarachnoid hemorrhage, but this appears to be an uncommon complication.[43]

The transvenous approach allows placement of a variety of embolic agents into the fistula to promote thrombosis, including steel or platinum coils, liquid adhesives, silk suture, or detachable balloons.[16, 46, 85, 114, 115] Balloons are used less frequently now because large catheters are required to deliver them and the veins must also be large.[46] Liquid adhesives have a higher risk of flowing out of the fistula and occluding the superior ophthalmic vein or other normal veins. Platinum coils, which can be delivered through micro-

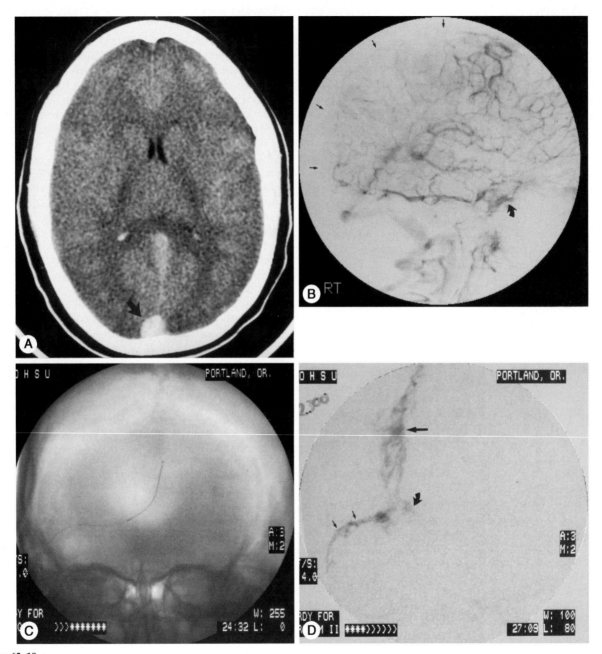

Figure 63–18

A 16-year-old girl with dural sinus thrombosis. *A.* Non–contrast-enhanced axial computed tomography demonstrates thrombus within the superior sagittal sinus (*arrow*). *B.* Right internal carotid artery angiogram, lateral projection, venous phase, demonstrates lack of filling of a superior sagittal sinus (*small straight arrows*). The venous drainage from the hemisphere is mostly anterior, toward the cavernous sinus (*curved arrow*). *C.* Skull radiograph showing the infusion catheter. The catheter has been placed transvenously through the right jugular vein and across the transverse sinus into the superior sagittal sinus for thrombolysis with urokinase. *D.* Superior sagittal sinus venogram, left anterior oblique projection, demonstrates partial reopening of the superior sagittal sinus (*large straight arrow*), torcula (*curved arrow*), and right transverse sinus (*small straight arrows*).

catheters in a controlled fashion, are now the most widely used embolic agent.[114]

There are several complications uniquely related to the transvenous approach, but they are uncommon. The most frequent and serious is diversion of flow to cortical veins or to the superior ophthalmic vein, which may result in hemorrhage, neurological deterioration, or loss of vision.[33, 43, 46, 53] Usually, these problems can be treated by additional therapy to close the fistula. For example, if the superior ophthalmic vein is acutely occluded and flow is diverted to cortical veins, the approach to the cavernous sinus through the inferior petrosal sinus may allow complete closure of the fistula. Not infrequently, after thrombosis of carotid cavernous fistulae, there is acute worsening of eye signs or symptoms, but this problem usually resolves without therapy. Occasionally angle-closure glaucoma may require cycloplegics, iridectomies, or lateral canthotomy.[33] Rupture of the inferior petrosal sinus, causing a subarachnoid hemorrhage, has been described in one case.[43]

Venous Sinus Thrombosis

Dural venous sinus thrombosis may occur in relation to trauma, tumor compression, or dural arteriovenous fistulae. It may also occur as a spontaneous event in patients with leukemia, coagulopathies, infection, or systemic illness, and even in seemingly normal individuals. The clinical spectrum may vary from asymptomatic patients to those with major neurological deficit and death.[6] The usual clinical findings include papilledema, headaches, seizures, and neurological deficit.[6] Computed tomography may identify hemorrhagic infarcts and the "delta sign," a low-density triangle within the torcula. Magnetic resonance imaging and angiography, particularly with directed venous imaging, is of value in the diagnosis. Cerebral angiography and dural venography, however, remain the optimal test for diagnosis and definition of the extent of occlusion.

The natural history of dural sinus thrombosis is difficult to define. Mortality rates range from 10 to 50 per cent, and this variation may reflect asymptomatic incidental thrombosis reported in some series. The rate of evolution of thrombosis, age, level of consciousness, and presence of cortical venous thrombosis have been suggested to be of prognostic significance, but this has not been substantiated in one large series.[12] Outcomes, also difficult to predict, vary from spontaneous recovery to rapid fatal progression. This variability makes comparison of treatment options impossible.

The medical therapy for sinus thrombosis is limited and is most relevant in treatment of the sequelae of the sinus occlusion. Mannitol, corticosteroids, and anticonvulsants are used when indicated. Systemic heparinization has been used and may have merit in preventing the propagation of the thrombus but does not have any therapeutic effect on opening the occluded sinus. The systemic fibrinolytic agents urokinase and streptokinase have been used with heparinization with favorable results but have been implicated in the development of major hemorrhagic complications.[6] Surgical thrombectomy has been described but has not gained wide acceptance. The benefit of selective sinus catheterization and local infusion of fibrinolytic agents into the dural sinus has also been described.[56] The authors prefer bolus infusion of urokinase followed by a continuous infusion, for up to several days, with an indwelling catheter until angiographic patency is identified (Fig. 63–18).

Summary

The clinical manifestations of carotid cavernous fistulae and dural arteriovenous fistulae, regardless of the type, depend on the pattern of venous drainage. The first step in determining treatment of dural arteriovenous fistulae is the angiographic analysis of the lesion. This step is done primarily to determine the venous drainage of the fistula in relation to the that of the brain. If cortical venous drainage is evident, the signs and symptoms may not be as apparent, but the risk of catastrophic hemorrhage is much higher. Many carotid cavernous fistulae, particularly indirect ones, may be managed in a conservative fashion. However, there are indications for urgent treatment to prevent a devastating hemorrhage or loss of vision. Direct carotid cavernous fistulae can usually be managed by transarterial embolization, most commonly with detachable balloons or platinum coils. The transvenous approach is most efficacious for treating indirect carotid cavernous fistulae. The treatment of dural arteriovenous fistulae may involve a combination of techniques, including endovascular and surgical procedures. The endovascular technique most likely to cure a fistula is occlusion of the vein or sinus that drains the fistula, with preservation of all veins or sinuses that drain normal venous blood from the brain. Frequently, a combined treatment of dural fistulae is most successful. Preoperative transarterial embolization is performed to slow flow through the fistula. Surgery can then be performed to remove the residual nidus or to provide access for occlusion of the draining vein by surgical occlusion or intraoperative embolization.

REFERENCES

1. Awad, I. A., Little, J. R., Akrawi, W. P., et al.: Intracranial dural arteriovenous malformations: Factors predisposing to an aggressive neurological course. J. Neurosurg., 72:839, 1990.
2. Barnwell, S. L., Halbach, V. V., Dowd, C. F., et al.: Dural arteriovenous fistulas involving the inferior petrosal sinus: Angiographic finding in six patients. A.J.N.R., 11:511, 1990.
3. Barnwell, S. L., Halbach, V. V., Dowd, C. F., et al.: Multiple dural arteriovenous fistulas of the cranium and spine. A.J.N.R., 12:441, 1991.
4. Barnwell, S. L., Halbach, V. V., Dowd, C. F., et al.: A variant of arteriovenous fistulas within the wall of dural sinuses. J. Neurosurg., 74:199, 1991.
5. Barnwell, S. L., Halbach, V. V., Higashida, R. T., et al.: Complex

dural arteriovenous fistulas: Results of combined endovascular and neurosurgical treatment in 16 patients. J. Neurosurg., 71:352, 1989.

6. Barnwell, S. L., Higashida, R. T., Halbach, V. V., et al.: Direct endovascular thrombolytic therapy for dural sinus thrombosis. Neurosurgery, 28:135, 1991.

7. Barnwell, S. L., and O'Neill, O. R.: Authors' unpublished data.

8. Barrow, D., Spector, R., Braun, I., et al.: Classification and treatment of spontaneous carotid-cavernous sinus fistulas. J. Neurosurg., 62:248, 1985.

9. Bitoh, S., and Sakaki, S.: Spontaneous cure of dural arteriovenous malformation in the posterior fossa. Surg. Neurol., 12:111, 1979.

10. Black, P., Uematsu, S., Perovic, M., et al.: Carotid-cavernous fistula: A controlled embolus technique for occlusion of fistula with preservation of carotid blood flow. Technical note. J. Neurosurg., 38:113, 1973.

11. Bonnol, J., and Brotchi, J.: Surgery of the superior sagittal sinus in parasagittal meningioma. J. Neurosurg., 48:935, 1978.

12. Bousser, M. G., Chiras, J., Bories, J., et al.: Cerebral venous thrombosis: A review of 38 cases. Stroke, 16:199, 1985.

13. Brothers, M. F., Kaufmann, J. C. E., Fox, A. J., et al.: N-Butyl 2-cyanoacrylate: Substitute for IBCA in interventional neuroradiology: Histopathologic and polymerization time studies. A.J.N.R., 10:777, 1989.

14. Castaigne, P., Bories, J., Brunet, P., et al.: Les fistules arterioveineuses meningees pures a drainage veineux cortical. Rev. Neurol. (Paris), 132:169, 1976.

15. Chaudhary, M. Y., Sachdev, V. P., Cho, S. H., et al.: Dural arteriovenous malformations of the major venous sinuses: An acquired lesion. A.J.N.R., 3:13, 1982.

16. Courthequx, P., Labbé, D., Hamel, C., et al.: Treatment of bilateral spontaneous dural carotid-cavernous fistulas by coils and sclerotherapy. J. Neurosurg., 66:468, 1987.

17. Cromwell, L. D., and Kerber, C. W.: Modification of cyanoacrylate for therapeutic embolization: Preliminary experience. A.J.R., 132:799, 1979.

18. Day, A. L., and Rhoton, A. L.: Aneurysms and arteriovenous fistulae of the intracavernous carotid artery and its branches. In Youmans, J. R., ed.: Neurological Surgery. 3rd ed. Philadelphia, W. B. Saunders, 1990, pp. 1807–1830.

19. Debrun, G., Davis, K., Nauta, H., et al.: Treatment of carotid cavernous fistulae or cavernous aneurysms associated with a persistent trigeminal artery: Report of three cases. A.J.N.R., 9:749, 1988.

20. Debrun, G., Lacour, P., Vinuela, F., et al.: Treatment of 54 traumatic carotid-cavernous fistulas. J. Neurosurg., 55:678, 1981.

21. Debrun, G., Vinuela, F., Fox, A., et al.: Indications for treatment and classification of 132 carotid-cavernous fistulas. Neurosurgery, 22:285, 1988.

22. Djindjian, R., Manelfe, C., and Picard, L.: Fistules arterio-veineuses carotide externe-sinus caverneux: Etude angiographique a propos de 6 observations et revue de la litterature. Neurochirurgie, 19:91, 1973.

23. Duckweiler, G., Dion, J., Vinuela, F., et al.: Intravascular microcatheter pressure monitoring: Experimental results and early clinical evaluation. A.J.N.R., 11:169, 1990.

24. Elster, A. D., Chen, M. Y. M., Richardson, D. N., et al.: Dilated intercavernous sinuses: MR sign of carotid-cavernous and carotid-dural fistulas. A.J.N.R., 12:641, 1991.

25. Endo, S., Koshu, K., and Suzuki, J.: Spontaneous regression of posterior fossa dural arteriovenous malformation. J. Neurosurg., 51:715, 1979.

26. Erba, S. M., Horton, J. A., Latchaw, R. E., et al.: Balloon test occlusion of the internal carotid artery with stable xenon/CT cerebral blood flow imaging. A.J.N.R., 9:533, 1988.

27. Eskridge, J. M., and Harling, R. P.: Preoperative embolization of brain AVMs using surgical silk and polyvinyl alcohol [Abstract]. A.J.N.R., 10:882, 1989.

28. Fardoun, R., Adam, Y., Mercier, P., et al.: Tentorial arteriovenous malformation presenting as an intracerebral hematoma. J. Neurosurg., 55:976, 1981.

29. Fournier, D., TerBrugge, K. G., Willinsky, R., et al.: Endovascular treatment of intracerebral arteriovenous malformations: Experience in 49 cases. J. Neurosurg., 75:228, 1991.

30. Fox, A. J., Pelz, D. M., and Lee, D. H.: Arteriovenous malformations of the brain: Recent results of endovascular therapy. Radiology, 177:51, 1990.

31. Fox, R., Pope, F., Narcisi, P., et al.: Spontaneous carotid cavernous fistula in Ehler-Danlos syndrome. J. Neurol. Neurosurg. Psychiatry, 51:984, 1988.

32. Gaensler, E. H., Jackson, D. E., and Halbach, V. V.: Arteriovenous fistulas of the cervicomedullary junction as a cause of myelopathy: Radiographic findings in two cases. A.J.N.R., 11:518, 1990.

33. Golnik, K., Newman, S., and Ferguson, R.: Angle-closure glaucoma consequent to embolization of dural cavernous sinus fistula. A.J.N.R., 112:1074, 1991.

34. Gonzalez, C. F., and Moret, J.: Balloon occlusion of the carotid artery prior to surgery for neck tumors. A.J.N.R., 11:649, 1990.

35. Graeb, D. A., and Dolman, C. L.: Radiological and pathological aspects of dural arteriovenous fistulas. J. Neurosurg., 64:962, 1986.

36. Grisoli, F., Vincentelli, F., Fuchs, S., et al.: Surgical treatment of tentorial arteriovenous malformations draining into the subarachnoid space. J. Neurosurg., 60:1059, 1984.

37. Guglielmi, G., Vinuela, F., Dion, J., et al.: Persistent primitive trigeminal artery-cavernous sinus fistulas: Report of two cases. Neurosurgery, 27:805, 1990.

38. Halbach, V. V., Hieshima, G. B., Higashida, R. T., et al.: Carotid cavernous fistulae: Indications for urgent treatment. A.J.N.R., 8:627, 1987.

39. Halbach, V., Higashida, R., Barnwell, S., et al.: Transarterial platinum coil embolization of carotid-cavernous fistulas. A.J.N.R., 12:429, 1991.

40. Halbach, V., Higashida, R., Dowd, C., et al.: Treatment of carotid-cavernous fistulas associated with Ehlers-Danlos syndrome. Neurosurgery, 26:1021, 1990.

41. Halbach, V., Higashida, R., Hieshima, G., et al.: Dural fistulas involving the cavernous sinus: Results of treatment in 30 patients. Radiology, 163:437, 1987.

42. Halbach, V. V., Higashida, R. T., Hieshima, G. B., et al.: Dural fistulas involving the transverse and sigmoid sinuses: Results of treatment in 28 patients. Radiology, 163:443, 1987.

43. Halbach, V., Higashida, R., Hieshima, G., et al.: Transvenous embolization of direct carotid cavernous fistulas. A.J.N.R., 9:741, 1988.

44. Halbach, V. V., Higashida, R. T., Hieshima, G. B., et al.: Treatment of dural arteriovenous malformations involving the superior sagittal sinus. A.J.N.R., 9:337, 1988.

45. Halbach, V., Higashida, R., Hieshima, G., et al.: Embolization of branches arising from the cavernous portion of the internal carotid artery. A.J.N.R., 10:143, 1989.

46. Halbach, V., Higashida, R., Hieshima, G., et al.: Transvenous embolization of dural fistulas involving the cavernous sinus. A.J.N.R., 10:377, 1989.

47. Halbach, V. V., Higashida, R. T., Hieshima, G. B., et al.: Transvenous embolization of dural fistulas involving the transverse and sigmoid sinuses. A.J.N.R., 10:385, 1989.

48. Halbach, V. V., Higashida, R. T., Hieshima, G. B., et al.: Treatment of dural fistulas involving the deep cerebral venous system. A.J.N.R., 10:393, 1989.

49. Halbach, V. V., Higashida, R. T., Hieshima, G. B., et al.: Venography and venous pressure monitoring in dural sinus meningiomas. A.J.N.R., 10:1209, 1989.

50. Halbach, V. V., Higashida, R. T., Hieshima, G. B., et al.: Dural arteriovenous fistulas supplied by ethmoidal arteries. Neurosurgery, 26:816, 1990.

51. Hanafee, W. N., Rosen, L., Weidnes, W., et al.: Venography of the cavernous sinus, orbital veins and the basal venous plexus. Radiology, 84:751, 1965.

52. Hansen, J. H., and Sogaard, I.: Spontaneous regression of an extra- and intracranial arteriovenous malformation: Case report. J. Neurosurg., 45:338, 1976.

53. Hashimoto, M., Yokota, A., Matsuoka, S., et al.: Central retinal vein occlusion after treatment of cavernous dural arteriovenous malformation. A.J.N.R., 10:S30, 1989.

54. Hays, R. J., Levinson, S. A., and Wylie, E. J.: Intraoperative measurement of carotid back pressure as a guide to operative management for carotid endarterectomy. Surgery, 72:953, 1972.

55. Higashida, R., Halbach, V., Tsai, F., et al.: Interventional neuro-vascular treatment of traumatic carotid and vertebral artery lesions: Results in 234 cases. A.J.R., *153*:577, 1989.

56. Higashida, R., Helmer, E., Halbach, V. V., et al.: Direct thrombo-lytic therapy for superior sagittal sinus thrombosis. A.J.N.R., *10*:54–56, 1989.

57. Higashida, R., Hieshima, G., Halbach, V., et al.: Closure of carotid cavernous sinus fistulae by external compression of the carotid artery and jugular vein. Acta. Radiol. Suppl., *369*:580, 1986.

58. Hiramatsu, K., Utsumi, S., Kyoi, K., et al.: Intracerebral hemor-rhage in carotid-cavernous fistula. Neuroradiology, *33*:67, 1991.

59. Horton, J. A., and Dawson, R. C.: Retinal Wada test. A.J.N.R., *9*:116, 1987.

60. Horton, J. A., and Kerber, C. W.: Lidocaine injection into exter-nal carotid branches: Provocative test to preserve cranial nerve function in therapeutic embolization. A.J.N.R., *7*:105, 1986.

61. Horton, J. A., Marano, G. D., Kerber, C. W., et al.: Polyvinyl alcohol foam-Gelfoam for therapeutic embolization: A syner-gistic mixture. A.J.N.R., *4*:143, 1983.

62. Houser, O. W., Baker, H. L., Jr., Rhoton, A. L., Jr., et al.: Intra-cranial dural arteriovenous malformations. Radiology, *105*:55, 1972.

63. Ishii, K., Goto, K., Ihara, K., et al.: High-risk dural arteriovenous fistulae of the transverse and sigmoid sinuses. A.J.N.R., *8*:1113, 1987.

64. Ishimori, S., Hattori, M., Shibata, Y., et al.: Treatment of carotid-cavernous fistula by Gelfoam embolization. J. Neurosurg., *27*:315, 1967.

65. Jack, C. R., Jr., Forbes, G., Dewanjee, M. K., et al.: Polyvinyl alcohol sponge for embolotherapy: Particle size and morphol-ogy. A.J.N.R., *6*:595, 1985.

66. Jorgenson, J. S., and Gutthoff, R. F.: Twenty-four cases of carotid cavernosus fistulas: Frequency, symptoms, diagnosis and treat-ment. Acta Ophthalmol., *63*(Suppl. 173):67, 1985.

67. Jungreis, C. A., and Horton, J. A.: Pressure changes in the arterial feeder to a cerebral AVM as a guide to monitoring therapeutic embolization. A.J.N.R., *10*:1057, 1989.

68. Jungreis, C. A., Horton, J. A., and Hecht, S. T.: Blood pressure changes in feeders to cerebral arteriovenous malformations dur-ing therapeutic embolization. A.J.N.R., *10*:575, 1989.

69. Kaech, D., Tribolet, N., and Lasjaunias, P.: Anterior inferior cerebellar artery aneurysm, carotid bifurcation aneurysm, and a dural arteriovenous malformation of the tentorium in the same patient. Neurosurgery, *21*:575, 1987.

70. Kataoka, K., and Taneda, M.: Angiographic disappearance of multiple dural arteriovenous malformations. J. Neurosurg., *60*:1275, 1984.

71. Keltner, J. L., Satterfield, D., Dublin, A. B., et al.: Dural and carotid cavernous sinus fistulas. Ophthalmology, *94*:1585, 1987.

72. Kendall, B.: Results of treatment of arteriovenous fistulae with the Debrun technique. A.J.N.R., *4*:405, 1983.

73. Kerber, W., and Manke, W.: Trigeminal artery to cavernous sinus fistula treated by balloon occlusion: Case report. J. Neurosurg., *58*:611, 1983.

74. Kosnik, E. J., Hunt, W. E., and Miller, C. A.: Dural arteriovenous malformations. J. Neurosurg., *40*:322, 1974.

75. Kihner, A., Krastel, A., and Stull, W.: Arteriovenous malforma-tions of the transverse dural sinus. J. Neurosurg., *45*:12, 1976.

76. Lach, B., Nair, S., Russell, N., et al.: Spontaneous carotid-cavern-ous fistula and multiple arterial dissections in type IV Ehlers-Danlos syndrome: Case report. J. Neurosurg., *66*:462, 1987.

77. Lanman, T. H., Martin, N. A., and Vinters, H. V.: The pathology of encephalic arteriovenous malformations treated by prior em-bolotherapy. Neuroradiology, *30*:1, 1988.

78. Lasjaunias, P., Berenstein, A., and Raybaud, C.: Intracranial venous system. *In* Lasjaunias, P., and Berenstein, A., eds.: Surgi-cal Neuroangiography. Vol. 3. Berlin, Springer-Verlag, 1990, pp. 223–296.

79. Lasjaunias, P., Chiu, M., Ter Brugge, K., et al.: Neurological manifestations of intracranial dural arteriovenous malforma-tions. J. Neurosurg., *64*:724, 1986.

80. Lister, J. R., and Sypert, G. W.: Traumatic false aneurysm and carotid-cavernous fistula: A complication of sphenoidectomy. Neurosurgery, *5*:473, 1979.

81. Mahaley, M. S., Jr., and Boone, S. C.: External carotid-cavernous fistula treated by arterial embolization: Case report. J. Neuro-surg., *40*:110, 1974.

82. Malik, G. M., Pearce, J. E., Ausman, J. I., et al.: Dural arteriove-nous malformations and intracranial hemorrhage. Neurosur-gery, *15*:332, 1984.

83. Manelfe, C., and Berenstein, A.: Treatment of carotid cavernous fistulas by venous approach. J. Neuroradiol., *7*:13, 1980.

84. Martin, N. A., King, W. A., Wilson, C. B., et al.: Management of dural arteriovenous malformations of the anterior cranial fossa. J. Neurosurg., *72*:692, 1990.

85. Monsein, L. H., Jeffery, P. J., Heerden, B. B., et al.: Assessing adequacy of collateral circulation during balloon test occlusion of the internal carotid artery with ^{99m}-Tc-HMPAO SPECT. A.J.N.R., *12*:1045, 1991.

86. Moody, E. B., Dawson, R. C., and Sandler, M. P.: ^{99m}Tc-HMPAO SPECT imaging in interventional neuroradiology: Validation of balloon test occlusion. A.J.N.R., *12*:1043, 1991.

87. Mullan, S.: Experiences with surgical thrombosis of intracranial berry aneurysms and carotid cavernous fistulas. J. Neurosurg., *41*:657, 1974.

88. Newton, T. H., and Cronqvist, S.: Involvement of the dural arteries in intracranial arteriovenous malformations. Radiology, *93*:1071, 1969.

89. Newton, H., and Hoyt, W.: Dural arteriovenous shunts in the region of the cavernous sinus. Neuroradiology, *1*:71, 1970.

90. Norman, D., Newton, T., Edwards, M., et al.: Carotid-cavernous fistula: Closure with detachable silicone balloons. Radiology, *149*:149, 1983.

91. Nukui, H., Shibasaki, T., Kaneko, M., et al.: Long-term observa-tions in cases with spontaneous carotid-cavernous fistulas. Surg. Neurol., *21*:543, 1984.

92. Obrador, S., Soto, M., and Silvela, J.: Clinical syndromes of arteriovenous malformations of the transverse-sigmoid sinus. J. Neurol. Neurosurg. Psychiatry, *38*:436, 1975.

93. Padayachee, T. S., Bingham, J. B., Graves, M. J., et al.: Dural sinus thrombosis: Diagnosis and follow-up by magnetic reso-nance angiography and imaging. Neuroradiology, *33*:165, 1991.

94. Parkinson, D.: Carotid cavernous fistula: Direct repair with preservation of the carotid artery. J. Neurosurg., *38*:99, 1973.

95. Parkinson, D.: A surgical approach to the cavernous portion of the carotid artery: Anatomical studies and case report. J. Neurosurg., *23*:474, 1965.

96. Pevsner, P. H., Klara, P., Doppman, J., et al.: Ethyl alcohol: Experimental agent for interventional therapy of neurovascular lesions. A.J.N.R., *4*:388, 1983.

97. Pierot, L., Chiras, J., Meder, J-F., et al.: Dural arteriovenous fistulas of the posterior fossa draining into subarachnoid veins. A.J.N.R., *13*:315, 1992.

98. Pugatch, R. D., and Wolpert, S. M.: Transfemoral embolization of an external carotid-cavernous fistula: Case report. J. Neuro-surg., *42*:94, 1975.

99. Quisling, R. G., Mickle, J. P., and Ballinger, W.: Small particle polyvinyl alcohol embolization of cranial lesions with minimal arteriolar-capillary barriers. Surg. Neurol., *25*:243, 1986.

100. Rao, V. R. K., Mandalam, K. R., Gupta, A. K., et al.: Dissolution of isobutyl 2-cyanoacrylate on long-term follow-up. A.J.N.R., *10*:135, 1989.

101. Repa, I., Moradian, G. P., Dehner, L. P., et al.: Mortalities associ-ated with use of a commercial suspension of polyvinyl alcohol. Radiology, *170*:395, 1989.

102. Rippe, D. J., Boyko, O. B., Spritzer, C. E., et al.: Demonstration of dural sinus occlusion by the use of MR angiography. A.J.N.R., *11*:199, 1990.

103. Sakaki, S., Fujita, J., Kohno, K., et al.: Dural arteriovenous mal-formation in the posterior fossa associated with intracerebellar hematoma: Case report. J. Neurosurg., *60*:1067, 1984.

104. Sanders, M. D., and Hoyt, W. F.: Hypoxic ocular sequelae of carotid-cavernous fistulae: Study of the causes of visual failure before and after neurosurgical treatment in a series of 25 cases. Br. J. Ophthalmol., *53*:82, 1969.

105. Schoolman, A., and Kepes, J.: Bilateral spontaneous carotid-cavernous fistulae in Ehlers-Danlos syndrome: Case report. J. Neurosurg., *26*:82, 1967.

106. Scialfa, G., and Scotti, G.: Superselective injection of polyvinyl

alcohol microemboli for the treatment of cerebral arteriovenous malformations. A.J.N.R., *6*:957, 1985.

107. Seeger, J., Gabrielsen, T., Gianotta, S., et al.: Carotid cavernous sinus fistulae and venous thrombosis. A.J.N.R., *1*:141, 1982.

108. Seidenwurm, D., Berenstein, A., Hyman, A., et al.: Vein of Galen malformation: Correlation of clinical presentation, arteriography, and MR imaging. A.J.N.R., *12*:347, 1991.

109. Spiegel, S. M., Vinuela, F., Goldwasser, M. J.: Adjusting polymerization time of isobutyl 2-cyanoacrylate. A.J.N.R., *7*:109, 1986.

110. Strother, C. M., Laravuso, R., Rappe, A., et al.: Glutaraldehyde cross-linked collagen (GAX): A new material for therapeutic embolization. A.J.N.R., *8*:509, 1987.

111. Sundt, T. M., Jr., and Piepgras, D. G.: The surgical approach to arteriovenous malformations of the lateral and sigmoid dural sinuses. J. Neurosurg., *59*:32, 1983.

112. Suzuki, J., and Komatsu, S.: New embolization method using estrogen for dural arteriovenous malformation and meningioma. Surg. Neurol., *16*:438, 1981.

113. Sze, G., Simmons, B., Krol, G., et al.: Dural sinus thrombosis: Verification with spin-echo techniques. A.J.N.R., *9*:679, 1988.

114. Taki, W., Yonekawa, Y., Iwata, H., et al.: A new liquid material for embolization of arteriovenous malformations. A.J.N.R., *11*:163, 1990.

115. Teng, M., Guo, W., Huang, C., et al.: Occlusion of arteriovenous malformations of the cavernous sinus via the superior ophthalmic vein. A.J.N.R., *9*:539, 1988.

116. Tsuruda, J. S., Shimakawa, A., Pelc, N. J., et al.: Dural sinus occlusion: Evaluation with phase-sensitive gradient-echo MR imaging. A.J.N.R., *12*:481, 1991.

117. Vinters, H. V., Lundie, M. J., and Kaufmann, J. C. E.: Long-term pathological follow-up of cerebral arteriovenous malformations treated by embolization with bucrylate. N. Engl. J. Med., *314*:477, 1986.

118. Vinuela, F., Fox, A., Debrun, G., et al.: Spontaneous carotid-cavernous fistulas: Clinical, radiological, and therapeutic considerations: Experience with 20 cases. J. Neurosurg., *60*:976, 1984.

119. Vinuela, F., Fox, A. J., Pelz, D. M., et al.: Unusual clinical manifestations of dural arteriovenous malformations. J. Neurosurg., *64*:554, 1986.

120. Wada, J., and Rasmussen, T.: Intracarotid injection of sodium amytal for the lateralization of cerebral speech dominance. J. Neurosurg., *17*:266, 1960.

121. Walker, A. E., and Allegre, G. E.: Carotid-cavernous fistulae. Surgery, *39*:411, 1956.

122. Wepsic, J. G., Pruett, R. C., and Tarlov, E.: Carotid-cavernous fistula due to extradural subtemporal retrogasserian rhizotomy: Case report. J. Neurosurg., *37*:498, 1972.

123. Wessbecher, F., Hartling, R., Nieves, M., et al.: Treatment of carotid cavernous fistulas: A new balloon delivery system. A.J.N.R., *13*:331, 1992.

124. Wilkins, R. H.: Natural history of intracranial vascular malformations: A review. Neurosurgery, *16*:421, 1985.

125. Yang, P. J., Halbach, V. V., Higashida, R. T., et al.: Platinum wire: A new transvascular embolic agent. A.J.N.R., *9*:547, 1988.

Aneurysms of the Vein of Galen

The vein of Galen is a centrally located, short venous structure formed by the confluence of the internal cerebral veins and the basal veins of Rosenthal. The vein of Galen passes posteriorly, emptying into the straight sinus at its junction with the inferior sagittal sinus. The structures drained by the vein of Galen include the thalamus, the medial temporal lobes, the occipital lobes, and the superior cerebellar vermis.

Aneurysms of the vein of Galen, also referred to as vein of Galen malformations, are rare lesions, accounting for only 1 per cent of all cerebral vascular malformations. This frequency has increased slightly over the last two decades with the introduction of more sensitive diagnostic tools, including computed tomography and magnetic resonance imaging.* In the truest sense, referring to these lesions as aneurysms or malformations is a misnomer. These "aneurysms" are a secondary effect of arteriovenous shunting through a fistula or drainage from a deep midline arteriovenous malformation that produces dilatation of the vein of Galen. In the majority of individuals, the clinical problems that develop with these lesions are not caused directly by the mass effect of the dilated vein of Galen but rather by the high flow through the shunt or shunts that are present.

Patients with vein of Galen aneurysms have traditionally been considered to have a bleak prognosis, with clinical manifestations that were difficult to treat.[30, 34, 38, 41, 46] However, the outlook for patients with these lesions has changed dramatically during the past decade.† Significant advancements have been made in understanding the pathophysiology associated with vein of Galen aneurysms, and improvements in both endovascular therapy and microneurosurgical techniques have contributed to a better outcome for these patients. However, significant morbidity and mortality remain associated with this diagnosis.

Historical Overview

Galen of Pergamum (129 to 199 AD) initially described a venous system at the base of the skull that was represented by one large venous sinus. This description was not obtained from humans and was therefore relevant only to lower animals. However, it served as the anatomical model for humans until the 1500's. Further anatomical dissections then revealed that this complex basal venous system actually comprises many separate structures, including the cavernous sinuses, the sphenoparietal sinuses, and the inferior and superior petrosal sinuses, as well as medial draining veins, such as the internal cerebral vein and the basal veins of Rosenthal, that drain into the vein of Galen and then into the straight sinus system.

It was not until 1895 that Steinheil first described a vein of Galen malformation and referred to it as a varix aneurysm.[67] This lesion subsequently became known as an aneurysm of the vein of Galen. In 1905, Ballance reported the use of bilateral carotid artery ligation to treat an infant with hydrocephalus; this child probably suffered from a vein of Galen aneurysm.[73] In 1937, Jaeger and colleagues provided the first thorough description of a patient with a vein of Galen aneurysm for whom treatment was attempted.[32] Oscherwitz and Davidoff described the first intracranial surgical approach to an aneurysm of the vein of Galen in 1947. This was followed in 1949 by the report from Boldrey and Miller detailing their treatment of a patient by exposure and clipping of the posterior cerebral arteries that supplied the galenic fistula.[6, 52]

Reviews and published analyses of patients with vein of Galen aneurysms include those of Hoffman

---

*See references 9 to 11, 16, 18, 30, and 34.
†See references 16, 18, 19, 34, 40, 47, and 71.

M. G. Hamilton • J. M. Herman • M. H. Khayata • R. F. Spetzler

and colleagues, who treated 29 patients at The Hospital For Sick Children in Toronto and reviewed an additional 128 patients, and of Johnston and associates, who described 13 patients and reviewed the reported experience of 232 others.[30, 34] Recent therapeutic advancements (modern neuroangiography, neuroendovascular treatment techniques, and modern microneurosurgery) have altered the management possibilities for these patients, and these innovations are the focus of most of this chapter.

Classification of Vein of Galen Aneurysms

Patients with vein of Galen aneurysms are a heterogeneous population that can generally be classified according to two criteria: the anatomy as seen on angiography, and the clinical presentation associated with the age at onset of signs and symptoms (Table 64–1). Each of these criteria provides information essential to management planning for these patients.

ANGIOGRAPHIC CLASSIFICATION

Lasjaunias proposed a simple anatomical classification system that differentiates "true" vein of Galen aneurysms (Yasargil types I to III) from the "secondary" vein of Galen dilatations caused by adjacent dural or parenchymatous arteriovenous malformation (Yasargil

Table 64–1

CLASSIFICATION SYSTEMS FOR VEIN OF GALEN ANEURYSMS

Clinical Classification
  Neonate: congestive heart failure, macrocephaly
  Infant: macrocephaly, seizures
  Neonates and young infants: mild congestive heart failure; macrocephaly
  Older child or adult: headache, hydrocephalus, subarachnoid hemorrhage, intraparenchymal hemorrhage, decreased cognitive function, progressive neurological deficit
  Spontaneous occlusion
Angiographic Classifications
  Lasjaunias*
    True vein of Galen aneurysms
      Mural type
      Choroidal type
    Secondary vein of Galen aneurysms
  Yasargil†
    Type I
    Type II
    Type III
    Type IV (secondary)
      Type IVA
      Type IVB
  Spetzler and Martin‡
    Relevant only to Yasargil type IV lesions (grade IV or V)

*See references 18, 37, and 40.
†See reference 73.
‡See references 24 and 63.

type IV).* The "true" vein of Galen aneurysms are classified into two subgroups based on the location of the fistula.[18] In mural vein of Galen aneurysms, the fistula is in the wall of the "prosencephalic vein" (see the section on embryology); the lesion is located most often in the inferolateral margin of the vein; and the malformation is typically supplied by collicular or posterior choroidal arteries (Fig. 64–1). In choroidal vein of Galen aneurysms, the fistula is seated in the cistern of the velum interpositum; the lesion is located in an extracerebral, subarachnoid position and communicates with the anterior aspect of the dorsal vein of the prosencephalon (see the section on embryology); and the malformation is typically fed bilaterally by choroidal arteries, the pericallosal arteries, and subependymal branches of the thalamoperforators (Fig. 64–2). Treatment difficulties and patient prognosis are linked to the type of malformation that is present.

Litvak and colleagues, and later Yasargil, classified vein of Galen aneurysms into four subgroups (types I through IV) that depend primarily on the location of the fistula.[41, 73] The type I vein of Galen aneurysm is a pure cisternal fistula between single or multiple pericallosal arteries and posterior cerebral arteries and the vein of Galen, with the actual nidus of the lesion represented by the ampulla of the vein of Galen (see Fig. 64–1). Type II aneurysms are fistulous connections between the thalamoperforators (basilar and first segment of posterior cerebral artery) and the vein of Galen. Type III aneurysms constitute a mixed form of type I and type II and represent the most common subtype of vein of Galen aneurysms. In type III lesions, pericallosal branches, branches of the posterior cerebral artery, and basilar and thalamoperforators form fistulous communications with the vein of Galen (see Fig. 64–2).

These first three lesion types have no intraparenchymal component and are synonymous with Lasjaunias' "true" aneurysm of the vein of Galen. The nidus is the fistulous connection of the vein of Galen, with no other nidus proximal to the vein of Galen. The type IV aneurysm is a true plexiform type of arteriovenous malformation, with one or more arteriovenous malformation nidi located within the mesencephalon or thalamus. Drainage is usually to an internal cerebral vein, medial atrial vein, or basilar vein. Two subgroups of the fourth type of malformation have also been described: type IVA is a pure plexiform malformation located in the parenchyma, and type IVB has a nidus within the parenchyma combined with a fistulous cisternal nidus.

Spetzler and Martin proposed a grading system to help establish treatment risk for cerebral arteriovenous malformations.[24, 63] This simple grading system assigns points based on three aspects of anatomy as seen on angiography: arteriovenous malformation size, presence or absence of deep (galenic) venous drainage, and whether the arteriovenous malformation is located in eloquent brain. The summation of the assigned points identifies whether the arteriovenous malformation is a grade I, II, III, IV, or V lesion. The treatment risk for

*See references 18, 35, 37, 38, 39, and 40.

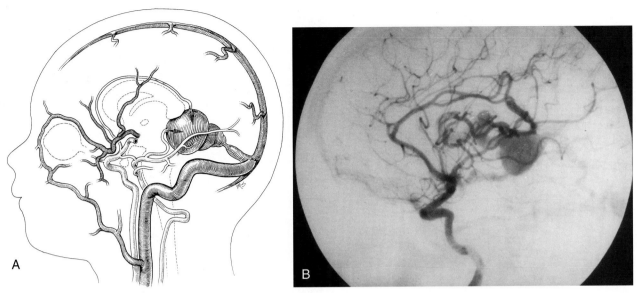

Figure 64–1

A. Diagram depicts a Yasargil type I direct arteriovenous fistula with vein of Galen aneurysm. The arterial connections are between a pericallosal artery branch or posterior cerebral artery branch and the vein of Galen. Notice the stenosis of the straight sinus. *B.* Lateral carotid artery angiography demonstrates Yasargil type I vein of Galen aneurysm with single fistulous connection. (*A* from Khayata, M. H., Casasco, A., Wakhloo, A. K., et al.: Vein of Galen malformations: Intravascular techniques. *In* Carter, L. P., Spetzler, R. F., and Hamilton, M. G., eds.: Neurovascular Surgery. New York, McGraw-Hill, Inc., 1994. Reprinted by permission.)

lesions of grades I through III is minimal, but the treatment risk for grade IV or V arteriovenous malformations approaches 20 per cent.[24, 63] Based on the Spetzler-Martin grading system, even a simple vein of Galen malformation would receive two points for size, one point for deep venous drainage, and one point for location in eloquent brain (minimum grade IV).

Because vein of Galen aneurysms are unique in character with respect to other cerebral arteriovenous malformations, the authors recommend that they be classified according to either the Lasjaunias or the Yasargil scheme.[18, 73] The Yasargil classification scheme provides more information about the vascular anatomy of the vein of Galen aneurysm than is possible with the Lasjaunias scheme and is therefore preferred by the authors. Yasargil type IV (Lasjaunias "secondary") lesions are true arteriovenous malformations and can also be effectively graded according to the Spetzler-Martin system (grade IV or V). This chapter focuses mainly on the Yasargil types I through III (Lasjaunias "true") vein of Galen aneurysms.

CLINICAL CLASSIFICATION

Patients with a vein of Galen aneurysm have clinical presentations that typically vary with the age at onset. In 1964, Gold and colleagues provided a clinical classification scheme that remains essentially valid today.[21] Their observations were based on only 34 patients who had been reported in the world literature and involved the correlation of three features: age at presentation, clinical syndrome, and pathophysiology. Three characteristic groups were identified: (1) the neonate presenting with severe congestive heart failure; (2) the

infant presenting with hydrocephalus or seizures; and (3) the older child or adult presenting with headaches or subarachnoid hemorrhage.

In 1973, Amacher and Shillito added another group to this classification system: neonates and young infants presenting with mild congestive heart failure and macrocephaly.[2] In 1990, a fifth clinical group was proposed by Wisoff and associates: patients of all ages with vein of Galen aneurysms that have spontaneously thrombosed.[5, 15, 71]

These clinical groups tend to correlate with specific angiographic patterns.[30, 71, 73] The basis for most clinical symptoms is not the mass effect produced by the aneurysm of the vein of Galen but rather the shunting of blood through the fistula, which produces either cerebral or coronary artery "steal."

Neonate. Newborns with a vein of Galen aneurysm tend to present with congestive heart failure.[1, 8, 12, 19, 29] About 40 per cent of patients with vein of Galen aneurysms are diagnosed during the neonatal period. Neonates presenting with congestive heart failure typically have multiple fistulae, and more than 25 per cent of their cardiac output is shunted through the fistulae. Angiographically, these can be Yasargil type I, II, or III vein of Galen aneurysms, although the type III pattern is more common.[30, 73] These neonates are gravely ill with severe myocardial and cerebral ischemia and can only rarely be successfully managed medically.

The vein of Galen aneurysm produces congestive heart failure (hypoxia, low cardiac output, tachycardia, pulmonary edema) that typically causes cyanosis and is refractory to medical therapy. Although the arteriovenous shunt develops in utero, it does not manifest with severe heart failure until after the child has been delivered because of the protective aspects afforded

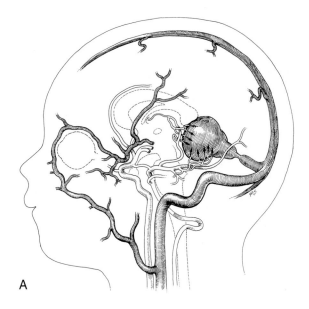

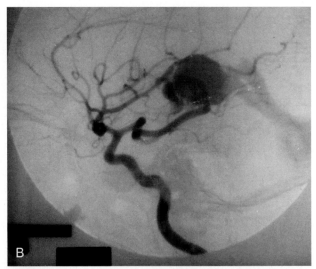

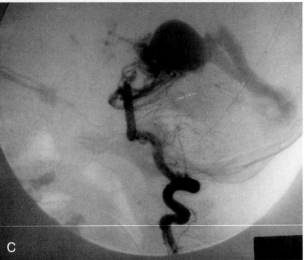

Figure 64–2

A. Yasargil type III vein of Galen aneurysm with multiple fistulae between the choroidals and the vein of Galen. This lesion can also be referred to as a "choroidal" type vein of Galen aneurysm. *B.* Lateral carotid artery angiography demonstrates arterial feeders supplying a Yasargil type III vein of Galen aneurysm. Notice the duplicated straight sinus. *C.* Lateral vertebral artery angiography of same patient as in *B* depicts the thalamoperforators supplying the aneurysm. (*A* from Khayata, M. H., Casasco, A., Wakhloo, A. K., et al.: Vein of Galen malformations: Intravascular techniques. *In* Carter, L. P., Spetzler, R. F., and Hamilton, M. G., eds.: Neurovascular Surgery. New York, McGraw-Hill, Inc., 1994. Reprinted by permission.)

by the significant hemodynamic differences that exist between the fetal and the neonatal circulations.[29] While in utero, the placenta receives about 40 per cent of fetal cardiac output, thereby reducing the absolute volume of the shunt. In addition, the circulatory overload is shared between two ventricles that function in parallel rather than in series.

In the neonate, the entire circulation is generated by each ventricle in series. With the loss of the placental bed and changes in pulmonary capillary bed resistance, compensatory increases in cardiac output and blood volume occur to maintain perfusion of the systemic vascular bed distal to the shunt. Pulmonary hypertension develops and maintains patency of the ductus arteriosus, producing right-to-left shunting and cyanosis.[11, 29] Coronary artery perfusion, reduced because the high cardiac output occurs in the presence of high cardiac ventricular pressures, produces myocardial ischemia and infarction. Untreated cardiac failure is a major cause of mortality and morbidity in this patient population.

In addition to producing severe congestive heart failure and myocardial ischemia, this rapid shunting through fistula emptying into the vein of Galen aneurysm is associated with cerebral steal, which produces cerebral venous hypertension, cerebral ischemia, and cerebral infarction.[29] Untreated cerebral damage may be manifested as atrophy and dystrophic calcifications in the cerebral parenchyma.

Infant. Infants presenting with a vein of Galen aneurysm typically have a smaller shunt than that of presenting neonates, and patients in this age group develop hydrocephalus or seizures. Frequently, the shunt consists of only one fistulous connection (Yasargil type I).

Head enlargement in infants can be caused by ventricular dilatation in the presence of a distensible skull.[13, 59] Previous assumptions that the ventriculomegaly was caused by obstructive hydrocephalus from compression of the aqueduct of Sylvius by the dilated vein of Galen have been challenged by pathological observation and by magnetic resonance imaging studies that have revealed the aqueduct to be patent in many of these patients.[4, 74] The fontanelle is full but seldom tense. Overt signs of increased intracranial pressure (e.g., lethargy, nausea, vomiting, decreased upward gaze) are rarely present. It now seems likely that ventriculomegaly in children with vein of Galen aneurysm results from increased pressure in the sagittal sinus or venous system that affects cerebrospinal fluid absorption.* There typically is no periventricular edema present on computed tomography or magnetic resonance imaging.

The volume of the cerebral ventricles is a dynamically regulated dimension that depends on the pressures within the cerebrospinal fluid–containing spaces, the anatomy of these spaces, the physics of the outflow pathways between compartments, and the pressures within these compartments.[51, 58] Although increased sagittal sinus pressure leads to pseudotumor cerebri in adults with nondistensible heads, it produces hydrocephalus in infants who have not yet undergone fusion of their sutures.[58] For cerebral spinal fluid to be absorbed, there must be a pressure difference of 5 to 7 mm Hg between the cerebrospinal fluid pathway (cortical subarachnoid space) and the sagittal sinus.[51, 57, 59] In the situation of a vein of Galen aneurysm in a neonate or infant, a number of variables can cause the ventricles to enlarge because intracranial pressure is, to some extent, open to atmospheric pressure: (1) sagittal sinus pressure is elevated; (2) there is an effective venous resistor; and (3) the fontanelle is open. Hydrocephalus from high venous pressure has been documented in craniosynostosis and achondroplasia.[61, 66] The macrocephaly and ventriculomegaly resolve without placement of a ventriculoperitoneal shunt if sagittal sinus pressure returns to normal after endovascular treatment.[3, 37, 74]

Seizures can also be a significant mode of presentation in this age group. Seizures are thought to represent the effects of the prolonged arteriovenous shunting on the cerebral parenchyma. This shunting, or steal, can produce ischemia, cerebral infarction, and deep striated calcifications. These dystrophic changes are irreversible and are a sign of untreated venous hypertension.[37] In addition, the cerebral injury that these calcifications represent predisposes the patient to the development of seizures.

Finally, the infant's developmental profile and cognitive abilities should be determined and followed. The number of children who present with cognitive difficulties (as expressed by decline in school performance) or who demonstrate loss of developmental milestones has probably been underappreciated.[71] The Minnesota Development Profile permits the child's progress to be followed. If this developmental profile deteriorates, urgent treatment may be required.

Neonate and Young Infant. This clinical category, established by Amacher and Shillito, includes those neonates with mild congestive heart failure (which is usually easy to control) and accelerated head growth starting at 1 to 6 months of age.[2] These children typically have fistulae that are intermediate in number between those of the neonate presenting with severe congestive heart failure and those of the infant presenting with head enlargement. The pathophysiology is, however, the same for children with this intermediate type of clinical presentation.

*See references 4, 14, 31, 33, 51, 61, 66, and 74.

Older Child or Adult. Children and adults with aneurysm of the vein of Galen usually present with subarachnoid hemorrhage, intracerebral hemorrhage, headaches, or cognitive dysfunction (e.g., decline in school performance). Less often, these patients present with hydrocephalus; they rarely present with congestive heart failure. As expected, these patients have a fistula with low flow, or they may have a Yasargil type IV vein of Galen aneurysm ("secondary" to a true cerebral arteriovenous malformation).

Embryology

The "true" vein of Galen aneurysm is a midline venous sac with direct arteriovenous fistulae located within its wall. The arterial feeders are typically bilateral and belong to the anterior and posterior arterial systems. This vascular pattern does not fit the anatomical relations of a normal vein of Galen. An explanation for the development of a vein of Galen aneurysm can be found by examining the precursor of the vein of Galen, a midline venous drainage system that drains the choroid plexus called the median prosencephalic vein of Markowski.[56] By about 3 months of development, the posterior part of this vein joins with the internal cerebral veins to form the vein of Galen; the remaining anterior part of the vein attenuates and finally disappears.[56]

According to Raybaud's hypothesis, the arterial pattern of the feeders of a vein of Galen aneurysm corresponds to those of the transient embryonic median prosencephalic vein of Markowski, a pattern that is reached by the sixth week of development but disappears when the prosencephalic vein changes at 11 weeks. Therefore, it has been inferred that a "true" vein of Galen aneurysm is the result of an insult of unknown mechanism that occurs between 6 and 11 weeks of development.[56] The fistulae of the vein of Galen aneurysm develop between pial arteries and an overlying arachnoid venous structure, with the resulting malformation being located totally extracerebrally.

Diagnosis

CLINICAL FEATURES

The clinical diagnostic features associated with a vein of Galen aneurysm depend on the age at which the patient initially presents (see the section on clinical classification). A child with heart failure, enlarging head, dilation of the orbital veins, and loud continuous intracranial bruit may harbor a vein of Galen aneurysm. At later ages patients can present with seizures, headaches, cognitive dysfunction, symptoms related to raised intracranial pressure secondary to hydrocephalus, or symptoms related to subarachnoid hemorrhage (e.g., headache, loss of consciousness, seizure) or intraparenchymal hemorrhage (e.g., headache, loss of consciousness, hemiparesis or hemiplegia). There are no pathognomonic clinical features for this disorder. Instead, the protean manifestations outlined above, placed in the proper context, can trigger an elevated index of suspicion for this disorder and prompt a series of investigations to establish the diagnosis.

Another clinical scenario occurs if the diagnosis of a vein of Galen aneurysm is established prenatally.[44, 62, 72, 74] Five of 43 patients in the series reported by Zerah and colleagues were diagnosed prenatally.[74] Sanders reported the prenatal diagnosis of a vein of Galen aneurysm with ultrasound, and prenatal diagnosis with magnetic resonance imaging has been reported by Yamashita and by Martinez-Lage and their co-workers.[44, 62, 72] An advantage of prenatal diagnosis lies in the opportunity it provides to plan the delivery of the baby in a medical center where immediate, definitive care can be administered.

DIAGNOSTIC INVESTIGATIONS

The investigation of a patient with a suspected vein of Galen aneurysm can be divided into three basic categories: imaging of the brain, imaging of the cerebral vasculature, and other investigations to assess the systemic effects associated with the vein of Galen aneurysm.

Brain Imaging. Cranial ultrasound can demonstrate the abnormality and may establish the diagnosis in many neonates. However, computed tomography (Fig. 64–3) and magnetic resonance imaging (Fig. 64–4) are

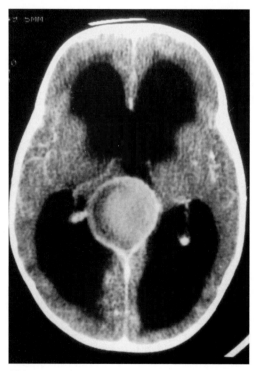

Figure 64–3

Axial computed tomography of patient with thrombosed vein of Galen aneurysm.

the two "gold standard" investigations for establishing the diagnosis of a vein of Galen aneurysm and documenting the presence of associated hydrocephalus. The computed tomography examination is significantly enhanced by the use of a contrast agent. Compared with computed tomography, magnetic resonance imaging provides superior information concerning the vein of Galen aneurysm and its effect on the surrounding brain. Magnetic resonance imaging is more sensitive than computed tomography for demonstrating ischemic changes in the brain parenchyma. In addition, standard magnetic resonance imaging also provides information concerning the patency and size of large arteries, veins, and venous sinuses.

Cerebral Vasculature Imaging. Delineation of the cerebral vasculature is essential after the diagnosis of a vein of Galen aneurysm has been established by computed tomography or magnetic resonance imaging. The "gold standard" investigation in this category is cerebral angiography (see Figs. 64–1 and 64–2), which confirms the diagnosis and provides the details of the vascular anatomy that are essential for treatment planning. Other investigations can be performed to assess the cerebral vasculature, including magnetic resonance angiography (Fig. 64–5), magnetic resonance venography (see Fig. 64–5), and Doppler ultrasound.[70] Although these latter diagnostic modalities are interesting, none approaches the value provided by high-quality cerebral angiography.[54, 55]

Arterial feeders into a vein of Galen aneurysm can be single or multiple. The feeders typically originate from pericallosal branches from the anterior cerebral artery as well as from posterior pericallosal, medial choroidal, lateral choroidal, and subventricular arteries from the posterior cerebral artery.[30, 34, 42, 73]

The arterial feeders come from vessels of two different embryological origins: one has prosencephalic origins, and the other has a mesencephalic origin. The first group includes the anterior cerebral artery, the posterior pericallosal artery, and the posterior lateral choroidal artery. The group with a mesencephalic origin includes the posterior medial choroidal artery, the thalamoperforators, and the superior cerebellar artery. Other arterial pedicles can feed these malformations, including lenticulostriate and sylvian branches.

The venous drainage in a vein of Galen aneurysm is usually through the straight sinus, which is frequently duplicated, into the lateral and sigmoid sinuses and, from there, on to the jugular bulb. According to Lasjaunias and associates, careful examination of the venous drainage system in cases of ventricular enlargement almost always reveals a point of narrowing or of relative stenosis in the outflow tracts[37, 38, 43] (see Figs. 64–1, 64–2, 64–4, and 64–5). This stenotic area produces vascular congestion, forcing the venous blood to find alternate drainage routes. Ideally, a viable alternate pathway would be in an anterior direction into the cavernous sinus, through to the pterygoid venous plexus. Developmentally, however, the cavernous sinus is not patent or fully formed until the infant is between 1 and 2 years old. Therefore, venous blood drains into the orbital veins and into the sphenoparietal sinuses

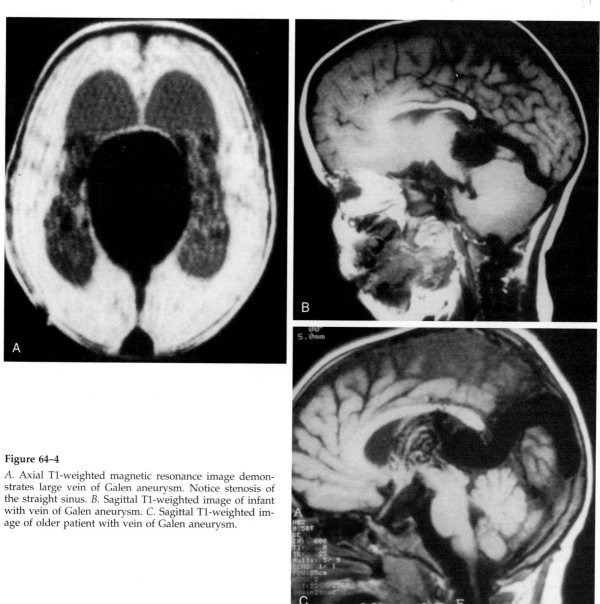

Figure 64–4

A. Axial T1-weighted magnetic resonance image demonstrates large vein of Galen aneurysm. Notice stenosis of the straight sinus. *B.* Sagittal T1-weighted image of infant with vein of Galen aneurysm. *C.* Sagittal T1-weighted image of older patient with vein of Galen aneurysm.

and middle cerebral veins. The orbital veins dilate and are clearly visible on clinical examination of these infants. Venous hypertension may be the pathophysiological event leading to cerebral ischemia and infarction, which produces deep cerebral calcifications.

Hoffman and colleagues described the anatomy of vein of Galen aneurysms on angiography and identified age-dependent differences that they categorized into the following four subgroups.[30]

In neonates, the feeding vessels entered the vein of Galen at its anterosuperior border. These vessels usually included both anterior cerebral arteries, the lenticulostriate arteries, the thalamoperforating arteries, both anterior and posterior choroidal arteries, and, less often, the superior cerebellar arteries. The vein of Galen aneurysms in this patient group were described as being of moderate size and draining into a large straight sinus and lateral sinuses. This description of multiple feeding arteries and multiple fistulae corres-

ponds to the usual neonatal clinical scenario of high-output cardiac failure because of the high shunt fraction through the aneurysm.

In infants, the major feeding vessels (often only one posterior choroidal artery) often entered inferiorly and laterally on the vein of Galen. This description of a single fistula or small number of fistulae corresponds with the clinical findings already outlined for infants with a vein of Galen aneurysm.

In infants and older children, the feeding vessels (typically one or both posterior choroidal arteries and one or both anterior cerebral arteries) usually entered the vein of Galen anteriorly and superiorly. In older children, the feeding vessels consisted of an angiomatous network (posterior choroidal arteries and thalamoperforating arteries) that entered directly into the vein of Galen, which was moderate in size. Again, the angiography patterns in these latter two groups correspond to the clinical situation seen in this age group.

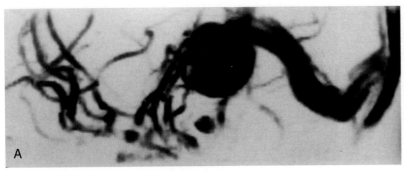

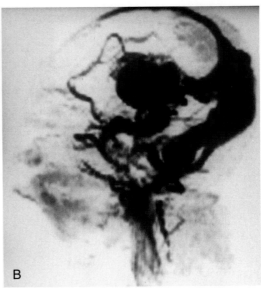

Figure 64–5

A. Magnetic resonance angiography depicts large vein of Galen aneurysm and its arterial input (lateral view). *B.* Magnetic resonance venography demonstrates the vein of Galen aneurysm and its venous drainage (lateral view).

Other Investigations. The investigations in this category are designed to assess the systemic abnormalities associated with vein of Galen aneurysm, such as congestive heart failure, pulmonary hypertension, and renal failure. They include studies of arterial blood gases, chest radiography, electrocardiography, echocardiography, serum electrolytes and creatinine, and urine electrolytes.

Differential Diagnosis

Not every enlargement of the vein of Galen is a vein of Galen aneurysm.* Many adjacent processes, such as pial fistulae, dural arteriovenous malformations or fistulae, or a parenchymatous arteriovenous malformation, cause the venous pouch to dilate and enlarge because of the high-flow conditions.[18, 69, 71] The Yasargil type IV vein of Galen aneurysm is, as discussed, merely a "secondary" dilatation of the vein associated with the drainage of a deep midline arteriovenous malformation.[18, 40, 73] In addition, a varix of the vein of Galen can exist without the presence of an arteriovenous shunt.[18, 40]

These other processes differ from true aneurysmal vein of Galen aneurysms in their clinical presentations, angiography features, treatment, and outcome. Pial fistulae tend to become symptomatic with hemorrhage and seizures and therefore represent a more urgent type of vascular malformation. Parenchymatous arteriovenous malformations are like arteriovenous malformations elsewhere in the brain, except that they drain into the vein of Galen. They become symptomatic with hemorrhage, seizures, and neurological deficits and have a natural history similar to those of other arteriovenous malformations. They should be treated like other arteriovenous malforma-

tions in the brain, by embolization, resection, or radiosurgery if appropriate.[17, 24, 28, 63, 68]

Natural History

Johnston's clinical series and review of the medical literature, completed in 1987, confirmed the accepted understanding that the prognosis for untreated patients with a vein of Galen aneurysm is grim.[34] Of 92 untreated patients (i.e., patients who received either no treatment or treatment only for congestive heart failure), 77.2 per cent died, 3.3 per cent were impaired, 12 per cent were normal, and 7.5 per cent were lost to follow-up (alive but with no details).[34] Furthermore, untreated neonates had a mortality rate of 96 per cent, identifying this subgroup as being at particularly high risk (Table 64–2). These results differ little from Hoffman's series of 29 untreated patients (also included in Johnston's group of 92 patients), in which 76.9 per cent died, 7.7 per cent were impaired, 7.7 per cent were normal, and the outcome of 7.7 per cent was unknown.[30]

Untreated patients typically die from a combination of cerebral and cardiac ischemic injury. Neonates succumb to their cardiovascular derangements and older children to central nervous system injury. Untreated cerebral shunting and venous hypertension produces arterial steal, ischemic injury, and cerebral infarction. All these latter events produce cerebral atrophy, dystrophic cerebral calcifications, and progressive neurological deterioration. More important, even with modern treatment, the mortality rate for this condition still approaches 79 per cent for neonates and 39 per cent for the entire population (see Table 64–2). The specifics of treatment as they affect patient outcome are presented in the next section.

---

*See references 18, 20, 23, 42, 50, and 69.

Table 64–2

NATURAL HISTORY OF VEIN OF GALEN ANEURYSM COMPARED WITH RESULTS OF SURGICAL TREATMENT (STRATIFIED BY AGE)

Age Group (No. of Patients)	Mortality (Number/Total [Percentage])		
	Natural History*	Any Surgery	Direct Surgery†
Neonate‡ (77)	55/58 (94.8)	15/19 (78.9)	15/19 (78.9)
Infant (75)	10/18 (55.6)	21/57 (36.8)	14/46 (30.4)
1–5 yr (34)	4/7 (57.1)	9/27 (33.3)	9/21 (42.9)
6–20 yr (18)	2/8 (25)	2/10 (20)	2/9 (22.2)
>20 yr (21)	5/8 (62.5)	2/13 (15.4)	1/9 (11.1)
TOTAL (225)	76/99 (76.8)	49/126 (38.9)	41/104 (39.4)

*Natural History refers to patients with no endovascular or surgical therapy; management of congestive heart failure was attempted in some of these patients.

†Direct Surgery excludes the patients who had only ventricular shunting operation.

‡Neonates classified as age 0–1 month; infants classified as age 1–12 months. Data from Johnston, I. H., Whittle, I. R., Besser, M., et al.: Vein of Galen malformation: Diagnosis and management. Neurosurgery, 20:747, 1987.

Treatment

OVERVIEW AND MEDICAL THERAPY

The timing of treatment and the selection of the most appropriate treatment method (Tables 64–3 and 64–4) depend on the patient's age and clinical presentation.[30, 34, 71] In newborns, the most common symptoms are cardiovascular. The initial treatment should therefore be aggressive medical stabilization. Congestive heart failure should be vigorously treated.[8, 11, 12, 19] The associated cardiomegaly and pulmonary congestion found on plain chest radiography normalizes after the heart failure is controlled.[1] In most cases, medical stabilization suffices as treatment in the acute phase and allows later definitive treatment when the infant is bigger and more stable.

If the neonate does not respond to maximal medical

Table 64–3

TREATMENT METHODS FOR MANAGEMENT OF PATIENTS WITH VEIN OF GALEN ANEURYSMS*

Endovascular treatment (embolization with glue, polyvinyl alcohol, coils, pellets, or balloons)
  Arterial route (preferred) (see references 18 and 74)
  Venous route
    Transfemoral/jugular (see references 7 and 16)
    Transtorcular (see references 26, 36, and 48)
  Multimodality endovascular (see references 9 and 43)
Microsurgical resection (see references 30, 34, and 73)
Multimodality combined endovascular and surgical treatment (see references 43 and 71)

*Includes medical therapy for congestive heart failure and seizures and ventricular shunting for the treatment of hydrocephalus, if indicated.

Table 64–4

NATURAL HISTORY OF VEIN OF GALEN ANEURYSM COMPARED WITH RESULTS OF VARIOUS MODES OF TREATMENT

	Reference Number	No. of Patients	Results (Percentage)			
			Lost	Normal	Impaired	Dead
Natural history						
	34	92	7.5	12	3.3	77.2
	30	29	7.7	7.7	7.7	76.9
Endovascular treatment Arterial						
	74	34	0	52.9	41.3	5.8
Venous Transfemoral/jugular						
	7	7	0	100	100	0
	16	3	0	100	100	0
Venous Transtorcular						
	26	15	0	80	80	20
	48	3	0	66.6	66.6	33.4
	36	3	0	66.6	33.3	0
Multimodality endovascular						
	9	8	0	37.5	37.5	25.0
	43	28	0	60.7	14.2	17.9
Open surgery						
	34	126	7.1	26.2	27.7	38.8
	30	70	0	44.3	20.0	35.7
	73	16	0	68.8	68.8	31.2
Multimodality treatment (surgery and endovascular)						
	71	35	0	31.4	37.2	31.4
	43	28	0	60.7	14.2	7.1

therapy, a dilemma arises as to whether to treat, knowing that the risks are higher in this critically ill patient, or to withhold treatment. The decision must be made on a case-by-case basis with full review of the clinical condition, the age of the patient, and the psychosocial situation.

If the newborn responds to medical therapy, close follow-up with serial head ultrasound examinations, computed tomography or magnetic resonance imaging studies, head circumference measurements, and developmental assessments is required. Ideally, intervention should be delayed until the infant is 6 months old. However, if there is any indication that the child is deteriorating according to the above criteria, urgent treatment may be indicated.

Neonates who have been stabilized for about 6 months and older children who present with a vein of Galen aneurysm should be treated to avoid the consequences of long-term venous congestion.* In infants, the venous circulation has transmedullary veins that equilibrate the superficial cortical and subependymal pressures. These veins are not encountered in older children, and they are therefore prone to develop chronic venous hypertension and, consequently, deep cerebral calcifications. These dystrophic calcifications are usually irreversible and forecast that the child will suffer from some degree of mental retardation. For this reason, venous hypertension and it sequela (i.e., dystrophic calcifications) should be prevented at all costs.

*See references 9, 12, 14, 18, 22, 31, and 73.

Older patients with "incidental" vein of Galen aneurysms should be thoroughly screened and followed carefully. If they are completely asymptomatic, these patients can be carefully followed by serial magnetic resonance imaging.[33]

Spontaneous closure or thrombosis of vein of Galen aneurysms, although uncommon, is a well-documented phenomenon, especially with low-flow lesions.[5, 15, 71] However, the presence of a low-flow lesion does not change the management criteria that have been outlined: if the vein of Galen aneurysm is symptomatic, it should be treated to avoid the long-term consequences of venous hypertension and cerebral ischemia.

INTERVENTIONAL TREATMENT STRATEGY

The dismal natural history associated with these lesions has spurred interest in protocols that combine sophisticated interventional neuroradiological embolization techniques and, if necessary, surgical resection. These endeavors have significantly improved the prognosis for neonates and infants with this lesion.* The poor medical condition of most neonates and infants who present with these malformations has limited the efficacy of operative treatment. Embolization can reduce blood flow though the aneurysm and can often ameliorate life threatening congestive heart failure; however, complete obliteration of the lesion with embolization alone is not always possible. In order to prevent risk of hemorrhage and late progressive enlargement of the lesion, staged surgical resection may be required. Therefore, vein of Galen aneurysms, like other high-grade arteriovenous malformations, are commonly treated with a multimodality strategy employing staged embolization and surgical resection.[36, 71]

The selection of treatment modalities is influenced by the clinical presentation and age of the patient and by the complexity of the aneurysm. Management of these lesions should be undertaken by a neurovascular team that includes a neurosurgeon and an experienced interventional endovascular neuroradiologist. Treatment aims are determined (e.g., complete obliteration of the aneurysm, palliative reduction of flow through the aneurysm, treatment of hydrocephalus), and then a management strategy is outlined that includes consideration of the various treatment modalities available to meet the treatment objectives. These modalities may include embolization (transarterial, via the femoral vein, or transtorcular), surgery, shunting for hydrocephalus, or a combination of these methods.

TREATMENT OF HYDROCEPHALUS

The results of most shunting procedures for ventriculomegaly in neonates and infants have been disappointing. It has long been known that the pressure inside the ventricles is invariably low. Shunting procedures have a high failure rate, and there is a high incidence of postshunting subdural hematoma collections.[37, 69, 74] Magnetic resonance imaging of patients with vein of Galen aneurysm demonstrates two interesting features in this context: there is no transependymal reabsorption of cerebrospinal fluid, and the aqueduct of Sylvius is frequently patent.[3, 4, 53, 74] The ventriculomegaly (not hydrocephalus) is thought to be caused by a secondary phenomenon related to the venous stenosis and the hemodynamic alterations that ensue. It is therefore best to avoid shunting these patients and to aim therapy at correction of the pathophysiological mechanisms of the ventriculomegaly (i.e., diminishing or eliminating shunting through the fistula at the vein of Galen aneurysm). This strategy by itself has been found to normalize head circumference.[37]

ENDOVASCULAR TREATMENT

Overview. Endovascular techniques have assumed a major role in the management of these patients. The sophisticated, high-resolution cerebral angiography and endovascular techniques developed for treating cerebral arteriovenous malformations and cerebral aneurysms have been applied to the management of vein of Galen aneurysms.* The transarterial approach is considered to be the most suitable endovascular approach for dealing with most Yasargil type I, II, or III vein of Galen aneurysms, although some authors believe that the transvenous approach is also suitable for many of these lesions.† Lasjaunias and colleagues have recommended that the transvenous route be reserved for patients in whom the arterial approach has failed.[37] Both transarterial and transvenous approaches have been used for Yasargil type IV vein of Galen aneurysms.[43] Each of these three endovascular techniques has particular advantages and disadvantages and can be used alone, in combination with the others, or in combination with surgery.[9, 43, 71]

Arterial Techniques. An informed patient and family are the best guarantees to obtain cooperation and ensure successful treatment. The limitations of the procedure should be presented, along with alternative treatments and expected short-term and long-term outcomes. Specifically, the potentials for hemorrhage, infection, thrombosis, embolism, hydrocephalus, worsening neurological deficit, and even death should be reviewed.

Children are especially likely to become agitated and confused and thereby jeopardize the entire procedure. For this reason, all endovascular procedures are performed with the patient under general anesthesia. An experienced neuroanesthesiologist is needed to ensure high-quality angiography.[25, 37, 48]

After anesthesia has been induced, the positions of the endotracheal tube and Foley catheter are checked with fluoroscopy. The patient's head is secured with

---

*See references 18, 27, 34, 35, 43, and 48.

*See references 7, 9, 16, 18, 26, 37, 38, 43, 48, and 74.
†See references 7, 16, 18, 26, 37, 43, and 48.

Velcro patches, and with each injection of contrast the respirator is disconnected to prevent movement artifact. Minimal amounts of diluted contrast medium (1:1 or 1:2 with normal saline) are used to avoid overloading the child's renal and circulatory systems, which may already be physiologically stressed. The maximum permissible amount of nonionic contrast material (300 mg per mL) is 5 mL per kg per session. Consequently, endovascular treatment should always be scheduled for the same time as the diagnostic arteriography procedure.

A 20-gauge pediatric needle is used to access the femoral artery, and a 4-French (1.3 mm) pediatric femoral sheath is introduced over a guide wire. Cutdowns are usually not required for vascular access. A 4-French dilator is passed ahead of the sheath to facilitate positioning in the femoral artery and to avoid undue trauma or spasm in the vessel wall. An ischemic leg is a potential although extremely uncommon risk. In about 10 per cent of cases, the pedal pulses disappear with no ischemic symptoms and return completely within 24 hours.[39]

After the femoral sheath is in place, it is connected to a continuous saline flush. The patient is then fully heparinized (100 IU per kg) for the duration of the procedure to prevent thromboembolic phenomena. At the end of the procedure, the heparin is reversed with the appropriate amount of protamine sulfate.

A 4-French catheter guide is navigated to the neck vessels and connected to a saline flush. A precurved microcatheter (either a flow-guided catheter or a steerable system with a guide wire) is introduced coaxially and navigated with the guidance of fluoroscopy (with road map capabilities) into the feeding vessels. After the catheter is in position, a superselective arteriogram is obtained to ensure that no normal branches are present.

A standard amount of N-butyl cyanoacrylate adhesive is mixed with Ethiodol. The N-butyl cyanoacrylate is injected from a full syringe. The glue molds the vein and fistula site and then backfills the pedicle. When the column of adhesive approaches the tip of the catheter, the injection is stopped. Suction is applied to remove any glue remaining at the tip, and the catheter is quickly removed by an experienced assistant. The process requires only a few seconds and has to be perfected by all members of the team before the procedure. Steroids (dexamethasone; 10 mg) are given before the embolization to reduce the inflammatory reaction that is usually produced by the glue, and after the procedure they are continued for a few more days.

Because some arteriovenous fistulae have high flow, several steps are needed to ensure that closure is adequate: (1) the catheter tip is aimed at the wall; (2) a sufficient pedicle length is allowed; (3) pure (or almost pure) N-butyl cyanoacrylate is used; and (4) hypotension is sometimes induced with nitroprusside. Special care should be taken when hypotensive agents are used in the presence of cardiac insufficiency. Coronary artery perfusion normally occurs during diastole, and coronary ischemia may occur if diastolic pressure is decreased too much in the presence of elevated cardiac ventriclar pressures.

The "mold" of glue obtained (Fig. 64–6), as seen on lateral radiography, involves the straight sinus, the arteriovenous fistula site itself, and the proximal pedicle.[18, 37] The process is repeated in the same sequence

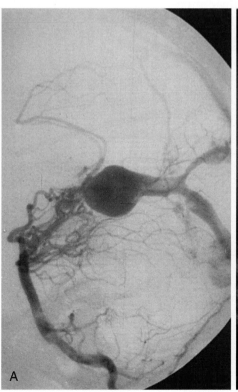
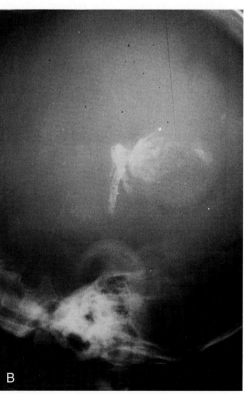

Figure 64–6

A. Lateral vertebral artery angiography depicts vein of Galen aneurysm before treatment. *B.* Lateral skull radiography after arterial embolization with *N*-butyl cyanoacrylate (NBCA) reveals the glue cast.

for each pedicle in the same session, or the treatments can be staged in two or three sessions.[18, 37, 40] Staging of the procedure is thought to allow hemodynamic adjustments to occur gradually, thereby avoiding sudden changes in intracerebral vascular pressure.[64, 65]

Alternatively, the arterial pedicle can be occluded with detachable balloons or coils to eliminate the fistula. The patient is extubated at the end of the procedure and is observed for 24 hours in the intensive care unit.

Venous Techniques. The transfemoral or transjugular venous route or, if this is not possible, the venous transtorcular route can be effectively used to treat these lesions.* In either case, a catheter is first placed in the appropriate artery by a transarterial approach to perform diagnostic arteriography and allow the progress of embolization to be assessed.[7, 16, 18, 23, 37]

To perform the transfemoral venous approach, a 20-gauge needle is used to enter the femoral vein contralateral to the side of the arterial catheter. A 4-French catheter is passed through a 5-French sheath and manipulated into the jugular bulb with the aid of a J-wire.[23] A steerable Tracker 18 microcatheter† is then introduced through the sigmoid and lateral sinuses into the straight sinus with the help of a guide wire with a diameter of 0.010 to 0.018 in.[7] After the catheter is inside the venous pouch, large and then smaller coils are introduced until the pouch is obliterated (Fig. 64–7). Staging the procedure over several sessions to avoid decreasing the pressure by more than 20 cm H_2O per session has been advocated to avoid the consequences of rapid hemodynamic changes.[7, 64, 65]

If the venous transfemoral approach is not possible, the transtorcular route can be used (Fig. 64–8). Mickle and colleagues reported the first use of the transtorcular approach in 1985.[49] The patient is positioned prone in a Mayfield frame.[26, 43, 48] The torcular is exposed with a high-speed drill. A pursestring suture is placed, and a venotomy is performed with a no. 11 scalpel blade. A 4-French introducer is then advanced into the venous pouch. The coils are delivered with the aid of digital subtraction angiography. Great care must be exerted to avoid passing the coils into the arterial feeders, which could produce a vessel perforation.

Another difficulty arises from the frequent association of venous stenosis with vein of Galen aneurysms. The stenosis can be present in the veins or major sinuses, and it can limit accessibility to the aneurysm from the venous femoral or transtorcular approaches. The decision about which technique to use first therefore depends somewhat on the vascular anatomy.

SURGICAL TREATMENT

General Aspects. During the acute treatment of a symptomatic neonate, surgery is usually reserved as a final management option. Newborns with a vein of Galen aneurysm commonly present with a compromised cardiac and respiratory status and therefore represent a high surgical risk. In 1982, Hoffman and co-workers reported that four of eight neonates with vein of Galen aneurysms who were surgically treated died.[30] Three patients were left with permanent impairment, and only one was neurologically normal. Massey and colleagues also reported experience with six neonatal patients who underwent surgical treatment for a vein of Galen aneurysm; only two patients survived.[45]

These poor surgical treatment results have spurred the development and use of less invasive methods for lesion obliteration. Significant success has been achieved with the use of advanced medical and endovascular therapies to stabilize neonates before surgical intervention. In many cases, surgery can be delayed or avoided if partial or complete obliteration with endovascular therapy can alleviate the progressive neurological or cardiovascular deterioration. It is the subgroup of neonates with progressive deterioration unresponsive to less invasive therapy for whom early surgery is indicated.

Yasargil reported that types I, II, and III vein of Galen aneurysms can be treated surgically with an acceptable risk of morbidity and mortality.[73] In contrast, he believed that types IVA and IVB vein of Galen aneurysms carry a significantly higher treatment risk for postoperative death or neurological deficit.[73] Other issues, such as patient age and cardiovascular status, also significantly affect the prospects for a good treatment outcome. With the aid of advancing endovascular techniques, the results of combined endovascular treatment and surgical resection are likely to continue improving.[43, 71]

Surgical Technique. Surgery should be delayed, if possible, until the medical condition and nutritional status of the child can be optimized. Many infants and neonates require a ventriculostomy or shunt to treat coexistent hydrocephalus either before or after resection of a vein of Galen aneurysm. In addition, preoperative embolization of accessible feeding vessels should be attempted to simplify resection of the lesion.[18, 43, 71]

The galenic region can be surgically accessed by the subtemporal, transcallosal, or supracerebellar-transtentorial approaches, either alone or in combination. The subtemporal route is useful for providing access to those aneurysms that are fed by one or both posterior choroidal arteries. Through this exposure, the choroidal arteries can be followed to the site of connection with the vein of Galen aneurysm, where they can be divided.

However, a posterior interhemispherical approach is most commonly used to adequately access a vein of Galen aneurysm and expose the feeding arteries (Fig. 64–9). The operation can be performed with the patient in the sitting, prone, or lateral position. The authors' preference is to place the patient in a modified park bench or lateral position with the head horizontal and the hemisphere of interest positioned inferiorly. The modified park bench position puts the patient at less risk for development of an air embolus than does the sitting position, and it produces less venous congestion than does the standard prone position. Placing the

---

*See references 7, 16, 26, 36, 43, 48, and 49.
†Manufactured by Target Therapeutics, Fremont, California.

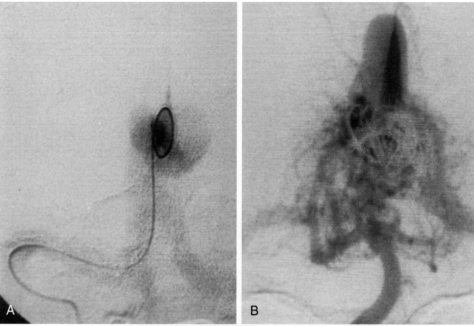

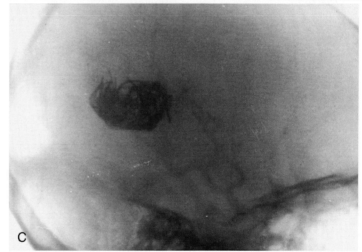

Figure 64–7

A. Anteroposterior angiography shows the catheter passing through the sinus system into the vein of Galen aneurysm. *B.* Anteroposterior vertebrobasilar angiography depicts coils in vein of Galen aneurysm. Flow through the lesion has been substantially reduced. *C.* Lateral skull radiography depicts the coils situated in the vein of Galen aneurysm. (*B* from Khayata, M. H., Casasco, A., Wakhloo, A. K., et al.: Vein of Galen malformations: Intravascular techniques. *In* Carter, L. P., Spetzler, R. F., and Hamilton, M. G., eds.: Neurovascular Surgery. New York, McGraw-Hill, Inc., 1994. Reprinted by permission.)

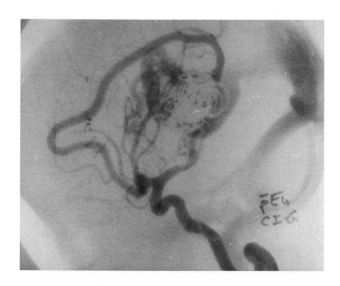

Figure 64–8

Lateral carotid artery angiography depicts the arterial feeders to a vein of Galen aneurysm that has been effectively embolized by the transtorcular route. Flow through the aneurysm is still present but is substantially reduced.

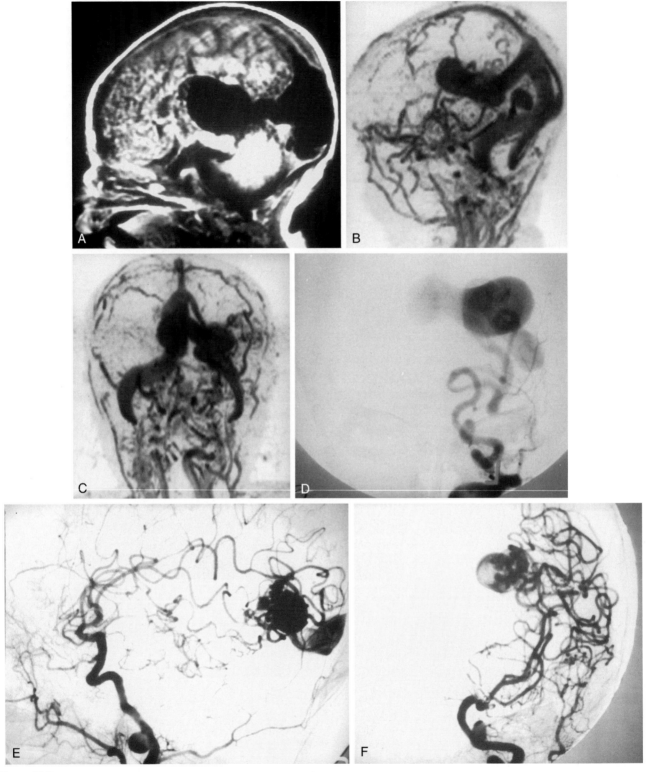

Figure 64–9

Newborn with congestive heart failure and hydrocephalus. *A.* Sagittal T1-weighted magnetic resonance imaging demonstrates the location and size of the vein of Galen aneurysm. Lateral *(B)* and anteroposterior *(C)* magnetic resonance angiography of the lesion demonstrate the multiple feeding vessels and multiple nidi. *D.* Anteroposterior projection of left internal carotid artery injection demonstrates the feeding arteries to the vein of Galen aneurysm. The aneurysm was a type I lesion with arterial branches from both the posterior cerebral and pericallosal arteries. There were two different nidi: one was located anteriorly and was supplied primarily by anterior branches from the posterior cerebral artery and basilar complex; the second portion was located more posteriorly and was supplied by pericallosal arteries. The infant was hemodynamically unstable and required obliteration of the aneurysm. The largest feeding vessels from the posterior circulation were accessed through a subtemporal approach. Two large supplying vessels were clipped and others were dissected and coagulated. After this was completed, a repeat angiography was obtained to document status of the residual nidus. Lateral *(E)* and anteroposterior *(F)* left internal carotid injections demonstrate residual vein of Galen aneurysm. A second-stage operative procedure was performed through a posterior interhemispherical approach, and the remaining feeding vessels and aneurysm were located and occluded.

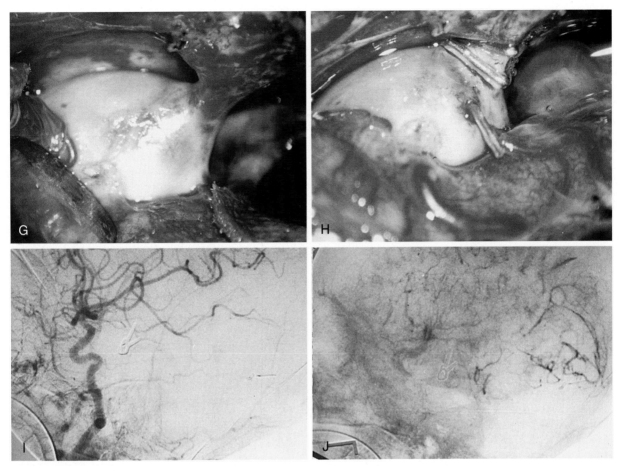

Figure 64–9 *Continued*

Intraoperative photography demonstrates the numerous feeding vessels and residual aneurysm before *(G)* and after *(H)* clip occlusion at the second-stage operative procedure. Early *(I)* and delayed *(J)* injections of the postoperative lateral internal carotid artery, completed after the second operative procedure, demonstrate complete elimination of the vein of Galen aneurysm. In addition, the infant required a ventriculoperitoneal shunt. At 1 year of age, he had mild developmental delay but was otherwise thriving. (From Herman, J. M., Hamilton, M. G., and Spetzler, R. F.: Vein of Galen malformations: Surgical indications and techniques. *In* Carter, L. P., Spetzler, R. F., and Hamilton, M. G., eds.: Neurovascular Surgery. New York, McGraw-Hill, Inc., 1994. Reprinted by permission.)

head in a horizontal plane allows the dependent hemisphere to fall away from the falx with minimal or no retraction and offers the surgeon a more comfortable hand position; instead of trying to move one hand over the other, as is required during the usual vertical position, the surgeon can use a more normal, side-by-side hand positioning. This added working space can be essential when dealing with deep feeding arteries.

The size and location of the scalp flap must be contoured to each specific vein of Galen aneurysm. A low paramedian craniotomy, similar to the interhemispherical suboccipital-transtentorial approach used on pineal region tumors, provides access to the posterior aspect of a vein of Galen aneurysm. This exposure is usually adequate to deal with a type II lesion, which is composed primarily of thalamoperforating arteries. However, for access to superior and anterior pericallosal feeding arteries, the craniotomy may need to be extended anteriorly. Contralateral exposure of the lesion can be obtained by opening the falx above the inferior sagittal sinus. Although this additional contralateral view allows access to the contralateral superior pericallosal arteries, it may allow only limited exposure of

inferior arterial feeders such as contralateral thalamoperforator or deep branches of the posterior cerebral artery. In these situations, it may be more appropriate to perform a bilateral craniotomy and approach the interhemispherical fissure from both sides.

The arachnoid of the callosal, dorsal ambient, and the quadrigeminal cisterns should be opened extensively to allow full exposure of the vein of Galen aneurysm. Opening of the ambient cistern laterally allows identification of the posterior cerebral and superior cerebellar arteries. Looking laterally in this cistern, the surgeon is usually able to identify the posterior cerebral artery first, with the superior cerebellar artery located immediately behind it. Both arteries should be followed to the aneurysm and divided. The distal segments of the anterior pericallosal arteries can be exposed over the splenium, which is usually displaced anteriorly and superiorly by the lesion. These arteries should also be followed to their point of connection with the vein of Galen aneurysm and divided. Ideally, dividing of these major arterial feeders allows more extensive exposure of the aneurysm and its residual anterior and inferior arterial feeders. Additional feeders from the posterior cerebral and the pericallosal arteries can be identified as the surgeon works around the margin of the aneurysm and then divided at their junction with the aneurysm.

After enough vascular input has been eliminated, the turgor of the vein of Galen aneurysm decreases, allowing further exposure of the more inferior aspect of the lesion. If the aneurysm remains distended after these branches have been divided, additional inferior feeders from the thalamoperforating or choroidal arteries still remain.

The most tedious and difficult portion of the Galen aneurysm resection often lies in the anterior and inferior region. Numerous venous and arterial connections may be present within a minimal working space. Gentle retraction of the vein of Galen, after it has been covered with Telfa, may provide improved access. Yasargil has recommended that veins in this area be coagulated and divided if they become too obstructive.[73] He states in addition that the internal cerebral veins may also be sacrificed in this situation, given that these vessels are usually unable to drain into normal venous areas because of high intracranial venous pressures. After the vascular supply to the aneurysm has been significantly reduced, the vein of Galen should collapse. The remaining aneurysm wall can then be obliterated with a clip or resected. With a large, complex aneurysm, it may be best to stage surgery in order to allow safe, progressive obliteration of the lesion.

Although type IV malformations (secondary to arteriovenous malformations that extend into the mesencephalon or thalamus) are usually inoperable, direct intraoperative injection of thalamoperforating feeding vessels with acrylic glue can be used with some success. Aberrant thalamic arteries are surgically isolated, cannulated with a small needle, imaged, and then injected with glue with the use of fluoroscopy guidance. Future development of this technique may allow for more complete obliteration of these complex lesions.

Treatment Outcome

The natural history of a patient with an untreated vein of Galen aneurysm is very poor. The overall mortality rate for untreated patients with a vein of Galen aneurysm is approximately 78 per cent, although, as noted, there is a definite difference between neonates and older patients. Untreated neonates experience a 96 per cent mortality rate, whereas the mortality rate for older patients is 25 to 63 per cent (see Table 64–3). Hoffman and colleagues reported that, of 13 untreated infants, 11 died and none of the survivors were neurologically normal; of 23 untreated older children and adults, 6 died, 6 were left significantly impaired, and the outcome of 11 children was unknown.[30] It is important to keep this dismal natural history in perspective when evaluating the treatment outcome for patients with a vein of Galen aneurysm. In addition, because of the intrinsic differences that exist between subgroups of patients, one should compare only similar populations. Unfortunately, this is frequently not possible in reviews of the literature because of limited information.

ARTERIAL ENDOVASCULAR TREATMENT

Arterial embolization has become the mainstay of endovascular therapy for vein of Galen aneurysms. In the series reported by Lasjaunias and associates, arterial endovascular techniques successfully eliminated 47 per cent of vein of Galen aneurysms.[37, 74] At the time of referral, 18 of the 43 patients were neonates, 14 were infants, and 11 were between 1 and 16 years of age. However, endovascular treatment was delayed with medical stabilization, and only 5 patients were still neonates when embolized. Only 34 of these 43 patients underwent embolization therapy. Four of the 34 patients had a transvenous approach after failure to sufficiently catheterize arterial feeders to the lesion. Of the 34 embolized patients, 52.9 per cent were normal, 41.3 per cent were impaired, and 5.8 per cent died after treatment (see Table 64–4). This compares with a mortality rate of 66.7 per cent for the 9 patients who were not embolized (80 per cent for neonates).

Although two patients in Lasjaunias' series died, neither death was thought to be directly associated with the actual embolization procedure. One death occurred secondary to multiorgan failure, and the other was secondary to bilateral subdural hematomas after ventricular shunting.[37] No femoral or neurological morbidity was noted with transarterial embolization. Major treatment morbidity was limited to three of the four patients who underwent the transvenous approach. One of these latter patients developed an intracerebral hematoma, one patient developed postembolization hydrocephalus, and one child was left with mild mental retardation. In addition, four patients developed delayed secondary distal dural sinus occlusion; one of them developed hydrocephalus, and the remaining three patients remained asymptomatic.

VENOUS ENDOVASCULAR TREATMENT

The venous transfemoral and transtorcular techniques have been reserved for patients for whom the arterial route is impossible or unsuccessful, or as an adjunct to arterial embolization.[9, 43, 74] Therefore, the number of patients who have been treated by only the venous route is small, and generalizations about benefits and risks cannot be clearly stated.[7, 16, 26, 36, 48] However, the reports from Rosenberg and Nazar and from Ciricillo, Lylyk, and Lasjaunias and their colleagues emphasize the potential risks associated with the venous approach.[9, 37, 43, 60]

The transfemoral or transjugular venous route has been reported by Casasco, Dowd, and Lasjaunias and their associates for a total of 14 patients[7, 16, 37] (see Table 64–4). Ciricillo and co-workers used the transfemoral venous approach with transarterial embolization in 7 patients.[9] Lylyk and colleagues used the transfemoral approach in combination with a transarterial or transtorcular approach in 12 patients, including 3 patients with Yasargil type IV lesions.[43] The experience of Lasjaunias and associates with this embolization technique has already been reviewed.[37]

In the series of 10 patients reported by Ciricillo and associates and by Dowd and colleagues, 6 experienced total occlusion of their vein of Galen aneurysm, and the remaining 4 patients had a significant reduction in flow after treatment. Six of the patients were treated primarily by the transfemoral route, 3 had failed transarterial treatment, and 3 had attempted transtorcular treatment (2 had both transtorcular and transarterial therapy). All 10 patients were reported to have stabilized or improved, although the final neurological status could not be determined from the reports. The one major complication reported was a vessel perforation that resulted in an intraventricular hemorrhage and required ventricular shunting for hydrocephalus.

In the series of Ciricillo and colleagues, all 7 patients (neonates) had venous treatment combined with arterial embolization: 3 were normal, 3 were disabled, and 1 died.[9] A total of 11 complications were documented: 3 hemorrhages, 5 intracerebral infarcts, 1 detached catheter, 2 embolus migrations, and 1 hydrocephalus. It is not possible to determine the outcome related to the transvenous technique in the report from Lylyk and associates, although no morbidity or mortality was reported for this patient group.[43]

The transtorcular technique was popularized by Mickle and Quisling.[48] The largest published series includes 15 patients reported by Mickle and Quisling's group[26] (see Table 64–4). Few pretreatment patient data were available in this report. Complete thrombosis of the fistula was accomplished in 6 patients, partial thrombosis was accomplished in 8 patients, and 1 patient had complete thrombosis of the vein of Galen with partial thrombosis of the fistula. Twelve of the 15 patients had significant improvement in symptoms, and 3 patients (all neonates) died. Specific information concerning the clinical status of the survivors was not published. Two of the deaths were related to uncontrolled congestive heart failure, and one occurred secondary to a subdural hematoma at the time of a ventriculostomy. The only complication reported was a cerebral venous thrombosis with resultant cerebral infarction ("minimal clinical symptoms").

Lylyk and colleagues used the transtorcular approach alone in 8 patients and in combination with transarterial or transfemoral embolizations in 3 patients.[43] Specific outcome was not available for this patient subpopulation, but the mortality rate for this endovascular approach was 27.3 per cent. Three patients died from intracranial hemorrhage secondary to perforation of the varix with the guiding wire catheter. King and colleagues used the transtorcular approach in 3 patients, with elimination of flow in 2 patients and significant reduction in the third.[36] All 3 patients survived, but 1 neonate experienced an intraventricular hemorrhage that produced seizures and hydrocepha-

lus. Finally, Rosenberg and Nazar reported 2 patients who died secondary to disseminated coagulopathy associated with transtorcular embolization.[60]

SURGICAL TREATMENT

Surgical techniques are quite efficacious, especially with a single-hole fistula. The technical difficulty increases with the more common situation of multiple, anteriorly located fistulae. However, other issues, such as patient age and clinical condition, are more predictive of surgical treatment risk; for example, neonates with congestive heart failure have a much higher surgical risk than do infants and older children. More patients with vein of Galen aneurysm have been treated with surgical management than with any other treatment methodology, thereby allowing for a comprehensive overview.

Johnston and associates reviewed the results of 126 surgically treated patients[34] (see Tables 64–2 and 64–4). The mortality rate for the whole population was 38.8 per cent. The mortality rate for surgically treated patients who had only a shunt insertion (n = 22) was 36.4 per cent, compared with a rate of 39.4 per cent for patients who had a surgical procedure directed at the vein of Galen aneurysm (n = 104). The data discussed here for the different age groups refer to all surgical treatments.

Operative results are the poorest for symptomatic neonates, with mortality rates as high as 78 per cent[2, 30, 34, 73] (see Table 64–2). Further, the severe morbidity rate for surviving neonates ranges between 60 and 90 per cent. Hoffman and colleagues reported that, of 15 surgically treated neonates, 1 was neurologically normal, 4 were neurologically impaired, and 10 (66.6 per cent) died.[30] Massey and associates described 70 patients with vein of Galen aneurysms.[45] Of the 6 neonates who underwent surgical treatment, 4 (66.6 per cent) died. Johnston and colleagues reviewed the results of 126 surgically treated patients; the mortality rate for neonates was 78.9 per cent[34] (see Table 64–2). Five patients (31.3 per cent) in Yasargil's series of 16 patients died; all 5 were newborns (a 100 per cent mortality rate for this age group).

Fortunately, treatment outcomes for vein of Galen aneurysm resection in an infant or older child are significantly better than those in neonates (see Table 64–2). Hoffman and colleagues reported that, of 30 surgically treated infants, 15 were neurologically normal, 4 were neurologically impaired, and 8 (26.7 per cent) died.[30] Of 29 older children or adults in Hoffman's series who were surgically treated, 15 were normal, 5 were left with a permanent neurological impairment, and 4 (13.8 per cent) died. In the review by Massey and associates describing 70 patients with vein of Galen aneurysms, 15 of 25 infants and 8 of 11 older children or adults survived surgical resection.[45] Johnston and associates reviewed the results of 126 surgically treated patients (see Table 64–2): the mortality rate for infants and older children ranged between 15.4 and 36.8 per cent.[34] In Yasargil's series of 16 surgically treated patients of various ages, all 11 of the older children survived and had "good" outcomes.[73]

MULTIMODALITY TREATMENT

Few authors have addressed the potential benefits of combined endovascular and surgical therapies (see Tables 64–3 and 64–4). Wisoff and Lylyk and their colleagues have emphasized the importance of considering different therapeutic alternatives for patients with vein of Galen aneurysm and, if necessary, using combination therapy to achieve the desired outcome.[43, 71] Wisoff and co-workers described the management of 35 patients by a multimodality approach with a 31.4 per cent mortality rate.[71] Only 7 of these patients had direct surgery as part of their treatment (17 shunts were inserted). Although the patient series reported by Lylyk and associates stressed the importance of considering different therapeutic alternatives, surgery was used in only 2 patients, and complete occlusion of the aneurysm was obtained in 46.4 per cent of patients.[43] The overall mortality rate for the 28 patients in Lylyk's series was only 17.9 per cent.

Summary and Conclusions

Vein of Galen aneurysms are uncommon lesions that involve midline arteriovenous fistulae, with single or multiple arterial feeders, associated with aneurysmal dilatation of the vein of Galen. Vein of Galen aneurysms represent a very complex subset of cerebral arteriovenous malformations. If they are left untreated, the massive shunting of blood can result in permanent cardiac or neurological injury and, often, death. The natural history of an untreated vein of Galen aneurysm is generally quite poor. In the reviews by Johnston and by Hoffman and their colleagues, the mortality rate of untreated patients (those receiving no embolization or surgery) was 77 per cent (see Tables 64–2 and 64–4).[30, 34] These patients represent a difficult management problem that is associated with a high treatment complication rate.

A number of angiographic and clinical classification systems have been proposed for these lesions (see Table 64–1). The simple scheme based on anatomical features seen on angiography defines two different types of lesions: "true" (congenital) vein of Galen aneurysms, with mural and choroidal subtypes, and "secondary" aneurysms, or vein of Galen dilatations caused by adjacent dural or true cerebral (parenchymatous) arteriovenous malformations.[18, 37] Yasargil expanded this classification system by defining three different types of "true" vein of Galen aneurysms with different vascular anatomy (types I to III) in addition to the "secondary" type of lesion (type IV).[73] Yasargil's classification system is probably more practical for treatment planning.

Patients with a vein of Galen aneurysm typically have different clinical presentations based on age at symptom onset. These age-related presentations define the clinical classification system[30] (see Table 64–1). Newborns tend to present with congestive heart failure; less often, with head enlargement secondary to ventriculomegaly; and rarely, with hemorrhage. Infants present with head enlargement secondary to ventriculomegaly or seizures, or, much less commonly, with congestive heart failure or hemorrhage. Older children and adults have the most varied modes of presentation, including subarachnoid hemorrhage, hydrocephalus, progressive neurological deficit secondary to steal phenomenon, and venous hypertension; they only rarely present with congestive heart failure.

Treatment for vein of Galen aneurysm is still evolving. Treatment methods include arterial and venous endovascular modalities, either alone or in combination with direct surgical treatment (see Table 64–4). Although outcomes in relation to the natural history have markedly improved, the mortality rate is still at about 35 per cent, and significant morbidity is seen in 30 to 35 per cent of patients. Results of surgical resection have been most favorable in the simpler lesions, which do not have thalamic involvement. Although endovascular therapy has made possible the alleviation of the acute symptoms and demonstrated early obliteration, complete removal of a lesion may require surgical resection.

REFERENCES

1. Al-Watban, J., and Banna, M.: Infantile cardiomegaly as a complication of vascular malformations of the brain: Report of two cases. Ann. Saudi Med., 8:373, 1988.
2. Amacher, A. L., and Shillito J., Jr.: The syndromes and surgical treatment of aneurysms of the great vein of Galen. J. Neurosurg., 39:89, 1973.
3. Andeweg, J.: Intracranial venous pressures, hydrocephalus and effects of cerebrospinal fluid shunts. Childs Nerv. Syst., 5:318, 1989.
4. Askenasy, H. M., Herzberger, E. E., and Wijsenbeek, H. S.: Hydrocephalus with vascular malformations of the brain: A preliminary report. Neurology, 3:213, 1953.
5. Beltremello, A., Preini, S., and Mazza, C.: Spontaneously healed vein of Galen aneurysms. Childs Nerv. Syst., 7:129, 1991.
6. Boldrey, E. B., and Miller, E. R.: Arteriovenous fistula (aneurysm) of the vein of Galen and circle of Willis. Arch. Neurol. Psychiatry, 62:778, 1949.
7. Casasco, A., Lylyk, P., Hodes, J. E., et al.: Percutaneous transvenous catheterization and embolization of vein of Galen aneurysms. Neurosurgery, 28:260, 1991.
8. Chan, S.-T., and Weeks, R. D.: Dural arteriovenous malformation presenting as cardiac failure in a neonate. Acta Neurochir. (Wien), 91:134, 1988.
9. Ciricillo, S. F., Edwards, M. S. B., Schmidt, K. G., et al.: Interventional neuroradiological management of vein of Galen malformations in the neonate. Neurosurgery, 27:22, 1990.
10. Clarisse, J., Dobbelaere, P., Rey, C., et al.: Aneurysms of the great vein of Galen: Radiological-anatomical study of 22 cases. J. Neuroradiol., 5:91, 1978.
11. Crawford, J. M., Rossitch E., Jr., Oakes, W. J., et al.: Arteriovenous malformation of the great vein of Galen associated with patent ductus arteriosus. Childs Nerv. Syst., 6:18, 1990.
12. Cumming, G. R.: Circulation in neonates with intracranial arteriovenous fistula and cardiac failure. Am. J. Cardiol., 45:1019, 1980.
13. Dandy, W. E.: Experimental hydrocephalus. Ann. Surg., 70:129, 1919.
14. De Lange, S. A., and De Vlieger, M.: Hydrocephalus associated

with raised venous pressure. Dev. Med. Child Neurol., 12(Suppl. 22):28, 1970.

15. De Morais, J. V., and Lemos, S.: Calcified aneurysm of the vein of Galen: Successful removal. Surg. Neurol., 174:304, 1982.

16. Dowd, C. F., Halbach, V. V., Barnwell, S. L., et al.: Transfemoral venous embolization of vein of Galen malformations. A.J.N.R., 11:643, 1990.

17. Drake, C. G.: Cerebral arteriovenous malformations: Considerations for and experience with surgical treatment in 166 cases. Clin. Neurosurg., 26:145, 1979.

18. Garcia-Monaco, R., Lasjaunias, P., and Berenstein, A.: Therapeutic management of vein of Galen aneurysmal malformations. *In* Viñuela, F., Halbach, V. V., and Dion, J. E., eds.: Interventional Neuroradiology: Endovascular Therapy of the Central Nervous System. New York, Raven Press, 1992, pp. 113–127.

19. Garcia-Monaco, R., de Victor, D., Mann, C., et al.: Congestive cardiac manifestations from cerebrocranial arteriovenous shunts: Endovascular management in 30 children. Childs Nerv. Syst., 7:48, 1991.

20. Garcia-Monaco, R., Rodesch, G., Terbrugge, K., et al.: Multifocal dural arteriovenous shunts in children. Childs Nerv. Syst., 7:425, 1991.

21. Gold, A. P., Ransohoff, J. R., and Carter, S.: Vein of Galen malformation. Acta Neurol. Scand. 40(Suppl. 11):5, 1964.

22. Haar, F. L., and Miller, C. A.: Hydrocephalus resulting from superior vena cava thrombosis in an infant. J. Neurosurg., 42:597, 1975.

23. Halbach, V. V., Higashida, R. T., Hieshima, G. R., et al.: Transvenous embolization of dural fistulas involving the transverse and sigmoid sinuses. A.J.N.R., 10:385, 1989.

24. Hamilton, M. G., and Spetzler, R. F.: The prospective application of a grading system for arteriovenous malformations. Neurosurgery, 34:2, 1994.

25. Hannedouche, A., Mann, C., Lasjaunias, P., et al.: Anaesthetic management for angiography and endovascular treatment in infants with vein of Galen arteriovenous malformations (VGAVM). Agressologie, 31:287, 1990.

26. Hanner, J. S., Quisling, R. G., Mickle, J. P., et al.: Gianturco coil embolization of vein of Galen aneurysms: Technical aspects. Radiographics, 8:935, 1988.

27. Herman, J. M., Hamilton, M. G., and Spetzler, R. F.: Vein of Galen malformations: Surgical indications and techniques. *In* Carter, L. P., Spetzler, R. F., Hamilton, M. G., eds.: Neurovascular Surgery. New York, McGraw-Hill (in press), 1994.

28. Heros, R. C., Korosue, K., and Diebold, P. M.: Surgical excision of cerebral arteriovenous malformations: Late results. Neurosurgery, 26:570, 1990.

29. Hoffman, H. J.: Malformations of the vein of Galen. *In* Edwards, M. S. B., and Hoffman, H. J., eds.: Current Neurosurgical Practice: Cerebral Vascular Disease in Children and Adolescents. Baltimore, Williams & Wilkins, 1989, pp. 239–246.

30. Hoffman, H. J., Chuang, S., Hendrick, E. B., et al.: Aneurysms of the vein of Galen: Experience at The Hospital for Sick Children, Toronto. J. Neurosurg., 57:316, 1982.

31. Hooper, R.: Hydrocephalus and obstruction of the superior vena cava in infancy: Clinical study of the relationship between cerebrospinal fluid pressure and venous pressure. Pediatrics, 28:792, 1961.

32. Jaeger, J. R., Forbes, R. P., and Dandy, W. E.: Bilateral congenital cerebral arteriovenous communications aneurysm. Trans. Am. Neurol. Assoc., 63:173, 1937.

33. Johnston, I.: Reduced C.S.F. absorption syndrome: Reapprasial of benign intracranial hypertension and related conditions. Lancet, 2:418, 1973.

34. Johnston, I. H., Whittle, I. R., Besser, M., et al.: Vein of Galen malformation: Diagnosis and management. Neurosurgery, 20:747, 1987.

35. Khayata, M. H., Casasco, A., Wakhloo, A. K., et al.: Vein of Galen malformations: Intravascular techniques. *In* Carter, L. P., Spetzler, R. F., Hamilton, M. G., eds.: Neurovascular Surgery. New York, McGraw-Hill (in press), 1994.

36. King, W. A., Wackym, P. A., Viñuela, F., et al.: Management of vein of Galen aneurysms: Combined surgical and endovascular approach. Childs Nerv. Syst., 5:208, 1989.

37. Lasjaunias, P., Garcia-Monaco, R., Rodesch, G., et al.: Vein of

38. Lasjaunias, P., Rodesch, G., Pruvost, P., et al.: Treatment of vein of Galen aneurysmal malformation. J. Neurosurg., 70:746, 1989.

Galen malformation: Endovascular management of 43 cases. Childs Nerv. Syst., 7:360, 1991.

39. Lasjaunias, P., Rodesch, G., Terbrugge, K., et al.: Vein of Galen aneurysmal malformations: Report of 36 cases managed between 1982 and 1988. Acta Neurochir. (Wien), 99:26, 1989.

40. Lasjaunias, P., Terbrugge, K., Piske, R., et al.: Vein of Galen dilatation: Anatomo-clinical forms and endovascular treatment. Fourteen cases explored and/or treated between 1983 and 1986. Neurochirurgie, 33:315, 1987.

41. Litvak, J., Yahr, M. D., and Ransohoff, J.: Aneurysms of the great vein of Galen and midline cerebral arteriovenous anomalies. J. Neurosurg., 17:945, 1960.

42. Long, D. M., Seljeskog, E. L., Chou, S. N., et al.: Giant arteriovenous malformations of infancy and childhood. J. Neurosurg., 40:304, 1974.

43. Lylyk, P., Viñuela, F., Dion, J. E., et al.: Therapeutic alternatives for vein of Galen vascular malformations. J. Neurosurg., 78:438, 1993.

44. Martinez-Lage, J. F., Santos, J. M. G., Poza, M., et al.: Prenatal magnetic resonance imaging detection of a vein of Galen aneurysm. Childs Nerv. Syst., 9:377, 1993.

45. Massey, C. E., Carson, L. V., Beveridge, W. D., et al.: Aneurysms of the great vein of Galen: Report of two cases and review of the literature. *In* Smith, R. R., Haerer, A., Russell, W. F., eds.: Vascular Malformations. New York, Raven Press, 1982, pp. 163–179.

46. Menezes, A. H., Graf, C. J., Jacoby, C. G., et al.: Management of vein of Galen aneurysms. J. Neurosurg., 55:457, 1981.

47. Merland, J. J., Laurent, A., Rufenacht, D., et al.: Arteriovenous malformations in the region of Galen's ampulla: Anatomical and clinical aspects and evolution of endovascular therapy 1979–1986. A review of 10 cases. Neurochirurgie, 33:349, 1987.

48. Mickle, J. P., and Quisling, R. G.: The transtorcular embolization of vein of Galen aneurysms. J. Neurosurg., 64:731, 1986.

49. Mickle, J. P., Quisling, R., and Ryan, P.: Transtorcular approach to vein of Galen aneurysms. Pediatr. Neurosurg., 20:163, 1994.

50. Olivecrona, H., and Riives, J.: Arteriovenous aneurysms of the brain: Their diagnosis and treatment. Arch. Neurol. Psychiatry, 59:567, 1948.

51. Olivero, W. C., Rekate, H. L., Ko, W., et al.: Relationship between intracranial and sagittal sinus pressure in normal and hydrocephalic dogs. Pediatr. Neurosci., 14:196, 1988.

52. Oscherwitz, K., and Davidoff, L. M.: Midline calcified intracranial aneurysm between occipital lobes: Report of a case. J. Neurosurg., 4:539, 1947.

53. Pertuiset, B., Ancri, D., Mahdi, M., et al.: A new haemodynamic factor in cerebral AVM: Aspiration from the venous system demonstrated in two cases of pedunculo-Galen AVM successfully cured by occlusion of the superior longitudinal sinus. Acta Neurochir. (Wien), 104:136, 1990.

54. Raimondi, A. J.: Vascular diseases. *In* Raimondi, A. J., ed.: Pediatric Neuroradiology. Philadelphia, W. B. Saunders, 1972, pp. 592–661.

55. Raimondi, A. J., and Cerullo, L. J.: Arteriovenous malformations of the Galenic system. *In* Nadjmi, E., ed.: Pediatric Cerebral Angiography. Stuttgart, Thieme, 1980, pp. 162–169.

56. Raybaud, C. A., Strother, C. M., and Hald, J. K.: Aneurysms of the vein of Galen: Embryonic and anatomical features relating to the pathogenesis of the malformation. Neuroradiology, 31:109, 1989.

57. Rekate, H. L.: Circuit diagram of the circulation of cerebrospinal fluid. Concepts Ped. Neurosurg., 9:46, 1989.

58. Rekate, H. L., Brodkey, J. A., Chizeck, H. J., et al.: Ventricular volume regulation: A mathematical model and computer simulation. Pediatr. Neurosci., 14:77, 1988.

59. Rekate, H. L., Olivero, W. M., McCormick, J., et al.: Resistance elements within the cerebrospinal fluid circulation. *In* Gjerris, F., Borgesen, S. E., Soelberg-Sorensen, P., eds.: Outflow of Cerebrospinal Fluid. Alfred Benzon Symposium 27. Copenhagen, Munksgaard, 1989, pp. 45–52.

60. Rosenberg, E. M., and Nazar, G. B.: Neonatal vein of Galen aneurysms: Severe coagulopathy associated with transtorcular embolization. Crit. Care Med., 19:441, 1991.

61. Sainte-Rose, C., LaCombe, J., Pierre-Kahn, A., et al.: Intracranial

venous sinus hypertension: Cause or consequence of hydrocephalus in infants? J. Neurosurg., *60*:727, 1984.

62. Sanders, R. C.: Prenatal ultrasonic detection of anomalies with a lethal or disastrous outcome. Radiol. Clin. North Am., *28*:163, 1990.

63. Spetzler, R. F., and Martin, N. A.: A proposed grading system for arteriovenous malformations. J. Neurosurg., *65*:476, 1986.

64. Spetzler, R. F., Martin, N. A., Carter, L. P., et al.: Surgical management of large AVM's by staged embolization and operative excision. J. Neurosurg., *67*:17, 1987.

65. Spetzler, R. F., Wilson, C. B., Weinstein, P., et al.: Normal perfusion pressure breakthrough theory. Clin. Neurosurg., *25*:651, 1978.

66. Steinbok, P., Hall, J., and Flodmark, O.: Hydrocephalus in achondroplasia: The possible role of intracranial venous hypertension. J. Neurosurg., *71*:42, 1989.

67. Steinheil, S. O.: Über einen Fall von Varix aneurysmaticus im Bereich der Gehirngefässe; Inaugural Diss., Würzburg 1895. Cited in Dandy, W. E.: Arteriovenous aneurysm of the brain. Arch. Surg., *17*:190, 1928.

68. Viñuela, F., Dion, J. E., Duckwiler, G., et al.: Combined endovascular embolization and surgery in the management of cerebral arteriovenous malformations: Experience with 101 cases. J. Neurosurg., *75*:856, 1991.

69. Viñuela, F., Drake, C. G., Fox, A. J., et al.: Giant intracranial varices secondary to high-flow arteriovenous fistulae. J. Neurosurg., *66*:198, 1987.

70. Westra, S. J., Curran, J. G., Duckwiler, G. R., et al.: Pediatric intracranial vascular malformations: Evaluation of treatment results with color Doppler US. Work in progress. Radiology, *186*:775, 1993.

71. Wisoff, J. H., Berenstein, A., Choi, I. S., et al.: Management of vein of Galen malformations. Concepts Ped. Neurosurg., *10*:137, 1990.

72. Yamashita, Y., Abe, T., Ohara, N., et al.: Successful treatment of neonatal aneurysmal dilatation of the vein of Galen: The role of prenatal diagnosis and trans-arterial embolization. Neuroradiology, *34*:457, 1992.

73. Yasargil, M. G.: Microneurosurgery: IIIB. AVM of the Brain, Clinical Considerations, General and Special Operative Techniques, Surgical Results, Nonoperated Cases, Cavernous and Venous Angiomas, Neuroanesthesia. New York, Thieme, 1988, pp. 323–357.

74. Zerah, M., Garcia-Monaco, R., Rodesch, G., et al.: Hydrodynamics in vein of Galen malformations. Childs Nerv. Syst., *8*:111, 1992.

Arteriovenous Malformations of the Spinal Cord

The first reports on spinal vascular malformations were published in the late 19th century.[16, 29, 59, 60, 67] In 1888, Gaupp described a vascular malformation of the spinal cord with the term "hemorrhoids of the pia mater spinalis."[59] Until the middle of this century, literature on this topic was limited to a few cases.[37] Wyburn-Mason found only 96 cases published in the literature before 1946.[164] Selective and superselective spinal angiography finally made possible a preoperative description of the hemodynamics and the angioarchitecture of spinal vascular malformations. During the past 15 years considerable evidence has emerged indicating that the enigmatically different structures of spinal arteriovenous malformations must be re-evaluated with regard to pathogenesis, classification, and therapy. In 1978, Jellinger summarized the confusing findings of pathological features and listed eight different classifications of the past decades.[76] Kendall and Logue and Merland and associates recognized the disease formerly described as retromedullary angioma to be a fistula.[79, 101] The arteriovenous shunts are found inside the dura of the spinal root, usually in the lumbar region, in the thoracolumbar region, or in the middle to lower thoracic regions.[101, 145] After increasing the use of selective spinal angiography, the majority of all spinal arteriovenous malformations turned out to be these dural arteriovenous fistulae.[40, 42, 43, 45, 48] With the arteriovenous shunt lying in the dura, the so-called dorsal retromedullary angioma represents a dilated medullary vein, draining the fistula blood in a direction retrograde to its normal flow. Interventional techniques and intraoperative flow and pressure measurements not only have proved this new concept to be correct but have also created a different and simple surgical technique and interventional therapeutic regimen.

The intradural perimedullary fistulae could be typed in three categories of size and by therapeutic options of surgical or combined interventional treatment. Their common characteristic feature is being supplied by medullary arteries and draining into medullary veins, with the fistulae lying outside the cord.*

Whereas dural arteriovenous fistulae constitute the majority of all arteriovenous malformations (60 to 80 per cent), they almost never lead to subarachnoid hemorrhage, and perimedullary fistulae (10 to 20 per cent) do so only rarely.[84, 105] Intramedullary angiomas (10 to 20 per cent), as the third type of arteriovenous malformation, are often complicated by subarachnoid hemorrhage and intramedullary hematomas. These are true angiomatous arteriovenous malformations, in which the nidus is located within the spinal cord and is filled by the anterior or the posterolateral spinal artery or both. They are treated by a conjoined interventional and operative neurovascular team and, owing to possible severe postoperative deterioration, may sometimes be handled in only a palliative way. In contrast, dural and perimedullary fistulae should be completely excised or occluded by interventional neuroradiology. In recognition of the results of many neurovascular teams and the authors' own angiographic interventional and intraoperative experience over the past 10 years, the authors believe that the classification presented in Table 65–2 meets the diagnostic and therapeutic features of almost all arteriovenous malformations of the spinal cord.

History and Incidence

Knowledge of the natural development of a sign or symptom presupposes knowledge of its incidence and prevalence in a normal population. Furthermore, the signs or symptoms should be followed throughout life and be unaffected by any therapeutic measures. Before the introduction of selective spinal angiography by

---

*See references 57, 63, 64, 99, 106, 130, and 131.

E. H. Grote • S. Bien

Djindjian, DiChiro, and Doppman in the 1960's and 1970's in vivo diagnosis of the spinal arteriovenous malformation was difficult. Antemortem diagnosis could be made on the basis of the myelographic image only. This method was published for the first time by Perthes in 1926. Before the use of myelography, antemortem diagnosis rested entirely on surmisal and could be confirmed only post mortem. The first publications refer exclusively to postmortem findings. In 1888, Gaupp reported on "hemorrhoids of the pia mater spinalis," probably the first account of a spinal dural fistula.[59] Accordingly, until 1943, Wyburn-Mason discovered no more than 112 published cases of a spinal vascular malformation, including his own 16 cases[164]; in the era of myelography between 1943 and 1962, Yasargil discovered 195 further cases, and again, after the introduction of selective spinal angiography, 151 cases from 1962 until 1970.[166, 168] A "natural history" of all spinal arteriovenous malformations cannot be written on that basis: The asymptomatic malformations were not and still are not recorded in any way. Even the symptomatic arteriovenous malformations had to reveal severe signs and symptoms for angiography to be indicated. The introduction of computed tomography and magnetic resonance imaging (the former in the 1970's, the latter in the 1980's) may have led to the fact that now even slightly symptomatic vascular malformations are discovered. One cannot calculate even approximately, however, the number of asymptomatic spinal vascular malformations occurring during a lifetime in a population. Autopsies are not performed on all individuals in a population group, and even when a postmortem examination is carried out, removal of the spinal cord is not part of the routine proceedings. The number of vascular spinal malformations found by accident has therefore remained very low, and the true prevalence and incidence are almost certainly higher than supposed. In a series of 31 necropsy cases that presented a clinical picture of transverse or diffuse myelitis, 9 cadavers were found to have a vascular malformation with myelomalacia.[30]

There exist many investigations of the relative frequency of vascular causes in diseases of the spinal cord versus tumors (Table 65–1).

There seems to emerge a large margin of variation with regard to the relative frequency that stretches from 2 to 11.5 per cent, without a clear tendency toward higher or lower relative frequency in correlation with chronological order. Yasargil found identical relative frequencies between spinal tumors and spinal vascular malformations, on the one hand, and between cerebral tumors and cerebrovascular malformations, on the other (4.42 and 4.43 per cent).[165] The relative frequency between spinal vascular malformations and cerebrovascular malformations was indicated as one in four, one in six, and one in eight, so that Berenstein and Lasjaunias suggested that the frequency of spinal cord arteriovenous malformations compared with brain arteriovenous malformations correlates with the mass or volume ratio between spinal cord and brain tissue.[18, 20, 76, 91]

Theoretically, there are various means by which a

Table 65–1

RELATIVE FREQUENCY OF VASCULAR CAUSES OF SPINAL CORD DISEASE VS. TUMORS

Source (Year)	No. of Tumors	% Arteriovenous Malformation
Rasmusen, et al. (1940)[123]	557	5.0
Nittner and Tönnis (1950)[111]	104	6.7
Newman (1935–1945)[109]	102	2.0
Newman (1946–1956)[109]	121	11.5
Klug (1958)[82]	148	3.4
Umbach (1962)[155]	192	7.0
Krayenbühl and Yasargil, (1963)[84]	568	3.3
Pia and Vogelsang (1965)[119]	161	8.0
Krayenbühl, et al.(1969)[85]	961	4.42

Data from Yasargil, M. G.: Surgery of vascular lesions of the spinal cord with the microsurgical technique. Clin. Neurosurg., 17:257, 1970; and Yasargil, M. G.: Diagnosis and treatment of spinal cord arteriovenous malformations. Prog. Neurochir., 4:355, 1971.

vascular arteriovenous malformation may become symptomatic:

1. It may bleed.
2. Because of its low flow resistance it may overstrain the transport capability of the artery and cause ischemic damage of the tissue fed by the same vessel.
3. Because of its dilated vessels it may have a crowding effect on its surroundings.
4. Because of its arteriovenous shunt volume it may overstrain the draining passages and cause venous congestion in the tissue that depends on the same draining ducts as does the arteriovenous malformation.

On the basis of these considerations, different clinical types of development of vascular malformations can be expected: (1) apoplectiform with hemorrhages and incomplete neurological reversal in case of destroyed parenchyma and (2) chronic or rapidly progressive with increasing ischemia or spatial extension.

These types of development can be confirmed in the literature. Aminoff and associates found in their group of patients a predominantly chronic progressive development, whereas Djindjian and co-workers described more frequently an apoplectiform course.[3, 5, 6, 48] This discrepancy may be explained by the makeup of their respective groups of patients: Aminoff and associates' group consisted for the most part of older men. Therefore, the share of dural fistulae, which as a rule do not bleed and are found predominantly in older men, was probably greater. Djindjian and co-workers had a younger group of patients, so in their cases the share of intramedullary arteriovenous malformations, which become symptomatic earlier and especially so by hemorrhage, was probably greater.

In a group of 60 patients who were not treated, Aminoff and Logue found a hemorrhage in 10 per cent.[5, 6] In addition, two clearly distinguishable types of development emerged: In 19 per cent of the patients there were grave disturbances of motor functions within 6 months after the onset of signs and symptoms (rapid progression), whereas in the other patients a markedly slower progression was observed (with

Table 65–2

FORMS OF PROGRESSION FOR PARTICULAR VASCULAR MALFORMATIONS

Malformation*	Onset	Development	Subarachnoid Hemorrhage	Predominant Localization	Feeding and Draining Vessels
A. Dural arteriovenous fistula	≥age 40	Chronic (rapid) progressive +/− acute deterioration	Seldom	Dorsolumbar Dorsal	Radicular arteries shunting in spinal veins of the dura of spinal root; small fistular region
B. Perimedullary fistula Type 1	Between ages 20 and 40	Rapidly progressive	Occasionally	Dorsolumbar Dorsal Rarely cervical	Spinal arteries are shunting in spinal veins intradurally and extramedullarily
Type 2 Type 3 C. Intramedullary arteriovenous malformation	Childhood; early adulthood	Lengthy progression; improvements alternate with acute deterioration	Often	Lumbar Dorsal Cervical	Spinal arteries feed an intramedullary arteriovenous malformation, draining into spinal veins intradurally and intramedullarily

*For the angioarchitecture of the following malformations, see Table 65–3.

grave motor disturbances after 3 years in 50 per cent); the remaining 50 per cent showed only a very slow progression or no progression at all in their disturbances. During the time of follow-up observation, 20 of 60 patients died. Only in three cases was the cause of death independent of the spinal vascular malformation; nine patients died of secondary complications of their paraparesis, and one patient died of a subarachnoid hemorrhage. In more than one third (7 of 20) the cause was related to the malformation but was not specified. Therefore, the number of deleterious progressions may possibly be higher than the proven mortality of 10 of 60 within a follow-up period of 8 years on average. An attribution of the different forms of progression to the classification of vascular malformations now in use could not be made. However, different forms of progression for the particular vascular malformations (e.g., spinal dural fistula, intramedullary arteriovenous malformation, perimedullary arteriovenous fistula) are now proved to a large extent (Table 65–2). However, the tendency toward progressive deterioration in the course of time is unmistakable. Only the amount of time that leads to severe disability is different for the particular groups of spinal vascular malformations. Diagnosis and therapy must take place as early as possible because the chances of recovery after therapy are clearly linked to the duration of the signs and symptoms and to the gravity of the disturbances before treatment.

Classification

Table 65–3 gives an overview of the arteriovenous malformations of the spinal canal with their relative

Table 65–3

ARTERIOVENOUS MALFORMATIONS OF THE SPINAL CORD: ANGIOARCHITECTURE, INCIDENCE, AND TREATMENT

Angioarchitecture	Therapy	Frequency (%)
A. Slow-flowing, slightly dilated radicular artery, with no participation of spinal arteries, draining into slightly dilated spinal veins; low blood flow velocity	Embolization with glue/operation	50–80
B. Simple, small arteriovenous fistula; one long, thin, slightly dilated spinal artery; slow blood flow velocity; one small, slightly dilated spinal vein	Operation (embolization)	
Middle-sized arteriovenous fistula with one or occasionally two supplying arteries, which are clearly dilated; distinctly increased blood flow velocity in the arteries and veins; venous pouch in the shunt region	Operation/embolization with particles	10–15
Giant arteriovenous fistula with multiple, large-caliber supplying arteries; high to very high blood flow velocity; very strongly dilated veins	Balloon embolization	
C. Spinal arteries (several) supply a nidus located in the spinal cord itself; supply through the anterior spinal artery, posterolateral spinal artery, or both; high blood velocity; drainage through spinal cord veins	Embolization/operation	15–40

incidence, their angioarchitecture, and the therapeutic options. Vascular malformations of a nonarteriovenous kind are the rare cavernomas and the isolated aneurysms of the spinal arteries or those that are associated with an arteriovenous malformation. The metameric combination of an intramedullary arteriovenous malformation with other vascular malformations was described by Cobb in 1915 and named after him.[34]

A comparable classification with a division into four types is proposed by Anson and Spetzler.[8] Their type I malformation corresponds to the dural arteriovenous fistula, their types II and III to the intramedullary malformation, and their type IV to the perimedullary fistulae (type IV-A to small type 1, type IV-B to type 2 medium-sized, and type IV-C to type 3 gigantic perimedullary fistulae).

DURAL ARTERIOVENOUS FISTULAE

Etiology and Anatomy

It is generally believed that dural arteriovenous fistulae are acquired lesions (Fig. 65–1). In cranial fistulae, recanalizations of a thrombosed sinus are widely accepted as pathogenetic mechanisms.[2, 4, 44, 75, 114] Whether an analogous conclusion is justified for the spinal location is not known.

Massive dilatation of the medullary vein may extend from the thoracolumbar region down to the sacral sac and up to the intracranial cavity.[12, 39] The main location is dorsal and retromedullary; normal veins draining the cord empty into these cavities. It was not recognized for a long time that this strongly dilated vein simply serves as a draining duct to a small fistula situated in the dura of the spinal root and that the signs and symptoms can be attributed mainly to the voluminal overstrain coming to bear on this vein and subsequent venous hypertension in the spinal cord. Pathophysiological notions and terminology were accordingly diffuse, including hemangioma of the pia mater, angioma venosum racemosum, the single coiled vessel malformation, retromedullary angioma, and long dorsal arteriovenous malformation.[43, 46, 79, 136, 164] The therapeutic consequence—removal of the dilated vein—did not lead to a durable improvement but worsened the venous draining situation for the spinal cord.[93]

Pathology and Pathophysiology

Selective spinal angiography showed that the arteriovenous communication (nidus) is usually situated in the dura in the intervertebral foramen. One or more small branches of a radicular artery supply the nidus (see Fig. 65–1B). No medullary arteries participate in supplying the fistula. The fistula is fed by thoracic or lumbar radicular arteries, which supply the segmental dura and the roots. However, the blood supply may also come from sacral or hypogastric arteries.* Also

described were cervical and intracranial fistulae (Fig. 65–2) with perimedullary venous draining and one case of a myelopathy due to large veins draining a carotidocavernous fistula.*

Flow velocities in the fistula-feeding vessels are low, and the supplying arteries are small. The authors have noted only one region of arteriovenous shunting, mostly fed by the adjacent-level radicular arteries. There have been two cases in the literature with two different fistulae fed by two different intercostal arteries.[122] In some cases, dural enlarged arteries from the next level below or above or the contralateral side contributed to the fistula. The arteries drain into intrathecal vessels that continue into portions of the subarachnoid plexus. Although the feeders have no significant caliber, the shunt volume leads to a considerable dilatation and arterialization of the perimedullary coronary plexus. The impression and misinterpretation that all these dilated veins were angiomas led to previous attempts to excise them over a great length after multiple-level laminectomy with the consequence of possible clinical deterioration. The draining of the fistula is affected by slow-flowing medullary veins, ascending or descending for long distances; occasionally, slow-flowing, dilated veins can be detected running from the lumbar fistula to the occipital foramen and, in rare cases, even to the posterior cranial fossa, or from an intracranial fistula (see Fig. 65–2) to the lumbar region.

The clinical findings in arteriovenous fistulae— slowly increasing myelopathy combined with signs and symptoms of lower neuron deficits—are caused by chronically increased venous pressure. The coronary plexus receives arterialized blood from the vein draining the dural shunt. This leads to an increased venous pressure, causing a reduced arteriovenous pressure gradient, intramedullary vasodilatation with exhaustion of autoregulation and chronic impairment by arterial pulsation, and hypoxic damage.[7, 43, 133, 145, 147] Because the arteriovenous shunts are located in the dura itself, subarachnoid hemorrhage is only very rarely a part of the clinical phenomena of the disease.

Compression effects from dilated vessels, steal phenomena, arachnoiditis, and subarachnoidal hemorrhages are pathophysiologically relevant in intramedullary arteriovenous malformations, but not in patients with spinal dural arteriovenous fistulae.†

Clinical Features

In 1926, Foix and Alajouanine described a syndrome that was designated as subacute necrotizing myelitis.[57] A 29-year-old man with a dural fistula diagnosed within 2½ years after the onset of the signs and symptoms died of the secondary effects of flaccid and complete paraplegia. In accordance with the almost pathognomonic description, the authors believe that this necrotizing myelitis was a spinal dural fistula.[37, 119, 152, 162] The majority of affected patients are in their fifth to

---

*See references 15, 23, 32, 45, 70, 121, and 144.

*See references 21, 33, 58, 62, 105, 108, 113, 120, 161, and 163.
†See references 68, 78, 85, 94, 109, 133, and 147.

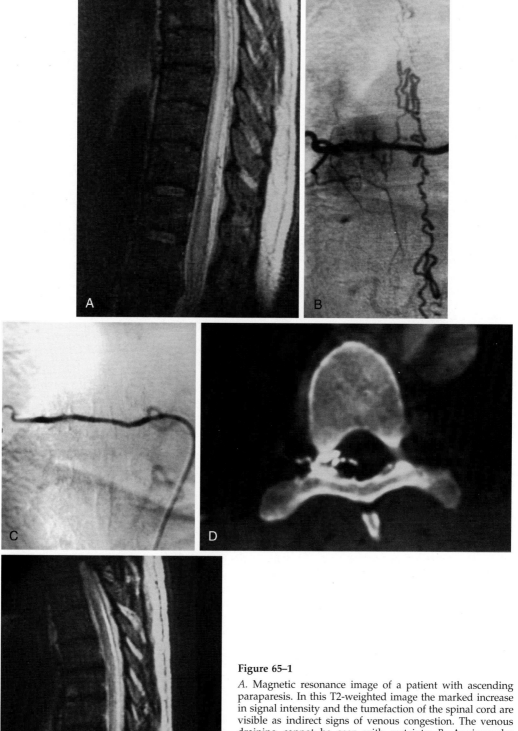

Figure 65–1

A. Magnetic resonance image of a patient with ascending paraparesis. In this T2-weighted image the marked increase in signal intensity and the tumefaction of the spinal cord are visible as indirect signs of venous congestion. The venous draining cannot be seen with certainty. *B.* Angiography shows a spinal dural fistula branching off the intercostal artery (D9 left). *C.* Control angiography after endovascular occlusion of the fistula with Histoacryl no longer shows any fistula shunts. *D.* On computed tomography 2 days after embolization, the embolization material is found in the region of the fistula at the dura of the root. *E.* One week after embolization the T2-weighted magnetic resonance image shows an almost complete reversal of the pretherapeutic increase in signal intensity.

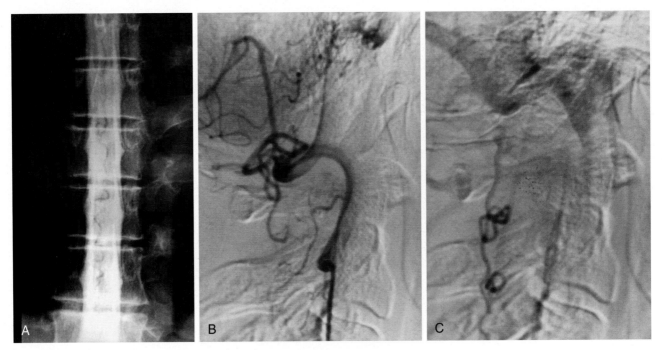

Figure 65–2

A. Typical myelogram of a vascular malformation. In the lower thoracic region there are some vessels with a winding course. Clinically, the patient had progressive ascending paraparesis. The spinal panangiography could not supply the proof of the suspected spinal dural fistula. *B.* Angiography of the left vertebral artery shows an intracranial dural fistula with very slow draining in the direction of the perimedullary zone. *C.* Only 10 seconds later the perimedullary draining in the cervical subarachnoid region became visible. The dorsolumbar vessels visualized in the myelogram became visible in the angiogram only about 40 seconds after the beginning of the injection.

seventh decades. Males are affected much more frequently than females in a ratio of five to one.[18] In most of the patients, past history reveals a duration of signs and symptoms of less than 2 to 3 years. The initial symptoms are typically back pain, leg numbness, and muscle weakness. Disturbance of bladder and bowel function is an uncommon initial symptom, but it is usually found at the time of diagnosis.[68, 107, 145] The symptoms and signs of dural arteriovenous fistulae are gradual in onset and progress slowly; rarely, serious symptoms and signs may occur within days, owing to thrombotic phenomena. The characteristic clinical course shows the development of a progressive myelopathy with combined sensory, motor, and sphincter disturbances. By the time of admission and diagnosis some degree of leg weakness and pyramidal signs are almost always present. An increase in tone in the lower limbs occurs as a first sign, followed by flaccid paresis (involvement of both upper and lower motor neurons).[83]

Other frequent findings are sensory disturbances, particularly in the buttocks and saddle area (caused by dorsal column impairment), as well as pronounced gait disturbance, sensory transverse lesions, and sphincter disturbances. Impairment of joint position sense and loss of vibration sense are further findings. The mixed picture of medullary, conal, and peripheral involvement is nearly pathognomonic and should lead to the diagnosis. Clinical findings are typically referred to the lumbar and sacral region despite varying localizations of the level of the nidus. One case of thoracic signs

and symptoms has been reported, however, initially presenting as pseudocoronary pain.

Investigations

Magnetic Resonance Imaging. Magnetic resonance imaging increasingly tends to replace myelography in the study of spinal cord diseases. In the case of dural arteriovenous fistulae, visualization of dilated spinal veins is possible but difficult, owing to the only slightly dilated vessels. The fistula itself cannot be visualized. The main information provided by this method is an increased intramedullary signal in T2-weighted images, reflecting the edema due to chronic venous hypertension (see Fig. 65–1).[95, 148] In most patients a long, serpiginous area of low signal was demonstrated intradurally but outside the medulla, owing to signal void in the draining vein.[41, 55, 95, 148]

Myelography. Despite the increase in the use of magnetic resonance imaging, myelography remains the primary diagnostic technique for vascular malformations and diseases of the spinal cord in many centers. In 1926, Perthes was the first to diagnose preoperatively a vascular spinal malformation by myelography.[116] Some reports have shown the detectability of vascular structures even with gas myelography.[89] A decisive improvement in partial resolution and detectability of even fine vascular structures was brought on by the introduction of contrast-enhanced myelography in the 1970's.[158] With the help of images obtained with good filling with contrast medium there now can be detected vascular structures of such small caliber that distinguishing normal vessels from pathologically dilated vessels feeding or draining an angioma or fistula can become difficult (Fig. 65–3; see also Fig. 65–2A). In 1983, Thron and associates found plainly recognizable vascular blanks in one third of their patients who underwent myelography not because of a vascular disease.[151] In another third, they found less clearly demonstrable vascular images, and only one third of the myelograms showed no vascular structures at all. On the other hand, even in the case of a detected spinal dural fistula the myelographic findings may be only minimally altered in a pathological sense with slightly dilated vessels or may even be normal. Terwey and co-workers studied 11 patients and found two instances of normal myelographic conditions and two instances of only minimally dilated vessels; in seven myelograms the dilatation of the thoracolumbar vessels was distinct.[148] Spinal angiography is therefore indicated in the case of all unclear vascular alterations on myelography, especially since spinal angiography performed by an experienced neuroradiologist entails low risk and avoids the possible serious consequences of an unrecognized dural fistula.

Spinal Angiography. Selective spinal angiography is the only way of diagnosing and localizing the nidus in dural fistulae. It requires detailed catheterization of thoracic and lumbar arteries. If angiographic results are routinely negative but there is a strong clinical suggestion of a fistula, it may be necessary to extend the investigation to the vertebral, the external carotid, or the sacral arteries. In the case of distinct clinical findings and a myelogram if all these arteries do not

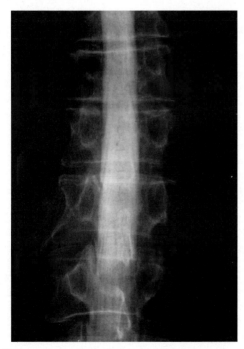

Figure 65–3

Normal vessels on myelography performed in a patient with lumbar disc disease. The panangiography carried out for clarification of the myelographic findings revealed no vascular malformation.

show a fistula, one should think of venous spinal hypertension due to tumor compression, of a congenital anomaly, or of an obstruction of the vena cava.[1, 28, 150]

The angiographic findings in cases of spinal dural arteriovenous fistulae usually show one or more small branches of radicular arteries in the region of an intervertebral foramen. The arterial branches merge into the nidus and drain into the subarachnoid coronary plexus through an intrathecally directed vessel. Physiologically, radiculomeningeal arteries cannot be displayed. If they are feeding vessels of a dural fistula of small caliber, their shunt leads to considerable filling of the draining veins (see Fig. 65–1B). In the past, this aspect of dilated and red veins led to misinterpretation as well as to false treatment.

Owing to the shunt volume, filling of draining veins ranges from very slow to fast. Even in the case of a higher shunt volume the venous system fills relatively slowly over quite a distance. In these cases, digital subtraction angiography is very helpful in demonstrating slow venous filling, starting in some cases as late as 10 seconds after displaying of radicular arteries; the diagnosis may be missed on normally timed film sequences.

Treatment

Possible treatments are surgical excision of the shunt or selective embolization of the fistula. The objective of every therapy must be lasting relief from the shunt volume generated by the arteriovenous fistula.

Surgical Technique

Direct surgical management provides simple and successful treatment of spinal dural arteriovenous fistulae.[104, 107, 133, 145] The aim of the surgical intervention is to excise the fistula. Preoperatively, patients with large neurological deficits that indicate progressive ischemia may receive dexamethasone at the standard dosage.

For correct intraoperative localization, accurate spinal marking should be performed when the fistula is displayed. Intraoperatively, exposure of the fistula may be achieved by hemilaminectomy or laminectomy and, if required, foraminotomy. After the dura is opened, it should be possible to demonstrate the enlarged vein originating in the dural layer near the nerve root (Fig. 65–4) and draining into the coronary venous plexus. Coagulation of abnormal vascular structures on the dural layer or excision of the whole area of abnormality or both may be done.

Sectioning of the draining vein alone, leaving the nidus in place, has been suggested. The authors believe that this may leave the chance for a reopening of the shunt. Stripping the whole length of the coiled perimedullary arterialized veins by division of adherent pia-arachnoid and interruption of venous draining vessels may lead to postoperative deterioration of neurological deficits, because these venous vessels drain the cord as well. The enlarged arterialized vessels are secondary and therefore treated correctly with interruption only of the fistula itself. After excision of the fistula, in contrast with the case of cerebral angiomas,

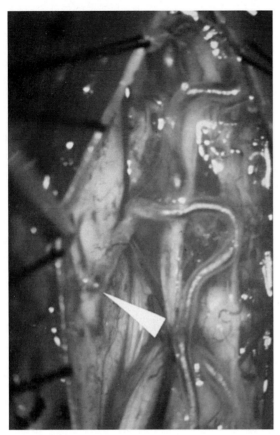

Figure 65–4

Dural arteriovenous fistula shown intraoperatively demonstrates nidus in the dura and beginning of a draining vein and dilatation of the dorsal vein.

it usually takes some minutes for the enlarged veins to turn from red to dark blue.

Intraoperative flow measurements with Doppler ultrasound[112] and direct intravascular pressure measurements have confirmed different flow characteristics of dural arteriovenous fistulae and dependence of venous blood flow on systemic arterial blood pressure.[68] Flow velocities in arteries feeding dural fistulae are much higher than those in arteries supplying the spinal cord. End-diastolic flow velocity depends on stream resistance and is therefore an indicator of the shunt volume (low resistance with high end-diastolic flow in high-flow fistulae, and vice versa). Because of increasing distance from the fistula and enlargement of the draining vessel, the flow velocity decreases. Correlating with the clinical finding of deterioration of neurological deficits by physical activity, systemic intraoperative hypertension was demonstrated to result in reduced spinal cord circulation, indicated by increased intravenous pressure.[68]

The intraoperative study of Hassler, Thron, and Grote proved convincingly the concept of the nidus in the dura.[68] The pressure in the draining vein was found to be 60 to 70 per cent of the systemic arterial blood pressure. This explains the sometimes-occurring formation of venous aneurysms. This high venous pressure dropped considerably after interruption from the nidus

(Fig. 65–5). Measurements clearly demonstrate the different flow characteristics of feeder, fistula, and draining vein and show circulation resistance and carbon dioxide reactivity of the medullary arteries to be normal (Fig. 65–6). Flow in the dilated veins was stagnating and undetectable after shunt interruption, so the veins stayed red and well filled for quite a time, indicating some outflow resistance, as usually noted on preoperative angiography as well.

Thrombosis may occur and probably is the cause of transient postoperative deterioration. As a consequence, low-dose heparin should be given.

The operation is simple and safe, and problems are solved permanently.[68] After nidus resection, reopening cannot occur, and operation under microsurgical conditions can certainly visualize and save the small cord-supplying arteries sometimes running parallel to the feeders.

Interventional Therapy

As an alternative to surgical therapy, injection of Histoacryl (enbucrilate) can be done after superselective catheterization of the radicular artery. If the occlusion of the fistula is attained endovascularly with definitive embolization material, an operation is not necessary. If the occlusion does not succeed completely, removal of the partially embolized fistula has to be performed. According to the most extensive series, endovascular occlusion was successful in about two thirds of the cases (40 of 63), whereas in 23 cases embolization was not complete or could not be done at all owing to catheterization problems in four instances as well as inflows into the anterior spinal artery.[107]

The actual procedure of the authors consists in having the patient undergo spinal angiography in the search for clinical evidence of a dural fistula. Such evidence can also be obtained based on computed tomography, magnetic resonance imaging, or myelography. Before the angiography, the patient is informed of the possibility of embolization. If the spinal angiography confirms the existence of the suspected dural arteriovenous fistula, embolization with Histoacryl is carried out in the same session after superselective catheterization (see Fig. 65–1C). The Histoacryl has to be diluted with Lipiodol (iodized oil) and injected in such a way as to occlude the starting segment of the radicular veins, the region of the shunt, and the final part of the artery (see Fig. 65–1D). The ascending, draining perimedullary vein must not be occluded. If this succeeds, the patient will undergo control angiography between 6 and 12 months later. If the occlusion is stable and no signs of revascularization or recanalization of the fistula or of venous arterialization are found, the patient will be followed clinically. Then, if there is no evidence of deterioration, further angiography is not necessary. If embolization succeeds only partially or not at all, or if it is contraindicated because of a spinal artery coming from the same level, the patient is scheduled for microsurgical intervention.

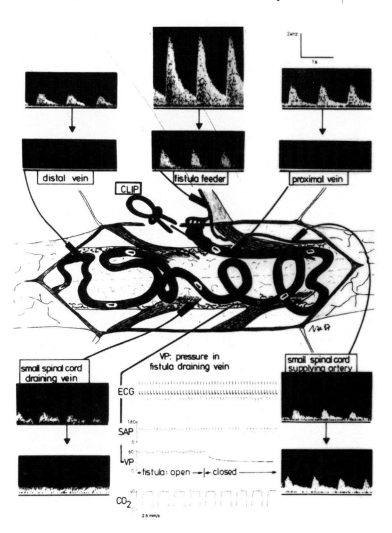

Figure 65–5

Flow velocities and pressure recorded before and after shunt occlusion in a low-flow fistula and in vessels supplying the spinal cord. In this case, a branch of the fistula feeder supplied the spinal cord as well. After fistula occlusion, no further flow was detectable in the draining vein and the flow velocity of the vessels supplying and draining the spinal cord increased. The pressure in the draining vein (VP) dropped from 56 to 24 mm Hg. ECG, electrocardiogram; SAP, systemic arterial pressure. (From Hassler, W., Thron, A., and Grote, E. H.: Hemodynamics of spinal dural arteriovenous fistulas. J. Neurosurg., 70:360–370, 1989.)

Results of Operation

Postoperative improvement of patients with neurological deficits depends on preoperative duration of signs and symptoms and on the degree of disability. The improvement involves the sensory and motor deficits. The genitosphincteric disturbances have a much more severe prognosis and persist more often.

Because of progressive ischemic lesions of the spinal cord caused by chronic venous congestion, the shunt should be eliminated as early as possible. In 65 per cent of severely disabled and 80 per cent of moderately disabled patients an appreciable improvement in gait disturbance has been reported.[145]

A total of 7 of 50 patients in the series of Symon and 1 of 30 in the series of Mourier showed some moderate and transient neurological deterioration after operation, presumably because of the thrombosis in the stagnating veins, which also drain the cord.[107, 145] This improvement may be due to the reduced blood flow in the veins after disconnecting the fistula. The upright position of the standing patient may accentuate this problem. If the patient begins to show deterioration of the neurological deficit that is not due to the operative procedure, the authors administer a full dose of heparin and recommend bed rest for several days.

Results of Interventional Therapy

Because of the slowly progressive development of signs and symptoms that remains clinically nonspecific over a long period of time, many patients are late in getting angiographic diagnosis and adequate therapy. The results of late therapy are in accordance with this: By shutting off the veins from the high load of arterialized volume, a standstill of the syndrome can always be achieved. Frequently, there still is an improvement in the motor disturbances and deep sensory function. In contrast, superficial sensation and pre-existing sphincter problems remained, or improvement was late and insufficient.[13, 18, 100] Spectacular improvements after treatment are possible but remain exceptions, especially if treatment occurred late and the disturbances were severe.[13, 37, 83, 107, 145]

The following results have been found in the more extensive endovascular series: Embolization was possible in 29 of 31 patients, and in 2 patients embolization was contraindicated because influx into the anterior spinal artery or the posterolateral artery depended on the same intercostal artery.[18] Of the patients who underwent embolization, 4 experienced interventional failure with subsequent surgery, whereas in 25 patients (81 per cent) a complete anatomical occlusion was ob-

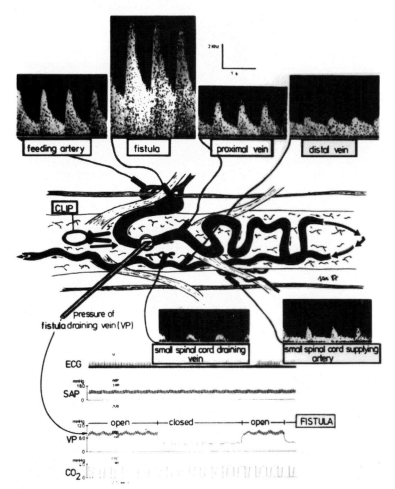

Figure 65–6

Flow velocities and pressure in a moderate-flow arteriovenous fistula system and in normal vessels supplying and draining the spinal cord. At the site of maximum pressure drop (fistula) the flow velocity was very high. In the large-diameter draining vein the flow velocity was low. With increasing distance from the fistula the flow velocity in the draining veins decreases. The small radicular arteries supplying the spinal cord show a typical flow pattern, with valve-closure incisura after the systolic peak. The small draining veins on the surface of the spinal cord have the characteristic half-moon–shaped flow spectra only during systole. After occlusion of the fistula the mean venous pressure (VP) in the draining vein dropped from 78 to 35 mm Hg. ECG, electrocardiogram; SAP, systemic arterial pressure; ABP, arterial blood pressure; ZVD, central venous pressure. (From Hassler, W., Thron, A., and Grote, E. H.: Hemodynamics of spinal dural arteriovenous fistulas. J. Neurosurg., *70*:360–370, 1989.)

tained. Of the 29 patients who were treated with embolization, 24 patients (83 per cent) improved; complications were not observed. In 1989, Mourier and colleagues reported on 70 patients, 40 of whom were treated endovascularly and 30 of whom had surgery.[107] Surgery was performed whenever embolization was contraindicated (7 patients) or inefficient (23 patients). An improvement in clinical condition could be observed in 50 per cent of the patients, but a complete recovery was not observed in any of the cases. In this series the results of embolization are comparable to the results of operation. Comparable results between endovascular therapy and surgical treatment of spinal dural fistulae were also reported by Barth and colleagues in 1984.[13] They point out, in particular, that greater improvement in the clinical condition occurred when treatment was instituted early.

Morgan and Marsh showed in patients at the Mayo Clinic that with an increasing distance from the first embolization more and more patients are in need of further therapy, be it surgical or endovascular.[104] They proved the regularly observable revascularization that occurs after endovascular therapy of spinal dural fistulae with polyvinyl alcohol or collagen. The observation that early clinical improvement is not lasting correlates well with the observation in angiography of a nondurable treatment of the fistula. Just as in other arteriovenous diseases, embolization with particles has been revealed not to be appropriate and should no longer be done. Revascularization of a dural fistula occluded in the arteriovenous shunt with polymerizing embolization materials has not yet been described.

Analytical assessment of the results published earlier is difficult because many dural fistulae were subsumed into the group of arteriovenous malformations. Because of the misunderstanding of its angioarchitecture, the draining vein was removed and not the fistula itself. The operation is technically simple: removal of the fistular region succeeds after hemilaminectomy because of precise angiographic localization. Arrest of the progression of the disease after removal of the fistula can be attained in more than 90 per cent of the cases. The speed and the degree of postoperative improvement in patients with neurological disturbances depend on the duration and the severity of the preoperative damages. A complete recovery can only rarely be obtained or may never be achieved. Deaths due to operation have not been reported.

PERIMEDULLARY FISTULAE

Perimedullary fistulae are arteriovenous short circuits situated ventrally or dorsally on the spinal cord.

They are usually thoracolumbar, occasionally thoracic, and rarely cervical and are characterized by a single shunt without a nidus between the spinal artery and the spinal vein.[100, 102, 128] In contrast with dural fistulae, they are located intradurally but extramedullarily. They are always supplied by spinal vessels, either by the anterior spinal artery or the posterolateral artery. The drainage is effected by very far-ascending spinal veins up to the craniocervical shunts and even into the posterior cranial fossa. These fistulae were described for the first time by Djindjian and associates in 1977.[51]

Perimedullary fistulae become symptomatic in early to middle adulthood as rapidly progressing ascending sensory and motor disturbances accompanied by disorders of the sphincter. Since they are situated intradurally, spinal subarachnoid hemorrhage is also one of the occasionally occurring signs. In most cases many years elapse between the onset of the symptoms and diagnosis and therapy.[106, 130, 131]

According to size, quantity of flow, and venous drainage, Merland and his group distinguished three types of perimedullary fistulae.* The type 1 perimedullary fistula is a simple, small arteriovenous fistula fed by a long, thin anterior spinal artery or posterolateral artery that is only minimally dilated. The mass of the fistula is small, as well as the flow velocity in the artery and the vein. Accordingly, the dilatation of the draining vein is insignificant. Since the feeding arteries are spinal vessels, embolization has to be carried out as close as possible to the aperture of the fistula. As a rule, this is not possible with the long and only minimally dilated arterial influxes of the type 1 perimedullary fistulae, so if the fistula is operatively accessible surgical elimination is the therapy of choice. Only in the case of ventrally situated type 1 perimedullary fistulae should embolization with particles be tried.

The type 2 perimedullary fistula is an arteriovenous fistula of medium size that is fed by one or two adductive arteries that are already clearly dilated. There is a distinctly increased flow; the fistula has a venous dilatation in the shunt region; the draining veins are clearly dilated and winding (Fig. 65–7A). If this fistula is situated dorsally and consequently is accessible to operation, surgical clipping and endovascular therapy (see Fig. 65–7B and C) are of equal efficacy, whereas the fistulae that are not operative have to be given over to an exclusively endovascular therapy. As a rule, the angioarchitecture of these middle-sized fistulae renders possible catheterization with microcatheters, so particles can be introduced far distally, immediately before the arteriovenous fistula. For embolization by balloon the diameter of the fistula is too small, just as the flow velocity is too slow.

The type 3 perimedullary fistula is a giant arteriovenous fistula with multiple feeding arteries of large caliber and high to very high flow, with very large shunt volume, and, accordingly, strongly dilated multiple veins of a winding course. Here, the therapy of choice is catheterization of the fistulae with a balloon catheter and their selective occlusion by balloon.[106, 129–131] Owing to the large number of vessels and the high flow, surgical alternatives for the most part do not exist.

INTRAMEDULLARY ARTERIOVENOUS MALFORMATIONS

Arteriovenous malformation of the spinal cord being rare, true intramedullary malformations form the smallest group. They are regarded as congenital, and children and young adults often become symptomatic because of subarachnoid hemorrhage and transverse lesions caused by hematomas. However, slow progression and regression of signs and symptoms are not unusual. Signs and symptoms occur not only because of hematoma and steal, as well as hypoxia, but also from the space-occupying lesion. These malformations can be found at any level of the spinal cord.

Clinical Features

In contrast with dural fistulae, intradural arteriovenous malformations have no significant male predominance. The first symptoms and signs occur in early adulthood or even earlier.[127] Berenstein and Lasjaunias found that in more than 50 per cent of the patients initial symptoms are present before the age of 16.[18] Symptoms and signs may be due to a hemorrhage (either subarachnoid or in the cord itself), to an arterial steal, or to the space-occupying nidus or vein.[153] Therefore, the symptoms and signs can be apoplectiform or progressive. In about one third of the patients with intramedullary arteriovenous malformations, hemorrhage is the first sign; in one half it is present at diagnosis.

Investigations

Magnetic Resonance Imaging. Only a few reports of magnetic resonance imaging of real intramedullary arteriovenous malformations have been published.* There is a typical appearance of these vascular lesions on magnetic resonance imaging. Because of the intramedullary location, a localized dilatation of the spinal cord can be demonstrated. The feeding and draining vessels appear as low-signal, round, long, and serpiginous structures because of signal void (high blood flow velocity) (Fig. 65–8). In coronal sections they appear as serpentine filling defects within the high signal of cerebrospinal fluid in T2-weighted images.[55] In high field magnetic resonance imaging studies, sometimes a surrounding area of low signal on T1- and T2-weighted images can be demonstrated. This picture corresponds to hemosiderin deposits as a residual finding after previous hemorrhages. In cases with venous hypertension, the signal of the spinal cord can be similar to that in cases with dural fistulae: hyposignal in T1-weighted images, hypersignal in T2-weighted images, and enlargement of the spinal cord due to the edema. Also, the complications of the arteriovenous malformations

---

*See references 51, 63, 64, 99, 106, 130, and 131.

*See references 9, 41, 55, 56, 86, and 103

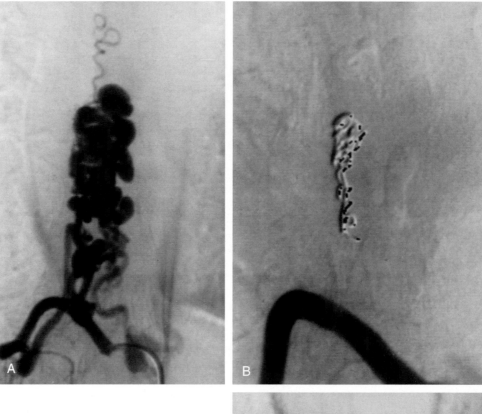

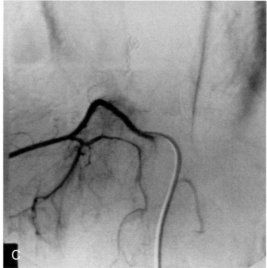

Figure 65–7

A. Perimedullary fistula type 2. Angiogram of the intercostal artery (D9). A distinctly dilated posterolateral artery is visualized that supplies a fistula dorsal to the spinal cord. *B.* After superselective catheterization, several coils were inserted for flow reduction; then the fistula was embolized with 1 mL of absolute alcohol. The control angiography reveals the complete occlusion of the fistula. *C.* Control angiography 1 year after endovascular therapy. In accordance with the clinically complete recovery from the pretherapeutically paraparetic syndrome there was a complete occlusion of the fistula.

could clearly be demonstrated[56]: a central cavity after operation, an extramedullary hematoma, spinal cord atrophy, and metameric lesions in Cobb's syndrome.

Magnetic resonance imaging is the only investigation that shows the arteriovenous malformation with its feeding and draining vessels and the spinal cord with its reactions (edema, hematoma) as well as the surrounding structures with their possible participation (metameric angiomatosis). Nevertheless, selective and superselective angiography is necessary before any treatment. Myelography may be replaced by magnetic resonance imaging, especially in the follow-up investigation after treatment.

Myelography. The typical appearance of dilated vessels and the problems in the differentiation of slightly dilated vessels from normal vessels have been described in earlier discussions of myelography. In cases of arteriovenous malformations, a "swelling" of the spinal cord can be seen caused by the intramedullary, space-occupying malformation or intramedullary hematomas (Fig. 65–9*A*).

Angiography. Despite the increased use of magnetic resonance imaging and its advantages in diagnosing an arteriovenous malformation, any patient should have a complete angiographic study before any treatment. Angiography is needed to determine the number and localization of the feeding arteries and associated or flow-related aneurysms, the extent and localization of the nidus, the localization and number of the draining veins (see Fig. 65–9*B* and *C*), whether there are anasto-

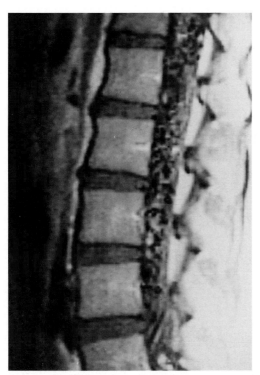

Figure 65–8

Magnetic resonance image of a large intramedullary arteriovenous malformation (see text).

moses to the normal spinal cord vessels, and the arterial supply of the spinal cord. Spinal angiography done by an experienced neuroradiologist, performed with nonionic contrast material, has a low risk of side effects.

Treatment

Interventional Therapy

Endovascular therapy for intramedullary arteriovenous malformations has been carried out as an alternative to surgical removal since the 1960's.* For endovascular occlusion of the arteriovenous malformation, particulate as well as liquid embolization materials have been used. Criscuolo and Rothbart have found 11 different embolization materials reported in the literature.[37] They can be reduced to two different embolization materials and to two different strategies. The representatives of the particulate embolization materials attain, by embolization, a reduction in the quantity of flow through the malformation. This method entails a reduction of steal and a lower ischemic risk for the spinal cord. The veins are relieved, and the consequences of the venous hypertension may recede. The risk of hemorrhage can be reduced or eliminated by these measures. If particles are used that are bigger than the vessels feeding the spinal cord but smaller than those feeding the malformation, risks for the spinal cord can be avoided. Since the particles do not

cause any inflammatory reactions, secondary damage of the spinal cord by tumefaction and edema is not to be expected. The decisive disadvantage of the particles is that they constitute no definitive embolization material. Revascularization of the malformation and recanalization of the embolized vessels are to be expected regularly. A definitive cure of the intramedullary malformation can, therefore, not be achieved. The patient has to be kept under continued clinical and angiographic supervision and is in need of regular further embolization. The main representative of the corpuscular embolization materials is polyvinyl alcohol,[17] which was introduced by Tadavarthy and colleagues and is available in different calibrated grain sizes.[146] The disadvantage of revascularization of embolized arteriovenous malformations was thought to be avoided by the use of liquid glues. The sticking properties of the substance alcyl-II-cyanoacrylate were first described in 1986 by Coover and Wicker.[35] It was widely used in the hemostasis of parenchymatous organs, in ophthalmology, and in plastic surgery. Kerber used cyanoacrylate for the first time in the treatment of intracranial arteriovenous malformations.[80] In 1976 he published the first case in which after catheterization with a "calibrated leak" balloon a partial elimination of an arteriovenous malformation could be achieved by isobutyl-2-cyanoacrylate. In 1977, he reported on the successful employment of the glue in vascular malformations of the spinal cord.[18] The indication that isobutyl, injected intraperitoneally in high doses, can induce sarcomas of the liver in experiments with rats prompted the manufacturer to withdraw the substance. Since then, N-butyl-2-cyanoacrylate has been used predominantly. The prospective advantage is a durable occlusion of the embolized regions and a cure if one succeeds in eliminating it completely endovascularly. A disadvantage may arise in the form of a possibly higher rate of complications caused by the occlusion of normal vessels and by the induced inflammatory reaction.[149] Comparison of the results of all published cases is not possible because before spinal dural fistulae were recognized entities, they were mistaken for angiomas of the spinal cord. This led to a result concerning the treatment of intramedullary arteriovenous malformations that was too positive, because prognosis after embolization seemed to be good. More recently Berenstein and Lasjaunias (with glues) and Merland and his team (with polyvinyl alcohol) have reported their results.[18, 99–102]

Merland and associates repeatedly presented good clinical results after particle embolization, with a stabilization of the clinical condition and avoidance of postoperative hemorrhage in all patients. Revascularization was to be expected regularly, however. For this reason the strategy of treatment consisted of annual repetition of control angiography and regular re-embolizations (see Fig. 65–9D). The 35 patients with thoracic angiomas were observed postoperatively for variable periods ranging from 1 to 15 years (average, 6 years).[27] Because of revascularizations the authors had to carry out 158 endovascular interventions. In comparison with the conditions at the beginning of the treatment,

*See references 10, 15, 18, 19, 27, 38, 46, 47, 49, 50, 52–54, 66, 72–74, 81, 129, and 143.

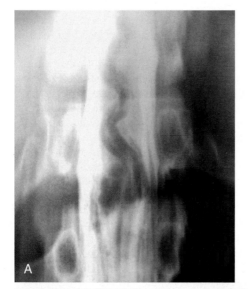

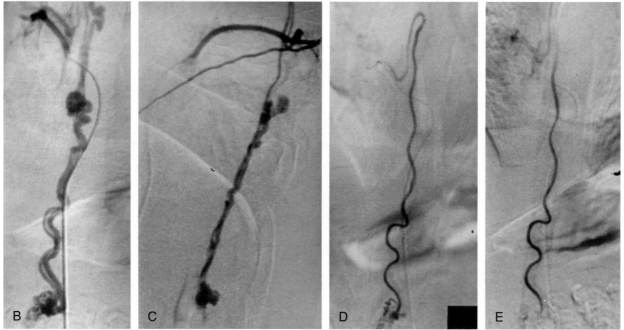

Figure 65–9

A. Myelotomography of a small arteriovenous malformation located in the conus of two dilated vessels. *B.* Angiography of the same patient. The injection of the intercostal artery (D8 right) (anteroposterior projection) shows a descending artery going down to the conus, the nidus, and the ascending vein. *C.* Lateral projection of the same vessel reveals the main supply of the arteriovenous malformation through the anterior spinal artery. *D.* After embolization with polyvinyl alcohol (Ivalon) the malformation is devascularized to a large extent. *E.* Control angiography after operative removal of the embolized malformation proves that its elimination has been complete.

they found a clinical improvement in 63 per cent of their patients; deterioration occurred in 20 per cent (7 patients) because of the embolization. A durable complete elimination could not be achieved in any of the cases. In 2 patients a subarachnoid hemorrhage occurred. Both of these patients, however, had evaded the schedule of treatment with its annual control angiography and re-embolization for a period of 3 years.

Berenstein and Lasjaunias, on the other hand, report on their experience with glues.[18] They treated 38 of 47 patients who had arteriovenous malformations with isobutyl-2-cyanoacrylate or *N*-butyl-2-cyanoacrylate. They attained a complete elimination of the lesion by endovascular technique in 53 per cent. The complication rate amounts to 10.6 per cent of permanent and 10.6 per cent of transitory deteriorations. After a complete elimination of the lesion there were no further subarachnoid hemorrhages. In 2 patients with partial

elimination there were further hemorrhages (follow-up supervision, 1 to 14 years; average, 7.5 years).

The results attained thus far after endovascular therapy show a distinct improvement in prognosis resulting from therapy compared with spontaneous progression.[3, 5, 6] Which one of the two endovascular strategies will prevail remains to be seen. Further follow-up studies are necessary.

Surgical Technique

Microsurgical therapy alone is sometimes technically difficult, owing to the intramedullary and ventral location. Even with great experience and a large number of cases, deterioration and rare deaths due to complications could not be avoided.[117, 118, 125, 169] Paraplegic patients do not have any benefits from surgery. In patients with cervical location the greatest number of improvements occurred.[117, 118, 169] Presumably, complete removal was achieved in 62 per cent.[76]

In microsurgical therapy a defocused neodymium: yttrium-aluminum-garnet laser attached to a microscope may help shrink the lesion and allow its separation from the cord (Fig. 65–10). With increasing experience in interventional neuroradiology, preoperative embolization may render the lesion a better surgical candidate.

Combined Therapy

Combined endovascular-microsurgical therapy is an established method in the management of intracranial arteriovenous malformations, but there exist only a few reports dealing with a combined interventional and surgical approach to spinal arteriovenous malformations.[87, 143] Some of the reports on endovascular therapy contain a reference to postembolization operation of intramedullary malformations[27, 66]; the extent of the benefit for the patient or of the facilitation of the operation for the neurosurgeon cannot currently be foreseen (see Fig. 65–9E).

Aneurysms

Only sporadic reports exist on isolated spinal arterial aneurysms. Estimation of their frequency is rendered still more difficult by the formerly very imprecise use

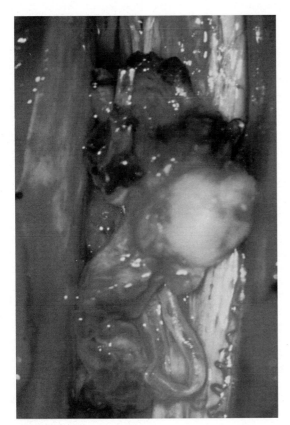

Figure 65–10

Intraoperative photograph showing flow-related aneurysm and partially resected angioma.

of the term "aneurysm" as well as by the mistaking of venous dilatations in fistulous diseases for aneurysms. If aneurysms exist in isolated form at all, they are certainly very rare. The combination of aneurysms and arteriovenous malformations has also been described (see Fig. 65–10). Sporadically, an increased risk of hemorrhage for these combinations has been reported.[25, 40, 71] A more extensive series noted the occurrence of 15 aneurysms combined with arteriovenous malformations in 14 of 70 patients with malformations.[25] Such a combination, then, is to be found in 20 per cent of the patients with intramedullary malformations, with 14 aneurysms occurring on the feeding artery. All these patients had a hemorrhage, so the increased risk of hemorrhage in relation to the other patients with intramedullary arteriovenous malformations but without aneurysms could be proved as significant. After treatment of the intramedullary malformation, four of the aneurysms receded or disappeared, but later they reappeared with the revascularization of the malformation.[26]

Metameric and Nonmetameric Syndromes

In 1915, Cobb described the progression and operative findings in the case of an 8-year-old boy with a combination of angioma of the spinal cord and skin nevi of the same metamere.[34] This combination of vascular malformations of the spinal cord, the dura, the vertebral bodies, and the segmental soft parts, including the skin, has since been designated as Cobb's syndrome. Even before Cobb's publication, however, there already existed some references to metameric arteriovenous malformations. In 1880, Berenbruch described the combination of several angiolipomas with an angioma of the spinal cord.[16] Since then the number of published cases has remained low. In the more extensive series of intramedullary arteriovenous malformations, however, there is a relative frequency of up to 38 per cent, which suggests that metameric angiomatosis is more frequent than was supposed until now.[27]

CAVERNOMAS

Although not of a truly arteriovenous origin, intramedullary cavernomas should be mentioned in this discussion on vascular disease of the spinal cord.

The first spinal cavernoma was reported in 1901.[92] It was in a 27-year-old girl who died 2½ days after an acute occurrence. Autopsy proved that an intramedullary cavernous angioma was situated in an intramedullary location at the level of the root of the seventh cervical nerve. Two years later a second case of an intramedullary cavernoma of the lumbar spinal cord was published.[65] This cavernoma attracted notice during autopsy for another cause of death and showed the signs of a microhemorrhage that had occurred and been resorbed. Until the past few years information about intramedullary or intradural extramedullary cavernomas has been rare.

Cavernomas constitute a group of vascular malformations. They consist of blood-filled caverns with venous vascular walls. The flow in the cavernoma ranges from very slow to stagnating.[97] Histologically, they are composed of vascular convolutions of different size with atypical vascular walls in which the elastica interna is missing and with calcifications and thromboses in the dilated vascular lumen.* Cavernomas are to be found everywhere in the central nervous system. Because of their slow blood flow velocity they usually escape direct angiographic representation.† Preoperative or premortal diagnosis was therefore very difficult or impossible in the era before computed tomography. Even in 1976, Voigt and Yasargil found only 164 accounts in the literature of intracranial cavernomas.[159] Simart and associates reported 26 cases from 1960 to 1986.[142] Since computed tomography, but especially since the beginning of the magnetic resonance imaging era, the number of reported cases has grown rapidly.[88, 90, 124, 132, 138] Intracranial cavernomas make up 5 to 18 per cent of intracranial vascular malformations.[76, 97, 167]

Despite the growing number of accounts about spinal cavernomas since the beginning of the magnetic resonance imaging era, the total amount of reported cases remains small. Reportedly, they make up 5 to 12 per cent of the spinal vascular malformations.[36, 76, 157] They seem more frequently to be situated in an intramedullary location; the authors found nine intramedullary and three intradural but extramedullary cavernous angiomas.‡ The case presented by Ortner and colleagues is, in the authors' opinion, an intramedullary arteriovenous angioma. Its clinical development is marked either by subarachnoid hemorrhage or by progressive ascending paraplegic syndrome.

In only a few cases does myelography show nonspecific findings of intramedullary or extramedullary expansion, whereas on angiography the lesion is invariably inconspicuous.[170] The diagnosis is very often possible preoperatively thanks to the very typical magnetic resonance image.[36, 96, 134, 170] In the authors' own four cases (Fig. 65–11), preoperative diagnosis could be made correctly from the magnetic resonance image. The typical manifestation is that of a webbed core of mixed spinal intensity with a moderate, occasionally strong absorption of contrast medium after an infusion of gadolinium. As a sign of previous hemorrhage in the T1-weighted image as well as in the T2-weighted image, a black ring around the cavernoma indicates disturbances of susceptibility caused by the iron in hemosiderin. The only therapy is microsurgical elimination of the cavernoma.

Summary

Arteriovenous malformations of the spinal cord are classified into three groups.

Dural arteriovenous fistulae represent 60 to 80 per cent of arteriovenous malformations of the spinal cord. They are believed to be acquired lesions. As a rule, there is only one nidus in or near the intervertebral foramen. The nidus is supplied by small branches of radicular arteries and drains into the venous perimedullary plexus. Typical clinical findings are initial back pain, progressive leg weakness, and sensory deficits. At the time of diagnosis, multiple neurological deficits are combined, resulting from impairment of the upper and lower motor neuron as well as the dorsal column. At this time, sphincter function is commonly disturbed. Symptoms of subarachnoid hemorrhage never occur, and thus subarachnoid adhesions have never been found on operative therapy.

Magnetic resonance imaging may reveal areas of increased signal intensity in T2-weighted sequences. Owing to ischemic cord lesion, visualization of congested vessels is not always possible. Myelography is an appropriate method for diagnosing spinal vascular anomalies and shows the dilated posterior veins as well as the dilated radicular veins. However, too much contrast medium may blur visualization. To confirm the diagnosis of spinal arteriovenous fistula, spinal selective angiography is required. In some cases, for visualization of the feeding artery and the fistula, it is necessary to extend the investigation to the vertebral artery or to branches of the internal iliac artery. To prevent lack of proof due to slow filling, late sequences of film have to be chosen. Surgical management is considered the most simple and effective method of treatment. Coagulation or excision of the dural fistula has been shown to cure the disease and prevent revascularization. Stripping and extirpation of coiled dorsal dilated veins is unnecessary and should be avoided, since the normal draining veins of the cord empty into them and deterioration may follow their resection.

Superselective angiographic studies and intraoperative measurements have proved the classification of dural arteriovenous malformation. In comparison with microsurgery, the same results can be obtained with an endovascular approach. After superselective catheterization the fistula has to be occluded with a nonresorbable, nonrevascularizable embolization material. With polyvinyl alcohol or other particles, such a definitive occlusion is not possible. Revascularization of the fistula and deterioration of neurological disturbances are always to be expected. With glue (*N*-butyl-2-cyanoacrylate or isobutyl-2-cyanoacrylate) definitive therapy is possible. The results after complete occlusion are as good as after surgery, and complications are comparably low. Embolization is indicated during angiography. If it fails or is contraindicated, the patient has to undergo surgery.

Intradural perimedullary fistulae are fed by spinal arteries and drained by spinal veins. They are lying on the surface of the spinal cord and have no nidus but a direct arteriovenous shunt. They have been subclassified in three types. Type 1 indicates a small, single fistula with a low flow velocity that is fed from one single small artery and drained through one small vein. The treatment of choice is surgery. Type 2 is a middle-sized fistula fed by several arteries with increased

---

*See references 14, 22, 24, 31, 77, 96, and 154.
†See references 61, 77, 137, 142, 156, and 160.
‡See references 36, 69, 96, 140, 154, 157, and 170.

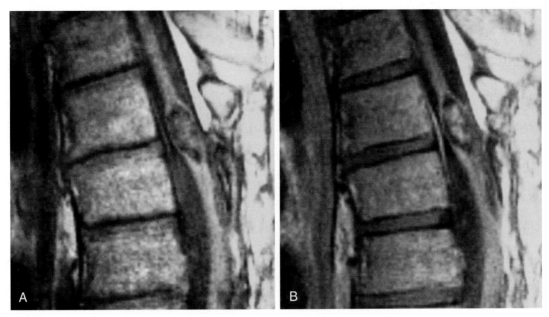

Figure 65–11

A. Magnetic resonance imaging (T1-weighted, inversion recovery, without gadolinium) shows typical aspect of an intramedullary cavernoma with signal distribution in spots and an enclosing black ring as a sign of previous hemorrhages. *B.* Magnetic resonance image after gadolinium enhancement with low increase in signal intensity in comparison with the precontrast image.

blood flow velocity and a dilated vein or veins. The treatment of choice can be surgery or embolization. Type 3 arteriovenous fistulae are giant fistulae with multiple feeding arteries and a high blood flow velocity, a marked venous dilatation in the region of the shunt, and multiple draining veins. The treatment of choice is the elective occlusion of the fistula with a balloon or coils.

True intramedullary arteriovenous angiomas are congenital and lead to early symptoms in children and young adults, often beginning with subarachnoid hemorrhage or an acute transverse lesion, owing to hematoma. However, repeated regression of symptoms may occur. The lesions are fed by anterior or posterolateral spinal arteries or both. Operative therapy in paraplegic patients has not shown any benefit. Removal of the angioma may be possible in two thirds of the cases; deterioration can occur even though the surgeon is experienced. With sophisticated means of interventional therapy, palliative partial occlusion may be possible so as to prevent further bleeding or to make the lesion amenable to selective microsurgical extirpation.

Although not of arteriovenous origin, intramedullary cavernomas should be mentioned. They tend to bleed in patients of young age, show a clear sensory level, and may be diagnosed by their typical appearance on magnetic resonance imaging. Microsurgical extirpation is advised, leading to improvement and cure.

REFERENCES

1. Aboulker, J., Bar, D., Mursault, L., et al.: L'hypertension véneuse intra-rachidienne par anomalies multiples du système cave: Une cause majeure du souffrance médullaire. Chirurgie, *103*:1003, 1977.
2. Aminoff, M. J.: Vascular anomalies in the intracranial dura mater. Brain, *96*:601, 1973.
3. Aminoff, M. J.: Spinal Angiomas. Oxford, Blackwell, 1976.
4. Aminoff, M. J., and Kendall, B. E.: Asymptomatic dural vascular anomalies. Br. J. Radiol., *46*:662, 1973.
5. Aminoff, M. J., and Logue, V.: Clinical features of spinal vascular malformations. Brain, *97*:197, 1974.
6. Aminoff, M. J., and Logue, V.: The prognosis of patients with spinal vascular malformations. Brain, *97*:211, 1974.
7. Aminoff, M. J., Barnard, R. O., and Logue, V.: The pathophysiology of spinal vascular malformations. J. Neurol. Sci., *23*:255, 1974.
8. Anson, J. A., and Spetzler, R. F.: Classification of spinal arteriovenous malformations and implications for treatment. B.N.I. Q., *8*:2, 1992.
9. Assouline, E., Gelbert, F., Dormont, D., et al.: MRI study of dural arteriovenous fistulae draining into the external spinal veins. J. Neuroradiol., *15*:1, 1988.
10. Ausman, J. I., Golde, L. H., Tadavarthy, S. M., et al.: Intraparenchymal embolization for obliteration of an intramedullary AVM of the spinal cord. J. Neurosurg., *47*:119, 1977.
11. Baker, H. L., Jr., Love, J. G., and Layron, D. D., Jr.: Angiographic and surgical aspects of spinal cord vascular anomalies. Radiology, *88*:1078, 1967.
12. Bailey, W. L., and Sperl, M. P.: Angiomas of the cervical spinal cord. J. Neurosurg., *30*:560, 1969.
13. Barth, M. O., Chiras, J., Rose, M., et al.: Résultat de l'embolisation des fistules artério-veineuses durales rachidiennes à drainage veineux péri-médullaire. Neurochirurgie, *30*:381, 1984.
14. Bartlett, J. E., and Kishore, P. R. S.: Intracranial cavernous angioma. A.J.R., *128*:653, 1977.
15. Bentson, J., Rand, R., Calcaterrra, T., et al.: Unexpected complications following therapeutic embolization. Neuroradiology, *16*:420, 1978.
16. Berenbruch, K.: Ein Fall von Multiplen Angiolipomen kombiniert mit einem Angiom des Rückenmarks. Inauguraldissertation, Tübingen, 1890.
17. Berenstein, A., and Kricheff, I. I.: Catheter and material selections for transarterial embolization: Technical considerations. Radiology, *132*:631, 1979.

18. Berenstein, A., and Lasjaunias, P.: Surgical Neuroangiography: V. Endovascular Treatment of Spine and Spinal Cord Lesions. Berlin, Springer, 1992.

19. Berenstein, A., Young, W., Ransohoff, J., et al.: Somatosensory evoked potentials during spinal angiography and therapeutic transvascular embolization. J. Neurosurg., 60:777, 1984.

20. Bergstrand, A., Hook, O., and Lidvall, H.: Vertebral hemangiomas compressing the spinal cord. Acta Neurol Scand 39:59, 1963.

21. Bien, S.: Intracranial dural AV fistula with perimedullary venous drainage presenting with an ascending paraplegia. Unpublished case, 1993.

22. Bien, S., Friedburg, H., Harders, A., et al.: Intracerebral cavernous angiomas in MRI. Acta Radiol., Suppl., 369:79–81, 1987.

23. Bien, S., Ott, D., and Riethmüller, A.: Spinal dural fistula fed by the spinal branch of the iliolumbar artery. A.J.N.R., 1995, submitted for publication.

24. Bien, S., Schumacher, M., Volk, B.: Neuroradiological and neuropathological findings in intracranial cavernous angiomas. *In* Walter, W., Brandt, M., Brock, M., et al.: Advances in Neurosurgery. Vol. 16, Modern Methods in Neurosurgery. Berlin, Springer-Verlag, 1988, pp. 187–195.

25. Biondi, A., Merland, J. J., Hodes, J. E., et al.: Aneurysms of spinal arteries associated with intramedullary arteriovenous malformations: I. Angiographic and clinical aspects. A.J.N.R., 13:913, 1992.

26. Biondi, A., Merland, J. J., Hodes, J. E., et al.: Aneurysms of spinal arteries associated with intramedullary arteriovenous malformations: II. Results of AVM endovascular treatment and hemodynamic considerations. A.J.N.R., 13:923, 1992.

27. Biondi, A., Merland, J. J., Reizine, D., et al.: Embolization with particles in thoracic intramedullary arteriovenous malformations: Long-term angiographic and clinical results. Radiology, 177:651, 1990.

28. Boeken, G.: Temporäre, belastungsabhängige Parästhesien bei Agenesie der Vena cava inferior. Dtsch. Med. Wochenschr., 113:1879, 1988.

29. Brasch, F.: Über einen schweren spinalen Symptomenkomplex, bedingt durch eine aneurysma-serpentinumartige Veränderung eines Theils der Rückenmarksgefässe. Berl. Klin. Wochenschr., 37:1210, 1900.

30. Brion, S., Netzky, M. G., Zimmerman, H. M.: Vascular malformations of the spinal cord. Arch. Neurol. Psychiatry, 68:339, 1952.

31. Brühlmann, Y., Tribolet, N., and Bereny, J.: Les angiomas caverneux intracerebraux. Neurochirurgie, 31:271, 1985.

32. Burguet, J. L., Dietemann, J. L., Wackenheim, A., et al.: Sacral meningeal arteriovenous fistula fed by branches of the hypogastric arteries and drained through medullary veins. Neuroradiology, 27:232, 1985.

33. Cahan, L. D., Halbach, V. V., Higashida, R. T., et al.: Variants of radiculomeningeal vascular malformations of the spine. J. Neurosurg. 66:333, 1987.

34. Cobb, S.: Haemangioma of the spinal cord associated with skin naevi of the same metamere. Ann. Surg., 62:641, 1915.

35. Coover, H. W., and Wicker, T. H.: Chemistry of methyl-2-cyanoacrylate. *In* Healey, J. E., Jr., ed.: A Symposium on Physiological Adhesives. Houston, University of Texas, 1966, pp. 3–10.

36. Cosgrove, G. R., Bertrand, G., Fontaine, S., et al.: Cavernous angiomas of the spinal cord. J. Neurosurg., 68:31, 1988.

37. Criscuolo, G. R., and Rothbart, D.: Vascular malformations of the spinal cord: Pathophysiology, diagnosis, and management. Neurosurg. Q., 2:77, 1992.

38. Decker, R. E., Stein, H. L., and Epstein, J. A.: Complete embolization of artery of Adamkiewicz to obliterate an intramedullary arteriovenous aneurysm. J. Neurosurg., 43:486, 1975.

39. DiChiro, G., and Doppman, J. L.: Endocranial drainage of spinal cord veins. Radiology, 95:555, 1970.

40. DiChiro, G., and Werner, L.: Angiography of the spinal cord: A review of contemporary techniques and applications. J. Neurosurg., 39:1, 1973.

41. DiChiro, G., Doppman, J. L., Dwyer, A. J., et al.: Tumors and arteriovenous malformations of the spinal cord: Assessment using MR. Radiology, 156:689, 1985.

42. DiChiro, G., Doppman, J. L., and Ommaya, A. K.: Selective arteriography of arteriovenous aneurysms of the spinal cord. Radiology, 88:1065, 1967.

43. DiChiro, G., Doppman, J. L., and Ommaya, A. K.: Radiology of spinal cord arteriovenous malformations. Prog. Neurol. Surg., 4:329, 1971.

44. Dichgans, J., Gottschaldt, M., and Voigt, K.: Arteriovenöse Duraangiome am Sinus transversus. Zbl. Neurochir., 33:1, 1972.

45. Djindjian, R. Angiography of the Spinal Cord. Baltimore, University Park Press, 1970.

46. Djindjian, R.: Embolization of angiomas of the spinal cord. Surg. Neurol., 4:411, 1975.

47. Djindjian, R., and Merland, J. J.: Place de l'embolisation dans le traitement des malformations arterio-veneuse medullaires: A propos de 38 cas. Neuroradiology, 16:428, 1978.

48. Djindjian, R., Hurth, M., and Hondart, R.: L'Angiographie de la Moelle Epinière. Paris, Masson, 1970.

49. Djindjian, R., Cophignon, J., Rey, A., et al.: Superselective arteriographic embolization by the femoral route in neuroradiology: Study of 50 cases: II. Embolization in vertebromedullary pathology. Neuroradiology, 6:132, 1973.

50. Djindjian, R., Cophignon, J., Theron, J., et al.: Superselective arteriographic embolization by the femoral route in neuroradiology: Study of 50 cases: I. Technique, indications, complications. Neuroradiology, 6:20, 1973.

51. Djindjian, M., Djindjian, R., Rey, A., et al.: Intradural extramedullary spinal arteriovenous malformation fed by the anterior spinal artery. Surg. Neurol., 8:85, 1977.

52. Djindjian, R., Houdart, R., Cophignon, J., et al.: Premiers essais d'embolisation par voie femorale dans un cas d'angiome medullaire et dans un cas d'angiome alimenté par la carotide externe. Rev. Neurol., 125:119, 1971.

53. Doppman, J. L., DiChiro, G., and Ommaya, A. K.: Obliteration of spinal cord arteriovenous malformation by percutaneous embolization [Letter]. Lancet, 1:577, 1968.

54. Doppman, J. L., DiChiro, G., and Ommaya, A. K.: Percutaneous embolization of spinal cord arterio-venous malformations. J. Neurosurg., 34:48, 1971.

55. Doppman, J. L., DiChiro, G., Dwyer, A. J., et al.: Magnetic resonance imaging of spinal arteriovenous malformations. J. Neurosurg., 66:830, 1987.

56. Dormont, D., Assouline, E., Gelbert, F., et al.: MRI study of spinal arteriovenous malformations. J. Neuroradiol., 14:351, 1987.

57. Foix, C. H., and Alajouanine, T. H.: La myélite necrotique subaigue: Myélite centrale angéio-hypertrophique à évolution progressive: Paraplegie amyotrophique lentement ascendante, d'abord spasmodique, puis flasque, s'accompagnant de dissociation albumino-cytologique. Rev. Neurol., 33:1, 1926.

58. Gaensler, E. H. L., Jackson, D. E., Jr., and Halbach, V. V.: Arteriovenous fistulas of the cervicomedullary junction as a cause of myelopathy: Radiographic findings in two cases. A.J.N.R., 11:518, 1990.

59. Gaupp, J.: Hämorrhoiden der Pia mater spinalis im Gebiet des Lendenmarks. Beitr. Pathol., 2:516, 1888.

60. Gebhardt, F.: Über das Verhalten der Reflexe bei Querdurchtrennung des Rückenmarks. Dtsch. Z. Nervenh., 6:127, 1895.

61. Giombini, S., and Morello, G.: Cavernous angiomas of the brain: Account of fourteen personal cases and review of the literature. Acta Neurochir., 40:61, 1978.

62. Gobin, Y. P., Rogopoulos, A., Aymard, A., et al.: Endovascular treatment of intracranial dural fistulas with spinal perimedullary venous drainage. J. Neurosurg., 77:718, 1992.

63. Gueguen, B.: Les fistules artério-veineuses extra-medullaires alimentées par des artères à destinée médulaire. Thèse médecine. Université de Paris, 1982.

64. Gueguen, B., Merland, J. J., Riche, M. C., et al.: Vascular malformations of the spinal cord: Intrathecal perimedullary arteriovenous fistulas fed by medullary arteries. Neurology, 37:969, 1987.

65. Hadlich, R.: Ein Fall von Tumor cavernosus des Rückenmarkes mit besonderer Berücksichtigung der neueren Theorien über die Genese des Cavernoms. Virchows Arch. Pathol. Anat. Physiol., 172:429, 1903.

66. Hall, W. A., Oldfield, E. H., and Doppman, J. L.: Recanalization of spinal arteriovenous malformations following embolization. J. Neurosurg., 70:714, 1989.

67. Harmann, I., and Balk, L.: A case of angioma of the spinal cord. B. M. J., 2:1707, 1900.
68. Hassler, W., Thron, A., and Grote, E. H.: Hemodynamics of spinal dural arteriovenous fistulas. J. Neurosurg., 70:360–370, 1989.
69. Heimberger, K., Schnaberth, G., Koos, W., et al.: Spinal cavernous haemangioma (intradural-extramedullary) underlying repeated subarachnoid haemorrhage. J. Neurol., 226:289, 1982.
70. Heindel, C. C., Dugger, G. S., and Guinto, F. C.: Spinal arteriovenous malformation with hypogastric blood supply. J. Neurosurg., 42:462, 1975.
71. Herdt, J. R., DiChiro, G., and Doppman, J. L.: Combined arterial and arteriovenous aneurysms of the spinal cord. Radiology, 99:589, 1971.
72. Hilal, S. K., Sane, P., Michelson, W. J., et al.: The embolization of vascular malformations of the spinal cord with low-viscosity silicone rubber. Neuroradiology, 16:430, 1978.
73. Horton, J. A., Latchaw, R. E., Gold, L. H., et al.: Embolization of intramedullary arteriovenous malformations of the spinal cord. A.J.N.R., 7:113, 1986.
74. Houdart, R., Djindjian, R., Hourth, M., et al.: Treatment of angiomas of the spinal cord. Surg. Neurol., 2:186, 1974.
75. Houser, O. W., Baker, H. L., Jr., and Roton, A. L., Jr.: Intracranial dural arteriovenous malformations. Radiology, 105:55, 1972.
76. Jellinger, K.: Pathology of spinal vascular malformations and vascular tumors. In Pia, H. W., and Djindjian, R.: Spinal Angiomas. Berlin, Springer, 1978, pp. 18–44.
77. Kamrin, R. B., and Buchsbaum, H. W.: Large vascular malformations of the brain not visualized by serial angiography. Arch. Neurol., 13:413, 1965.
78. Kaufmann, H. H., Ommaya, A. K., DiChiro, G., et al.: Compression vs "steal": The pathogenesis of symptom in arteriovenous malformations of the spinal cord. Arch. Neurol., 23:173, 1970.
79. Kendall, B. E., and Logue, V.: Spinal epidural angiomatous malformations draining into intrathecal veins. Neuroradiology, 13:181, 1977.
80. Kerber, C.: Intracranial cyanoacrylate: A new catheter therapy for arteriovenous malformations. Invest. Radiol., 10:536, 1975.
81. Kerber, C. W., Cromwell, L. D., and Sheptak, P. E.: Intraarterial cyanoacrylate: An adjunct in the treatment of spinal/paraspinal arteriovenous malformations. A.J.R., 103:99, 1978.
82. Klug, W.: Die Angiome der Wirbelsäule und ihres Inhaltes. Zbl. Neurochir., 18:279, 1958.
83. König, E., Thron, A., Schrader, V., et al.: Spinal arteriovenous malformations and fistulae: Clinical, neuroradiological and neurophysiological findings. J. Neurol., 236:260, 1989.
84. Krayenbühl, H., and Yasargil, M. G.: Die Varicosis spinalis und ihre Behandlung. Schweiz Arch. Neurochir. Psychiat., 92:74, 1963.
85. Krayenbühl, H., Yasargil, M. G., and McClintock, H. G.: Treatment of spinal cord vascular malformations by surgical excision. J. Neurosurg., 30:427, 1969.
86. Kulkarni, M. V., Burks, D. D., Price, A. C., et al.: Diagnosis of spinal arteriovenous malformation in a pregnant patient by MR imaging. J. Comput. Assist. Tomogr., 9:171, 1985.
87. Latchaw, R. E., Harris, R. D., Chou, S. N., et al.: Combined embolization and operation in the treatment of cervical arteriovenous malformations. Neurosurgery, 6:131, 1980.
88. Lemme-Plaghos, L., Kucharczyk, W., Brant-Zawadzki, M., et al.: MR imaging of angiographically occult vascular malformations. A.J.N.R., 7:217, 1986.
89. Liliequist, B.: Spinal cord angiomas diagnosed by gas myelography. Neuroradiology, 12:15, 1976.
90. Lobato, R., Perez, C., Rivas, J., et al.: Clinical, radiological and pathological spectrum of angiographically occult intracranial cascular malformations: Analysis of 21 cases and review of the literature. J. Neurosurg., 68:518, 1988.
91. Lombardi, G., and Migliavacca, F.: Angiomas of the spinal cord. Br. J. Radiol., 32:810–814, 1959.
92. Lorenz, O.: Cavernöses Angiom des Rückenmarkes. Tötliche Blutung. Inaug.-Dissertation, Jena, 1901.
93. Luessenhop, A. J., and Cruz, T. D.: The surgical excision of spinal intradural vascular malformations. J. Neurosurg., 30:552, 1969.
94. Malis, L. I.: Arteriovenous malformations of the spinal cord. In Youmans, J. R., ed: Neurological Surgery. 2nd ed. Philadelphia, W. B. Saunders, 1982, pp. 1850–1874.
95. Masaryk, T. J., Ross, J. S., Modic, M. T., et al.: Radiculomeningeal vascular malformations of the spine: MR imaging. Radiology, 164:845, 1987.
96. Mastronardi, L., Ferrante, L., Scarpinati, M., et al.: Intradural extramedullary cavernous angioma: Case report. Neurosurgery, 29:924, 1991.
97. McCormick, W. F., Hardman, J. M., Voulter, T. R.: Vascular malformations ("angiomas") of the brain, with special reference to those occurring in the posterior fossa. J. Neurosurg., 28:241, 1968.
98. Meder, J. F., Chiras, J., Barth, M. O., et al.: Myelographic features of the normal external spinal veins. J. Neuroradiol. 11:315, 1984.
99. Merland, J. J., and Reizine, D.: Malformations vasculaires vertébromédullaires. Encycl Med Chir Paris: Radiodiagnost II 31671 G10, 5-1987.
100. Merland, J. J., and Reizine, D.: Treatment of arteriovenous spinal cord malformations. Semin. Intervent. Radiol., 4:281, 1987.
101. Merland, J. J., Riché, M. C., and Chiras, J.: Les fistules artérioveineus intra-canalaires, extra-médullaires à drainage veineux medullaire. J. Neuroradiol., 7:271, 1980.
102. Merland, J. J., Assouline, E., Rüfenacht, D., et al.: Dural spinal arteriovenous fistulae draining into medullary veins: Clinical and radiological results of treatment (embolization and surgery) in 56 cases. In Valk, J.: Neuroradiology 1985/1986. Amsterdam, Elsevier Science, 1986, pp. 283–289.
103. Modic, M. T., Weinstein, M. A., Pavlicek, W., et al.: Magnetic resonance imaging of the cervical spine: Technical and clinical observations. A.J.R., 141:1129, 1993.
104. Morgan, M. K., and Marsh, W. R.: Management of spinal dural arteriovenous malformations. J. Neurosurg., 70:832, 1989.
105. Morimoto, T., Yoshida, S., and Basugi, N.: Dural arteriovenous malformation in the cervical spine presenting with subarachnoidal hemorrhage: Case report. Neurosurgery, 31:118, 1992.
106. Mourier, F., et al.: Intradural perimedullary arteriovenous fistulae: Results of surgical and endovascular treatment in a series of 35 cases. Neurosurgery, 32:885, 1993.
107. Mourier, K. L., Gelbert, F., Rey, A., et al.: Spinal dural arteriovenous malformations with perimedullary drainage. Acta Neurochir. (Wien), 100:136, 1989.
108. Narita, Y., Watanabe, Y., Hoshino, T., et al.: Myelopathy due to large veins draining recurrent spontaneous carotidocavernous fistula. Neuroradiology, 34:433, 1992.
109. Newman, M. J. D.: Racemose angioma of the spinal cord. Q. J. Med., 28:97, 1959.
110. Newton, T. H., and Adams, J. E.: Angiographic demonstration and nonsurgical embolization of spinal cord angioma. Radiology, 91:873, 1968.
111. Nittner, K., and Tönnis, W.: Symptomatologie, Diagnostik und Behandlungsergebnisse der Rückenmarks- und Wirbelangiome. Zbl. Neurochir., 10:317, 1950.
112. Nornes, H., Grip, A., and Wikeby, P.: Intraoperative evaluation of cerebral hemodynamics using directional Doppler technique: I. Arteriovenous malformations. J. Neurosurg., 50:145, 1979.
113. Oda, Y., Konishi, T., Suzui, H., et al.: Partially thrombosed radiculomeningeal arteriovenous fistula in spinomedullary junction. Neurol. Surg. (Tokyo), 17:63, 1989.
114. Olutola, P. S., Eliam, M., Molot, M., et al.: Spontaneous regression of a dural arteriovenous malformation. Neurosurgery, 12:687, 1983.
115. Ortner, W. D., Kubin, H., Pilz, P.: Ein zervikales kavernöses Angiom. Fortschr. Röntgenstr., 118:475, 1973.
116. Perthes, G.: Über das Rankenangiom der weichen Häute des Gehirns und Rückenmarks. Dtsch. Z. Chir., 203:93, 1927.
117. Pia, H. W.: Operative treatment of arteriovenous malformations of the spinal cord. In Carrea, R., and Le Vay, D., eds.: Neurological Surgery, with Special Emphasis on Non-invasive Methods of Diagnosis and Treatment. Amsterdam, Excerpta Medica, 1978, pp. 203–209.
118. Pia, H. W.: Operative treatment of spinal angiomas. In Pia, H. W., and Djindjian, R., eds.: Spinal Angiomas. Berlin, Springer, 1978, pp. 137–160.
119. Pia, H., and Vogelsang, H.: Diagnose und Therapie spinaler Angiome. Dtsch. Z. Nervenheilkd., 187:74, 1965.

120. Picard, L., Bracard, S., Moret, J., et al.: Spontaneous dural arteriovenous fistulas. Semin. Intervent. Radiol., 4:219, 1987.

121. Picard, L., Vert, P., Renard, M., et al.: Aspects radio-anatomiques des angiomes médullaires. Neurochirurgie, 15:519, 1969.

122. Pierot, L., Vlachopoulos, T., Attal, N., et al.: Double spinal dural arteriovenous fistulas: Report of two cases. A.J.N.R., 14:1109, 1993.

123. Rasmusen, T. B., Kernohan, J. W., and Adson, A. W.: Pathologic classification with surgical consideration of intraspinal tumors. Ann. Surg., 111:513, 1940.

124. Requena, I., Arias, M., López-Ibor, L., et al.: Cavernomas of the central nervous system: Clinical and neuroimaging manifestations in 47 patients. J. Neurol. Neurosurg. Psychiatry, 54:590, 1991.

125. Rey, A., Djindjian, M., Djindjian, R., et al.: Surgical treatment of intramedullary and anterior spinal angiomas. In Pia, H. W., and Djindjian, R., eds.: Spinal Angiomas. Berlin, Springer, 1978, pp. 161–170.

126. Riché, M. C., Melki, J. P., and Merland, J. J.: Embolization of spinal cord vascular malformations via the anterior spinal artery. A.J.N.R., 4:378, 1983.

127. Riché, M. C., Modenesi, F. J., Djindjian, M., et al.: Arteriovenous malformations (AVM) of the spinal cord in children: A review of 38 cases. Neuroradiology, 22:171, 1982.

128. Riché, M. C., Reizine, D., Melki, J. P., et al.: Classification of spinal cord vascular malformations. Radiat. Med., 3:17, 1985.

129. Riché, M. C., Scialfa, G., Gueguen, B., et al.: Giant extramedullary arteriovenous fistula supplied by the anterior spinal artery: Treatment by detachable balloons. A.J.N.R., 4:391, 1983.

130. Ricolfi, F.: Les fistules géantes perimedullaires. Thése médecine. Université de Paris, 1989.

131. Ricolfi, F., Gobin, Y., Aymard, A., et al.: Endovascular treatment of giant perimedullary spinal arteriovenous fistulae (14 cases). In Du Boulay, G., et al., eds: Proceedings of the XIV Symposium Neuroradiologicum. New York, Springer-Verlag, 1991.

132. Rigamonti, D., Drayer, B., Johnson, P., et al.: The MRI appearance of cavernous malformations (angiomas). J. Neurosurg., 67:518, 1987.

133. Rosenblum, B., Oldfield, E. H., Doppman, J. L., et al.: Spinal arteriovenous malformations: A comparison of dural arteriovenous fistulas and intradural AVM's in 81 patients. J. Neurosurg., 67:795, 1987.

134. Saito, N., Yamakawa, K., Sasaki, T., et al.: Intramedullary cavernous angioma with trigeminal neuralgia: A case report and review of the literature. Neurosurgery, 25:97, 1989.

135. Samson, D., and Marshall, D.: Carcinogenic potential of isobutyl-cyanoacrylate. J. Neurosurg., 65:571, 1986.

136. Sargent, P.: Hemangioma of the pia mater causing compression paraplegia. Brain, 48:259, 1925.

137. Savoiardo, M., and Passerini, A.: CT, angiography and RN scans in intracranial cavernous hemangiomas. Neuroradiology, 16:256, 1978.

138. Schefer, S., Valavanis, A., and Wichmann, W.: Morphology and classification of cerebral cavernomas or MRI. Radiologe, 31:283, 1991.

139. Schrader, V., König, E., Thron, A., et al.: Neurophysiological characteristics of spinal arteriovenous malformations. Electromyogr. Clin. Neurophysiol., 29:169, 1989.

140. Schröder, J. M., and Brunngraber, C. V.: Über ein intramedulläres cavernöses Angiom. Acta Neurochir. 12:41, 1965.

141. Shepard, R. H.: Observations on intradural spinal angioma: Treatment by excision. Neurochirurgia, 6:58, 1963.

142. Simard, J. M., Gardia-Bengochea, F., Ballinger, W. E., et al.: Cavernous angioma: A review of 126 collected and 12 new clinical cases. Neurosurgery, 18:62, 1986.

143. Spetzler, R. F., Zabramski, J. M., and Flom, R. A.: Management of juvenile spinal AVMs by embolization and operative excision. J. Neurosurg., 70:628, 1989.

144. Stein, S., Ommaya, A. K., Doppman, J. L., et al.: Arteriovenous malformation of the cauda equina with arterial supply from branches of the internal iliac arteries. J. Neurosurg., 36:649, 1972.

145. Symon, L., Kuyama, H., and Kendall, B.: Dural arteriovenous malformations of the spine: Clinical features and surgical results in 55 cases. J. Neurosurg., 60:238, 1984.

146. Tadavarthy, S. M., Moller, J. H., and Amplatz, K.: Polyvinyl alcohol (Ivalon): A new embolic material. A.J.R., 125:609, 1975.

147. Teng, P., and Papatheodoru, C.: Myelographic appearance of vascular anomalies of the spinal cord. Br. J. Radiol., 37:358, 1964.

148. Terwey, B., Becker, H., Thron, A. K., et al.: Gadolinium-DTPA enhanced MR imaging of spinal dural arteriovenous fistulas. J. Comp. Assoc. Tomogr., 13:30, 1989.

149. Theron, J., Cosgrove, R., and Melanson, D.: Spinal arteriovenous malformations: Advances in therapeutic embolization. Radiology, 158:163, 1986.

150. Thron, A.: Vascular Anatomy of the Spinal Cord: Neuroradiological Investigations and Clinical Syndromes. New York, Springer, 1988.

151. Thron, A., Mironov, A., and Voigt, K.: Wie verläßlich ist die Diagnose spinaler Angiome im Myelogramm? Radiologe, 23:451, 1983.

152. Thron, A., König, E., Pfeiffer, P., et al.: Dural vascular anomalies of the spine: An important cause of progressive radiculomyelopathy. In Cervos Navarro, J., and Ferszt, R., eds.: Stroke and Microcirculation. New York, Raven Press, 1987.

153. Tobin, W. D., and Layton, D. D.: The diagnosis and natural history of spinal cord arteriovenous malformations. Mayo Clin. Proc., 51:637, 1976.

154. Ueda, S., Saito, A., Inomori, S., et al.: Cavernous angioma of the cauda equina producing subarachnoidal hemorrhage: Case report. J. Neurosurg., 66:134, 1987.

155. Umbach, W.: Klinik und Verlauf bei 192 spinalen Prozessen mit besonderer Berücksichtigung der Gefäßtumoren. Acta Neurochir., 10:167, 1962.

156. Vaquero, J., Leunda, G., Martinez, R., et al.: Cavernomas of the brain. Neurosurgery, 12:208, 1983.

157. Villani, R. M., Arienta, C., and Caroli, M.: Cavernous angiomas of the central nervous system. J. Neurosurg. Sci., 33:229, 1989.

158. Vogelsang, H., Schmidt, R., and Grunwald, F.: Die thorakale Myelographie mit wasserlöslichen Kontrastmitteln (metrizamide). Fortschr. Röntgenstr., 128:342, 1978.

159. Voigt, K., and Yasargil, M. G.: Cerebral cavernous hemangiomas or cavernomas: Incidence, pathology, localization, diagnosis, clinical features and treatment: Review of the literature and report of an unusual case. Neurochirurgia, 19:59, 1976.

160. Wakai, S., Ueda, Y., Inoh, S., et al.: Angiographically occult angiomas: A report of thirteen cases with analysis of the cases documented in the literature. Neurosurgery, 17:549, 1985.

161. Willkinsky, R., TerBrugge, K., Lasjaunias, P., et al.: The variable presentations of craniocervical and cervical dural arteriovenous malformations. Surg. Neurol., 34:118, 1990.

162. Wirth, F. Jr., Post, K., CiChiro, G., et al.: Foix-Alajouanine desease: Spontaneous thrombosis of spinal cord arteriovenous malformation: A case report. Neurology, 20:1114, 1970.

163. Wrobel, C. J., Oldfield, E. H., DiChiro, G., et al.: Myelopathy due to intracranial dural arteriovenous fistulas draining intrathecally into spinal medullary veins. J. Neurosurg., 69:934, 1988.

164. Wyburn-Mason, R.: The Vascular Abnormalities and Tumours of the Spinal Cord and Its Membranes. London, Henry Kimpton, 1943.

165. Yasargil, M. G.: Surgery of vascular lesions of the spinal cord with the microsurgical technique. Clin. Neurosurg., 17:257, 1970.

166. Yasargil, M. G.: Diagnosis and treatment of spinal cord arteriovenous malformations. Prog. Neurochir., 4:355, 1971.

167. Yasargil, M. G.: Cavernous and occult angiomas. In Yasargil, M. G., ed.: Microneurosurgery. Vol. III. Stuttgart, Georg Thieme, 1988.

168. Yasargil, M. G.: Intradural spinal arteriovenous malformations. In Vinken, P. J., and Bruyn, G. W., eds.: Handbook of Clinical Neurology. Vol. 20. Amsterdam, North Holland, 1973.

169. Yasargil, M. G., Symon, L., and Teddy, P. J.: Arteriovenous malformations of the spinal cord. In Symon, L., Brihaye, J., Guidetti, B., et al., eds.: Advances and Technical Standards in Neurosurgery. Vol. II. Wien, Springer, 1984, p. 61.

170. Zentner, J., Hassler, W., Gawehn, J., et al.: Intramedullary cavernous angiomas. Surg. Neurol., 31:64, 1989.

Index

Note: Page numbers in *italics* refer to illustrations; numbers followed by b refer to boxed material; numbers followed by t refer to tables.

ISBN 0-7216-5143-7